Fifth Edition

Nursing Assessment and Health Promotion

Strategies Through the Life Span

Ruth Beckmann Murray, RN, MSN, EdD
Professor
Coordinator, Psychiatric/Mental Health Nursing Graduate Major
School of Nursing
St. Louis University
St. Louis, Missouri

Judith Proctor Zentner, RN, MA, CFNP
Director of Health Services
Hickory Hill Furniture Corporation
Valdese, North Carolina

APPLETON & LANGE
Norwalk, Connecticut

ISBN   0-8385-6637-5   NB2I

9 780838 566374   90000

93 94 95 96 97 / 10 9 8 7 6 5 4 3 2

Prentice Hall International (UK) Limited, *London*
Prentice Hall of Australia Pty. Limited, *Sydney*
Prentice Hall Canada, Inc., *Toronto*
Prentice Hall Hispanoamericana, S.A., *Mexico*
Prentice Hall of India Private Limited, *New Delhi*
Prentice Hall of Japan, Inc., *Tokyo*
Simon & Schuster Asia Pte. Ltd., *Singapore*
Editora Prentice Hall do Brasil Ltda., *Rio de Janeiro*
Prentice Hall, *Englewood Cliffs, New Jersey*

Library of Congress Cataloging-in-Publication Data

Murray, Ruth Beckmann.
    Nursing assessment & health promotion strategies through the life
span / Ruth Beckmann Murray, Judith Proctor Zentner.—5th ed.
      p.   cm.
    Includes bibliographical references and index.
    ISBN 0–8385–6637–5
    1. Nursing. 2. Health promotion. 3. Life cycle, Human.
4. Developmental psychology. I. Zentner, Judith Proctor.
II. Title. III. Title: Nursing assessment and health promotion
strategies through the life span.
    [DNLM: 1. Health Promotion—nurses' instruction. 2. Human
Development—nurses' instruction. 3. Nursing Assessment. WY 100
M983nb]
RT42.M8 1993
613—dc20
DNLM/DLC
for Library of Congress   92–48926
                                                            CIP

♻ text printed on recycled paper

Editor-in-Chief: Barbara Ellen Norwitz
Development Editor: Donna Frassetto
Production Editor: CRACOM Corporation
Designer: Michael J. Kelly

PRINTED IN THE UNITED STATES OF AMERICA

This book is dedicated to

Our students—for their inspiration
Our families—for their patience

Contributors

Mildred Heyes Boland, RN, MSN
Assistant Professor, Retired, College of Nursing
University of Arizona
Tucson, Arizona

Joyce Patricia Dees Brockhaus, RN, PhD
Child/Family/Marital Therapist (private practice)
Associate Clinical Professor, Department of Psychiatry
St. Louis University School of Medicine
St. Louis, Missouri

Robert Herold Brockhaus, PhD
Professor, School of Business and Administration
St. Louis University
St. Louis, Missouri

Ellen K. Duvall, RN, MSN, MAEd
Instructor
Burge School of Nursing
Springfield, Missouri

Dorothy Fox, RN, PhD
Associate Administrator, Nursing Education, Quality and Research
Henry Ford Hospital
Detroit, Michigan

Mary Ellen Grohar-Murray, RN, MSN, PhD
Associate Professor of Medical-Surgical Nursing
School of Nursing
St. Louis University
St. Louis, Missouri

Joan Haugk, RN, BSN, MSW
In private counseling practice
St. Louis, Missouri

Ruth Ann Launius Jenkins, RN, MSN, PhD
Associate Dean, Graduate Studies
University of Missouri
St. Louis, Missouri

Ruth Murray, RN, MSN, EdD
Professor
Coordinator, Psychiatric/Mental Health Nursing
Graduate Major, School of Nursing
St. Louis University
St. Louis, Missouri

Peggy H. McDowell, RN, CFNP, CPNP
President, Health for Industry, Inc.
Newton, North Carolina

Norma Nolan Pinnell, RN, MSN
Instructor of Medical-Surgical Nursing, School of Nursing
Southern Illinois University
Edwardsville, Illinois

Eleanor Palermo Sullivan, RN, PhD
Dean, Professor, School of Nursing
College of Health Sciences
University of Kansas
Kansas City, Kansas

Carolyn Samiezadé-Yazd, RN, BSN
Researcher in Transcultural Nursing
St. Louis, Missouri
and
Graduate Student in
Maternal-Child Health
School of Nursing
University of Missouri
St. Louis, Missouri

Nina Kelsey Westhus, RN, MSN
Doctoral Student
School of Nursing
St. Louis University
St. Louis, Missouri

Judith Proctor Zentner, RN, MA, CFNP
Director of Health Services
Hickory Hill Furniture Corporation
Valdese, North Carolina

Contents

We believe the nurse must consider all dimensions of development and the total health of the person and family. The physical, mental, emotional, sociocultural, and spiritual needs and characteristics are interrelated. Your emphasis must be on comprehensive assessment of the whole person and on health promotion rather than on patchwork remedies or fragmented understanding.

This has been an emphasis in each of our previous editions. We are gratified to see nursing's emphasis dramatically follow our projection. As we have moved from young adults to middle-aged adults and as our children have moved from the preschool era to young adulthood, we have experienced a good deal of the life-span development as well as the inclusion of comprehensive health promotion in nursing practice. Now in the fifth edition we have retained and updated the most important of these concepts.

We do not cover many diseases, their treatment, or specific manual assessment techniques. These are covered in many books that can be used in conjunction with this text. Instead we present knowledge of the highly complex normal and well person along with common health problems. Before you can understand the ill person and the family, you must understand the well person in the usual family and community setting. Only then can your assessment be thorough and your intervention individualized.

Before reading any chapters, you should orient yourself by studying Figure P–1, which shows the many factors that must be considered in nursing for health promotion. *Next,* read the text introduction. You can *gain further orientation* by (1) reading the table of contents, (2) looking at the list of objectives that precedes each chapter, (3) glancing at chapter headings, and (4) noting the key terms, which appear in boldface followed by italic definitions in the text.

We invite you to be an active participant as you read. Our ideas are presented with conviction and directness. But we want you to integrate and modify our ideas into your specific circumstances. Each of you will have to adapt this information to your setting—be it independent practice, health maintenance organization, hospital, clinic, or home.

ACKNOWLEDGMENTS

A book is the result of collaborative thinking and efforts on the part of many people; authors do not work in isolation.

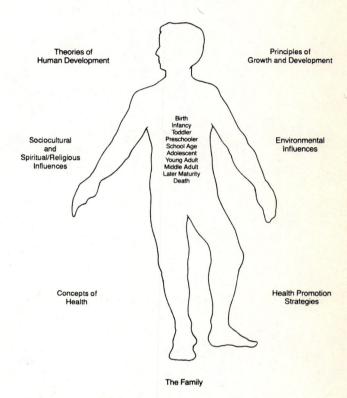

Figure P-1. Organizational approach.

We appreciate the feedback from students, colleagues, and reviewers; we have incorporated their ideas and maintained the basic direction of the book, based on their comments. We are grateful, also, to a number of people who have helped in manuscript preparation.

To our typists, JoAnn Jenkins, Anne Willen, and Stephanie Breedon, who each came to our rescue, we are grateful. Their conscientious work with handwritten material is commendable and appreciated. Without the conscientious assistance of Ruth's sister, Elizabeth Henry (this is the second time she has helped with the tasks of manuscript preparation), and the conscientious assistance of a dear friend, Helena Servis, the manuscript would not have been completed. They lovingly gave up time to assist with paste-up of the updated reference lists, reference numbering, and a variety of other such tasks. Another friend, Kathryn Lehmann, also assisted the authors with reference lists.

Equally important was the support and assistance given by our families. Postal deliveries by Judy's husband, Reid, and the words of encouragement by various family members enabled us in our work.

Our thanks, too, to the staff of Appleton & Lange, including William Brottmiller, Vice President, Sales and Marketing, who began with us on this project; Barbara Norwitz, Editor-in-Chief for Nursing; and Donna Frassetto, Development Editor; each of whom gave valu-able guidance and were our advocates at the publisher level; and to Joy Moore, CRACOM Corp., who most ably shepherded our book through the production process.

Ruth Beckmann Murray
Judith Proctor Zentner

This text introduces you to the person and the family during the entire life span—from birth to death. Birth is considered the first developmental stage, death the last. Initially you will explore the influences on the developing person and an overview of theories of human development. After holistic study of the person and family in each era, you will review basic concepts of health and health promotion strategies.

During the assessment a great deal of knowledge is needed. Not only is physiologic knowledge necessary, but also the whole range of psychosocial circumstances affecting the person, of whatever age, is equally important. These areas are addressed in this book. Major influences on the person such as culture, environment, religion, social class, and family are included. Relevant nursing diagnoses are also included in each chapter.

Each person is unique. But the uniqueness occurs in the predictable patterns discussed in this text. You can allay fears, give sound information, and make objective predictions with this knowledge. For example, a mother may be unduly distressed by the stubborn be-

havior of her toddler whom you are assessing. Your explanation that this behavior is characteristic of that age, with suggestions on how to deal positively with the behavior and what behavioral changes to expect in the future, can change a crisis into a workable situation. Also, your knowledge of normal mental and physical health at this and other developmental stages can help you detect deviations from the norm.

Your understanding of normal growth and development is used as a reference point not only for assessment but also for intervention measures appropriate to the person's or family's development. In this text, nursing intervention focuses on measures that maintain health as well as major points of care for common health problems.

Although nurses have always had to cope with death, usually it has been on a superficial basis. An indepth study of the phases of dying, along with specific care measures, will enhance your ability to foster a naturalness about this last event in life.

Part I

Influences on the Developing Person and Family Unit

1. *Sociocultural Influences on the Person and Family*
2. *Environmental Influences on the Person and Family*
3. *Spiritual and Religious Influences on the Person and Family*

Chapter 1

Sociocultural Influences on the Person and Family

The culture and subcultures into which we are born encompass us and direct us for life. We learn an identity, values, beliefs, norms and habits of life, language(s), relationships, time, space, work, play, right, wrong, and physical and mental health practices.

KEY TERMS

Culture	Ritual	Empacho	Ethnocentrism
Subculture	Status	Mollera caido	Culture shock
Ethnic	Roles	Resfriada	Pluralistic society
Ethnicity	Dialect	Cotarro constipado	Mongolian spots
Hispanic	Mores	Poverty	Lactose intolerance
Latino	Customs	Acute	Caring
Regional culture	Science	Chronic	Cupping
Socioeconomic level	Ethic	Internal locus of control	Coinage
Value system	Evil eye	Maldición	
Religious culture	Acculturation	Transcultural nursing	
Family culture	Susto	Cultural relativity	

OBJECTIVES

Study of this chapter will enable you to:

1. Define *culture* and *subculture* and describe various types of subcultures.
2. Discuss the general features of any culture and how they affect the persons under your care.
3. Identify the dominant cultural and social-class values in the United States and how they influence you as a health care worker as well as the client and family.
4. Compare the cultural values of the traditional Greek, the Spanish-speaking American living in the southwestern United States, and the Japanese in relation to the family unit, male and female relationships, childrearing patterns, the group versus privacy, time orientation, work, and use of leisure, education, and change.
5. Contrast attitudes toward health and illness of persons living in the main cultures of the United States, Greece, Spanish-speaking-American neighborhoods in the southwestern United States, Japan, and the Middle East.
6. Interview a person from another culture and contrast his or her values with those described in this chapter.
7. Discuss the influences of culture and socioeconomic level on the health status of the person and group.
8. Describe how knowledge of cultural and socioeconomic level values and attitudes toward daily living practices, health, and illness can contribute to the effectiveness of your health care.
9. Discuss ways to meet the needs of a person with cultural values and a socioeconomic level different from your own.
10. Apply knowledge about the teaching-learning process to a health education program for a person or family from another culture or socioeconomic level.
11. Assess and care for a person or family from another culture and socioeconomic level and identify your own ethnocentric tendencies.

When people talk or act differently from you, consider that to them you may also seem to talk or act differently. Many such differences are cultural and should be understood rather than laughed at or ignored.

The great divide between humans and animals is culture. Culture includes using language, art forms, and games to communicate with others; cooperating in problem solving; deliberately training children; developing unique interpretations; forming organizations; and making, saving, using, and changing tools. Humans are heir to the accumulation of wisdom and folly of preceding generations and, in turn, they teach others their beliefs, feelings, and practices. The client, family, and you are deeply affected by the culture learned during the early years, often more so than by that learned later. An understanding of cultural and socioeconomic class systems and their influence on development of behavior is essential to understanding yourself and the person under your care.

DEFINITIONS

Culture is the sum total of the learned ways of doing, feeling, and thinking, past and present, of a social group within a given period of time. These ways are transmitted from one generation to the next or to immigrants who become members of the society. **Culture** is a group's design for living, a shared set of socially transmitted assumptions about the nature of the physical and social world, goals in life, attitudes, roles, and values. **Culture** is a complex integrated system that includes *knowledge, beliefs, skills, art, morals, law, customs, and any other acquired habits and capabilities of the human being. All provide a pattern for living together.*

A **subculture** *is a group of persons within a culture of the same age, socioeconomic level, ethnic origin, education, or occupation, or with the same goals, who have an identity of their own but are related to the total culture in certain ways.* Mexican-Americans, Latinos or Spanish-speaking Americans, American Indians, African-Americans, and Asians or Asian-Americans such as Chinese, Filipino, or Japanese people represent subcultures within the overall culture of the United States of America. Ethnic, regional, socioeconomic, religious, and family subcultures also exist. A description of each follows.

The term **ethnic** *pertains to a group of people, distinguished from other people by race or nationality, who possess common physical and mental traits as a result of heredity, cultural traditions, language or speech, customs, and common history.* **Ethnicity** *frequently refers to nationality (11).* In the United States, there are many European ethnic subcultures; for example, German, Italian, Polish, Slavic (representing a number of Slovakian countries), Scandinavian (Danish, Norwegian, Icelandic, Finnish, or Swedish), Swiss, French, Dutch, or Russian. There are also ethnic subcultures from the United Kingdom: English, Irish, Welsh, or Scotch.

Hispanic, referring to Spain, Hispania, or Spanish, is often a term reserved for **Latinos** or Spanish or Latin Americans who have mixed ancestry, without identifying country of origin. Most of those who are called Latino or Hispanic speak Spanish or Portuguese. However, *among the Latino or Hispanic population there are wide differences in genetic background, culture, tradition, life-style, and health behavior, depending on culture of origin, ancestry, and current socioeconomic status. The person who is designated Latino or Hispanic may be olive or dark complexioned and have come from Spain, Mexico, Puerto Rico, Cuba, Dominican Islands, or any Central American or South American country.* Those of Mexican-American origin constitute the largest group of Latinos or Hispanics. The term **Latino** has been coined in preference to the term Hispanic. For statistical purposes, specific birthplace should be recorded. *For a general discussion of culture in this text the term Latino or Spanish-speaking will be used (52, 87, 249).*

Regional culture *refers to the local or regional manifestations of the larger culture.* Thus the child learns the sectional variant of the national culture—for example, rural or urban, Yankee, southern, midwestern. Regional culture is influenced by geography, climate, natural resources, trade, and economics; variations may be shown in values, beliefs, housing, food, occupational skills, and language.

Socioeconomic level *is a cultural grouping of persons who, through group consensus and similarity of financial position or wealth, occupation, and educa-*tion, *have come to have a similar status, life-style, interests, feelings, attitudes, language usage, and overt forms of behavior.* The people belonging to this group meet each other on equal terms and have a consciousness of cohesion (33). Socioeconomic level is not only economic in origin. Other factors also contribute to superior status, such as age; gender; personal endowment; the influence of the person or family in the community of residence, various organizations, or politically; and reliance on tradition versus adoption of norms of dominant American culture.

The more the economic level of a group becomes fixed, the more predictable are its patterns of attitudes and behavior. Children learn the patterns of their own group and the group's attitude toward another level. The attitude patterns make up a culture's **value system,** *its concept of how people should behave in various situations as well as which goals they should pursue and how.* The value systems of the general culture and of the subculture or socioeconomic level may conflict at times. Further, in the United States or other westernized countries, all except the affluent members of several generations may at times change their economic or prosperity levels, but the values of the original level are likely to be maintained.

Religious culture also influences the person, for a *religion constitutes a way of living, behaving, and thinking and therefore is a kind of culture.* Religious influences on values, attitudes, and behavior are discussed in Chapter 3.

Family culture *refers to family life, which is part of the cultural system.* The family is the medium through which the large cultural heritage is transmitted to the child. *Family culture consists of ways of living and thinking that constitute the family and sexual aspects of group life.* These include courtship and marriage patterns, sexual mores, husband-wife relationships, status and relationships of men and women, parent-child relationships, childrearing, responsibilities to parents, and attitudes toward unmarried women, illegitimate children, divorce, homosexuality, or various health problems (59).

The family gives the child status. The family name gives the child a social position as well as an identity; the child is assigned the status of the family and the reputation that goes with it. Family status has a great deal to do with health and behavior throughout life because of its effect on self-concept (58).

Family rituals are the collective way of working out household routines and using time within the family culture, and are indicators of family values. **Ritual** *is a system of definitely prescribed behaviors and procedures. It provides exactness in daily tasks of living and has a sense of rightness about it.* The more often the behavior is repeated, the more it comes to be approved and therefore habitual. Thus rituals inevitably develop in family life as a result of the intimacy of relationships and the repetition of continuity of certain interactions. Rituals change from one life cycle to another—for example, at marriage, after childbirth, when children go to school, and when children leave home. Rituals are important in child development for several reasons.

1. They are group habits that communicate ways of doing things and attitudes related to events, including family etiquette, affectionate responses between family members, organization of leisure time, and education for group adjustment.
2. They promote solidarity and continuity by promoting habitual behavior, unconsciously performed, that brings harmony to family life. Many rituals will continue to the next generation, increasing the person's sense of worth, security, and family continuity or identity.
3. They aid in maintaining self-control through disciplinary measures.
4. They promote feelings of euphoria, sentimentality, or well-being—for example, through holiday celebrations.
5. They dictate reactions to threat, such as at times of loss, illness, or death (58).

Family influences are dealt with more extensively in Chapter 4.

In nursing, consider the person's culture or subculture and standard rituals as you plan care.

CHARACTERISTICS OF CULTURE

Culture as Learned

Culture has three basic characteristics. First, *culture is learned*. People function physiologically in much the same way throughout the world, but their behavior is learned and therefore relatively diverse. Because of culture, a child is ascribed or acquires a certain **status** *or position of prestige*. The child also learns or assumes certain **roles,** *patterns or related behaviors expected by others, and later by oneself, that define behavior and adjustment to a given group.* The behavior, values, attitudes, and beliefs learned within the culture become a matter of tradition, even though the culture allows choices within limits and may even encourage certain kinds of deviancy. The way in which a person experiences the culture and society and what he or she learns during development are of great significance. Culture determines the kinds of experiences the person encounters and the extent to which responses to life situations will be either unhealthy, maladaptive, and self-defeating, or healthy, adaptive, constructive, and creative (5, 142, 183). What the person has learned from the culture

determines how and what you will be able to teach him or her, as well as your approach during care.

Culture as Stable but Changing

The second characteristic of culture is that *it is subject to and capable of change in order to remain viable and adaptive, although it is basically a stable entity.* The culture of a society, like a human body, is dynamic but maintained at a steady state by self-regulating devices. In the United States and westernized countries throughout the world, there is often much overt change occurring. Yet underneath the manifested life-style changes, certain basic values of the group are unlikely to be changed because behavior is defined by the culture. *Stabilizing features are traditions, group pressure, and the ready-made solutions to life's problems* that are provided for the group, enabling individuals to anticipate the behavior of others, predict future events, and regulate their life within the culture. *Everyone within the same culture does not behave in exactly the same way.* Norms and customs that persist may have a negative influence on the group (183). Food taboos during illness and pregnancy, pica, a high-animal-fat diet, or crowding of people into a common dwelling that provides an apt incubator for spread of contagious disease are examples.

A culture makes adaptation possible through its ideas, inventions, and customs. Together with physiological adaptive processes, culture is a powerful force. Humans, for example, are able to live in a wide variety of climates because the body has adjusted gradually to permit survival. People also heat and cool the environment for comfort, control predators and parasites, and domesticate animals and plants for personal needs. We have constructed a variety of lifestyles and patterns of social relationships to guarantee our survival and free ourselves from the limits of physical environments. Prescribed cultural norms are the most effective adaptive mechanisms that humans use. They affect physical, social, and mental well-being; aid adaptation to diverse situations, environments, and recurring problems; and teach about other environments to which we may have to adapt. In addition, some adaptive modifications are achieved through genetic, physiologic, and constitutional capacities that have been transmitted for generations through natural selection or cultural conditioning. Physical mutation and survival of the fittest may also promote permanent changes in a group if they enable a person to compete successfully and live, promoting adaptation.

Another stabilizing, limiting aspect of culture is the use of language. Although language forms vary from culture to culture, the terms for *mother* and *father* sound very much alike across cultural lines, perhaps because certain vocalizations are easy for a child to articulate and learn.

Learning cultural and family language is primarily by ear. In addition, use of language is determined considerably by age and gender—for example, baby talk, child talk, adult talk, girl talk, and boy talk. Subcultural groups, particularly the family, people from various geographic areas, or people from different ethnic or racial backgrounds differ in conversational conventions—that is, permitted topics of conversation; proper situations for discussing certain topics, such as during mealtime or before bedtime; level of vocabulary used; reaction to new words used; number of interruptions permitted; who can be interrupted; and who talks most (58).

The meeting ground between cultures is in language and **dialect,** *a variety of a language spoken by a distinct group of people in a definite place.* All immigrants to the United States brought their own ethnic/racial and cultural heritage and language. No doubt all had problems being acculturated to mainstream America, but generally their different lifestyles and accents were considered interesting and eventually accepted (193). Until recently, African-Americans were the least-accepted and -understood group of "immigrants," brought to America by force and separated from their culture in Africa. They were expected to express their cultural and racial identity through the Caucasian culture and image of what it meant to be Black. Thus standard English, the language spoken by the educated community was superimposed on the many African languages that were forced together. An artificial subculture characterized by Aunt Jemima and Uncle Remus was created (54).

Beginning with the "Black is Beautiful" movement in the 1960s, African-Americans have continued to express identity and dialect, as well as other cultural components. In fact, dominant American culture has incorporated some of the components of African-American culture. Understanding African-American subculture and dialect can help you to talk with, understand, and care for the person, just as an understanding of the subculture and dialect of any ethnic group enhances acceptance and care of that person. Non-Blacks often do not understand Black dialect. Although it may coincide with standard American English, it has its own grammatical rules (and errors), slang, cadence, and intonation. Black dialect will vary from region to region and with the age, gender, and economic level of the user. Some African-Americans avoid using Black dialect, especially those more highly educated and in higher socioeconomic levels. And keep in mind that dialect usage changes, as all language usage changes, with time. A word that is first specific to a minority ethnic group can later be adopted by members of the mainstream culture (54, 67).

Black dialect has words for which there are no analogies in standard American English, such as *hawk,* a severe, bone-chilling wind (originally blowing off the Great Lakes). There may be a simplification of consonants, such as *des* for desk, or deletion of *l* (*hep* for

help). The verbs *am, is,* and *are* often are omitted in dialect, being unnecessary for a complete sentence. The verb form *be* may be deleted (I pretty today), or *be* can indicate extended or repeated action, and *been,* completed or past action. "He *be* hurtin'" means "He has been in pain for some time." "He *been* hurtin'" means "He was in pain." A sentence without an auxiliary verb indicates an activity going on now that does not usually occur—for example, "She workin'." "She *be* workin'" indicates the person is doing the work she usually does. Possession can be expressed without the use of plurals ('s)—for example, "my baby clothes," instead of "my baby's clothes," or "De Chicago Cub won today." The letter *g* is commonly dropped as an end sound. Two syllables may be shortened into one, and *th* pronounced like *v* or *d.* To avoid grammatical redundancy, the *s* is omitted in plural noun forms if some other word in the sentence indicates plural—for example, "She have three brother." *Man* may be used instead of the name of the person addressed or to convey emphasis. The word *ain't* can be used to negate verbs in the past tense: "Dey ain't like dat" can mean "They *didn't* like that" rather than "They *aren't* like that." An undifferentiated form of the possessive pronoun occurs, as in "He a nice girl." (25, 54, 67, 193).

You will find a variety of regional dialects in the United States—for example, "Brooklynese," southern mountain, "Tex-Mex" along the Texas–Mexico border, Texas cotton country, Missouri Ozarkian, and Pennsylvania Dutch. Variations can include aspects of pronunciation (*park, pahk, pawk),* usage (quarter *of, 'til, to* nine), or vocabulary (*sack* or *bag; submarine sandwich* or *po' boy*). Language differences may give a false impression about the intelligence of a person, for some people have difficulty switching from dialect to standard American English. Listen carefully to the language spoken, be accepting of the dialect, and validate meanings of words when necessary.

Von Bertalanffy (231) and others discuss how language emphasizes the values of a culture. For example, neither the language of the Nootka Indians on Vancouver Island nor that of the Hopi has a separate subject and predicate or parts of speech, as does English. These languages instead describe an event as a whole with a single term. He points out that Americans are complex, abstract, and fragmentary in their descriptions of the world around them. The Indo-European languages, of which English is one, emphasize time. Cultures using these languages keep records, use mathematics, do accounting, use clocks and calendars, and study archeology to learn of their historical past. In contrast, past, present, and future tenses do not exist in the Hopi language; the validity of a statement is not based on time or history but on "fact," memory, expectations, or customs. The Navaho language has little mention of clock time and instead emphasizes type of activity, duration, or aspects of movement. Moreover, von Bertalanffy shows how Indo-European languages, like English, describe nonspatial relationships with spatial metaphors—for example, *long* and *short* for duration; *heavy* and *light* or *long* and *short* for intensity; *rise* and *fall* for tendency. In the Hopi language psychologic metaphors are used to name mental processes; for example, *heart* can be used for *think* or *remember*. Lopez writes that the Hopi language has limited tenses, makes no reference to time as an entity distinct from space, and is rich in verbs (in contrast to English, which is rich in nouns). It is a language that projects a world of movement and changing relationships (126).

Eskimos have numerous concepts about the varieties of space, whereas Americans have more words for the concept of time. The Eskimo language is seasonal—terms for many varieties of snow emerge in winter and for whaling in spring. Whole areas of the language are disappearing in the younger generations because the words refer to activities no longer much practiced, such as traveling with dogs, or the intercession of a shaman (true for people in many lands). Certainly in the Arctic (and among farmers in the United States), the order of the language, the ecology of its sound and thoughts, derives from the mind's intercourse with the landscape. To learn a language is to know how its speaker perceives the land (126).

Thus various cultures have different conceptualizations with which to perceive the same matter or reality. The kinds of conceptualizations influence the values, behavior, stability, and progress of a culture (231). Assessment of the person's intellectual ability must consider culture as well as age. People from non-Western cultures may learn differently and at a different rate because of different language and perceptual skills and value orientations (11). Most cultures are less technical and verbal than ours.

Analyses of the habits and practices of various peoples show that traditional language and behavior patterns practiced between parent and child within a culture are related to the interactions within that culture between employer and employee, among peers, and between nurse and patient, making for predictability and stability. Stability of culture promotes adaptability and economy of energy (80, 142).

Cultures also change, sometimes imperceptibly, so that norms, the usual rules for living, are modified to meet the group's needs as new life challenges arise. Cultures change primarily in response to technologic innovation, by borrowing from another culture, or through mass media and education. For example, the harnessing of electrical power and the subsequent invention and use of electrical appliances and tools changed ways of life in the United States: in work, recreation, food preservation, communication, education, vocabulary, women's roles, health care, and the entire value system.

Cultures also change for other reasons:

1. Competition among groups for geographical regions in order to meet members' sustenance and safety needs.
2. Use of deferred gains for members to induce them to work for the good of the culture, as in communist countries.
3. Change in political leadership, as in China, Russia, Iran, or Central America.
4. Increased scientific and industrial complexity.
5. Increased or decreased population growth.
6. Change in economic practices and standards, such as the change from feudalism to industrialism seen in some African and Asian countries.
7. Use of behavior modification techniques by groups in power.
8. Promotion of values, life-styles, and products through mass-media programming and advertisements (80).

Culture is continually shaped by forces and people outside our awareness. Toffler (224) describes how the United States is moving into a postindustrial society. He identifies some of the problem areas of such a society:

1. The need for more professional knowledge.
2. Greater expectations by the public.
3. More goods considered to be public goods.
4. Lack of measurements to show what is actually needed and thus where money and resources should be directed.
5. A changing demography with more urban concentration.
6. Increased life expectancy.
7. Changing values.

Toffler (224) described the concept of "future shock," a force he predicted would ensure adaptational breakdown unless people came to grips with rapid social change. He described the frequent shifting of families from one place to another, alterations in bureaucratic structures that may speedily engulf the worker in change, and diversity of options and continuing novelty in many life situations. A disposable, transient culture makes it difficult for people to establish roots or pass on culture as a guideline to future generations. Many of his predictions are now part of the norm in the United States. Not all people have adjusted to the continual rapid change.

Because of this "future shock syndrome," risk of illness can be predicted from the amount of change present. If a person is in the equivalent of the Alarm Stage of the stress syndrome continually, body defenses weaken (see Chapter 17). Extreme examples of persons caught in rapidly changing environments are the combat soldier, the disaster victim, the culturally dislocated traveler, the homeless, the migrant worker. Other examples include the aged who are uprooted and the person who moves from a rural to an urban environment.

Resulting problems in health care include rising costs, maldistribution of health personnel and specialized services, greater demand by the consumer for professional competence, more regulation of health care services, movement to standardized care across different regions, and accountability and more procedures for ensuring it (224).

When significant numbers of people begin to respond differently to one or more facets of a culture, this factor may cause others in the society to realize that a particular custom or norm is no longer useful. Such customs might pertain to marriage, burial, childrearing, or moral codes. If a group of people (or isolated persons) can consistently adapt while at the same time following the norm imperfectly, they may establish a new norm, which may be gradually adopted by others until it becomes the generally established pattern. Thus the culture and the people in it can be changed in spite of initial resistance. Such changes can have a positive or negative influence on health (142).

Each culture is a whole, but not every culture is integrated in the same way to the same extent. Some cultures are so tightly integrated that any change threatens the whole. Other cultures are characterized by traditional patterns that are easy to manipulate and change.

Cultural Components and Patterns

The third characteristic of culture is that *certain components or patterns are present in every culture,* regardless of how "primitive" or "advanced" it may be (80). Understanding them can help you understand yourself, your client and the health care system in which you work.

Communication Systems. The language itself or the complexities of mass media, computers, and satellites are the basis for interaction and cohesion between persons, and a vehicle for the transmission and preservation of culture. In addition to vocabulary and word taboos, gestures, facial expressions, and voice qualities— intonation, rhythm, speed, pronunciation—vary among families or groups within a culture and carry specific meanings. Because millions of U.S. residents watch television nightly, it has become the most powerful cultural communication force in the United States today. Television could be used more effectively for mass health teaching, just as it is used now for mass advertising (80). Television is a powerful force in other countries as well.

Methods and Objects Used to Provide for Physical Welfare. Methods include getting food; establishing personal care habits; making, using, saving, and improving tools; and manufacturing. Objects include instruments and machines used to change land terrain for farming, home building, or industrialization, and equipment used to diagnose and test disease.

Means or Techniques of Travel and Transportation of Goods and Services. Travel and transportation are particularized to a culture. Whether walking, use of dog or horse, or a complex system of cars, trucks, railways, and airplanes, they will affect a person's ability to obtain health care, among other services and goods.

Exchange of Goods and Services. Exchange may occur through barter, trade, commerce; involve occupational roles; and affect work and payment in a health care system.

Forms of Property. Real estate and personal property are defined by a culture in terms of their necessity and worth. Respecting a person's property in the hospital or home shows that you respect him or her personally.

Sexual and Family Patterns. Patterns may vary considerably from culture to culture and affect how you care for and teach a person. Such patterns include wedding ceremonies, divorce proceedings, forms of kinship, guardianship roles, inheritance rights, the family's division of labor, and roles assigned to men, women, and children.

Societal Controls and Institutions of Government. Controls include **mores,** *morally binding attitudes, and* **customs,** *long-established practices having the force of unwritten law.* Other controls include public or group opinion, laws, political offices and the organization of government, regulation of time, and institutionalized forms of conflict within the society or between tribes, states, or nations, such as war. These factors all influence the health care system in which you work. Increasingly, practitioners must become familiar with the political system and skilled in using it for improving health care.

Artistic Expression. Architecture, painting, sculpture, music, literature, and dance are universal art forms, although what is considered art by one culture may not be so considered by another. Knowledge of these factors can be useful in therapy and rehabilitation.

Recreational and Leisure-Time Interests and Activities. These are defined by each cultural group, are essential for health and must be considered in the nursing history and in medical diagnosis.

Religious and Magical Ideas and Practices. These exist in the form of various beliefs, taboos, ethical codes, rituals, mythology, philosophy, or the organized institution of the church and serve to guide the behavior of a cultural group during health and illness.

Knowledge Basic to Survival and Expansion of the Group. In developed countries **science,** *systematized knowledge based on observation, study, and experimen-*

tation, is basic to technologic innovation and improving material living standards. In the United States, education has traditionally been considered a bridge that enables individuals to move to higher socioeconomic levels. In modern Western cultures science is highly valued as a basis for health care. Medical science influences people biologically and socially. Less-developed countries also have a knowledge base; although it may be less scientific from our view, it is equally important.

Cultural Structuring of Basic Human Patterns. This includes rules for all social interaction, competition, conflict, cooperation, collaboration, and games. Also, the intimate habits of daily life, both personally and in groups, the manner in which one's house and body are perceived, and the many "taken-for-granted" activities between people are basically structured.

• • •

All the foregoing components and patterns influence and are influenced by adaptation to climate, use of natural resources, geography, sanitation facilities, diet, group biologic and genetic factors, and disease conditions and health practices.

COMPARISON OF CULTURES

Cultural Values in the United States

Perhaps the best indicator of what we really are and value is to observe what we watch on television, who we consider to be our heroes, how we spend our money, and how we use our time. Values also are influenced by the historical time in which a person was reared (the decade of childhood), and thus the person's age, as well as religion or philosophy, socioeconomic level, and ethnic/racial background.

The United States has been characterized as a melting pot, in that many cultural groups make up the population and have contributed to the value system. Over the years, many ethnic minorities have resettled in the United States and obtained citizenship. Many immigrants worked in bondage for 3 to 7 years in the United States in order to pay for their passage. In the late 1700s, the 1800s, and through the 1940s, numerous Germans, as well as other Europeans, emigrated to North America in search of religious or political freedom, for economic reasons, as refugees, and as a result of wars. Germans, for example, even arrived having been sold as mercenaries to fight with the British or the colonists in the Revolutionary War (196). There are approximately 50 million Americans directly descended from German immigrants. Census records indicate that there have been more immigrants of German ancestry than of any other nation, except perhaps England. Thus German values

and lifeways have seeped into all of American life, contributing to the mainstream value system (196).

Since the turn of the century, the United States has witnessed major immigrations of Chinese, Cuban, Filipino, Indochinese, Japanese, Korean, Mexican, Vietnamese, and other people. Causes include war and other military engagements, postwar reparations, economic disaster, and the Communist takeover of such countries as Cuba, Vietnam, Cambodia, and Korea. As a result of economic hardship in Mexico, the United States has also experienced an influx of immigrants from our southern neighbor.

Several orientations and value systems may be simultaneously present in a given society or culture, but only one orientation dominates over a given period of time. The middle-class (or mainstream) orientation and values dominant in the United States are presented in Box 1–1. Some listed values show a conflict between ideal and manifested values and behavior, based on values held by different generations, and the erosion of some basic values over the years.

A recent Gallup Poll of people from three different economic levels revealed some value differences between the groups. Table 1–1 lists value ratings for the three income levels; the numbers in parentheses represent the national averages in the United States (70).

A Louis Harris poll of adults in the United States revealed the following values in order of priority (189):

1. Happy family life (97%)
2. Clean environment (95%)
3. Close friends (85%)
4. Successful career (80%)
5. Satisfying sex life (71%)
6. Good income (60%)

Leininger's research indicated the following values to be held by rural southern African-Americans and Caucasians:

1. Religion (follow the Bible); spiritual health is related to other aspects of health and involves a total way of living and acting.
2. Doing right, following a code of conduct.
3. Work ethic, sense of responsibility in work.
4. Care and concern for others, sharing food and other goods, being able to receive help in return.
5. Involvement, participating in activities to assist others, being aware of and feeling responsible for needs in the community.
6. Presence of self or remaining with another in times of trouble or need.
7. Health preservation; concern about others' health first, then personal health; use of traditional medicine if ill (114).

African-American cultural values differ from the dominant cultural values in several ways, as shown in Table 1–2 (97).

■ BOX 1-1.
Dominant Values in the United States

1. Family unity* and stability, yet opportunity for each member to be self-fulfilled, which may result in divorce. Marriage is no longer considered permanent nor the only way of life. Romantic love is the basis for a couple's relationship and marriage.
2. Sanction of sexual activity in relationships where there is affection, even if there is no commitment to marriage.
3. Less investment in having children, and less willingness to sacrifice for children.
4. Decreased emphasis on former rules of conduct and social intercourse.
5. Sense of freedom to indulge self, a commitment to self-aggrandizement, with a decreasing emphasis on the work ethic and less concern about the effect of one's behavior on others.
6. Conformity to the group simultaneously with emphasis on rugged individualism and personal pleasure.
7. Competitive and aggressive behavior and exploitation of others rather than cooperation and contemplation.
8. Personal achievement,* occupational and financial success,* and status consciousness.
9. Youth, beauty, health,* self-reliance, strength.*
10. Social, geographical, economic, and occupational mobility.
11. Pursuit of recreational activities; a leisure ethic in contrast to past work ethic* and quality workmanship.*
12. Equality of people,* but recognition of social differentiation and inequality based on personal abilities, education,* and opportunity.
13. Future orientation; interest in long-term goals and willingness to defer immediate satisfaction.
14. Economic security for the present and future, to be able to purchase material goods and education that signal prestige.
15. Speed, change, progress, activity,* time schedules,* and efficiency.*
16. Science* and the use of machines and various social institutions.
17. Materialism, consumerism, and use of disposable items, practicality.
18. Exerting our will over the land and environment, and securing resources from it or changing it to meet our needs, with some efforts to conserve the environment and recycle some materials.
19. Sense of patriotism,* awareness of democracy* and freedom;* yet for some, an apathy about our country and what it has stood for.
20. Sense of humanitarianism, concern for others in trouble or disaster;* moral concern although there is much publicity about crime, amoral behavior, or the meanness in the world.
21. Sports events,* cultural arts,* the theatre,* music.*

*Values that have been influenced historically by German values and lifeways (196, 197).
See references 10, 52, 58, 80, 183, 230.

TABLE 1-1. VALUE DIFFERENCES ACCORDING TO ECONOMIC LEVEL

Value	Income Level		
	$40,000 and over	$25,000– 39,999	Under $25,000
1. Good family life (89%)	85%	89%	93%
2. Good self-image (85%)	83%	84%	87%
3. Good physical health (84%)	76%	87%	87%
4. Sense of accomplishment; lasting contribution (69%)	68%	71%	68%
5. Working for betterment of society (67%)	62%	68%	71%
6. Following a strict moral code (60%)	60%	63%	61%
7. Nice home, car, other belongings (41%)	36%	37%	46%

Adapted from Gallup, George, *The Gallup Poll: Public Opinion 1989.* Wilmington, DE: Scholarly Resources, Inc., 1989, 55–58.

Although research indicates that value differences exist for different racial/ethnic groups and economic levels, Lewis and Looney in their research found similarities as well as differences between the most competent working class African-American families and affluent Caucasian families in the same geographic area (118). And Billingsley provides information about interrelationships between Caucasian and African-American families (13).

In the 1990s, we see increasing nostalgia for the apparent, though not necessarily real, serenity of past eras and for pastoral images. There is a return by some people in the United States to Victorian Age values, such as emphasis on family life, domesticity, and home as a haven; historic preservation; appreciation for Victorian architecture, and use of Victorian Age products—authentic or imitation. Others are returning to the clothing styles, music, dance steps, entertainment themes, and perhaps the values of the 1950s. It is a way for the adult generation to expose their children to a way of life that young adults, adolescents, and children have not experienced.

In the past (and to some degree still for the elderly and middle-aged adults), the Puritan or Protestant ethic described by sociologist Max Weber was the prime influence on American culture, even for those Americans who were not Protestants. An **ethic** *is defined as an outlook or view made up of assumptions that are not often noticed and still less often questioned or tested.* These assumptions are blindly and passively accepted because they have been handed down from generation to generation and had their origins in an unimpeachable, but long forgotten, authority. With new knowledge, the assumptions are often found invalid, but assumptions about living undergo a slow process of change. The Protestant ethic encompasses a harsh, pes-

TABLE 1-2. COMPARISON OF SELECTED AFRICAN-AMERICAN VALUES AND DOMINANT CULTURAL VALUES

Value	African-American Culture	Dominant Caucasian Culture
Psychologic connectedness	Individual secondary to group; individuality cannot be separated from group. Progress of group more important than that of individual. All members of group share disappointments or concerns of group. Both positive and negative feelings shared by group.	Primacy of the individual. Each person master of own destiny. Each citizen to carry own weight and be rewarded according to abilities and effort expended. Person esteemed for achievements. Group benefits from combined efforts of individual members; person only peripherally accountable for group's faults.
Rhythm: openness to feelings and emotionality	Rhythm: a natural flow of emotional release that can be looked into by others close to self; a source of all actions, song, dance, poetry, drama, sculpture. Engage in unrestrained emotionality without interference of the cognitive; behavior is "real."	Emotional outbursts regarded as unsightly. Behavior cognitively examined for motives in order to understand another. Left-brain dominance fostered. Behavior governed by codes of conduct.
Social values	Home and family are centers of values rather than workplace.	Workplace, achievement, and material innovation valued.
Time perspective	Time divided into natural units—day and night, seasons. Meetings and get-togethers scheduled around natural cycles. Emphasis on time is not a behavior of choice, but clock time is utilized in order to receive appropriate rewards (pay) or avoid punishment (low grades). Exactness about time not expected or required.	Time dissected into seconds, minutes, and hours. Activities and meetings are scheduled. Exactness about time expected and often required.
Direct experience	Person experiences reality through direct involvement; learning constantly occurs in interaction with environment. Learning not confined to classroom but gained through living. Book knowledge not as important as being able to put knowledge "to the test" of behaving.	Knowledge from experience and books valued. Abstract learning emphasized.
Oral tradition	Themes in the language are: (1) emotional vitality, (2) realness, (3) resilience, (4) interrelatedness, (5) value of direct experience, and (6) distrust and deception. Black English provides organization to communicate unique cultural ideas. Body posture validates the language used.	Standard English follows different grammatical rules and syntax.
Spirituality	Reality of the spirit acknowledged and accepted as a basic part of self. Each person expected to know God personally. Many have a strong attachment to religion. Prayer and supernatural forces outside realm of cognitive/conscious awareness often attributed causal properties.	Spirituality often overlooked by mainstream psychological thought. Often less open expression about spirituality even if person has deep faith.
Creative improvisation	All creation is believed to return to former being. A group may perform as an act while each member creates his or her own reality. Everyone united by thematic material of eternity and thus behavior should be able to be understood and new relationships formed. No mental state is static or entrenched. Everything is part of a larger process.	Concept not present in Western thought.

simistic view of the human race. It upholds the five following assumptions.

1. Man is basically imperfect and must struggle against imperfection.
2. Man was placed on earth to struggle and so struggle must be valued. Any sign of surrender or softness denotes weakness in the person and is bad.
3. Self-sacrifice and aspiring to good conduct are essential to overcome evil and gain personal salvation.
4. Emotions cannot be overtly expressed. Displaying anger is basically un-Christian. One should love one's neighbor, but expressing love openly is suspect, especially if related to sexuality, for sex is considered an animal pleasure and therefore a taboo topic. Even too intense an expression of nonsexual love can be a sign of weakness and one must be strong and self-controlled in order to struggle. Anxiety must be avoided or denied, for it shows that the struggle is not going well.

5. The world is seen as useful to man and should provide for material satisfaction. Thus the exploitation of land, even ruthlessly, is acceptable. Mastery of the environment is emphasized. Conservation of natural resources is secondary, for the resources of the world (which are supposedly inexhaustible) were put there to be used (237).

Earlier in this century Puritanical values and rigid Christian morality upheld the tenet of God's judgment. A strong conscience was developed in fear of punishment and social disfavor. Society was stable because traditions were adhered to and proverbs were taken seriously. Hard work, plain living, thrift, self-control, responsibility, willpower, honesty, and initiative were emphasized. Family, gender, and community roles were clearly defined: father was the patriarch, mother was subservient to him, and children were obedient to all. Education also emphasized discipline, order, and obedience to authority. People were tradition-bound and hard-working, and they provided stability in society. Your understanding that many elderly and middle-aged persons still live by these values can help you better accept them and plan their care.

You need only look around at what Toffler calls our superindustrial society to realize that the Protestant ethic has lost its hold (224). Yet parts of this ethic are being revived by some of the growing fundamentalist religious groups.

The value system of the United States is worldly, in spite of its religious roots, for the most highly valued activities involve competitive, practical, secular pursuits rather than contemplation, devotion, cooperation, or esthetic satisfaction. Thus the ideal society, originally the Kingdom of God on earth, has for many people been secularized into a good society with ideals of liberty, justice, general prosperity, materialism and consumerism, and equality of opportunity (58).

The United States is undergoing major cultural shifts, according to Naisbitt (162, 163), which include moving from:

1. Industrialization to an information society.
2. Forced technology to a combination of high technology and high touch or interaction.
3. Short-term to long-term considerations in business, the economy, health practices, and social services.
4. Centralization to decentralization of management and services.
5. Institutional to self-help practices.
6. Representative democracy to participatory democracy.
7. Use of hierarchies to the practice of networking (interacting with others), to solve problems and achieve goals.
8. Either/or to multiple options in solving problems or seeking services.

Naisbitt also notes the rise of more women as leaders, a renaissance of the arts, sweeping worldwide religious movements, and the decline of the welfare state.

Several of these trends are important to nursing: the emphasis on an information society, high technology/high touch in care, the long-term perspective, decentralization of services, use of self-help practices, use of networking, seeking of multiple options, the rise of more women in leadership positions, and decline of the welfare state.

Because of these cultural shifts, we see another phenomenon in the United States. There is an increasing number of a new class of migrant workers—mostly well-educated professionals and highly paid blue-collar workers who move around the country, following job relocations and business and economic trends. Frequent migrations prevent the family from establishing roots. Changing addresses may help the family and children be more flexible, if there is a strong family cohesion and identity, or it may create a sense of anomie, isolation, and identity diffusion. The family must realize that its problems will move with them, and often a change in life-style and higher cost of living awaits them in the new job/residential area. In the transition, there may be loss of friends, familiarity, and finances, and sometimes treasured items as well (3).

Other cultural life-styles are often perceived as problematic by mainstream America. Various cultural groups may have values and behaviors or a life-style that are in conflict with the dominant values of society. For example, American Indian and Alaskan native people value nature. Mainstream America believes that environmental resources are to be used. A persistent sense of family responsibility is traditional to American Indians, for example. Although family members leave the reservation to find work, they are expected to return to visit relatives or for emergencies and life-cycle, or tribal, events. When cultural values of sharing, cooperation, and mutual dependence conflict with the demands of a job, American Indians face a difficult choice. If the call to attend a funeral or help a sick relative comes when a worker cannot take time off, the decision may be to give up the job. Employers are not always understanding of the values underlying the behavior (93, 248).

Western movies showing rampaging Indians killing American pioneers are not fully accurate; through the media, attitudes have been shaped negatively. Most Caucasians in the United States can trace their ancestry to the White settlers of the 1600s, 1700s, and 1800s, immigrants who were escaping the brutality of feudal and industrial slavery, oppression, and wars in Europe. In turn, when they moved into the wilderness areas of this country, they were relatively helpless in the strange continent. In contrast to the movies, myths, and legends about the murderous American Indian, these early settlers survived because of the goodwill and assistance of various Indian people. That most American Indians, like most Caucasians, are peaceful and helpful to others must be taught to the public. Values such as assistance to others; family harmony; gentleness to and love of the natural environment; inclusion in community roles and respect for and care of the elderly; and cooperation instead of competition are values that would be useful for all of our society to learn and practice. American Indian tribes were quite ahead of our Women's Liberation Movement in many ways. For example, marriage customs do not treat women and children as property, and homosexuality has been better accepted. In some tribes, such as the Iroquois, women have had a central role in community and governmental affairs (76, 187, 188).

For many second- and third-generation Latin or Spanish-speaking Americans, educational and socioeconomic advances have paralleled a reduction in the size of their households and the development of individual and family rather than community orientation. But for the majority, loyalty to the family and a preference for large kin groups that act as support networks are very strong. Thus the competitiveness against others that is part of the educational system is avoided, and children may not make the high grades in school that are likely to ensure continued educational and employment success.

Many non-Jewish, Caucasian U.S. ethnic cultures inherited work and family values from European Catholic peasant societies—values that seem to set family interests against individual achievement. Generations of underemployment, fear of losing what little wealth the family had managed to accumulate, and the constant struggle to feed ever-growing families encouraged European immigrants to favor economic security over risk taking.

The southern Appalachian person may have a value system that is almost on the opposite end of the continuum from the upper-middle-class professional as shown by Table 1–3 (103, 104).

Issues of violence are to this generation in the United States what the issue of sex was to the Victorian world. Today's young adults have grown up with the ever-present possibility of instantaneous death or permanent maiming by thermonuclear, chemical, or biological warfare agents. The threat and fear of violence are therefore constant facts of life. Fear of violence has led to a fascination with violence that further surrounds people with its symptoms. U.S. society is preoccupied with, almost mesmerized by, the violence of individual assault, homicide, teen gangs, and organized crime, urban rioting, and political assassinations. Violence on television and in the movies shows the potential for brutality and aggression in all (80).

People react differently to constant exposure to violence: they may tolerate it, develop disease symptoms,

project their own aggression onto others, develop a neurotic preoccupation with it, or act violently themselves in order to discharge rage. We see examples of each reaction in our society in the form of physical, emotional, and social illness.

Persad (179) discusses how concepts of aggression and dependency vary from culture to culture. In U.S. culture, aggression is regarded as an innate force that has survival value and that requires appropriate channels for its expression; it is considered an integral part of social success. If aggression is not dealt with appropriately, however, the person becomes psychopathic. In some cultures, aggression is considered the result rather than the cause of psychopathy. Americans teach their children to be independent and emphasize the importance of the adolescent or young adult leaving home. Psychiatric therapy in the United States is often directed toward these goals. In Asian and many Asian-American cultures, however, indirect communication, modesty, cooperation with the team, and conformity to the group are valued rather than assertiveness of the individual. Touch or physical contact between business colleagues is avoided. Young adults may be castigated for abruptly leaving home or striving for independence. Consideration for family elders is more important than one's desires to pursue personal goals. In our culture, a well-developed ego is considered necessary for maturity. In Asian cultures, personal preoccupation with the ego is considered absurd. In the Saudi Arabian culture, behavior that is normal for a U.S. businessperson is considered offensive, such as abrupt or interrupting speech, asking about a man's wife, or emphasizing a time schedule (179).

Comparison of Cultures: Greek, Latino or Spanish-Speaking, Japanese, and Middle Eastern

Tables 1–4 through 1–10 contrast Greek culture, Spanish-speaking American culture in the southwestern United States, and Japanese culture. Although many nationality groups fit under Spanish-speaking, and each nationality group has its unique values and customs, the values, norms, customs, and behaviors described in the following tables are applicable to people who have a Spanish or Latino background, whether they are from Spain, Mexico, Puerto Rico, the Caribbean Islands, or Central or South America. There are variations in these values as the person or family is integrated into mainstream American culture. Furthermore, values may be lived differently, outwardly, if the person resides in Greece, Mexico, or Japan rather than the United States. Middle Eastern culture is described in the following section.

Yet much of the behavior of a third- or fourth-generation family or person from a country reflects the original cultural and/or ethnic values. That fact explains dif-

TABLE 1-3. BASIC VALUES OF CULTURES WITH SELECTED CULTURAL EXAMPLES

Value	Range of Beliefs	Example of Cultural or Subcultural Group Adhering to Value
Human Nature (What is innate nature of man?)	The person is basically *evil but capable of achieving goodness* with self-control and effort.	Puritan ancestors. Protestants of Pentecostal or Fundamentalist background. Appalachian subculture.
	The person is a *combination of good and evil,* with self-control necessary but lapses in behavior understood.	Most people in the United States.
	The person is basically *good.*	Some religious groups, such as Society of Friends. Some philosophical groups, such as humanistic psychologists or members of Ethical Society.
Man-Nature (What is relation of man to nature or super-natural?)	The person is *subjugated* to *nature* and cannot change whatever is destined to happen.	Spanish-speaking cultures. Appalachian subculture.
	The person is to gain *mastery over nature;* all natural forces can be overcome.	Middle- and upper-class and highly educated people in the United States.
Time (What is temporal focus of human life?)	*Past time* is given preference; most important events to guide life have happened in the past.	Historic China.
	Present time is the main focus; people pay little attention to the past and regard the future as vague.	Spanish-speaking cultures. Appalachian subculture.
	Future is the main emphasis, seen as bigger and better; people are not content with the present.	Educated, professional, and middle-class people in the United States.
Activity (What is the main purpose in life?)	*Being orientation.* The person is important just because he or she is and may spontaneously express impulses and desires.	Appalachian subculture. While no culture allows complete expression of impulses and all cultures must have some work done, the Mexican fiesta and Mardi Gras in New Orleans are manifestations of this value.
	Becoming-in-being orientation. The person is important for what he or she is, but must continue to develop.	Most religious cultures. American Indian subcultures.
	Doing orientation. The person is important when active or accomplishing something.	Most people in the United States.
Relational (What is one's relation to other people?)	*Individualistic relations.* These emphasize autonomy; the person does not have to fully submit to authority. Individual goals have primacy over group goal.	Most Gemeinschaft societies, such as folk or rural cultures. Yankee and Appalachian subcultures. Middle-class America, with emphasis on nuclear family.
	Collateral relations. These emphasize that the person is part of a social and family order and does not live just for oneself. Group or family goals have primacy.	Most European-American ethnic groups, especially Italian-American, Spanish-speaking culture. American Indian tribal subcultures. Most cultures adhere to somewhat through sibling relations in family.
	Lineal relations. These emphasize the extended family and biological and cultural relationships through time. Group goals have primacy.	Cultures that emphasize hereditary lines. Upper-class America. Oriental cultures. Middle East cultures.
	Relations are impersonal, focused on role behavior.	Business interactions, upper middle class, and those moving up the social ladder.

Data from references 103 and 104.

ferences among groups of people and should not be considered abnormal. Discussion centers on the family unit, male and female relationships, childrearing, the group versus privacy, time orientation, work and use of leisure time, education, and attitudes regarding change. The following discussion then compares the attitudes of U.S. residents toward health and illness with the corresponding attitudes in each of these cultures (6, 7, 11, 20, 27, 61, 68, 84, 87, 133, 134, 153, 156, 159, 166, 171, 178, 185, 186, 199, 214, 215, 218, 219, 222).

Table 1–3 summarizes Kluckhorn's presentation of five basic value questions, the range of beliefs derived from these questions, and examples of some (sub)cultural groups adhering to these beliefs (104). You may wish to assess your clients and their families according to these values as well as the characteristics presented in

TABLE 1-4. A COMPARISON OF CULTURES: THE FAMILY UNIT

Component	Greek	Spanish-speaking	Japanese
Basis for marriage	Social and family welfare. All of society patterned on family.	Family welfare central.	Value family and household lineage. Family gives sense of purpose.
Type of family system	Paternalistic. Extended family. Monogamy. Marriage bond strong.	Paternalistic. Extended. Monogamy. Marriage bond strong. Family cares for ill, needy.	Traditional value on authority of father and elderly. Family strongly identified with father. Subordinate position of women and arranged marriage still accepted by older generation. Home, family, children are focus of women.
Family size	Want many children.	Large so parents not alone in old age.	Family planning, including use of abortion to control size in modern family.
Pattern of interaction	Authoritarian; man dominant in conversation and decision making. Man head of house and disciplinarian. Sex roles traditional male and female. Mother powerful in own way; credited with sustaining child with moral strength. Children subordinate. Oldest son responsible for family if husband not present. Child not focus of family activity. No special activities for child, even birthday a time to wish family long happiness with child rather than focus on child. Family together most of time with child learning to enjoy adult behavior and anticipate adulthood. Peer contacts through family.	Authoritarian. Man head of house; woman subordinate socially. Sex roles traditional male and female. Child not sole focus of attention. Avoid admiration of child for fear of "evil eye." Child proud of home responsibilities. Age and authority figures highly respected. Family loyalty strong. Obedience emphasized. Family ties may extend beyond biologic relatives, including godparents, the boss. Modesty about body care and functions and sexuality.	Family revered as an institution. Close family relationship although may not express spontaneous companionship and warmth. Major decisions made by family. Subordination of individual to family interest. Traditional autocratic family system stronger in rural areas, with eldest son inheriting family property and hesitant to rebel against father. Young generation choosing own marriage partner, establishing own household, and daughter-in-law gaining freedom from mother-in-law's dominance. Increasing premarital and extramartial sexual affairs.

Tables 1–4 through 1–10. *Although neither a comprehensive study nor a stereotype of everyone in these cultures,* these comparisons indicate that subtle as well as obvious differences, along with some similarities, exist among different groups' values and behavior. *Understand that these cultural patterns will be followed by different persons in each culture to varying degrees,* denied by some, and not identified yet taken for granted by others. Chapter 4 will discuss some of these values in relation to the family culture of the United States.

Focus: Middle Eastern Culture*

More people from the Middle East[†] are migrating to the United States because of political unrest in the region and somewhat easier travel possibilities. Many first-generation immigrants come here to study and then become permanent residents in America. These people strongly maintain their culture and religious values and practices;

this makes them a unique set of clients to be cared for. Even though many of these clients identify with their country of origin, many also identify with a family, such as the Seyeds of Iran, or a city or a village they lived in, or a religion.

Roles. In Middle Eastern countries, Islam is a dominant religion, and roles and families are also dictated by the religion of Islam, as well as by the culture of the country. Men tend to have earning positions in the household, and thus they either cannot or refuse to help with household duties. Women, on the other hand, tend to be in control of household affairs. These roles are divided but complementary. There are some women in Islamic culture who maintain professional roles through the performance of a professional job outside the home. But in a traditional society and environment, roles tend to hold a status quo; the woman is at home and the man is the wage earner.

Muslim society tends to be paternalistic. Children carry throughout their entire life the last name of their father as their legal name. Even upon marriage, women will continue to maintain the last name of their father's

---

* This section is written by Caroline Samiezadé-Yazd, B.S.N.
† We are referring here to Lebanon, Syria, Jordan, Arabia, Egypt, Central Asia, Turkey, Afghanistan, Iran, and Palestine.

TABLE 1-5. A COMPARISON OF CULTURES: CHILDREARING PATTERNS

Component	Greek	Spanish-speaking	Japanese
Process of childbirth	Considered normal process, not to be feared.	Considered normal process. Husband little involved. Prefer woman's presence. Special practices surrounding process.	Considered normal process.
Philosophy of childrearing	Effectiveness sought as parent, not as pal. Chld raised to be strong, hard, firm, straight, for that is ideal personality. Wishes of elders put before child's wishes.	Effectiveness sought as parent, not as a pal. Child taught to do as parents do, to listen to parents' advice, learn from their experience, and not advance further than their parents.	Traditionally child to be dutiful, disciplined, responsible, respectful to elders. Young urban generations not bound as firmly by traditions.
Practices of childrearing	Mother firm, not overprotective. Baby kept in straight position when carried or in bed. Follow rigid schedule, consistent.	Consistent, traditional, faith in own judgment. Tradition of beast feeding needs reinforcement if in Anglo health care setting.	Mother enveloping child in warmth during early years, but when child older, relationship more distant. Oldest son reared differently from other brothers, and brothers from sisters, so every child aware of his or her place.
Responsibility for child care	Primarily mother, but older children involved in daily activities, including care of younger siblings. Attitude of love and responsibility among siblings; new baby not seen as competition.	Husband ultimately responsible as head of household. Any family member, including siblings and cousins, responsible at times.	Mother primarily, but all of family involved.
Discipline	Consistent. Obedience very important and taught to child at early age. Child praised when good and told when bad; taught that it is important to be good and not shame family. Use group pressure to set limits on behavior.	Consistently correct child when behavior is bothersome and warned not to act in a way to provoke father. Instill fear of consequences. Instill pride in self-control and fear of being shamed. Seldom told he or she is "good" or "bad."	Firm, consistent, lack strong emotional expression. Emphasis on responsibility, duty, loyalty, patience, and orderliness. Promote feeling of insecurity when doing wrong.
Training of child	Taught to value interdependence, cooperation. Sibling rivalry when new baby arrives but does not last long. Mother delighted with new baby but shares self equally with older child, including offer of free breast during feeding. Older child invited to share excitement about baby. Parents never clown for child's amusement or give many material things.	Taught to value interdependence, companionship. Little sibling jealousy. Freely show affection and attention. May use child as translator for family if they are not bilingual.	Taught to value interdependence but responsible for own behavior. Taught to carry out obligation regardless of personal cost and to control behavior to avoid personal shame and disgrace of group. Develop strong sense of responsibility, loyalty to family or work group. Poor communication between generations because of differences in experiences, education, language comprehension, and values, fostering problems in modern society.

family. Men have a great need to feel in control of situations relating to self and the family, and this may be viewed in Western culture as excessive control of women or family members. The controlling male brings great compliance into the family system through his role of leader.

Therefore, in the health care setting it is best to ask the man's permission or opinion when it relates to family members. If this aspect is neglected, the man may feel insulted, and mistrust may develop in the relationship. In Western culture, this practice is viewed as a type of ownership by the man over his family. It is not viewed in this way by Muslims. The man rather per-

ceives this as protecting the family for which he is responsible. This protection can be seen especially with a new mother and baby. In the absence of the husband, the health care provider can communicate through the woman's father or father-in-law, a designated brother or uncle of the husband, or the husband's mother.

In the Middle East, a large portion of a traditional village's female population is illiterate. Therefore, the role of mother and ability to bear and raise children is a major source of sense of self-esteem and identity. This affords one of the greatest opportunities for a woman to realize her potential as a person. Because women are very respected for their role as mother, children, even

TABLE 1-6. A COMPARISON OF CULTURES: INTERACTION WITH OTHERS VERSUS PRIVACY

Component	Greek	Spanish-speaking	Japanese
Basic values of person and behavior	Strong sense of self-esteem. Inner core of personality not to be exposed or shamed. Value equality, individuality. Aloneness not sought, but borne with fortitude. Pride in glorious past of Greece.	Anxiety about being alone and concern for people who are alone. Not considered proper to compete, push self forward in group through achievements. Better to submit than provoke anger in another. Self-restraint emphasized. Violence atypical.	Strong sense of self-respect and important to be treated respectfully by others. Privacy not valued, apparently unwanted, and seen as loneliness. Group relationships sought and valued.
Personal possessions	Value in shared living and sharing possessions, especially with family and friends.	Sharing of possessions. One's own house nebulous; frequent unannounced visiting among family and friends.	Possessions not highly valued. Shared living space and possessions in family.
Status of person	Valued for what he or she is rather than position or achievement. Family unit valued, not individual.	Valued for what he or she is, depends on family. Child has mother and father's surname, respectively; hyphenated name common.	Belonging to right clique or faction important to status and future success. Try to join influential group at early age.
Interaction among persons	Resentment when treated impersonally, mechanically, or like a number on a chart. No word for "group," but born into group of family and friends. Extended family working together for benefit of each other. Units of cooperation retained from past, not created. Work to achieve common goal with those to whom individual feels loyalty. Speech important because it establishes interactions; expressive of feelings.	Much neighborhood socializing, especially among women to borrow, help, consult, discuss, or exchange gifts. Interchange of gifts and services frequent. Accepting as gracious as giving, and person not satisfied until he or she has returned a gift to show appreciation; return gift not necessarily same kind or form. Strangers not completely accepted unless related to established family by marriage. Interdependence between family and close friends does not extend to broader community.	Suppression of emotion in many situations. Most docile with strong urge to conform. Pleasant, polite, correct but aloof behavior to others in all classes. Avoids handshake or body contact. Restrained, formal, hierarchal relationships in family, company, and political party rather than horizontal, comradely behavior. Ceremonious, at ease, and apologetic to acquaintances and friends but less so with strangers. Man unappreciative of domineering woman. Wish to avoid confrontation; strive to save face in conflictual situation.
Social activities	Family basic social group. Circle of friends important. Enjoy social affiliations, great loyalty to all groups to which one belongs. Food important with social activities.	Few formalized social groups. Suspicious of outsiders. Dependency on others accepted. Family basic social group. Women thought of as one social group, men another. Remain close to own social group for job or marriage partner. Use of diplomacy, tact, concern, respect for other's feelings. May appear to agree when does not. Child may avoid eye contact or not verbalize feelings, out of deference to elder.	Fondness for crowds and physical proximity of people. Participation and spectator roles in social activities and sports enjoyed.

into adulthood, place their mother's needs as paramount. Often this is done before considering even the wife's or family's needs, which places an internal strain within the family structure.

Parenthood. Women do not practice contraception in the Middle East as often as in the West because the traditional role of the female is to bear children. Many misconceptions center around conception; for instance, that conception will not occur during breast-feeding. Such misconceptions are held even by the most educated people. When contraception is used, it must be, by Islamic law, a form that will not destroy an already united egg and sperm, such as birth control pills or a condom,

TABLE 1-7. A COMPARISON OF CULTURES: TIME ORIENTATION

Component	Greek	Spanish-speaking	Japanese
Concept of time	Present important but prepare for something in future that is sure part of the life. No automatic faith in future. Distasteful to organize activities according to clock. Life regulated by body needs and rhythms, daily pattern of light and dark, and seasons.	Present important but validated by past. Expect future to be like present. Perform with distinction in present rather than emphasize efficiency, quantity. Life not regulated by clock but by body needs and rhythms, light and dark, seasons, religious holidays.	Time neither an absolute nor objective category but a process—the changing of nature with man as part of it. Planning for future valued. Present considered important, and past priceless.
Use of time	Time used spontaneously; not time-conscious. Elastic attitude toward time; governed by cycles of nature. "Tomorrow" thought of as tomorrow, next week, or never. Activities and appointments usually not starting on time, person not hurried.	Time used spontaneously; not time-conscious. Little emphasis on long-range planning. "Right now" means now or later. May arrive after scheduled appointment time.	Appreciation and effective use of time. Calmness and time for daily ceremony highly valued. Ceremony carried out in spite of rush of work.

because Muslims hold to the belief that life begins at conception. Arabs and Iranians may use abortion as a form of birth control, although it is not openly recommended or talked about and is clearly prohibited by Islamic law. Selective abortions are used in the case of an illegitimate child, as an attempt by the individual to maintain the society's integrity, since illegitimate children and unsanctioned sexual practices carry grave consequences with them (144).

Sexuality and childrearing practices differ from those of the West. Middle Eastern clients possess a feeling of fatalism; they do not plan excessively for future events but rather leave them to the will of God. Many women do not seek prenatal care in the Middle East; only when the baby is ready to be born do they go to the hospital or call a midwife to come to the home for the birth. Often women do not plan the layette or select a name until after the infant is born. Traditional as well

TABLE 1-8. A COMPARISON OF CULTURES: WORK AND USE OF LEISURE TIME

Component	Greek	Spanish-speaking	Japanese
Concept of work	Work thought of as life, a joy and dignity, not drudgery. Work interrupted primarily for religious reasons, not as claim to idleness or leisure. Women work as hard as men. Tenacious and resourceful at making the best of what they have and coping with difficulty. Person not to be hurried but works efficiently at own pace.	Work considered inevitable part of daily life. Not done just to keep busy or earn more money if present needs met. No moral corruption in being idle. Work at own pace and no specially defined working hours if possible. Everyone expected to cooperate and do his or her part. Work shared to decrease loneliness. Work roles of sexes and age groups distinct but each aware of tasks performed by others. Able to take over work roles of other family members. Child a part of work of home and family and feels important. No special rewards.	Enjoyment of work more important than money earned. Industriousness and hard work emphasized. Strong ties between person, the job, and the company. Work hard for success. Job mobility frowned on; loyalty to company. Independence in work traditionally valued but younger workers adjusting to Western concept of employment. Seek perfection on job; high sense of responsibility for job; quiet achievement. Consensus management emphasized.
Concepts of leisure	Leisure an attitude, a dimension of all life and work. Not confined to certain time but a continual expression of internal freedom, at work or rest.	Leisure synonymous with free time. No emphasis on leisure for own sake. Intersperse work with rest, socialize during work. Free time spent visiting.	Some leisure time used in solitude. Much leisure time spent in traveling with peers. Freer expression of emotion in recreational pursuits.

TABLE 1-9. A COMPARISON OF CULTURES: EDUCATION

Component	Greek	Spanish-speaking	Japanese
Value on education	Highly prized, especially professional education. Curiosity and creativity valued. Educated person accorded much respect. Use of creative intellect and being a cultured citizen valued, but can be achieved through life's experiences and work as well as by education.	Learns that which interests him or her. Absent from school if learning little or if something more interesting going on elsewhere. Not seen as only way to achieve.	Respect for school and teacher. Education highly valued, with emphasis on scientific information. Parents involved in education. Eager to learn. Memorization emphasized. Believe in value of practical experience as well. Choice of college influences status in life. Much competition in education.
Educational methods	Emphasize quickness, curiosity, cleverness, realism, reason. Education applied to matters of life.	No emphasis on excelling or competing against other family members for high grades or honors. Use of native language may interfere with success in school.	Educational reform by U.S. occupation after World War II counter to traditional methods: replaced rote memorization with progressive methods, de-emphasized moral training and unquestioning acceptance of authority, granted equal status to women, broadened opportunity for women.

as modern Middle Eastern women tend to breast-feed for extended periods of time; it is written as a requirement in the Koran to breast-feed for 2 years (106).

Children in the Middle East are viewed not only as a commodity but also as a blessing to the family. They are something to be cherished; therefore, families invest a great deal emotionally into their children and tend to practice lenient discipline measures. Children are usually not physically hit or verbally abused. Rather they are distracted away from whatever they are doing that is bad and encouraged to do good things.

Many Middle Eastern clients tend to base the success of their parenthood not on the cognitive skills of children, but rather on the weight gain, health, and normality of their children. They do not accept deviation of health status in others compared to the normal population. This author knew a woman from Kuwait who had a younger sister with Down's Syndrome. Upon introduction of her family, she said "This is my mother and this is my abnormal sister." She does not feel her sister is worthy enough to be called by her name.

Need for Affiliation. An important aspect of caring for Middle Eastern clients is to recognize their need for affil-

TABLE 1-10. A COMPARISON OF CULTURES: ATTITUDES REGARDING CHANGE

Component	Greek	Spanish-speaking	Japanese
Value of change	Not valued for itself. Progress hoped for but not taken for granted. Change does not necessarily bring progress or improvement.	Change condemned if simply because it is change. Patience and postponing personal desires emphasized. Appreciate gentle approach. Little faith in progress or control over own destiny.	Physical world considered transient. Person appreciative of but does not cling to things; thus change accepted.
Pace of change	Deliberate.	Deliberate. Slow. Fearful or suspicious of change.	Able to adjust lifestyle to rapid economic, industrial, and urban changes.
Effect of change	No value on unlimited progress. Wants what is better than present but what is known and can be achieved. A plan to an American is synonymous with a dream to a Greek. Use material goods. Do not discard useful articles. Repair objects to maintain usefulness. Traditional Greek culture changing, becoming Westernized, affecting behavior of young.	Value system seen as constant. Feel many individuals not amenable to change by human endeavor. Adjust to environment. Use material goods to capacity. Generally remain near traditional home, maintain stable relationships with people. Change in main culture affecting behavior of young, causing insecurity in elders.	Urgency of Western-like activity a new phenomenon. Breaking traditional patterns and solidarity; increased individualism, competition, and individual insecurity. Youth seeking new values to replace old dogmas. Parent's generation generally reveres authority of family and state—now rejected by younger generation.

iation and belonging, which is central and critical to survival. The strength and importance of the individual is directly related to family members and friends; they are an integral part of life. Although men and women may be segregated, socialization is extensive. Middle Eastern people are known for their hospitality, and they emphasize family relations. Visiting among members of the extended family and their friends is a social obligation on all occasions, and children of all ages are included as part of the visits.

Cleanliness. Although Middle Easterners may live in crowded family situations within their homes, they use basic measures to insure cleanliness. The client's body and clothes must be clean of bodily secretions, and most of these clients' homes are very clean and are always being cleaned. The expression, "You can eat off the floor," is literally true, because the family does eat from the floor, as well as sit, lie down, and sleep on the floor. These homes generally have no furniture or are sparsely or very selectively furnished. When you walk into such a home, you are required to remove your shoes in order to keep the carpet clean so events of the home may take place on a clean area. This produces for the Middle Easterner a definite feeling of separation between the external world and the internal world of their home.

Health Care. Muslims and Middle Eastern people often have home cures for common health problems. If it does not harm the client, let the person carry out the home or cultural remedies. It will serve to build trust in the relationship and show respect for the client. They believe that cures can be obtained through the use of home remedies, such as herbs, concentrated sugar preparations, and hot/cold foods. Although they believe in the superiority of Western medicine, they do not always trust it; therefore, they practice home-remedy medicine side by side with modern Western medical practices. When prescribing medical treatment or dispensing medicine, these clients believe that intrusive measures are of more value than nonintrusive measures. For example, intravenous medication is better than that given intramuscularly, injections are better than pills, and colored pills are better than white ones. Another example of a cultural practice is that at the time of delivery, parents want to say a prayer in the newly born child's ears. Muslims believe that the first sounds a child hears should be from the Koran in praise and supplication to God. This practice does not hurt the baby, but allowing its practice will go a long way to build trust into the relationship with the parents and family.

In the health care setting, the extensive visiting by family and friends can become very difficult for the institution to accommodate because visiting is usually restricted by policy. But for the Middle Eastern client, this visiting becomes extremely important in how the person perceives the disease and adapts to it. Lack of visitors can imply to the client that he or she is gravely ill and close to death when this may not be the case at all, but instead is the result of the hospital policy about visitors. Visiting should be allowed on a liberal basis. Visits from family members are also important because Middle Eastern clients do not expect personal care from health care providers; the role of the family members is to physically care for the person who is in the hospital.

Communication. Islam dictates that family affairs remain in the family; they are not affairs for the rest of the world. This can be seen in many situations, with modesty as one example. Women dress differently outside the home than they do inside the home. The body tends to be covered and only the face, hands, and feet show. For Muslim women residing in the West, this manner of dress is usually modified but still retains the quality of conservative fashion.

Respecting the client's modesty during health care or implementation of procedures is essential. Because of modesty, there is a difference in the information that a person gives to various people. Very personal information is shared only with intimate contacts; nonintimate or general information can be shared with almost anyone. Thus assessment must be done gradually and respectfully. Certain information may never be obtained.

Communication in the Middle East is an elaborate system. It can be either very intimate in terms of content and word usage, or it can be very stilted, using only proper nouns and formal forms of verbs. The choice depends on whom you are talking to and the subject. A person may knowingly say the opposite of what he or she is thinking to avoid being rude. There are communication methods to avoid, especially in nonintimate conversations, because they are perceived as offensive and rude. First, outwardly showing anger or insulting someone is considered bad manners. Emotion can be shown with intimate persons but not with nonintimate contacts. Second, do not be abrupt or interrupt, especially with elders or when another is speaking. Third, in preliminary casual conversation that is part of business or professional association, if you are a man, do not ask the man about the female members of his family, including his wife, sisters, or daughters after they reach the age of puberty. For a woman to ask about female members is acceptable.

As in all populations, communication and teaching become critical issues related to health outcome. Individuality should never be viewed as noncompliance. There are generally reasons for a Muslim's behavior or choice of action. Not carrying out a health care professional's teachings does not mean the Muslim is begin uncooperative. You should reassess the situation in terms of its cultural totality.

Language Barriers. Interpreters or family members can be used to assist with teaching when the client's language is not known. However, family members may withhold information that they feel is too threatening for the client to hear or inappropriate to disclose about the client. If interpreters are used, they should be of the same language, religion, and country of origin. A mistake was made in one agency by having a female Muslim from Iraq translate in Arabic to a new Muslim mother from Arabia, without first having obtained the husband's consent. When the father of the baby discovered this arrangement for his wife to learn newborn care through the Iraqi woman, he became angry and would not allow the situation to take place. Involve family members when doing client teaching and always attempt to involve both the husband and wife together in discussions. If in the event the health care provider needs to talk to a woman about her husband, extreme tact should be used at all times in the discussion.

Language barriers can cause a great amount of misunderstanding to occur. Listen to the themes of the content being discussed rather than to the exact words being used. It can take many years for a foreign person to learn a language, and usually building a vocabulary is the most difficult part of any language mastery. As an example, this author's husband has been in the United States for 9 years and is a doctoral student as well as a college instructor; he still is learning vocabulary that I take for granted. Ironically, with many foreigners, even though their vocabulary is not strong, their grammar and word usage is perfect.

When you do teaching with an individual or a family, remember that foreign people may appear to be understanding your communication, when in reality they are not understanding what you are saying, in order to avoid embarrassment and save face. Some Middle Eastern persons are very good at convincing others that they know what to do when in reality they do not understand enough to take responsibility for their own or their family's health needs or care. It is best in these situations, if a translator cannot be procured, to use short simple sentences containing easy-to-understand vocabulary and speak slowly and clearly. It is also best to communicate with the client using the same sentence each time. Saying, "How are you today?" one day, and then, "How are you feeling?" the next time may not be confusing to some one who speaks fluent English. But for someone who is struggling with the language it can be very confusing. It is also best to avoid slang and unconventional English because most Middle Easterners, when learning English, learn and cling to the security of proper English.

You may also rely on nonverbal means of teaching. Although there may be cultural differences in body language, some nonverbal communication may express similar emotions in any culture, such as fear, pain, or sadness. Teaching can also occur by physically moving the body of the person or showing what you want the person to learn by demonstrating in yourself. Pictures can be drawn to illustrate points of learning, or bilingual flash cards can be made to aid teaching. The cards should be bilingual so that the teacher and the learner each know what the card says and therefore have some basis for communication. These cards can be used at other times when translators or family are not available to communicate basic needs of the client, such as on night shift when the client wants to use the bathroom. Although this appears to be a simplistic means of communication, it can be very efficient and serve to decrease frustration and anxiety in both the client and health care professional.

Differences in Values. Middle Eastern clients do not emphasize a time schedule; this Western value and practice is imposed on Middle Eastern people. Time factors for these people tend to be in terms of what is important at that moment rather than projecting rigidly into the future as to what is important.

This can cause conflicts in a health care setting where tests or health care appointments are scheduled at particular times and the client does not feel it is a priority. The client may view taking a bath and being clean as more of a priority and that the test can wait or be rescheduled for later.

Middle Eastern clients expect health care practitioners to find effective cures without asking many questions or using numerous diagnostic tests, which are often needed for a correct diagnosis. They believe if a doctor or nurse asks too many questions or orders too many tests that the practitioner is naive, lacks experience, should not be trusted, or is narrow in perspective and understanding. These clients prefer older male doctors, preferably heads of departments in their specialty area, rather than younger or female doctors. The exception is that a female obstetrician or gynecologist is required for a female client who is pregnant or has a gynecological disorder. Generally, Middle Eastern clients do not trust doctors completely because they feel doctors are too expensive, ask too many questions, and often lack experience.

Due to strict Islamic law, Muslims are not allowed to engage in deviant sexual practices, premarital sex, or adultery or to use illegal drugs or alcohol. Thus the incidence of associated diseases (i.e., AIDS, sexually transmitted diseases, alcoholism, fetal alcohol syndrome) is virtually nonexistent.

These clients prefer the same caretaker each day; the same caretaker increases trust and acceptance in the relationship and decreases suspicion of the health care provider by the client and the family. Having the same caretaker also helps decrease mistrust of the world of medicine that these clients really do not understand thoroughly. A nurse can capitalize on this situation by being the same caregiver and consistently offering help.

The Middle Eastern client believes that if somebody compliments a person about something that is good or of value, such as jewelry or a new baby, or even looks at it with admiration, this behavior will bring out the evil eye. The **evil eye** *is a form of jealousy and mistrust of the admirer by the owner of the object being complimented.*

In the health care setting, avoid suspicion of the evil eye in Middle Eastern clients by directing compliments to the owner or to God (Allah), rather than to the object itself. Such action converts the possibility of the evil eye and misfortune into a blessing instead.

Legal Documents. The last area of client concerns is legal documents. It is recommended that birth certificates be signed by both the father and mother of the baby. In the United States, statistical agencies of state governments feel that only the mother is the verifiable parent of a child. This can be very insulting to a patrilineal father. By having both parents sign the birth certificate, the problem of the father being insulted is remedied and both the state and family have their interests met.

Consent forms are generally not used in the Middle East. First, the client does not feel he or she has the knowledge to assume responsibility for health decisions and therefore leaves this responsibility to the health care professional who has been trained to make these decisions. Secondly, in Islam, especially in front of witnesses, a man's word and agreement are considered binding and written documentation is therefore not necessary. When a consent form needs to be signed after an agreement has been made, it can be interpreted with mistrust and suspicion toward the health care provider. To avoid this, one physician found that, if the consent form was just presented in an institutionally oriented, matter-of-fact way, mistrust was minimized, and clients carried through with the required procedures.

Religious Beliefs. Middle Eastern clients may be Muslims, or they may adhere to other religions. Life-style and health care practices will be influenced by their religious beliefs. Chapter 3 discusses additional practices to be considered in the person's care, based on religious beliefs.

Without your understanding of Middle Eastern culture, these patients can be very frustrating to work with, but when you understand the culture and reasons for the cultural values, and realize that these values have meaning for the individual, Middle Eastern clients become enjoyable and rewarding clients to work with. When you have established trust with the person and family, you will see other aspects of their lives open up to you. This new view can be rewarding.

Attitudes Toward Health and Illness

How health is identified, physically and emotionally, varies from culture to culture, as do ideas about the factors related to health and disease. American definitions are emphasized in Chapter 16.

Dominant U.S. Culture. Attitudes in the United States toward health are influenced considerably by society's emphasis on mastery of the environment as opposed to adjustment to it. Illness is seen as a challenge to be met by mobilizing resources: research, science, funds, institutions, and people. Americans tax themselves to finance health and welfare organizations and persons devoting time and effort to these organizations are given special status by the community. Because independence is highly valued, the weak are expected to help themselves as much as possible. Self-care is emphasized. The strong help the weak as long as their problems are caused by events beyond their control; otherwise the physically, socially, or emotionally weak, deformed, or unsightly are devalued.

A person is evaluated on productivity, or "doing good." Because the ability to be productive depends in part on health, individual health is highly valued. Health in the broadest sense is considered necessary for successful interaction with others, educational accomplishment, ability to work, leadership, childrearing, and capacity to use opportunities. Thus development of medical, nursing, and other health sciences and technology is considered important. The physical cause of illness is generally accepted. Only recently have the psychologic and sociocultural causes of disease also been emphasized.

For example, a nationwide study that compared life expectancy, disease incidence, alcohol and tobacco use, access to medical care, absence from work due to illness, and mortality rates found that Utah has the healthiest citizens and that they live $2\frac{1}{2}$ years longer than the national average. Further, people who live in the Rocky Mountains and Midwest are healthier than residents of the Southeast and East Coast, possibly related to lifestyle and environmental factors (228). The media have reported that Hawaii is the healthiest state in the Union because of access to health care, and West Virginia the least healthy because of lack of access to health care.

A 13-year study of over 8,000 adults by the Center for Disease Control showed that the effects of poverty may explain the high rate of premature deaths among African-Americans. No more than 31% of the difference between the death rate of Caucasians and African-Americans in the United States can be attributed to hereditary or environmental factors, including the high-risk factors of smoking, drinking, diabetes, obesity, and hypertension. Impoverished Americans use the health care system less often and are more likely to suffer from preventable acute diseases. The study suggests that eradicating poverty and providing accessible quality care are important to health and longevity (184).

Studies of Alaskan Natives show a strikingly lower

death rate from cardiovascular disease than for other Alaskans, while the death rate from infections, respiratory diseases, and neoplasms were higher. Diet, lifestyle, and accessibility to health care appear to be reasons for these differences (126).

The importance of health has been accentuated by industrialization, high-level technology, greater social controls, and mass communications, as well as by a high level of responsibility and stress placed on the individual. Americans at times react to the complexities of society by retreating into ill health, physically, emotionally, or socially. Levels of pathology that could be tolerated in preindustrial societies cannot be tolerated in complex modern life. Americans are more likely than people in other societies to interpret a person's difficulty in fulfilling social-role expectations as illness. Thus the person who is ill is less likely to be tolerated or kept in the family. When ill, the person is supposed to leave home, isolate self from the family, and be cared for in a strange place, the hospital, by strange people who are authorities on illness. One's capacity for meeting social-role expectations is developed primarily through family socialization and education, but it is protected and restored through the health care system. The ill person is expected to want to return to normal roles and leave behind the feelings of alienation, regression, and passivity that are part of the deviance of illness. The impersonal agency of the hospital exerts pressures that discourage staying dependent and ill.

Greek Culture. In Greece health is important and desired, but it is not a preoccupation. One should not pamper the self. Straight living gives a healthy body; thus fortitude, hardness, and a simple standard of living are pursued. Excesses in living—in eating, drinking, or smoking—are avoided, and, in general, the level of public health is high. Because children are prized, their health needs take precedence over adults' needs.

Going to bed is a sign of weakness except for recognized disease. People do not go to a physician unless there is something seriously wrong; but then they expect the physician, who is a father figure, to have the answers for their problems. Home remedies and the services of an herbalist are tried first as treatment. Prayers are said and vows are made. Illness is thought to arise from evil or magical sources that can be counteracted through magical practices. Entering the hospital is a last resort. The whole family is involved when a member is sick; each person has a specific role and a role gap exists during illness (11, 84, 244).

The organs of highest significance are the eyes, for they reflect the real person. Next in importance are the lips because of the words that come out of them. A girl's hair and a man's mustache are important symbols of sexual identity and attractiveness. The genital organs are not freely talked about but are respected for their reproductive functions. The body is meant to be covered and exposed only when necessary. Dress and ornamentation are essential to complete one's body image (11, 84, 244).

Childlessness is unfortunate and in the past the woman was held responsible. Women dislike any examination or treatment of the reproductive organs and will accept gynecologic problems rather than seek medical care for fear fertility will be affected. Special care is given to women during pregnancy, when special regulations about hygiene, rest, activity, and a happy environment are followed (11, 84, 244).

The handicapped are not easily accepted because of the emphasis on a whole, strong, firm body. To be crippled, blind, or lame means that one is not a whole person, is dependent, and is unable to do anything for oneself (84, 244).

Greek-Americans adhere to some or many of the aforementioned values and practices, depending on closeness to cultural ties.

Latino Culture. Attitudes among Latinos in the American Southwest (or other Spanish-speaking people) are very unlike attitudes in mainstream America. Spanish-American people considers the self to be a whole person; thus "better health" has no meaning. Good health is associated with the ability to work and fulfill normal roles, for one gains and maintains respect by meeting one's responsibilities. Criteria of health are a sturdy body, ability to maintain normal physical activity, and absence of pain. A person does not have to have perfect health; as long as the family is around, he or she is all right. Thus preventive measures are not highly valued. A person does seek to care for oneself, however, through moderation in eating, drinking, work, recreation, and sleep, and by leading a good life (171).

Acculturation, *the process of change occurring as a result of contact between cultural groups,* is demonstrated by a minority group's adoption of the larger group's cultural mores. Lack of assimilation on the part of Latinos has been described as a strong barrier to their optimal use of health services. It is assumed that Latinos who retain Spanish as their first language, who are proud of their ethnic heritage, and who do not follow American norms and values are much less likely than their more assimilated counterparts to use health services or engage in preventive health behaviors. Marks et al., as a result of their study of elderly Latino women in Los Angeles, believe that cultural factors may have little impact on the health-care-seeking behavior of Hispanics. Access to and availability of services, feelings toward screening processes, values about privacy, and sociodemographic factors are stronger determinants of Latino health practices (132).

Latino people believe that hardship and suffering are part of destiny, and that reward for being submissive to God's will and for doing good will come in the next life. Ill health is accepted as part of life and is thought to be caused by an unknown external event or object, such as natural forces of cold, heat, storms, water, or as the result of sinning—acting against God's will. Latinos, for example, think that one cause of illness is bad air, especially night air, which enters through a cavity or opening in the body. Thus a raisin may be placed on the cord stump of the newborn and surgery is avoided if possible; both practices help prevent air from entering the body. Avoiding drafts, keeping windows closed at night, keeping the head covered, and following certain postpartum practices have the same basis. Other causes of disease (according to Hispanic beliefs) include overwork, poor food, excess worry or emotional strain, undue exposure to weather, uneven wetting of the body, taking a drink when overheated, and giving blood for transfusion. Underlying this thinking is the hot-cold theory of disease that stems from the Hippocratic humoral theory and was carried to the Western Hemisphere by the Spanish and Portuguese in the sixteenth and seventeenth centuries. Basically all diseases are classified as hot and cold. Arthritis is a cold disease and an ulcer is a hot disease, for instance. It is considered dangerous to be outdoors at night if one's body is warm. Pregnancy and menstruation are considered warm body states. The hot-and-cold theory of disease does not always refer to physical temperature or foodstuff, but also to the effects that certain substances have or are thought to have on the body. Beliefs about which foods are warm and cold vary from one geographic region and culture to another. For example, prenatal vitamins may be a hot food and will not be taken during pregnancy, a hot condition, unless swallowed with fruit juice, a cold food. All foods, herbs, and medicines are classified as hot or cold. Avocado is a cold food and aspirin and cornmeal are considered hot. A goal is to balance the body: a hot disease is cured with a cold food and a cold disease is cured with a hot food, herb, or medication. Thus aspirin could be taken for arthritis—which also fits into the Western medical system (6, 20, 171).

Evil eye, *mal ojo, is a cause of disease that results when a person looks admiringly at the child of another.* Usually children are not openly admired, but precautions against illness include patting the child on the head or a light slap. (Do you know people in other subcultures with similar beliefs? Such causes are commonly stated when illness occurs.) A common illness in this culture, **susto,** with *symptoms of agitation and depression, results from traumatic, frightening experiences and may result in death.* Psychosocial forces causing disease are also seen in **empacho,** *a gastrointestinal disease that results from eating food that is disliked, or from overeating, or from eating hot bread.* **Mollera caido** *(fallen fontanels) is caused by a child falling or someone pulling the nipple out of the mouth too quickly, and results in crying, vomiting, sunken eyes, and inability to grasp the nipple.* Hydration is essential in treatment. **Resfriade** *(chilled) results from getting wet and*

not changing to dry clothes. In turn, **cotarro constipado** *(head cold or sinusitis)* may result. Disease may also result from organs or parts of the body moving from the normal position. Little attention is paid to colds, minor aches, or common gastrointestinal disorders (6, 20, 171, 242).

The role of the family is important in time of illness. The head of the house, the man, determines whether illness exists and what treatment is to be given. The person goes to bed when too ill to work or move. Treatment from a lay healer is sought if family care does not help. A physician is called only when the person is gravely ill; this is combined with visiting so the sick person does not get the rest and isolation advised by health care professionals in the majority culture. The sick person does not withdraw from the group; doing so would only make him or her feel worse. Acceptance of fate amounts to saying "If the Lord intends for me to die, I'll die." The discomfort of the present is considered, but not in terms of future complications. Being ill brings no secondary advantage of care or coddling. Communicable diseases are hard to control, for resistance to isolation is based on the idea that family members, relatives, and familiar objects cannot contaminate or cause illness. Taking home remedies, wearing special articles, and performing special ceremonies are accepted ways of getting and staying well. The person feels he or she will keep well by observing the ritual calendar, being brotherly, being a good Catholic and member of the community. If the health care provider uses any procedure, such as an x-ray, it is considered to be the treatment and hence the person should be cured (6, 20, 171, 242).

Accidents are feared because they disrupt the wholeness of the person. In addition, Latinos fear surgery, the impersonality of the hospital and nurses, and any infringement on modesty.

The hospital represents death and isolation from family or friends. The "professional" (Anglo) approach of the majority culture is regarded as showing indifference to needs and as causing anxiety and discomfort.

Anthony-Tkach describes specific health care practices of Spanish-speaking people and families and nursing implications, including for childbirth, childrearing, and prevention of communicable diseases. She also discusses customs related to use of folk medicine, use of surnames, and customs of interaction (6).

Japanese Culture. Attitudes in Japan toward health strongly reflect the belief in a body-mind-spirit interrelationship. Spiritual and temporal affairs in life are closely integrated; thus health practices and religion are closely intertwined, influenced considerably by the magicoreligious practices of Shinto, Japan's ancient religion. Bathing customs stem from Shinto purification rites, for example, and baths are taken in the evening before eating not only for cleanliness but for ceremony and relaxation as well.

There is a strong emphasis on healthy diet (low fat, low sugar), physical fitness, an intact body, physical strength, determination, family and group relationships, and long life. Self-discipline in daily habits is highly valued, as are the mental, spiritual, and esthetic aspects of the person. All of these values and traits promote health and remain equally important to the sick person to promote recovery.

As a child, the individual is taught to minimize reactions to injury and illness. Hence to the Westerner a sick person may appear stoic. Part of the reserve in expressing emotion and pain is also influenced by childrearing and interaction practices, which emphasize correct behavior and suppression of emotion. Yet the sick person, as much as one who is well, expects to be treated with respect and resents being addressed abruptly or informally by first name. The person also resents people entering the hospital room without knocking. The Japanese male resents being dominated by women and he may feel uncomfortable with an American female health care professional because he interprets her behavior as overbearing. The person is eager to cooperate with the medical care program but wishes to be included in planning and decisions regarding care. The so-called professional approach of the average U.S. health care provider is likely to insult the average Japanese, although he or she may be too polite to say so (219).

By studying life patterns of people in various cultures (especially those of patients for whom you care) and by taking into account the factors discussed in the following chapters on religion and family, you can better understand and handle varying levels of health, health problems, and attitudes toward care of different groups.

You may obtain additional information about people from the following (sub)cultures and their specific nursing needs from references at the end of the chapter:

1. African-American (29, 42, 43, 54, 67, 77, 86, 96, 97, 100, 102, 114, 118, 137, 139, 185, 193, 198, 212, 216, 218, 222, 242, 247)
2. American Indian (26, 40, 88, 93, 105, 133, 139, 180, 187, 188, 194, 208, 218, 234, 236, 242, 248, 251)
3. Amish (92, 241)
4. Appalachian (65, 72, 98, 165, 191, 206, 226, 235, 245)
5. Asian-American (12, 23, 28, 32, 49, 50, 53, 55, 69, 120, 121, 124, 133, 139, 141, 157, 201, 213, 214, 217, 218, 219, 238, 246, 250, 252)
6. Eskimo (14, 18, 40, 57, 126, 133, 139, 147, 155)
7. German-American (62, 81, 139, 190, 196, 197, 205, 209)
8. Greek-American (11, 84, 139, 199, 244)
9. Gypsy (4)
10. Irish-American (11, 78, 81, 139, 169, 253, 254)
11. Italian-American (11, 45, 81, 133, 139, 253, 254)
12.

Japanese-American (11, 49, 79, 120, 124, 133, 158, 166, 219)
13. Jewish (11, 20, 61, 139, 161, 171, 253)
14. Middle Eastern (8, 9, 74, 82, 122, 123, 128, 139, 143–146, 149, 151, 167, 240)
15. Migrant farmer (11, 95, 174, 233)
16. Polish-American (101, 125, 139, 168, 203)
17. Puerto Rican (49, 64, 117)
18. Southeast Asian refugees (12, 36, 66, 75, 124, 201, 222)
19. Spanish-speaking or Latino (1, 6, 7, 29, 40, 47, 51, 59, 73, 87, 89, 91, 107, 131–134, 139, 153, 156, 159, 185, 186, 202, 218)
20. Vietnamese (35, 53, 124, 139, 222, 232)

SOCIOECONOMIC CLASS SUBCULTURE

Research about social stratification indicates that a person's class position is influenced by economic and social status and political power of the family and affects formation of values, attitudes, and lifestyle. Each class tends to have a more or less well-specified set of values and role expectations regarding practically every area of human activity: sex, marriage, male-female and parent-child responsibilities and behavior, birth, death, education, dress, housing, home furnishings, leisure, reading habits, occupational status, politics, religion, and status symbols. In turn, health status in the United States is closely linked to income level. Poor people are more likely to have poor health and chronic illness (83, 184). Social class includes a group consciousness. Most persons can be objectively placed within a certain class (80), but they are sometimes accorded a status by others around them that might be different. Furthermore, they may see themselves at yet a different status level, based on race, sex, religion, ancestry, ethnic origin, or wealth in material goods. What seems natural and logical in determining status to some people may be rejected by others.

As you gain general knowledge about values and lifestyles of people in various economic levels, realize also that no one person encompasses all that the literature describes. Knowledge about lifestyles is generally useful to a nursing practice, but *avoid stereotyping people* because of this knowledge.

Profile of Socioeconomic Levels

The Upper-Upper or Corporate Level

This level consists of a relatively small number of people who own a disproportionate share of personal wealth and whose income is largely derived from ownership. Their work, profession, or business provides prestige, status, honor, wealth, and power. This group has both money and power and it can control how its assets are used as well as various other economic and political aspects of society. The decisions made by this group affect everyone else. Coles (39, 41) refers to them as the *affluent*. These are the people who have had lineage, inherited wealth, and power for several generations. They are acknowledged by the general public and themselves as leaders locally, nationally, and internationally. They feel obliged to tend their own financial and material resources well, to obtain the best possible education, and to take care of their health so that they can meet their obligation of giving of themselves personally and philanthropically to society (39, 41, 85, 181). The affluent family is almost clanlike. All members, including the women and youth, belong to elite clubs or organizations and also participate in and contribute considerably to the community and society as a whole through financial contributions and volunteer activities to various social, welfare, health, and political organizations. Yet the very rich remain anonymous to most Americans.

This person or family lives in an exclusive residential area in a house whose atmosphere is spatial, elegant, and formal, and that affords privacy from the masses. This person or family may own several estates in different areas of the country (or world) that are located in the best areas, are furnished with family heirlooms and works of art, and are used in different seasons or for different purposes. The family may have a number of people to help it maintain its life-style, such as a maid, butler, gardener, and other staff members (39, 41, 46, 85, 181).

The children are reared by a governess or maid as well as by the parents. The mother usually is selective in her teaching, guiding, and care. Certain aspects of rearing are done only by the mother, others only by the maid. The children may feel closer to the parent surrogates than to the parents. They, like the parents, live with choices, for they have more animate and inanimate objects and possessions than others and many opportunities to follow the arts; to learn certain sports, such as horseback riding, tennis, swimming, or skiing; and to travel worldwide. But even the children know the importance and value of the objects and opportunities that surround them. They recognize the importance of self-control, behaviorally and in their various activities and sports, and of following family wishes and upholding the family name. They seek privacy, reverie, and disciplined activity even though in the public view. They are able to move smoothly from one activity to another without being driven to excel. Yet they expect to be competent at their chosen academic, recreational, and social pursuits (39, 41, 46, 71, 85, 181).

Although the upper economic level is adult oriented, children know at an early age that they are special and parents try to instill a feeling that the children must do well because they have special responsibilities to society on reaching adulthood. The child, like the parent, associates with others from the same level, observing the average person from the sidelines, never really understanding what life is like for the average citizen or why people from lower economic levels live as they do. Although both adults and children take a lot for granted and feel entitled to the fine things in life, they feel a sense of responsibility, are discrete in behavior, and try to live up to their ideals. Destiny is abundance and limitless possibility. They are confident that life will be rewarding. Even crisis, such as illness or surgery, can be made into something basically pleasant, for the best of specialized health care professionals and comprehensive facilities can be obtained, and convalescence frequently involves a trip to and rest at a secluded place (39, 41, 46, 71, 85, 181).

Values that members of this group hold include the family, its home, its name, and position; lineage and tradition; privacy; power and prestige; contribution to society; economic achievements; affluence; education; travel; consumption of material goods and possession of cultural artifacts and art pieces; and philanthropy.

The Lower-Upper Level

This group consists of people whose wealth is more recently acquired and who have become well-known (actors, famous doctors or lawyers, athletes), or they may be less famous but have large incomes, homes, and life-styles that show off their money. They have social position and prestige because of what they *do*. The upper-upper-level person has position and prestige because of *who* he or she is; the person does not lose them even if encountering financial setbacks. The lower-upper-level person may slide down into middle-level anonymity if wealth is lost. The lower-upper-level (or newly rich) person or family also has an abundance of possessions and opportunity, but may be less humble about or more self-conscious of it than the upper-upper-level person. Although this person or family may attend the same activities, travel to the same areas, or send children to the same schools as the upper-upper-level family, this person or family is seen by the long-established wealthy as being different (39, 41). Often a fine line separates these two levels in a community; such intangibles as social charm or likeability, family background, religion, area and value of residence, and schooling often make the difference. Money is only loosely related to social standing in many communities (39, 41, 46, 183). Both women and men of this level are working—entering a profession, starting a business, or doing consultant work—for fun, for a sense of identity, to be worthwhile, to provide structure to the day or to life, to avoid the image of being intellectual (they are usually college educated), or to avoid being important only through the spouse.

The Upper-Middle Level

This group is described as *those who are well off* and is considered to be the backbone of the community. Income is high but varies, depending on occupation and geographic area. Each spouse is college educated and at least one is a professional—doctor, dentist, engineer, business manager, or lawyer. The main work of these people is intellectual instead of manual, requires professional training, and offers upward mobility. The workplace is as important to the spouse as to the employed member. They may begin family life in an apartment, but when financially able, they move to a large house in a better part of town or a suburb. They may have a maid and gardener, own more than one car, travel nationally and abroad, belong to a semi-elite country club, and frequently send their children to private schools and colleges (41, 80, 183). Both family stability and community leadership are valued. The children have a number of opportunities educationally and culturally; in return, they are expected to be successful academically and socially. The children are often involved in a number of prestigious out-of-home activities and organizations, as are parents, and the children may actually have fewer home responsibilities than the upper-class child. Childrearing is permissive; children are given explanations instead of punishment. The parents will exert more direct influence on the child's schooling than will parents of the middle or working class (41, 183, 230). The work ethic is different for this group from the work ethic of the rich. Thus, children may do tasks to earn an allowance and may work at various jobs, such as babysitting, lawnmowing, or fast-food service, in the teen years to earn extra money. (By contrast, parents at higher economic levels do not expect their children to work.) This group has a relatively carefree life-style because money is not a major issue. Movement, gaiety, leisure activities, fun in indoor or outdoor sports, dancing, theatre, museums, travel or educational experiences, acquiring a deeper self-knowledge, and remaining youthful are major foci. One image is that of the serious-minded sportsman (33, 183, 230).

This group values education, hard work, career success and achievement, intellect, high goals, initiative, responsibility, ability to withstand stress, honesty, the ability to understand and work with concepts, upward social and economic mobility, security, democracy and patriotism, consumption of material goods and material comfort, family stability and prestige, patience in relationships, community leadership and involvement, leisure activity and travel, and involvement in societal changes and progress.

The Middle Level

The middle economic level sometimes is divided in two categories: those who reached the American dream and those who have a comfortable existence. Members of the *American dream* group have education above the high school level in a professional or specialized school and include business people with small or medium-sized enterprises, self-employed business people, artists, skilled workers, office and sales workers, and public or private school teachers. Nurses and other health care professionals typically are in this level. These people have a special status because of education and occupation (many *work with* people), although they do not have much wealth. Typically they work in occupations that involve thinking rather than hard physical labor. They live in a pleasant residential section or suburb, in a nicely furnished house, have two cars, sometimes including a van or four-wheel-drive vehicle. The family eats out weekly and vacations annually. This family is usually a nuclear family. It has linkages through kin for social and family goals as well as close friendships with neighbors. The family is active in community activities and organizations, and members may have some positions of power. They pursue some sports or other leisure activities as a family unit, but the family members frequently go to separate activities several evenings a week.

Members of the *comfortable existence* group tend to have less education and less material goods than the first group, but they live comfortably. They have more than the necessities and are somewhat active in the community (33, 58, 71, 183, 220).

Parents in this group are child-oriented; family life often revolves around children and their interests. At work, the person typically deals with manipulation of symbols, ideas, or interpersonal relationships, has to be self-directed, and must use initiative to get ahead. Thus, families (single- or two-parent) have high aspirations for children and take pride in their accomplishments. Parents emphasize education, self-actualization, creativity, interpersonal sensitivity, and they value and encourage verbal and problem-solving skills. The middle (and upper) economic level(s) uses an elaborate code of speech, which is characterized by precision, differentiation of ideas, and extensive use of modifiers and clauses. Its verbosity may bury the meaning, and the abstractness of such speech causes lack of understanding among the working and lower economic levels (58, 183). Parents teach the importance of hard work, self-reliance, thrift, patience, planning ahead, and postponing immediate rewards for later rewards.

These parents are typically more responsive to the advice of experts and research results. They accept the advice of experts, since it is based on their values and therefore offers what they want. Thus, for example, the parents change childrearing practices, perhaps several times on one child and, because of education, are more likely to feel insecure in childrearing and view it as problematic. They discuss childrearing practices with neighbors and friends, consult the physician, nurse, or child's teacher about what they are doing wrong (seldom do they see themselves doing anything right), and join various community organizations, such as the P.T.A., where they can learn even more about childrearing. Parents are consistently more concerned about the child's feelings and try to understand the dynamics of the child's behavior and mix discipline with permissiveness. Discipline is often in the form of withdrawal of privileges or of disapproval, threats, or appeals to reason. Punishment is based on the parent's interpretation of the child's intent behind his or her action. If the child loses control, punishment results. If the outburst represents a release of feeling, the child is less likely to be punished. Additionally, the parent is more likely than a working-class parent to feel and be supportive, accepting, and egalitarian to the child. Children are expected to be expressive verbally and emotionally, be happy and cooperative, confide in parents, want to learn, have self-control, share readily, be self-directed, and stay well and healthy (33, 38, 52, 58, 80, 119, 183, 220).

The parents do many activities together, and roles are not as sharply differentiated. Both parents are supportive of the children, especially of same-sexed children, and the father's role as disciplinarian is secondary to that of supportive figure. This is in accordance with his wife's wishes. Father tends to agree with mother and plays a role close to that desired by her. The parent has greater stability of income and takes for granted much of what a poor parent works hard to achieve. As a result, this parent is freer to give attention to the child (52, 58, 80, 119, 183, 220).

Overall, the people in this group use the internist, family-practice physician, and pediatrician for routine health care, but the services of specialists are used when indicated. They respect health professionals and want thorough and scientific diagnosis and treatment. They see themselves as knowledgeable about health, and appreciate and will try to use additional information. They tolerate, although they do not like, high medical costs (58).

The group's values correspond closely to those of the dominant society previously described.

The Lower-Middle or Working Level

This group is often perceived as those who are *just getting by*. Generally both spouses have graduated from high school and may attend community college. They both have jobs as industrial or blue-collar workers, clerical or service workers, agricultural wage earners, technicians, skilled or semiskilled workers, telephone operators, or waitresses (58, 183). Many of this group work with machines, tools, or objects. Chances for advancement are minimal unless the person pursues further education. Job security is threatened by the effects of automation in the workplace. Opportunity for job advancement is minimal without additional education or an apprenticeship. Many workers who are a part of this economic level are proud of their work, do it very well, and know that they make an important contribution to society. Society must have carpenters, plumbers, secretaries, farmers, garbage collectors, and all of the other workers who are in this group (170).

The family rents either a small home with two or three bedrooms or an apartment and takes good care of its home and belongings, including an older car. It has

some conveniences but may not own many luxuries. The family depends on the extended family instead of social agencies for economic and emotional support and may be active in church but not in the P.T.A. or other community organizations. The husband is typically head of the house and the woman is considered responsible for the home and child care. The family enjoys recreational activities as a family unit, such as bowling or movies, and eating at fast-service or local "home-style" restaurants (38, 58, 183, 230).

The members of this group have watched and feel concern about the steady degradation and erosion of values and customs they consider essential to their perception of a real America (170). They value patriotism, religion, authority, the work ethic, honesty, neatness, decency, proper behavior, respectability, self-reliance, thrift, postponing personal gratification, independence, conformity, consumerism, competition, achievement, education, the home, saving for the future, and law and order. They believe people with money are not happy, and they are grateful for their parents' sacrifices. They accept their position and are basically proud of their hard work, homes, and accomplishments, even with less education. They believe that on-the-job, collective action is important. They believe that the poor are lazy, deserve their poverty, and should not be given welfare. (A natural economic depression and forced unemployment are the only two causes for poverty without moral blame.) Being higher in the social scale than the poor and some minorities gives them a social identity and a measure of social worth. They feel that equality of all people, including the poor, minorities, and women, is threatening and would pose problems of social adjustment. Another danger of equality is that friends or neighbors might surpass them. The present inequality allows the affluent or supervisors to be an elite group, to take care of people, to be friendly, helpful leaders. Equality of income would deprive people of their incentive to work. These people are stable breadwinners, churchgoers, voters, and family men and women. They may have two jobs and little leisure. Leisure is usually focused on activities that help the person temporarily forget the life situation and work. Many do not like their jobs but fear not finding another; therefore they keep the job because of family responsibilities and the hold on respectability that the job brings. What they want most is a decent standard of living (33, 38, 52, 58, 170, 183).

The adult in this level typically has less education, reads less, and is therefore less responsive to research results and the advice of experts. Further, expert advice usually is not relevant to this value system. Childrearing is taken for granted and is not perceived as something that you do with a preset plan, nor as something that is problematic—or to be discussed with others. These parents rely heavily on the extended family, retaining traditional methods of parenting and keeping the same goals that they perceived in their homes and parents. Desirable characteristics in the child, according to the parent, include the following: the child should be neat, clean, honest, obedient, respectful to parents, pleasant to adults, conform to externally imposed standards, trustworthy, and respect the rights of others (38, 52, 58, 80, 170, 183).

That the parent has the above values and views on childrearing can be related to how he or she was raised and educated and the present occupational role. The person typically deals with the manipulation of things and is subjected to standardization and direct supervision and authority; and getting ahead depends on collective action rather than individual initiative. Congruence exists between the adult's occupational requirements and values about the behavior of children. The occupational experience affects the parent's concept of what is desirable behavior—on or off the job, for adults or children. The parents value conformity of behavior; they have learned to conform to get ahead. Thus they punish nonconforming behavior, including what experts would call the natural curiosity of the child, as well as behavior that is extreme or disturbing. The preferred discipline technique is physical punishment rather than emphasis on reasoning. The child should not break rules that are externally imposed, but should remain orderly and obedient. And so the child of the working-class parent is prepared for a position in society as an adult, and in the future as a parent will impose constraints on his or her children in much the same manner (38, 58, 183).

In this level, work and social roles and the roles of mother and father are more sharply differentiated, and the man and woman lead separate social lives. The mother is the more supportive parent, wanting the father to help with discipline. Frequently, the father views himself as the economic provider but sees no reason to help shoulder the responsibility of childrearing. He thinks it is important that the child be taught not to transgress, and since the mother has the primary responsibility for child care, discipline should also be her job. Because he is less involved in childrearing, the father also has less real authority and status in family affairs. In the process, the male and female children learn what it is to be a father and mother, and as adults, their expectations and behavior are influenced, at least some degree by what they unconsciously learned as children. If they have the opportunity of enough education and advantage to move into the middle level, they may slowly change their values and childrearing practices as they outwardly imitate other middle-class parents around them. Yet very often, values do not change and even overt behavior is nearer to that of their parents than that of their newly found middle-class friends (38, 52, 58, 80, 183, 230).

Health care is sought when a person is too sick to work—the group's definition of illness. Prevention is emphasized less than in the foregoing economic levels.

People may try home or folk remedies first and then go to a general practitioner. The neighborhood health center will be used if one exists. Dental care is more likely to be neglected than other medical care. People in this level respond well to an approach that is respectful, personable, prompt, and thorough. They do not understand why health care should be so costly, and they may omit very expensive treatments or drugs whenever possible (33, 38, 58).

The Upper-Lower Level

This group is perceived as those who are *having a real hard time*. The family is often only one step away from poverty and welfare. An individual has fewer chances of acquiring education. Thus people work at menial tasks, usually in nonunion jobs, but are proud to be working. Wages and job benefits are a concern (38). These people may work as domestics, gardeners, hospital or school maintenance or cafeteria workers, junk collectors, garbage collectors, or street cleaners. Often neither husband nor wife has completed high school and sometimes one may not have completed junior high. The family lives in a substandard flat in an older building, usually with an absentee landlord. The family is patriarchal; the woman works but also has all house and child responsibilities. Children are an asset; they leave school early and help support the family (183). The family enjoys picnics in the park and other free diversions. The family's only long trips are for funerals of relatives (183). Often the family had its beginning in lack of motivation for education, resulting in high school dropout for pregnancy or lack of academic success, early parenthood, a poor first job, a rapid succession of children, or an early separation or divorce. As life progresses, the chance to advance becomes even less likely (33, 38, 136, 183, 230).

Values of people in this level are similar to those of the lower-middle level, with greater emphasis on thrift and conformity to external authority.

The Poor

Poor people, the underclass, include those who are in acute poverty and those in chronic poverty. First, poverty has two definitions. **Poverty** *is having inadequate pre-tax money or source of income to purchase a minimum amount of goods and services.* Poverty is also a power issue. *It is the relative lack of an individual's access to and control over environmental resources.* Poverty reflects class and racial stratification and hopelessness and is seen in increasing homelessness and health problems that result from the conditions of poverty (150). The person or family in **acute poverty** *has reduced economic means for a limited time because of given circumstances* but anticipates being able to return to work and a better life-style. The person or family in **chronic poverty** *has a long family history of being unemployed and without adequate economic means* *and is unlikely to see much opportunity for improvement* (37, 174).

The lines are not always so clearly drawn, however. Because of the unemployment problems of the 1980s and 1990s, more people who were in the middle economic level now are economically classified as poor. A single parent raising several children, although middle class by birth, may become acutely poor when a job is not available or a prolonged illness or other crisis occurs (60). Currently, one in every five American children live in poverty (17% of Caucasian children; 40% of Hispanic children; 50% of African-American children). In the late 1980s, one child in every four was born into poverty. Poor children are often sick at birth, are more likely to suffer physical deformities and display mental deficiencies, either because of inadequate nutrition or poor prenatal and early child care. Seventy percent of poor children live with only one parent, often a teen and usually the mother. Among African-Americans, more than one-half, and in some regions two-thirds, of the children live with one parent. The children develop deep emotional scars and feel low self-esteem, a sense of failure, mistrust of self and others, and anger. The older children get the greater their difficulties. In school, they perform badly on tests and often drop out. Then they are less employable, more susceptible to drug and alcohol abuse, more likely to serve a jail term, and more likely to have children who will repeat the cycle (37, 94, 135, 136, 150, 174, 183, 184, 195, 230).

Some poor children will defy the odds, and through initiative, a strong will, defiance against their situation, good parenting, and an encounter with an extraordinary teacher or adult over the years will break out of the cycle (136).

Other people are joining the ranks of acutely poor in the 1990s because of governmental policies and economic trends. Some people work full-time but earn minimum wage or less. Acutely poor families include the middle- or working-class family where both spouses work to maintain their standard of living, and one or both becomes unemployed. Or the main provider becomes unemployed; the second salary, once providing extras, is now inadequate. In many industries, layoffs have put one, if not both spouses, out of work. The longer the person is unemployed, the more difficult it becomes to find a job using specific educational or job skills. Unless the individual is willing to take any kind of job, there may be no available job.

Another group of people, many of whom have joined the ranks of recent and acutely poor, is the small farmer. Having only the skills, the muscle, and knowledge involved in farming; having overinvested in the land and farm operation; had having lost money because of weather conditions and consequent poor crops, falling prices for grain and livestock, and increasing costs for machinery, land, seed, and fertilizer; the farm family, once able to provide for basic needs, may rather suddenly lose the farm land and home and everything in it. Homelessness and destitution may follow. In a rural area, economic losses to farmers in turn affect the businessmen in small towns. The circle of poverty become larger.

Poverty is widespread among the elderly. Elderly people who once considered themselves to be middle class or even affluent may now barely be able to pay for the essentials of life or may be living in poverty conditions (152, 176). Reder (192) states that poverty among the elderly is more prevalent than among other adults, twice as high for elderly women as men. Elderly minorities, those who are single, those with fewer years of education, and the very old, over 85 years, are especially vulnerable. The poverty rate for elderly African-Americans is three times higher than for elderly Caucasians; one of every four Spanish-speaking elderly are in poverty. In 1985, poverty levels had declined slightly from 1976 for Caucasians and African-Americans, but not for people of Latin origin (239).

Although the poor or underclass person has traditionally not finished high school, perhaps not even elementary school, and is an unskilled or semiskilled worker, often employed in temporary or seasonal jobs, the person with a doctorate degree may also be unemployed and living in poverty. Often the woman is better able to get a job than the man, but neither may have the necessary job skills for our competitive and technologically changing society. The poor person may live in a mixed residential area, on welfare in the city or rural area, or in an inner city or ghetto tenement infested by rats and roaches and without hot water. Recreation for the man may consist of talking with peers on the street corner or at a cheap bar, sitting alone in a park, or watching television. The woman's chief leisure activity may be attending church and visiting relatives. The family unit may be nuclear or extended and frequently there are a number of offspring (37, 94, 135, 150).

Much of the results of the research of the 1960s on people in the lower socioeconomic class and "the culture of poverty" reflected the bias or race of the researchers or focused on institutionalized populations or people in trouble, without reflecting on the many variables that influence people. Typically only negative traits were assigned to the poor person or family—traits at the opposite end of the continuum from the desired middle-class characteristics. The victim of social oppression and racism was blamed for his or her problems. Fortunately, later research findings give a more balanced view, which should help health workers to better understand and offer the same quality of care to poor people as to the people in middle and upper levels (37, 174). *Characteristics and behavior of a poor person or family are adaptive for the economic and social situation and constraints on life-styles* (135).

Patterns of childrearing and family relationships of

the very poor affect the next generation of parents. These characteristics include:

1. Misbehavior is regarded in terms of overt outcome; reasons for behavior are infrequently considered.
2. Lack of goal commitment, impulsive gratification, fatalism, and lack of belief in long-range success result from effects of chronic poverty upon a person's motivations and life-style.
3. Communication between family members is more physical than verbal.
4. Families are frequently large; each member acts to get whatever gratification he or she can. Previously unmet needs in the parent causes self-centeredness; the parent is poorly equipped to meet the dependency needs of many children. The child, as adult, will continue the cycle of previously unmet needs and inability to gratify another as parent.
5. Mother is the chief child-care agent; father is mainly a punitive figure. The milieu of the home is authoritarian, even though father may be frequently out of the home.
6. Discipline is harsh, inconsistent, and physical, makes use of ridicule, and is based on whether or not the child's behavior annoys the parent.
7. Aggressive behavior is alternately encouraged and restrained, depending primarily upon the consequences to the parent of the child's behavior. Such inconsistency causes the child to learn how to get away with certain behavior and does not teach impulse control.
8. Sex is viewed as an exploitative relationship. Questions about sex and sexual experimentation are met with a repressive, punitive attitude (37, 58, 94, 135, 136, 150, 174, 176).

Poor parents often have low self-esteem. Studies indicate that parents with low self-esteem provoke feelings of shame, guilt, defensiveness, decreased self-worth, and being bad in children by overestimating their ability to conform, by inappropriately or forcefully punishing or restraining them, denying necessities, and withdrawing love. Such childhood experiences cause low self-esteem in children and these feelings continue into adulthood, so that as parents these individuals inflict the same feelings they suffered as a child (44, 58, 119).

Authoritarian or harsh childrearing practices, which may be a euphemism for discipline, have as their explicit objective the development of toughness and self-sufficiency for survival. Yet in spite of the authoritarian, direct approach, parents are warm and expressive. An attachment exists between parent and child. In their own home children are also likely to be expressive, although they may seem restrained with strangers (37). Children are often given adult responsibilities early; they are not the focus of the family in the way that middle-class children are. They must fend more for themselves (24, 242).

Most minority and ethnic cultures value kinship ties and the emotional, social, and economic support that the extended family provides, in contrast to dominant middle-class America, which values individualism and independence. Much visiting goes on between relatives in the lower and working levels; assistance is sought and appreciated. All get along better by sharing meager resources or by working together to gain resources. The grandmother (and grandfather if living) is valued as caretaker for the child if the mother works. But the grandmother is also valued because she is the carrier of the culture; she is wise and can teach the young a great deal. The grandparent also benefits from being valued as a person (24, 37, 242).

Ability to delay gratification appears related to the situation. If a minority person is being tested by a Caucasian or has experienced broken promises—either by the researcher or others—he or she does not delay gratification. That is, the person requests an immediate reward in the experiment instead of being willing to wait. Moreover, ability to wait is related to **internal locus of control,** *a feeling that the self has some control over events.* Frequently poor people learn early that they are at the mercy of the system, whether the system is legal-political, economic, educational, or health (24, 37). Then, too, if hungry, cold, or without necessities, small wonder that a person takes whatever possible to appease hunger or feel more comfortable. Children learn to delay gratification if they can trust that what is needed will be there when needed. Poor children may seldom have this opportunity because of economic problems in the family. If meager resources are used to meet today's needs, it is difficult or impossible to plan ahead, save, or anticipate that planning and saving have merit. The poor person is present-oriented, in contrast to the future perspective of people in the middle and upper levels, because of necessity, cultural values, or inability to trust what is not tangible (37, 174).

Often the poor person appears to need an authoritarian, directive approach. The poor person (or the parents) may work in a situation in which he or she takes orders; the poor person's expectancy is to be *told* rather than *invited to talk with* someone about his or her ideas, problems, tentative solutions, or insights. Or the person may not understand the health care provider's professional jargon but is too polite or fearful to ask for an explanation. Also, if previous attempts to share ideas were met with rejection or ridicule by a parent, teacher, or health care professional, the person learned that it was safer not to respond. Finally, the poor person values action—getting something accomplished—more than words or promises (24, 37, 135, 150).

Impaired verbal communication and problem-solving ability may be present, not because the poor person is cognitively deficient but for other reasons. Many ethnic or minority groups speak a dialect in the home; the child then has difficulty understanding standard English or being understood. Essentially the child must become bilingual to be successful in school (42). The poor person uses a restricted code that is characterized by short sentences, lack of specificity, and lack of subordinate clauses for elaboration of meaning. The poor person speaks directly to the point. Such language is said to be concrete and to indicate lack of abstract thinking. In contrast to middle-class elaborate and sometimes vague speech, the speech of the poor person is logical and expressive. Thought is not buried in verbosity and vagueness. The blunt speech may be uncomfortable to listen to, both in words and ideas (42, 150, 183). The same words in professional and folk terminology may have a different meaning. For example, some African-Americans use the term "high blood" to mean that they believe there is too much blood in the body. Ingestion of large amounts of salty foods is believed to be helpful for an astringent effect. The health care professional must clarify that high blood pressure is different so that the person does not increase the hypertensive state further by excessive eating of salty foods (68).

Linguists have found that dialects do have grammatical structure (25, 54). Use of a dialect does not necessarily inhibit abstract thinking. Children must be taught problem solving and abstract thinking, however. If parents are seldom at home because of work, if the subculture values action more than words, if parents talk little with their children or brush aside questions, and if children associate more with peers than with adults, they are not likely to be stimulated to try new speech forms or new thought patterns. School teachers try, but unfortunately they often have classes too large to give the needed individual instruction, to form a motivating relationship, or to assess fully what a child does not know. Parents often wish to help children learn more; in fact, most poor parents repeatedly emphasize that their children must get an education so that they can achieve more than their parents did. Unfortunately, good intentions and admonitions are not enough. Poor parents often lack the education, energy, time, or resources to help their children advance educationally or even keep up minimally. The farther behind a child gets, the less the likelihood of ever catching up with cognitive skills. The cycle is repeated each generation. Yet most poor parents are receptive to suggestions on how to make the best possible use of their limited resources or what specific measures to follow to enhance child development (37, 42, 43, 93).

There is a clear relationship between poverty and ill health. Long-term ill health may contribute to poverty. Poverty predisposes to certain illnesses or causes a person to suffer adverse consequences of illness. As income level drops, health status declines: in the United States, 4.6 percent of people with incomes over $35,000 annually report fair and poor health in contrast to 21.1 per-

cent of people with incomes below $10,000 annually. Number of bed disability days is three times higher for people with annual incomes under $5,000 as compared to people with incomes above $25,000. As of 1983, 4.5 percent of Caucasian women with live births had no prenatal care or prenatal care only in the third trimester, in contrast to 9.7 percent of African-American women (195). Illness and use of physician services were compared for three income levels. The impact of multiple health problems, measured by days spent in bed, is greater for children from low income-families, and these children were less likely to receive physician care (164). The ill child who is poor is less likely to attend school. The poor have a higher infant and maternal mortality rate, and a higher number of deaths from accidents. Preventive measures are less likely to be carried out in the family; children are less likely to be immunized (184, 195).

A poor person defines oneself as ill when unable to work for days or weeks, and first uses folk or home remedies when ill or may go to a cultural healer. Reluctantly, and only when absolutely necessary, does he or she enter the scientific health care system. A person in *abject* poverty may not go for professional, scientific care at all because of lack of knowledge, money, transportation, or an inadequate sense of self-worth. A poor person is suspicious of health care professionals or feels that there is a distance between the practitioner and self. These feelings can be overcome only by a gentle, respectful, courteous, prompt approach and straightforward speech. Although many people feel that much financial assistance is available for the poor and sick, such assistance is limited. Moreover, poor people are unfamiliar with or unlikely to use community agencies wisely without your assistance. Because they often do not have the resources to practice preventive physical or dental care, they may be very ill—even irreversibly—on entry to the health care system (24, 37, 114, 135, 150, 176, 195).

Living in poverty takes its toll physically, emotionally, and mentally. A person who lives in chronic poverty is more likely to have behavioral characteristics opposite to the dominant culture because of not being involved with or learning from the dominant culture. Such behaviors, however, should not be viewed as innately bad, predetermined, irreversible, or the fault of the victims (37, 184). Even in Sweden, which guarantees birth-to-death care, an 11-year study showed the lower the economic level, the greater the risk of heart disease, cancer, and death from all causes (83).

INFLUENCES OF CULTURE ON HEALTH

Because every culture is complex, it can be difficult to determine whether health and illness are the result of cultural or other elements, such as physiological or psychological factors. Yet there are numerous accounts of the presence or absence of certain diseases in certain cultural groups and reactions to illness that are culturally determined. Cultural influences may include food availability, dietary taboos, methods of hygiene, and effects of climate—all factors related to culture. Several examples of the influences of culture on health and illness follow. The examples are necessarily limited. The influence of other cultural folkways on health has been studied. Race, social class, ethnic group, and religion influence distribution of disease and death.

Health status differs by race. Kennedy describes political, economic, and environmental factors that influence the health of elderly Black Americans. Black/White relationships influence general health, welfare, and well-being of people (100). Non-Caucasians are more likely to be admitted to state and county mental hospitals, less likely to receive prenatal care, and the children are less likely than Caucasians to be immunized. Of Caucasians who are diagnosed with cancer, 49 percent survived to five years in contrast to 38 percent of African-Americans. The incidence of Caucasian women who die from complications of pregnancy, childbirth, and the puerperuim was 5.9 per 100,000 for live births in 1983, in contrast to 16.3 for non-Caucasian women. However, since 1970, the recorded maternal death rate has dropped for Caucasians but not for non-Caucasians. Obesity continues to be a problem despite emphasis on slimness: incidence has increased for both men and women from 1960 to 1980. African-Americans had a greater increase in obesity from 1975 to 1980 for both sexes compared to Caucasians; 26.7 percent of Caucasian men compared to 30.9 percent of African-American males and 27.5 percent of Caucasian women compared to 49.8 percent African-American women. A greater percentage of African-Americans than Caucasians smoke: 42.6 percent of African-American men, 34.7 percent of Caucasian men, 32.5 percent of African-American women, and 29.8 percent of Caucasian women smoke. However, Caucasians are more likely to be heavy smokers; more than 25 cigarettes are smoked daily by 36.3 percent Caucasian and 11.6 percent of African-American men and by 21.7 percent of Caucasian and 5.3 percent of African-American women. From 1960 to 1980, high blood cholesterol counts dropped for many Caucasian men, but rose for African-American men, and dropped for both Caucasian and African-American women. In most age groups, African-Americans are more likely than Caucasians to have hypertension. American Indians have the poorest health status of all ethnic groups in the United States; their income averages less than one-half the poverty level (195).

Although some studies have demonstrated that poor people feel helpless, powerless, alienated, present-oriented, distrustful, and socially isolated, other studies show that these traits may not be due to cultural reasons but may be responses to situational circumstances. The larger society plays a major role in perpetuating poverty, and the poor find it difficult if not impossible to achieve the values and behaviors of the dominant society. The poor share many of the primary values of the larger society but develop negative secondary values when the dominant cultural values cannot be actualized (135).

Culturally induced belief in magic can cause illness and death. The profound physiologic consequences of intense fear, including inability to eat or drink, may be responsible. Yet there may be no physiological changes except in the terminal moments. If the behavior of friends and relatives—what they say or do—strongly reinforces the person's conviction of imminent death, the victim becomes resigned to fate and soon meets it (130).

Gomes and Carozos (73) describe the sudden death of a 21-year-old Mexican-American male following a **maldición** (*hex*) uttered by his mother. Toxicology and drug screening were negative in autopsy; only chronic bronchitis was evidenced. There was no indication of suicide. The mother admitted to having delivered a curse upon the son the evening before his death and that he trembled and sobbed all night. When she called an ambulance to take the son to a local hospital, he died enroute. The woman's husband died of a heart attack while crossing the street 10 days later. It was then that relatives and neighbors designated her as a *bruja* or witch. She blamed the local hospital for both deaths.

Immigration is a complex crisis that exacts a great toll from the migrant in terms of mental and physical health, occupational and socioeconomic status, and total lifeways. Of all migrants, the lot of the refugee is the most difficult. Memories of torture, losses, and culture shock are major components. The crisis of immigration appears to be manifested as follows:

> During the first year, the refugees experience relief, euphoria, and relatively high levels of happiness and life satisfaction.
> During the second year, exile shock occurs, with high levels of depression and unhappiness.
> During the third year, emotional improvement and increased adaptability are manifested (201).

Smith describes conditions of Inuit Indians in the Canadian Arctic, people in refugee camps, Ethiopians in the Sudan, and Cambodians on the Thailand-Cambodian border. Health agencies give service but do not seek justice on behalf of the people they are serving. Yet the health of people is influenced far more by politics and power, and by distribution of land and wealth, than by treatment or preventive health measures. If a population loses control and feels powerlessness or despair, the essence of the people, as well as their health, will begin to disintegrate (211).

Nursing Applications

Importance of Cultural Concepts for Nursing

Mainstream Americans have not been adept at understanding people from other countries and cultures, although the United States has been an open society to foreigners and immigrants. Those of minority cultures in the United States and people from other lands typically, and of necessity, have carefully observed and become familiar with the mainstream Caucasian culture in the United States.

Because of the rise of scientific medical practices and specialization, many consumers of health care in the United States are voicing a preference for caring behaviors and cultural practices. Especially the poor, middle-to-lower socioeconomic groups, and rural populations find the cosmopolitan approach to medical care too complex, too questionable, too difficult to understand and attain, and too expensive. Further, human dignity and normal developmental processes may be sacrificed in the process (110).

A poor person or a person from an ethnic minority does not seek medical help until the problem is a serious one, for various reasons: finances, child-care problems, fear of hospitals and medical personnel, fear of becoming a "guinea pig," and fear of death. Often the person relies first on various family and cultural remedies and folk healers. Or the person may rely on religious beliefs for healing. The response to poor or indifferent health care or inhumane treatment is to stay away (135).

Transcultural (cross-cultural) nursing, developed by Madeleine Leininger in the mid-1960s, is increasingly a focus in nursing education and practice. **Transcultural nursing** *is the study and comparative analysis of different cultures/subcultures throughout the world in relation to caring, health, illness, beliefs, values, and practices, so that this knowledge can be used in the nursing process to provide culture-specific and cultural-universal nursing care to people* (109–113). The goal is to develop a body of knowledge so that transcultural nursing concepts, theories, and practices are an integral part of nursing education, service, and research. Essential to practice is awareness of cultural values, sensitivity to different beliefs and practices, and the concept of **cultural relativity** (*behavior that is appropriate or right in one culture may not be so defined in another culture*) versus **ethnocentrism** (*behavior based on the belief that one's own group is superior*) (110).

Attitudes Related to Culture

If you live or work in a culture different from your own, you may suffer **culture shock,** *feelings of bewilderment, confusion, disorganization, frustration, and stupidity, and the inability to adapt to differences in language and word meanings, activities, time, and customs that are part of the new culture* (240).

Brink and Saunders describe four phases of culture shock:

1. Honeymoon Phase, characterized by excitement, exploration, and pleasure. This phase may be experienced by a short-term visitor.
2. Disenchanted Phase, during which the person feels stuck, depressed, irritated, and that the environment is unpredictable and no longer exotic. The normal cues for social intercourse are absent and the person is cut adrift. The person may become physically ill.
3. Beginning Resolution Phase, when new cultural behavior patterns are being adopted. Friends are found. Life becomes easier and more predictable.
4. Effective Function Phase, in which the person has become almost bicultural and may experience reverse culture shock on return home (21).

An antidote for culture shock is to look for similarities between your native and new cultures. In order to adapt to a new culture, be interested in the culture and be prepared to ask questions tactfully and to give up some of your own habits. Learn the language, customs, beliefs, and values to the greatest extent possible. Seek a support system—someone with whom you can be yourself and validate, and who can help you to adapt (21, 240). Leininger (109) and Weiss (240) give a number of specific suggestions for adapting to another culture. Brislen, Cushner, and Young also discuss techniques that assist individuals in making the transition from one culture to another (22).

In the United States, you are working in a **pluralistic society** *in which members of diverse ethnic, racial, religious, and social groups maintain independent lifestyles and adhere to certain values within the confines of a common civilization*. Knowledge of other cultures helps you examine your own cultural foundations, values, and beliefs, which, in turn, promotes increased self-understanding. But avoid ethnocentricity, believing that your own ways of behavior are best for everyone. For example, emphasizing daily bathing to a group that has a severely limited water supply is useless, for the water will be needed for survival. Recognize that your patterns of life and language are peculiar to your culture.

Anderson described how Caucasian health professionals labeled Chinese parents as noncompliant because they were not as forceful as Caucasian parents in having the chronically ill child carry out prescribed exercises when the exercises caused pain. In turn, the Chinese parents were less responsive to the health professionals. Health professionals are often unaware of the complex factors that influence client responses to treatment and care. Clients may not follow the treatment because they have different priorities (5). In fact, many cultural groups do not respond like the average middle-class American. American Indians value cooperation and patience, and respond quietly, even passively. Don't misinterpret this behavior as apathy about health or health care. They believe each living thing follows a

Research Abstract

Rosenbaum, J., Mental Health Care Needs of Soviet-Jewish Immigrants, in Care: Discovery and Uses in Clinical and Community Nursing, *ed. M. Leininger. Detroit: Wayne State University Press, 1988, 107–121.*

The purpose of this study was to identify the general lifeways of Soviet-Jewish immigrants who have settled in North America since the mid-1970s, and to suggest application of this information to improve mental health care practices. The theoretical framework for the study was Leininger's Transcultural Theory and Theory of Care.

Technologic, economic, educational, political, religious, and philosophical factors, and kinship, social, and cultural values were studied in relation to mental health care needs and conditions of the immigrants. Data were collected using Leininger's transcultural interviewing and health assessment form, and through interviews with social workers who assisted immigrants who settled in the Detroit metropolitan area.

The study focused on the following research questions:

1. What are specific cultural care values, beliefs, and practices of the Soviet-Jewish immigrants to North America?
2. What factors help determine mental health patterns of the immigrants?
3. What childrearing practices appear to positively or negatively affect mental health of the immigrants?
4. What are the practical implications from the ethnographic and ethnonursing data for providing culture-specific care?

The study revealed several mental health concerns and needs related to immigrants' cultural values and lifeways. Immigrants demonstrated a strong need for affiliation, dependence, and oral gratification. Their actions revealed issues related to trust versus mistrust, optimism versus pessimism, and activity versus passivity. They distrusted authority, but looked to authority to care for them and make decisions. They also expressed conflicting feelings of optimism versus pessimism toward new surroundings, with a tendency to hopelessness and despair. Resettlement was stressful because they were separated from the familiar.

Often adults were unemployed despite professional or skilled work backgrounds, causing further loss of self-esteem. Discontinuity existed in cultural values related to obedience, conformity, education, and health care; adjustment time and care varied. Mental health difficulties included loneliness, depression, unemployment, language barriers, and uncertainty in a new country.

Several values were identified that can guide mental health nursing care for these clients. These values include world view, social and educational aspects, religion, and kinship. Prevailing cultural values that should be included in care are intellectual and educational achievement, shared suffering, family and cultural pride, and expression of feelings in a trusting environment.

Nurses must also reduce the gap between the previous Soviet care values and Western professional care values. Insight-oriented, problem-solving approaches have not been part of the therapy process in the former Soviet Union. Immigrant clients will not be willing to express feelings about emotional or sexual issues until trust is established, although they may express suffering or pain. Family involvement, behavior modification methods, and educational groups may promote security and affiliative needs. Nursing care should promote acculturation and cultural repatterning, identification and reduction of stress holistically, health teaching, and encouragement of choices and decision making.

Promoting rapport with confidence and trust in the health care provider encourages repatterning. Nonconfrontational communication can be taught when trust is established. Promoting contact with the Jewish community can reestablish cultural lifeways and identity and reduce immigrants' feelings of isolation. Assistance with contact; obtaining transportation, health care, and education; and encouragement of participation in community activities also may be necessary.

cycle; illness is defined in relation to a personal inner cycle and seasonal cycles, in contrast to the emphasis on germ theory by the health care system. Thus the medicine man is seen as more helpful than the physician (88, 105, 187, 218, 251).

All people have some prejudice; it emerges in such expressions as "Those upper-crust people always . . . " or "Those welfare people never. . . . " Examine your thinking for unconscious prejudice, understand your own class background, and distinguish your values from those held by people under your care. Try to withhold value judgments that interfere with your relationship with the patient and with objective care. *There are too many unknown factors in people's lives to set up stereotyped categories.* A family may be in the middle class or upper class in terms of income, education, and goals, for example, and yet live in an upper-lower-class neighborhood because they refuse to emphasize material wealth. A farmer, according to our criteria, may be categorized

in the upper-lower economic level and yet regard himself or herself as very much a part of the middle class. A person who lives in an economically depressed section of the United States and is poor may have an adequate public education, a middle-class value system, and upper-class graciousness.

If you feel you are stooping by helping poor people, you may be labelled a "do-gooder" and be ineffective. Recognize the behavior of poor people not as pathologic but as adaptive for their needs. Realize, too, that not only the poor need your help. A rich person also may need a great deal of help with care, health teaching, or counseling. Having money does not necessarily mean one is knowledgeable about preventive health measures, nutrition, and disease processes. Persons of all classes deserve competent care, clear explanations, and a helpful attitude.

The misinterpretation of behavior typical of a social class does not always go in one direction, from upper to lower. Suppose that you are a nurse with a working-class background whose patient is a 50-year-old corporation president, a member of the newly rich class, admitted for coronary disease. This person seems obsessed with finding out when he or she can resume professional duties, exactly how many hours can be worked daily, and chances for a recurrence. An understanding of socioeconomic position, along with possible motives, values, and status (which this individual feels must be maintained), will enable you to work with the seeming obsession rather than simply label the client an "impossible patient."

Try to accept people as they are regardless of culture or social class. Picture the world through the eyes of others—those you care for. In this way, you can maintain your own personal standards without being shocked by theirs.

Box 1–2 provides a questionnaire that can help you to assess your own cultural attitudes and perceptions.

Assessment

Learning about another's cultural background can promote feelings of respect and humility as well as enhance understanding of the person and the family—needs, like and dislikes, behavior, attitudes, care and treatment ap-

proaches, and sociocultural causes of disease. According to Tripp-Reimer, Brink, and Saunders, a thorough cultural assessment guide would include the following components (227):

1. Values: Health, human nature, man-nature, time, activity, relational, and other.
2. Beliefs: Health (health maintenance, causes and treatment of illness), religious, other.
3. Customs: Communication (verbal and nonverbal), decision making, food/diet, grief/dying, religious, family roles, and sick role/patient.
4. Social structure: Family, political involvement, education, ethnic affiliation, physical environment, religion, use of economic resources, health care facilities, use of art and history, and cultural change.

Orque's Ethnic/Cultural System Framework shows how basic human needs are influenced by various aspects of a culture: (1) value orientation, (2) family life processes, (3) diet, (4) religion, (5) language and communication processes, (6) healing beliefs and practices, (7) the social groups's interactive patterns, and (8) art and history of the social group (171).

Cultural differences should be anticipated not only in foreigners and first-generation immigrants but also in persons even further removed in time from their country of origin and in persons from other regions within your country. A person's behavior during illness is influenced by cultural definitions of how he or she should act and the meaning of illness. Understanding this situation and seeking reasons for behavior help avoid stereotyping and labeling a person as uncooperative and resistant just because the behavior is different. As you consider alternate reasons for behavior, care can be individualized. People from different cultural backgrounds classify health problems differently and have certain expectations about how they should be helped. If cultural differences are ignored, your ability to assess and help the clients and their ability to progress toward a personally and culturally defined health status may be hampered. You should be able to translate your knowledge of the health care system into terms that match the concepts of your clients.

Knowledge about socioeconomic levels and cultural groups may help explain late or broken agency appointments that result from fear or inferiority feelings, lack of transportation, or someone to care for the children at home rather than from lack of interest in health. A reservation American Indian, poor African-American, or recent immigrant, for instance, may not be accustomed to keeping a strict time schedule or appointments if unemployed, for a strict clock-time orientation is not valued as highly as in the industrialized work force. Take time to talk with the person and you will learn of fears, problems, aspirations, and concern for health and family, and human warmth.

As you assess clients, remember that people differ

■ BOX 1-2.
Self-Assessment of Cultural Attitudes

In order to become more aware of your attitudes toward and feelings about people of other racial/ethnic backgrounds, ask yourself the following questions:

1. What is your earliest remembrance of racial or ethnic differences?
2. What are the messages you have received in your life about African-American, Asian-American, American Indian, or Latino people?
3. What messages have you received in your life about Caucasians of different nationality backgrounds?
4. How much experience did you have with any person from a racial/ethnic minority group different from your own while you were growing up?
5. In what way have these experiences affected your behavior toward people from the group(s)?
6. Describe people from other racial/ethnic minority groups with whom you have felt comfortable or uncomfortable.
7. What features or characteristics are dominant in people from other racial/ethnic minority groups with whom you have had contact?
8. What have you observed about the racial/ethnic composition of your community?
9. What have you observed about the interaction of people from diverse cultural backgrounds at your school, church, or workplace or in organizations you attend.
10. Do you consider yourself to be nonracist or racist?

not only culturally but also biologically (Table 1–11). Studies on biologic baselines for growth and development or normal characteristics have usually been done on Caucasian populations. These norms may not be applicable to nonwhites. Biologic features, such as skin color, body size and shape, and presence of enzymes, are the result of biologic adjustments made by ancestors to the environment in which they lived (15, 172, 198).

Various physical differences are known to exist. **Mongolian spots,** *the hyperpigmented, bluish discoloration* occasionally seen in Caucasian neonates, are normal for many Asians, American Indians, and African-Americans. Type of ear wax varies and may determine the presence of ear disease in preschoolers. Dry ear wax is recessive and is found primarily in American Indians and Asians. Wet ear wax is found in most African-Americans and Caucasians. Also, people with dry ear wax have fewer apocrine glands and perspire less; they usually do not have as much body odor. Thus presence of body odor may be indicative of disease. Pelvic shape of the woman, shape of teeth and tongue, fingerprint pattern, blood type, keloid formation, and presence of the enzyme lactase vary among groups. Persons with certain blood types are more prone to certain illnesses (15, 172, 198). Adults who have **lactose intolerance** are *missing lactase, the enzyme for digestion and metabolism of lactose in milk and milk products;* they become ill on ingestion of these foods. Symptoms include flatulence, distention, abdominal cramping, diarrhea, and colitis. Milk intolerance because of enzyme deficiency occurs in over 80 percent of Chinese, Japanese, and Eskimo adults and in 60% to 80% of American-Indian, African-American, Jewish, and Mexican-American adults. Only people of northern European Caucasian extraction and members of two African tribes tolerate lactose indefinitely, and even some aged Caucasians will have lactose deficiency. Do not automatically teach everyone to drink milk. Calcium can be obtained in other ways: seafoods (cook fish to yield edible bones), leafy vegetables, yogurt, buttermilk, aged cheese (lactose has been changed to lactic acid during aging), or homemade soup (add vinegar to the water when cooking a soupbone to decalcify the bone). Most ethnic groups have adapted ways of cooking to ensure calcium intake from nondairy sources; listen carefully to their dietary descriptions. If the lactase-deficient person wishes to ingest considerable milk foods, an enzyme product to add to milk, called Lact-Aid, may be purchased from drug or health food stores (90, 182, 200). An acidophilus milk, which contains a controlled culture of lactobacillus acidophilus bacteria, is also easily digested.

Other biological variations exist. Susceptibility to disease varies with blood type. Rh-negative blood type is common in Caucasians, rarer in other groups, and absent in Eskimos. Myopia is more common in Chinese; color blindness is more common in Europeans and East Indians. Nose size and shape correlate with ancestral homeland. Small noses (seen in Asians or Eskimos) were produced in cold regions, high-bridged noses (common to Iranians and American Indians) were com-

TABLE 1-11. ASSESSMENT OF SKIN COLOR

Characteristic	White or Light-skinned Person	Dark-skinned Person
Pallor: Vasoconstriction present	Skin takes on white hue, which is color of collagen fibers in subcutaneous connective tissue.	Skin loses underlying red tones. Brown-skinned person appears yellow-brown. Black-skinned person appears ashen-gray. Mucous membranes, lips, nailbeds pale or gray.
Erythema, Inflammation: Cutaneous vasodilation	Skin is red.	Palpate for increased warmth of skin, edema, tightness, or induration of skin. Streaking and redness difficult to assess.
Cyanosis: Hypoxia of tissues	Bluish tinges of skin, especially in earlobes, as well as in lips, oral mucosa, and nailbeds.	Lips, tongue, conjunctiva, palms, soles of feet are pale or ashen gray. Apply light pressure to create pallor; in cyanosis tissue color returns slowly by spreading from periphery to the center.
Ecchymosis: Deoxygenated blood seeps from broken blood vessel into subcutaneous tissue	Skin changes color from purple-blue to yellow-green to yellow.	Oral mucous membrane or conjunctiva will show color changes from purple-blue to yellow-green to yellow. Obtain history of trauma and discomfort. Note swelling and induration.
Petechiae: Intradermal or submucosal bleeding	Round, pinpoint purplish red spots on skin.	Oral mucosa or conjunctiva show purplish-red spots if person has black skin.
Jaundice: Accumulated bilirubin in tissues	Yellow color in skin, mucous membranes, and sclera of eyes. Light-colored stools and dark urine often occur.	Sclera of eyes, oral mucous membranes, palms of hand and soles of feet have yellow discoloration.

mon in dry areas; and the flat, broad noses characteristic of some Blacks were adaptive in moist, warm climates (15, 172, 198).

If a client does not speak English as a first language, learn key words of his or her language. Use language dictionaries or a card file of key words. Breach the language barrier so that your assessment is more accurate and care measures will be understood by the person. Muecke offers practical suggestions to overcome language differences (157).

To aid assessment, learn about the significant religious practices and the everyday patterns of hygiene, eating, types of foods eaten, sleeping, elimination, use of space, and various rituals that are a part of the person's culture. Because the client and the practitioner may have different perspectives of health and illness, the following questions can enhance understanding about the client's viewpoint:

1. What do you think caused your problem?
2. Why do you think it started when it did?
3. What do you think this illness does to you? What problems has it caused for you?
4. What do you fear most about your illness?
5. How severe is your illness?
6. What kind of treatment have you already tried? What else would help?
7. What would you like for health care providers to do for you? What results do you wish for from treatment? (5)

Nursing Diagnoses

The nursing diagnoses in Box 1–3 may be applicable to your work with people in various cultures. Leininger discusses the importance of including non-Anglicized cultural concepts in the North American Nursing Diagnosis Association (NANDA) taxonomy, rather than focusing on Anglo-American Western cultural values. Further, the diagnostic categories should include positive health descriptors and assets of cultures in dealing with human conditions (115).

Intervention

Caring *is assistive, supportive, or facilitative actions toward another person or group with evident or anticipated needs in order to ameliorate or improve a human condition or lifeway* (110, 113). Nurses in different cultures tend to know and emphasize different care constructs such as support, comfort, and touch. Caucasian nurses in the United States generally believe that care involves use of technological aids, medicines, and psychophysiological comfort measures. Generally, Caucasian and some non-Caucasian clients agree. In several non-Western cultures, nurses and clients perceive care as protective with a sociocultural emphasis. For example, nurses in Turkey and Israel emphasize restorative

caring functions because of war activities. Samoan caregivers are expected to protect the person from breaking cultural or social rules in order to prevent illness or harm. Chinese nurses perceive surveillance and protection as dominant caring modes. Depending upon the culture, Leininger states, the concept *care* can mean many different things (110–112).

Comfort	Restoration
Support	Direct assistance
Attention	Helping the dependent
Compassion	Tenderness
Touch	Trust
Love	Instruction
Stimulation	Succorance
Presence	Empathy
Protection	Medical/Technical
Surveillance	Assistance
Personalized help	Maintaining well-being
Nurturance	
Stress alleviation	

Learn what the client has as a priority in care. Include the person's ideas in planning and giving care. Often you may have to negotiate with the individual or family in order to carry out the essential medical treatments and nursing care, as well as include the cultural practices, the medicine man or spiritualist, or spiritual healing rituals they hold most dear.

Respecting the person's need for privacy or need to have others continually around is essential. Understand that some clients or families will not be expressive emo-

---

■ **BOX 1-3.**
Selected Nursing Diagnoses Related to Transcultural Nursing*

Pattern 5: Choosing

Ineffective Individual Coping
Decisional Conflict
Health Seeking Behaviors

Pattern 6: Moving

Altered Health Maintenance

Pattern 7: Perceiving

Powerlessness

Pattern 8: Knowing

Knowledge Deficit

*Many of the NANDA nursing diagnoses are applicable to an individual in any culture who is ill.
From North American Nursing Diagnosis Association, *NANDA Nursing Diagnosis Taxonomy I* (Rev.). St. Louis: North American Nursing Diagnosis Association, 1990.

tionally or verbally. Respect this pattern, recognizing that nonverbal behavior is also significant. Be aware, too, that word meanings may vary considerably from culture to culture so that the person may have difficulty understanding you and vice versa. Be sure the gesture or touch you use conveys the message you intend. If you are unsure, avoid nonverbal behavior to the extent that you can.

Interference with normal living patterns or practices adds to the stress of being ill. You will encounter and need to adapt care to the following customs: drinking tea instead of coffee with meals, eating the main meal at midday instead of in the evening, refusing to undress before a strange person, doing special hair care as described by Grier (77), avoiding use of the bedpan because someone else must handle its contents, maintaining special religious or ethnic customs, refusing to bathe daily, refusing a pelvic exam by a male doctor, moaning loudly when in pain, and showing unreserved demonstrations of grief when a loved one dies.

A client with a strict time orientation must take medicines and receive treatments on time or feel neglected. You are expected to give prompt and efficient, but compassionate, service to the patient and family. Time orientation also affects making appointments for the clinic and plans for medication routine or return to work after discharge, and influences a person's ideas about how quickly he or she should get well. Clients with little future-time orientation have difficulty planning a future clinic appointment or a long-range medication schedule. They cannot predict now how they will feel at a later date and may think that clinic visits or medicines are unnecessary if they feel all right at the moment.

For some clients, the hurrying behavior of the nurse is distressing; it conveys a lack of concern and lack of time to give adequate care. In turn, the person expresses guilt feelings when it is necessary to ask for help. Although you may look very efficient when scurrying, you are likely to miss many observations, cues, and hidden meanings in what the person or family says.

Examine your own attitude about busyness and leisure in order to help others consider leisure as part of life. The disabled person, whose inability to work carries a stigma, must develop a positive attitude about leisure and may seek your help.

Your knowledge of cultures will enable you to practice holistic nursing care, including cultural values and norms as part of the nursing process. Holistic healing practices combine the best of two worlds: the wisdom and sensitivity of the East and the technology and precision of the West. Although holistic practitioners use conventional therapies in many cases, the emphasis remains on the whole person: physical, emotional, intellectual, spiritual, and sociocultural background. The focus is on prevention and overall fitness, and on the individual taking responsibility for his or her own health

and well-being. Multiple techniques are used to restore and maintain balance of body energy. These techniques include exercise, acupuncture, massage, herbal medicine, nutritional changes, manipulation of joints and spine, medications, stress management, and counseling. The nurse-client relationship is the key to holistic nursing care, for the person has come to expect a caring interaction from the healer. The *curandera* (herb healer) of the Spanish-speaking Southwest makes a tea from herbs, for example, and the patient slowly sips the tea. The pain is gone. The client's faith is a major factor in herbal cures—faith in God, the plants, and the curandera. The curandera also has faith in recovery as she shows caring, looks at and listens to the patient, and heals.

Herbs used by various cultural groups are increasingly found to have medicinal value; they are chemically similar to drugs used by scientific practitioners. Also, a culture's favored drink may have implications for health. Health practitioners in a remote Mexican village found that the only available beverage was an alcoholic drink made from the juice of a local plant. A safe water supply was brought in, but the people did not fare well on it. The local drink was a rich source of essential vitamins and minerals not otherwise present in the local diet. Although it may have appeared desirable to change a cultural pattern for certain health reasons, the unanticipated consequences proved detrimental to health in another way.

A woman in labor who is a product of a parochial background with reliance on lay medical help, and who is suspicious of the impersonal hospital and professional-looking nurses, asks to have a knife placed under the bed to help "cut labor pains." While implementing scientific health care, you can be more prepared to act on this belief that psychologically helps the patient.

Folk medicine practices help people gain a sense of control over their fate. Often the practice does no real harm but can be misinterpreted. In one example, a Vietnamese mother used the ancient Chinese practice of *cao gio* ("scratching the wind") to care for her child's cold. In this practice, the child's chest or back is covered with mentholated oil and then rubbed with a coin or hard object. The striations left on the child's skin, while causing no harm or injury, were interpreted by a health care provider as signs of child abuse. The health care provider reported the family, as required by law, based on her perceptions. The parents were charged, and the father, in fear of jail term and in humiliation, hung himself (68, 222). Be aware of possible folk medicine practices and their terminology, and explore these practices prior to making conclusions about the client.

Some recent immigrants may adhere closely to traditional practices. Others may not. Your care cannot be based on assumption or stereotype. Immigrants may combine traditional cultural and Western practices. Many Chinese Americans practice Western-oriented activities of exercise, religious practices, lifestyle, and illness behavior activities. In the health behavior activities of dietary practices and the sick behavior measures, use of a mixture of Chinese and Western practices have been reported by over 50% of the Chinese Americans. Chinese Americans described more Western practices the longer they lived in the United States. Four influencing variables, (1) the familiarity of the participant with Western health care systems, (2) language, (3) occupation, and (4) religion, are significant to their described health beliefs, dietary practices, and sick behavior measures (28, 160, 238, 250). Yep shares information on how nurses can better care for clients from an Asian culture (250):

1. Talk to the person in a way that shows respect. Call the person by title and last name. Do not talk down to the person or family.
2. Older people may not be fluent in English, even if they have lived in the United States for many years. Speak slowly to the client; invite the family to help interpret to the client and communicate feelings or questions to the health professional. The client is unlikely to admit that he or she is not understanding.
3. Asian clients probably will not want to bother the practitioners with their complaints and problems. Most Asians believe suffering is part of life and must be accepted. However, the client is likely to complain to family members. Include family in your assessment, and question the client repeatedly and in several different ways in order to assess pain.
4. Illness may be viewed as the result of an imbalance between yin and yang, an evil spirit, improper food, or by something bad in the family.
5. Having the family bring familiar foods will make the hospital stay more comfortable for the Asian client. Some are accustomed to having rice at every meal.
6. Most Asians highly respect and even fear authority; doctors and nurses represent authority. Thus the client expects a formal relationship and may become confused by an informal approach.
7. Explanations should be given slowly and repeatedly in simple language; the client is likely to be too intimidated by the authority figure to ask questions. The family should also be given the explanations so they can clarify for the client, if necessary.
8. Older Asian people may associate hospitals with death; it's the last place to go. On the other hand, hospitals also represent power and dominion. Hospital routines may not be understood. For example, an Asian person views his or her blood as finite in supply, vital energy, and a life source; thus repeated blood samples may cause much fear.
9. Asian adults do not touch much and are not usually demonstrative about affection. A smile conveys caring much better than a touch, as does performing little extras for the client without being asked, such as filling the water pitcher.
10. Utilize the family as an important resource. Request they visit frequently and for long hours, if they desire. They can assist in care; in fact, the client may expect them to. Cooperation with treatment and care routines will be fostered through communication with and involvement of the family (250).

These points are pertinent to people in other cultures as well. Among the nearly one million Southeast Asian Vietnamese, Hmong, Cambodian, and Laotian refugees in the United States, adjustment difficulties are manifested in anxiety, family abuse, Post-Traumatic Stress Disorder, intergenerational conflict, psychotic episodes, suicidal threats, substance abuse, and other antisocial behaviors that may be masked by physical symptoms. High levels of dysfunction occur for the first and second years, often into the third year of resettlement. If culturally focused health care is given, with appropriate psychotherapeutic intervention and *low* doses of antidepressant medication, emotional health shows improvement in the third or fourth years (201).

Nursing intervention is key for the refugees, in that the nurse focuses on the needs of the whole person as well as medical and psychiatric symptoms, in contrast to the emphasis of physicians. Often 24-hour caretaking is required by the ill person; thus other family members may also become debilitated and are unable to go to work and school. The refugees may be desperate for help and seek medical care, diagnostic tests, and medication prescriptions from multiple physicians and care centers, each quite unaware of the others. This results not only in duplication of services and increased costs, but often in conflicting instructions, sacks full of medication in the home, confusion and fragmentation for the person, and no alleviation of the problems (201).

Culturally, these clients acknowledge a belief in a supernatural or magical etiology of their illness and consult regularly with indigenous healers. Nearly all display evidence of healing methods such as **cupping** (*applying a heated jar to the skin to form a vacuum to suction out illness*) and **coinage** (*rubbing a coin or spoon over the skin to rub out illness*) for physical symptoms. Polypharmacy is the norm. They use substances from many sources: herbal medications, over-the-counter and prescription drugs from the United States as well as other countries, and remedies sent by relatives in Southeast Asia and France. Use of prescription drugs ranges from total noncompliance to self-regulated drug use (201).

Mental illness carries shame and stigma in the Southeast Asian community; social support systems tend to disappear as the patient becomes less manageable. Hospitalization is often for threatened or attempted suicide. Barriers to health care, in addition to cultural and family attitudes, include lack of transportation to or inaccessibility of services, job schedules, family demands, and financial limitations. A culturally appropriate mental-status examination form is a priority to determine effects of folk beliefs and healing modalities (12, 201).

Some cultures, such as the traditional Filipino, believe that illness is the result of evil forces and that treatment involves protection from or removal of these evil forces. For example, the body is viewed as a container that collects debris, so flushing involves stimulating perspiration, vomiting, flatus, or menstrual bleeding to remove evil forces from the body. Use of heat and control of cold through herbs, teas, water, and fire help maintain a balanced internal temperature. Protection involves a gatekeeping system against the invasion of natural and supernatural forces. Mental illness may be thought to be the result of a witch casting a spell; carrying an oval stone or wearing a cross, if the person is a Christian, will act as an antidote or protection. Using direct eye contact with the sick person is also believed to remove a witch's spell (141). Snyder describes folk healing among older Asian-Americans and Hawaiians in Honolulu and the implications for health education and nursing care (213). Die and Seelback describe the importance of the family and church or temple for elderly Vietnamese immigrants in securing health and other services (53).

You can incorporate indigenous folk medicine and practitioners into professional and scientific health care practices. The two are not automatically exclusive. For example, in one Navaho nursing care service, the medicine man is an active participant, and Navaho mothers are encouraged to use their infant cradle boards and to be home for the blessing ceremonies (110).

As you intervene, teach, or counsel, adjust your communication approach with and behavior toward clients from another cultural background, since people from most ethnic/racial groups feel uncomfortable initially when interacting with someone who is different. While you may be communicating in a way that is natural to you, someone from another culture may perceive that behavior as too forward or aggressive, too passive, or unempathic. While you cannot assume a different mask for each person you interact with, be aware that the client may misinterpret your well-intentioned behavior. Use general knowledge about a culture while you simultaneously see the individual and unique differences of people. Unfortunately, many nurses are not bilingual. The client who uses English as a second language may not speak or understand English adequately for you to effectively assess, teach, or intervene in other ways.

In male-dominated households (Spanish-speaking, Asian, Middle Eastern), the male head of house must be included in all decisions and health teaching if you expect to solicit cooperation. In most such families, and African-American and Jewish families, there is also an older female relative such as an aunt, mother-in-law, or grandmother who is the designated health care provider for that family. She must also be included in decision making and health teaching. Speaking to the important family elder with respect will gain you a staunch ally; the desired behavior change will almost certainly be assured (68, 221, 222).

Relations between the client and the family may at times seem offensive or disharmonious to you. Differentiate carefully between patterns of behavior that are culturally induced and expected and those that are unhealthy for the persons involved.

The changing society may cause families to have a variety of problems. Be a supportive listener, validate realistic ideas, prepare the family to adapt to a new or changing environment, and be aware of community agencies or resources that can provide additional help. When a client has no family nearby and seems alone and friendless, you may provide significant support.

Develop a personal philosophy that promotes a feeling of stability in your life so that you, in turn, can assist the client and family to explore feelings and formulate a philosophy for coping with change. Toffler speaks about ways in which a person can learn to cope with rapid change. One important way is to develop some ritual or pattern in your personal life that you can practice regardless of where you are, and thus maintain some sense of continuity and stability (224).

One way to have a lasting effect on the health practices of a different cultural group is through health teaching that includes a philosophy of prevention. Present-day China compared with China during the 1940s is an example of how public health standards can be effectively raised through an emphasis on prevention. Increasingly your role includes health education, as discussed in Chapter 17. Outsiders cannot make decisions for others, but people should be given sufficient knowledge concerning alternate behavior so that they can make intelligent choices themselves.

Various pressures interfere with attempts at health teaching. Behind poor health habits lie more than ignorance, economic pressure, or selfish desires. Motivation plays a great part in continuing certain practices even though a person has been taught differently by you. Motivation, moreover, is influenced by a person's culture, status, and role in that culture and by social pressures for conformity. Starting programs of prevention can be difficult when people place a low value on health, cannot recognize cause-and-effect relationships in disease, lack future-time orientation, or are confused about the existence of preventive measures in their culture. Thus preventive programs or innovations in health care must be shaped to fit the cultural and health profiles of the population. Long-range prevention goals stand a better chance of implementation if combined with measures to meet immediate needs. A mother is more likely to heed your advice about how to prevent further illness in her sick child if you give the child immediate attention.

Be mindful of how people view you. If they cannot understand you, if you threaten their values, or if they view you as an untouchable professional, you will not cross the cultural barrier.

You may also talk with members of the National Association of Hispanic Nurses, the American Indian/Alaskan Indian Nurses Association, and the Black Nurses Association in order to gain information about how to give care that includes cultural values and customs.

With knowledge about cultures and ways to care for people from different cultures, you can be an advocate for a client from a different culture to ensure accessibility and appropriateness of services. In turn, you can help the health care system to be more culturally sensitive to care of clients, or several agencies can work together for that goal. One example is the Portland, Oregon, Minority Project, which has worked to identify and articulate key elements of cultural competence in social service agencies that serve minority children and families. Agency philosophy and structure are key elements. Agencies that are culturally competent change their philosophy to give more empowerment to the client and family and to reflect a goal of ethnic, cultural, or racial diversity in clients and staff. When agency structure has been changed to be less hierarchial with less status and power differentials, and board membership reflects a cultural mix, the agency is viewed as more culturally competent because it encourages a variety of cultural and group methods of decision making. Agency staff are also aware that continued advocacy with referral agencies is necessary to serve minority populations (210).

Cannon et al. describe the importance of value clarification as you care for people from diverse cultures (30). The information in this chapter will aid you in the process of value clarification as well as in the nursing process with clients and families through the life span, as you promote health and care for the ill individual.

REFERENCES

1. Ailinger, R., A Study of Illness Referral in a Spanish Speaking Community, *Nursing Research,* 26, no. 1 (1977), 53–56.
2. Allman, R., Preparing Global Citizens, *Kappa Delta Pi Record,* Winter, 1991, 53–54.
3. America's New Migrant Workers, *Newsweek* (August 3, 1987), 34–35.
4. Anderson, G., and B. Tighs, Gypsy Culture and Health Care, *American Journal of Nursing,* 73, no. 2 (1973), 282–285.
5. Anderson, J., Health Care Across Cultures, *Nursing Outlook,* 38, no. 3 (1990), 136–139.
6.

7. Anthony-Tkach, C., Care of the Mexican-American Patient, *Nursing and Health Care,* 2, no. 8 (1981), 424–432.
7. Baca, J., Some Health Beliefs of the Spanish Speaking, *American Journal of Nursing,* 69, no. 10 (1969), 2172–2176.
8. Beare, P., Nursing Education Comes into Its Own in Saudi Arabia, *Nursing and Health Care,* 8, no. 5 (1987), 272–274.
9. Beeman, W.O., What Is (Iranian) National Character? A Sociological Approach, *Iranian Studies.* (Winter, 1976), 22–48.
10. Bender, D., ed., *American Values: Opposing Viewpoints.* San Diego: Greenhouse Press, 1989.
11. Bernadino, S., *The Ethnic Almanac.* Garden City, NY: Doubleday, 1981.
12. Bickwell, S., The Incorporation of Family Primary Care for Southeast Asian Refugees in a Community-Based Mental Health Facility. *Archives of Psychiatric Nursing,* 3, no. 3 (1989), 173–177.
13. Billingsley, A., *Black Families and the Struggle for Survival: Teaching Our Children to Walk Tall.* New York: Friendship Press, 1974.
14. Birkert-Smith, K., *Eskimos.* New York: Crown Publishers, 1971.
15. Block, B., and M. Hunter, Teaching Physiological Assessment of Black Persons, *Nurse Educator,* 6, no. 1 (1981), 24–27.
16. Bouws, B., Working with Albanian Families, *American Journal of Nursing,* 74, no. 5 (1974), 902–905.
17. Branch, M., and P. Paxton, *Providing Safe Nursing Care for Ethnic People of Color.* New York: Appleton-Century-Crofts, 1976.
18. Briggs, J.L., *Never in Anger, Portrait of an Eskimo Family.* Cambridge, MA: Harvard University Press, 1970.
19. Brink, P., ed., *Transcultural Nursing: A Book of Readings.* Englewood Cliffs, NJ: Prentice-Hall, 1978.
20. Brink, P., Value Orientations as an Assessment Tool in Cultural Diversity, *Nursing Research,* 33, no. 4 (1984), 198–203.
21. ——, and J. Saunders, Culture Shock: Theoretical and Applied, in *Transcultural Nursing: A Book of Readings,* ed. P. Brink. Englewood Cliffs, NJ: Prentice Hall, 1978, pp. 128–138.
22. Brislen, R., K. Cushner, and M. Young, *Intercultural Interactions: A Practice Guide.* Beverly Hills, CA: Sage Publishers, 1986.
23. Brower, H.T., Culture and Nursing in China, *Nursing and Health Care,* 5, no. 1 (1984), 26–31.
24. Bullough, V.L., and B. Bullough, *Health Care for the Other Americans.* New York: Appleton-Century-Crofts, 1982.
25. Burling, R., *English in Black and White.* New York: Holt, Rinehart & Winston, 1973.
26. Bushy, A., and K. Rohr, The Plains Indians: Cultural Considerations in the use of Apnea Monitors. *Neonatal Network,* 6, no. 4 (1990), 59–66.
27. Cadena, M., The Mexican-American Family and the Mexican-American Nurse, in *Family Health Care,* eds. D. Hymovich and M. Barnard. New York: McGraw-Hill, 1979.
28. Campbell, T., and B. Chung, Health Care of the Chinese in America, *Nursing Outlook,* 21, no. 4 (1973), 245–249.

29. Campinha-Bacote, J., Voodoo Illness, *Perspectives in Psychiatric Care,* 28, no. 1 (1992), 11–17.

30. Cannon, R., et al., A Values Clarification Approach to Cultural Diversity, *Nursing and Health Care,* 5, no. 3 (1984), 161–164.

31. Catalano, R., The Health Effects of Economic Insecurity, *American Journal of Public Health,* 81, no. 9 (1991), 1148–1152.

32. Chang, M., Nursing in China: Three Perspectives, *American Journal of Nursing,* 83, no. 3 (1983), 389–395.

33. Charon, J., *The Meaning of Sociology.* Englewood Cliffs, NJ: Prentice-Hall, 1990.

34. Childs, A., and G. Melton, eds., *Rural Psychology.* New York: Plenum Press, 1983.

35. Ching, C., Vietnamese in America: A Case Study in Cross-Cultural Health Education, *Health Values: Achieving High-Level Wellness,* 8, no. 3 (1984), 16–20.

36. Coakley, T.A., P. Ehrlich, and E. Hurd, Southeast Asian Refugees: Health Screening in a Family Clinic, *American Journal of Nursing,* 80, no. 11 (1980), 2032–2036.

37. Cohen, S., et al., *Culture of Poverty Revisited.* New York: Mental Health Committee Against Racism, n.d.

38. Coleman, R., and L. Rainwater, *Social Standing in America.* New York: Basic Books, 1985.

39. Coles, R., The Children of Affluence, *The Atlantic Monthly,* September 1977, 53–66.

40. ———, *Eskimos, Chicanos, Indians.* Boston: Little, Brown, 1978a.

41. ———, *Children of Crisis: Vol 5—Privileged Ones, The Well Off, and Rich in America.* Boston: Little, Brown, 1978b.

42. Comer, J., *Beyond Black and White.* New York: Quadrangle Books, 1972.

43. ———, and A. Poussaint, *Black Child Care.* New York: Simon & Schuster, 1975.

44. Coopersmith, S., *The Antecedents of Self Esteem.* San Francisco: W.H. Freeman, 1967.

45. Cordasco, F., ed., *Studies in Italian American Social History.* Totowa, NJ: Rowman and Littlefield, 1975.

46. Danner, P., *An Ethic for the Affluent.* Lanham, MD: University Press of America, 1980.

47. Darabi, K., and V. Ortuz, Childbearing Among Young Latino Women in The United States, *American Journal of Public Health,* 77, no. 1 (1987), 25–28.

48. Davis, M., Getting to the Root of the Problem, *Nursing '77,* 7, no. 4 (1977), 60–65.

49. Davitz, L., Y. Sameshima, and J. Davitz, Suffering as Viewed in Six Different Cultures, *American Journal of Nursing,* 76, no. 8 (1976), 1296–1297.

50. DeGracio, R., Filipino Cultural Influences, *American Journal of Nursing,* 79, no. 8 (1979), 1412–1414.

51. deLeon Siantz, M., Who is the Hispanic Child? *Pacesetter: Council on Psychiatric and Mental Health Nursing,* 17, no. 1. (1990), 1, 5.

52. DeMott, B., *The Imperial Middle.* New York: William Morrow, 1990.

53. Die, A., and W. Seelback, Problems, Sources of Assistance, and Knowledge of Services Among Elderly Vietnamese Immigrants, *The Gerontologist,* 28, no. 4 (1988), 448–452.

54. Dillard, J.L., *Black English: Its History and Usage in the United States.* New York: Random House, 1973.

55.

56. Dorio, J., and M. Nelson, China's Caring Is the Same, *Nursing Outlook,* 31, no. 2 (1983), 100–104.

56. Dorson, R., *American Folklores.* Chicago: The University of Chicago Press, 1977.

57. Dumond, D.E., *The Eskimos and the Aleuts.* London: Thames and Hudson, 1977.

58. Duvall, E., and B. Miller, *Marriage and Family Development* (6th ed.). New Yorker: Harper and Row, 1985.

59. Ehling, M.B., The Mexican American (el chicano), in *Culture and Childrearing,* ed. A.L. Clark. Philadelphia: F.A. Davis, 1981.

60. Ehrenreich, B., and K. Stallard, The Nouveau Poor, *The New Day,* 14, no. 4 (1982), 1.

61. *Ethnicity and Health Care.* New York: National League for Nursing, 1976.

62. Evans, R.J., *German Family Life.* London: Croom Helm, 1982.

63. Farhood, L., and R. Day, Nursing Interventions in Wartime, *Journal of Psychosocial Nursing,* 24, no. 7 (1986), 25–29.

64. Fitzpatrick, J., *Puerto Rican Americans: The Meaning of Migration to the Mainland.* Englewood Cliffs, NJ: Prentice-Hall, 1971.

65. Flaskerud, J., Perceptions of Problematic Behavior by Appalachians, Mental Health Professionals, and Lay Non-Appalachians, *Nursing Research,* 29, no. 3 (1980), 140–149.

66. Floriani, C., Southeast Asian Refugees: Life in a Camp, *American Journal of Nursing,* 80, no. 11 (1980), 2028–2030.

67. Folb, E., *Runnin' Down Some Lines: The Language and Culture of Black Teenagers.* Cambridge, MA: Harvard University Press, 1980.

68. Folk Medicine, *California Nursing Today* (January, 1986), 2, 13, 20.

69. Fraser, J., *The Portrait of a Chinese People.* New York: Summit Books, 1980.

70. Gallup, G., *The Gallup Poll: Public Opinion 1989.* Wilmington, DE: Scholarly Resources, Inc., 1989, 55–58.

71. Gilbert, D.A., *Compendium of American Public Opinion.* New York: Facts on File Publications, 1989.

72. Glenn, M., *Appalachia in Transition.* St. Louis: Bethany Press, 1970.

73. Gomez, E., and N. Carazos, Was Hexing the Cause of Death? *American Journal of Social Psychiatry,* 1, no. 1 (April, 1981), 50–52.

74. Good, B.J., The Heart of What's the Matter, *Culture, Medicine, and Psychiatry,* 1 (1977), 25–58.

75. Gordon, V., I. Matonsek, and T. Lang, Southeast Asian Refugees: Life in America, *American Journal of Nursing,* 80, no. 11 (1980), 2031–2036.

76. Graham, J., *Another Mother Tongue.* New York: Beacon Press, 1990.

77. Grier, M., Hair Care for the Black Patient, *American Journal of Nursing,* 76, no. 11 (1976), 1781.

78. Griffin, W.D., *A Portrait of the Irish in America.* New York: Macmillan, 1983.

79. Grossberg, K.A., ed., *Japan Today.* Philadelphia: Ishi Institute for Study of Human Issues, 1981.

80. Haferkamp, H., ed., *Social Structure and Culture.* Berlin: Walter de Gruyter & Co., 1989.

81. Hand, D., *Magical Medicine: The Folklores and Ritual of*

the People of Europe and America. Berkeley, CA: University of California Press, 1980.

82. Hathout, M., Comment on Ethical Crisis and Cultural Differences, *The Western Journal of Medicine,* 139, no. 3 (1983), 380–381.

83. Health Status Is Linked to Occupational Class, Even in Sweden, *The Nation's Health,* January 1989, 14.

84. Hecker, M., and F. Heike, eds., *The Greeks in America, 1528–1977.* Dobbs Ferry, NY: Oceana Publishers, 1978.

85. Henry, B., and E. Di Giacomo-Geffers, The Hospitalized Rich and Famous, *American Journal of Nursing,* 80, no. 8 (1980), 1426–1429.

86. Hill, R. *The Strengths of Black Families.* New York: Emerson Hall, 1972.

87. Hispanic Latino—What's In a Name? *American Journal of Public Health,* 77, no. 1 (1987), 15–17.

88. Hobus, R., Living in Two Worlds: A Lakota Transcultural Nursing Experience, *Journal of Transcultural Nursing,* 2, no. 1 (1990), 33–36.

89. Holck, S., et al., Lung Cancer Mortality and Smoking Habits: Mexican-American Women, *American Journal of Public Health,* 72, no. 1 (1982), 38–42.

90. Hongladarom, G., and M. Russell, An Ethnic Difference—Lactose Intolerance, *Nursing Outlook,* 24, no. 12 (1976), 764–765.

91. Horn, B., Cultural Concepts and Postpartal Care, *Nursing and Health Care,* 2, no. 11 (1981), 516–517, 526–527.

92. Hostetler, J.A., *Amish Society* (3rd ed). Baltimore MD: The John Hopkins University Press, 1980.

93. Hutchinson, S., The American Indian Senior Citizens View of Women, *Bulletin of American Association of Social Psychiatry,* 1, no. 3 (1980), 13–15.

94. Hutto, R., Poverty's Children, *American Journal of Nursing,* 69, no. 10 (1969), 2166–2169.

95. Jacobson, M., M. Mercer, L. Miller, et al., Tuberculosis Risk Among Migrant Farm Workers on the Delmarva Peninsula, *American Journal of Public Health,* 77, no. 1 (1987), 29–31.

96. James, S., When Your Patient Is Black West Indian, *American Journal of Nursing,* 78, no. 11 (1978), 1908–1909.

97. Jones, J., and C. Block, Black Cultural Perspectives, *The Clinical Psychologist,* 37, no. 2 (1984), 58–62.

98. Keefe, S., *Appalachian Mental Health.* Lexington, KY: University Press of Kentucky, 1988.

99. Kelly, L., Another Look at the Future of Health Care. *Nursing Outlook,* 34, no. 4 (1991), 150–151.

100. Kennedy, T., *You Gotta Deal With It: Black Family Relations in a Southern Community.* New York: Oxford Press, 1980.

101. Kimball, S., The Polish Presence in Illinois, *Alumnus—Southern Illinois University at Edwardsville,* Fall, 1986, 5–7.

102. Kitnano, H., *Race Relations* (4th ed.) Englewood Cliffs, NJ: Prentice-Hall, 1991.

103. Kluckhorn, F., Family Diagnosis: Variations in Basic Values of Family Systems, *Social Casework,* 32 (February–March 1958), 63–72.

104. Kluckhorn, F., and E. Strodtbeck, *Variations in Value Orientations.* New York: Row, Petersen, 1961.

105. Kniep-Hardy, M., and M. Burkhardt, Nursing the Navaho, *American Journal of Nursing,* 77, no. 1 (1977), 95–96.

106. *Koran.* Translation and commentary by A. Yusef Ali. 2:223.

107. Kosko, D., and J. Flaskerad, Mexican American Nurse Practitioner, and Lay Control Group Beliefs About Cause and Treatment of Chest Pain, *Nursing Research,* 36, no. 4 (1987), 226–231.

108. Latimer, G., A Threat to American Values: The Disparity Between Urban Cities and Rural Towns, *Nation's City Weekly,* 11 (August 8, 1988), 4.

109. Leininger, M., *Transcultural Nursing.* New York: Masson, 1979.

110. ——, Caring: A Central Focus of Nursing and Health Care Services, *Nursing and Health Care,* 1, no. 10 (1980), 135–143.

111. ——, *Transcultural Care Diversity and Universality: A Theory of Nursing.* Thorofare, NJ: Charles B. Slack, Inc., 1985.

112. ——, ed., *Care: Discovery and Uses in Clinical and Community Nursing.* Detroit: Wayne State University Press, 1988a.

113. ——, ed., *Care: The Essence of Nursing and Health.* Detroit: Wayne State University, 1988b.

114. ——, Southern Rural Black and White American Lifeways with Focus on Care and Health Phenomena, in *Care: The Essence of Nursing and Health,* ed. M. Leininger. Detroit: Wayne State University Press, (1988c), 133–159.

115. ——, Issues, Questions, and Concerns Related to the Nursing Diagnosis Cultural Movement from a Transcultural Nursing Perspective, *Journal of Transcultural Nursing,* 2, no. 1 (1990a), 23–32.

116. ——, The Significance of Cultural Concepts in Nursing, *Journal of Transcultural Nursing,* 2, no. 1 (1990b), 52–59.

117. Leonard, M.A., and C.A. Joyce, Two Worlds United, *American Journal of Nursing,* 71, no. 6 (1971), 1152–1155.

118. Lewis, J., and J. Looney, *The Long Struggle: Well-Functioning Working Class Black Families.* New York: Brunner/Mazel, 1983.

119. Lidz, T., *The Person: His and Her Development Throughout the Life Cycle* (2nd ed.). New York: Basic Books, 1983.

120. Lin, E., W. Carter, and A. Kleinman, An Exploration of Somatization Among Asian Refugees and Immigrants in Primary Care, *American Journal of Public Health,* 75, no. 9 (1985), 1081–1084.

121. Lin, Y.C., China: Health Care in Transition, *Nursing Outlook,* 31, no. 2 (1983), 94–99.

122. Lipson, J.G., and A. Meleis, Issues in Health Care of Middle Eastern Patients, *The Western Journal of Medicine,* 139, no. 6 (1983), 854–861.

123. ——, Culturally Appropriate Care: The Case of Immigrants, *TCN,* 7, no. 3 (1985), 48–56.

124. Lomund, B., *Asian Americans: Social and Psychological Perspectives,* vols. I and II. Los Angeles: Science and Behavior Books, 1980.

125. Lopata, H., *Polish Americans: Status Competition in an Ethnic Community.* Englewood Cliffs, NJ: Prentice-Hall, 1976.

126. Lopez, B., *Arctic Dreams.* Toronto: Bantam Books, 1986.

127. Loughlin, B., Pregnancy in the Navajo Culture, *Nursing Outlook,* 13, no. 3 (1965), 55–58.

128. Luna, J., Transcultural Nursing Care of Arab Muslims, *Journal of Transcultural Nursing,* 1, no. 1 (1989), 22–26.

129. Lykins, R., Children of the Third Culture, *Kappa Delta Pi Record,* Winter, 1985, 39–43.

130. MacDonald, A., Folk Health Practices Among North Coastal Peruvians: Implications for Nursing, *Image,* 13, no. 6 (1981), 51–56.

131. Manfredi, M., Primary Health Care and Nursing Education in Latin America, *Nursing Outlook,* 31, no. 2 (1983), 105–108.

132. Marks, G., et al., Health Behavior of Elderly Hispanic Women: Does Cultural Assimilation Make a Difference? *American Journal of Public Health,* 77, no. 10 (1987), 1315–1319.

133. Marsella, A., and P. Pedersen, *Cross Cultural Counseling and Psychotherapy.* New York: Pergamon Press, 1981.

134. Martines, E., *The Mexican American.* Boston: Houghton Mifflin, 1973.

135. Mason, D., Perspectives on Poverty, *Image,* 13, no. 3 (1981), 82–88.

136. Mayer, S., and C. Jencks, Growing Up in Poor Neighborhoods: How Much Does It Matter? *Science,* 243 (March 17, 1989), 1441–1445.

137. McCabe, G., Cultural Influences on Patient Behavior, *American Journal of Nursing,* 60, no. 8 (1960), 1101–1104.

138. McEvoy, L., and G. Land, Life Style and Death Patterns of the Missouri RLD's Church Members, *American Journal of Public Health,* 71, no. 12 (1981), 1350–1356.

139. McGoldrick, M., J. Pearce, and J. Giordano, eds. *Ethnicity and Family Therapy.* New York: Guilford Press, 1985.

140. McGregor, F., Uncooperative Patients: Some Cultural Interpretations, *American Journal of Nursing,* 67, no. 1 (1967), 88–91.

141. McKenzie, J., and N. Chrisman, Healing Herbs, Gods, and Magic: Folk Health Beliefs Among Filipino-Americans, *Nursing Outlook,* 26, no. 5 (1977), 326–329.

142. Mead, M., ed. *Cultural Patterns and Technological Change.* New York: Greenwood Press, 1985.

143. Meleis, A., The Arab American in the Health Care System, *American Journal of Nursing,* 81, no. 6 (1981a), 1880–1883.

144. ——, Arab American Women and Their Birth Experience, *MCN,* 6, no. 3 (1981b), 171–176.

145. ——, and A.R. Jansen, Ethical Crisis and Cultural Differences, *The Western Journal of Medicine,* 138, no. 6 (1983), 889–893.

146. ——, and C. LaFever, The Arab American and Psychiatric Care, *Perspectives in Psychiatric Care,* 22, no. 2 (1984), 72–86.

147. Middaugh, J., Cardiovascular Deaths Among Alaskan Natives, *American Journal of Public Health,* 80, no. 3 (1990), 282–283.

148. Millar, W., and T. Stephens, The Prevalence of Overweight and Obesity in Britain, Canada, and the United States, *American Journal of Public Health,* 77, no. 1 (1987), 38–41.

149. Mills, A., Saudia Arabia: An Overview of Nursing and Health Care, *Focus on Critical Care,* 13, no. 1 (1986), 50–56.

150. Moccia, P., and D. Mason, Poverty Trends: Implications for Nursing, *Nursing Outlook,* 34, no. 1 (1986), 20–24.

151. Mohseni, M., and A.A. Alemi, A Causal Concept of Disease in an Iranian Community, *Journal of Biosocial Science,* 10 (1978), 347–351.

152. Moon, R., Things I Wish I'd Known Before I Moved to a Small Town, *Medical Economics,* 63 (February 3, 1986), 80.

153. Moore, J., *Mexican-Americans* (2nd ed). Englewood Cliffs, NJ: Prentice-Hall, 1976.

154. Moore, L.G., P.W. VanArsdale, J.E. Glittenberg, et al., *The Biocultural Basis of Health Care.* St. Louis: C.V. Mosby, 1980.

155. Morgan, L., *And the Land Provides: Alaskan Natives in a Year of Transition.* Garden City, NY: Anchor Press/Doubleday & Co., 1974.

156. Moses, M., Viva in Causa, *American Journal of Nursing,* 73, no. 5 (1973), 843–848.

157. Muecke, M., Overcoming the Language Barrier, *Nursing Outlook,* 22, no. 4 (1970), 53–54.

158. Mummah, R., Sakaguchi San and I Had a Contract: A Nurse Helps a Patient Surmount Seemingly Insurmountable Setbacks, *Nursing '78,* 8, no. 12 (1978), 36, 38.

159. Murillo, N., The Mexican American Family, in *Chicanos: Social and Psychological Perspectives,* eds. C.A. Hernandez, M.J. Haug, and N.W. Wagner. St. Louis: C.V. Mosby, 1976.

160. Murphy, P., Tuberculosis Control in San Francisco's Chinatown, *American Journal of Nursing,* 70, no. 5 (1970), 1044–1046.

161. Naimann, H., Nursing in Jewish Law, *American Journal of Nursing,* 70, no. 11 (1970), 2378–2379.

162. Naisbitt, J., *Megatrends.* New York: Warner Books, 1982.

163. Naisbitt, J., and P. Aburdene, *Megatrends 2000: Ten New Directions for the 1990s.* New York: William Morrow, 1990.

164. Nevachek, P., and B. Starfield, Morbidity and Use of Ambulatory Care Services Among Poor and Nonpoor Children, *American Journal of Public Health,* 78, no. 8 (1988), 927–933.

165. Newman, M., *The Political Economy of Appalachia.* Lexington, MA: D.C. Heath, 1972.

166. Norbury, P., ed., *Introducing Japan.* New York: St. Martin's Press, 1977.

167. Nichols, P., Transplanted to Saudi Arabia, *American Journal of Nursing,* 89, no. 8 (1989), 1048–1050.

168. Obedinski, E., and H. Stankiewiczand, *Polish Folkways in America.* Lanham MD: University Press of America, 1987.

169. O'Grady, J., *How the Irish Became American.* Boston: Twayne Publishers, 1981.

170. Olson, S., Year of the Blue Collar Guy, *Newsweek,* November 8, 1989, 16.

171. Orque, M., B. Bloch, and L. Monrroy, *Ethnic Nursing Care: A Multi-cultural Approach.* St. Louis: C.V. Mosby, 1983.

172. Overfield, T., Biological Variations: Concepts from Physical Anthropology, *Nursing Clinics of North America,* 12, no. 1 (1977), 19–26.

173. Park, J., Children Who Follow the Sun, *Today's Education* (January–February 1976), 53–56.

174. Parker, S., and R.J. Kleiner, The Culture of Poverty: An Adjustive Dimension, *American Anthropologist,* 72 (1970), 516–527.

175. Patrick, D., Y. Sittampalam, S. Somerville, et al., A Cross-Cultural Comparison of Health Status Values, *American Journal of Public Health,* 75, no. 12 (1985), 1402–1407.

176. Patrick, P., et al., Poverty, Health Services, and Health Status in Rural America, *The Milbank Quarterly,* 66 (Spring, 1988), 105.

177. Paynich, M., Cultural Barriers to Nurse Communication, *American Journal of Nursing,* 64, no. 2 (1964), 87–90.

178. Pedersen, P., J. Draguns, W. Lonner, J. Trible, eds., *Counseling Across Cultures,* Honolulu, University of Hawaii Press, 1981.

179. Persad, E., Some Cultural Factors in Psychiatric Training, *Canadian Mental Health,* 19, nos. 3–4 (1971), 11–15.

180. Phillips, S., and S. Lobar, Literature Summary of Some Navajo Child Health Beliefs and Rearing Practices within a Transcultural Nursing Framework, *Journal of Transcultural Nursing,* 1, no. 2 (1990), 13–20.

181. Phipps, L. Confusion of a Young WASP, *New York,* 21, no. 34 (1991), 24–31.

182. Pipes, P., *Nutrition in Infancy and Childhood* (4th ed.). St. Louis: Times Mirror/Mosby, 1988.

183. Popenoe, D., *Sociology* (8th ed.). Englewood Cliffs, NJ: Prentice-Hall, 1991.

184. Poverty Kills, *St. Louis Post-Dispatch,* February 18, 1990, sec. A, p. 1.

185. Prather, J.L., *A Mere Reflection: The Psychodynamics of Black and Hispanic Psychology.* Ardmore, PA: Dorrance, 1977.

186. Prattes, O., Beliefs of the Mexican-American Family, in *Family Health Care,* eds. D. Hymovich and M. Barnard. New York: McGraw-Hill, 1979, pp. 128–137.

187. Primeaux, M., Caring for the American Indian Patient, *American Journal of Nursing,* 77, no. 1 (1977a), 91–94.

188. ——, American Indian Health Care Practices, *Nursing Clinics of North America,* 12, no. 1 (1977b), 55–65.

189. Priorities. *Newsweek,* April 2, 1990, p. 5.

190. Prittie, T., *Germany.* New York: Time, Inc., 1981.

191. Rafferty, M., *The Ozarks: Land and Life.* Tulsa: The University of Oklahoma Press, 1980.

192. Reder, N., In Search of Welfare Solutions, *The National Voter,* 37, no. 1 (May, 1987), 9–12.

193. Reed, C., *Dialects of American English.* Amherst: University of Massachusetts Press, 1977.

194. Reidhead, V., Odyssey to Navajo-Hopi Land, *Discovery* (Fall 1986), 8–11.

195. Report Shows What It Means to Health to be Disadvantaged, *The Nation's Health* (May–June 1987), 1, 20.

196. Ripples, L.J., *Of German Ways.* New York: Barnes and Noble, 1970.

197. ——, *The German-Americans.* Boston: Twayne Publishers, Division of G.K. Hall, 1976.

198. Roach, L., Assessment: Color Changes in Dark Skin, *Nursing '77,* 7, no. 1 (1977), 48–51.

199. Rosenbaum, J., Cultural Care of Older Greek Canadian Widows within Leininger's Theory of Culture Care, *Journal of Transcultural Nursing,* 2, no. 1 (1990), 37–47.

200.

201. Rumbaut, R., How Well Are Southeast Asian Refugees Adapting? *Business Forum,* 10, no. 4 (1985), 26–31.

202. Samet, J., et al., Respiratory Disease Mortality in New Mexico's American Indians and Hispanics, *American Journal of Public Health,* 70, no. 5 (1980), 492–497.

203. Sanders, I., and E. Morawska, *Polish American Community Life: A Survey of Research.* Boston: Boston University Press, 1975.

204. Sargis, N., J. Jennrich, and K. Murray, Housing Conditions and Health: A Crucial Link, *Nursing and Health Care,* 8, no. 3 (1987), 335–338.

205. Schalk, A., *The Germans.* Englewood Cliffs, NJ: Prentice-Hall, 1971.

206. Schmidt, C., Five Becomes a Team in Appalachia, *American Journal of Nursing,* 75, no. 8 (1975), 1314–1315.

207. Scholz, J., Cultural Expressions Affecting Patient Care, *Dimensions of Oncology Nursing,* 4, no. 1 (1990), 16–26.

208. Schroeder, A., ed., *The Changing Ways of Southwestern Indians: A Historic Prospective.* Glorieta, NM: The Rio Grande Press, 1973.

209. Seidell, J., K. Bakx, P. Deurenberg, et al., The Relation Between Overweight and Subjective Health According to Age, Social Class, Slimming Behavior, and Smoking Habits in Dutch Adults, *American Journal of Public Health,* 76, no. 2 (1986), 1410–1415.

210. Services to Minority Populations: Developing Cultural Competence for Agencies, *Focal Point,* 2, no. 4 (Summer, 1988), 5–7.

211. Smith, S., Speaking Out: People Without Land, *American Journal of Nursing,* 89, no. 2 (1989), 208–209.

212. Snow, L., Traditional Health Beliefs and Practices Among Lower Class Black-Americans, *The Western Journal of Medicine,* 139 (1983), 830–838.

213. Snyder, P., Health Service Implications of Folk Healing Among Older Asian Americans and Hawaiians in Honolulu, *The Gerontologist,* 24, no. 5 (1984), 471–476.

214. Sowell, T., *Ethnic America: A History.* New York: Basic Books, 1983.

215. Spector, R.E., *Cultural Diversity in Health and Illness* (3rd ed). New York: Appleton & Lange, 1991.

216. Stack, C., *All Our Kin: Strategies and Survival in a Black Community.* New York: Harper & Row, 1970.

217. Stern, P., Solving Problems of Cross-Cultural Health Teaching: The Filipino Childbearing Family, *Image,* 13, no. 6 (1981), 47–50.

218. Sue, D., *Counseling the Culturally Different: Theory and Practice* (2nd ed). New York: John Wiley, 1990.

219. Tao-Kim-Hai, A., Orientals Are Stoic, in *Social Interaction and Patient Care,* eds. J. Skipper and R. Leonard. Philadelphia: J.B. Lippincott, 1965, pp. 142–155.

220. Tarshis, B., *The Average American Book.* Saddle Brook, NJ: American Book-Stratford Press, 1979.

221. Thiederman, S., Ethnocentrism: A Barrier to Effective Health Care, *The Nurse Practitioner* (August, 1986), 52–59.

222. Thiederman, S., Folk Medicine, *California Nursing Today,* January, 1986, 12, 13, 20.

223. Thornton, J., Developing a Rural Nursing Clinic, *Nurse Educator,* no. 3, (Summer, 1983).

224. Toffler, A., *Future Shock.* New York: Bantam Books, 1970.

225. ——, *The Third Wave*. New York: Bantam Books, 1980.

226. Tripp-Reimer, T., and M. Friedl, Appalachians: A Neglected Minority, *Nursing Clinics of North America,* 12, no. 1 (1977), 41–54.

227. Tripp-Reimer, T., P. Brink, and J. Saunders, Cultural Assessment: Content and Process, *Nursing Outlook,* 32, no. 2 (1984), 78–82.

228. Utah Has Healthiest Citizens, *Cappers Weekly,* November 21, 1989, p. 1.

229. Urban, H., Humanist, Phenomenological, and Existential Approaches, in *Clinical Psychology Handbook* (2nd ed.), eds. M. Hersen, A. Kazdin, and A. Bellak. New York: Pergamon Press, 1991, pp. 200–219.

230. Vander Zanden, J., *The Social Experience: An Introduction to Sociology* (2nd ed.). New York: McGraw-Hill, 1990.

231. von Bertalanffy, L., *General System Theory*. New York: George Braziller, 1968.

232. Vuong, G.T., *Getting to Know the Vietnamese*. New York: Frederick Unger, 1976.

233. Walker, G.M., Utilization of Health Care: The Laredo Migrant Experience, *American Journal of Public Health,* 69 (1979), 667–672.

234. Wallace, L.T., Patient Is an American Indian, *Supervisor Nurse* (May 1977), 22–23.

235. Wang, J., Caretaker-Child Interaction Observed in Two Appalachian Clinics, in *Care: The Essence of Nursing and Health,* ed. M. Leininger, Detroit: Wayne State University Press, 1988, pp. 195–216.

236. Wax, M., *Indian American: Unity and Diversity*. Englewood Cliffs, NJ: Prentice-Hall, 1971.

237. Weber, M., *The Protestant Ethic and the Spirit of Capitalism,* trans. Talcott Parsons. New York: Charles Scribner's Sons, 1930; students' edition, 1958.

238. Webster, R., Asian Patients in the CCU, *Nursing* 4, no. 31 (March 28–April 10, 1991), 16–19.

239. Weiss, M., *The Clustering of America*. New York: Harper & Row, 1988.

240. Weiss, O., Cultural Shock, *Nursing Outlook,* 19, no. 1 (1971), 40–43.

241. Wenger, A., and M. Wenger, Community and Family Patterns of the Old Order Amish, in *Care: Discovery and Uses in Clinical and Community Nursing,* ed. M. Leininger. Detroit: Wayne State University, 1988, pp. 39–54.

242. White, E., Giving Health Care to Minority Patients, *Nursing Clinics of North America,* 12, no. 1 (1977), 27–40.

243. White, J., and P. Thana, *The Psychology of Blacks*. New York: Prentice-Hall, 1990.

244. White, P., To Be Indomitable, To Be Joyous: Greece, *National Geographic,* 157, no. 3 (1980), 360–393.

245. Wigginton, E., *The Foxfire Books,* Vols. 1–5. Garden City, NY: Anchor Press/Doubleday, 1979.

246. Williams, P., A Comparison of Philippine and American Children's Concepts of Body Organs and Illness in Relation to Five Variables. *International Journal of Nursing Studies,* 15 (1978), 193–202.

247. Willie, C., The Black Family and Social Class, *The American Journal of Orthopsychiatry,* 44, no. 1 (1974), 50–60.

248. Wisdom of the Elders: Mississippi Choctaws, *AARP News Bulletin,* 27, no. 11 (December, 1986), 5.

249. Yankauer, A., Hispanic/Latino—What's in a Name? *American Journal of Public Health,* 77, no. 1 (1987), 15–17.

250. Yep, J., An Asian Patient: How Does Culture Affect Care? A Family Member Responds, *Journal of Christian Nursing,* 6, no. 5 (1991), 5–8.

251. Yuki, T., Caring for the Urban American Indian Patient, *Journal of Emergency Nursing,* 7, no. 3 (1981), 110–113.

252. Zabilka, G., *Customs and Culture of the Philippines*. Rutland, VT: Charles E. Tuttle, 1970.

253. Zborowski, M., Cultural Components in Response to Pain, in *Sociological Studies of Health and Sickness,* ed. Dorrian Apple. New York: McGraw-Hill, 1960, pp. 118–133.

254. Zola, I.K., Culture and Symptoms: An Analysis of Patients Presenting Complaints, *American Sociological Review,* 31, (October, 1966), 615–631.

Chapter 2

Environmental Influences on the Person and Family

Earth does not belong to us; we belong to the earth.
—Chief Seattle

KEY TERMS

Perfect or complete combustion	Sulfuric acid	Radioactive substances	Sound overload
Imperfect or incomplete combustion	Nitrogen oxide	Formaldehyde	Decibels
	Nitrogen dioxide	Radon	Recycled
Carbon monoxide	Particulate matter	Sewage	Hazardous waste
Hypoxic state	Hydrocarbons	Biologic oxygen demand	Pica
Sulfur oxide compounds	Ozone	Pesticides	Teratogenic
	Photochemical smog	Food additives	Mutagenic
Sulfur dioxide	Acid rain	Zoonoses	Therapeutic milieu

OBJECTIVES

Study of this chapter will enable you to:

1. Explore the scope of environmental pollution, both outdoors and indoors, and the interrelationship of different kinds of pollution with one another and with people.
2. Observe sources of air pollution in your community and identify resulting hazards to human health.
3. List types of water pollution and describe resultant health problems.
4. Describe substances that cause soil pollution and the effect of those substances on the food web and on other facets of health.
5. Discuss types of food pollution and ways to prevent food contamination.
6. Listen to noise pollution in various settings and discuss its long-term effects on health.
7. Contrast different types of surface pollution and resultant health problems.
8. Discuss health hazards encountered in the home and on the job and the major effects of these contaminants.
9. Discuss and practice ways that, as a citizen, you can reduce environmental pollution.
10. Discuss your professional responsibility in assessing for illness caused by environmental pollutants and in taking general intervention measures.
11. Demonstrate an ability to help establish a therapeutic milieu for a client.

Although ecology is a well-publicized subject, often the physical environment in which we live is taken for granted and overlooked as a direct influence on people and their health. You may wonder why a book discussing major influences on the developing person, family unit, and their health contains a chapter about humans and their environment. Yet where we live and the condition of that area—its air, water, and soil—determine to a great extent how we live, what we eat, the disease agents to which we are exposed, our state of health, and our ability to adapt. This chapter focuses primarily on noxious agents to which many people in the United States are exposed in the external environment. Because of the interdependence of people, only those living in isolated rural areas escape the unpleasant effects of our urban, technologically advanced society. Yet even the isolated few may encounter some kind of environmental pollution, whether through groundwater contaminated from afar, food shipped into the area, smog blown from a nearby city, or contaminated rain or snow. Further, the pollutants that are discussed are observed world wide (35).

Nursing in the past was concerned primarily with the client's immediate environment in the hospital or home. Today nursing is extended to include assessment of the family and community as well as the individual. Interventions are directed toward promoting a healthy environment for individuals and families, well or ill, and maintaining public health standards and federal regulations. Understanding some specific environmental health problems and their sources and effects will enable you to function both as a citizen and as a professional nurse to help prevent or correct those problems. Teach about prevention of and effects from the pollutants described in this chapter as you care for people in the agency, home, or community. There are links between various pollutants and between pollutants and disease (149).

HISTORICAL PERSPECTIVE

The natural components of the environment were once considered dangerous. In most instances people dealt successfully with any environmental problems encountered. In their quest to conquer nature, early people discovered fire and the wheel. Fire was essential to survival; but with its advent, natural or man-made sparks and pollutants were sent into the atmosphere—the beginning of environmental pollution.

The fire and the wheel played major roles in early civilization and industrialization of the world. With the industrial revolution came many technological advances that gave people increased power and comforts. These advances also introduced artificial, chemical, and physical hazards into the environment. Soon after the start of the industrial revolution, the population of cities grew; disease spread with the crowding of people, and food distribution became more complex. It became apparent that the natural components of the environment were not as dangerous as the man-made components.

The entire environment has been and is a vital part of our existence. Human skill in manipulating the environment has produced tremendous benefits; but none has been without a price, the high price of pollution. Pollution of our environment is not only a health threat but also offends esthetic, spiritual, social, and philosophic values. Environmental pollution is a complex, significant problem requiring multiple solutions (Fig. 2–1).

Antipollution legislation in the United States can be traced back to the early 1900s. In 1906 the first federal Food and Drug Act was passed, and in 1914 drinking water standards were enacted to serve as guides for water supplied on interstate carriers. Congress passed the federal Water Pollution Control Act in 1948. Most of these legislative moves were poorly funded and supported, however, and so had little effect on growing pollution problems. Finally in the early 1960s Congress began taking a firm and leading role in combating environmental pollution. The Clean Air and Solid Waste Disposal Act of 1965 and the Clean Water Restoration Act of 1966 are examples of this attempt to fight pollution (38, 60, 62). The United States Environmental Protection Agency (EPA) was created in 1970 to consolidate,

strengthen, and coordinate federal efforts. Several important laws were passed after the formation of the EPA (e.g., Clean Water Act [1972], Pesticides Control Act [1972], Safe Drinking Water Act [1974], Resource Conservation and Recovery Act [1976], and Toxic Substances Control Act [1976]). The Toxic Substances Control Act was the first attempt to provide comprehensive regulation of potentially dangerous chemical substances. The Resource Conservation and Recovery Act gave the EPA the power to track hazardous wastes from generation site to final disposal (60, 131, 153).

During the 1980s the EPA reversed some earlier decisions and postponed implementation of some of their requirements. Nevertheless, enactment of important laws did occur, including Asbestos School Hazard Detection and Control Act (1980), Consumer-Patient Radiation and Health Safety Act (1981), Nuclear Waste Policy Act (1982), International Environmental Protection Act (1983), and Asbestos Hazard Emergency Response Act (1986) (38, 60). In the 1990s attempts are being made to develop environmental impact statements based on health-risk assessment (87), and legislation such as the Clean Air Act of 1990 has tightened previous regulations (80).

The following is divided into discussions of air, water, soil, food, noise, and surface pollution. However, these categories overlap. To illustrate, when a person inhales harmful particles from the soil that have become airborne, soil pollution becomes air pollution; and soil or surface pollution becomes water or food pollution if the harmful particles are swept into the water, consumed first by fish and then by people.

AIR POLLUTION

> . . . This most excellent canopy, the air, look you, this brave o'erhanging firmament, this majestical roof fretted with golden fire—why, it appears no other thing to me than a foul and pestilent congregation of vapors.
>
> *Hamlet* (II, ii, 314–315)

Problems of Air Pollution

Air pollution is not a new problem; people have known for centuries that air can carry poisons. Miners would take canaries with them into the mines—a dead bird meant the presence of lethal gas. Natural processes such as forest and prairie fires, volcanic eruptions, or wind erosion have long contaminated the air. A dramatic example of natural air pollution in the United States was caused by the 1980 eruption of Mount St. Helens in the state of Washington. Gases and dust from the volcano were spewed into the atmosphere, and local communities were covered with volcanic ash. Human activities such as burning fossil fuels, surface mining of coal, incineration of solid wastes, or manufacturing processes

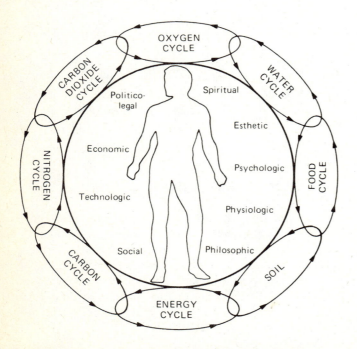

Figure 2-1. Human interrelationship with the environment.

are recognized as sources of pollution. The current problem of toxic air pollution came sharply into focus in late 1984 when more than 2500 people died and as many as 100,000 were left with permanent disabilities as a result of a gas leak from a Union Carbide Corporation fertilizer plant in India (225).

Air pollution and water pollution act interchangeably; together they present a world problem. All people on the earth share the oceans and the air. Significant local pollution of either can greatly affect distant areas, especially if the oceans cannot, by the processes of precipitation, oxidation, and absorption, cleanse the atmosphere before harmful effects occur. Given enough time, the oceans can cleanse the atmosphere; but if the amount of pollution exceeds the ocean's capacity to neutralize the waste, harmful materials are dispersed into the atmosphere, and we realize the effects by breathing contaminated air (42).

Sources of Air Pollution

The five most common pollutants found in the air are carbon monoxide, sulfur oxides, nitrogen oxides, suspended particles, and hydrocarbons. The sources of these air pollutants vary, and the effects on humans differ according to length and degree of exposure to the pollutant. Air pollution is most harmful to the very young, the very old, and persons with respiratory and cardiac disease (24, 27, 29, 55, 74, 153) (Table 2–1).

Carbon Monoxide

A major cause of air contamination is imperfect or incomplete combustion. **Perfect or complete combustion** exists only in chemistry books and is the *result of hydrogen and carbon uniting completely with oxygen, thereby relinquishing heat, water vapor, light, and carbon dioxide to the air.* **Imperfect or incomplete combusion** refers to the *additional liberation of carbon monoxide, sulfur oxides, and nitrogen oxides into the air.* Industry, forest fires, burning cigarettes, and motor vehicles are sources of **carbon monoxide,** a *colorless*

and odorless poisonous gas produced during the incomplete combusion of carbon. The greatest source of carbon monoxide in our cities is the motor vehicle. Between 1975 and 1987 total annual carbon monoxide emissions decreased by 24% (44). However, dangerous levels of carbon monoxide can accumulate in garages, tunnels, and heavy traffic. Research has shown that some people in New York City have blood concentration levels of 5.8% carbon monoxide as compared to the 1.5% considered safe (131). Carbon monoxide combines with the hemoglobin of red blood cells in place of oxygen and can produce a **hypoxic state,** a *decreased amount of oxygen* in the body. The severity of this state depends on the ratio of carbon monoxide to oxygen in the air inhaled. The deficiency of oxygen in the blood caused by carbon monoxide primarily affects respiration and the function of the brain and heart. Carbon monoxide in high concentrations can cause death; in small amounts it can cause dizziness, headache, fatigue, and impaired perception and thinking. Carbon monoxide pollution can be especially dangerous for persons who suffer from heart disease, respiratory disease, or anemia because they already have a physiologically impaired oxygen-carrying capacity (27, 117) and for the fetus because carbon monoxide can cause retardation of growth and brain development.

Sulfur Oxides

When coal or oil-containing sulfur is burned by factories and power plants, the sulfur in the fuels is oxidized. These **sulfur oxide compounds** (*sulfur dioxide* and *sulfur trioxide*) pollute the air in many sections of the country. **Sulfur dioxide (SO_2)** is a *heavy, poisonous gas that causes a choking sensation when inhaled.* **Sulfur trioxide (SO_3)** reacts with water vapor to form a mist of **sulfuric acid (H_2SO_4),** a *heavy, corrosive, colorless liquid.*

Pushed by Congress, electric utilities have developed methods to cut drastically the emissions caused by burning coal. Clean coal technology includes advanced methods of cleaning flue gases and techniques for re-

TABLE 2-1. COMMON AIR POLLUTANTS

Pollutant	Source	Effects
Carbon monoxide	Car exhaust; forest fires; burning cigarette	Reduces oxygen levels in blood; contributes to photochemical smog
Sulfur oxides	Burning coal or oil containing sulfur	Irritation of mucous membranes of eyes, nose, and throat; injury to lungs; damage to plant life; contribution to corrosion
Nitrogen oxides	Burning fossil fuel	Increase in respiratory illness; irritation to mucous membranes; alteration in night vision
Suspended particles	Wind erosion; fires; incineration of solid wastes; surface mining	Respiratory diseases
Hydrocarbons	Toxic chemicals may also be wind-borne.	Birth defects, neurologic impairment, cancer
	Decomposition of organic matter; incomplete combustion of gasoline	Involved in formation of ozone and photochemical smog

moving pollutants from coal before and after it is burned (45). Because of these changes and other regulations, the level of sulfur dioxide in the air decreased 37% between 1975 and 1986 (44, 59).

Worldwide it is estimated that more than 600 million people live in cities where average sulfur dioxide levels in the air are higher than safety guidelines set by the World Health Organization (186). Elevated levels of sulfur oxide have been linked to human illness and death. Irritation of the sensitive mucous membranes of the eyes, nose, and throat; injury to the mucous membranes that line the lungs; and aggravation or precipitation of respiratory problems such as bronchitis may occur (27, 153). Besides directly affecting our health, sulfur dioxide and its by-product, sulfuric acid, indirectly jeopardize health by damaging plant life and contributing to rust on metals.

Nitrogen Oxides

Other *gaseous end products* are the **nitrogen oxides.** The majority of the annual emissions of nitrogen oxides stem from burning fossil fuels, from motor vehicles and other transportation modes, from burning natural gas, oil, and coal in power plants, and from industrial combustion of fossil fuels. Chemical reactions in the air convert much of the nitrogen oxides to **nitrogen dioxide,** *a visible, red-brown, toxic, foul-smelling gas.* Between 1975 and 1986 the level of nitrogen dioxide in the air decreased 14% (3, 44, 59, 201, 224). Exposure to nitrogen dioxide causes irritation of the mucous membranes of the throat, altered night vision, and breathing difficulties. Research has also suggested that high levels of nitrogen dioxide contribute to an increase in respiratory disease, cancer, and heart disease (29).

Suspended Particles

Another air contaminant is **particulate matter,** *minute particles such as dust, dirt, soot, smoke, aerosols, and fly ash* that are suspended in the air. Most of the suspended particle pollutants are produced by industrial processes and power and heating plants (201). Particulate matter suspended in vapors and fumes may hover for annoying and dangerous periods of time, depending on atmospheric conditions. These pollutants may contaminate surfaces, scatter or distribute light rays unevenly, and, most dangerously, enter people's lungs. The severity of the lungs' response depends on the percentage of particulate matter or fumes and vapors in the air mixture and on preexisting lung disease.

Breathing asbestos particles can cause cancer and asbestosis. Asbestos once was widely used for fireproofing and insulating homes and public and private buildings. It was used in vinyl floor tiles and floorings, patching compounds and textured paints, shingles and siding, and appliances. Most of these uses are now prohibited or regulated by EPA standards. However, the individual who unknowingly has items containing asbestos in the home or workplace is not always protected. When asbestos material becomes damaged or starts to deteriorate, asbestos fibers are released into the air. In addition, particles are released into the atmosphere as brake linings and clutch facings wear and from manufacturing and fabricating facilities and mining (55, 61, 62, 117). Inhaled beryllium, used in making metal alloys, also causes a debilitating form of lung infection (117).

Cigarette smoke has been identified as an air pollutant, causing increased carbon monoxide content in the blood. In addition, numerous other chemicals make up the particulate matter in tobacco smoke, which can produce cardiovascular, respiratory, and other symptoms in both nonsmokers and smokers. Nonsmoking pregnant women exposed to tobacco smoke for at least 2 hours daily are twice as likely to deliver a low-birthweight infant as pregnant women not exposed to smoking. Secondhand smoke can produce respiratory disease and cancer in nonsmokers and smokers. Sufficient exposure to any type of particulate pollution can lead to pulmonary emphysema, a condition in which the alveoli of the lungs become distended or ruptured (2, 6, 44, 76, 104, 108, 144, 174, 180).

Hydrocarbons

Hydrocarbons (*volatile organic compounds*) *consist of only hydrogen and carbon.* Approximately 85% of the hydrocarbons found in the atmosphere come from natural sources, including forests, coal, gas, and petroleum fields, and decomposition of organic matter. Incomplete combustion and evaporation of gasoline from motor vehicles account for most of the emissions caused by human activities. Industrial and chemical manufacturing processes also contribute to this form of pollution. Hydrocarbons appear to have little direct effect on plants or animals but are involved in atmospheric reactions that form secondary air pollutants (122, 153).

Nitrogen oxides and hydrocarbons react in the presence of sunlight to produce ozone, photochemical smog, and peroxylacetyl nitrate. **Ozone (triatomic oxygen, O_3)** is a *pungent, colorless, toxic gas*. In the upper atmosphere ozone forms a protective barrier that prevents excessive ultraviolet light from reaching the earth. In the lower atmosphere ozone is *formed in the air by chemical reactions between nitrogen oxides and hydrocarbons* such as vapors from gasoline and chemical solvents (57).

Ozone is a dangerous pollutant. It affects the eyes, respiratory tract, and nervous system and produces nausea, drowsiness, eye irritation, respiratory distress, irritation of the mucous membranes of the nose and throat, exhaustion, headaches, and decreased tolerance to physical exercise. School-age children, the elderly, and individuals with chronic heart and lung diseases are the most severely affected by ozone. New research has also found that ozone can impair the immune system of animals. In plants ozone causes a significant reduction in photosynthesis, causing vegetation to turn yellow (56, 57, 74, 117, 131, 208, 231).

Peroxylacetyl nitrate (PAN) is damaging to plants and causes leaf mottling and reduced growth, which affects the food supply. **Photochemical smog** *occurs when the chemical reactions between nitrogen oxides and hydrocarbons are stimulated by sunlight.* Photochemical smog was first noted in the Los Angeles area. Since then, it frequently has been observed in many other cities. Photochemical smog produces some of the same effects on humans as ozone—eye irritation, lung damage, and decreased tolerance to physical activity (64, 117).

The EPA has developed the Pollutant Standards Index (PSI) as a means of reporting daily air pollution concentrations. The PSI converts the pollutant concentrations measured in a community's air to a number on a scale of 0 to 500. Intervals of the PSI scale are related to the potential health effects of the daily measured concentrations of the five major pollutants previously described. The intervals and terms used to describe the air quality levels are as follows: 0 to 50—good; above 50—moderate; above 100—unhealthful; 201 to 300—first stage alert, very unhealthful; 301-400—second stage alert, hazardous; 401–500—third stage alert, significant harm (209). When the pollution index is greater than 100, individuals with existing heart or respiratory ailments should reduce physical exertion and outdoor activity.

Four additional air pollution problems should be mentioned: (1) depletion of the upper atmosphere ozone layer; (2) increasing levels of atmospheric carbon dioxide; (3) acid rain; and (4) radioactive substances. As noted, a thin layer of ozone surrounds the earth and blocks much of the sun's ultraviolet radiation from reaching the earth's surface. The ozone layer is in danger of being depleted by the continued use of fluorocarbons (Freon) and chlorofluoromethanes that release chlorine into the stratosphere to combine with ozone. The continued use of fluorocarbon-propelled aerosol products and supersonic transport planes adds to that danger (74, 117).

In Caucasians short-wavelength ultraviolet sunlight is thought to cause melanoma and nonmelanoma skin cancer that would increase in incidence if there were a reduction of the ozone layer. In addition, studies have shown that an increase in ultraviolet radiation damages the immune system of humans (74, 189).

Increasing Carbon Dioxide

The atmospheric content of carbon dioxide has increased significantly in the past century. Carbon dioxide is added to the atmosphere by burning fossil fuels. The increased level of atmospheric carbon dioxide alters the heat balance of the earth. Sunlight passes through the carbon dioxide, but the radiation of heat away from the earth is slowed, producing what is known as the *greenhouse effect*. Such changes might eventually result in polar ice caps' melting, flooding of large coastal plain areas, and disruption of food production (66, 117). Some scientists fear the opposite may occur—the *refrigerator effect*. The carbon dioxide concentration would eventually prevent enough of the sun's rays from reaching earth that cooler temperatures would occur, again affecting food production and health factors (66, 131).

Acid Rain

Acid rain is the *end product of chemical reactions that begin when sulfur dioxide and nitrogen oxides enter the atmosphere from coal-, oil-, and gas-burning power plants, iron and copper smelters, and automobile exhausts.* These gases undergo changes and eventually react with moisture to form sulfuric acid and nitric acid. One half to two thirds of the pollution falls as acid rain or snow; some of the remainder is deposited as sulfate or nitrate particles that combine with dew and mist to form dilute acids (227). Most of northeastern United States, portions of the upper Midwest, Rocky Mountains, and West Coast, and parts of Ontario, Quebec, Nova Scotia, and Newfoundland in Canada now receive strongly acidic precipitation (145, 166). The United Kingdom, continental Europe, Poland, and central Russia have reported environmental damage from acid rain or snow. Although the full effect on the environment is not understood as yet, increased acidity in soil, streams, or ponds can be documented. Certain freshwater ecosystems are particularly sensitive to acid; fish, frogs, and some aquatic plants die. Acid rain leaches compounds out of soil, damaging the root systems of plants. Forests die. Crops are damaged. With continued episodes of acid rain, limestone and marble statues and buildings are dissolved, and homes and other structures weather more quickly (43, 75, 145, 158, 166, 227). It will be years before the full effect of acid precipitation is known. At present, the only solution is to decrease the emissions of sulfur and nitrogen oxide into the atmosphere.

Radioactive Substances

Radioactive substances are *produced by mining and processing radioactive ore and by nuclear-fission and radiation procedures* used in industry, medicine, and research. Pollution from radioactive materials poses a serious threat to our ability to reproduce and to our gene structure. It is also related to an increase in leukemia and other cancers, as demonstrated in persons working with radioactive materials over long periods without adequate safeguards, and in survivors of the bombings in Hiroshima and Nagasaki, Japan. A small fraction, 1% to 3%, of all cancers in the general population is attributable to natural radiation. Occupational irradiation produces an increase over the natural incidence (27, 44, 190).

Indoor Air Pollution

Some significant indoor air pollutants are carbon monoxide, asbestos particles, formaldehyde, nitrogen oxides, and radon. In the home carbon monoxide is released by unvented gas stoves, kerosene space heaters, wood stoves, and tobacco smoke. As mentioned previously, asbestos particles can be released as fireproofing materials, insulation, ceiling tiles, floor tiles, and other building materials begin to deteriorate.

Formaldehyde, a *colorless gas characterized by a strong, pungent odor*, escapes into the air from foam insulation, particle board, plywood, and fiberboards. Formaldehyde gas in newly insulated homes has reached concentrations high enough to cause dizziness, drowsiness, nausea, vomiting, rashes, nosebleeds, and diarrhea. It is extremely hazardous and probably is a carcinogen. Nitrogen oxides are released from unvented gas stoves and space heaters. As they accumulate in the home, these pollutants can affect sensory perception and produce eye irritation.

Radon, a *natural radioactive gas produced by the decay of uranium 238*, is the most serious health threat of the common indoor pollutants. It seeps into basements through cracked floors and diffuses out of brick and concrete building materials. The EPA estimates that radon is responsible for 5,000 to 20,000 deaths from lung cancer each year (23, 27, 44, 55, 150, 155, 165, 167, 219).

Particles such as dust, soot, ash, or cigarette smoke may be inhaled into the lungs. Many household products such as cleansers, drain openers, or paint removers have toxic ingredients and cause respiratory irritation and eye or skin irritation on contact. Some are carcinogenic when fumes or particles are inhaled over time (16, 128). Fungi and bacteria from humidifiers and air conditioning systems can cause allergies or Legionnaires' disease and aggravate asthma.

Indoor air pollution can be controlled by several measures: proper venting of gas stoves, heaters, and wood stoves; painting over materials that emit radon and formaldehyde; and daily airing of the house. Houseplants, especially spider plants, can be used to absorb air pollutants in the home.

All forms of air pollution are physically irritating and present a potential hazard to long-range health either by direct harm to the mucous membranes of the respiratory tract or by the indirect effects of continuously breathing contaminated air. Only in becoming aware of these factors as personal health threats will we seriously consider alternatives to using two or three cars, seek to know the serious hazards in our jobs, become concerned about houses downwind from an industrial site or the amount of ultraviolet light we receive, and use natural products instead of chemicals for many household tasks.

WATER POLLUTION

Pollution of the water from the natural processes of aquatic animal and plant life, combined with man-made waste, constitutes another hazard to the delicate state of human health. Man-made water pollution has two major origins, *point sources* and *nonpoint sources.* Point sources are those that discharge pollutants from a well-defined place (e.g., outlet pipes of sewage treatment plants and factories). Nonpoint sources consist of runoff from city streets, construction sites, farms, and mines.

Types of Water Pollution

The most common water pollutants are common sewage, pathogenic organisms, plant nutrients, synthetic chemicals, inorganic chemicals, sediment, radioactive substances, oil, and heat.

Common Sewage
Traditional waste from domestic and industrial sources, or **sewage,** is a significant problem. Of particular concern are on-site sewage disposal systems such as septic tanks, cesspools, and outdoor toilets (75, 109). When sewage is drained or dumped into water sources, oxygen is required to render the waste harmless. The waste uses oxygen needed by aquatic plant and animal life. With increasing amounts of sewage, the problem is even more serious because of the inability of the water to deal successfully with the waste. When bacteria in the water can no longer decompose the waste, widespread aquatic death results. Waste then accumulates, and the water becomes useless as a personal or industrial resource.

Pathogenic Organisms
Pathogenic organisms pollute water when sewage carrying them enters a river, lake, or stream. A human or animal drinking this water can become ill. Occasionally a whole community or area is affected negatively if a large source of water becomes contaminated with diseased microbes. Although medical science has made major strides in the prevention and treatment of these diseases, it is still possible for outbreaks of infectious gastroenteritis and hepatitis, typhoid fever, giardiasis, cholera, or other infectious diseases to occur. Farm workers and persons living in rural and urban fringe areas where population density is high or public utilities are limited are at greater risk from this form of pollution (10, 39, 109, 112). Health problems from polluted water are occurring worldwide, including in Israeli kibbutzim (185).

Plant Nutrients

Nutrients that nourish plant life, especially phosphates and nitrates, are produced by sewage, livestock and human excrement, soil erosion, industrial wastes, and chemical fertilizers. In rural areas these nutrients can contaminate groundwater and rural drinking water supplies. Infant illness and death from nitrate-induced methemoglobinemia are significant problems (39). In areas where drinking water is treated, these nutrients also produce problems. The nutrients are not easily removed by treatment centers because they do not respond to the usual biologic processes. Moreover, treatment centers may inadvertently change these substances into a more usable mineral form that stimulates excessive plant growth. This increased growth of bacteria and algae becomes a problem by interfering with treatment processes, marring the landscape, producing an unpleasant odor and taste in the water, and disturbing the normal food web in a body of water. Because humans depend on many lower forms of life for food, this process could eventually affect their well-being (Fig. 2–2).

Synthetic Chemicals

Synthetic chemicals used in everyday household chores, especially those found in detergents, pesticides, and other cleaning agents, affect the water. They may be poisonous to aquatic life even in small proportions. When resistant to local treatment measures, they can produce an unpleasant taste and odor in the water. The extent of the long-term problem is not known, but the possibility of human poisoning over a long period by the consumption of small doses of these chemicals taken in drinking water cannot be ignored. This problem is discussed later in the chapter.

Inorganic Chemicals

Inorganic chemicals are mineral substances from mining or manufacturing processes that can destroy land animals (including people) and aquatic life when ingested. Industries sometimes improperly and illegally empty large quantities of toxic materials into sources of local water supply. This group of pollutants corrodes water-treatment equipment and makes waste treatment an even more expensive problem.

Sediment

Particles of dirt or sand resulting from soil erosion have been identified as a significant water pollutant. Soil particles suspended in water interfere with the penetration of sunlight and therefore reduce photosynthesis of aquatic plants and animals (175). When sediment settles, it covers food sources on the bottom of lakes and streams, smothers bottom-dwelling organisms, disrupts the reproductive cycle of fish and other organisms, fills

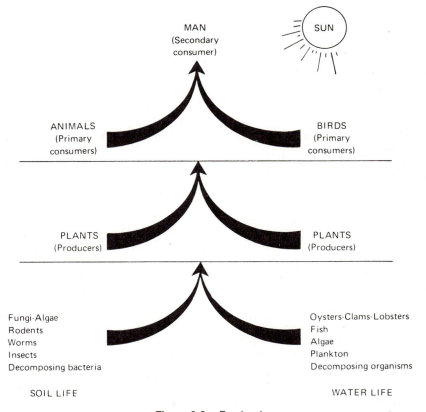

Figure 2-2. Food web.

streams, and prevents natural reservoirs from filling during rainy seasons. Because of its sheer volume, sediment also increases the cost of water treatment.

Radioactive Material

Natural or synthetic radioactive material can contaminate water. Potential sources of radioactive pollutants in water include waste from nuclear power plants, industrial or research facilities using radioactive materials, or uranium mines (39). Incidence of stomach cancer among Navaho Indians is four times the national average, probably because half of the nation's supply of uranium was mined in or near the Navaho Reservation during the 1950s and 1960s. Water and, in turn, food supplies have been contaminated with radioactive materials; uranium tailings remain even though the mines are closed (196).

Oil

Oil found in natural water is usually the result of man's deliberate actions, not from accidents. Accidental spills account for only a small percent of all oil spilled into the ocean. The rest is from natural seepage, dumping of waste oil, flushing of ships' bilges, and discharging oil from refineries. Numerous biologic effects result from the presence of oil in natural waters: contact with the oil ruins the waterproofing and insulating qualities of birds; oil contaminates or destroys the natural food of birds; and residuals from the oil are being found in the food web of humans (75).

Heat

Heat becomes a problem because it reduces the ability of the water to absorb oxygen. If significant amounts of water are heated through industrial use, the water becomes less efficient in providing oxygen for aquatic life and in assimilating waste. Even more dangerous, the ecologic balance of lakes and rivers can be permanently upset through prolonged alteration of water temperature. The food that people eat either comes directly from water or has fed on aquatic life somewhere in the food web. Faced with an expanding world population, we must increasingly be aware of the significance of every organism in the food web (see Fig. 2–2) and its relationship to us.

One of the most frightening results of water pollution is the threat to the oceans. The collective practice of the world's nations of ocean dumping of sewage may permanently pollute the oceans. The Ocean Dumping Act was amended in 1977 so that ocean dumping would not be allowed after December 31, 1981. Yet ocean dumping of garbage, sewage, toxic chemicals, radioactive wastes, and medical wastes not only continues but is increasing. When the Act was amended in the 1970s, most people were concerned about the environment. In the 1980s the major concern was the cost of enforcing environmental standards. Now the results from failure to

enforce the Ocean Dumping Act are apparent. Paper, boxes, cans, glass bottles, egg cartons, fishing nets, plastic products, syringes, vials of blood, and other debris clutter the shore line. Some beaches have closed because of the health hazard. In addition to the danger to humans, the pollution is endangering wildlife; dolphins, gulls, turtles, shellfish, fish, and sea lions mistake the waste for food or become entangled in the debris (44, 62, 75, 124, 135).

Problems in Water Purification

The common denominator of all major water pollution is called **biologic oxygen demand (BOD),** *the amount of free oxygen that extraneous substances absorb from water* (75). The natural water purification process involves the action of bacteria, which use oxygen to decompose organic matter. If too much waste is dumped into a given body of water, this natural cleansing process cannot take place or at least does not take place fast enough. Further, once the water in the underground aquifer is contaminated, it is nearly impossible to guarantee a safe water supply.

The ultimate problem of water pollution stems from our using natural resources in greater and greater amounts because of additional industrialization, population growth, a greater dependence on appliances, and a subsequent increase in the need for sewage disposal. The problem of dissolving waste has put a strain on waste-disposal systems. Even excessive amounts of treated waste now obstruct the waterways. Current engineering research is attempting to solve some of the problems of water pollution by developing different types of waste-disposal systems.

When water contains pollutants in ever-increasing amounts, it becomes a threat to human health. At present, the quality of water service for countless people must be improved; many inhabitants of rural areas and small towns obtain their drinking water from polluted sources. In several areas of the United States wastewater is being used for irrigation. This water contains low levels of organic chemicals. Although it is considered safe for human use, the water is not meant for drinking purposes. However, indirect human consumption does occur when surface waters are used for water supply (62, 63, 75, 109, 215, 216). Keeping drinking water separate from water for other uses would help conserve water supplies and ensure greater purity, for water used for other purposes could be refiltered at less expense (157).

Pollution of marshes and shorelines has severely impaired breeding habitats for many types of shellfish and deep-water species, thereby subsequently affecting the nations' food supply. Polluted water cannot be used for recreational purposes; backpackers, campers, swimmers, windsurfers, and waterskiers have all felt the impact of water pollution. In addition to the health risk, the odor of decay and the unsightliness of polluted water destroy the beauty of any natural setting.

Misuse of our water has far-reaching consequences, threatening people all over the world from every age group and culture. We must take personal responsibility for stopping needless pollution of the water by exercising careful personal use of agents that can ultimately destroy it and by using legal procedures to prevent undue dumping of wastes into lakes, rivers, and streams. Some health problems associated with contaminated water could be eliminated by proper legislation, and needless sickness and death could be avoided. Such legislation as the Clean Water Act of 1987 and the revised Safe Drinking Water Act of 1986, which promote water quality standards and impose a system of control on all sources of pollution, are effective and worthy of support. More importantly, the health of future generations and their chance to enjoy the beauty, taste, and power of the water depend on those of us who are so carelessly polluting it. Water, like oxygen, is essential to life, development, and health.

SOIL POLLUTION

As early as 1950 the federal Food and Drug Administration announced that the potential health hazards of compounds containing chlorinated hydrocarbons such as dichlorodiphenyltrichloroethane (DDT) had been underestimated (127). The Federal Environmental Pesticide Control Act, passed in 1972 and amended in 1975 and 1978, requires that all pesticide products sold or distributed in this country must be registered with the United States EPA (58).

Substances used to kill weeds, rats, mice, worms, fungi, and insects are called **pesticides.** Soil pollution can occur as a result of excessive or improper use of pesticides (insecticides, herbicides, fungicides) or crop fertilizers. Many chemicals used in these preparations are highly toxic and can remain in the soil for long periods of time without being degraded, thus setting the stage for pollution of food, water, and, ultimately, people (27, 195).

Although farmers are their largest users, pesticides are also used by industry; federal, state, and local governmental agencies; and individuals in their homes and gardens. The actual toxic effects of the different compounds vary, and some products have never been completely tested.

Reports from epidemiologic studies indicate that various acute illnesses and physiologic changes have been observed in individuals who were exposed to agricultural chemicals (i.e., farmers, workers in pesticide manufacturing plants, agricultural workers, and commercial pest-control operators). Exposure to the chemicals can occur in several ways: inhalation of pesticide dust or spray, direct skin contact, ingestion of food and water containing residues, and contact with contaminated equipment. Inhalation exposure can occur in a subtle manner at times (e.g., by inhaling the dust from storage bags during the filling or emptying process or from cultivated soil previously treated with pesticides). Symptoms occurring as the result of such exposure may not be attributed to the pesticides. Therefore many episodes of acute poisoning go undiagnosed. Direct skin contact can occur when solutions are spilled accidentally or when the moist spray touches exposed skin.

The physiologic effects from pesticide exposure are varied. Some pesticides are cholinesterase inhibitors; others are known central nervous system stimulants or depressants, producing forgetfulness, decreased attention and interest span, hyperirritability, anxiety, depression, nervousness, and insomnia. Skin diseases, eye and respiratory conditions, and digestive disorders have also been identified. In some instances these health problems have occurred after a single exposure to the toxic chemical. Reproductive problems, birth defects, and increased risk of cancer and leukemia have been associated with low-level chronic exposure to pesticides (11, 20, 27, 61, 83, 162, 168, 209, 222).

Pesticides have an immediate toxic effect on birds, bees, and rodents, thus curtailing the necessary agents of cross-pollination and insect destruction, which, in turn, can affect the food supply. Surface water can be contaminated during spraying or dusting, and rain can wash pesticides or fertilizers into streams and lakes, again affecting food supply. Earthworms are capable of concentrating toxic chemicals from the soil and storing these chemicals in their fatty tissues. Because earthworms provide food for other animals that are also capable of concentrating these chemicals, they may become an important source of undesirable chemical residues in higher animals and humans (61, 140).

The EPA's pesticide control program has three major components: registration of pesticides, training of pesticide applicators, and monitoring and research. All pesticides must be registered with the agency before being marketed. The agency approves labeling and sets maximum safe levels for pesticide residues in human and animal food. The EPA has developed an applicator training program, certifying individuals permitted to apply restricted-use pesticides. In addition, the agency sponsors research on pesticides and monitors pesticide levels in the environment. Both acute and long-term pesticide effects are considered in the epidemiologic studies (62).

In spite of the EPA's efforts, evidence indicates that the EPA receives insufficient funding, and standards are not being followed; long-term effects are yet unknown. According to a report from the National Research Council of the National Academy of Sciences, industrial wastes are being dumped on or pumped into the earth's crust, and few studies are being done to determine whether the sites are safe. It may be possible to contain wastes safely and to lessen toxicity in wastes in the natural systems of the earth if the chemical nature of the waste and the geologic nature of the disposal area are understood. Geologic mapping is needed as a guide to safe disposal sites and for research on reactions between chemicals and rock or soil, fracture patterns in rocks, fluid flow, and hydrodynamics of deep basins (98).

The widespread contamination by dioxin in Missouri in 1983 following massive flooding illustrates the complexity and extent of the problem. Chemicals were used without awareness of harmful effect. Unregulated use of chemicals and dumping of various chemicals by industries had occurred for some time and had only become apparent later. Furthermore, chemicals did not remain where originally used or dumped. Flood waters, underground water, and wind transported chemicals or their residues from one soil site to another. People are now learning that their past and present symptoms and diseases are related to or caused by hazardous pollutants in the environment to which they did not know they were being exposed (184).

Dioxin is considered a toxic synthetic compound by some scientists; others believe it is not as toxic as originally thought. A complex organic chemical compound, it is insoluble in water but dissolves in organic solvents mixed with water. It is strongly attracted to lipids: fatty tissues in the body, oils, or related lipid substances. It becomes strongly attached to soil particles. The chemical remains in lipids or soil for many years and during a flood or soil erosion can move through water with solvents, soil particles, or colloids to which it is attached. Dioxin is also part of many other chemical compounds (e.g., chlorophenols, herbicides, and the antiseptic hexachlorophene). It can be generated by incineration of industrial, commercial, and municipal wastes that contain chlorinated aromatics, chlorophenols, or polychlorinated biphenyls (PCBs) (48, 184, 214).

Dioxin produces a wide range of harmful effects in animals:

1. Liver damage
2. Birth defects
3. Spontaneous abortions and sterility
4. Some types of cancer
5. Nerve and brain damage; decreased sensory perception
6. Disturbed enzyme production
7. Reduced immunity to infections
8. Chloracne, a disfiguring and painful affliction of the skin that may last many years
9. Damge to the gastrointestinal tract, with weight loss
10. Damage to the immune system

Many effects are chronic and long term (184, 214).

Dioxin is not only a problem for residents along rivers outside of St. Louis, Missouri, the scene of much publicity in 1983. Dioxin is a contaminant in Agent Orange, the herbicide sprayed in Vietnam. Many U.S. service personnel and their families were exposed and are suffering a variety of health problems. Where additional sites of dioxin contamination may be found is not yet known, but dioxin is being found in many areas of the United States (48, 214).

FOOD POLLUTION

Some of the same chemicals found in pesticide preparation are used as **food additives.** These purposely used additives are not designed to be toxic but rather to *preserve, improve, and protect nutritional value.*

Although the average person in the United States consumes a significant amount of additives every year, it is difficult to determine the potential health risk over a life span. Certain food additives interfere with intestinal mucosa absorptive ability and therefore affect availability of nutrients and drugs. Also, some nontoxic substances or chemicals used as food additives are metabolized into toxic substances in the body. Adverse reactions to synthetic flavors and colors include gastrointestinal, respiratory, neurologic, skeletal, and skin disorders. Removal of artificial flavors and colors from the diet has been found to reduce hyperkinesis and certain learning disabilities in children with these disabilities (21, 27, 125, 203, 220, 225).

Unexpected side effects have resulted from *antibiotic and hormone residues from drugs given to animals for growth promotion and disease prevention.* In people these residues have resulted in (1) allergy and increased drug toxicity or resistance to pathogens when the *same* family of antibiotics is later administered therapeutically and (2) change of normal bacterial flora in a body area so that invasion by pathogens is more likely, causing infection or disease (28). Synthetic estrogen, diethylstilbestrol (DES), was used in cattle feed to promote rapid weight gain. Studies have linked DES to increases in a rare genital tract tumor in young women whose mothers were given DES while pregnant. As a result of these studies, use of DES has been restricted. An attempt to ban its use and the use of other sex hormones as feed supplements is underway (205).

A considerable amount of pesticides is ingested by most families in the United States from eating fruits and vegetables grown in Mexico and the United States where large amounts of chemicals are used repeatedly to control insects, weeds, rodents, and other agricultural pests. The U.S. consumer wants to purchase fruits and vegetables that are without blemish and appear as perfect as a picture. Blight, rust, fungus, or other causes of discoloration can most quickly be controlled by chemical application. However, the farmers are caught in a pesticide treadmill. Each year it takes more and different poisons to accomplish the same task, and the insects continue to produce hybrid strains that are resistant to the chemicals. Even those banned by the EPA in the United States are likely to be used in other countries usually are shipped by U.S. chemical manufacturers. Examples of disease-producing chemicals that contaminate foodstuffs include:

1. Chlordane
2. Toxaphine
3. 2,4-D
4. DBCP
5. Paraquat (a small amount on the skin causes asphyxiation)
6. EDBC (a fungicide which breaks down into a potent carcinogen ETU)
7. Aldicarb (methyl isocyanate which converts to hydrogen cyanide gas, which killed and injured people at Bhopal, India)
8. Parathion (an organophosphate pesticide so lethal that a tablespoon on the skin is fatal)

The pesticide market is so large that production is estimated to equal 1 pound of chemicals annually for every person—men, women, and children—on earth. Although DDT, chlordane, Dieldren, and 2,4,5-T are banned in the United States and Europe, they are sold to many developing countries that are increasingly a source of some of our food products. People in Third World countries do not know how to use chemicals to avoid widespread contamination, and the number of deaths and injuries attributed to agrichemicals in those countries is increasing. For example, in rural Brazil, DDT levels 10 times that considered safe have been found in mother's milk. Ten percent of that population suffers symptoms of mild chronic poisoning. Levels of DDT 90 times higher than that in U.S. milk have been found in milk sold in Guatemala. Stomach and colon cancers have increased five times in African countries where large amounts of agrichemicals have been used. Drinking paraquat has become a popular form of suicide in Sri Lanka and Central and South America, although careless handling causes the most deaths of agricultural workers. In addition to causing human misery, the pesticides and herbicides are ravaging the ecosystems by killing birds, plants, and marine life.

Pesticide use could be reduced greatly by using better agricultural techniques:

1. Crop rotation
2. Intercropping, alternating small plots of different plants
3. Avoidance of monocropping—planting huge fields of only one crop season after season
4. Polyculture—diversifying species within the same crop type
5. Providing habitat for beneficial insects
6. Selecting plants for their resistance to pests
7. Timing planting of crops to avoid pest attacks or to plant them in their optimal climate

8. Development of biologic controls (some insects and pests are natural predators on other insects and pests)
9. Developing improved hardware for safer application when pesticides and herbicides are applied (139, 140).

Farmers in the United States are decreasing pesticide use (202). However, the problem of a toxin remaining in the food chain often remains even after a toxic chemical has been banned because the toxins bioaccumulate in the environment. Chlordane, used widely in the Midwest in the 1970s as a soil insecticide for corn, was banned for that use because studies showed it produced cancer. However, it was allowed until recently to remain in the market as a termiticide. Through goundwater contamination, it has accumulated in the sediments of rivers and lakes. In the spring of 1987, residents of Missouri and other nearby states that receive river flow from Missouri were warned not to eat fish from a number of the Missouri rivers and lakes because the fish were contaminated with chlordane (148).

In St. Louis and the surrounding area, the soil, water, and air remain contaminated from the processing of uranium oxide for the world's first nuclear reaction 45 years ago. Several radioactive waste sites are in the St. Louis metropolitan area. Nearby people live and children play without knowledge of the radioactive levels, the impending danger, or the long-term effects in health development. Only recently have the sites and their potential dangers become known (111).

This situation is not too different from that of residents of the Great Lakes regions: 37 million people who live near the Great Lakes have as much as 20% higher levels of toxic chemicals in their bodies than other U.S. residents. Over the years they have ingested many toxins (benzine, hexachloride, PCBs, DDT, toxaphene, mercury) from contaminated water and fish (154).

The effects on present and future generations of the 900 identified leaking hazardous waste sites in the United States remain unknown. Other sites, as yet unidentified, may be contaminating soil and, in turn, water, food, and air (154).

In addition to the additives, synthetic pesticides, and other man-made chemicals that may appear in trace amounts in processed foods, natural toxic compounds are in huge concentrations in the food supply; for example, apples, cabbage, celery, lettuce, peaches, pineapple, and turnips are all considered natural carcinogens. Regulatory agencies pay little attention to the dangers of these natural toxic chemicals (229).

Other food pollution hazards are *radioactive materials* such as strontium 90, which has been traced in milk; mercury found in swordfish; worms; and mold, which may be present without noticeable change in the food's appearance, taste, or smell. Food handlers may introduce their infectious diseases into food by touching it or the equipment with soiled hands or by coughing onto it. Prolonged storage of highly acidic foods in aluminum cookware or aluminum foil may cause more aluminum than usual to enter the body. Using unlined copper utensils for cooking or storing food may also be harmful (89, 170, 225). Food sources may become contaminated by the chemicals and metals used in fertilizers and pesticides. In the future, diseases from food additives may assume as much significance in humans as do the **zoonoses,** *diseases transmitted between animals and humans,* such as trichinosis, brucellosis, tuberculosis, psittacosis, salmonellosis, typhus, roundworms, and rabies.

Because of the endless contamination possibilities from bacteria, toxins, viruses, parasites, and protozoa, the Food and Drug Administration and the Department of Agriculture enforce laws passed by Congress, impose various regulations of their own, and, in general, monitor the food industry nationwide. Various state and local authorities also attempt to regulate standards within their respective jurisdictions (60, 62). Yet these agencies cannot possibly determine every breach of regulation.

Astute observations must be made about standards in the food store. Demanding to know the growing, cleansing, processing, and handling procedures is not out of line. Reporting suspected breaches is your responsibility for health.

NOISE POLLUTION

Sensory stimulation plays a major role in psychologic and physiologic development and is therefore directly related to physical and mental health. Sound is but one form of sensory stimulation. **Sound overload,** *unwanted sound that produces unwanted effects,* and sound deprivation can be hazards to health (27, 44, 81, 118, 224).

Sound overload can produce temporary or permanent hearing loss by affecting the tympanic membrane and by slowly deteriorating the microscopic cells that send sound waves from the ear to the brain. The effects produced on each person's hearing vary, depending on the sound intensity and pitch, the location of the source in relation to the person, the length of exposure, and the person's age and history of previous ear problems. Millions of Americans have either measurable hearing deficits or are exposed to occupational noise levels capable of producing permanent hearing loss (27, 81, 118, 159).

One means of determining the potential hazard of any sound is to measure its loudness. The *measurement of sound loudness is stated in* **decibels.** The faintest audible sound is designated 1 decibel; ordinary conversation, measured at 40 to 60 decibels, is considered adequately quiet. The EPA identifies 55 decibels as the level above which harmful effects occur. Studies have shown that moderately loud sounds of 75 to 80 decibels such as

those produced by a clothes washer, tabulating machine, or home garbage-disposal unit can be discomforting to human ears and can, over a period of time, produce temporary or permanent hearing loss. Table 2–2 presents examples of common sound pollutants and their decibel readings. Sound louder than 130 decibels (e.g., that produced by a nearby jet plane, gunshot blast, or a rocket at the launching pad) may cause actual pain (27, 44, 209). Persons who work regularly with any of the machines listed should realize the potential longrange effects of such noise levels.

The Noise Control Act was passed in 1972 and amended in 1978 as the Quiet Communities Act. Under this act the EPA set noise emission standards for the transportation vehicles and products that are major sources of noise. The act also provides for research into the psychologic and physiologic effects of noise on people. State and local governments have been given primary responsibility for enforcing these standards (147).

Effects of Noise Pollution

Sound overload affects everyone at some time by intruding on privacy and shattering serenity. In addition to hearing loss, it can produce impaired communication and social relationships, irritability, chronic headache, depression, fatigue, and tension. Noise has also been associated with elevated blood cholesterol levels, atherosclerosis, and accident proneness. Research indicates

TABLE 2-2. COMMON SOUND POLLUTANTS AND THEIR DECIBEL READINGS

Sound	Decibels
Library whisper	30
Vacuum cleaner	72
Dishwasher	76-96
Minibike	76
Loud street noise	80-100
Alarm clock	80
Heavy city traffic	90-95
Food blender in home	93
Pneumatic hammer	95
Air compressor	95
Power lawnmower	95
Farm tractor	98
Chain saw	100
Outboard motor	102
Jet flying at 1000 feet	103
Ambulance siren	105
Riveting gun	110
Motorcycle	115
Jackhammer	120
Live rock music	120
Jet plane at takeoff	150
Rocket engine	180

that less obvious physiologic changes in the digestive, cardiovascular, endocrine, and nervous systems also can occur. These changes can produce blood vessel constriction, pallor, dilated pupils and visual disturbance, increased and irregular heart rate, hypertension, headache, gastrointestinal spasm with nausea and diarrhea and eventual peptic ulcer, hyperactive reflexes, and muscle tenseness. These responses do not subside immediately but continue up to five times longer than the actual noise (26, 209). Humans do not adapt to excessive sound, as was once thought, but learn to tolerate it. Even when a person is asleep, noise cannot be shut out completely. He or she awakens exhausted by the efforts to sleep in the midst of excessive external stimuli. Awareness of environmental stress factors can aid an individual to reduce or cope with them.

Although not every harmful form of sound can be avoided, certain measures such as wearing protective ear coverings, shortening exposure time, having regular hearing examinations, and seeking immediate medical attention for any ear injury or infection decrease the possibility of permanent damage or hearing loss. Noise can be brought under control without excessive cost. You can educate the public about the hazards of excess noise and ways to reduce noise in the home environment. Some suggestions to reduce noise are to hang heavy drapes over windows closest to outside noise sources, use foam pads under blenders and mixers, use carpeting in areas of heavy foot traffic, use upholstered instead of hard-surfaced furniture, and install sound absorbing ceiling tile in the kitchen.

The hospital, considered a place to recuperate and rest, may actually contribute to symptoms because of the noise levels in certain areas. One study showed that noise levels in infant incubators, the recovery room, and acute care units were high enough to act as a stressor and stimulate the hypophyseal-adrenocortical axis. Peripheral vasoconstriction affecting blood pressure and pulse, threats to hearing loss in patients receiving aminoglycosidic antibiotics, and sleep deprivation were noted. Noise pollution in the operating room, causing vasoconstriction, pupil dilation, fatigue, and impaired speech communication, has also been found.

SURFACE POLLUTION

Until the mid-1960s U.S. residents were not concerned with problems of waste disposal or recycling. Raw materials were plentiful, and the open-dump method of disposal was convenient and economical. In the early 1970s, however, people became more concerned with the decreasing supply of natural resources and the health problems created by open dumps.

The Solid Waste Disposal Act was passed by Congress in 1965. The primary focus of this act was on the disposal of waste, not collection or street cleaning. In 1970 Congress passed the Resource Recovery Act, which shifted the emphasis of federal involvement from disposal to recycling, resource recovery, and the conversion of waste into energy. Subsequent laws such as the Resource Conservation and Recovery Act of 1976 have been passed to facilitate further the safe disposal of waste (60, 62).

The total quantity of solid waste is large and increasing. Every day the average American generates approximately $3\frac{1}{2}$ pounds of trash. Over 160 million tons of solid wastes per year, not including sludge, construction debris, factory wastes, and dumped cars, are produced in the United States (80). Most present disposal methods for this waste pollute land, air, or water. This pollution appears many places: in open air, foul-smelling dumps, smoking incineration centers, junkyards, and poorly covered landfills.

Solid-Waste Disposal Methods

Solid waste is discarded in four basic ways: (1) in open dumps, (2) in landfills, (3) by incineration, and (4) as salvage.

Open Dumps

The open dump (now illegal in most states) is the oldest, most convenient, and most economical method. It creates many health problems, however, and is esthetically undesirable. Dumps serve as breeding grounds for rodents, flies, and other insects such as cockroaches; they also attract seagulls, notorious as thieves and litterers. Houseflies carry poliomyelitis, tuberculosis, diarrhea, dysentery, hepatitis, and cholera. Rats carry plague, tapeworm, Rocky Mountain spotted fever, and rat-bite fever. Water running off from these dumps pollutes local streams and lakes. Rain and surface water can seep through the wastes and pollute underground water. Any attempt to burn the surface waste in the dumps emits large quantities of foul-smelling fumes that increase air pollution and thus respiratory problems among local inhabitants. Dumps invite accidents and fires in addition to lowering the value of surrounding property (124, 127).

Landfills

Landfills are the final destination for 80% to 86% of the trash generated in the United States. Of the total amount of trash in a landfill, 35.6% is paper; 20.1% is yard wastes; 8.9% is food wastes; 8.7% is metal; 7.3% is plastics; and 8.4% is glass. Many of these materials are biodegradable; they are reduced to their basic components through natural actions of the environment (18, 71, 80, 124).

Landfills are not the answer to the problem of surface pollution. In fact, landfills are closing at the rate of almost one a day. Some older landfills are closing because they are full. Others are being closed because they leak toxic fluids. Even though landfills, especially sanitary landfills, are more acceptable than open dumps, they can produce dangerous health hazards. Local groundwater can be contaminated by chemical mixtures that leak out of the landfill area. In addition, as the trash ferments, methane gas is produced. When this gas accumulates, explosions and spontaneous combustion can occur. The methane gas can also migrate underground and kill nearby vegetation (72, 117, 124).

When handled properly, landfills can be economical, sanitary, and aesthetically acceptable. Landfills should be placed far from water sources, and the waste should be quickly covered to avoid foul smells, spontaneous combustion, breeding of rats and flies, and scavenging by rodents.

Incineration

A significant amount of household solid wastes is combustible and therefore suitable for incineration. Decentralized incineration is usually poorly controlled and frequently produces gaseous emissions and particulates that pollute the air and damage our health. Central incineration conducted by federal, state, or local governmental bodies is expensive, although necessary for large urban areas. The controlled-combustion process used in these centers prevents the emission of harmful gases and uses the by-product, heat, for an energy source. Through incineration, the volume of waste can be reduced by 90% of its original bulk. The remaining material can be removed to landfills or compressed for use in soil conditioners or construction material (44, 117, 123).

Salvage

The composition of solid waste has changed in past years; today it includes larger amounts of paper, plastics, aluminum cans, and other packaging and wrapping materials. Many such materials will not decompose or rust; therefore they present new problems in disposal. If these products are *salvaged,* they can be **recycled,** *treated by mechanical, thermal, or biologic means so that they can be used again,* thus promoting resource recovery and reuse (28, 36, 123).

Hazardous-Waste Disposal

The EPA has defined **hazardous waste** as *discarded material that may pose a threat or hazard to human health or the environment.* These wastes can be solids, liquids, sludges, or gases. They are toxic, ignitable, corrosive, infectious, reactive (react with air, water, or other substances, resulting in explosions and toxic fumes), or radioactive. It is estimated that 10% to 15% of all garbage produced in the United States is considered hazardous (40, 117, 124). According to the EPA, the United States generates approximately 300 million tons of hazardous waste annually (124).

Although most hazardous wastes are generated by the manufacturing industries, the Armed Forces, with their obsolete explosives, herbicides, and nerve gases, contribute significantly to the total volume. Hospitals, medical research laboratories, mining operations, service stations, retailers, and householders also contribute to the problem of hazardous-waste production. Only a small percent of the hazardous waste currently generated is disposed of in an environmentally sound manner. The rest threatens our water and air quality and our water and land ecosystems. The EPA has identified approximately 1200 sites where improper disposal of hazardous wastes has occurred. These sites are on a priority list for cleanup action (44, 224).

Hazardous wastes can become a threat to human health in various ways: direct exposure of persons at or near the disposal site; direct exposure to persons as a result of accidents during transportation of the wastes; exposure to polluted air during improperly controlled incineration; and contamination of groundwater and food (44, 224).

An example of the problems associated with hazardous-waste disposal occurred in the small community of Wilsonville, Illinois. In 1977 Wilsonville residents learned that a national disposal firm was burying dirt contaminated with polychlorinated biphenyls (PCBs) a cancer-causing substance, in a landfill near their town. After a long legal battle, the landfill was closed and the hazardous wastes were to be removed. Removal of the waste did not begin until late 1982. Because the company had no way of disposing of the material completely, it was transferred to a landfill in the Midwest (88). Thus a task that will take several years to complete will decrease the danger at Wilsonville but may pose a threat to another community. In an attempt to prevent such happenings and to protect U.S. citizens from the dangers of hazardous waste, The Comprehensive Environmental Response, Compensation and Liability Act was passed in 1980. One objective of this act was to establish a fund—Superfund—for the purpose of responding to emergency situations involving hazardous substances and of performing remedial cleanups. In 1986 a new Superfund was established and the program strengthened (61, 62).

Nuclear Waste

One type of hazardous-waste product that has attracted considerable attention is radioactive waste. Some fission products that must be stored are cesium-137, strontium-90, iodine-131, and plutonium-239. Some decay rapidly in hours or days, whereas others require thousands and millions of years to lose their radioactive potency (13, 141). No satisfactory method of permanent disposal has been developed; the cost and fear of leakage from the storage area have been stumbling blocks (85).

The use of nuclear energy or power produced by fission reactors has caused much concern and debate among the people of the United States. The concerns center around two major issues: the long-term disposal of radioactive wastes and the safety of the actual reactors.

When a utility shuts down a reactor at the end of its period of usefulness, the utility is faced with the problem of what to do with intensely radioactive materials. At present, only three means of disposal exist: dismantlement of the reactor with the debris shipped to a burial site; entombment of the reactor in a concrete structure; and protective storage that would prevent public access for 30 to 100 years. Even though nuclear power is a quarter-century old, the problem of safe disposal of radioactive waste has not been solved.

The seriousness of problems associated with the safety of nuclear reactors for generating electricity is well illustrated by the following highly publicized events. In Pennsylvania in March 1979, an accident occurred at the nuclear reactor site known as Three Mile Island. In retrospect, the accident was preventable and was less severe than originally reported (120). The major health effect of the accident was on the mental health of the people in the region. It is estimated that residents near the site were exposed to 0.10 rad, the equivalent of four x-ray studies (134). Another accident occurred in April of 1986 at a nuclear power plant at Chernobyl in the former Soviet Union. A fire in the plant's nuclear reactor sent a cloud of deadly radiation into the air. Some people in the plant died immediately, and hundreds of people in the vicinity developed radiation sickness. Contamination was so severe that the escaped radiation was detected around the world by monitoring devices (117, 171).

The fear, anger, and confusion felt by the Three Mile Island and Chernobyl communities are shared nationally and internationally. The majority of citizens now have serious second thoughts about the safety and reliability of nuclear power (120, 224). Diminishing resources lead to the need for alternative energy sources such as coal and the sun. The problems in this area must be explored.

Hospital Waste

The amount of solid waste produced by hospitals should be a primary concern to health workers. The average citizen accumulates and disposes of many pounds of solid waste daily. The average hospital patient also accumulates many pounds of solid waste daily. Hospitals add tons of pathologic materials yearly to the waste load. This increase in hospital wastes can be attributed to the increase in disposable products: syringes, needles, surgical supplies, styrene dishes and utensils, various plastic products, linens, uniforms, and medication containers. Many hospitals use disposable products because they are considered cheaper, easier to store, and less likely to produce cross-infection. Yet hospitals often fail to consider the cost or inconvenience of transporting or

discarding large quantities of these contaminated objects. Much of a hospital's solid waste, often contaminated by infectious organisms, in the past was removed to open dumps or sanitary landfills without proper initial sterilization, thus spreading pathogens to land, water, and air (129). Most hospital workers did not consider the implications of casually using disposable items (206) (Fig. 2–3). However, the laws have been tightened on the disposal of infectious and related waste. The mandates and consequent fines for not following the mandates have made a significant difference in this issue.

One study conducted in an urban area with 16 participating hospitals revealed that the nurse influences decisions about the purchase of patient care items more than any other hospital worker. If these decisions are largely your responsibility, know how much trash your hospital creates, where the waste goes, the decontamination procedures used before disposal, the cost of disposal, why your agency uses disposable products, and how much your agency contributes to environmental pollution. Form an interdepartmental committee, perhaps of administrators, nurses, doctors, and patients. Report your findings to them, and together consider all the advantages and drawbacks of various products. Consider cost, convenience, infection control, and quality. Give each new product a careful clinical trial and adopt it for use only after careful consideration about contributions to patient care. Avoid using disposable items if nondisposables will do the job as well. Pass this information on to the patients and families. Encourage health workers in homes to demonstrate and teach proper disposal of such items as syringes and dressings, especially at this time of increasing incidence of infectious diseases, including AIDS. Work to reduce the huge volume of solid waste that is taking space and depleting natural resources (102), and for disposal of infectious wastes in non-air-polluting incinerators, which many cities and hospitals do not have.

The effectiveness of nonpolluting incinerator conversion of trash into hot gases, which then transforms water into steam, has been demonstrated for over 10 years by St. Louis University Hospital, St. Louis, Missouri. The Hospital's incinerator conversion project, which heats and cools the entire St. Louis University Medical Center and also sterilizes all hospital equipment, received national attention at the U.S. Department of Energy's Technology Transfer 80's Program. The hospital received a national award for the project from the Department of Energy in November 1984.

Lead Poisoning

Lead is another surface pollutant. The two principal routes of exposure to lead are ingestion and inhalation. Sources contributing to the ingestion of lead are lead-based paint chips or flakes, lead solder in plumbing,

Figure 2-3. Hospitals accumulate large amounts of infectious wastes, which pose a health hazard if not stored and disposed of properly. (Photograph by Patrick Watson.)

lead solder in seams of food cans, lead from dietary sources that were contaminated while being grown or cooked, lead from improperly glazed earthenware or ceramic ware, and lead-contaminated "moonshine." Sources contributing to the inhalation of lead are leaded gasoline, contaminated dust or soil particles, cigarette smoke, and industrial sites such as battery plants. Since the airborne levels of lead significantly decreased (87% between 1975 and 1986) with the phaseout of leaded gasoline, other sources of lead are being closely studied (27, 38, 117, 131, 209).

Although lead poisoning is seen most frequently in children from inner cities, no economic or racial subgroup of children is exempt from lead toxicity. Children in some ethnic groups are exposed to lead through folk remedies used by their families; other children living in the "lead belt" (i.e., cities of the Northeast and Midwest) are especially at risk (32, 121).

Another urgent problem arises when young children, mainly in urban slums, form the *habit of eating nonfood substances, including peeling paint, plaster, or putty containing lead, a behavior called* **pica.** The precise cause of pica is not completely understood, but it may be related to nutritional, cultural, and emotional factors. Acute or chronic lead poisoning, and insidious disease, results from this eating pattern and is a major source of brain damage, mental deficiency, and behavior problems. The pathologic changes that occur affect the nervous, renal, and hematopoietic systems. Kidney damage is usually reversible, but chronic lead poisoning in childhood may lead to gout or kidney disease later in life. Damage to the hematopoietic system is evident by the reduction in the number and quality of red blood cells produced, thus leading to severe anemia. The most serious effects are on the nervous system (12, 31, 38, 78, 90).

Studies show the following trends:

1. Blood lead levels are higher in African-Americans than Caucasians among all socioeconomic and urbanization levels.

2. Young children from both African-American and Caucasian families with incomes less than $6000 have a significantly higher prevalence of elevated blood lead than those from households with incomes of $6000 or more.

3. Almost one fifth of African-American children from low-income families, the group with the highest proportion of elevated blood lead levels, should be referred for medical follow-up.

4. Mean blood lead level in young children increases with the degree of urbanization where they live (90).

Although the trend apparently is toward reduced lead screening, child health programs should consider routine screening of all children from 1 to 5 years of age. Reduction of leaded gasoline and establishment of auto-emissions standards set by the EPA have been steps in the right direction, for the mean blood level in the United States fell significantly between 1976 and 1980 (90).

OCCUPATIONAL HAZARDS

Increasingly we learn of the health hazards that many workers face daily at their jobs. Monotony, paced work, and performance pressures are major sources of stress in many jobs and can contribute to disease pathology. The muscle strains, backaches, fractures, burns, eye injuries, and other accidental emergencies are taken for granted by the public. But workers may not suffer the consequences of the hidden environmental hazards—the chemicals or radiation they work with directly or indirectly—until years later. Often in the past the cause of the physical illness remained unsolved. Not only do miners and factory workers become ill because of their work environment, hospital workers also may suffer. Those who work regularly with certain anesthetics, for example, may develop cancer, leukemia, or lymphoma. Those who work with high levels of radiation risk sterility or defective offspring if adequate protection is not maintained. Nurses may suffer infections, back and muscle injuries, varicose veins, and any of the other physical or emotional effects of stress.

The Occupational Safety and Health Act of 1970, the Coal Mine Health and Safety Act of 1969, and the Toxic Substances Control Act of 1976 are some of the laws passed by Congress that have been responsible for making occupational safety and health a public health concern rather than a private matter. Through these laws the federal government works to prevent work-related accidents and disease, to correct hazardous working conditions, to promote good health for working men and women, and to improve compensation. The Occupational Safety and Health Act established the Occupational Safety and Health Administration, which conducts inspections of industries to force compliance and re-

search to establish the hazardous levels of various chemicals. Relatively few of the many chemicals in industry have been researched, but the standards and prevention and treatment measures are published periodically in the *Federal Register,* which can be obtained from the Department of Labor.

The Occupational Safety and Health Act has forced industries to become more active in seeking health services for employees and has assisted the occupational health nurse to offer additional services related to disease prevention and education of employees (183). Health screening is also being emphasized, for contamination from some substances can be detected early enough to prevent disease. In one community where smelter employees were manifesting symptoms of nerve damage, for example, high levels of arsenic were found in their urine, fingernails, and hair (191). Earlier screening could have prevented arsenic poisoning. In one area respiratory disease and hospital admissions were directly linked to operation of the local steel mill. Some precautions could be taken (163).

It takes approximately two decades for health effects of industry to be evident. In the 1940s Louisiana had a large petrochemical industry. In the 1950s and 1960s a higher cancer incidence was being documented. About that time, companies moved from the North to the mouth of the Mississippi River to avoid property taxes and costs associated with pollution regulation. Pesticides, chlorine, rubber, antifreeze, detergents, plastics, and a variety of chemicals were manufactured. In 1986 Louisiana ranked third in the United States in chemical production after New Jersey and Texas. There has been an increasing death rate from cancer in each of those states, surpassing that of other industrial states (24).

To promote early screening and prevent long-term effects of noise pollution on hearing, the *Federal Register* publishes updated guidelines on occupational hearing conservation. Basically, each hearing program must consist of five parts:

1. Employee education (each employee must be told the significance of the program)
2. An analysis of the noise in the workplace, now required every 2 years or as noise levels change
3. Engineering and administrative controls (environmental noise must be altered if possible)
4. Audiometric testing (all employees exposed to 85 decibels or more [over a period of 8 hours] must be tested yearly and before employment)
5. Personal protective equipment (a variety of hearing protectors must be available)

Along with these guidelines are specific requirements for those who administer and interpret tests, circumstances under which tests are administered, and the instruments for measuring noise levels and hearing (194).

Another group of health hazards is related to the large cosmetics industry in the United States. Aerosol preparations, hair dyes, and feminine sprays increasingly are related to skin and other diseases, including cancer. As with other occupational chemicals, effects of the use of these products are usually not known until years after their regular usage. The World Health Organization estimates that 75% to 85% of all cancers are environmentally caused. No one knows how much occupational factors contribute to these causes.

Laryngeal cancer has been found among workers exposed to asbestos, cutting oil, wood dust, grease, and oil; among workers in the paper, metal, construction, leather, food, and textile industries; and among barbers, sheet metal workers, electricians, and naphthalene cleaners (67).

Often occupational hazards are taken for granted. They are seen as part of the job. Employees in laundry and dry cleaning establishments, for example, suffer hazards of excess heat, humidity, and noise; falls and accidents from slipping on wet floors; back injury and muscle strains from lifting; and circulatory problems from standing. Janitorial workers may have contact with dangerous chemicals in cleaning agents. Asthma is an occupational hazard for animal workers, veterinarians, farmers, bakers, carpenters, welders, and many other workers.

Industrial nurses and safety engineers emphasize wearing protective clothing and using protective equipment. Yet there are problems. The employee may not want to be bothered with cumbersome protective clothing; or the protective clothing and equipment given to a female worker may be too large and heavy and thus be illfitting and not protective, for they are designed for the male employee. (However, a few companies do specialize in protective clothing designed for females.) Hard hats, safety shoes and gloves, and ear muffs that fit improperly may actually contribute toward an accidental injury.

To compound the problem of prevention, length of exposure to an industrial substance often determines if it will cause disease. The amount of exposure to the worker often depends on the production phase involved. Additionally, each substance appears likely to produce a disease such as cancer in a specific body part; such information becomes available after workers become ill. Sex is also a factor, for some substances affect the reproductive organs of the female (or fetus) but do not affect the male. Some substances do not affect the male reproductive organs, but the father's genes may contribute to fetal damage.*

Each year an estimated 10,000 American workers die of work-related injuries. In 1980 women comprised

43% of the American workforce; they were more likely than men to work in certain industries and occupations (retail trade, personal services, and professional and related services) and less likely than men to work in others (agriculture, mining, construction, and transportation). The risks men and women workers face, therefore, can be expected to differ (46, 47). Risks also differ according to racial or ethnic background (177).

In a review of death certificates of 348 Texas women whose death resulted from injury at work, the median age of the women at death was 37 years (range, 17 to 92 years), resulting in a premature loss (death before age 65) of 9078 potential years of life. Homicide was the leading cause of death (53%), followed by injuries from motor vehicles, falls, fires and flames, machinery or tools, explosions, and other causes. Injuries from firearms caused 70% of the homicides. The remaining homicides were caused by injuries from cutting or piercing instruments, strangulation, drowning, and other means. The retail trade industry had the highest workplace homicide rate. Three retail trade subindustries had especially high workplace homicide rates: gasoline service stations, food-bakery-and-dairy stores, and eating-and-drinking places. Of the occupations, female drivers of heavy trucks had the highest fatal occupational injury rate, with motor vehicle incidents accounting for 89% of their fatal injuries. Three occupations had markedly elevated workplace homicide rates: stock handlers and baggers, food counter and fountain workers, and supervisors and proprietors in sales occupations. Of the 85 confirmed workplace homicides, 47% occurred during robberies, 7% during arguments between victims and customers, 21% under other known circumstances, and 25% under unknown circumstances. The offenders were either of unknown relationships or strangers to the victims in 71% of the homicides; spouses or other intimate acquaintances in 16% of the homicides; customers in 8% of the homicides; and coworkers in 5% of the homicides. Injuries from firearms caused 81% of the confirmed workplace homicides. Similar results have been found in studies in Wisconsin and Maryland. However, these studies probably underestimate fatal occupational injuries of women (47).

Studies of causes of occupationally related death in California and Texas showed a higher percentage of homicides, particularly for police, security guards, taxi drivers, supervisors or clerks in gas stations, waiters in food and dairy stores and eating and drinking places. In California homicide rates for females were highest among service occupations (eating and drinking places). Firearms accounted for 77% of all work-related homicides. Workers 65 years or older were at higher risk for homicide than younger workers. Homicides are more likely to occur between 3 P.M. and 3 A.M. (46, 115).

Controlling exposures of high-risk individuals and developing strict standards for reducing such exposures (e.g., handgun control laws) might greatly reduce as-

*Information about health hazards for women employees and preventive or corrective measures is available from the Woman's Occupational Health Resource Center, American Health Foundation, 320 East 43rd Street, New York, NY 10017.

saults and prevent senseless loss of life in the workplace. Employees in food-bakery-and-dairy stores are a high-risk group. The number of homicide-related robberies in convenience stores can be reduced by making the cash register area more visible from the street; by making it known that as little money as possible is kept in the cash register; by using a drop safe into which, at night, all bills of value greater than $1 are placed; and by keeping the store clean of potential hiding places. Bulletproof barriers between the driver and passenger compartments in taxicabs, enclosed cashier booths in gasoline service stations, and protective vests for law-enforcement officers and private-security personnel are other possible techniques to prevent workplace homicides. However, the extent to which these techniques are already practiced and their efficacy at preventing these homicides are unknown (46, 115).

Hazards of the factory or mine can extend beyond the workplace and endanger the workers' families and other residents of the community. Workers carry out dust particles on skin and clothing; wind currents also deposit particles. Even if workers shower before leaving work, the total removal of all dust particles of some chemicals or elements is difficult. As a result, some communities become known for a high incidence of certain types of cancer or skin or respiratory disease.

Knowing that the worker may come in contact with a variety of harmful substances and that presenting symptoms may often seem unrelated to the occupation should help you be more thorough and careful in assessment. Also, as a citizen you can work for enforcement of preventive measures for known hazards and for continued research.

Table 2–3 summarizes common industrial agents (various substances, elements, or chemicals) and their major known effects. Refer to the references at the end of the chapter for more information (9, 16, 24, 30, 34, 50, 51, 67, 70, 71, 96, 98, 99, 111, 117, 132, 136–138, 148, 160, 164, 172, 182, 191–193, 199, 206, 207, 228).

Excessive heat, cold, humidity, sunlight, noise, and/or vibration are health hazards in many occupations. Examples are listed below. These hazards are further aggravated by smoking or alcohol or drug abuse (160).

Agriculture	Highway/street
Airlines	workers
Auto mechanics	Laundry
Construction	Lumbering/sawmill
Cosmetology	operations
Dry cleaning	Meat butchering/
Exterminators	wrapping
Factory assembly line	Mining
production	Painting
Firefighting	Police/security guard
Fisherman	Postal workers
Forestry	Shipping industry
Foundry/smelter	Shipyard workers
Gardener/nursery	Transportation
Gasoline station	Welding
attendant	Wood workers

Other occupational hazards exist for women and men. Clerical and other workers who regularly use video display terminals and computers have higher stress– related illnesses, more eyestrain, and greater emotional burnout (191).

Nursing Applications

Personal Responsibility

Consider the environment, the various social institutions, and the population as a complex of interacting, interdependent systems. Environmental problems are a concern to everyone and are of equal consequence to every part of the world. Each of us shares the earth, so we are all responsible for its well-being. Environmental pollution is our collective fault and requires our collective solutions. In the United States alone discarded materials amount to billions of tons yearly, and the quantity is growing annually.

A fourfold environmental protection system is useful for continuously identifying, analyzing, and controlling environmental hazards:

1. Surveillance—maintaining an awareness of what people and industries are doing to the air, water, and land and of the effect of these actions on health; monitoring exposure
2. Development of criteria for the detection of pollution; detection
3. Research, including data from various records
4. Compliance—getting local government and industry to accept and implement new standards (71, 127, 182).

Citizen Role

An informed public can help establish such a system, but the financial support and legislative and administrative guidance of federal, state, and local governments provide the most feasible solutions. Encourage your local, state, or federal government officials to pass legislation that would protect the environment (e.g., installation of scrubbers in factories to decrease the release of sulfur dioxide, use of low-sulfur or "washed" coal, and installation of antipollution devices on automobiles and air crafts). Support production of biodegradable products from potato scraps, corn, molasses, beets, and castor oil. These non-petroleum ingredients can be transformed into a strong, flexible plastic that will degrade completely.

The Resource Conservation and Recovery Act of 1976 (PC 94-580) provides for recycling of our natural resources, safe disposal of discarded materials, and

TABLE 2-3. EFFECTS OF SOME COMMON INDUSTRIAL AGENTS UPON THE WORKER

Agent	Type of Industry or Occupation	Body Area Affected
Acetaldelhyde	Chemical; paint	All body cells, especially brain and respiratory tract
Acetic anhydride	Textile	Exposed tissue damage, especially eye and respiratory tract (ulceration, irritation)
Acetylene	Welding; plastic; dry cleaning	Respiratory tract asphyxiant; explosive, especially when combined with certain substances
Acrolein	Chemical	Skin, eye, respiratory tract
Allyl chloride	Plastic	Skin, respiratory tract, kidney
Ammonia	Chemical; leather; wool; farmers; refrigeration workers	Eyes, skin, respiratory tract (ulceration, irritation)
Anesthetic gases (leakage from equipment, exhalation of patients)	Surgical nurses; medical, hospital, dental, veterinary workers	Reproductive organs (spontaneous abortions, infertility, congenital abnormalities and cancer whether male or female exposure) Neurologic system (drowsy, irritable, headache) Respiraory tract (infections, cancer)
Aniline	Paint; rubber; dye manufacture	Skin, hematopoietic system, respiratory system
Arsenic	Mines; smelters; leather; chemical; oil refinery; ship builders; insecticide and pesticide makers and sprayers; pottery workers; agriculture; brass and bronze makers	Skin (ulcerations, cancer) Lung, liver (cancer) Neurologic damage, gastrointestinal symptoms Reproductive system (birth defects, chromosome alterations); if acute exposure, death in 1-7 days
Asbestos	Brake mechanics; mines; textiles; insulation; paint; sheet metal workers; shipyard workers; construction; plastics; pipe fitters; maintenance workers; millers; present on city streets	Respiratory tract (cancer, asbestosis, bronchitis, emphysema) Gastrointestinal tract (cancer) More harmful to people who smoke
Benzene	Rubber; chemicals; explosives; paints and paint strippers; shoemakers; dye users; office workers; chemists; hospital workers; solvent cleaner users; coke oven workers; furniture finishers; artists; degreasers	Skin, liver, brain (carcinogenic), respiratory system Hematopoietic system (anemia, leukemia); reproductive system (chromosome mutations in males, menstrual irregularities, stillbirths)
Beryllium	Foundry; metallurgic; aerospace; nuclear; household appliance; production, metal cans; shipbuilding	Skin and eye (inflammation, ulcers); respiratory tract (acute inflammation and berylliosis—chronic lung infection); systemic effects on heart, liver, spleen, kidneys
Butyl alcohol	Lacquer; paint	Eye, skin, respiratory tract
Cadmium	Smelters; storage battery workers; silver industry; plastics; dental; pigment makers; artists; electrical workers; households (silver cleaner, ice cube trays); plating; alloys	Gastrointestinal tract (irritation, cancer); reproductive system (decreased sperm, impotence) Respiratory tract, hematopoietic system
Carbon disulfide	Rubber; viscose rayon workers; plastics; soil treaters; wax, glue, or resin makers; medical; laboratory workers; agriculture	Gastrointestinal tract, heart, liver, kidney, brain Reproductive system (decreased sperm, decreased libido, impotence, infertility, menstrual changes, stillbirth, spontaneous abortion)
Carbon tetrachloride	Solvent; dry cleaning; paint; chemical laboratory; household (fire extinguishers)	Skin, gastrointestinal tract, liver, kidney, bladder Brain, respiratory tract (irritation and carcinogen)
Chemotherapy (antineoplastic) medications	Medical; nurses	Skin and cornea (irritation, ulcers); reproductive system (fetal damage, cancer); liver and other organs (may be carcinogenic) (some need special handling; effects vary with specific agent)
Chlorine	Industrial bleaching; laundry; chemical industries; swimming pool maintenance	Eyes; respiratory tract and skin (irritation, ulcerations, infections, cancer) Skin discoloration (orange)
Chloroform (chlorinated hydrocarbons)	Chemical; plastics; dry cleaners; drug workers; electronic equipment workers; insect control	Heart degeneration, liver, kidney, reproductive system (infertility male and female), brain, skin
Chromium	Chrome plating; chemical; industrial bleaching; glass and pottery; linoleum makers; battery makers; metal cans and coatings	Irritating to all body cells, skin, eye, respiratory tract (cancer, ulcerations), liver, kidney
Cleaning agents, solvents	Maintenance workers; painters; households	Respiratory tract (irritation, allergy, asthma, cancer) Eyes (irritation, ulcers) Skin (ulcers, dermatosis, cancer)

Agent	Type of Industry or Occupation	Body Area Affected
Coal combustion products (soot, tar, coal tar products)	Gashouse workers; asphalt, coal tar, or pitch workers; coke oven workers; mines; plastics; roofers; waterproofers; metal coating workers; ship building	Skin, respiratory tract, larynx, gastrointestinal tract Scrotum, urinary tract, bladder (carcinogenic to all areas), hyperpigmentaton of skin
Cotton, flax, hemp, lint	Textile	Respiratory tract (byssinosis—chest tightness, dyspnea, cough, wheezing; chronic bronchitis) Cigarette smokers especially affected
Creosol	Chemical; oil refining	Denatures and precipitates all cellular protein Skin, eye, respiratory tract, liver, kidney Brain
Dichloroethyl ether	Insecticide; oil refining	Respiratory tract
Dimethyl sulfate	Chemical; pharmaceutical	Eye, respiratory tract, liver, kidney, brain
Dyes	Dyeworkers	Urinary bladder (cancer)
Ethylene oxide	Hospital workers (sterilization); workers using epoxyresins	Skin, eyes (infection, ulcers, burns) Neurologic system (drowsy, weak); leukemia; lymphoma; respiratory tract (dyspnea, cyanosis, pulmonary edema, cancer) Gastrointestinal tract (vomiting, (cancer) Reproductive organs (chromosome damage, spontaneous abortion, fetal damage, infertility—male and female)
Exhaust fumes	Mechanics; gas station and garage workers	Respiratory tract; urinary bladder (cancer)
Formaldehyde	Laboratory workers; medical (cold sterilization); mechanics; textile; home insulators; mobile home owners; households (wet-strength paper towels, permanent press clothing, foam insulation)	Liver, lung, skin (infection, ulcers, cancer) Eye, nose, throat (irritation) Neurologic system (headache, fatigue, memory loss, nausea) Reproductive tract (gene mutation)
Freon	Refrigeration; aerosol propellants	Respiratory tract; cardiovascular system
Fungus, parasites, microorganisms	Food; animal; outdoor workers; clinical laboratory workers	Skin; respiratory tract (infection, including hepatitis B)
Germicidal agents	Health care providers; maintenance/cleaning workers	Skin (contact allergy, dermatosis)
Hydrogen chloride	Meat wrappers	Respiratory tract (irritation and asthma)
Hydrogen sulfide	Mines; oil wells; refineries; sewers	Respiratory tract (respiratory paralysis in high concentrations); eye
Iron oxide	Mine, iron foundry; metal polishers and finishers	Respiratory tract (cancer); larynx
Lead	Auto; smelters; plumbing; paint; metallurgic; battery workers; paint; plumbers; plastics; pottery; ceramics; gasoline station attendants; electronics; manufacture; shipbuilding; shoemakers; households; exposure in 120 industries	Hematopoietic, cardiovascular (hypertension) Liver; kidney; central nervous system and brain (behavioral change); muscles; bone; gastrointestinal tract; reproductive system (decreased sperm count, chromosome mutation, causes fetal damage or spontaneous abortion during first trimester of pregnancy, infertility—male and female, stillbirth, impotency, menstrual irregularities)
Leather	Leather; shoe	Nasal cavity and sinuses; urinary bladder (carcinogenic)
Lye	Households (drain openers, oven and other cleaners)	Eyes (corneal ulceration) Skin (ulcerations) Respiratory tract (irritation)
Manganese	Mine; metallurgic; welders; shipbuilding	Respiratory tract, liver, brain
Mercury	Electrical and laboratory workers; dye makers; explosives; drug workers; plastics; paint; pesticide workers; households; exposure in 80 different types of industries	Toxic to all cells; skin (ulcers, dermatosis, hyperpigmentation); respiratory tract; liver Brain damage; reproductive system (infertility—male and female, spontaneous abortions, birth defects); reduced vision; psychic changes Exposure of pregnant women causes congenital defects and retardation in child
Methylene chloride	Paint removers	Respiratory tract (irritant, carcinogen), skin, eye, liver, brain, cardiac, gastrointestinal tract
Mica	Rubber; insulation	Respiratory tract
Nickel	Metallurgic; smelter; electrolysis workers	Skin, respiratory tract (infection and cancer), reproductive tract

(continued)

TABLE 2-3. EFFECTS OF SOME COMMON INDUSTRIAL AGENTS UPON THE WORKER (Continued)

Agent	Type of Industry or Occupation	Body Area Affected
Nitric acid	Chemical industries; electroplaters; jewelers; lithographers	Skin (ulcerations, orange discoloration) Eye (ulcerations)
Nitrobenzene	Synthetic dyes	Skin, hematopoietic system, brain
Nitrogen dioxide	Chemical; metal; arc welding; explosives; silos	Eye, respiratory tract, hematopoietic system
Organophosphates (pesticides; insecticides)	Agriculture; pesticide manufacturers and sprayers; exterminators	Reproductive system (congenital anomalies) Brain dysfunction and neurologic damage (memory loss, disorientation, ataxia, liver and convulsions); kidney (cancer) Respiratory tract (infections, cancer)
Pentachlorophenol	Wood preservatives industry	Liver, kidney, nervous system, reproductive system, carcinogenic
Petroleum products	Rubber; textile; aerospace; workers in contact with fuel oil, coke, paraffin, lubricants Dry cleaning; diesel jet testers	Skin, respiratory tract, larynx, scrotum (carcinogenic to each), dermatosis, hyperpigmentation to skin
Phenol	Plastics	Corrosive to all tissue, liver, kidney, brain Skin (ulceration)
Polyurethane	Plastics and most other industries	Respiratory tract (asthma, cancer) Dermatosis
Printing ink	Printers	Respiratory tract (irritation) Urinary bladder (cancer)
Radiation	Health care providers: doctors, nurses, dentists, radiologists, and x-ray technicians (diagnostic, fluoroscopy, treatment, isotopes), physical therapists (diathermy), microbiologists and laboratory technicians (electron microscope); office workers (some types of computers and office machines); radar systems (police, weather, airport workers); nuclear generating stations; AM, FM, TV broadcasting stations; atomic workers; food workers; fiber workers; households (microwave ovens, some computers)	Reproductive system (chromosome irritation, sterility in men and women, birth defects, impotence, cancer) Hematopoietic system (leukemia) Thyroid (cancer) Other body systems, bone and skin (cancer)
Rubber dust	Rubber	Respiratory tract (chronic disease, cancer), dermatosis.
Silica	Mine; foundry; ceramic or glass production	Respiratory tract (silicosis, pneumoconiosis, emphysema)
Sulfur dioxide	Oil refining; ore smelting; brewery workers; flour bleachers; paper; sulfuric acid workers	Respiratory tract (acute exposure causes laryngospasm, circulatory arrest, death)
Talc dust	Mine	Respiratory tract (cancer); calcification of pericardium
Tetraethyl lead	Chemical	Hematopoietic system, brain
Thallium	Pesticide; fireworks or explosives	Skin, eye, respiratory and gastrointestinal tracts, kidney, brain
Toluene	Metal coatings; rubber; paint; clerical workers; printers; cosmetologists; plastics	Skin; respiratory tract, liver, hematopoietic system; brain (may cause drunken state and accidents); reproductive system (infertility, birth defects, chromosome damage in male); kidneys
Trichloroethylene	Chemical-metal degreasing; contact cement; paint; plastics; upholstery cleaners	Skin, liver, kidney, brain (carcinogen), cardiac system
Vinyl chloride	Plastic; rubber; insulation; organic-chemical synthesizers; polyvinyl-resin makers	Skin, respiratory tract (asthma); cancer in the liver, kidney, spleen and brain; reproductive system (chromosome mutation, stillbirth, spontaneous abortion); exposure of pregnant woman to polyvinyl chloride causes defective fetus
Wood products	Furniture	Respiratory tract (asthma)
Zinc	Plating; in brass, bronze, other alloys	Respiratory tract, neurologic system, hematopoietic system

management of hazardous wastes, those that contribute to increased mortality or pose a substantial present or potential threat to human health or environment. But these goals are not possible without individual effort. Refer to Table 2–4 for disposal of hazardous products. Box 2–1 summarizes conservation solutions for a number of areas (22, 41, 96, 130, 204, 218).

As a citizen, you should conserve natural resources to the best of your ability and learn about the environmental pollution in your own area. Remember that metallurgic and chemical companies are the greatest sources of hazardous waste. Campaign for minimized waste and for safe disposal of unavoidable waste. Encourage the development of additional burial sites for long-term

TABLE 2-4. COMMON TOXICS AND HOW TO DISPOSE OF THEM

Product	Danger	Disposal
Pest-control chemicals (insecticides; moth-balls, flea and roach powder, weed killer)	Poisonous carcinogenic	Offer leftovers to a nursery or garden shop or local business. Pesticides may be accepted by a chemical waste company or county agricultural agency.
Oil-based paints	Flammable	Call your local health department; ask if it has a policy for disposal of paint (some agencies have free cleanup days). Paint you cannot use can go to a neighbor, friend, or local organization or theatre group.
Solvents (paint thinner, turpentine, rust remover, nail polish remover, furniture stripper)	Flammable and poisonous; respiratory, eye, and skin irritant	Use all of them or give them away. Paint thinner can be reused by letting the liquid set (in a closed jar) until paint particles settle out. Strain off and reuse the clear liquid. Wrap the residue in plastic and put in trash.
Waste motor oil	Poisonous if ingested	Recycle at a gas station or auto service center.
Car batteries	Corrosive to skin and eyes	Check area gas stations. Some will take old batteries. A few offer cash for them.

safety and the monitoring of present sites for escape of wastes (64, 213).

Life-Style Changes

Box 2–1 summarizes activities to conserve, reduce pollution, and change life-style that can be accomplished by the citizens to conserve natural resources (22, 41, 96, 130, 204, 218). For some people, following the suggestions in the box will mean major changes—in shopping, in not carelessly disposing of articles, or in transportation—or it could mean planting a patio or rooftop garden or limiting the number of pets.

Quiet surroundings are a natural resource, too. Make your own quieter through personal habits. Help plan for local recreation sites that offer natural surroundings. Campaign for adequate acoustical standards in homes, apartments, hospitals, and industrial buildings and for noiseless kitchen equipment. Participate in local government planning to decrease town and city noise in relation to transportation routes, zoning, and industrial sites.

Support for Conservation

Join citizens' crusades for a clean environment or a conservation organization and attend workshops given by the Cancer Society, Sierra Club, Conservation Foundation, and League of Women Voters to learn more about problems, preventive measures, and means of strengthening legislation. Support antipollution and noise-control laws. Support your city and health agencies in their attempts at pollution control and recycling (19, 181, 210). Be an involved citizen!

The various national wildlife organizations are studying the environment and alerting citizens about hazardous wastes and toxins in the environment. These organizations such as National Wildlife Federation, Au-

dubon Society, Sierra Club, Nature Conservancy, and Coalition for the Environment in St. Louis have worked closely with Congress and state legislators to pass protective legislation, have held public hearings to initiate protective measures, and have conducted citizen education. Often neither the legislators nor the citizens are as attentive as they should be. Support given to this type of organization and to legislative efforts is important as a citizen. In the process you are contributing to the health of your family, your community, and your nation.*

Professional Responsibility

Although nursing responsibilities have been interwoven throughout this chapter, consider that your primary responsibilities are detection through thorough assessment, making suggestions for intervention, and health teaching.

Assessment and Nursing Diagnosis

Screening for occupational diseases resulting from exposure to contaminants is most accurately done by occupational health nurses and physicians rather than by employees in corporate medical groups (228). Increasingly there are improved radiologic and blood chemistry diagnostic tests to detect diseases that are related to the occupation, including a blood test to detect pesticide contamination. Keep abreast of medical advances (207, 228).

---

*For more information on specific measures for wasting less and practicing ecologically sound living, see Saltonstall, *Your Environment and What You Can Do About it* (179) and the booklets published by the United States Department of Labor and the EPA that are listed in the references.

■ BOX 2-1.
Conservation Solutions

Energy Solutions

- Use public transportation; carpool; bike; walk rather than driving a car if feasible.
- Invest in ample insulation, weatherstripping, caulking for home and workplace.
- Use electricity and hot water efficiently. Buy energy saving household appliances.
- Reduce demand for energy by turning off lights, radio, television when no one is using them; run dishwasher and washer and dryer only when they have full loads.
- Make the most of oven heat—bake foods in batches; turn oven off shortly before baking is finished and use remaining heat to complete the job.
- Dry clothes outdoors on a line.
- Use clothes dryer efficiently; separate loads into heavy- and lightweight items since lighter ones take less time.
- In winter turn down thermostat a few degrees, especially at night and when house is empty. In summer if using air conditioning, turn thermostat up a few degrees. Regularly service the furnace and air conditioner.
- Close off and do not heat or cool unused rooms; use insulating shades and curtains on cold winter nights and hot summer days.

Food Solutions

- Eat foods lower on the food chain—vegetables, fruits, and grains; decrease consumption of meat and animal products.
- Read the labels on food; buy foods that have not been heavily processed. Learn which additives are harmful.
- Support laws that ban harmful pesticides, drugs, and other chemicals used in food production. Support markets that offer contaminant-free food.
- Avoid food from endangered environments, such as rain forests.

Water Solutions

- Install sink faucet aerators and water-efficient showerheads, which use two to five times less water with no noticeable decrease in performance.
- Take showers, not baths, to reduce water consumption.
- Do not let water run when it is not actually being used while showering, shaving, brushing teeth, or hand washing clothes.
- Use ultra low-flush or air-assisted toilets, saving 60% to 90% water. Composting toilets use no water and recycle organic waste.
- Buy phosphatefree, biodegradable soaps and detergents; ask your supermarket to carry them if it does not.
- Do not run the tap until the water is cold to get a drink. Instead, keep water in a refrigerator bottle.
- Economize water when washing the car, sprinkling the lawn, removing debris from surfaces; repair leaks.

Toxins and Pollutants Solutions

- Read labels; buy the least toxic products available; find out the best disposal methods for toxic products. Use nonharmful substitutes.
- Avoid purchasing clothes that require dry cleaning, which uses toxic chlorinated solvents. Dry clean only when necessary.
- Avoid contact with pesticides by thoroughly scrubbing or peeling foodstuffs; if possible, maintain your own garden without use of pesticides.
- Test your home for radon, especially if you live on the east coast or in Wisconsin, Minnesota, North Dakota, Colorado, or Wyoming.
- Ask your service station to use CFC recovery equipment when repairing auto air conditioners.
- Use more energy-efficient cars.
- Keep your automobile in top working condition with a regular tune-up; make sure antipollution controls are working properly.
- Operate your vehicle properly; do not idle or rev engine; drive at steady pace; obey speed limits.
- Support legislative initiatives that encourage industry to modify manufacturing processes to eliminate the production of hazardous wastes and to reuse and recycle wastes when possible.

Waste Reduction and Recycling Solutions

- Buy products in bulk or with the least amount of packaging. (A major contributor to acid rain is sulfur dioxide, one of the chemicals used to process virgin paper. In the very low-oxygen environment of the trash dump, paper or plastic may take 40 or more years to degrade.)
- Buy products that are recyclable, repairable, reusable, and biodegradable; avoid disposables. (Every 3 months enough aluminum cans are thrown away to rebuild an entire commercial fleet.)
- Separate your recyclable garbage such as newspaper, glass, paper, aluminum, and organic waste if you have a garden. Send to the landfill what cannot be reused. (Only 10% of garbage is recycled in the United States.)
- Recycle newspapers through paper drives. Each Sunday thousands of trees are made into newspapers that are not recycled.
- Use recycled products. Landfills are rapidly being exhausted, and the cost of recycling must be recovered.
- Buy recycled paper for all uses. (It takes 16,320 kilowatt-hours of electricity to produce 1 ton of paper from virgin wood pulp. It takes 64% fewer kilowatt-hours (5919) to produce 1 ton of recycled paper from waste paper.)

■ **BOX 2-1.** Continued

- Use curbside pickup for recyclables if available.
- If you do not have a recycle center, ask your city council to establish one. Find local groups that can use your recyclables.

Housekeeping Solutions

- Use simple substances for cleaning. An all-purpose cleaner, safe for all surfaces, is 1 gallon hot water, $\frac{1}{4}$ cup sudsy ammonia, $\frac{1}{4}$ cup vinegar, and 1 tablespoon baking soda. After use, wipe surface with water to rinse.
- Keep drains open by using the following mix once weekly: 1 cup baking soda, 1 cup salt, $\frac{1}{4}$ cup cream of tartar. Pour $\frac{1}{4}$ cup of the mixture weekly into the drain; follow with a pot of boiling water. If drain is clogged, pour in $\frac{1}{4}$ cup baking soda followed by $\frac{1}{2}$ cup vinegar. Close drain until fizzing stops. Then flush with boiling water.
- Use low phosphate or phosphate-free detergents to wash clothes and dishes.
- Use natural furniture and floor polish products; such products use lemon oil or beeswax in a mineral oil base.
- Use nontoxic products to control pests. Control ants by sprinkling barriers of talcum powder, chalk, bone meal, or boric acid across their trails. Control cockroaches by dusting lightly with borax. Control ticks and fleas on pets by applying a herbal rinse. Boil $\frac{1}{2}$ cup of fresh or dried rosemary in a quart of water. Steep herb 20 minutes, strain, and cool. Then sponge on pet. Air dry.
- Maintain air circulation and clean ventilation systems and ducts to remove fungi, mold, pollen, toxic residues, sprays, and other contaminants. Avoid hair spray and cleaning sprays.
- Manage household hazardous waste: buy only what is needed; do not store with household products: give unused product to someone else who may be able to use it rather than disposing of it. Do not pour oil, grease, or hazardous chemicals down the drain.

Tree-Saver Solutions

- Plant trees; as trees grow, they remove carbon dioxide from the atmosphere through photosynthesis, slowing buildup of carbon dioxide. (Carbon dioxide causes over 50% of the greenhouse effect.)
- Join efforts to save forests from being cleared or burned. When forests are burned, carbon is released, adding to carbon dioxide buildup and global warming.

Preservation of Life and Environment Solutions

- Do not burn leaves or garbage; instead, compost organic materials.
- Do not buy endangered plants, animals, or products made from overexploited species (furs, ivory, reptile skin, or tortoise shell).
- Avoid buying wood from the tropical rain forests unless it was propagated by sustainable tree farming methods.
- Buy products from companies that do not pollute or damage the environment.
- Join, support, volunteer your time to organizations working on environmental causes.
- Contact your elected representatives through letters, telegrams, calls, or visits to communicate your concerns about conservation and environmental issues.

You can play a significant role in the early detection of lead poisoning, for example. Assessment of a child's health should include observation for physical signs such as tremors, abdominal discomfort, decreased appetite, and vomiting and questions related to a pica behavior. Ask the mother about her child's interest in play, ability to get along with playmates, coordination, and level of developmental skill attainment. Phrase your questions and comments carefully, in a nonjudgmental manner, so that the mother will not feel that her fitness as a parent is being judged. If the persons for whom you are caring live in unsatisfactory, low-income housing, work for improvement through local legislation. Emphasis must be placed on repair and deleading of dwelling places, not just on moving the present dweller to a new house or apartment. You can encourage the formation of screening and case-finding programs, already started in many cities, and you can assist with their activities. Be as thorough in assessment as possible. An example of

questions usually not asked on standard health history forms that you could use in assessment of the employed client is presented in Fig. 2–4. Box 2–2 refers to nursing diagnoses. Exposure to lead is also seen in other areas such as indoor firing ranges. Such recreation raises blood lead levels (212).

Intervention

Health teaching and advocacy can increase client and community awareness and contribute to prevention of illness from pollutants or hazards. Encourage people to read labels and current literature (Box 2–3).

Natural or man-made chemical pollution in soil, water, and food products can produce various adverse effects, ranging from slight health impairments to death. Although local public health officials are responsible for maintaining safe nitrate levels in the water supply, your responsibilities are to aid in the education of the public concerning the health hazards of such pollutants and to

1. Occupational history (start with last job first).

	COMPANY	DATE EMPLOYED	JOB
(a)	_____	_____	_____
(b)	_____	_____	_____
(c)	_____	_____	_____
(d)	_____	_____	_____

2. In these jobs, have you ever been exposed to:
   Excessive radiation or radioactive material?
   Excessive noise? _____ Excessive heat or light? _____

3. Have you worked in dusty trades? _____
   With any specific chemicals? _____
   In any vapors or fumes? _____
   If your answer is yes to any questions in (2) and (3), please elaborate. _____
   _____
   _____

4. Has a job ever made you "sick"? _____ If so, which job? _____
   Explain how you were sick. _____

5. Have you ever worn any protective equipment or a specific support? _____
   If so, what? _____

6. Have you ever had a serious work injury? _____ If so, please describe.
   _____

7. Have you had several minor work injuries? _____ If so, please describe.
   _____

8. Have you ever applied for, or received, workers' compensation? _____

9. Have you ever had a pension for disability? _____

Figure 2-4. Occupational history form.

use the epidemiologic method in your work. Be aware of such symptoms as fatigue, listlessness, and sleepiness that may indicate an untoward reaction to this particular form of pollution.

You may have an opportunity to teach people who earn a living as pesticide applicators and handlers. They should follow the following precautions:

1. Wear rubber or neoprene gloves while handling pesticides to avoid skin contact.
2. Keep pesticide-soiled clothing separate from other family laundry.
3. Empty all cuffs and pockets before doing laundry so trapped pesticide granules do not dissolve in wash water.
4. Daily wash all clothing worn while applying pesticides. The longer the garments are stored before laundering, the more difficult it is to remove the pesticide.
5. Prerinsing is an effective way to dislodge pesticide residue.
6. Wash only a few items at a time, and wash for a 12 to 14-minute cycle. Use the recommended amount of heavy-duty detergent. Liquid detergents are more effective than powders in removing oil-based pesticides.
7. The hotter the water (preferably 140° F), the more effectively pesticide is removed.
8. It may be necessary to discard heavily contaminated clothing.
9. To remove possible pesticide residues from the washing machine tub, run the washer through a complete cycle using detergent and a full level of hot water (187).

Another dangerous problem associated with chemical pollution is its possible carcinogenic effect (as seen on Table 2–3). Incidence of specific forms of cancer can be higher or lower, depending on exposure to specific compounds, a common example being the high incidence of lung cancer in the United States and England because of heavy tobacco use. Be aware and knowledgeable about the incidence of chemically produced cancer in your particular locale. Health teaching can then be directed at trying to eliminate or control the responsible carcinogenic chemical. Radiation is also carcinogenic. Encourage the use of protective clothing and sunscreen lotions to prevent overexposure to the sun. Prevent overexposure to ionizing radiation by making certain that unnecessary x-ray studies are not taken, by keeping a record of the frequency of such studies, and by using a lead shield when x-ray examinations are given.

The biochemical response to chemical pollution or radiation can influence the cells in various ways. **Teratogenic** (*producing malformations*) and **mutagenic**

■ **BOX 2-2**
Selected Nursing Diagnoses Related to Environmental Considerations[a]

Pattern 1: Exchanging

Potential for injury

Pattern 3: Relating

Social isolation

Pattern 5: Choosing

Health seeking behaviors

Pattern 6: Moving

Altered health maintenance

Pattern 7: Perceiving

Powerlessness

Pattern 8: Knowing

Knowledge deficit

[a]Many of the NANDA nursing diagnoses are applicable to the person who is ill as a result of environmental pollution or hazards, or occupational causes.
From North American Nursing Diagnosis Association, *NANDA Nursing Diagnosis Taxonomy I* (Rev). St. Louis: North American Nursing Diagnosis Association, 1990.

■ **BOX 2-3**
Educate the Consumer: Signal Words on U.S. Labels

Caution: fatal dose is more than 1 ounce (32 ml); low-level toxicity
Corrosive: may chemically "eat" through standard containers
Danger: a few drops can be fatal; highly toxic; requires specific protective measures
Ignitable: may pose a fire hazard
Nontoxic: only an advertising word; can mean anything from safe when swallowed to less than 50% of tested animals died within 2 weeks of testing
Reactive: may be explosive or produce poisonous substances
Toxic: a poison to humans or environment
Warning: fatal dose is somewhere between 1 tablespoon (16 ml) and 1 ounce (32 ml); moderately toxic

(*producing hereditary changes*) are two such changes in cells. Be aware that these changes can occur in both the client and the health care provider who are exposed to radiation. Genetic counseling might be indicated for couples who have been exposed to radiation. Citizens should know of the possibility for dealing effectively and therapeutically with biochemical changes, whether prenatally or in any stage of growth and development (27, 44, 84, 117, 224).

In 1977 the National Institute for Occupational Safety and Health (NIOSH) issued a document, "The Right to Know: Practical Problems and Policy Issues Arising From Exposure to Hazardous Chemicals and Physical Agents in the Workplace." It proceeded from the premise that workers have a right to know about risks to which they have been exposed. For political and economic reasons and because of constraints from the Department of Health and Human Services, NIOSH officials were reluctant to create a regulation based on the document. However, pressure from workers, consumer and conservation groups, and unions persisted.

Under the Hazardous Communication Rule passed in 1983, workers must be informed about any hazardous chemicals to which employees are exposed in the workplace. However, the rule is limited; it covers only manufacturing companies, and employers may claim a chemical is a trade secret and release the name only to a

health professional who has a right to know. Health care professionals, the unions, and conservation and consumer groups must continue to advocate for all workers so that the rule will be applied in a broader perspective (14, 178). Stromberg (200) discusses legislation that regulates the workplace and carcinogenic agents, benefits to workers, and the nurse's role. Her information may be useful to you. You, the nurse, are also a worker, and nurses are exposed to a variety of health hazards, including musculoskeletal injuries, infectious diseases, antineoplastic agents administered to cancer clients, laser injuries, smoke inhalation, and stress (101, 223).

As a professional and as a citizen, you can encourage officials and consumers in your community to develop innovative technologies to cope with the hazardous effects of aspects of our current lifestyle. For example, the city of Muskegan, Michigan, constructed an innovative facility that recycles wastewater so that it can be used safely and economically to irrigate farmland. Sewage residues given conventional treatment become more toxic with each step. Wastewater and sewage residues that are gradually percolated through natural soil filters use fewer chemicals to treat sewage and generate less sludge. The resulting water residues are high in plant nutrients and can be recycled as fertilizer. Land-treatment facilities use energy only for pumping, allow communities to reuse water, and can make money for the community (126).

Join the Nurses Environmental Health Watch, a nonprofit organization, with chapters in most states. The organization seeks to educate nurses and the public about current issues influencing health and the environment, including environmental toxins and pollutants, nuclear energy and energy alternatives, resource recovery and recycling, chemical and biologic warfare, and occupational hazards for nurses. A quarterly newsletter, *Health Watch,* includes items about national and local activities and resources on environmental issues. Educational forums are sponsored by local chapters.

In the past 100 years disease and death have been reduced because of preventive public health measures in the form of environmental control such as water and waste management, rodent and insect control, development of housing codes. Now we are again faced with problems and diseases that have an environmental impact. Prevention can begin with informed consumer groups who have educational and work projects as their goals. It can begin with your responsibility for the client's environment.

Client's Immediate Environment

Besides a feeling of responsibility for the community and physical environment in which the client lives, you also have a responsibility for that individual's immediate environment while receiving health care. The client's *surroundings should constitute a* **therapeutic milieu** *free of hazards and conducive to recovery, physically and emotionally.*

The client's surroundings should be clean and adequately lighted, ventilated, heated, and safe. Precautions should always be taken to prevent injury such as burns from a hot water bottle. Falls should be prevented by removing obstacles and electric cords from walking areas and having the person wear well-fitted shoes and use adequate support while walking. Lock the bed or wheelchair while the client is moving to and from them. In the home be sure that electric cords and scatter rugs are not so placed that the person could fall. Wipe up spilled liquids immediately. Use sterile technique and proper handwashing methods to ensure that you bring no pathogenic organisms to the client. Avoid excessive noise from personnel and equipment to the degree possible. Various equipment used in client care must also be monitored for safe function (143).

The esthetic environment is also important for rest. Arrange articles on the bedside table in a pleasing manner if the client is unable to do so. Keep unattractive equipment and supplies out of sight as much as possible. Electric equipment should be in proper repair and function. Minimize offensive odors and noise. Place the person's bed or chair by a window or door so that the person can watch normal activity rather than stare at the ceiling or walls. As a nurse, involve yourself in making the entire ward and the clients' rooms look pleasing. Consider color combinations and the use of drapes, furniture, clocks, calendars, pictures, and various artifacts to create a more homelike atmosphere. The committee in charge of decorating and building should include at least one nurse. You may need to volunteer to ensure that nursing and, indirectly, clients are represented in such programs.

The client's surroundings should not only be safe and attractive, but the emotional climate of the unit and entire institution affects clients and staff as well. The client and family are quick to respond and react to the attitudes and manner of the staff. Here are some questions you might ask yourself. How do I treat delivery workers who bring gifts and flowers to clients? Do I participate in the joy such remembrances bring to the client? Do I help arrange the flowers into a pleasant pattern or just stick them quickly into whatever can be found? Do I treat visitors as welcome guests or as foreign intruders? The emotional climate should radiate security and acceptance. A warmth should prevail that promotes a sense of feeling of trust, confidence, and motivation within the client as he or she and the staff work together to cope with problems. The emotional relationship between the client and the health care staff should help the client reach the goal of maximum health.

In a truly **therapeutic milieu** the staff members also feel a sense of harmony among themselves. There are mutual trust and acceptance between staff and supervisors, and supervisors recognize work well done by the staff. As a result, staff members feel motivated to continue to learn and to improve the quality of client care. Staff members are not likely to give individualized, comprehensive, compassionate care in an agency where they are not treated like individuals or where their basic needs are not met.

Be aware of environmental pollution in the health care environment. "No Smoking" should be the rule, not only when oxygen is in use but also in most health care settings. Conference or dining rooms or lounges for health care providers may have either a "No Smoking" rule or a limited "Smoking" area. Sometimes there are designated smoking areas outside the building so that employees or visitors who smoke must go outdoors. In the past it was difficult to teach a client the adverse effects of smoking and nicotine when an odor of cigarette smoke hung on the uniform. Moreover, health care providers benefit from practicing what they teach others. Health care providers and clients may also come in contact with agents listed in Table 2–3. Constant vigilance is necessary to detect harmful agents and prevent or reduce their usage. Early assessment of harmful effects to reduce the symptoms and proper interventions for dermatoses, allergens, or other symptoms is essential.

Be aware that a "sick building syndrome" exists. However, it is the people in the building that suffer. The source of the problem is an inadequate ventilation system that creates poor mechanical air flow. Equipment such as the ozone from the photocopier and furnishings such as fiberboard or carpet that contains formaldehyde add to the problem when there are no windows or windows do not open. Volatile organic compounds (benzene, chloroform, and formaldehyde) may be given off by paints, vinyls, printed documents, telephone cable, solvents, and some furniture. Biologic agents, including mold, dust, mites, algae, fungus, and pollen, may be in the humidifier or vent system. Tobacco smoke, which contains volatile organic compounds and other gases and particles, is dirtier than the usual air the smoker inhales. Carbon dioxide levels may be well above that considered healthy. Common complaints are headaches, fatigue, coughing, sneezing, nausea, difficulty with concentration, bleary eyes, and irritation of the nose and throat. The symptoms clear when the person leaves the building. Vents must be cleaned and furniture arranged so that airflow can be maintained. Fresh air should be circulated indoors. Coworkers should unite to find and correct the problem. The Occupational Health and Safety Administration has standards for various settings, and employees and clients have a right to a workplace free of recognized hazard (116, 119, 133, 142).

There are times when the treatment for the client may also affect the health care provider—for example, radiotherapy. Proper precautions should be taken to protect the provider from excess exposure and to protect any body areas of the client that should not be exposed. Constant monitoring of the dosage and duration of exposure to radiation, whether from a portable x-ray machine or a radium implant, is essential.

When the following safety rules are followed, nurses can be assured of personal safety (132):

1. Quantities of radioactive materials used in *diagnostic* tests are very small and do not constitute a health hazard.
2. If a client has had *therapeutic* doses of radioisotope, he or she becomes potentially dangerous, and strict precautions should be observed. The hazard varies with the type and dosage of the isotope used and the circumstances of the particular client. Avoid radiation exposure as much as possible and avoid contamination from radioactive body fluids.
3. Check the client's chart for the type of isotope given and its dosage.
4. Special orders are usually written for each client in respect to handling contaminated linens, utensils, and other sources of contamination.
5. Contaminated materials should be kept in containers specified by the radiologist.
6. Nursing care should be given adequately, but the time element is important; the radiologist should prescribe the time that can safely be spent with the client. Follow the principle that the farther one is away from the source of radiation, the less the danger (inverse square law).
7. Hands should be kept clean; wash thoroughly after caring for the client under radioisotope treatment.
8. Rubber gloves should be worn to handle contaminated objects. Never touch the face; be sure to wash the gloved hands thoroughly before removing the gloves.

9. In case of a client's death, either the radiologist or the physician (or both) should be notified and their directions specifically followed.
10. Never touch a dislodged radium needle. The radiologist should be called at once if it seems to be out of place.

Clients who are receiving radiotherapy should be assessed for the following side effects:

1. Malaise, weakness, fatigue, headache
2. Redness, edema, itching, denuding, and atrophy of skin
3. Inflammation, dryness, pain, and impaired physiologic function of mucous-lined areas of the body, including the oral cavity, esophagus, and vagina; alterations in taste are common
4. Sloughing of epithelial cells in various body areas such as the esophagus, stomach, intestine, and genitourinary tract, resulting in ulceration, chronic inflammation, pain, necrosis, and impaired physiologic functions of the organ system affected (vomiting, diarrhea, cystitis)
5. Depression of bone marrow, resulting in reduction of white and red blood cells and platelets, which, in turn, causes infections, anemia, and hemorrhagic tendencies
6. Inflammatory and fibrotic damage to the lungs and heart, causing pneumonitis, pericarditis, and occasionally myocarditis
7. Temporary or permanent loss of hair, depending on dosage and duration of exposure

Intervention for these side effects includes skin and mouth care; dietary modifications; use of mild analgesics, antiemetics, and antidiarrheal drugs; and reverse isolation technics. Refer to a medical-surgical text for specific interventions for the client who is suffering side effects from radiotherapy.

If you are caring for a person in the home, you are limited in the amount of change you can make. You can point out such hazards as electric cords in the walking area, however. You can suggest furniture rearrangement if you think that the person could function more easily with the change. You can put a clock in sight, pull the drapes, or put needed materials within the client's reach if feasible.

Specific ways of meeting the client's environmental needs also differ for various developmental stages. The components of a therapeutic milieu are different for the baby than for the middle-aged man. However, a safe, secure environment, physically and psychologically, must be present for both. Accurately determining the factors that make up the environment and making appropriate changes may be the first step in promoting health.

Research Abstract

Pender, N., et al., Predicting Health-Promoting Lifestyles in the Workplace, **Nursing Research, 39,** *no. 6 (1990), 326–331.*

Employees often enroll in workplace health-promotion efforts; however, erratic participation and dropouts occur. Lack of consistency in health-promoting efforts minimizes potential impact on health. Life-style in the context of health is broadly defined as a constellation of activities with significant impact on health status that are an integral part of one's pattern of living.

A wellness-oriented framework was used in this investigation. The Health Promotion Model was proposed as a paradigm to explain and predict the health-promoting component of life-style. The Health Promotion Model focuses on health promotion without threat of disease identified as a behavioral determinant. It is based on Bandura's social cognitive theory in which cognition, affect, actions, and environmental events are proposed as operating interactively in determining behavior. Seven cognitive and perceptual factors included in the model are considered amenable to change: importance of health, perceived control of health, perceived self-efficacy, definition of health, perceived health status, perceived benefits of health-promoting behavior, and perceived barriers to health-promoting behaviors. Modifying factors that interact causally with cognitive and perceptual processes in the determination of healthrelated behavior are demographic characteristics, biologic characteristics, interpersonal influences, situational factors, and behavioral factors, including prior experience with health actions.

Six companies in the Midwest, each with more than 250 employees, collaborated in this investigation. Health professionals at each company were responsible for health-promotion programs, including physical fitness, nutrition, and stress management at on-site exercise facilities. Mandatory orientation sessions were given before the period of self-directed program involvement.

Of the 745 health-promotion program enrollees contacted in the six companies, 633 enrollees (85%) agreed to participate, and 589 (93%) of those consenting to participate provided complete data for both concurrent and time-lagged phases of the study. Study participants were full-time clerical, operations, and managerial employees. The majority, 54%, were male; 83% were white, 10% Black, 5% Hispanic, and 2% Asian; and 65% were currently married. They ranged in age from 20 to 65 years with a mean age of 38 years. Family income for the sample ranged from less than $20,000 to more than $60,000. Eighty-three percent of the sample had attended college, and 50% of the total sample had completed college. Forty percent of the sample were in the first 6 months of participation in their respective workplace fitness programs; 60% had participated for more than 6 months.

Means for health-promoting life-style dimensions at the time of first testing revealed that employees enrolled in workplace health-promotion programs tended to score highest on the subscales of self-actualizaton and exercise and lowest on the subscales of health responsibility and stress management, with scores on the interpersonal support and nutrition subscales falling in between. Enrollees increased significantly on overall life-style scores from initial testing to 3-month testing and on the subscale scores of health responsibility from initial to 3-month testing, of nutrition from first to 3-month testing, and of stress management from first measure to second measure. No significant differences over time were found on the self-actualization and interpersonal support subscales. Only the exercise subscale showed a significant decrease from initial testing to 3-month testing. This reported decrease in exercise was in agreement with records of exercise frequency maintained by fitness program personnel at the participating corporations.

Perceived personal competence, definition of health, perceived health status, and perceived control of health accounted for 31% of the variance in health-promoting life-style patterns. Employees who reported more health-promoting life-styles perceived themselves as competent in handling life situations, defined health as a high-level wellness rather than merely the absence of illness, evaluated their health positively, and perceived their health as affected by significant others but not by chance. Those who were female, older, and in the maintenance phase of the company fitness program also had healthier life-style patterns. These variables and the perception of health as internally controlled were predictive of health-promoting life-styles 3 months later. Employees improved significantly in reported life-style in the areas of assuming responsibility for health, nutrition, and stress management over a 3-month period of enrollment in the programs, attesting to the positive impact of such programs on employee health practices. The decrease in reported exercise behavior over 3 months despite the ease of access to fitness facilities at the worksite underscores the need to assist employees to integrate physical fitness activities into patterns of daily living and sustain these patterns over time.

It is past time for all of us to ask ourselves some basic questions. How much energy and natural resources do we need to sustain life, to maintain the high standard of living in the United States? How much are we willing to pay for benefits that will not poison us with side effects? How does population growth affect the use and abuse of natural resources? Will strictly controlled energy allocation be necessary because people refuse to abide by suggested limits? Must people continue to grow up with strontium 90 in their bones, DDT in their fat, and asbestos in their lungs? What more can each of us do personally and professionally to maintain a health-fostering environment?

REFERENCES

1. Agahian, B., et al., Arsenic Levels in Fingernails as a Biological Indicator of Exposure to Arsenic, *American Industrial Hygiene Association Journal,* 51, no. 12 (1990), 646–651.
2. Ahlborg, G., and L. Bodin, Tobacco Smoke Exposure

and Pregnancy Outcome Among Women. A Prospective Study at Prenatal Care Centers in Orebro County, Sweden, *American Journal of Epidemiology,* 133, no. 4 (1991), 338–347.

3. Air Trends, *Chemecology,* 17, no. 3 (1988), 2–4.

4. American Lung Association, *Clean Air is Up to You!* 1991.

5. Ames, B.N., Dietary Carcinogens, Environmental Pollution, and Cancer: Some Misconceptions, *Medical Oncology and Tumor Pharmacotherapy,* 7, nos. 2–3 (1990), 69–85.

6. Anthony, H.M., Reactive Changes in the Blood of Smokers and the Development of Arterial Diseases and COPD: A Review, *Review of Environmental Health,* 8, nos. 1–4 (1989), 25–86.

7. Anzovin, S., ed., *Preserving the World Ecology.* New York: H.W. Wilson, 1990.

8. Archer, V.E., Air Pollution and Fatal Lung Disease in Three Utah Counties, *Archives of Environmental Health,* 45, no. 6 (1990), 325–334.

9. Archer, V., and J. Lee, eds., Health Hazards in the Occupational Environment, *Family and Community Health,* 7, no. 3 (1984), 1–88.

10. Baker, D., Giardia! *National Wildlife,* 23, no. 5 (1985), 19–21.

11. Baker, J.L., Agricultural Chemical Management Practices to Reduce Losses Due to Drainage, *American Journal of Industrial Medicine,* 18, no. 4 (1990), 477–483.

12. Barker, P., and D. Lewis, The Management of Lead Exposure in Pediatric Populations, *Nurse Practitioner: American Journal of Primary Health Care,* 15, no. 12 (1990), 8–10, 12–13, 16.

13. Barlett, D., and J. Steele, *Forevermore: Nuclear Waste in America.* New York: W.W. Norton, 1985.

14. Bayer, R., Notifying Workers at Risk: The Politics of the Right-to-Know, *American Journal of Public Health,* 76, no. 11 (1986), 1352–1356.

15. Bennett Information Group, *The Green Pages.* New York: Random House, 1990.

16. Beware Sick-Building Syndrome, *Newsweek* (January 7, 1985), 58–60.

17. Biagini, R.E., et al., Antibodies to Morphine in Workers Exposed to Opiates at a Narcotics Manufacturing Facility and Evidence for Similar Antibodies in Heroin Abusers, *Life Science,* 47, no. 10 (1990), 897–908.

18. Biodegradable Plastics: Friend or Foe of Waste Management? *Chemecology,* 19, no. 8 (1990), 2–3.

19. Blueprint for Clear Skies, *Sierra* (July-August, 1989), 16–17.

20. Bode, L.E., Agricultural Chemical Application Practices to Reduce Environmental Contamination, *American Journal of Industrial Medicine,* 18, no. 4 (1990), 485–489.

21. Bradstock, M., et al., Evaluation of Reactions to Food Additives: The Aspartame Experience, *American Journal of Clinical Nutrition,* 43 (1986), 464.

22. Brand, C., Fifty Ways to Save Water, *St. Louis Society Audobon Newsletter* (April, 1988), 3.

23. Briasco, M.E., Indoor Air Pollution: Are Employees Sick from Their Work? *AAOHN Journal,* 38, no. 8 (1990), 375–380.

24. Brown, M., The Toxic Cloud, *Greenpeace,* 12, no. 4 (1987), 17–23.

25. Brownson, R., et al., An Analysis of Occupational Risks for Brain Cancer, *American Journal of Public Health,* 80, no. 2 (1990), 169–172.

26. Bruce, R.D., Noise Pollution, *Community Health Nursing.* Philadelphia: F.A. Davis, 1985.

27. Bullough, B., and V. Bullough, *Nursing in the Community.* St. Louis: C.V. Mosby, 1990.

28. Burton, L., and H. Smith, *Public Health and Community Medicine for the Allied Medical Professions* (2nd ed.). Baltimore: Williams & Wilkins, 1975.

29. Caplan, R., *Our Earth. Ourselves.* New York: Bantam Books, 1990.

30. Castleman, M., Toxics and Male Infertility, *Sierra,* 70, no. 2 (1985), 49–52.

31. Centers for Disease Control, Childhood Lead Poisoning—United States Report to the Congress by the Agency for Toxic Substances and Disease Registry, *MMWR,* 37, no. 32 (1988), 481–485.

32. Chadzynski, L., *Manual for the Identification and Abatement of Environmental Lead Hazards.* Washington, DC: Division of Maternal and Child Health, 1986.

33. Chemical Industry Reduces Generation of Hazardous Waste, *Chemecology,* 18, no. 8 (1989), 9.

34. Choi-Lao, A., Trace Anesthetic Vapors in Hospital Operating Room Environments, *Nursing Research,* 30, no. 3 (1981), 156–160.

35. Christup, J., Return to Sender, *Greenpeace,* 13, no. 6 (1988), 8–13.

36. Clark, M., The Garbage Health Scare, *Newsweek* (July 20, 1987), 56.

37. Cleaning Up after Incinerators, *Science News* (December 9, 1990), 381.

38. Clemen-Stone, S., D. Gerber Eigsti, and S.L. McGuire, *Comprehensive Family and Community Health Nursing* (3rd ed.). St. Louis: Mosby-Year Book, 1991.

39. Coffel, S., *But Not a Drop to Drink!* New York: Rawson, 1989.

40. Cohen, G., and J. O'Connor, *Fighting Toxics: A Manual for Protecting Your Family, Community, and Workplace.* Washington, DC: Island Press, 1989.

41. Collins, E., The Perils of Plastic, *Health* (June 1990), 36–37.

42. Commoner, B., *Making Peace with the Planet.* New York: Pantheon Books, 1990.

43. Communist Governments Leave Dark Cloud of Pollution in Their Wake, *Chemecology,* 19, no. 4 (1990), 2–3.

44. Cookfair, J., *Nursing Process and Practice in the Community.* St. Louis: Mosby-Year Book, 1991.

45. Corcoran, E., Trends in Energy: Cleaning Up Coal, *Scientific American,* 264, no. 5 (1991), 106–116.

46. Davis, H., Workplace Homicides of Texas Males, *American Journal of Public Health,* 77, no. 10 (1987), 1290–1293.

47. ———, P. Honchar, and L. Suarez, Fatal Occupational Injuries of Women, Texas 1975–84, *American Journal of Public Health,* 77, no. 12 (1987), 1524–1527.

48. Dioxins: A Polychlorinated Perplexity, *Health and Environment Digest.* Navarre, NM: Freshwater Foundation, 1990, 1.

49. The Earth's Ozone, *Chemecology,* 16, no. 8 (1987), 1–3.

50. Effects of Toxic Agents on Reproduction, *Occupational Health and Safety,* (April 1979), 36–43.

51. Egginton, J., Menace of Whispering Hills, *Audobon,* (January 1989), 28–35.

52. Elkington, J., et al., *Going Green: A Kid's Handbook to Saving the Planet.* New York: Tilden Press Book, 1990.

53. ENR, *A Homeowner's Guide to Recycling Yard Wastes.* Springfield, Ill: Illinois Department of Energy and Natural Resources, 1990a.

54. ——, *Recycle: Be Part of the Solution, Not Part of the Problem.* Springfield, Ill: Illinois Department of Energy and Natural Resources, 1990b.

55. Environmental Protection Agency, *Asbestos Fact Book.* Washington, DC: Office of Public Affairs, May 1986.

56. ——, *Ozone in the Lower Atmosphere: A Threat to Health and Welfare.* Washington, DC: U.S. Government Printing Office, December 1986.

57. ——, *Ozone Fact Sheet.* Washington, DC: Office of Public Affairs, July 1987.

58. ——, Pesticides and the Consumer, *EPA Journal,* 13, no. 4 (1987), 2–47.

59. ——, *Environmental Progress and Challenges: EPA's Update.* Washington, DC: Environmental Protection Agency, 1988.

60. ——, *An Introductory Guide to the Statutory Authorities of the United States Environmental Protection Agency.* Chicago: United States Environmental Protection Agency, 1988.

61. ——, *Our Air, Our Land, Our Water.* Chicago: United States Environmental Protection Agency, 1988.

62. ——, *Your Guide to the U.S. EPA.* Chicago: United States Environmental Protection Agency, 1988.

63. Fattal, B., et al., Health Risks Associated with Wastewater Irrigation: An Epidemiological Study, *American Journal of Public Health,* 76, no. 8 (1986), 977–979.

64. Fighting to Save a Fragile Earth, *International Wildlife,* 20, no. 2 (1990), 4–21.

65. Fischhoff, B., Report from Poland: Science and Politics in the Midst of Environmental Disaster, *Environment,* 33, no. 2 (1991), 13–17, 37.

66. Fisher, D., *Fire and Ice: The Greenhouse Effect, Ozone Depletion and Nuclear Winter.* New York: Harper & Row, 1990.

67. Flanders, W., and K. Rothman, Occupational Risk for Laryngeal Cancer, *American Journal of Public Health,* 72, no. 4 (1982), 369–372.

68. Fleiss, J.L., and A.J. Gross, Meta-analysis in Epidemiology, with Special Reference to Studies of the Association Between Exposure to Environmental Tobacco Smoke and Lung Cancer: A Critique, *Journal Clinical Epidemiology,* 44, no. 2 (1991), 127–139.

69. Fox, B.C., et al., Heavy Contamination of Operating Room Air by Penicillium Species: Identification of the Source and Attempts at Decontamination, *American Journal of Infection Control,* 18, no. 5 (1990), 300–306.

70. Freidman, T., Staying at Home Can be Dangerous to Your Health, *Common Cause* (June 1982), 13–17.

71. Froines, J., C. Dellenbaugh, and D. Wegman, Occupational Health Surveillance: A Means to Identify Work-Related Risks, *American Journal of Public Health,* 76, no. 9 (1986), 1089–1096.

72. Fuortes, L., A Sick House Syndrome, Possibly Resulting from a Landfill Geologic Effluvia, *Veterinary and Human Toxicology,* 32, no. 6 (1990), 528–530.

73. Gallaher, M.M., et al., Cryptosporidiosis and Surface Water, *American Journal of Public Health,* 79, no. 1 (1989), 39–42.

74. Gay, K., *Ozone.* New York: Franklin Watts, 1989.

75. ——, *Water Pollution.* New York: Franklin Watts, 1990

76. Glantz, S.A., and W.W. Parmley, Passive Smoking and Heart Disease: Epidemiology, Physiology, and Biochemistry, *Circulation,* 83, no. 1 (1991), 1–12.

77. Gorham, E., An Ecologist's Guide to the Problems of the 21st Century, *The American Biology Teacher,* 52, no. 8 (1990), 480–483.

78. Government Steps Up Efforts to Prevent Lead Poisoning, *Chemecology,* 20, no. 1 (1991), 10–11.

79. Graham, N.M., The Epidemiology of Acute Respiratory Infections in Children and Adults: A Global Perspective, *Epidemiology Review,* 12, (1990), 149–178.

80. Green Watch, *Good Housekeeping* (April 1991), 71, 73–74, 78–80, 84, 88, 90–92, 94.

81. Grossman, J., The Quest for Quiet, *Health,* (February, 1990), 57.

82. Gustafson, D.I., Field Calibration of Surface: A Model of Agricultural Chemicals in Surface Waters, *Journal of Environmental Science and Health. Part B. Pesticides, Food Contaminates, Agricultural Wastes and Environmental Letters,* 25, no. 5 (1990), 665–687.

83. Hallenbeck, W.H., *Pesticides and Human Health.* New York: Springer-Verlag, 1985.

84. Hamilton, M., ed., *The New Genetics and the Future of Man.* Grand Rapids, Mich: William B. Eerdmans, 1972.

85. Hanrahan, J., Testing Ground, *Common Cause Magazine* (January-February 1989), 13–19, 38.

86. Harris, L. Checking Up on Environmental Health, *Registered Nurse,* 2, no. 1 (1990), 26–27, 29, 31.

87. Harvey, P.D., Educated Guesses: Health Risk Assessment in Environmental Impact Statements, *American Journal Of Law and Medicine,* 16, no. 3 (1990), 399–427.

88. Hazelwood, M., Wilsonville: What Went In, Must Come Out, *Alton Evening Telegraph,* October 9, 1982, Sec. B, p. 8.

89. Henderson, D., Cookware as a Source of Additives, *FDA Consumer,* 16, no. 2 (1982), 11-B.

90. Hickey, S., Report: Lead Poisoning Worse Than Predicted, *The Nation's Health,* 12, no. 10 (1982), 7.

91. Hirst, E., Boosting U.S. Energy Efficiency Through Federal Action, *Environment,* 33, no. 2 (1991), 7–11, 32–35.

92. Holdgate, M., The Environment of Tomorrow, *Environment,* 33, no. 6 (1991), 14–20, 40–42.

93. *Home Personal Action Guide.* Washington, DC: Humane Society, 1990.

94. Household Waste Need Not Trash the Environment, *Chemecology,* 20, no. 5 (1991), 2–3.

95. Howe, H.L., Predicting Public Concern Regarding Toxic Substances in the Environment, *Environmental Health Perspective,* 87 (1990), 275–281.

96. Hutchinson, S., How To Protect Yourself Against the Environment, *National Wildlife,* 28, no. 5 (1990), 30–42.

97. *Indoor Air Pollution and S. 1198 Fact Sheet.* Washington, DC: Consumer Federation of America, 1985.

98. Industrial Wastes and the Earth, *The Nation's Health,* 12, no. 10 (1982), 7.

99. Inh, R.W., and N. Asal, Mortality Among Laundry and

Dry Cleaning Workers in Oklahoma, *American Journal of Public Health,* 74, no. 11 (1984), 1278–1280.

100. Is Poland Lost? Pollution and Politics in Eastern Europe, *Greenpeace,* 13, no. 6, 1988, 14, 19.

101. Jacobson, E., New Hospital Hazards: How to Protect Yourself, *American Journal of Nursing,* 90, no. 2 (1990), 36–41.

102. Jennings, B., and S. Gudermuth, Hospital Solid Waste: A Challenge for Nurses, *Missouri Nurse,* 47, no. 2 (1973), 5–7.

103. Jo, W.K., C.P. Weisel, and P. Lioy, Chloroform Exposure and the Health Risk Associated With Multiple Uses of Chlorinated Tap Water, *Risk Analysis,* 10, no. 4 (1990), 581–585.

104. John, E.M., D.A. Savitz, and D.P. Sandler, Prenatal Exposure to Parents' Smoking and Childhood Cancer, *American Journal of Epidemiology,* 133, no. 2 (1991), 123–132.

105. Johnson, C.J., and B.C. Kross, Continuing Importance of Nitrate Contamination of Groundwater and Wells in Rural Areas, *American Journal of Industrial Medicine,* 18, no. 4 (1990), 449–456.

106. Johnstone, H., *Facts on Domestic Wastes and Industrial Pollutants*. New York: Franklin Watts, 1990.

107. ———, *Facts on Nuclear Waste and Radioactivity*. New York: Franklin Watts, 1990.

108. Jones, C.J., et al., Elevated Nicotine Levels in Cervical Lavages from Passive Smokers, *American Journal of Public Health,* 81, no. 3 (1991), 378–379.

109. Jorgensen, E., ed., *The Poisoned Well: New Strategies for Groundwater Protection*. Washington, DC: Island Press, 1989.

110. Kang, H., et al., Dioxin and Dibenzofurans in Adipose Tissue of US Vietnam Veterans and Controls, *American Journal of Public Health,* 81, no. 3 (1991), 344–349.

111. Kaufman, S., Radioactive Wastes in St. Louis: The Waste Pile Grows to 45 Years High, *Alert,* 18, no. 1 (1987), 4, 8.

112. Kent, G.J., et al., Epidemic Giardiasis Caused by a Contaminated Public Water Supply, *American Journal of Public Health,* 78, (1988), 139–143.

113. Kerenyi, N.A., E. Pandula, and G. Feuer, Why the Incidence of Cancer Is Increasing: The Role of 'Light Pollution,' *Medical Hypotheses,* 33, no. 2 (1990), 75–78.

114. Kjellstrom, T., and L. Rosenstock, The Role of Environmental and Occupational Hazards in the Adult Health Transition, *World Health Statistics Quarterly,* 43, no. 3 (1990), 188–196.

115. Kraus, J., Homicide While at Work: Persons, Industries, and Occupations at High Risk, *American Journal of Public Health,* 77, no. 10 (1987), 1285–1289.

116. Kreiss, K., The Sick Building Syndrome: Where is the Epidemiologic Basis? *American Journal of Public Health,* 80, no. 10 (1990), 1172–1173.

117. Kronenwetter, M., *Managing Toxic Wastes*. New York: Julian Messner, 1989.

118. Kryter, K., *The Effects of Noise on Man* (2nd ed.). Orlando: Academic Press, 1985.

119. Laliberte, R., The Truth about Sick-Building Syndrome: Breathing Uneasy, *Health* (September, 1990), 63–65, 82.

120. Last, J.M., *Public Health and Human Ecology*. East Norwalk, Conn: Appleton & Lange, 1987.

121. Lead in the Modern Workplace, *American Journal of Public Health,* 80, no. 9 (1990), 907.

122. Leahy, J.G., and R.R. Colwell, Microbial Degradation of Hydrocarbons in the Environment, *Microbiology Review,* 54, no. 3 (1990), 305–315.

123. Lee, S.D., Risk Assessment and Risk Management of Noncriteria Pollutants, *Toxicology and Industrial Health,* 6, no. 5 (1990), 245–255.

124. Lee, S., *The Throwaway Society*. New York: Franklin Watts, 1990.

125. Lehmann, P., What Are Those Additives in Food? *Consumer's Research Magazine,* 65, no. 3 (1982), 13–17.

126. Licht, J., and J. Johnson, Sludge is an Awful Thing to Waste, *Sierra* (March-April, 1986), 29–32.

127. Linton, R., *Terracide*. Boston: Little, Brown, 1970.

128. Lipske, M., How Safe Is the Air Inside Your Home? *National Wildlife,* 25, no. 3 (1987), 35–39.

129. Litsky, W., J. Martin, and B. Litsky, Solid Waste: A Hospital Dilemma, *American Journal of Nursing,* 72, no. 10 (1972), 1841–1847.

130. MacEachern, D., *Save Our Planet*. New York: Dell Trade Paperback, 1990.

131. Mader, S., *Biology: Evolution, Diversity, and the Environment* (2nd ed.). Dubuque, Iowa: Wm C Brown, 1987.

132. Mancino, D.J., Radiation in the Nurse's Workplace, *Imprint,* 30, (1983), 35–39.

133. Marino, P., et al., A Case Report of Lead Paint Poisoning During Renovation of a Victorian Farmhouse, *American Journal of Public Health,* 80, no. 10 (1990), 1183–1185.

134. Marshall, G., Don't Be Shocked, *Nursing Times,* 77, no. 17 (1981), 721–722.

135. Marx, W., Cry of the American Coast, *Reader's Digest* (December 1988), 110–115.

136. Mattia, M.A., Hazards in the Hospital Environment: Anesthesia Gases and Methylmethacrylate, *American Journal of Nursing,* 83, no. 1 (1983), 73–76.

137. ———, Hazards in the Hospital Environment: The Sterilants, Ethylene Oxide and Formaldehyde, *American Journal of Nursing,* 83, no. 2 (1983), 241–243.

138. ———, and S. Blake, Hospital Hazards: Cancer Drugs, *American Journal of Nursing,* 83, no. 5 (1983), 758–762.

139. McConnell, R., A. Anton, and R. Magnotti, Crop Duster Aviation Mechanics: High Risk for Pesticide Poisoning, *American Journal of Public Health,* 80, no. 10 (1990), 1236–1239.

140. McCormick, J., Diet for a Poisoned Planet, *Greenpeace,* 12, no. 3 (1987), 17–20.

141. McCuen, G., *Nuclear Waste: The Biggest Clean-Up in History*. Hudson, Wisc: GEM Publications, 1990.

142. Mendel, A., and A. Smith, Consistent Pattern of Elevated Symptoms in Air Conditioned Office Buildings: A Reanalysis of Epidemiologic Studies, *American Journal of Public Health,* 80, no. 10 (1990), 1193–1199.

143. Meth, I., Electrical Safety in the Hospital, *American Journal of Nursing,* 80, no. 7 (1980), 1344–1348.

144. Miller, A., Climate—Economic Models and Policy on Global Warming, *Environment,* 33, no. 6 (1991), 3–5, 43.

145. Miller, C., and L. Berry, *Acid Rain: A Sourcebook for Young People*. New York: Julian Messner, 1986.

146. Miller, G.H., The Impact of Passive Smoking: Cancer Deaths among NonSmoking Women, *Cancer Detection Previews,* 14, no. 5 (1990), 497–503.

147. Miller, M., and C. Silverman, eds., *Occupational Hearing Conservation.* Englewood Cliffs, NJ: Prentice-Hall, 1984.

148. Miller, M., Chlordane in Missouri, *Alert,* 18, no. 1 (Spring 1987), 1, 6–7.

149. Moore, C., Does Your Cup of Coffee Cause Forest Fires? *International Wildlife,* 19, no. 2 (1989), 39–44.

150. Mossman, K.L., and M. Sollitto, Regulatory Control of Indoor Rn, *Health Physics,* 60, no. 2 (1991), 169–176.

151. Murray, A.B., and B.J. Morrison, It is Children with Atopic Dermatitis Who Develop Asthma More Frequently if the Mother Smokes, *Journal of Allergy and Clinical Immunology,* 86, no. 5 (1990), 732–739.

152. Myers, N., The Heat Is On: Global Warming Threatens the Natural World, *Greenpeace,* 14, no. 3 (1989), 8–13.

153. Nathanson, J., *Basic Environmental Technology: Water Supply, Waste Disposal and Pollution Control.* New York: John Wiley & Sons, 1986.

154. A Nation Troubled by Toxins, *National Wildlife,* 25, no. 2 (1987), 33–40.

155. Nero, A., Controlling Indoor Air Pollution, *Scientific American,* 258, no. 5 (1988), 42–48.

156. Novotny, T.E., et al., Prevalence of *Giardia lamblia* and Risk Factors for Infection Among Children Attending Day-Care Facilities in Denver, *Public Health Reports,* 105, no. 1 (1990), 72–75.

157. Okum, D., Drinking Water for the Future, *American Journal of Public Health,* 66, no. 7 (1976), 639–643.

158. On the Trail of Acid Rain, *National Wildlife,* 25, no. 2 (1987), 8–12.

159. Orloske, A.J., and J.S. Leddo, Environmental Effects on Children's Hearing: How Can School Systems Cope? *Journal of School Health,* 51, no. 5 (1981), 12–14.

160. Ossler, C., Men's Work Environments and Health Risks, *Nursing Clinics of North America,* 21, no. 1 (1986), 25–36.

161. Patterson, P., Keeping a Lid on OR Waste, *Today's OR Nurse,* 12, no. 10 (1990), 54.

162. Pesticides and the Human Condition, *Chemecology,* 17, no. 8 (1988), 2–4.

163. Pope, C., Respiratory Disease Associated with Community Air Pollution and a Steel Mill, Utah Valley, *American Journal of Public Health,* 79, no. 5 (1989), 623–628.

164. Precautionary Measures in the Preparation of Antineoplastics, *American Journal of Hospital Pharmacy* (September 1980), 1184–1186.

165. Precipitation Affects Indoor Radon Levels, *Chemecology,* 19, no. 8 (1990), 9.

166. Pringle, L., *Rain of Troubles: The Science and Politics of Acid Rain.* New York: MacMillan, 1988.

167. Probart, C.K., Issues Related to Radon in Schools, *Journal of School Health,* 59, no. 10 (1989), 441–443.

168. Putting Risk in Perspective: Pesticide Benefits Far Outweigh Risk, *Chemecology,* 19, no. 6 (1990), 2–3.

169. Ratoff, J., Acid Rain's Most Visible Symptom, *Science News* (March 3, 1990), 143.

170. ———, What's the Source of Acid Rain? *Science News* (March 3, 1990), 143.

171. ———, and D.E. Thomsen, Chernobyl May Be Worst Nuclear Accident, *Science News,* 129, (1986), 276.

172. Reich, S.D., Pharmaceutics: Antineoplastic Agents as Potential Carcinogens—Are Nurses and Pharmacists at Risk? *Cancer Nurse,* 4, no. 6 (1981), 500–502.

173. Reider, E., et al., Are You at Risk for Food Poisoning? *Good Housekeeping* (August 1991), 161–162.

174. Reuben, D., Mind If I Give You Cancer? *Reader's Digest* (May 1991), 119–122.

175. Risks of Living Near Love Canal, *Science,* 217, no. 4562 (1982), 808–810.

176. Roan, S., *Ozone Crisis.* New York: John Wiley & Sons, 1989.

177. Robinson, J., Exposure to Occupational Hazards Among Hispanics, Blacks, and Non-Hispanic Whites in California, *American Journal of Public Health,* 79, no. 5 (1989), 629–630.

178. Rule Finalized Last November: Suit Challenges OSHA Limits on Workers' Right to Know Hazards, *The Nation's Health* (July 1984), 1, 5.

179. Saltonstall, R., *Your Environment and What You Can Do About It: A Citizens' Guide.* New York: Walker & Co, 1970.

180. Samet, J.M., New Effects of Active and Passive Smoking on Reproduction? *American Journal of Epidemiology,* 133, no. 4 (1991), 348–350.

181. Schneider, C., Turning Down the Heat, *National Parks* (July-August 1989), 16–17.

182. Seligman, P., et al., Occupational Lead Poisoning in Ohio: Surveillance Using Workers' Compensation Data, *American Journal of Public Health,* 76, no. 11 (1986), 1299–1302.

183. Serafini, P., Nursing Assessment in Industry, *American Journal of Public Health,* 66, no. 8 (1976), 755–760.

184. Shaeffer, M., Alert on Dioxin (a series of articles), *Alert Newsletter—Coalition for the Environment,* 13, no. 1 (1983).

185. Shuval, H., et al., Transmission of Enteric Disease Associated with Wastewater Irrigation: A Prospective Epidemiological Study, *American Journal of Public Health,* 79, no. 7 (1989), 850–852.

186. 600 Million Live in Cities with Air Pollution Risk, *The Nation's Health* (July 1987), 9.

187. Sohn, M., Special Care Is Required with Pesticide Applicator's Clothing, *Union Banner,* (May 23, 1990), 11.

188. Solbe, J.F., *Effects of Land Use on Fresh Waters: Agriculture, Forestry, Mineral Exploitation, Urbanisation.* Chichester, England: Ellis Horwood, 1986.

189. Some Cancers May Increase due to Ozone Depletion, *The Nation's Health,* 12, no. 6 (1982), 7.

190. Spradley, B.W., *Community Health Nursing: Concepts and Practice* (3rd ed.). Glenview, Ill: Scott, Foresman/Little, Brown, 1990.

191. Stellman, J., Occupational Health Hazards of Women— An Overview, *Preventive Medicine,* 7 (1978), 281–293.

192. ———, *Women's Work, Women's Health: Myths and Realities.* New York: Pantheon Press, 1978.

193. ———, The Effects of Toxic Agents on Reproduction, *Occupational Health and Safety* (April 1979), 36–43.

194. Stewart, A.P., Oral presentation at an Industrial Hearing Conservationist Training Course, November 10–12, 1982, Carrboro, NC.

195. Stigliani, W., et al., Chemical Time Bombs, *Environment,* 33, no. 4 (1991), 4–9, 26–30.

196. Stomach Cancer in Navahos and Uranium Link Suspected, *The Nation's Health* (July 1987), 9.

197. Stranahan, S., It's Enough to Make You Sick, *National Wildlife,* 28, no. 2 (February-March 1990), 8–15.

198. Strobel, G., Biological Control of Weeds, *Scientific American,* 265, no. 1 (1991), 72–78.

199. Strobino, B., J. Kline, and Z. Stein, Chemical and Physical Exposure of Parents: Effects on Human Reproduction and Offspring, *Early Human Development,* 1, no. 4 (1978), 371.

200. Stromberg, M., Carcinogens: Are Some Risks Acceptable? *American Journal of Nursing,* 86, no. 7 (1986), 815–817.

201. Study Highlights Economic, Environmental Growth Since Earth Day 1970, *Chemecology,* 19, no. 4 (1990), 10–11.

202. Survey—Farmers Using Fewer Pesticides, *Farm Week,* (May 15, 1989), 9.

203. Takashi, S.T., et al., Mutagens in Food as Causes of Cancer, *Nutrition and Cancer: Etiology and Treatment.* New York: Raven Press, 1981.

204. Taming Toxics in Your Home, *National Wildlife,* 28, no. 3 (1990), 29.

205. Taylor, S.L., Food Allergies and Sensitivities, *Journal of American Diet Association,* 86 (1986), 599.

206. Technology Produced Occupational Hazards for Nurses, *The American Nurse* (April 1987), 7–8.

207. Test Can Detect Pesticide Poisoning in Farmers, *St. Louis Post-Dispatch,* February 1, 1987, Sec C, p 12.

208. A Tiny Solution to a Big Problem: Use of Bacteria Promising for Hazardous Waste Disposal, *Chemecology,* 19, no. 7 (1990), 2–3.

209. Turk, J., and A. Turk, *Environmental Science.* Philadelphia: W.B. Saunders, 1988.

210. Udall, J., Turning Down the Heat, *Sierra* (July-August 1989), 26–39.

211. United States Department of Labor, Occupational Safety and Health Administration, *Handling Hazardous Wastes.* Washington, DC: U.S. Government Printing Office, 1975.

212. Valway, S., et al., Lead Absorption in Indoor Firing Range Users, *American Journal of Public Health,* 79, no. 8 (1989), 1029–1032.

213. Vo, C., Not in My Backyard, *National Wildlife,* 26, no. 5 (1988), 24–27.

214. Von Stackelberg, P., Whitewash: The Dioxin Cover-Up, *Greenpeace* (March-April 1989), 7–11.

215. Waste Treatment that Pays Off in Water, Energy and Plants, *Chemecology,* 17, no. 8 (1988), 5–6.

216. Wastewater Recycling and Reuse, *American Journal of Public Health,* 76, no. 8 (1986), 960–961.

217. Water Pollution Control Federation, *Hazardous Waste: What You Should and Shouldn't Do.* Alexandria, Va: Water Pollution Control Federation, 1986.

218. Weaver, D., Our Global Community and You, *Missouri Resource Review,* (Winter-Spring 1990), 18–27.

219. What Is Making These People Sick? *Chemecology,* 20, no. 1 (1991), 2–3.

220. Whelan, E., Diseases and Misinformation. In Nutrition Myths and Misinformation: Special Report, *Nutrition and the MD,* 11 (1985), 1.

221. Whitaker, M., 'It was Like Breathing Fire . . . ,' *Newsweek* (December 17, 1984), 26–32.

222. Whyatt, R.M., Setting Human Health-Based Groundwater Protection Standards When Toxicological Data Are Inadequate, *American Journal of Industrial Medicine,* 18, no. 4 (1990) 505–510.

223. Williamson, K., et al., Occupational Health Hazards for Nurses, Part II, *Image,* 20, no. 3 (1988), 162–168.

224. Wold, S., *Community Health Nursing: Issues and Topics.* Norwalk, Conn: Appleton & Lange, 1990.

225. Woods, M., Nature Makes Its Own Toxins, *Chemecology,* 20, no. 5 (1991), 12–13.

226. Wright, A.L., et al., Relationship of Parental Smoking to Wheezing and Nonwheezing Lower Respiratory Tract Illnesses in Infancy, *Journal Pediatrics,* 118, no. 2 (1991), 207–214.

227. Young, L., *Sowing the Wind: Reflections on the Earth's Atmosphere.* New York: Prentice Hall Press, 1990.

228. Zoloth, S., et al., Asbestos Disease Screening by Non-Specialists: Results of an Evaluation, *American Journal of Public Health,* 76, no. 12 (1986), 1392–1395.

Chapter *3*

Spiritual and Religious Influences on the Person and Family

Faith is the soul riding at anchor.
—H. W. Shaw

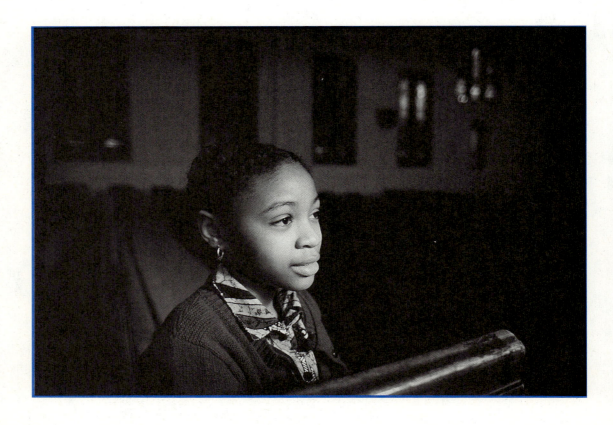

KEY TERMS

Religion

Spiritual dimension

Hinduism and Sikhism

Buddhism, Jainism, and Shintoism

Confucianism and Taoism

Islam

Judaism

Christianity

   Roman Catholicism

Greek/Eastern Ortho-
   dox faith

Protestantism

Seventh Day Adventists

Church of Jesus Christ
   of Latter-Day Saints

Jehovah's Witnesses

Church of Christ, Scientist

Unity School of Christi-
   anity

Society of Friends

Mennonites

Amish

Moravians

Waldenses

Neo-Pentecostalism

North American Indian
   religions

   Shamanism

Spirit world

Supreme Being

Culture hero

Agnostic

Atheistic

Cults

Devil or Satan worship

Voodo illness

Spiritual distress

OBJECTIVES

Study of this chapter will enable you to:

1. Define the terms *religious* and *spiritual* and the connotations of each.
2. Contrast the major tenets of Hinduism, Sikhism, Buddhism, Jainism, Shintoism, Confucianism, Taoism, Islam, Judaism, Christianity, and American Indians.
3. Compare the major tenets of the various branches of Christianity: Roman Catholicism, Eastern Orthodoxy, various Protestant denominations, other Christian sects.
4. Gain an overview of the variety of religions in the United States.
5. Discuss how religious beliefs influence life-style and health status in the various religious groups and subgroups.
6. Identify your religious beliefs, or lack of them, and explore how they will influence your nursing practice.
7. Discuss your role in meeting the spiritual needs of client and family.
8. Describe specific nursing measures that can be used to meet the needs of persons with different religious backgrounds.
9. Work with a client who has religious beliefs different from your own or refer the client to an appropriate resource.

> Until an illness occurs, the person may give no thought to the meaning of his or her life or spiritual beliefs. But when he or she feels vulnerable and fearful of the future, solace is sought. Religion can provide that solace.

A person sneezes. You say, "God bless you." Why? Perhaps unconsciously you are coordinating the medical-physical with the religious-spiritual. But you may feel afraid to work professionally with the combination. This fear comes in part from the long-lived schism between science and religion.

The attitude that medical science is superior to the spiritual or to religion has affected us all. Yet spiritual dimensions and religion are there as they always have been. Each culture has had some organization or priesthood to sustain the important rituals and myths of its people. Primitive man combined the roles of physician, psychiatrist, and priest. The Indian medicine man and the African witch doctor combine magic with religion; with their herbs, psychosuggestion, and appeals to the gods, they realize that man is a biopsychospiritual being (113).

> I had the cancer patient visualize an army of white blood cells attacking and overcoming the cancer cells. Within 2 weeks the cancer had diminished and he was rapidly gaining weight. He is alive and well today.

Is this a priest or a faith healer talking? No, this is a prominent tumor specialist talking today. An internationally known neurosurgeon says, "In a very real sense, medicine is now—as it has always been—faith healing." Dr. Elisabeth Kübler-Ross, internationally known for studies of dying, states that there is definitely life after death (53). Thus some health workers are trying to reunite the biopsychospiritual being.

The 1980s and the 1990s have shown an increased awareness of the link between health and religion, and the subject is being discussed more openly.

DEFINITIONS

Religion is defined on various levels: *a belief in a supernatural or divine force that has power over the universe and commands worship and obedience; a system of beliefs; a comprehensive code of ethics or philosophy; a set of practices that are followed; a church affiliation; the conscious pursuit of any object the person holds as supreme. In short, religion signifies that a group of people have established and organized practices that are related to spiritual concerns.*

This definition, however, does not portray the constancy and at times the fervency that can underlie religious belief. In every human there seems to be a **spiritual dimension,** *a quality that goes beyond religious affiliation, that strives for inspiration, reverence, awe, meaning, and purpose even in those who do not believe in any god. The spiritual dimension tries to be in harmony with the universe, strives for answers about the infinite, and especially comes into focus as a sustaining power when the person faces emotional stress, physical illness, or death. It goes outside a person's own power.*

In the midst of our specialized health care you have an opportunity to go beyond the dogma to bring together the biopsychospiritual being through the study of the religions and religious symbols of your clients. Those are world religions, not your personal or country's basic religion. Mass media, rapid transportation, and cultural exchanges have nullified the provincial approach.

WORLD RELIGIONS

Studying world religions poses a semantic difficulty in that an expression in the Chinese-based religion of Confucianism may have no equivalent in the English language. Thus language has dictated what people think, how they act, and how their religious beliefs are carried out (67).

Concepts, however, are often basically the same but are rephrased in each religion's own linguistic style. The saying "Love one another as I have loved you" will appear to the Hindu as "This is the sum of religion, do not unto others what causes pain to you"; to the Taoist as "Return goodness for hatred"; and to the Muslim as "No one is a believer unless he desires for his brother what he desires for himself."

Each religion also has other characteristics in common:

1. Basis of authority or source(s) of power
2. A portion of scripture or sacred word
3. An ethical code that defines right and wrong
4. A psychology and identity so that its adherents fit into a group and the world is defined by the religion
5. Aspirations or expectations
6. Some ideas about what follows death

The major world religions can be divided into categories in an attempt to group characteristics even further (67). The *alpha* group includes Christianity, Judaism, and Islam. All adhere to a Biblical revelation of a supernatural, monotheistic God. People in these religions are "doers." They obey because God commands; they make covenants with God for protection; they have a historical fixed scripture that is canonized for public use, and they often proselytize. Into the *gamma* group go Tao-

ism,* Confucianism, and Shintoism. In these religions people believe either that everything is in the being of God or that there is no Godhead (still a definite belief). These people try to be in harmony with the world around them. Their most immediate concern is in relationships with others. Scripture is a family affair. They can be characterized as simple in faith, spontaneous, and straightforward in feelings of affection for people, flowers, and birds. The final grouping is the *beta* group, which includes Buddhism and Hinduism. These religions have their roots in Indian soil and teach that everything is in the being of God. Adherents are interested in "being" rather than "doing." They have a collective literature for private devotion. Control of mind and body is desired, as some of the yoga practices show. The beta and gamma groups do not define God as clearly as the alpha group. The beta and gamma groups look inside themselves for answers: common sense rather than commands from God determines good.

The following discussion presents a more detailed insight into each major world religion through personality sketches. Each person has a fictitious name and represents not a single person but a composite of knowledge gained from the authors' interviewing, reading, and personal experience. Although these personalities are presented as acting and thinking in a certain way, remember that the person's culture, family background, and personality affect how that person lives out a religious experience. Thus a particular Hindu and a given Roman Catholic may be more in agreement religiously than two Lutherans. You cannot make generalizations about a religion from knowing a single follower.

 ## *Hinduism and Sikhism*

Rama tells us that nothing is typically **Hindu** and that anyone who puts religion in neat packages will have difficulty comprehending his outlook. Rama is named after Ramakrishna, the greatest Hindu saint of the nineteenth century. The history of Rama's religion goes back to approximately 1500 BC, when the **Vedas**— *divine revelations*—were written. His main religious texts are the **Upanishads,** or *scriptures,* and the **Bhagavad Gita,** a *summary of the former with additions.* The *most expressive and universal word of God is* **Om,** *or* **Aum**—providing the most important auditory and visual symbol in Rama's religion.[†]

Rama speaks of some of the worship popular in India today: of the family and local deities; of the trin-

---

*Pronounced "dowism."
[†]See the symbol at the beginning of this section. A transliteration of the script is *a, u, m.* It is written in English as *Om,* or *Aum. Om, God,* and *Brahman* are synonymous and mean a *consciousness* or *awareness* rather than a personified being.

ity—**Brahma,** the *creator;* **Vishnu,** the *preserver and god of love;* and **Shiva,** the *destroyer.*

Rama tells of his own shrine in his home where, in the presence of various pictures of **incarnations** (*human forms of God*) and with incense burning, he meditates. He also thinks of Buddha, Muhammed, and Jesus as incarnations and sometimes reads from the scriptures inspired by their teachings, although they represent other major religions.

In spite of this vast array of deities and the recognition that all religions are valid, Rama believes in one universal concept—**Brahman,** the *Divine Intelligence, the Supreme Reality.* Rama believes all paths lead to the understanding that this "reality" exists as part of all physical beings, especially humans. Rama's entire spiritual quest is directed toward uniting his *inner and real self,* the **atman,** with the concept of Brahman. So although Rama has gone through several stages of desire—for pleasure, power, wealth, fame, and humanitarianism— the last stage, his desire for freedom, for touching the infinite, is his main goal.

Rama is interested in health and illness only as a guide to this goal. He feels that the human love for the body is a cause for illness. He says, for example, that we overeat and get a stomachache. He views the pain as a warning—in this case, to stop overeating. He does not oppose medical treatment if absolutely necessary, but he believes that medicine can sometimes dull the pain and then the person overeats again, thus perpetuating the cause of the problem. Medical or psychiatric help, Rama says, is at best transitory. The cause of the pain must be rooted out.

In order not to dwell on physical concerns, Rama strives for moderation in eating and in other body functions. He considers only the atman as real and eternal and the body as unreal and finite. The body is a temple, a vehicle, no more. He tries to take care of it so that it will not scream at him because of overindulgence or underindulgence. Rama is a vegetarian. He believes that meat and intoxicants would excite his senses too much. Yet the Hindu diet pattern is flexible; definite rules are not set. If Rama is sick, he tries to bear his illness with resignation, knowing its temporary nature. He believes that the prayer of supplication for body cure is the lowest form of prayer, whereas the highest form is devotion to God. To him, death and rebirth are nearly synonymous, for the atman never changes and always remains pure. He compares the atman to the ocean: as ocean water can be put into various containers without changing its nature, so can the atman be put into various physical and human containers without changing its nature.

Thus if death is imminent, Rama believes that the body, mind, and senses weaken and become lifeless but that the never-changing atman is ready to enter into a new form of life, depending on the person's knowledge, deeds, and past experiences. Full acceptance of death is encouraged. Death is a friend to be faced bravely, calmly, and confidently.

Rama says that as a devotee of God he is following a *training course* called **yoga.** As a preliminary, however, he must establish certain moral qualifications. He must strive for self-control, self-discipline, cleanliness, and contentment. He must avoid injury, deceitfulness, and stealing. His overwhelming desire to reach God can be implemented through one or a combination of the four yoga paths: (1) **inana yoga** through *reading and absorbing knowledge,* (2) **bhakti yoga** through the *devotion of emotion and love,* (3) **karma yoga** through *work dedicated to God,* and (4) **raja yoga** through *psychologic experiments on oneself.* Rama combines the first three by reading and memorizing portions of the ancient scriptures, by meditating daily at his shrine, and by dedicating the results of his professional work to God.

Rama mentions that various forms of yoga have spread around the world to form hybrid groups with varied purposes. One branch that has appeared in medical centers is **hatha yoga,** meaning *sun and moon,* symbolizing an inner balance that is achieved through *muscle and breathing exercises.* Ultimately the body is prepared for meditation through these exercises.

From the bhakti emphasis comes **Sikhism,** founded by Nanak who was born in 1469. The Sikhs had nine other gurus, or spiritual mentors, who sequentially taught that God was the one and only reality. The fifth guru compiled the scripture. Starting as a pacifist group, the Sikhs evolved to warriors.

Also from bhakti influence has come the **Hare Krishna** movement in the United States, starting in 1965 when A.C. Bhaktivedanta came to New York City. The first Krishna temple was established on the Lower East Side (26). Rama reports that there are now reportedly 150,000 Krishnas in the United States, almost all of them converts from Catholicism, Judaism, or Protestantism. At New Vrindaban Krishna community in Moundsville, West Virginia, a palace has been built solely by community members. It contains $500,000 worth of gold, silver, onyx, marble, stained glass, teak, and crystal chandeliers. In contrast, the lifestyle is austere: work, study, and praise, beginning at approximately 3:30 A.M., no meat eating, no stimulants, no intoxicants, and no sex except for procreation (55).

For Rama, religion is not something to be picked up and put down according to a schedule or one's mood. It is a constant and all pervading part of his life and the life of his country. India's literature and art are witness to this fact. It also influences family life and structure. Basically marriage is for life, and people marry someone in the same social level. The husband is treated with respect, and the mother is thought of as ideal. Children have reverence for both father and mother, and back talk is unthinkable. Friends are to be treated as brothers and sisters, and visitors are always treated congenially.

Buddhism, Jainism, and Shintoism

Umeko Sato is a member of the *Buddhist sect* **Soka Gakkai.** This sect is a powerful religion in Japan, with a government party, a university, and a grand temple representing it. Now more than 60 years old, this organization that comprises 10% of Japan's population, known previously as a militant proselytizer, has toned down this phase and is living more graciously with other sects and creeds. Based on the **Lotus Sutra,** *part of the Buddhist scriptures,* its doctrine advocates the three values of happiness: profit, goodness, and beauty. Sato is attracted by the practicality of the teaching, the mottoes that she can live by, the emphasis on small group study, and present world benefits, especially healing.

Although Sato's beliefs at some points seem in direct contrast to the original Buddhist teachings, she is happy to explain the rich multireligious tradition that her family has had for generations. She emphasizes that she is affected by the ***Confucian*** emphasis on the family unit, by Christianity's healing emphasis, by ***Shintoism,*** the state religion of Japan until 1945, and by Buddhism, which originated about 600 BC in India with a Hindu named Siddhartha Gautama.

Currently approximately 90% of Japan's 120 million people adhere both to Buddhism and to Shintoism, although the nation has never been known as devout. Less than 1% are Christian. Another small religious group is known as **Jainism.** The "Jains" hark back to the sixth century BC, about the same time as Buddha. Their fundamental tenet is *ahimsa,* a refusal to injure any living thing. Jains believe every living thing has a soul.

There are two groups of Jains. A small group of approximately 100 are called *sky clad* because they wear no clothes. They renounce clothing and all earthly possessions. The other, larger group is called *white clad* because they wear white clothes. Together the groups contain monks, nuns, laymen, and laywomen who all take vows to guide them in all aspects of daily life.

Although the Jains are found in Japan and other countries, including the United States, they probably are known best for their bird hospital in Old Delhi, India, which treats 20,000 birds each year.

Gautama, shortly after a historic enlightenment experience during which he became the Buddha, preached a sermon to his followers and drew on the earth a wheel representing the continuous round of life and death and rebirth. Later eight spokes were added to illustrate the sermon and to provide the most explicit visual symbol of Buddhism* today. Sato repeats Buddha's four noble truths: (1) life is disjointed or out of balance, especially in birth, old age, illness, and death;

(2) the cause of this imbalance is ignorance of one's own true nature; (3) removal of this ignorance is attained by reaching **Nirvana,** the *divine state of release,* the *ultimate reality,* the *perfect knowledge* via (4) the eightfold path.

The eight spokes of the wheel represent the eightfold path used to reach Nirvana. Sato says that followers subscribe to right knowledge, right intentions, right speech, right conduct, right means of livelihood, right effort, right mindfulness, and concentration. From these concepts has arisen a moral code that, among other things, prohibits intoxicants, lying, and killing of any kind (which explains why Buddhists are often vegetarians). She further explains that the Mahayana branch of Buddhism took hold in Japan as opposed to the Theravada branch. The **Theravada branch** emphasizes an intellectual approach through wisdom, man working by himself through meditation and without ritual. The **Mahayana branch** emphasizes involvement with mankind, ritual, petitionary prayer, and concern for one's sibling. Sato believes that the Mahayana branch provides the happier philosophy of the two, and she tells of the ritual of celebration of Gautama's birthday. But most Japanese believe in **Amitabha Buddha,** a god rather than a historical figure, who is replacing the austere image of Gautama as a glorious redeemer, one of infinite light. Also, the people worship **Kwannon,** a goddess of compassion.

Sato explains that she cannot omit mention of the one austere movement within the Mahayana branch, the **Zen sect.** Taking their example from Gautama's extended contemplation of a flower, Zen followers care little for discourse, books, or other symbolic interpretations and explanations of reality. Hours and years are devoted to meditation, contemplation of word puzzles, and consultation with a Zen master. In seeking absolute honesty and truthfulness through such simple acts as drinking tea or gardening, the Zen student hopes to experience enlightenment.

Sato next turns to her former state religion, **Shintoism.** Whereas Buddhism produced a solemnizing effect on her country, Shintoism had an affirmative and joyous effect. Emperor, ancestor, ancient hero, and nature worship form its core. Those who follow Shintoism, she says, feel an intense loyalty and devotion to every lake, tree, and blossom in Japan and to the ancestral spirits abiding there. They also have a great concern for cleanliness, a carryover from early ideas surrounding dread of pollution in the dead.

Sato says that her parents have two god shelves in their home. One contains wooden tablets inscribed with the name of the household's patron-deity and a symbolic form of the goddess of rice and other texts and objects of family significance. Here her family performs simple rites such as offering a prayer or a food gift each day. In a family crisis, perhaps an illness, the family con-

---

*See the symbol at the beginning of this section.

ducts more elaborate rites such as lighting tapers or offering rice brandy. The other god shelf, in another room, is the Buddha shelf; and if a family member dies, a Buddhist priest, the spiritual leader, performs specified rituals there.

Sato strongly emphasizes that if illness or impending death causes a family member to be hospitalized, another well family member will stay at the hospital to bathe, cook for, and give emotional support to the ill person. Sato believes that recovery largely depends on this family tie. If death occurs, Sato will be reminded of the Buddhist doctrine teaching that death is a total nonfunction of the physical body and mind and that the life force is displaced and transformed to continue to function in another form. Every birth is a rebirth, much as in the Hindu teaching, and rebirth happens immediately after death, according to some Buddhists. Others believe that rebirth occurs 49 days after death, during which time the person is in an intermediary state. The difference in quality of death, birth, and existence depends on whether the person lived a disciplined or undisciplined life.

Buddhist religion teaches the living how to die well. The elderly, or feeble, are to prepare themselves mentally for a state that would be conducive for a good rebirth. The person is to remain watchful and alert in the face of death, to resist distraction and confusion, to be lucid and calm. Distinct instructions are given in what to expect as life leaves the body, as the person enters an intermediary state, and as Nirvana is about to occur.

So although Sato has grasped a new religious path for herself, her respect for tradition remains.

In giving care to a person with Umeko Sato's background, be aware of the varied religious influences on life. The sect's emphasis on the here and now rather than on the long road to Nirvana may place a high value on physical health so that the person can benefit from the joys and beauty of this life. The person may readily voice impatience with the body's dysfunction. You can also respond to the great concern for cleanliness, the desire to have family nearby, and the need for family rites that are offered for the sick member. Should a family member be dying, you may see some ambivalence. The family member may want to prepare himself or herself in the traditional way, but someone with Sato's background, with emphasis on present world benefits and healing, may deny that there is a valid preparation for death.

 Confucianism and Taoism

Wong Huieng is a young teacher in Taiwan simultaneously influenced by **Taoism,** the *romantic and mystical,* and **Confucianism,** the *practical and pragmatic.* To provide insights into these Chinese modes of think-

ing, although it is more representative of Taoism, Wong Huieng uses the yin-yang symbol.* The symbol is a circle, representing **Tao** or the *absolute,* in which two tear shapes fit perfectly into one another, each containing a small dot from the other. Generally yang is light or red, and yin is dark. Ancient Chinese tradition says that everything exists in these two interacting forces. Each represents a group of qualities. Yang is positive or masculine—dry, hot, active, moving, and light. Yin is feminine or negative—wet, cold, passive, restful, and empty. For example, fire is almost pure yang and water almost pure yin—but not quite. The combination of yin and yang constitutes all the dualisms a person can imagine: day–night, summer–winter, beauty–ugliness, illness–health, life–death. Both qualities are necessary for life in the universe; they are complementary and, if in harmony, good. Yang and yin energy forces are embodied in the body parts and affect food preferences and eating habits.

Huieng translates this symbol into a relaxed philosophy of life: "If I am sick, I will get better. Life is like going up and down a mountain; sometimes I feel good and sometimes I feel bad. That's the way it is." Though educated, she is not interested in climbing up the job ladder, accumulating wealth, or conquering nature. Her goal is to help provide money to build an orphanage in a natural wooded setting.

Huieng thinks of death as a natural part of life, as the peace that comes when the body is worn out. She admits, however, that when her father died, human grief took hold of her. Before his death, her mother went to the Taoist temple priest and got some incense that was to help cast the sickness from his body. After death, they kept his body in the house for the required time, 49 days. The priest executed a special ceremony every 7 days. Her mother could cry only 1 hour daily, 2:00 until 3:00 in the morning. Now her mother talks through the priest to her father's ghost. Although Huieng regards this practice as superstitious and thinks that painting a picture of a lake and mountain is a more fitting way to erase her grief, she looks at the little yellow bag, containing a blessing from the priest, hanging around her neck, and finds it comforting if not intellectually acceptable.

Now Huieng turns to her practical side and talks about **Confucius,** the first saint of the nation. Although **Lao-tzu,** the *founder of Taoism,* is a semilegendary figure said to have vanished after he wrote the bible of Taoism, **Tao-te-ching,** Confucius has a well documented existence.

Confucius, born in 551 BC, wrote little. His disciples wrote the **Analects,** *short proverbs, embodying his teachings.* He is revered as a teacher, not as a god. Huieng does not ask him to bless her but tries to emu-

*See the symbol at the beginning of this section.

late him and his teachings, which she has heard since birth. The temple in his memory is a place for studying, not for praying. And on his birthday, a national holiday, people pay respect to their teachers in his memory.

Five important terms in Confucius' teaching are **Jen,** a *striving for goodness within;* **Chun-sui,** *establishing a gentlemanly or womanly approach with others;* **Li,** *knowing how relationships should be conducted and having respect for age;* **Te,** *leading by virtuous character rather than by force;* and **Wen,** *pursuing the arts as an adjunct to moral character.* Huieng stresses that in *Li* are the directives for family relationships. So strongly did Confucius feel about the family that he gave directives on proper attitudes between father and son, elder brother and junior brother, husband and wife. Also, Huieng believes she cannot harm her body because it was given to her by her parents. Her concept of immediate family includes grandparents, uncles, aunts, and cousins. Her language has more words for relationships between relatives than the English language does.

Huieng believes that in caring for her body, she cares for her family, the country, and the universe. Essentially, to her, all people are family.

Important in your understanding of a person with Wong Huieng's background is the dualism that exists in such thinking. Acceptance of the particular version of mysticism and practicality and of the yin and yang forces that are seen as operating within self will help in building a foundation of personalized care.

The person may have more respect for older than younger staff members and may respond well to teaching. There may be a strong desire to attain and maintain wellness. These factors are directly related to the religious teaching; you can use them to enhance care. Additionally, talk slowly to the person if language is an issue. Rely on family members to help you understand the person's feelings. Permit familiar foods. Remember that foods are also divided into appropriate groups for types of illness. Address the person by the proper name. Do not use excessive touch signals unless they are invited. Remember this person may be in awe of health care authority and may be intimidated.

 *Islam**

Omar Ali is **Muslim,** a member of Islam, the youngest of the major world religions. "There is no God but Allah; Muhammed is His Prophet"[†] provides the key to Omar's beliefs. He must say this but once in his life as a requirement, but he will repeat it many times as an affirmation.

Muslims believe in a final judgment day when everyone will be judged and either sent to Paradise or to the fire of hell, depending on how justly he or she lived life according to God's Laws. They believe everyone, except children before the age of puberty, are responsible for their own good and bad actions and deeds and that no one can intercede on behalf of another.

Omar has also been influenced by the 3000-year-old **Zoroastrianism,** *which is a religion of pre-Islamic Iran* that flourishes in Bombay today. Likewise, it was a monotheistic religion even though dualism was also espoused.

Omar is an Egyptian physician whose religious tradition was revealed through Muhammed, born approximately AD 571 in Mecca, then a trading point between India and Syria on the Arabian peninsula. Hating polytheism and paganism in any form, Muhammed wrote *God's revelation to him* in the **Quran,*** *scriptures.* Omar believes in the biblical prophets, but he calls Muhammed the greatest—the Seal of Prophets.

Through the *Quran* and the **Hadith,** the *traditions,* Omar has guidelines for his thinking, devotional life, and social obligations. He believes he is a unique individual with an eternal soul. He believes in a heaven and hell, and while on earth he wants to walk the straight path.

To keep on this path, Omar prays five times a day: generally on rising, at midday, in the afternoon, in the early evening, and before retiring. Articles needed are water and a prayer rug. Because the *Quran* emphasizes cleanliness of body, Omar performs a ritual washing with *running* water over the face, arms, top of head, and feet before each prayer. Omar explains that in the bedridden client this requirement can be accomplished by pouring water out of some sort of receptacle. If a Muslim's entire body is considered ritually unclean, he must wash the entire body. If water is unavailable or the person cannot bathe, clean soil may be used in place of the ritual washing. After this washing the Muslim needs either a ritually clean cloth or a prayer rug and a clean place to pray. He may not face a dirty area such as the bathroom when making his prayer, even if this area is in the line toward Mecca. The Moslem must physically readjust himself in this case to comply with Islamic regulations. Then, facing Mecca, he goes through a series of prescribed bodily motions and repeats various passages in praise and supplication.

Omar also observes **Ramadan,** a fast month,[†] during which time he eats or drinks nothing from sunrise to sunset; after sunset he takes nourishment only in moderation. He explains **fasting** (abstinence from eating) as a discipline aiding him to understand those with little food and more importantly, as a submission to Allah. At

---

*A portion of this section was contributed by Caroline Samiezadé-Yazd, R.N., B.S.N.
[†]These words are a translation of the sacred calligraphy in the symbol shown at the beginning of this section. The prophet's name is sometimes spelled *Muhammad.*

---

*Sometimes spelled *Koran.*
[†]Coming during the ninth month of the Muslim year, always at a different time each year by the Western calendar, and sometimes spelled *Ramazan.*

the end of Ramadan, he enters a festive period with feelings of goodwill and gift exchanges. The sick, the very old, pregnant and lactating mothers, children, and Muslims who require the ingestion or injection of substances throughout the day hours are exempt without penalty from practice of this belief.

Omar has made one pilgrimage to Mecca, another requirement for all healthy and financially able Muslims. He believes the experience created a great sense of brotherhood, for all the pilgrims wore similar modest clothing, exchanged news of followers in various lands, and renewed their mutual faith. The twelfth day of the Pilgrimage month is the **Feast of Sacrifice, (*Eida-Fita*)** when all Muslim families kill a lamb in honor of Abraham's offering of his son to God.

In line with the *Quran's* teaching, Omar does not eat pork (including such items as bologna, which might contain partial pork products), gamble, drink intoxicants, use illicit drugs, or engage in religiously unlawful sexual practices such as premarital sex, homosexuality, or infidelity. The emphasis on strict moral upbringing—dating, dancing, drinking, and sex outside marriage are forbidden—puts the Muslim on a common ground with conservative Christians. Abstinence from drug use also eliminates many potential health and social problems.

Omar worships no images or pictures of Muhammed, for the prophet is not deified. Nor does he hang or display pictures of any prophet or any god or worship statues or religious symbols. He gives a portion of his money to the poor, for Islam advocates a responsibility to society.

Omar points out that not all Arabs are Muslims and not all Muslims are Arabs. Arabs come from a number of nations stretching from Morocco to the Persian Gulf. Persons who are Arab Muslims speak Arabic and uphold the tenets of Islam. Omar emphasizes the importance of gaining specific knowledge about their complex social structure. The centrality of religion and the family are closely related and reflect many aspects of health care.

Omar mentions that parts of the basic Islam faith are used by a United States–based group commonly known as the Black Muslims (Nation of Islam). Known to have stringent, seclusionist rules, the Black Muslims have taken some new positions since 1976 and seem to be moving toward more orthodox Islam. Members may now get politically involved; membership is open to Caucasians; dress codes have changed; and some of the myths about the American founder, W.D. Fard, have been erased.

Omar outlines the ideas of his religion as it applies to his profession. He believes that he can make a significant contribution to health care but that essentially what happens is God's will. Submission to God is the very meaning of Islam. This belief produces a very fluid feeling of time and sense of fatalism. Planning ahead for a Muslim is not a value as it is in Western culture; to defy God's will brings on the evil eye.

Muslim clients are excused from many, but not all, religious rules, but many will still want to follow them as closely as possible. Even though in a body cast and unable to get out of bed, a client may want to go through prayers symbolically. The person might also recite the first chapters of the *Quran,* centered on praise to Allah, which are often used in times of crises. Family is a great comfort in illness, and praying with a group is strengthening, but the Muslim has no priest. The relationship is directly with God. Some clients may seem fatalistic, completely resigned to death, whereas others, hoping it is God's will that they live, cooperate vigorously with the medical program. Muslims do not discuss death openly because if they did, the client and family may lose all hope and the client could die as a result. Instead, Muslims tend to communicate grief in gradual stages rather than immediately and all at once. Further, they make it a point never to let the affected person lose hope. The family, even in the gravest of situations, will not attempt to prepare for the death even when it is imminent. After death, a body must be washed with running water by a Muslim and the hands folded in prayer. Muslims do not perform autopsies, embalmment, or use caskets for burials. Instead, they wrap a white linen cloth around the dead person and place the body into the ground facing Mecca. Knowledge of these attitudes and traditions can greatly enhance your care.

 Judaism

Seth Lieberman, strongly influenced by the social-concern emphasis in Judaism, is a psychiatrist. In the Jewish community each member is expected to contribute to others' needs according to his or her ability. Jews have traditionally considered their community as a whole responsible for feeding the hungry, helping the widowed and orphaned, rescuing the captured, and even burying the dead. Jewish retirement homes, senior citizens' centers, and medical centers are witnesses to this philosophy.

Seth cannot remember when his religious instruction began—it was always there. He went through the motions and felt the emotion of the Sabbath eve with its candles and cup of sanctification long before he could comprehend his father's explanations. Book learning followed, however, and he came to understand the fervency with which his people study and live the law as given in the **Torah,** the *first five books of the Bible;* and in the **Talmud,** a *commentary and enlargement of the Torah*. His *spiritual leader* is the **rabbi.** His *spiritual symbol* is the **menorah.***

---

*See the symbol at beginning of this section. The seven-branched candelabrum stands for the creation of the universe in 7 days; the center light symbolizes the Sabbath; and the candlelight symbolizes the presence of God in the Temple.

His own *entrance into a responsible religious life and manhood* was through the **Bar Mitzvah,** a ceremony which took place in the synagogue when he was 13. (Girls are also educated to live responsible religious lives, and a few congregations now have a similar ceremony, the **Bas Mitzvah,** for girls.)

Although raised in an *Orthodox* home, Seth and his family are now *Reform.* He mentions another group, the *Conservatives.* The **Orthodox** *believe God gave the law;* it was written exactly as He gave it; it should be followed precisely. **Reform** *Jews believe the law was written by inspired men* at various times and therefore is subject to reinterpretation. Seth says he follows the traditions because they are traditions rather than because God demands it. **Conservatives** *are in the middle,* taking some practices from both groups. Overriding any differences in interpretation of ritual and tradition is the fundamental concept expressed in the prayer "Hear, O Israel, the Lord our God, the Lord is One." Not only is He one, He loves His creation, wants His people to live justly, and wants to bless their food, drink, and celebration. Judaism's double theme might be expressed as "Enjoy life now, and share it with God." Understandably then, Seth's religious emphasis is not on an afterlife, although some Jewish people believe in one. Although Jews have had a history of suffering, the inherent value of suffering or illness is not stressed. Through their observance of the law, the belief of their historical role as God's chosen people, and their hope for better days, Jews have survived seemingly insurmountable persecution.

Seth works with physically, emotionally, and spiritually depressed persons. He believes that often the spiritual depression is unnoticed, misunderstood, or ignored by professional workers. He cites instances in which mental attitudes have brightened as he shared a common bond of Judaism with a client.

He offers guidelines for working with a Jewish person in a hospital or nursing home. Although Jewish law can be suspended when a person is ill, the client will be most comfortable following as many practices as possible.

Every Jew observes the **Sabbath,** a *time for spiritual refreshment, from sundown on Friday to shortly after sundown on Saturday.* During this period Orthodox Jews may refuse freshly cooked food, medicine, treatment, surgery, and use of radio, television, and writing equipment lest the direction of their thinking be diverted on this special day. An Orthodox male may want to wear a **yarmulke** or *skullcap* continuously; use a *prayerbook called* **Siddur,** and use **phylacteries,** *leather strips with boxes containing scriptures,* at weekday morning prayer. Also, the ultra-Orthodox male may refuse to use a razor because of the Levitical ban on shaving.

Some Orthodox Jewish women observe the rite of **Mikvah,** an *ancient ritual of family purity.* From marriage to menopause (except when pregnant) these women observe no physical-sexual relations with their husbands from 24 hours before menstruation until 12 days later when a ritual immersion in water renders them ready to meet their husbands again.

Jewish dietary laws have been considered by some scholars as health measures: to enjoy life is to eat properly and in moderation. The Orthodox, however, obey them because God so commanded. Food is called **treyfe** (or *treyfah*) if it is *unfit* and **kosher** if it is *ritually correct.*

Foods forbidden are pig, horse, shrimp, lobster, crab, oyster, and fowl that are birds of prey. Meats approved are from those animals that are ruminants and have divided hooves. Fish approved must have both fins and scales. Also, the kosher animals must be healthy and slaughtered in a prescribed manner. Because of the Biblical passage stating not to soak a young goat in its mother's milk, Jews do not eat meat products and milk products together. Neither are the utensils used to cook these products nor the dishes from which to eat these products ever intermixed.

Guidelines for a satisfactory diet for the Orthodox are as follows:

1. Serve milk products first, meat second. Meat can be eaten a few minutes after milk, but milk cannot be taken for 6 hours after meat.
2. If a person completely refuses meat because of incorrect slaughter, encourage a vegetarian diet with protein supplements such as fish and eggs, considered neutral unless prepared with milk or meat shortening.
3. Get frozen kosher products marked Ⓤ, K, or *pareve.*
4. Heat and serve food in the original container and use plastic utensils.

Two important holy days are *Rosh Hashanah* and *Yom Kippur.* **Rosh Hashanah,** the *Jewish New Year,* is a time to meet with the family, give thanks to God for good health, and renew traditions. **Yom Kippur,** the *day of atonement,* a time for asking forgiveness of family members for wrongs done, occurs 10 days later. On Yom Kippur, Jews fast for 24 hours, a symbolic act of self-denial, mourning, and petition. **Tisha Bab,** the *day of lamentation,* recalling the destruction of both Temples of Jerusalem, is another 24-hour fast period. **Pesach** or **Passover** (8 days for Orthodox and Conservative, 7 days for Reform) *celebrates the ancient Jews' deliverance from Egyptian bondage.* **Matzo,** an *unleavened bread,* replaces leavened bread during this period.

The Jewish person is preoccupied with health. Jews are future-oriented and want to know diagnosis, how a disease will affect business, family life, and social life. The Jewish people as a whole are highly educated, and although they respect the doctor, they may get several medical opinions before carrying out a treatment plan.

Although family, friends, and rabbi may visit the ill especially on or near holidays, they will also come at other times. Visiting the sick is a religious duty. And although death is final to many Jews except for living on in the memories of others, guidelines exist for this time. When a Jewish person has suffered irreversible brain damage and can no longer say a **bracha,** a *blessing to praise God,* or perform a **mitzvah,** an *act to help a fellow,* he or she is considered a "vegetable" with nothing to save. Prolonging the life by artificial means would not be recommended. But until then the dying client must be treated as the complete person he or she always was, capable of conducting his or her own affairs and entering into relationships.

Jewish tradition says never to leave the bedside of the dying person, which is of value to the dying and the mourners. The dying soul should leave in the presence of people, and the mourner is shielded from guilt of thinking that the client was alone at death or that more could be done. The bedside vigil also serves as a time to encourage a personal confession by the dying, which is a *rite de passage* to another phase of existence (even though unknown). This type of confessional is said throughout the Jewish life cycle whenever one stage has been completed. Confessional on the deathbed is a recognition that one cycle is ending and that another cycle is beginning. Recitation of the *Shema* in the last moments before death helps the dying to affirm faith in God and focus on the most familiar rituals of life.

Death, being witnessed at the bedside, helps to reinforce the reality of the situation. Immediate burial and specified mourning also move the remaining loved ones through the crisis period. (Note, however, that if a Jew dies on the Sabbath, he or she cannot be moved, except by a non-Jew, until sundown.) After the burial, the mourners are fed in a meal of replenishment called *se'udat havra'ah.* This step symbolizes the rallying of the community and the sustenance of life for the remaining. Also, Jews follow the custom of sitting *shiva* or visiting with remaining relatives for 1 week after the death (50).

Judaism identifies a year of mourning. The first 3 days are of deep grief; clothes may be torn to symbolize the tearing of a life from others. Seven days of lesser mourning follow, leading to 30 days of gradual readjustment. The remainder of the year calls for remembrance and healing. During that year a prayer called the mourner's *Kaddish* is recited in religious services. It helps convey the feeling of support for the mourner (50). At the annual anniversary of death, a candle is burned, and special prayers said.

So from circumcision of the male infant on the eighth day after birth to his deathbed and from the days of the original menorah in the sanctuary in the wilderness until the present day, the followers of Judaism reenact their traditions. Because many of these traditions remain an intrinsic part of the Jew while striving to maintain or regain wellness, the preceding guidelines offer a foundation for knowledgeable care.

Christianity

Beth Meyer, a *Roman Catholic,* Demetrius Callas, an *Eastern Orthodox,* and Jean Taylor, a *Protestant,* are Christian American nurses representing the three major branches of Christianity. Although Christianity divided into Eastern Orthodox and Roman Catholic in AD 1054, and the Protestant Reformation provided a third division in the sixteenth century, these nurses share some basic beliefs, most importantly that Jesus Christ as described in the *Bible* is God's son. Jesus, born in Palestine, changed "BC" to "AD." The details of His 33 years are few, but His deeds and words recorded in the *Bible's* New Testament show quiet authority, loving humility, and an ability to perform miracles and to visit easily with people in varied social positions.

The main symbol of Christianity is the cross,* but it signifies more than a wooden structure on which Jesus was crucified. It also symbolizes the finished redemption—Christ rising from the dead and ascending to the Father in order to rule with Him and continuously pervade the personal lives of His followers.

Christians observe **Christmas** as *Christ's birthday;* **Lent** as a *season of penitence and self-examination preceding* **Good Friday,** *Christ's crucifixion day;* and **Easter,** *His Resurrection day.*

Beth, Demetrius, and Jean rely on the New Testament as a guideline for their lives. They believe that Jesus was fully God and fully man at the same time, that their original sin (which they accept as a basic part of themselves) can be forgiven, and that they are acceptable to God because of Jesus Christ's life and death. They believe God is three persons—the Father, the Son, and the Holy Spirit (Holy Ghost), the last providing a spirit of love and truth.

Beth, Demetrius, and Jean differ in some worship practices and theology, but all highly regard their individuality as children of God and hope for life with God after death. They feel responsible for their own souls, the *spiritual dimension of themselves,* and for aiding the spiritual needs of their patients.

Roman Catholicism, according to Beth, is a religion based on the dignity of man as a social, intellectual, and spiritual being made in the image of God. She traces the teaching authority of the church through the scriptures: God sent His Son to provide salvation and redemption from sin. He established the Church to continue His work after ascension into heaven. Jesus chose apostles to preach, teach, and guide. He appointed Saint

---

*See the symbol at the beginning of this section.

Peter as the Church's head to preserve unity and to have authority over the apostles. The mission given by Jesus to Saint Peter and the apostles is the same that continues to the present through the pope and his bishops. Beth notes that in the last several years, women in the Roman Catholic Church, both nuns and laywomen, are speaking out more on issues and are asking for more recognition and respect as God's spokespeople.

Beth believes that the seven *Sacraments* are grace-giving rites that give her a share in Christ's own life and help sustain her in her efforts to follow His example. The Sacraments that are received once in life are Baptism, Confirmation, Holy Orders, and usually Matrimony.

Through **Baptism** Catholics believe the *soul is incorporated into the life of Christ and shares His divinity.* Any infant in danger of death should be baptized, even an aborted fetus. If a priest is not available, you can perform the sacrament by pouring water on the forehead and saying, "I baptize thee in the name of the Father, of the Son, and of the Holy Spirit." The healthy baby is baptized some time during the first weeks of life. Adults are also baptized when they convert to Catholicism and join the church.

Confirmation is the *sacrament in which the Holy Spirit is imparted in a fuller measure to help strengthen the individual in his or her spiritual life.* **Matrimony** *acknowledges the love and lifelong commitment between a man and a woman.* **Holy Orders** *ordains deacons and priests.*

The Sacraments that may be received more than once are Penance (Confession), the Eucharist (Holy Communion), and the Anointing of the Sick (Sacrament of the Sick). Beth believes that **Penance**, an *acknowledgment and forgiveness of her sins in the presence of a priest,* should be received according to individual need even though it is required only once a year by church law. The Mass, often called the **Eucharist,** is the liturgical celebration whose core is the sacrament of the Holy Eucharist. Bread and wine are consecrated and become the body and blood of Christ. The body and blood are then received in Holy Communion.

The Eucharist is celebrated daily, and all Roman Catholics are encouraged to participate as often as possible; they are required by church law to attend on Sundays (or late Saturdays) and specified holy days throughout the year unless prevented by illness or some other serious reason.

Beth is glad that the Anointing of the Sick has been modified and broadened and explains the rite to client and family to allay anxiety. Formerly known as Extreme Unction or the last rites, this sacrament was reserved for those near death. Now **Anointing of the Sick,** *symbolic of Christ's healing love and the concern of the Christian community,* can provide spiritual strength to those less gravely ill. Following anointing with oil, the priest offers

prayers for forgiveness of sin and restoration of health. Whenever possible, the family should be present to join in the prayers.

If the client is dying, extraordinary artificial measures to maintain life are unnecessary. At the hour of death the priest offers communion to the dying person by means of a special formula. This final communion is called *Viaticum.* In sudden deaths the priest should be called and the anointing and Viaticum should be administered if possible. If the person is dead when the priest arrives, there is no anointing, but the priest leads the family in prayers for the person who just died.

Beth divides the Roman Catholic funeral into three phases: the **wake,** a *period of waiting* or vigil during which the body is viewed and the family is sustained through visiting; the **funeral mass,** a *prayer service* incorporated into the celebration of the Mass; and the **burial,** the *final act* of placing the person in the ground. (This procedure may vary somewhat, for some Catholics are now choosing cremation.) The mourners retain the memory of the dead through a Month's Mind Mass, celebrated a month after death, and anniversary masses. Finally, the priest integrates the liturgy for the dead with the whole parish liturgical life.

Beth is convinced that her religious practice contributes to her health. She believes that the body, mind, and spirit work together and that a spirit rid of guilt and grievances and fortified with the strength of Christ's life has positive effects on the body. She believes that suffering and illness are allowed by God because of our disobedience (original sin) but that they are not necessarily willed by God or given as punishment for personal sin.

While in the hospital, a Roman Catholic may want to attend Mass, have the priest visit, or receive the Eucharist at bedside. (Fasting an hour before the sacrament is traditional, but in the case of physical illness, fasting is not necessary). Other symbols that might be comforting are a Bible, prayer book, holy water, a lighted candle, crucifix, rosary, and various relics and medals.

The Greek Orthodox faith is discussed by Demetrius. The Eastern Orthodox Church, the main denomination, is divided into groups by nationality. Each group has the **Divine Liturgy,** the *Eucharistic service,* in the native language and sometimes in English also. Although similar in many respects to the Roman Catholic faith, the Eastern Orthodox faith has no pope. The seven sacraments are followed with slight variations. Baptism is by triple immersion: the priest places the infant in a basin of water and pours water on the forehead three times. He then immediately confirms the infant by anointing with holy oil.

If death is imminent for a hospitalized infant and the parents or priest cannot be reached, you can baptize the infant by placing a small amount of water on the forehead three times. Even a symbolic baptism is acceptable, but only a living being should receive the sacrament. Adults who join the church are also baptized and confirmed.

The **unction of the sick** has never been practiced as a last rite by the Eastern Orthodox; *it is a blessing for the sick.* Confession at least once a year is a prerequisite to participation in the Eucharist, which is taken at least four times a year: at Christmas, at Easter, on the Feast Day of Saint Peter and Saint Paul (June 30), and on the day celebrating the Sleeping of the Virgin Mary (August 15).

Fasting from the last meal in the evening until after **Communion,** another term for the Eucharist, is the general rule. Other fast periods include each Wednesday, representing the seizure of Jesus; each Friday, representing His death; and two 40-day periods, the first before Christmas and the second before Easter.

Fasting to Demetrius means avoiding meat, dairy products, and olive oil. Its purpose is spiritual betterment, to avoid producing extra energy in the body and instead think of the spirit. Fasting is not necessary when ill. Religion should not harm one's health.

Demetrius retains the Eastern influence in his thinking. He envisions his soul as blending in with the spiritual cosmos and his actions as affecting the rest of creation. He is mystically inclined and believes insights can be gained directly from God. He tells of sharing such an experience with a patient, Mrs. A., also Greek Orthodox.

Mrs. A. had experienced nine surgeries to build up deteriorating bones caused by rheumatoid arthritis. She faced another surgery. On the positive side, the surgery promised hope for walking; on the negative, it was a new and risky procedure. Possibly she would not walk; possibly she would not live. Demetrius saw Mrs. A. when he started working at 3:30 P.M. She was depressed, fearful, and crying. Later, at 6:30 P.M., he saw a changed person—fearless and calm, ready for surgery. She explained that she had seen Jesus in a vision, and that He said, "Go ahead with the surgery. You'll have positive results. But call your priest and take Communion first." Demetrius called the priest, who gave her Communion. She went into surgery the next day with supreme confidence. She now walks.

In addition to Communion, other helpful symbols are prayer books, lighted candles, and holy water. Especially helpful to the Orthodox are **icons,** *pictures of Jesus, Mary, or a revered saint.* Saints can intercede between God and the person. One of the most loved is **Saint Nicholas,** a *third-century teacher and father figure* who gave his wealth to the poor and became an archbishop. He is honored on Saint Nicholas Day, December 6, and prayed to continuously for guidance and protection.

Every Sunday morning Demetrius participates in an hour-long liturgy. Sitting in an ornate sanctuary with figures and symbols on the windows, walls, and ceiling, facing the tabernacle containing the holy gifts and scrip-

ture, Demetrius finds renewal. He recites, "I believe in one God, the Father Almighty, Maker of Heaven and Earth, and of all things visible and invisible. And in one Lord Jesus Christ, the only begotten Son of God."

Protestantism is divided into many denominations and sects. Jean Taylor is a member of the *Church of God* (Anderson, Indiana). She identifies the church by its headquarters because there are some 200 independent church groups in the United States using the phrase "Church of God" in their title. Her group evolved late in the nineteenth century because members of various churches felt that organization and ritual were taking precedence over direction from God. They banded together in a drive toward Christian unity, toward a recognition that any people who followed Christ's teachings were members of a universal Church of God and could worship freely together.

This example speaks of one of the chief characteristics of Protestantism: the insistence that God has not given any one person or group of persons sole authority to interpret His truth to others. Protestants use a freedom of spiritual searching and reinterpretation. Thus new groups form as certain persons and their followers come to believe that they see God's teaching in a new and better light. Jean believes that reading the Bible for historical knowledge and guidance, having a minister to teach and counsel her, and relying on certain worship forms are all important aids. But discerning God's will for her life individually and following that will are her ultimate religious goals.

Jean explains that she "accepted Christ into her life" when she was 8 years old. This identified her as personally following the church's teaching rather than just adhering to family religious tradition. A later experience, in which the Holy Spirit gives the person more spiritual power and discernment, is called *sanctification.*

Jean defines her corporate worship as free liturgical, with an emphasis on congregational singing, verbal prayer, and scripture reading. A sermon by the **minister,** the *spiritual leader,* may take half the worship period. As with many Protestant groups, two sacraments or ordinances are observed: (1) baptism (in this case, **believer's** or **mature baptism** by *total immersion into water*) and (2) Communion. To Protestants, the bread and wine used in Communion are symbolic of Christ's body and blood rather than the actual elements. One additional ordinance practiced in Jean's church and among some other groups is **foot-washing,** *symbolic of Jesus' washing His disciples' feet.* These ordinances are practiced with varied frequencies.

Because of the spectrum of beliefs and practices, defining Protestants, even within a single denomination or sect, is almost impossible. Some Protestant groups, retaining their initial emphasis on individual freedom, have allowed no written creed but expect members to follow an unwritten code of behavior. Jean does suggest some guidelines, however, She lists some of the **main Protestant bodies** in the United States, beginning with the most formal liturgically and sacramentally, the *Protestant Episcopal* and *Lutheran* churches. The in-betweens are the *Presbyterians, United Church of Christ, United Methodists,* and *Disciples of Christ (Christian Church)*. The liturgically freest and the least sacramental are the *Baptists* and *Pentecostals.*

Among these groups, some of the opposing doctrines and practices are as follows: living in sin versus living above sin; predestination versus free will; infant versus believer's baptism; and loose organization versus tightly knit organization. Some uphold **fundamental precepts,** *holding to the Scriptures as infallible,* whereas others uphold **liberal precepts,** *using the Scriptures as a guide, with various interpretations for current living.*

With this infinite variety, Jean believes that learning the individual beliefs of her Protestant client is essential. When and if a client wants Communion; if an infant should be baptized; and what will be most helpful spiritually to the patient—these factors are learned by careful listening. Generally Jean believes that prayer, a scriptural motto such as "I can do all things through Christ who gives me strength," or a line from a hymn can give strength to a Protestant. Some patients will also want anointing with oil as a symbolic aid to healing.

Jean has discovered that there are wide differences in Protestantism, sometimes even within the same denomination, about the theology and rituals of death. Some Protestant theologies have come to grips with the realities and meaning of death; others block authentic expression of grief by denying death and focusing on "If you are a Christian, you won't be sad."

Some Protestants view death as penalty and punishment for sins; others see death as a transition when the soul leaves the body for eternal reward; and still others view death as an absolute end. All agree that death is a biologic and spiritual event, a mystery not fully comprehended.

Rituals surrounding death vary widely. Some churches believe that the funeral service with a closed casket or memorial service with no casket present is more of a testimony to the joy and victory of Christian life than the open-casket service. Others believe that death is a reality to face instead of deny and that viewing the dead person promotes the grief process and confrontation with death in a Christian context.

Jean believes that for most Protestants the minister represents friendship, love, acceptance, forgiveness, and understanding. His or her presence seems to help the dying face death with more ease. She also believes that Protestants are becoming more active in ministering to the bereaved through regularly scheduled visits during the 12 to 18 months after the funeral, although there are no formal rituals.

OTHER GROUPS OF INTEREST

Practices or beliefs unique to certain groups should be part of every health provider's knowledge.*

Other Protestant Denominations

Seventh-Day Adventists rely on Old Testament law more than do other Christian churches. As in Jewish tradition, the Sabbath is from sundown Friday to sundown Saturday. Like the Orthodox Jew, the Seventh-Day Adventist may refuse medical treatment and use of secular items such as television during this period and prefer to read spiritual literature. Diet is also restricted. Pork, fish without both scales and fins, tea, and coffee are prohibited. Some Seventh-Day Adventists are **lacto-ovo-vegetarians:** *they eat milk and eggs but no meat.* Tobacco, alcoholic beverages, and narcotics are also avoided. Because Adventists view the body as the "temple of God," health reform is high on their list of priorities and they sponsor health institutes, cooking schools, and food-producing organizations. They have pioneered in making foods for vegetarians, including meatlike foods from vegetable sources. Worldwide they operate an extensive system of over 4000 schools and 400 medical institutions and are active medical missionaries (75, 105). Much of their inspiration comes from Ellen G. White, a nineteenth century prophetess who gave advice on diet and food and who stressed Christ's return to earth.

The **Church of Jesus Christ of Latter-Day Saints (Mormons)** takes much of its inspiration from the **Book of Mormon,** *translated from golden tablets found by the prophet Joseph Smith.* The Mormons believe that this book and two others supplement the *Bible.* Every Mormon is an official missionary. There is no official congregational leader, but a **seventy** and a **high priest** *represent successive steps upward in commitment and authority.*

The Articles of Faith of the Church of Jesus Christ of Latter-Day Saints, as given by Joseph Smith, include statements of belief:

1. God and His Son, Jesus Christ, and the Holy Ghost
2. The same organization that existed in the Primitive Church
3. Worship of God according to personal conscience while obeying the law of the land
4. People being punished for their own sins and not for Adam's transgression
5. All people being saved, repentance, and obedience to the laws and ordinances of the Gospel
6. Being honest, true, chaste, benevolent, virtuous, hopeful, persistent, and doing good to all people

Specific Mormon beliefs are that the dead can hear

---

*See *Nursing '77,* December 1977, pp. 64–70, for more detailed study.

the Gospel and can be baptized by proxy. Marriage in the temple seals the relationship for time and eternity. This celestial marriage permits husband and wife to become gods. This process, called *exaltation* or *eternal progression,* allows the pair to populate other worlds by having newly created human souls as their offspring. After a special ceremony in the temple, worthy members receive a white garment. This garment, continuously worn under the clothes, has priesthood marks at the naval and at the right knee and is considered a safeguard against danger. The church believes in a whole-being approach and provides education, recreation, and financial aid for its members. A health and conduct code called *Word of Wisdom* prohibits tobacco, alcohol, and hot drinks (interpreted as tea and coffee) and recommends eating, though sparingly and with thankfulness, herbs, fruit, meat, fowl, and grain, especially wheat.

The Mormon believes that disease comes from failure to obey the laws of health and from failure to keep the other commandments of God. However, righteous persons sometimes become ill simply because they have been exposed to microorganisms that cause disease. They also believe that by faith the righteous sometimes escape plagues that are sweeping the land and often, having become sick, the gift of faith restores the obedient to full physical well-being.

Statistics indicate that the Mormon population succumbs to cancer and diseases of the major body systems at a much lower rate than the general population in this country. The death rate for patients suffering from cancer is less than 50% that of the general population; 50% less for those with diseases of the nervous, circulatory, and digestive systems; 33% less for kidney diseases, and 10% less for those with respiratory diseases. Mental illness occurs only half as often among Mormons as among the general population (115).

An explanation for these differences from the norm might be that the Mormons literally believe that the body is the "temple of God." They have programs of diet, exercise, family life, and work to help that "temple" function at optimum level.

Although the two groups just discussed—the Seventh-Day Adventists and the Mormons—generally accept and promote modern medical practices, the next two groups hold views that conflict with the medical field. The first group, **Jehovah's Witnesses,** refuses to accept blood transfusions. Their refusal is based on the Levitical commandment, given by God to Moses, declaring that no one in the House of David should eat blood or he or she would be cut off from his or her people, and on a New Testament reference (in Acts) prohibiting the tasting of blood. Jehovah's Witnesses in need of surgery may be fortunate enough to be near a surgeon who uses no blood transfusions because of reduced operating time. Other surgeons are becoming more willing to do surgery without using blood, using intravenous fluids

similar to the body's fluid composition instead. The new plasma expanders can also be used.

Masulis (58) discusses the ethical dilemmas facing the nurse and other health care professionals when caring for the child of a family that is Jehovah's Witness. She believes the Jehovah's Witness argument against receiving blood transfusions (ingesting blood) (Genesis 9:3-6; 1 Samuel 14:31-35; Acts 15:19-21, 28-29) is based on false analogy. Transfused blood does not function as food and is not equivalent to ingested blood.

Every Jehovah's Witness is a minister. Members meet in halls rather than in traditional churches, and they produce massive amounts of literature explaining their faith.

The second group, **Church of Christ, Scientist (Christian Scientists),** turn wholly to spiritual means for healing. Occasionally they allow an orthopedist to set a bone if no medication is used. Parents do not allow their children to get a physical examination for school; to have eye, ear, or blood pressure screening; or to receive immunizations. In addition to the *Bible,* Christian Scientists use as their guide Mary Baker Eddy's *Science and Health With Key to the Scriptures,* originally published in 1875. The title of this work indicates an approach to wholeness, and those who follow its precepts think of God as Divine Mind, of spirit as real and eternal, of matter as unreal illusion. Sin, sickness, and death are unrealities or erring belief. Christian Scientists do not ignore their erring belief, however, for they have established nursing homes and sanitoriums, the latter recognized in the United States under the federal Medicare program and in insurance regulations. These facilities are operated by trained Christian Science nurses who give first-aid measures and spiritual assistance.

A Christian Science graduate nurse must complete a 3-year course of training at one of a number of accredited sanitoriums. The training includes, among other subjects, classes in basic nursing arts, care of the elderly, cooking, bandaging, nursing ethics, care of reportable diseases, and theory of obstetric nursing. The training is nonmedical, and in the work of a Christian Science nurse no medication is administered. The nurse supports the work of the **practitioner,** *who devotes full time to the public practice of Christian Science healing.* Healing is not thought of as miraculous but as the application of natural spiritual law.

The practitioner helps people apply natural spiritual law. Such a person is not a clergyman and does not necessarily hold special church office. Becoming a practitioner is largely attained through self-conducted study and a short course of intensive study from an authorized teacher of Christian Science, but daily study, prayer, application, and spiritual growth are the foundation of practice. The practitioner will treat anyone who comes for help and is supported, like other general practitioners, by clients' payments.

A Christian Scientist who is in a medical hospital has undoubtedly tried Christian Science healing first, may have been put there by a non-Scientist relative, or may be at variance with sacred beliefs. If brought in while unconscious, the person would want to be given the minimum emergency care and treatment consistent with hospital policy. The person may also appreciate having a Christian Science practitioner called for treatment through prayer.

Yet sometimes the Christian Scientist person or family may feel so desperate about personal or a loved one's health status that they seek traditional medical care—sometimes too late. The article by Case (14) describes how a Christian Scientist family, following their traditional beliefs and guidance of the sect elders, sought medical care too late to save the life of their son. The parents describe their anguish as they learned that earlier antibiotic treatment for bacterial meningitis could have saved their son's life and that Christian Science practitioners had no effective care measures. They also discuss the conflicts and guilt related to leaving Christian Science and seeking spiritual solace elsewhere. They discuss appreciation of the nonjudgmental and supportive approach of the nursing and medical team as they rendered treatment, explained, and tried to save the son's life.

Two more groups of special interest because of their positive personal and health emphasis are the **Unity School of Christianity** and the **Society of Friends (Quakers).** Whereas most Roman Catholics acknowledge the earthly spiritual authority of the pope and most Protestants regard the *Bible* as their ultimate authority, the *Friend's* authority resides in direct experience of God within the self. A Friend obeys the **light within,** *the* **inner light** *or the* **divine principle;** *this spiritual quality causes the Friend to esteem self and listen to inner direction.*

All Friends are spiritual equals. Without a minister and without any symbols or religious decor, unprogrammed corporate worship consists of silent meditation with each person seeking divine guidance. Toward the end of the meeting, people are free to share their inspiration. The meeting closes with handshaking. Always interested in world peace, Friends have been instrumental in establishing organizations that work toward human brotherhood and economic and social improvements resulting in better health. Friends have staffed hospitals, driven ambulances, and served in medical corps, among numerous other volunteer services.

The **Unity School of Christianity** believes that health is natural and sickness is unnatural. Followers think illness is real, but they believe it can be overcome by concentrating on spiritual goals. Late in the nineteenth century Charles and Myrtle Fillmore started this group after studying, among other religions, Christian Science, Quakerism, and Hinduism. Thus it blends several established concepts in a new direction. Today

Unity Village in Missouri has a publication center that publishes several inspirational periodicals, is beautifully landscaped and open for guests to share in the beauty, and houses its real force, Silent Unity. **Silent Unity** *consists of staff who are available on a 24-hour basis to answer telephone calls, telegrams, and letters from people seeking spiritual help.* They offer prayer and counseling to all faiths with no charge.

Some religious groups have retained life-style and geographic solidarity and theologic unity. These groups originated in other countries and immigrated to America.

The **Mennonites,** for example, some of whom settled in Pennsylvania, are part of a group called the Pennsylvania Dutch, who are of German, rather than Dutch or Holland, descent. The Mennonites generally emphasize plain ways of dressing, living, and worshipping. They do not believe in going to war, swearing oaths, or holding offices that require the use of force. Many of them farm the land or are inclined toward service professions. They are well known for their missionary efforts. Another group, the **Amish,** is a split from the Mennonite family.

A group with northern headquarters in Bethlehem, Pennsylvania, and southern headquarters in Winston-Salem, North Carolina, is the **Moravians.** These people have also been noted for their missionary work. A restored Moravian village is open for touring in Winston-Salem, and during Christmas and Easter special services are shared with non-Moravian friends.

The **Waldenses,** a Presbyterian group, have their headquarters in Rome but largely populate the town of Valdese, North Carolina. Each summer an outdoor drama portrays their pilgrimage to freedom.

Unitarian Universalists comprise yet another group of interest. The principle founder and leader in the early nineteenth century was William Ellery Channing. A Unitarian is considered a member of a universal church from which no person can be excommunicated except by the "death of goodness" in that person's heart. Freedom, democracy, positive faith, and saving the world from tyranny and oppression are major themes. Jesus is usually viewed by the members as a great prophet but not as part of the Trinity.

Another facet of Christianity in the United States is **Neo-Pentecostalism.** This is not a group but a trend or phenomenon that has gained support from small groups in all major denominations—some Roman Catholics, Presbyterians, and Lutherans—and from those churches traditionally closer to the Pentecostal spirit.

The heart of the Pentecostal spirit is an enthusiastic personal relationship with Christ. Those who are a part of this trend tell about getting out of dead, organized religion or of getting out of a religious tradition that no longer has meaning. They are anxious to share their insights. The hallmark of this experience is "speaking in tongues" or "glossolalia." Christians trace this experience back to the first century AD. In 1914, however, the phenomenon became institutionalized with the organization of the Pentecostal Assembly of God Church. This group placed its emphasis of a right relationship with God on glossolalia. Three other Pentecostal denominations have come into being: Church of God (Cleveland, Tennessee), Foursquare, and United Evangelical Brethren (21).

Neo-Pentecostalism is thought of as the *renewed interest in glossolalia; it is sometimes called the Charismatic Movement.*

Just what is **glossolalia?** Oral Roberts (82) describes it as the *prayer language of the spirit;* he believes that it is a release of thoughts so deep within the person that ordinary words do not suffice. Sounds made by the person are not in any known language, and the conscious mind, through prayer, should interpret the glossolalia after the experience so that the person can use the gained insight in everyday living (82).

Followers of the Neo-Pentecostal phenomenon have sometimes remained as part of the mainline churches in which their experience originated. Others have formed new organizational fellowships that are evolving into new mainline churches. For example, followers of a certain television evangelist will go to that person's religious training center or college. In turn, that religiously trained person will start a congregation following the tenets of that leadership. Eventually all those congregations will bind together in an overall identity membership.

North American Indian Religions

The **North American Indian religions** developed for centuries with very little influence from outside the continent. Power, supreme being, guardian spirits, totems, fasting, visions, **shamanism** (*belief in a priest who can influence good and evil spirits*), myth telling, and ritualism are all part of a varied belief system.

The location of the tribal group influenced its belief system. Indians of the Far North, Northeast Woodlands, Southeast Woodlands, Plains, Northwest Coast, California and the Intermountain Region, and the Southwest make up the main tribal divisions.

Yet all belief systems have certain features in common: (1) **spirit world**—*a dimension that permeates life but is different; (2)* **Supreme Being**—*God who represents other lesser deities; (3)* **culture hero**—*a spirit who competes with the Great Spirit, and who sometimes is a trickster; (4) spirits and ghosts such as atmospheric spirits (wind) or underworld powers (snakes); (5) guardian spirits acquired by visions seen during fasting; (6) medicine men and medicine societies; (7) ritual acts such as the Sun Dance; (8) prayers and offerings.*

A direct descendant from the Oglada Sioux outlines the belief of the Makaha (2). The Great Spirit, or Wakan Tanka, which is in all and throughout all, manifests itself in the following sixteen powers:

Notice that people (who have souls) ranked at the bottom. This explains the reverence for aspects of nature and animals.

Harmony or spiritual balance is what North American Indians want to achieve in their relations with the supernatural powers.

When caring for an American Indian, it is wise to obtain access to the spiritual leader from that particular region and his or her tribe. Many healing rituals are kept secret, so the health care provider can be most effective by making the appropriate connection, rather than by trying to intervene in the belief system.

New Age Movement

Recently much media attention has been given to the **New Age Movement.** Despite the name, some of the philosophies and practices of this movement are generally old ideas and practices, such as the use of positive thinking. The New Age Movement also has claimed some of the terms that nursing has used. For example, our philosophy for the past 20 years in writing nursing textbooks has been holistic health. Unfortunately, some nurses who are leery of the New Age Movement are now renouncing these terms (22, 39). Yet, giving care to the whole person is a basic and essential concept of nursing.

Basically New Age thinking is pantheistic and does not dwell on sin or evil. In this view human beings are considered all divine, all good. All is God, so God is in everything. In Christian theism, humans are sinful and saved by God through Jesus. Carried to extreme, the pantheistic philosophy would have people healing themselves because they are God and the Christian theism would have God doing all work without human cooperation or help. Both approaches, however, make use of optimism, holism, and synergism. New Age practices such as positive thinking, biofeedback, autosuggestion, and meditation can remain helpful adjuncts to healing as long as they do not become the "only way" for healing to take place (22, 39).

Agnosticism and Atheism

This chapter has concentrated so far on worship of God, the divine or other positive spirits, with an emphasis on traditional teaching. Some people live by ethical standards, considering themselves either **agnostic,** *incapable of knowing whether God exists,* or **atheistic,** *believing that God does not exist*.

Cults

In the 1970s various *cults* gained publicity. Some older cults are based on fundamental religions, but they are unique in their own way. The Snake People, for example, incorporate the holding of snakes into their services. Newer cults have arisen from communal groups whose goals are stated as religious. Some cults spring from the philosophy and schedule of a self-chosen leader who entices youth in search of identity from their parents and formalized church. The youth involved may evolve into robots; parents have had to "kidnap" their children to get them home and "deprogram" them to recognize their original personalities (30).

You may be involved in the long-term therapy of such a youth. Attention has focused on cults that are attracting not only the young but also the elderly. In the early 1980s there were thought to be 2000 cults throughout the world with a membership of 3 million (79), and the emphasis is growing.

Devil or **Satan Worship** is also practiced as a cult. The Satanic Bible was reportedly written by Anton Szandor LaVey who was part of the Church of Satan in San Francisco. The group is supposedly inactive but has splinter groups working, which are called *covens*. Reportedly there are various categories of worshippers: dabblers; self-styled, traditional satanists; and occult cult worshippers. The basic beliefs encompass power or energy in souls and bodies of animals and humans that can be absorbed through rituals. Rituals can be very powerful and macabre when they involve murder, dismembering body parts of animals and humans, and eating these organs. One young man spoke of how he became a precocious student of Satan. He read dozens of books on Satan as "Light-Bearer, the strongest and wisest angel in heaven, robbed of his rightful worship by a jealous God." He spoke of putting a hex on others, drinking ghoulish concoctions, and being obsessed with certain

rites as he moved through the hierarchy to priesthood (110).

Signs associated with Satanism are the sign "666"; an upside-down cross; the word *SATAN;* a picture of a horned beast; skulls; hoods; goat heads; reversed words (*NATAS*); ashes; and obsession with black such as a black room, black candles (3, 19, 32).

Adolescents are most likely to investigate Satanism. Usually they are unsure of their identity, need a group to accept them, and can find a sense of power in the rituals. Occasionally a teenager or college student will appear to have one life of being an outgoing honor student and another life of occult Satanism. Class lines, religion, and intelligence levels are crossed easily in cults (19).

Counselors and psychiatrists and some ministers and priests have had to deal with devil possession in treating clients. Although we do not often speak in these terms in our scientific age, devil possession is a recurring theme in clients' self-diagnosis and one that you should listen for with the new wave of interest in psychic occultism and witchcraft and their various practices.

Summary of American Religions

The *Encyclopedia of American Religions* (1978, two volumes) by J. Gordan Meltan (63) would be a good addition to the reference shelf in any health care facility in the United States. It is the first reference work to gather detailed information on all 1200 American religions from the well-known to the lesser cults. This work encompasses all religionists from mystical Hassidic Jews, metaphysicians, psychics, and witches to believers in the imminent end of the world, magic, unidentified flying objects (UFOs), traditional Catholics, Lutherans, and Methodists. The author places all 1200 groups into 18 families with common heritages and life-styles and identifies these families as:

Liturgical	Liberal
Reformed-Presbyterian	Holiness
Pietist Methodist	European Free Church
Pentecostal	Independent
Baptist	Fundamentalists
Adventist	Latter-Day Saints
Communal	Metaphysical
Psychic and New Age	Magick
Eastern	Middle Eastern
Lutheran	

OTHER TRENDS IN THE SPIRITUAL DIMENSION

Only when Christianity combines its beliefs with the already existing beliefs of other religions does the blend have a chance of working in the nondominant culture in the United States. For example, Mormonism and Charismatics have had the most impact on American Indians' religion, and since the 1960s these groups have become more visible on Indian Reservations. Likewise, the Peyote religion, in which the followers eat the peyote cactus, has added some Christian content such as God, Mary, Jesus, and heavenly angels—all with Indian symbolism.

In churches across the country, what formerly was known as "voodoo" is now called "spiritualism" and is testimony to blending of African and Catholic traditions.

Voodoo illness involves the belief that illness or death may occur as a result of a supernatural force. Various terms are used interchangeably with voodoo, including *rootwork, hex, black magic, witchcraft, spell,* or *conjuring.* Rootwork is part of the voodoo system associated with putting a hex on a person so they have good or bad experiences. There is a "misery hex" and a "lucky hex." Bags with dirt and roots may be hidden on a person's property. Mediating these experiences is a root doctor who can cast or remove spells (10, 40, 52). J. Campinha-Bacote describes the history of voodoo illness, the nonacceptance of Western medicine by voodoo believers, how the nurse may assess for this cultural phenomenon, and relevant nursing interventions for these clients, who are usually of African-Haitian, West African, or African-American descent (10).

In another trend, religion is being thought of by "mainline" Americans as a private affair. People may have strong personal beliefs but not want to rely on established institutions to control their religious life. Also, more religious programming is brought into the home, car, or work, via television, VCR, tapes, radio, and compact discs. People can listen in almost any setting via headphones without disturbing others.

A trend in mainline churches is to evaluate the role of women in the clergy and to consider gender-neutral and nonsexist language for the liturgy. For centuries Western religious thought has maintained the concept of the great chain of being—God, angels, men, women, animals, plants, inanimate objects—in which those above rule those below. This hierarchic concept was reflected in the traditional subordinate role for women in many churches. Along with a stronger role for women in our society has come an expanded role in many churches. For example, of 166 Christian denominations surveyed, 84 now ordain women.

As more women begin to lead the service and liturgy, the language issue will become more focused. Some people are unable to relate to the idea of God as male or God as the father. Proponents of nonsexist language for the liturgy are attempting to address these issues. One male author writes that he could never relate to God until he faced the issue that his feelings of relationship to God were exactly the same as to his biologic father. He advocated that a positive spiritual life for him could come only after he separated the emotional background from the spiritual and cleared the emotional areas first (101). The same principle is applicable to women who may speak of God as parent (91, 92, 101).

Another trend in the 1990s is to use the 12-step program (originally developed by Alcoholics Anonymous) for overcoming several addictions and for building spiritual strength. This approach refers to "God" but may view God as a higher power, deity, spiritual force, or even the collective power of the group (104).

Also families may be meeting their needs in nontraditional ways. One family of four—two parents and two children—decided at a family conference that their historical church was not providing an adequate spiritual diet for them. Rather than all look for another church together, they decided to pursue what was developmentally and spiritually appropriate for each. In time one child joined the Methodist Church, the other child an Interdenominational Church, one parent a Charismatic Church, and the other parent an Episcopal Church.

Another trend can be seen on university and college campuses. In spite of talk of the cynical and materialistic 1990s, a fervency of religious spirit, along with well-planned and well-executed spiritual programs, has been funneled through such groups as Inter-Varsity and Campus Crusade for Christ as well as mainline Catholic, Muslim, Jewish, and Methodist groups.

Health care professionals, as well as religious leaders and lay people, are increasingly concerned about the erosion of values and the need to practice moral values and ethical principles. Smedes, a professor of ethics at Fuller Seminary, writes that the United States is experiencing a crisis of morals. The crisis is not that people engage in wrong acts—people have always done that; it lies, instead, in the loss of a shared understanding of what is universally considered to be right behavior toward others and doubt about whether there is a moral right or wrong. Organized religion, families who follow moral precepts, and schools that teach moral values have a key role in formation of moral values. The F.B.I. has studied the relationship of proportion of church members and nonchurch members to crime rates in various communities. Cities with higher proportions of church members have lower rates of crime than more secular cities. For example, the West Coast has a higher crime rate than other parts of the nation and has by far the lowest church attendance rates. We may be healthier in all dimensions and development may proceed more normally for our population if our nation continues to embody religious teachings (102).

Nursing Applications

You can use the foregoing—basic beliefs, dietary laws, and ideas of illness, health, body, spirit, mysticism, pragmatism, pain, death, cleanliness, and family ties—as a *beginning.* Even more basic than understanding these concepts is respecting your client as a person with spiritual needs who has a right to have these needs met, whether he or she has formal religious beliefs. No one will respect your spiritual aid if you do not appear competent and thoughtful in your work. You are not expected to be a professional spiritual leader, for which lengthy training and experience would be required. You can, however, aid clients. You are the transition, the key person between the client and spiritual help.

If you feel inadequate, you may want to imitate several nurses who also felt the same. They decided that they could not meet the spiritual needs of others because they had not met—or even identified—their own. They had a series of discussions focusing on their own needs and used the book *Spiritual Care: The Nurses Role* (98), along with the accompanying workbook (95). When they had a clear vision of their own value system and made plans to meet their own needs, they could begin to focus on others. They also discussed appropriate and inappropriate spiritual intervention and learned to be comfortable making appropriate referrals when they believed that their lack of time or expertise did not allow them to intervene (7).

Also, by one of the same authors is *The Spiritual Needs of Children* (96) and *Spiritual Dimensions of Mental Health* (97), both excellent guidebooks.

In considering another's spiritual needs, the nurse should never overwhelm or be antagonistic. The goal should be to allow the (Holy) Spirit to touch another person through the caregiver.

Assessment

Although you can learn a great deal by picking out points in case studies, remember that they provide only a basis. You will have to accept each client's individual spiritual development. For example, the sacraments have a very different meaning to John than to a child. To a 10-year-old child the meaning of baptism might be carrying an ugly little baby on a pillow to the front of the church, pouring water on its head, and trying to believe that the baby emerges as a beautiful child of God.

Robert Coles (16) recounted anecdotes from Hopi, Christian, Muslim, Jewish, agnostic, and atheistic children. His conclusion was that they all have an immediacy of spiritual issues in their lives. An adolescent or young adult caught up in sorting out various facets of learned idealism and trying to fit them into more realistic daily patterns may temporarily discard religious teaching. He or she may reject the guidance of a spiritual leader because the latter is associated with the parents' beliefs; yet the adolescent is nevertheless searching and needs guidance. An elderly person suffering the grief of a recently lost mate may repeatedly question how a God of love could allow this loss. Some physiologically mature people are not religiously mature; they may expect magic from God. The spiritually maturing individual ex-

CASE SITUATION: Spiritual Distress

John Santini is a 40-year-old, middle-class, Caucasian bank president. He lives in a small town with his wife and four children. He also deals in real estate, works with civic and Roman Catholic church groups, and is developing an advertising company. He seems constantly busy. He discusses business over lunch and competes with friends when playing golf or tennis.

One evening he started vomiting and defecating blood and learned, after being hospitalized locally, that he had a bleeding duodenal ulcer. He was taken in an ambulance to a metropolitan hospital 200 miles away where a specialist successfully performed a partial gastrectomy, surgical removal of part of the stomach.

For the first time in his life, John was stopped. He was away from family and friends and was confined. Good and bad memories flooded his mind. He began to evaluate his activities, his emphasis on material gain and competition, how his children were growing so fast, how his religious activities were superficial, and how, without skilled surgery, he might have died.

At first he tried being jovial with the staff to strike out these new and troubling thoughts. But he could not sleep well. He was dreaming about death in wild combinations with his past life. He began to mention these dreams, along with questions about how the surgery would affect his life span, diet, and activities. He mentioned a friend who seemed severely limited from a similar surgery. He also said he was worried about the problems his teenagers were beginning to face and about his own ability to guide them properly.

The staff members never forced John to express more than he wished but answered the questions that were medically based and asked him if he would like to see the chaplain since his own priest was not available. John agreed. An appointed nurse then informed the chaplain of John's physical, emotional, and spiritual history to date. In the course of several sessions the chaplain helped John work through a revised philosophy of life that put more emphasis on spiritual values, family life, and healthy use of leisure.

periences the fruits of faith in God in behavioral terms of love, trust, and security. The external spiritual stimuli of God's word, sacraments, and relationships with other believers create an inner peace and love through which the person experiences God within and then reaches out to others in supporting relationships.

One author noted that the elderly, at a time when they were attending fewer organized religious functions, seemed to have improved inner spiritual strength (78). This is attributed to "transcendental operations" in which knowledge comes from personal ways of knowing rather than from a given external circumstance.

Furthermore, realize that people can use the same religious terms differently; *saved, sanctified, fell out, slain by the spirit,* and *deathbed conversion* all connote religious experiences. You should listen carefully, and you may have to ask questions to determine accurately the individual person's meaning.

Spiritual beliefs and beliefs about purpose in life and life after death are important dimensions of high-level wellness. Beliefs are related to feelings about self-worth, goals, interactions with others, philosophy of life, interpretations of birth, life events, and death. The value and meaning of life is not judged by its length but by the purpose for which the person lives, the principles by which they live, the reflection about a being greater than self, and the love and joy obtained from relationships with others. All of these factors may directly affect health status.

Assessment for spiritual needs of any client, not just the terminally ill or dying, should be part of the nursing history. Four areas of concern can be covered later in the interview as part of psychosocial assessment if necessary and after the client feels safe with the nurse. These areas are:

1. The person's concept of God or deity
2. The person's source of strength and hope
3. The significance of religious practices and rituals
4. The perceived relationship between spiritual beliefs and current state of health

During this part of the assessment, be prepared for any answer. The agnostic or atheist may answer with as much depth and meaning from his or her perspective as someone with a specific religious background. The person who is part of a formal religion may not answer freely, reserving such conversation for the spiritual leader or hesitating until the nurse is better known to the client.

When determining medical background such as drug or food allergies, you could also ask about religious dietary laws, special rituals, or restrictions that might be an important part of the client's history. Recording and helping the client follow beliefs could speed recovery.

Perhaps you could share with the chaplain the responsibility for asking some of the following questions as you give client care. No specific set of questions will be right for every client, but the following questions might draw helpful responses as you make a nursing assessment-diagnosis in the spiritual realm (105):

1. Who is your God? What is He/She/It like? (Or, what is your religion? Tell me about it.)
2. Do you believe that God or someone is concerned for you?
3. Who is the most important person to you? Is that person available?
4. Has being sick (what has been happening to you) made any difference in your feelings about God? In the practice of your faith? If it has, could you explain how it has changed?
5. Do you believe that your faith is helpful to you? If it is, how? If it is not, why not?
6. Are there any religious beliefs, practices, or rituals that are important to you now? If there are, could you tell me about them? May I help you carry them out by showing you where the chapel is? By telling the dietary department about your vegetarian preference? By allowing you specific times for prayer or meditation?
7. Is there anything that would make your situation easier? (Such as a visit from the minister, priest, rabbi, or chaplain? Someone who would read to you? Time for reading your religious book or praying? Someone to pray with you?)
8. Is prayer important to you? (If so, has being sick made a difference in your practice of praying?) What happens when you pray?
9. Do you have available religious books or articles such as the Bible, prayer books, phylacteries, or crucifix that mean something to you?
10. What are your ideas about illness? About life after death?
11. Is there anything especially frightening or meaningful to you right now?
12. If these questions have not uncovered your source of spiritual support, can you tell me where you do find support?

Be sure to look for the client's strengths, not weaknesses. Remember that you must not preach or reconstruct. Allow the client to assume his or her own spiritual stance.

Because your relationship with the client may be of short duration, be sure to document well the results of this interview. Later, when you or others care for the client, you should watch for religious needs that may be expressed through nonreligious language. You must again let the client know what options are open for spiritual help. If you hide behind busyness and procedures, you may lose a valuable opportunity to aid in health restoration.

Your greater understanding of social-class and cultural differences gleaned from Chapter 1 should help you comprehend some of the religious differences. For instance, a poor Protestant American who has grown up with the barest survival materials, who has no economic power, no money for recreation, no hope for significant gain, and no positive attitude about this life may center his or her whole being in the church. It provides as best it can for his or her emotional, recreational, and spiritual needs. When the person sings about heaven in terms of having beautiful clothes, a crown, and a mansion, he or she is singing with a much different meaning than the wealthy Protestant American who is really more concerned about mansions *here* than *over there*.

In a wider sense an Egyptian Christian and an American Christian, although voicing the same basic beliefs, will differ in their approaches to religion. The Egyptian, influenced by the Islamic attitudes of his or her country might say, "No matter what happens; it's God's will. I can do no more about it." The American Christian may be more influenced by the individual drive to guide his or her life, a philosophy prevalent in this culture. Another cultural difference centers on the influence of the family with an ill member. The Egyp-

tian, accustomed to having family and friends around nearly constantly, will expect a continuation of such activity during illness. Their presence provides spiritual and emotional support. The American, more mobile and used to the American hospital system of limiting visitors in number and time, may be better able to detach self from the emotional and religious support given by the presence of family.

Religion influences behavior and attitudes toward:

1. Work—whether you work to expiate sin, because it is there to do, or because of a conviction that it is a God-given right and responsibility
2. Money—whether you save money to deny yourself something, do installment buying, buy health insurance, consider money the root of all evil, or believe that it should be used for the betterment and development of persons and society
3. Political behavior—ideas about the sanctity of the Constitution, effects of Communism, importance of world problems, spending abroad versus spending for national defense, school or residential desegregation, welfare aid, and union membership
4. Family—kinds of interaction within the family, honoring of parents or spouse, children, or siblings
5. Childrearing—interest in the child's present and fu-

Research Abstract

Wells, C., and S. Zarit, Informal Support From Black Churches and the Well-Being of Elderly Blacks, **The Gerontologist, 31, no. 4 (1991), 490–495.**

In addition to family support, elderly African-Americans rely on assistance from the church before using services from other formal agencies more so than do the Caucasian elderly. There is a potential for expansion and development of social service programming and provision of informal services in the church to address needs of the elderly.

The structure and function of African-American churches, congregations in which decision-making is controlled by African-Americans, enhance the church's ability to provide a range of formal and informal services and to confirm personal identity and promote community unity.

The purpose of this study was to examine perceptions of the amount and type of support available to older African-Americans from their families and churches and the contribution of church-based support and religiosity to well-being.

The sample included 98 persons from African-American churches in urban, central Pennsylvania who ranged in age from 65 to 104 years of age. Sixty percent stated they were in good health, and 75% of the sample were women. Only 2% were never married; 5% were divorced or separated, and 53% were widowed. The subjects had 10 years of education and an annual median income of $8,000 to $10,000.

Subjects were interviewed, and seven instruments were used to measure social support, religiosity, well-being, health status, and functional ability. A multivariable analysis of variance (MANOVA) was used to test for differences in levels of perceived church versus family support.

Results showed the overlap in family and church networks. Approximately 40% of those named as important or close to the subjects were church members, primarily non-family members. Fifty percent of the network were family members. Perceptions of support from the family members were higher than perceptions of support from church members for all dimensions of support except social integration. Neither religiosity nor involvement in organized religious activities predicted well-being, but overall support from church members did. Elderly who perceived high support from both family and church scored highest on well-being. The majority of church programs were spiritual in nature. A variety of nonspiritual programs such as preventative health screenings, social outings and activities, respite care, personal care, home-delivered meals, assistance with household and health problems, and transportation to the church, doctors, or store was also offered by the churches.

Because of the emotional attachment to the church rather than to formal organizations, the church can operate as a major force in getting minority elderly to participate more fully in formal delivery of health services. The church is a link to health and social professional workers and agencies in the community when they attempt to reach elderly African-Americans. These findings validate the historical importance of the church for African-Americans who attend church, the use of ministers as linking agents, and the church as a service site.

ture, attitudes toward punishment or rewards for behavior, values of strict obedience as contrasted with independent thinking, or how many children should be born

6. Right and wrong—what is sin, how wrong is gambling, drinking, birth control, divorce, smoking, and abortion.

Consider how essentially the same situation can be diversely interpreted by two teenagers of different faiths. One, a fundamentalist Protestant, may spend an evening dancing and playing cards and suffer crushing guilt because she participated in supposed sinful acts. The other, a Jewish teenager, may participate in the same activities and consider it a religiously based function. Your knowledge of and sensitivity to such differences are important, for essentially similar kinds of decisions—right and wrong as religiously defined—will be made about autopsy, cremation, and organ transplants. (See reference 48 for additional information.) Furthermore, although religious bodies may hand down statements on these issues, often the individual person will alter the group's stand while incorporating individual circumstances into the decision.

Ideally, religion provides strength, an inner calm and faith with which to work through life's problems. But you must be prepared to see the negative aspect. To some, religion seems to add guilt, depression, and confusion. Some may blame God for making them ill, for letting them suffer, or for not healing them in a prescribed manner. One Protestant believed she had made a contract with God: if she lived the best Christian life she could, God would keep her relatively well and free from tragedy. When an incurable disease was diagnosed, she said, "What did I do to deserve this?" Another Protestant, during her illness, took the opposite view of her contract with God. She said, "I wasn't living as well as I should and God knocked me down to let me know I was backsliding."

Healing, too, has varied meanings. Some will demand that God provide a quick and miraculous recovery, whereas others will expect the process to occur through the work of the health team. Still others combine God's touch, the health providers' skill, and their own emotional and physical cooperation. Some will even consider death as the final form of healing.

Sometimes you must deal with your own negative reactions. Your medical background and knowledge may cause you dismay at some religious practices. For instance, how will you react as you watch a postoperative Jehovah's Witness client die because she has refused blood? How will you react to a Christian Scientist client who, in your opinion, should have sought medical help a month ago to avoid present complications? Here is one response given by a Christian Science nurse: "People can be ruined psychologically by going against a long-held belief. They may live and get better physi-

cally but will suffer depression, guilt, and failure in not holding to their standard." Basically they prefer to die. Should you dictate otherwise? You may need to think through and discuss such situations with a spiritual leader.

Nursing Diagnosis

The spiritual needs of clients have become a part of the evolving nursing diagnosis system of classification under the value-belief category. **Spiritual distress,** *when the person experiences or could experience a disturbance in the belief system that is his or her source of strength,* is the main diagnostic category. This problem may be related to not being able to practice spiritual rituals or may be caused by a conflict between the spiritual beliefs and the health regimen.

Other issues may be present also. For example, clients may question their belief system, may be discouraged or despairing, may feel spiritually empty, or may be ambivalent, first asking for spiritual assistance, then rejecting it.

The person's situation may be pathologic (losing a body part), treatment-related (abortion), or situational (death of significant person); however, all these areas are affected by spiritual beliefs. *As nurses become more attuned to these situations, perhaps meeting the client's spiritual needs will not be unattached from other care.* At the same time, the spiritual dimensions must be thought of as something in addition to the psychosocial dimension. Specific measures must be taken for spiritual care, which are not necessarily included in psychosocial care. One study showed that nursing educators were using only psychosocial intervention for spiritual care (75).

Intervention

Spirituality is an integral part of holistic health. Spiritual support to the ill and dying person can be given in various ways. Your warmth, empathy, and caring human relationship are essential. Respect for the person's belief, willingness to discuss spiritual matters, and providing for rituals and sacraments of religion are important. Be open to religious and philosophical beliefs other than your own. Some nurses may be uncomfortable discussing spiritual matters, yet it is for the client that the nurse will try to overcome personal reluctance to discuss spiritual concerns, just as nurses have worked to overcome reluctance to discuss sexuality concerns. Often the intimacy of spiritual concerns are discussed by the client during the intimacy of physical care. Helping the person ask questions and seek solutions does not mean that you have to supply the answers.

With the dying client, the aspects of spiritual support considered most helpful are (1) calling the person directly by name, (2) talking directly to the person (realize everything may be heard by the dying person), and

(3) supporting the family by staying with them as they say goodbye. Let family members know they can touch their dying loved one, offer your condolences, and offer to help them in any appropriate way.

The nurse who has struggled with personal spiritual needs, beliefs, and concerns, including the thought of her or his own death, can better help another work through concerns and needs. Being aware of sources for spiritual growth and support is important for self and the client. Knowledge about various religions and their spiritual leaders and about cultures and the related values can prepare you for providing spiritual support.

Be alert to subtle clues that indicate desire to talk about spiritual matters, need for expressions of love and hope, desire for your silent presence, and acceptance of behavior when the client labels self as bad.

Certain norms for providing spiritual care must be followed:

1. Do not impose personal beliefs on clients or families. A sickbed or deathbed is not a proper time for proselytizing.
2. Respond to the person out of his or her own background. Use knowledge about that background, but avoid acting in stereotypes. (For example, all Catholics believe _____ or all Hindus do _____.)
3. If you cannot give the spiritual support being asked for by the person, enlist someone who can.

Often there is little communication between health care providers and pastoral care representatives. You can fill that gap. Such rapport can mean that the *whole* person is served rather than segmented parts. Chaplains are especially helpful to clients and to nurses when they assist with the expression of anger, death, and the expression of grief (28). Nurse and chaplain, however, need to know what to expect from each other; there is no substitute for talking about these expectations and agreeing on strategies.

The following chart lists nine combinations of behavior that call for conferring with or referring to a spiritual leader unless contraindicated by the care plan:

1. Withdrawn, sullen, silent, depressed
2. Restless, irritable, complaining
3. Restless, excitable, garrulous, wants to talk a lot
4. Shows by word or other signs undue curiosity, anxiety about self
5. Takes turn to worse, critical, terminal
6. Shows conversational interest, curiosity in religious questions, issues; reads Scriptures
7. Specifically inquires about chaplain, chapel worship, Scripture
8. Has few or no visitors; has no cards, flowers
9. Has had, or faces, particularly traumatic or threatening surgical procedure

With all these aspects to consider, a team approach that includes the client, family, health care providers, and chaplain or other spiritual leader is imperative. Because Americans want weekends away from the job, the weekend hospital staff often has double responsibility. Furthermore, weekends are when most people attend corporate worship. Preparing the client for chapel service or seeing that the Sabbath ritual is carried out, puts a special responsibility on you, the nurse. Be especially sensitive to acceptance of the person's spiritual belief and try to provide the important factors, be they rituals, diet, quiet, group work, various articles, or family relationships.

Validate the appropriateness of proposed interventions with the client; for example, ask if the person wishes you to pray with him or her about the concerns that have been voiced. The person can then accept or reject your offer.

If a client is confined to a room, you can prepare a worship center or shrine by arranging flowers, prayer book, relics, or whatever other objects have spiritual meaning.

You should keep one or more calendars of various religious holidays. The Eastern Orthodox Easter usually does not coincide with the Roman Catholic and Protestant Easter. Jewish holidays usually do not fall on the same dates of the Western calendar in successive years. Remember, also, that holidays are family days and that ill people separated from the family at such times may be especially depressed.

Maintaining a list of available spiritual leaders, knowing when to call them, and knowing how to prepare for their arrival are other important responsibilities. If a client cannot make the request, consult with the family. One woman said, "If my sister sees a priest, she will be sure she is dying." Once a health care provider took the initiative to call an Eastern Orthodox priest who, unfortunately, represented the wrong nationality; the client's main source of comfort was to have come from discussion and prayers in the native language.

As you prepare the client and the setting for a spiritual leader, help create an atmosphere that reflects more than sterile procedure. Privacy has previously been emphasized by drawing curtains and shutting doors. Although acceptable to some, this approach may produce a negative response in others. Perhaps more emphasis should be given to cheerful surroundings: sunshine, flowers, lighted candles, openness, and participation by family and staff in at least an introductory way. Perhaps the client and spiritual leader could meet outdoors in an adjoining garden. The Shintoist and Taoist would especially benefit from the esthetic exposure. If the client is a child on a prolonged hospitalization, a special area might be designated for religious instruction.

Brief the spiritual leader on any points that might

provide special insight and be sure that the client is ready to receive him or her. Prepare any special arrangements such as having a clean, cloth-covered tray for Communion. Guard against interruption by health care providers from other departments who may be unaware of the visit. Finally, incorporate the results of the visit into the client's record.

Many will benefit from the sacraments, the prayers, Scripture reading, and counseling given by the spiritual leader, but others will want to rely on their own direct communication with God. The Zen Buddhist, Hindu, Muslim, and Friend might be in the latter category. All may wish reading material, however. Most will bring their sacred book with them, but if they express a desire for more literature, offer to get it. Some hospitals furnish daily and weekly meditations and copies of the King James Version of the *Bible* (which has been updated). You might suggest the *Bible* paraphrased in modern language by Kenneth Taylor, called *The Living Bible* (Tyndale House, 1971). The same edition is available as *The Children's Living Bible* (Tyndale House, 1972) with appropriate illustrations. *The Way* (Tyndale House, 1972) has the same wording as *The Living Bible* with guidelines and illustrations for youth. The *Amplified Bible* (Zondervan Publishing House, 1965) is especially good for translating the original Greek into comparable English meaning. The *New International Version* (Zondervan Bible Publishers, 1978) was a new translation that resulted from over 100 scholars working from the best available Hebrew, Aramaic, and Greek texts.

Occasionally it may be helpful to give Scripture references for various stated spiritual needs. For example, reference to love and relatedness can be found in Psalm 23; reference to forgiveness in Matthew 6:9–15; reference to meaning and purpose in Acts 1:8.

A positive interfaith magazine is *Guideposts* (Guideposts Associates). A novel with religious insights is *Christy* (Avon Books, 1968) by Catherine Marshall. A spiritually based autobiography is *Joni* (World Wide Publication, 1976) by Joni Eareckson. A delightful biography about a spiritually mature preschool-school-age child is *Mister God, This Is Anna* (Ballantine Books, 1974) by Fynn. *In Search of God: The Story of Religion* by Marietta Maskin is written for youth but is also recommended for adults who work with youth. Many other spiritually inspiring books and journals are availabe for use by clients and health care providers. Do not overlook the opportunity to share the ministry of books.

If you feel comfortable doing so, you can at times say a prayer, read a Scripture, or provide a statement of faith helpful to the client. If you do not feel comfortable in providing this kind of spiritual care, you can still meet the client's spiritual needs through respectful conversation, listening to the client talk about beliefs, referral to another staff member, or calling one of the client's friends who can bolster his or her faith. If spiritual lead-

ers are not available, you could organize a group of health workers willing to counsel with or make referrals for clients of their own faiths.

Shared prayer, if it is accepted by the client, counteracts the loneliness of illness or dying by offering the person intimacy with a Supreme Being and another person without the need for confession. It can be a means of bringing both human and divine love. It holds transcendent qualities and conveys both present and future hope. Prayer can focus on the conditions or emotions that the client is unable to talk about, allowing the person to handle the matter or vent in another way. Prayer should promote closeness, through closed eyes and hands that touch. Prayer should not strip the person of defenses. Nor should prayers be recited as a way to avoid the person or avoid questions raised by the person.

Use of life review can foster developmental, emotional, and spiritual maturity (not only in the elderly and dying person). Encourage the person to reminisce about past life experiences. Memories can be pleasurable or painful, but recalling them with a skilled listener can help resolve those ridden with shame, guilt, anger, or other feelings. Past sources of strength can also be identified, and sometimes they are useful in the present situation.

Several authors describe how counseling and mental and spiritual methods can be combined to help the client heal hurtful or traumatic memories, forgive self or others, work through unresolved grief, promote healing within self, and establish healthier relationships with others. Both non-Christian and Christian nurses may find these articles helpful (84, 93, 107).

Atheists should not be neglected because they do not profess a belief in God. They have the same need for respect as everyone else and may need you to listen to fears and doubts. The person does not need your judgment.

Moreover, just as health teaching is often omitted for health care providers who are clients, so is spiritual guidance often omitted for spiritual leaders who are clients. You must recognize that each person, regardless of religious stand or leadership capacity, may need spiritual help.

Various groups refuse medical or hospital treatment for illness, including members of Fundamentalist or Holiness groups, Jehovah's Witnesses, Amish, and Christian Scientists. Realize that if adults refuse treatment for themselves or their children, they are not deliberately choosing death. They are rejecting something objectionable, based on their beliefs. If at all possible, offer acceptable alternative treatments. Jehovah's Witnesses accept intravenous normal saline solution, Ringer's lactate solution, dextrose, Haemaccel, and hydroxyethyl starch solution. Members of rural Fundamentalist sects and the Amish are often willing to go to chiropractors and will allow physicians to set fractures and suture lacerations. Nurses may teach nutritional therapy or various stress management or relaxation techniques (56). Sometimes parents will accept the services of a home health nurse even though they refuse hospital and formal medical treatment.

Although a hospital setting has been used as a point of reference throughout this chapter, you can improvise in your setting—nursing home, school, industry, clinic, home, or other health center—to provide adequate spiritual assistance.

Evaluation

Exactly what constitutes spiritual intervention needs further research. In an attempt to identify which practices are used by individuals to establish or maintain a relationship with God, three groups within the Judeo-Christian religion completed a 23-item questionnaire presented by Ellen Duvall, a graduate nursing student at Texas Christian Women's University, as part of her graduate thesis. The questionnaire listed 16 practices that individuals in the Judeo-Christian religion might do to establish or maintain a relationship with God; study participants were asked to check if the practice was "helpful" or "not helpful" to them. The questionnaire focused on religious practices that do not require the clergy. The three groups, one Protestant, one Catholic, and one Jewish, were randomly selected from churches and synagogues listed in the Yellow Pages of a Midwestern city. The Protestant church so selected was Pentecostal, and the Jewish synagogue was Orthodox. At least 25 individuals from each group completed the questionnaire.

Table 3–1 lists the practices from her questionnaire and the number and percentage of subjects that identified the practice "helpful" from each of the three groups.

Subjects who had had contact with nurses were also asked if they believed a nurse could be helpful to them in establishing or maintaining a relationship with God. Only 5 of 24 Jewish subjects responded "yes." One subject added the comment, "No one, nurse or otherwise, can help in my relationship with God." However, 42 (91%) of the Protestant respondents and 26 (72%) of 36 Catholic respondents checked "yes." The subjects indicating a nurse could be helpful were asked to rate "helpful" or "not helpful" to five possible nursing interventions. The Catholic and Protestant responses are in Table 3–2.

This study was limited by the small number of subjects in each of the three groups. The responses, however, can give direction for more investigation to other Catholic, Protestant, and Jewish groups. Additional studies also need to determine which practices are helpful to individuals in hospitals, hospices, and nursing homes.

Outcomes that we must strive for are those that (1) enhance trust, (2) allow people to carry on spiritual practices not detrimental to health, (3) decrease feelings

TABLE 3-1. PRACTICES RATED HELPFUL BY INDIVIDUALS IN THE JUDEO-CHRISTIAN RELIGION TO ESTABLISH AND/OR MAINTAIN A RELATIONSHIP WITH GOD

Using Religious Literature	Catholics (%)	N	Protestants (%)	N	Jews (%)	N
Reading from the Bible by yourself	21 (68)	31	48 (98)	49	23 (92)	25
Reading from the Bible with others	18 (56)	32	48 (96)	50	20 (83)	24
Discussing Bible passages with others	21 (66)	32	50 (100)	50	23 (96)	24
Reading from religious writings of people of your religious group or denomination	22 (71)	31	45 (92)	49	20 (87)	24
Reading religious books, magazines, and/or religious newspapers	29 (83)	35	45 (92)	49	21 (88)	24
Using Prayer						
Praying silently, using your own words	37 (100)	37	48 (96)	50	25 (100)	25
Praying silently, using written or memorized prayers	36 (95)	38	7 (14)	49	11 (69)	16
Praying aloud with your religious leader	31 (91)	34	44 (90)	49	23 (85)	27
Praying aloud when a group of your faith is listening and praying with you	29 (85)	34	46 (94)	49	21 (84)	25
Praying aloud when you are alone	31 (84)	37	48 (98)	49	16 (64)	25
Praying aloud with one or two others	22 (65)	34	46 (94)	49	12 (48)	25
Praying aloud when people not of your faith are in the vicinity and may overhear you	10 (33)	30	35 (73)	48	8 (33)	24
Attaining Spiritual Support With Help of Others						
Listening to me talk through my problems	33 (97)	34	47 (94)	50	19 (76)	25
Reading Bible passages to me	13 (41)	32	44 (88)	50	4 (20)	20
Praying with me	28 (78)	36	47 (98)	48	12 (52)	23
Saying prayers for me (when I was not with the person)	36 (95)	38	47 (94)	50	12 (48)	25

N, the number of people who responded to each item.
Adapted from Duvall, E., Practices Used by People of the Judeo-Christian Religion to Relate to God, unpublished thesis, 1983.

TABLE 3-2. NURSING INTERVENTIONS RATED HELPFUL

Having a Nurse:	Catholic (%)	N	Protestant (%)	N
Read to me Bible passages I have chosen	15 (75)	20	36 (88)	41
Read or recite Bible passages of the nurse's choice	12 (55)	22	31 (78)	40
Listen to me talk through my problems	22 (92)	24	32 (80)	40
Pray with me at my bedside	20 (83)	24	37 (93)	40
Tell me that the nurse is praying for me (when not with me)	23 (96)	24	36 (92)	39

N, the number of people responding to each item as either helpful or not helpful.
Adapted from Duvall, E., Practices Used by People of the Judeo-Christian Religion to Relate to God, unpublished thesis, 1983.

of anxiety and guilt, and (4) cause satisfaction with their spiritual condition. To ensure these responses, spirituality enhancement must be part of what nurses do. It should be considered part of quality assurance. Sister Rosemary Donley suggests that this incorporation—with the addition of more mystery and more grace—will help foster support for the poor, the minorities, the very rich, that is, those who are sometimes blamed for their illnesses (25).

REFERENCES

1. Abbott, W.M., and J. Galleger, eds., *The Documents of Vatican II*. New York: The America Press, 1966, pp. 37–39, 158, 363.
2. Adams, B., *Prayers of Smoke*. Berkeley, Cal: Celestial Arts, 1990.
3. Area Officers Schooled by Expert on Satanism, *Union Banner* (May 17, 1989), Sec. 1, p. 1.
4. Bakken K., *The Call to Wholeness: Health as a Spiritual Journey*. New York: Crossroad Publishing, 1990.
5. Berkowitz, P., and N. Berkowitz, The Jewish Patient in the Hospital, *American Journal of Nursing*, 67, no. 11 (1967), 2335–2337.
6. Butler, R., The Roman Catholic Way in Death and Mourning. In Grollman, E., ed., *Concerning Death: A Practical Guide for the Living*. Boston: Beacon Press, 1974, pp. 101–118.
7. Buys, A., Discussion Series Sensitizes Nurses to Patient's Spiritual Needs, *Hospital Progress*, 62 (October 1981), 44–45.
8. Caillat, C., Jainism. In Eliade, Mircea, ed., *The Encyclopedia of Religion*, 7. New York: Macmillan, 1987, pp. 507–514.
9. Campbell, T., and B. Chang, Health Care of the Chinese in America, *Nursing Outlook*, 21, no. 4 (1973), 245–249.
10. Campinha-Bacote, J., Voodoo Illness, *Perspectives in Psychiatric Care*, 28, no. 1 (1982), 11–12.
11. Carpenito, L., *Handbook of Nursing Diagnosis* (4th ed.). Philadelphia: J.B. Lippincott, 1991, pp. 264–267.
12. Carson, V., Meeting the Spiritual Needs of Hospitalized Psychiatric Patients, *Perspectives in Psychiatric Care*, 18, no. 1 (1980), 17–20.
13. ——, et al., The Effect of Didactic Teaching on Spiritual Attitudes, *Image: Journal of Nursing Scholarship*, 18, no. 4 (1986), 161–164.
14. Case, R., We Let Our Son Die, *Journal of Christian Nursing*, 4, no. 2 (1987), 4–8.
15. Clark, C.C., et al., Spirituality: Integral to Quality Care, *Holistic Nursing Practice*, 5, no. 3 (1991), 67–76.
16. Coles, R., *The Spiritual Life of Children*. Boston: Houghton Mifflin. 1991.
17. Conrad, N.L., Spiritual Support for the Dying, *Nursing Clinics of North America*, 20, no. 2 (1985), 415–426.
18. Davies, A.P., *The Unitarian Faith*. Washington DC: A. Powell Davies Memorial Committee, 1979.
19. Davis, R., Protect Your Family From Cults, *Home Life* (April 1991), 32–34.
20. Davis, T., The Truth about the Mormon Family, *Home Life* (May 1991), 48–49.
21. DeVol, T., Ecstatic Pentecostal Prayer and Meditation, *Journal of Religion and Health*, 13, no. 4 (1974), 285–288.
22. Dieter, M.E., The Gospel and New Age Thought, *Vital Christianity*, 111, no. 7 (1991), 27.
23. Dixon, D., *World Religions for the Classroom*. West Mystic, Conn: Twenty-Third Publications, 1975.
24. Dobmeier, T., Professionalizing Spiritual Care, *Journal of Christian Nursing*, 1, no. 2 (1990), 32.
25. Donley, Sr. R., Spiritual Dimensions of Health Care: Nursing's Mission, *Nursing and Health Care*, 12, no. 4 (1991), 178–183.
26. Eck, D., *Roots in Who Are They?* Los Angeles: The Bhaktivedanta Book Trust, 1982.
27. Eich W., When is Emergency Baptism Appropriate?, *American Journal of Nursing*, 87, no. 12 (1987), 1680–1681.
28. Eickhoff, A., The Chaplain-Nurse Relationship, *Nursing Management*, 13, no. 3 (1982), 25–26.
29. Ellis, D., Whatever Happened to the Spiritual Dimension? *The Canadian Nurse* (September 1980), 42–43.
30. Enroth, R., *Youth, Brainwashing, and the Extremist Cults*. Grand Rapids, Mich: Zondervan Publishing House, 1977.
31. Fleeger, R., and J. Van Heukelein, The Patient's Spiritual Needs—A Part of Nursing Diagnosis, *The Nurses Lamp*, 28, no. 4 (1977).
32. Gibney, F., Jr., Ritual Murder in Mexico, *Newsweek* (April 24, 1989), 55.
33. Glustrom, S., *When Your Child Asks: A Handbook for Jewish Parents*, (rev. ed.). New York: Bloch Publishing, 1991.
34. Gordon, A. The Jewish View of Death: Guidelines for Mourning. In Kubler-Ross, E., ed., *Death, the Final Stage of Growth*. Englewood Cliffs, NJ: Prentice-Hall, 1975, pp. 44–51.

35. Guoli, G., Zorastrianism. In Eliade, M., ed., *The Encyclopedia of Religion,* 15th ed. New York: Macmillan, 1987, pp. 579–591.

36. Gurka, A., How Did Anne Help? *Journal of Christian Nursing,* 6, no. 5 (1991), 23.

37. Hackney, E.J., personal letter on Zen Buddhism, January 19, 1973.

38. Hauerwas, S., *Nursing the Silences: God, Medicine, and the Problem of Suffering.* Grand Rapids, Mich: Eerdman's Publishing, 1990.

39. Hensley, D.E., Old or New? Understanding the New Age Movement, *Vital Christianity,* 111, no. 7 (1991), 21–23.

40. Hillard, J.R., Diagnosis and Treatment of the Rootwork Victim, *Psychiatric Annals,* 12, no. 7 (1982), 709–714.

41. Hover, M., If a Patient Asks You to Pray With Him, *RN* (April, 1986), 17–18.

42. Hultkrantz, A., North American Religions: An Overview. In Eliade, M., ed., *The Encyclopedia of Religion,* 10. New York: Macmillan, 1987, pp. 526–535.

43. Impoco, J., Japanese Religious Group Changing, *Hickory Daily Record,* December 16, 1987, Sec. D, p. 13.

44. Jordan, M., The Protestant Way in Death and Mourning. In Grollman, E., ed., *Concerning Death: A Practical Guide for Living.* Boston: Beacon Press, 1974, pp. 81–100.

45. Jorgensen, J.G., Modern Movements. In Eliade, M., ed., *The Encyclopedia of Religion,* 10. New York: Macmillan, 1987, pp. 541–544.

46. Karns, P.S., Building a Foundation for Spiritual Care, *Journal of Christian Nursing,* 6, no. 5 (1991), 11–13.

47. Kepler, M., The Religious Factor in Pediatric Care, *Clinical Pediatrics,* 9, no. 3 (1970), 128–130.

48. ———, Human Values in Medicine: Some Helping Organizations, *Journal of the American Medical Association,* 15, no. 3 (1973), 305–307.

49. Kertzer, M., *What Is a Jew?* (rev. ed.). New York: Macmillan, 1969.

50. Kushner, H., *When Bad Things Happen to Good People,* New York: Schocken Books, 1989.

51. Lang, B., The Death that Ends Death in Hinduism and Buddhism. In Kubler-Ross, E., ed., *Death, The Final Stage of Growth.* Englewood Cliffs, NJ: Prentice-Hall, 1975, pp. 52–57.

52. Lex, B., Voodoo Death: New Thoughts on an Old Explanation, *American Anthropologist,* 76 (1974), 819–823.

53. Life After Death? "Beyond Shadow of Doubt," Psychiatrist Says, *St. Louis Globe-Democrat,* November 15–16, 1975, Sec. A, p. 15.

54. Luna, L.J., Transcultural Nursing Care of Arab Muslims, *Journal of Transcultural Nursing,* 1, no. 1 (1989), 22–26.

55. Marshall, G., Growing up in Krishna, *Parade: St. Louis Post-Dispatch,* February 24, 1980, pp. 4–10.

56. Martin, J., A Home Health Aide Responds: Seek Understanding, *Journal of Christian Nursing,* 4, no. 2 (1987), 10–16.

57. Marty, M.E., Native Americans, *Christian Churches in the United States,* 1985, pp. 114–115.

58. Masulis, K., When Parents Refuse Treatment for Their Children, *Journal of Christian Nursing,* 4, no. 2 (1987), 10–16.

59. McConkie, B.R., *Mormon Doctrine.* Salt Lake City: Bookcraft, 1966.

60. McGilloway, O., and F. Myco, eds., *Nursing and Spiritual Care.* London: Harper & Row, 1985.

61. McIntyre, S., Ritual as Spiritual Practice, *Woman of Power,* 19 (Winter 1991), 19–21.

62. Mead, F., *Handbook of Denominations in the United States* (8th ed.). Nashville: Abingdon Press, 1985.

63. Melton, J.G., *The Encyclopedia of American Religions,* I & II. Wilmington, NC: McGrath, 1978.

64. Moody, R., *Life After Life.* New York: Bantam Books, 1976.

65. Munley, A., *The Hospice Alternative: A New Context for Death and Dying.* New York: Basic Books, 1983.

66. O'Driscoll, P., Muslims Fight Stereotypes of Their Faith, *USA Today* (April 7, 1989), 1–2.

67. Okamoto, A., Religious Barriers to World Peace, *Journal of Religion and Health,* 15, no. 1 (1976), 26–33.

68. Olson, M., The Out-of-Body Experience and Other States of Conscious, *Archives of Psychiatric Nursing,* 1, no. 3 (1987), 201–207.

69. Papovitz, L., Life/Death/Life, *American Journal of Nursing,* 86, no. 4 (1986) 416–418.

70. Peck, M.L., The Therapeutic Effect of Faith, *Nursing Forum,* 20 (1981), 2153–2166.

71. Penrose, V., et al., Spiritual Need in Sickness: I Lack Myself, *Nursing Mirror,* 154 (March 10, 1982), 38–39.

72. Petersen, M., *A World of Wisdom.* Salt Lake City: Church of Jesus Christ of Latter-Day Saints, n.d.

73. Peterson, E., and K. Nelson, How to Meet Your Client's Spiritual Needs, *Journal of Psychosocial Nursing,* 25, no. 5 (1987), 35–39.

74. Piles, C., Providing Spiritual Care, *Nurse Educator,* 15, no. 1 (1990), 36–41.

75. Piles, C., Putting Spiritual Care into the Curriculum, *Journal of Christian Nursing,* 6, no. 3 (1989), 18–21.

76. Pill, R., The Christian Science Practitioner, *Journal of Pastoral Counseling,* 4, no. 1 (1969), 39–42.

77. Porath, T., Humanizing the Sacrament of the Sick, *Hospital Progress,* 53, no. 7 (1972), 45–47.

78. Reed, P.G., Spirituality and Mental Health in Older Adults: Extant Knowledge for Nursing, *Family and Community Health,* 14, no. 2 (1991), 14–25.

79. Religious Cults and the Elderly, *Information on Aging.* Institute of Gerontology at Wayne State University, Michigan, July 1982, p. 2.

80. Repass, D.D., Stolen Words, *Vital Christianity,* 11, no. 7 (1991), 29.

81. Richards, L., *A Marvelous Work and a Wonder.* Salt Lake City: Deseret Book Company, 1975.

82. Roberts, O., *A Daily Guide to Miracles.* Tulsa: Pinoak Publications, 1975.

83. Rosten, L., ed., *Religions of America* (rev. ed.). New York: Simon & Schuster, 1975.

84. Rush, B., Healing A Hidden Grief, *Journal of Christian Nursing,* 3, no. 2 (Summer 1986), 10.

85. Russell, D.L., personal letter on Christian Science beliefs and practices, December 1, 1975.

86. Ryan, J., The Neglected Crisis, *American Journal of Nursing,* 84, no. 10 (1984), 1257–1258.

87. Sachen, K.L., and V.J. Carson, Responding to the Spiritual Needs of the Chronically Ill, *Nursing Clinics of North America,* 22, no. 3 (1987), 603–611.

88. Salladay, S.A., World Views Apart: Nursing Practice and

New Age Therapies, *Journal of Christian Nursing,* 6, no. 4 (1991), 15–18.

89. Satprakashananda, S., ed., *The Use of Symbols in Religion.* St. Louis: The Vedanta Society, 1970.

90. Saunders, E.D., *Buddhism in Japan.* Philadelphia: University of Philadelphia Press, 1964, pp. 265–286.

91. Schroeder, J.A., Towards a Feminist Eucharistic Theology and Piety, *Dialog,* no. 30 (Summer 1991), 221–226.

92. Schutzius, M.J., Missing Voices of Women in our Church, *Probe,* 25, no. 4 (1987), 1.

93. Seamonds, D., Healing of Memories: What Is It? Is It Biblical? *Journal of Christian Nursing,* 3, no. 2 (Summer 1986), 4–9.

94. Shannon, M., Spiritual Needs and Nursing Responsibility, *Imprint,* 27 (December 1980), 23. .

95. Shelly, J.A., *Spiritual Care Workbook.* Downer's Grove, Ill: Inter-Varsity Press, 1978.

96. ——, *The Spiritual Needs of Children: A Guide for Nurses, Parents and Teachers.* Downer's Grove, Ill: Inter-Varsity Press, 1982.

97. ——, and S.D. John, *Spiritual Dimensions of Mental Health.* Downer's Grove, Ill: Inter-Varsity Press, 1983.

98. ——, and S. Fish *Spiritual Care: The Nurses Role* (3rd ed.), Downer's Grove, Ill:Inter-Varsity Press, 1988.

99. Singh, K., Sikhism. In Eliade, M., ed., *The Encyclopedia of Religion,* 13. New York: Macmillan, 1987, pp. 315–320.

100. Slimmer, L., Helping Students to Resolve Conflicts Between Their Religious Beliefs and Psychiatric-Mental Health Treatment Approaches, *Journal of Psychiatric Nursing and Mental Health Services,* 18 (July 1980), 37–39.

101. Sloat, D.E., Why Can't I Relate to God? *Journal of Christian Nursing,* 6, no. 6 (1988), 11–15.

102. Smedes, L., *Caring and Commitment.* San Francisco: Harper & Row, 1988.

103. Smith, H., *The Religions of Man.* New York: Harper & Row, 1965.

104. Stafford, T., The Hidden Gospel of the 12 Steps, *Christianity Today,* 35, no. 8 (1991), 14–19.

105. Stroll, R., Guidelines for Spiritual Assessment, *American Journal of Nursing,* 79, no. 9 (1979), 1574–1577.

106. Suzuki, D.T., E. Fromm, and R. DeMartino, *Zen Buddhism and Psychoanalysis.* New York: Grove Press, 1960, p. 5.

107. Tawless, J., Visualizing the Healer, *Journal of Christian Nursing,* 3, no. 2(Summer 1986), 12–14.

108. Those Who Preserve the Ritual Bath, *St. Louis Post-Dispatch,* January 9, 1977, Sec. H, p. 3.

109. Tinney, J.S., Black Muslims, *Christianity Today,* 20 (March 12, 1976), 51–52.

110. Ujhely, G., On Being Possessed by the Devil, *Perspectives in Psychiatric Care,* 10, no. 5 (1972), 202–209.

111. *Unity School of Christianity.* Unity Village, Mo: Unity School of Christianity, n.d.

112. Utt, R., *The Builders: A Photo Story of Seventh-Day Adventists at Work Around the World.* Mountain View, Cal: Pacific Press Publishing Association, 1970.

113. Walker, H.B., Why Medicine Needs Religion, *International Surgery,* 56, no. 8 (1971), 37B–40B.

114. Wasson, E., personal letter and paper from Christian Science Committee on Publication for Missouri, January 8, 1973.

115. Wilson, J., *Religion in American Society.* Englewood Cliffs, NJ: Prentice-Hall, 1981.

116. Wood, V., personal letter on Religious Society of Friends, January 29, 1973.

117. Yep, J., An Asian Patient: How Does Culture Affect Care? *Journal of Christian Nursing,* 6, no. 5 (1991), 6–9.

PERSONAL INTERVIEWS

118. Andrews, C., pastor, St. Nicholas Greek Orthodox Church, St. Louis, January 26, 1973.

119. Bregman, A., rabbi, Temple Israel, St. Louis, January 27, 1973.

120. Crump, R., pastor, Rock Hill Church of God, St. Louis, January 30, 1973.

121. Danker, W., professor of world mission, Concordia Seminary, St. Louis, January 26, 1973.

122. Dickes, H., a seventy in the Church of Jesus Christ of Latter-Day Saints, St. Louis, January 20, 1973.

123. Duvall, E., R.N., M.S.N., Instructor, Burge School of Nursing, Springfield, Mo., September 19, 1992.

124. Gowing, P., regional professor, southeast Asia, Graduate School of Theology, Singapore, January 10, 1973.

125. Griswell, J., pastor, Seventh-Day Adventist Central Church, St. Louis, January 31, 1973.

126. Guirguis, Y., and L. Guirguis, Egyptian Christians, January 13, 1973.

127. Katsarus, G., Greek Orthodox, January 19, 1973.

128. Khalifa, S., S. Eltoumi, E.Z. Eltoumi, M. Ahmed, and F. Ahmed, Egyptian Muslims, January 13, 1973.

129. Kimelman, Dr. N., Mrs. N. Kimelman, Dr. H.G. Mellman, and J. Tarlow, American Jews, January 29 and February 2, 1973.

Part II

Basic Concepts Related to the Developing Person and Family Unit

Chapter 4

The Family: Basic Unit for the Developing Person

The American family does not exist. Rather, we are creating many American families of diverse styles and shapes.
—J. Footlick

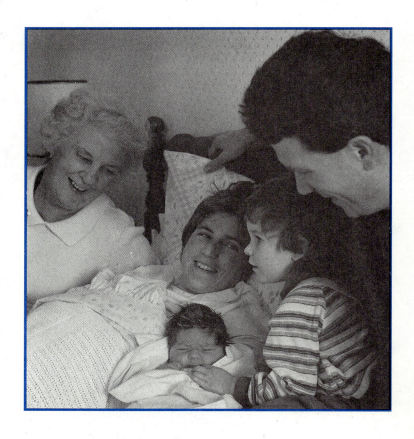

KEY TERMS

Family	Stepfamily	Social functions	Disengagement stage
Compadrazgo	Patrifocal/Patriarchal family	Personality	Family interaction
Padrinazgo	Matrifocal/Matriarchal family	Adaptive responses in the family	Dyads
Compadre	Roles	Establishment stage	Single-parent family
Nuclear family	Physical functions	Expectant stage	Stepfamily
Extended family	Affectional functions	Couvade syndrome	Stepgeneration parents
Single-parent family		Parenthood stage	Family cultural pattern

OBJECTIVES

Study of this chapter will enable you to:

1. Define *family* and discuss the family as a system and the implications for the developing person.
2. Summarize theoretic approaches for studying the family.
3. Describe the purposes, tasks, roles, and functions of the family and their relationship to the development and health of its members.
4. Describe family adaptive mechanisms and their purposes.
5. List stages of family life and developmental tasks for the establishment, expectancy, parenthood, and disengagement phases.
6. Discuss your role in helping the family achieve its developmental tasks.
7. Relate the impact of feelings about the self and childhood experiences on later family interaction patterns.
8. List and describe the variables affecting the relationship between parent and child and general family interaction, including single-parent, stepparent, and adoptive families.
9. Identify ways in which your family life has influenced your present attitudes about family.
10. Discuss the influence of twentieth-century changes on family life and childrearing practices.
11. Predict how a changing culture may affect the development and health of the family system.
12. Explore your role in promoting physical and emotional health of a family and assess community services that might assist you.
13. Assess and work with a family to enhance its welfare while simultaneously giving health care to one of its members.

It's an uncanny feeling—to suddenly know that I am answering my son's question with the same words—even the same tone—as my father used with me 30 years ago.

Even though I have a happy, successful marriage, two loving children, a nice home, and a profession in which I feel competent, I constantly fight a feeling of inferiority. A contributing factor must be that my parents never encouraged or complimented me. When I took a test, they emphasized the 2 wrong, not the 98 right.

I always admired my aunt. If my cousin, her son, had told her he wanted to build a bridge to the moon, she would have furnished the nails.

These three people are speaking of aspects of a social and biological phenomenon that is often taken for granted: the family. So strongly can this basic unit affect our development and health that we may live successfully or unsuccessfully because of its influence. Much that the person learns about loving, coping, and the various aspects of life is first learned in the family unit.

Between society and the individual person, the family exists as a primary system and social group, for most people share many of life's experiences with the family. Thus the family has a major role in shaping the person; it is a basic unit of growth, experience, adaptation, health, or illness.

The traditional family persists as a norm in the imagination, but today norms hardly exist with the fragility of marriage, the high incidence of divorce (and remarriage), the many styles of family life, the diversity of roles held by members, and the increasing number of homeless families. Thus today's children are being shaped differently—sometimes negatively—by the family unit. For many youngsters, the pain of family life, a changing family scene, having no permanent home, and being separated from other family members is compounded by poverty and neglect.

This chapter is not an exhaustive study of families or family life. Rather, it is an overview of the various forms, stages, and functions of contemporary American families and of how nursing can use this knowledge. Although various aspects of the family are discussed separately, keep in mind that family purposes, stages of development, developmental tasks, and patterns of interaction are all closely interrelated, all influenced by historical foundations, and all continually evolving into new forms. Thus the family should be viewed as a system, affected by the culture, the environment, religious-spiritual dimensions, and other variables, which in turn affects the person and society.

DEFINITIONS

Family

The **family** *is a small social system and primary reference group made up of two or more persons living together who are related by blood, marriage, or adoption or who are living together by agreement over a period of time.* The family unit is *characterized by face-to-face contact, bonds of affection, love, loyalty, emotional and financial commitment, harmony, simultaneous competition and mutual concern, a continuity of past, present, and future, shared goals and identity, and behaviors and rituals common only to the specific unit* (5, 54, 57).

The **family** may also be defined as *domestic partners, people who have chosen to share each other's life in an intimate and committed relationship of mutual caring.* This definition permits the extension of legal benefits usually accorded traditionally married heterosexuals such as health and life insurance and pension benefits, property rights, hospital and prison visitation rights, and bereavement leave to homosexual or same-gender families or unmarried partners. Family may be defined differently by different cultures. For example, **compadrazgo** *is a form of social alliance embedded in the Latino culture.* It involves family-type links with roots back to the feudal European days. Compadrazgo can be identified as follows:

1. It is a family kin tie, but it is *not biologically or legally ascribed.* Once entered into, it assumes *dimensions of affection and responsibility similar to that of a family.*
2. It *has a ritualistic aspect;* the relationship is initiated via a religious blessing.
3. It is *coparenthood* in contrast to **padrinazgo** (*godparent*), *with a relationship like parent, grandparent, aunt, and sister.* Individuals call one another **compadre,** *a title imbued with great warm feeling and deep respect.* The relationship is only good, ideal, supportive, and caring.
4. *Caring in this relationship includes a reciprocity, expressed by gift giving, hospitality, economic aid, and assurance about assistance in the future* (27).

The family is a group whose members rely on each other for daily services. With the family, the person can usually let down his or her guard and be more himself or herself than with other people. The family is comprised of a household (or cluster of households) that persists over years or decades and that is characterized by value, role, and power structures; communication patterns; affective socialization, family coping, and health care functions; and developmental stages and tasks (34, 89). Internal and external structures exist in a family. *Internal structure* includes family composition, rank order, subsystems, and boundary. *External struc-*ture includes culture, religion, social class status and mobility, environment, and extended family. *Instrumental function* refers to how routine activities of daily living are handled. *Expressive function* refers to nonverbal and verbal communication patterns, problem solving roles, control aspects, beliefs, alliances, and coalitions (5).

Healthy families are characterized by (1) a sense of togetherness that promotes capacity for change; (2) a balance between mutual and independent action on the part of family members; (3) availability of nurturance and resources for growth and sustenance; (4) stability and integrity of structure; (5) adaptive functioning; and (6) mastery of developmental tasks leading to interdependence, progressive differentiation, and transformation to meet the requisites for survival of the system (74, 87).

Sometimes families live together daily. Sometimes the adult partners are employed in different geographic areas, or one member is hospitalized or in prison. They maintain contact by telephone, correspondence, and visits. In the two-career family the partners share the same residence on weekends or on a consistent basis. These families carry out their functions and characteristics in their own unique way.

In this stressful time families may have difficulty in maintaining these characteristics. Your support, teaching, and counseling may assist them in maintaining health.

Family Composition

The family takes several forms. It may be **nuclear** (*mother, father, child*), **extended** (*nuclear plus other relatives of either or both spouses live together*), **single parent** (*mother or father, living with either biologic or adopted children, but not tied legally or emotionally to a partner*), or **step-** (*one divorced or widowed adult with all or some of his or her children and a new spouse with all or some of his or her children, plus children born to this union so that parents, stepparents, children, and stepchildren live together*). Any of these family structures may be **patrifocal** or **patriarchal** (*the man has the main authority and decision-making power*) or **matrifocal** or **matriarchal** (*the woman has the main authority*). Or the family may comprise a childless couple; siblings, especially in middle or late life; friends in a commune; or a man and woman living together without being married, with or without children. The family may be **same-gender** or **homosexual,** either a **gay** or **lesbian** couple that is childless, has custody of and is caring for biologic children from a previous heterosexual marriage, or has adopted children that they consider their own. Alternately, one of the lesbian women may, through artificial insemination or one-time contact with a selected man, bear a child, and the other woman in the relationship also takes on the parenting role, clearly acknowledging that she is not the mother; or the gay couple may contract with a woman to carry a baby to term for them. Currently the homosexual who has had a biologic child more frequently is exerting custody, visiting, and caretaking rights and responsibilities with the child after establishment of the same-gender relationship. Various references describe the same-gender family (12, 13, 21, 35, 37, 43, 49, 58, 59, 84, 86).

The family may be *symbolically duplicated in the work setting:* a woman may be perceived as a grandmother, mother, or sister, or a man may be perceived as a grandfather, father, or brother to an employee. The family member who is no longer present because of divorce or who is dead or missing may remain clearly in the other members' memory; they may refer to the person on special occasions. Or the deviant of the family—the alcoholic or runaway—may influence other family members to act in an opposite manner.

The family may also be a *series of separate but interrelated families.* The middle-aged parents are helping the adolescent and young adult offspring to be emancipated from the home while simultaneously caring for increasingly dependent parents and sometimes up to four pairs of grandparents plus older aunts and uncles. All related family members may not live under the same roof (in fact, they never did in America), but the extended family exists psychologically—in spirit. Often the responsibility is nearly overwhelming to the middle-aged adults who may have little time or resources to spend on themselves. The conflict inherent in having to care for a number of relatives and in-laws can contribute to marital disharmony and poor relationships between the generations. The middle-aged person's caregiving role is discussed in Chapter 13.

The elderly person is sometimes aware of such a situation and will try to make minimum demands. Often he or she believes more attention is deserved and may make extra demands or chastise the middle-aged offspring for not doing more for elder family members.

A real entity is psychic life of the family; the *extended* family affects thoughts and actions, provides sustenance, and contributes to identity. Present day mobility of people, ease of communication over distance, freedom to evolve and think independently, freedom to develop in ways less restricted by strong or rigid ethnic or cultural mores, and ease of transportation allow families in the United States to be geographically distant yet emotionally close and often quite involved with each other—to the point of giving assistance.

The mass media presents a picture of family life dissolving in the United States. Although the divorce rate is approximately 50% to 70%, most divorced people remarry. Because of longer life expectancy and the young age at which people marry, the young couples of today enter and remain in marriage longer than did their grandparents. Family authorities estimate that the divorce rate, extremely high in the 1970s and early 1980s, may begin to decline by the 1990s. People are beginning to realize that divorce does not necessarily improve life; the allure of creativity, growth, and expanding oneself emotionally through divorce is not necessarily realistic. Some families speak of trying harder, resolving to stay committed to each other in conflictual times.

OVERVIEW OF FAMILY THEORETIC APPROACHES

Theoretic approaches to the study of families include developmental, structural-functional, interactional, and role theories. These approaches are summarized in Table 4–1. Refer to several references at the end of the chapter for more extensive explanation (1, 3, 34, 89, 96).

PURPOSES, TASKS, ROLES, AND FUNCTIONS OF THE FAMILY

Although the institution of the family is being scrutinized and predictions are made that it may pass into oblivion, the family has demonstrated throughout history that it is a virtually indestructible institution. Family structure, roles, and responsibilities have been influenced by technology and the resulting social changes. But technologic advances alone do not determine family structure and function. Family systems are endlessly adaptive and very resistant to outside pressure. In a society in which objects are often disposable and people feel uneasy and dispensable, individuals seek secure relationships. The family can be a source of security, although for some people it is not, with long-term detrimental consequences.

The U.S. family has passed through major transitions. The family was once a relatively self-contained, cohesive domestic work unit; it has become a group of persons dispersed among various educational and work settings. Various agencies have absorbed many purposes once handled solely by the family group. Schools educate; hospitals care for the sick; mortuaries prepare the dead for burial; churches give religious training; government and private organizations erect recreational facilities; nursing homes care for the aged; and various manufacturing firms bake, can, or bottle food and make clothes.

Purposes and Tasks of the Family

When the family changed from a production unit to a consumption unit, it also lost some degree of authority to regulate its members' behavior. The emphasis now is on democratic sharing, togetherness, the child's poten-

TABLE 4-1. SUMMARY OF FOUR FAMILY THEORIES AND APPROACHES

Family Theory	Definition of Family	View of Person	Approach/Focus
Developmental theory: compilation of several frameworks	Series of interacting personalities, intricately organized into paired positions (father, husband, daughter, sister); norms for reciprocal relations prescribe role behavior for each position; predictable natural history designated by stages	Person is a member of group; each new member adds to complexity of interaction.	**Study family** in terms of role behaviors for each family life-cycle stage, along with the changing ages of each person; study quality and type of interaction as age and member composition of family changes. **Focus:** Analyze developmental needs and tasks of each family life-cycle stage; analyze family behaviors and changing developmental tasks and role expectations in terms of increasing complexity, analyze children, parents, and family unit as a whole. Cultural influences at each stage of family life cycle are considered.
Structural-functional theory: focus on family as a system	Social system open to outside influences and transactions; maintains boundaries by responding to demands of system or acting under family constraints, passively adapting to external forces rather than acting as an agent of change in itself	Person is seen as reactive in fulfilling roles and as having status in the social system.	**Study family** in relation to other social structures or social systems and in terms of roles. **Focus:** Determine how family patterns are related to other institutions and overall society; study family functions (reproduction, socialization of children, provision of physical needs, economics).
Interactional theory: rejection of role theory and psychodynamic theory	Defined in terms of individual members, a unity of interacting personalities with assigned position and roles, expectations, and norms of behavior; seen as closed unit with little relationship to outside institutions, associations, or cultures	Person is seen as fulfilling roles and as an interacting being.	**Study family** in terms of overt interactions, fulfillment of interacting roles. **Focus:** Analyze roles, interstatus relations, authority matters, action-taking communication processes, conflicts, problem solving, decision making.

Role theory: life is structured according to roles that are ascribed or assumed by the person in interaction with others; roles are learned through socialization	Defined in terms of members' role interaction; roles contribute in the following way to the family unit:
	  Circumscribe behavior
	  Define social position, responses, expectations
	  Influence group associations
	  Are purpose of interaction
	  Provide norms for the family or group
		Person is seen in terms of roles, which are specialized or shared and depend on gender, age, social norms, status, complementarity. Roles change through development and negotiation, which depend on flexibility, stability, and congruence of expectations. Person experiences role reciprocity, complementarity, or strain.
		
		Role reciprocity—mutual exchange; sharing affects decision making and cohesion; personal and family needs met; high mutual dependence in division of labor; potential for growth; commitment to family and reducing conflict
		Role complementarity—family members differentiate and define roles in relation to each other; opportunity for growth; sometimes not a sense of mutual gratification; can confirm identity of one at expense of other; if rigid roles, transitions are difficult
			Study family in terms of role interactions, differentiation, allocation, role change, and role strain.
			Focus: Analyze role reciprocity, complementarity, and strain.

TABLE 4-1. SUMMARY OF FOUR FAMILY THEORIES AND APPROACHES (Continued)

Family Theory	Definition of Family	View of Person	Approach/Focus
Role theory (cont.)		*Role strain*—occurs when individuals have difficulty meeting others' or own expectations and the obligations of the role and is manifested as: 1. *Role conflict*—unclear, incomplete, contradictory elements in role; performing one role makes it impossible to perform another; conflicting norms 2. *Role overload*—must consider impact of distribution of power; the greater the control over negotiation of roles, the more person can avoid role strain; person with less power assumes more unwanted burdens; person with more power has less dependency needs and can make role demands	

tial as an individual, and the fun aspects of parenthood. Enjoyment and relaxation in every human relationship are considered important. Technology is seen as the reason for this view and the way to attain the happy state, but the person who believes too strongly in what technology can accomplish may have unrealistic expectations about living and thus undergo considerable stress in marriage and child-rearing.

Yet the family is still considered responsible for the child's growth and development and behavioral outcomes; indeed, the family is a cornerstone for the child's competency development. Because the family is strongly influenced by its surrounding environment and by the child itself, the family should not bear full blame for what the child is or becomes. Few parents deliberately set out to rear a disturbed, handicapped, or delinquent offspring, although such failures occur.

The family is expected to perform the following tasks. The tasks may be basically the same for most types of family composition, but how they are manifested often is related to the type of family structure: nuclear, extended, single-parent, same-gender, patrifocal, or matrifocal. Culture of the family group (racial, ethnic, geographic, socioeconomic, religious) also influences how the following tasks are achieved. *Basic tasks* are as follows:

1. Provide for physical safety and economic needs of its members and obtain enough goods, services, and resources to survive.
2. Create a sense of family loyalty and a mentally healthy environment for the family's well-being.
3. Help members to develop physically, emotionally, intellectually, and spiritually and to develop a personal and family identity.
4. Foster a value system built on spiritual and philosophical beliefs and the cultural and social system that is part of the identity.
5. Teach members social skills and to communicate effectively their needs, ideas, and feelings and to respect each other.
6. Provide social togetherness simultaneously with division of labor, patterning of sexual roles, and performance of family roles with flexibility and cooperation.
7. Reproduce and socialize the child(ren), inculcating values and appropriate behavior, providing adult role models, and fostering a positive self-concept and self-esteem in the child(ren).
8. Provide relationships and experience within and without the family that foster security, support, encouragement, motivation, morale, and creativity.
9. Help the members to cope with crises and societal demands; create a place for recuperation from external stresses.
10. Maintain authority and decision making, with the parents representing society to the family as a whole and the family unit to society.
11. Promote integration into society and the ability to use social organizations for special needs when necessary.
12. Release family members into the larger society—school, church, organizations, work, and politics.
13. Maintain constructive and responsible ties with the neighborhood, school, and local and state government (1, 5, 10, 29, 65).

The family often has difficulty in meeting these tasks and needs assistance from external resources. The family's ability to meet its tasks depends on the maturity of the adult members, the support given by the social system—nursing and health care, educational, work, religious, social, welfare, governmental, and leisure institutions. The family that is most successful as a unit has a working philosophy and value system that is understood and lived, uses healthy adaptive patterns most of the time, can ask for help and use the community services available, and develops linkages with nonfamily units and organizations (29).

Roles of the Family

The family apportions **roles,** *prescribed behaviors in a situation,* in a way similar to society at large (57). In society there are specialists who enforce laws, teach, practice medicine, and fight fires. In the family there are also such performance roles: breadwinner, homemaker, handyman (or handywoman), the expert, political advisor, chauffeur, and gardener. There are also emotional roles: leader, nurturer, sustainer, protection, healer, arbitrator, scapegoat, jester, rebel, dependent, "sexpot," and "black sheep." Members may fill more than one role. The fewer people there are to fulfill these roles, as in the nuclear family, the greater the number of demands placed on one person. If a member leaves home, someone else takes up his or her role. Any member of the family can satisfactorily fulfill any role in either category unless he or she is uncomfortable in that role. The man who is sure of his masculinity will have no emotional problems diapering a baby or cooking a meal. The woman who is sure of her femininity will have no trouble gardening or taking the car for repair. Today many men and women no longer are restricted to carrying out only traditional gender roles. They enjoy sharing roles, working together to get the tasks done without worrying about what is man's or woman's work.

The emotional response of a person to the role he or she fulfills should be considered. Someone may perform the job competently and yet dread doing it. The man may be a carpenter because his father taught him the trade, although he wants to be a music teacher. Changes in performance roles also necessitate emotional changes (e.g., in the man who takes over household duties when his wife becomes incapacitated).

The child learns about emotional response to roles in the family while imitating adults. The child experiments with various roles in play and eventually finds one that is emotionally comfortable. The more pressure put on the child by the parents to respond in a particular way, the more likely that child is to learn only one role and be uncomfortable in others, as evidenced by the athletic champion who may be a social misfit. The child becomes less adaptive socially and even within the family as a result.

Exercising a capacity for a variety of roles, either in actuality or in fantasy, is healthy. The healthy family is the one in which there is opportunity to shift roles inter-

mittently with ease (57). Through these roles family functions are fulfilled.

Functions of the Family as a Social System

The family is a system. It functions as a unit to fulfill its purposes, roles, and tasks. It provides shelter, stability, security, and a setting for nurturance and growth. It is a safe place to experiment with the dynamics and role behaviors required in a system. It has an energy that provides a support system for individual members. As the social system changes, the family system must also adapt if it is to meet individual needs and prepare its members to participate in the social system.

The organization of a family system is hierarchal, although it may not be directly observable. The usual family hierarchies are built on kinship, power, status, and privilege relationships that may be related to individual characteristics of age, sex, education, personality, health, strength, or vigor. We can infer a hierarchy by observing each person's behavior and communication. For instance, who talks first? Last? Longest? Who talks to whom? When? Where? About what? If one family member consistently approaches the staff about the client's health care, he or she probably holds an upper position in the family and has the task of being "expert." Your attempt to communicate with family members may meet with resistance if the communication inadvertently violates the family communication hierarchy (73).

Hierarchal relations in the family system determine the role behavior of family members. These hierarchal role relationships typically have great stability, and ordinarily family members can be counted on to behave congruently with their roles. When there are differences in behavior from situation to situation, they are almost inevitably in response to the family's expectations for that particular situation or circumstance (73). Families develop a system of balanced relationships. When one member leaves the family or experiences a change such as illness, other family members also must adapt. Roles and relationships are based on reciprocal interaction, with each member of the family contributing to the total unit in a unique and functional way. If a member should fail to meet the expectations of the roles established by his or her position in the hierarchy for the moment, the remaining members of the family generally react by using pressure (e.g., persuasion, punishment, argument, being ignored) on the "deviant" person (73). Ackerman (1) states that all family functions can be reduced to two basic ones: (1) ensuring the physical survival of the species and (2) transmitting the culture, thereby ensuring essential humanness. The union of mother and father, of parent and child, forms the bonds of identity that are the matrix for the development of this humanness.

Physical functions of the family are met by the parents' *providing food, clothing, and shelter, protection against danger, provision for bodily repairs after fatigue* *or illness, and reproduction.* In "primitive" societies these physical needs are the dominant concern. In Western societies many families take them for granted (1, 57).

Affectional functions are equally important. Although many traditional family functions such as education, job training, and medical care are being absorbed by other agencies, *meeting emotional needs and promoting adaptation and adjustment are still two of the family's major functions.* The family is the primary unit in which the child tests emotional reactions. Learning how to reach and maintain emotional equilibrium within the family enables him or her to repeat the pattern in later life situations. The child who feels loved is likely to contract fewer physical illnesses, learn more quickly, and generally have an easier time growing up and adapting to society (1, 57).

Satir (81) believes a healthy family has five dominant attitudes:

1. No distinctions are made about worth of people; all members are perceived as equal.
2. All persons are seen as unique and developing.
3. When a disturbing situation arises, members understand that many factors were involved—people were not simply trying to be difficult.
4. Members accept that change is continuous.
5. Members freely share their thoughts and feelings with a minimum of blame and feel good about each other and themselves.

Other important attitudes are:

1. The feeling of unity between man and woman and a separateness from their families of origins so that interfamily interference with the marriage is avoided
2. An ability to invest in the marriage to a greater degree than in other relationships
3. A feeling of balance or complementarity, for perfect equality is probably impossible
4. A movement from a romantic "falling in love" to a warm, loving, companionable, accepting relationship
5. An ability to maintain variety and frequent interactions with each other (81).

Social functions of the modern family include *providing social togetherness, fostering self-esteem and a personal identity tied to family identity, providing opportunities for observing and learning social and sexual roles, accepting responsibility for behavior, and supporting individual creativity and initiative.* The family actually begins the indoctrination of the infant into society when it bestows a name and hence a social position or status in relation to the immediate and kinship-group families. Simultaneously, each family begins to transmit its own version of the cultural heritage and its own family culture to the child. Because the culture is too vast and comprehensive to transmit to the child in its entirety and

all at once, the family selects what will be transmitted. In addition, the family interprets and evaluates what is transmitted. Through this process, the child learns to share family values (1, 5, 57).

Thus socialization is a primary task of the parents, for they teach the child about the body, peers, family, community, age-appropriate roles, language, perceptions, social values, and ethics. The family also teaches about the different standards of responsibility society demands from various social groups. For example, the professional person such as a physician, nurse, or lawyer, those in whom people confide and to whom they entrust their lives and fortunes, are held more accountable than the farmer or day laborer. There is also a difference in the type of contact that society has with a particular group: for example, the mail or milk deliverer does not enter the home, but the exterminator is free to enter a home and look into every corner.

The parent generation educates by literal instruction and by serving as models. Thus the child's **personality,** *a product of all the influences that have and are impinging on him or her,* is greatly influenced by the parents (54).

FAMILY ADAPTATION

Adaptive responses in the family represent the *means by which it maintains an internal equilibrium so that it can fulfill purposes and tasks, deal with stress and crisis, and allow for growth of individual members.* Some capacity for functioning may be sacrificed to control conflict and aid work as a unit. But the best functioning family keeps anxiety and conflict within tolerable limits and maintains a balance between effects of the past and new experiences. Just as other social systems adapt, so must the family system (34).

Ideally, the family achieves equilibrium by talking over problems and finding solutions together. Humor, nonsense, shared work, and leisure all help relieve tension. The family members know that certain freedoms exist within their confines that are not available elsewhere.

Successful and happy families define their most important priority as the spouse and the family; the business or career of both or either one of the partners comes second. Children may come second before the business or career; hobbies and volunteer activities are further removed priorities. Each spouse needs to serve as a comforter, listener, companion, and counselor to the other, to be supportive and fully committed, and to avoid being negative. That does not mean one person is a doormat, for each is supportive to the other. The spouses may wish to set aside one night a week, or a month, to be only with each other, sharing uninterrupted time and activity. Each parent may wish to have a day date with each child monthly, spending time together at lunch, shopping, or in some mutually favorite activity (83).

Yet even the most stable family will briefly use various adaptive mechanisms to cope with stress, which, in turn, promotes more stress. However, these mechanisms are not overused in healthy families (50, 57).

Adaptive Mechanisms in Family Life

Emotional conflicts in the family may be avoided, minimized, or resolved through scapegoating, coalitions, withdrawal of emotional ties, repetitive verbal or physical fighting, use of family myths, reaction formation, compromise, or designation of a family healer. Two or more of these mechanisms may be used within the same family. If these mechanisms are used exclusively, however, they become defensive and are unlikely to promote resolution of the conflict so that the same issue will arise repeatedly (50, 57).

Scapegoating or Blaming. Scapegoating or blaming involves labeling one member as the cause of the family trouble and is expressed in the attitude, "If it weren't for you. . . . " Or one member may offer himself or herself

as a scapegoat to end an argument by saying, "It's all my fault." Such labeling controls the conflict and reduces anxiety, but it prevents communication that can get at the root of the problem. Growth toward resolution of the problem is prohibited.

Coalitions or Alliances. Coalitions or alliances may form when some family members side together against other members. Antagonisms and anger result. Eventually the losing party tries to get control.

Withdrawal of Emotional Ties. Loosening the family unit and reducing communication may be used to handle conflict, but then the family becomes rigid and mechanized. Family members are also likely to seek affection outside the family so that the home becomes a hotel with everyone superficially nice. In some families there is no show of emotion, for such emotion signifies loss of control or giving in to unacceptable impulses.

Repetitive Fighting. Verbal abuse, physical battles, loud complaints, curses, or accusations may be used to relieve tension and allow some harmony until the next round. The fight may have the same theme each time stress hits the family. The healthy family allows some

---

Research Abstract

Friedemann, M., Families of Unemployed Workers: Need for Nursing Intervention and Prevention, Archives of Psychiatric Nursing, *1, no. 2 (1987), 81–89.*

Most research on unemployment has focused on the unemployed male, the family members' resultant depression, and the economic stress for the entire family. The framework for this study was the double ABCX Model of Coping with Family Stress: *A* is the stressor; *B* is existing resources; and *C* is the perception of the stressor, which interacts with *X,* the crisis. This model proposes a joint effort of the family in coping with unexpected happenings to restore family balance. If there are insufficient existing resources or if the family is dysfunctional in behavior patterns, the family system itself may induce new stress, which affects all family members negatively. The process by which stress is transferred to the child is unclear.

The purpose of this study was to determine how children suffer in families in which the father is unemployed and whether they are more vulnerable to emotional instability. It was hypothesized that if the family success in coping depends on quality of family relationships, social support, and various additional internal and external resources, parents who experience symptoms of severe family disruption may become depressed and unable to meet their child's needs. As a result, the child may become insecure and dependent, which would be observable in the child's interaction with peers.

The sample was 52 Caucasian, two-parent families from three school districts in southeastern Michigan, where the unemployment rate was 20%. All families had a child in kindergarten who was 5 or 6 years old (32 boys and 20 girls). The study procedure involved observing each child at play for 10 minutes, three different times, at 2-week intervals. Behavioral acts were divided into leader, follower, and loner

and were scored for peer acceptance or rejection. Parents were surveyed for depression and interviewed for information about family economics and coping methods.

Results indicated a relationship between peer acceptance and income setback. Children of families with high income setbacks scored lower in peer acceptance than families with less severe setbacks. Fathers with high financial stress and low incomes usually were more depressed than those from other families. The mother's depression score was not related to economic variables; her depression was lower if the mother had close friends. Depression scores were higher for couples with troubled marital relationships and families with high economic stress were more likely to have troubled marital relationships. Girls of depressed fathers had higher scores for leadership acts and lower scores for loner acts than other girls. The mother's depression had negligible effects on the girls or boys. Children from multiproblem families showed one or two behavior patterns in the peer groups: (1) quiet, withdrawn, short attention span, occasional daydreaming, and minimal involvement in play with low peer acceptance or (2) active and assertive play, leader role, director of the group, attention seeking from peers, with high peer acceptance. Children of relatively problemfree families were more relaxed in play and had one or several preferred friends. Often unemployed fathers spent more time playing with their children and enjoyed doing so.

Nurses should be aware of the effects of unemployment on children and the need for social support for mothers when the father is unemployed. Unemployment often leads to other problems; the total amount of stress a family experiences consists of the total of all existing stressors.

"blowing up" as release from everyday frustrations, but it does not make a major case out of every minor incident or temporary disagreement.

Family Myths or Traditional Beliefs. These myths or beliefs can be used to overcome anxieties and maintain control over others. Such statements are as follows: "Children are seen, not heard." "We can't survive if you leave home." "Talking about feelings will cause loss of love." In contrast, the healthy family members encourage growth and creativity rather than rigid control.

Reaction Formation. Reaction formation is seen in a family in which there is superficial harmony or togetherness. Traumatic ideas are repressed and transformed into the opposite behavior. Everybody smiles, but nobody loves. No one admits to having any difficulties. Great tension is felt because true feelings are not expressed.

Resignation or Compromise. Temporary harmony may occur when someone gives up or suppresses the need for assertion, affection, or emotional expression to keep peace. The surface calm eventually explodes when unmet needs can no longer be successfully suppressed.

Designation of One Person as Family Healer or Umpire. This mechanism involves using a "wise one" (most often in the extended family) or a minister, storekeeper, bartender, or druggist to arrange a reconciliation between dissenting parties. Part of the dynamics sometimes underlying the helper role is that the referee gets great satisfaction from finding someone worse off than self. The healer feels a sense of heightened self-esteem or omnipotence. A variant of the healer role is that of family "protector," who takes on all the stresses to save other members stress or conflict. One person ends up fighting the battles for everyone else in the family.

To remain adaptive, families maneuver to secure compliance of all members with the family rules through verbal and nonverbal communication to each other. Usually one member is designated as the one who must maintain a specific pattern of dependent behavior, sometimes negative or unhealthy, to keep all other family members comfortable. If the designated member tries to change behavior and become more independent, he or she receives no support. The feedback received is that he or she is disrupting the status quo and the other family members are uncomfortable. Thus sick behavior will be maintained at the expense of the development of the designated person and of the family.

Maladaptation

Signs of strained or destructive family relationships include:

1. Lack of understanding and communication between spouses
2. Each family member alternately acting as if the other did not exist or harassing through arguments
3. Lack of family decision making
4. Parents' possessiveness of the children or the mate
5. Children's derogatory remarks to parents or vice versa
6. Extreme closeness between husband and his mother or family or the wife and her mother or family
7. Parent being domineering about performance of household tasks
8. Few outside friends for parents or children
9. Scapegoating or blaming each other for difficulties
10. High level of anxiety or insecurity present in the home
11. Lack of creativity
12. Pattern of immature or regressive behavior in parents or children. (5, 34, 93)

You may find yourself in the role of family healer. Help the family to develop harmonious ways of coping and avoid the protector or omnipotent role. The text by Kramer (50) gives in-depth information pertinent to assessment of and intervention with families.

STAGES OF FAMILY DEVELOPMENT

Like an individual, the family has a developmental history marked by predictable crises. The developmental crises are normal, but they are also disturbing or frightening because each life stage is a new experience. The natural history of the family is on a continuum: from marriage or cohabitation; choosing whether to have children; rearing biologic or adoptive offspring, if any; and releasing children into society to establish homes of their own. In later life the aging parent or grandparents are a couple once again, barring divorce or death. The nurturing of spouse or children goes on simultaneously with a multitude of other activities: work at a job or profession, managing a household, participation in church and community groups, pursuit of leisure and hobbies, maintaining friendships and family ties. Or the person may decide to remain single but live with a person of the same or opposite sex; then the purposes, tasks, and roles of family life must also be worked out.

Initial or Establishment Stage

Courtship and engagement precede establishment of the family unit. Developmental tasks to accomplish during this courtship period include contending with partner-selection pressures from parents; giving over autonomy while retaining some independence; preparing for marriage, including a mutually satisfying sex life; and becoming free of parental domination. In the **establishment stage,** *the couple establishes a home of its own; main psychologic tie is no longer with family of orientation (parental family).* They commit themselves to living together, usually through marriage. (Readiness for marriage in U.S. society is discussed in relation to young adulthood in Chapter 12.) They must work out patterns of communication, daily living, sexual relations, a budget, and a philosophy of life. Relationships with family and friends are also different after marriage and must be worked out (29, 60, 93).

Today families may choose to have no children, one child and adopt others, or have two or three children instead of a larger family. Some women believe that motherhood is not necessary for fulfillment. Certainly the man's chief fulfillment is not necessarily from fatherhood. Some people are wise enough to know that children do not automatically bring happiness to a marriage. Children bring happiness to parents who want them and who are selfless enough to become involved in the adventure of rearing them. Children bring trauma to a troubled marriage.

Limitation of family size and birth spacing yield substantial family health benefits. Certain associations in death, disease, and disability are apparent. Maternal deaths increase when maternal age is below 20 or above 40 years and after the third pregnancy for women of all age groups except those over 40. Increased maternal disease, obstetric complications, maternal deaths, and postnatal mortality occur with six or more pregnancies. Unwanted pregnancy increases maternal disease and death, especially if the pregnancy is terminated by abortion that results in infection or hemorrhage. Other effects of unwanted pregnancy include excessive nausea and vomiting, spontaneous abortion, toxemias, complications of labor and delivery, emotional illness prenatally or postnatally, marital friction, and divorce. Infant mortality rate increases for birth order above three in the lower social class and rises among women under 17 years of age. The safest years for a normal delivery are between ages 20 and 29. Infants of youngest mothers of highest parity are at greatest risk for disease and death regardless of social class. Mothers are less likely to have premature or low-birthweight infants and therefore healthier infants when spacing is greater than 2 years but less than 6 years (85).

The establishment phase ends when the woman becomes pregnant or when the couple works out its living patterns and philosophy of life (which may include a decision not to have children).

Expectant Stage

During the **expectant stage,** or *pregnancy,* which is a developmental crisis, many domestic and social adjustments must be made. The couple (or the single mother and her significant other) is learning new roles and gaining new status in the community. Attitudes toward pregnancy and the physical and emotional status of the mother and father (and of significant others) will affect parenting abilities. Now the couple thinks in terms of family instead of a pair. They explore beliefs about

childrearing and plan for the expanded family in terms of space, budget, and necessary supplies (29).

The woman may initially dislike being pregnant because it interferes with her personal plans, or she may feel proud and fulfilled. Sexual desire may either increase or decrease. She may be more or less interested in her surroundings. Usually she is more preoccupied with herself, her new feelings, and changing body image, and she experiences fantasies and fears about the baby and the childbirth experiences.

The man experiences a variety of feelings on learning of the pregnancy, feelings that change during the pregnancy. The reality of the pregnancy increases with time. One study showed that 70% of the men experienced ambivalent feelings initially, but fatherly feelings developed. The men also felt guilty about the wife's pregnancy and her physical symptoms, anxious and depressed about their own adequacy, proud of their virility, and fearful of approaching the wife sexually. Concerns identified by fathers were as follows: caring for the infant, adequacy as a father, financial security, and concern related to the baby's effect on the marital dyad (45, 52, 54, 56).

Early and thorough prenatal care for the woman is essential. Both the woman and the man may experience similar physical and emotional symptoms such as nausea, indigestion, backache, distention, irritability, and depression. Symptoms may result from hormonal changes or feelings about the pregnancy in the woman. In the man they are part of the **couvade syndrome,** *which may be a reaction based on identification with or sympathy for the woman, ambivalence or hostility toward the pregnancy, or envy of the woman's childbearing ability.* The symptoms of couvade syndrome are (1) symbolically a means for the father to participate in the client's development and birth, (2) an early indication of interactions that will continue with the child, and (3) a means of affording the pregnant woman and new infant protection (22, 38, 45). The physical symptoms, complex feelings, and changes in body image that accompany pregnancy are described by several authors (22, 24, 46, 67, 78, 79, 85).

Major decisions for the couple are whether to attend childbirth preparation classes and whether the man should be present in the labor and delivery rooms. The woman may feel eager to have the man with her, or she may fear that he will think of her as sexually unattractive or be repulsed. The man may be curious about what is happening and want to attend his child's birth, or he may feel guilty about not wanting to when he feels others expect him to be there. He may be embarrassed about his wife's behavior and appearance during labor and delivery, or he may fear that he cannot cope with the childbirth event if present. Sexual fantasies triggered by labor and delivery may threaten the man who has tenuous emotional equilibrium. If the man has considerable unconscious conflicts or a weak self-image as a man, he may wish not to be involved in childbirth preparation, labor, or delivery. Some men and women cannot participate in childbirth preparation classes and should not be made to feel guilty about their decision. Participation may not enhance the couple's self-esteem and may create additional emotional crisis. Participation in Lamaze classes and childbirth does not change the woman's perception of her partner as ideal man, husband, or father, but it does improve her self-image as ideal woman, wife, and mother (45). In addition, the woman more likely will be in good physical condition for labor if she has had preparation.

Although the woman needs extra "mothering" from the partner (or others) during pregnancy, the man also needs extra attention and nurturing or he may be unable to continue to support the mother-to-be emotionally (45). You can listen to the woman's and man's concerns and help them understand that what they are experiencing is normal. Various teaching aids explaining pregnancy and what to expect during the birth experience are also useful. Your care should be family centered, directed toward both parents-to-be. You can help the woman to gain maternal feelings and the man to see the importance of his role as provider and nurturer.

The man must be prepared for fathering just as the woman is for mothering. Fathers also go through the five operations (mimicry, role play, fantasy, introjection-projection-rejection, and grief work) identified by Rubin (78) as necessary to attain the maternal role.

For additional information about prenatal influences on the mother and baby, see Chapters 6 and 7. Information about parenting and developmental tasks for the expectancy phase is also presented in Chapter 12. Several authors give further information on the fathers' reactions and responsibilities (42, 52, 54, 56, 85).

The family that prepares for adoption of a child does not have the tasks associated with the physical aspects of pregnancy, but it does have to accomplish the other tasks of readiness.

Parenthood or Expansion Stage

In the **parenthood or expansion stage,** there is *birth or adoption of a child,* and the couple assumes a status that it will never lose as long as each has memory and life—that of parent. The *stages of parenthood* are:

1. Anticipatory stage. The woman is pregnant, and the couple is learning the new roles and perceptions associated with pregnancy discussed earlier.
2. Honeymoon stage—the time following birth when the parents feel excited about the new relationship but also uncertain about the meaning of parental love. A parent-child attachment is being formed. During this time difficult adjustments must be made. Because the parents lose sleep, husband-wife intimacy diminishes, and there is less freedom for the couple to follow their own interests.
3. Plateau or consolidation stage—the years during the child's development when the parents are active in the role of mother and father. During this time the parents deal with problems in the family, community, church, school and immediate social sphere. They are concerned with family planning, socialization and education of the child, and participating in community organizations.
4. Disengagement or contraction stage—the termination of the parent-child family unit that occurs when the last child marries or leaves home permanently and the parents let go of their major childrearing responsibilities to allow the offspring to be autonomous (76, 77).

Americans value creativity and individuality; thus no set patterns of parenthood exist. Parents rely on their own uniqueness, wisdom, and skills, how their parents raised them, or on books. Youth are poorly prepared to make the transition to parenthood. Yet how parents treat a child is the single most important influence on the child's physical, emotional, and cognitive development and health.

The couple may accept the idea of parenthood but reject a particular child because of the child's sex, appearance, time of the birth in their life cycle, or the child's threatening helplessness; or the couple may reject the idea of parenthood but genuinely love the baby who was unplanned. Often parents have difficulty because pregnancy, childbirth, and parenting are romanticized in our society, and the romantic ideal differs considerably from the reality of 24-hour responsibility and submersion of their personal desires for many years to come.

How the parents care for and discipline the child is influenced considerably by the parents' own maturity; how they were cared for as children (as shown by studies on child abuse); their feelings about self; culture, social class, and religion (see Chapters 1 and 3); their relationship with each other; their perceptions of and experiences with children and other adults; their values and philosophy of life; and life stresses that arise. Moreover, the historical eras in which the parents were reared and in which they are now living and the prominent social values of each era subtly influence parental behavior.

Each critical period in the child's development reactivates a critical period in the parent. Demands made on the parent vary with the age of the child. The infant needs almost total and constant nurturance. Some parents thrive during this period and depend on each other for support. Other parents feel overwhelmed by the infant's dependency because their own dependent needs are stimulated but unmet. The baby's cry and behavior evoke feelings of helplessness, dependency, and anger associated with their unacceptable dependency needs and feelings and then guilt and fatigue. The toddler struggles with individuality and autonomy, exploring and vacillating between dependency and independency. At this stage the child is intense and often unreasonable in demands and refusal to obey commands. The parents may enjoy this explorative, independent behavior of the child, even though the toddler leaves the parent feeling tired and frustrated; or the primitive behavior of the child may stimulate primitive impulses in the parent, who may feel threatened by the will of the toddler. The parent who has difficulty controlling angry impulses may find the toddler's temper outbursts totally unacceptable. Parents who have difficulty caring for the dependent infant may do very well with the independent preschooler or adolescent, or the reverse may be true. The parent may be able to resolve personal conflicts and move to a more advanced level of integration as he or she works with the developing child, or the parent may be unable to cope with the aroused feelings (7).

Some parents believe that they must possess a child and will try to fit that child into a mold—their image. Other parents see their task of parenthood as stewards—to be a guide, a helping friend, a standard setter for the child. They invest themselves in the creative potentialities of their young—nurturing, educating, and protecting the child. They love but do not smother; guide but do not control; discipline but do not punish; offer freedom but do not abandon. They see the child as a lamp to light rather than a vessel to fill (8, 60).

Parents who possess their children believe they have the right to dictate the terms of their child's life. Then the child has only half a life; parental need to control is greater than real love for child. Too much pressure is placed on the growing child, disturbing his or her emotional development (8, 60).

Just as detrimental are the parents who abandon the child to rear itself—parents who spend too little time with and give too little affection to the child. Such children spend considerable time with television and peers; they learn that the adult world does not want them. In one study children who spent most of their time with peers were more influenced by the lack of the parents' presence, attention, and concern than by the attractiveness of the peer group. The peer-oriented child held negative views of self and peer group and expressed dim views of the future. The peer-oriented children rated parents lower in both expression of affection and support and in exercise of discipline control than did children who spent more time with adults. Peer-oriented children reported engaging in more antisocial behavior such as doing something illegal, playing hooky from school, or lying (8, 60).

Parents should rethink their priorities when they have children. Parents must invest time in such a way that it brings quality to their relationship with the child. Children need the encouragement of doing things and talking through things with adults (8, 60).

Developmental tasks for the couple, which are reworked with the birth of each child, are to:

1. Provide for the physical and emotional needs of the child, conveying love and security freely regardless of the child's appearance or temperament.
2. Reconcile conflicting roles—wife-mother, husband-father, worker-homemaker or family man, and parent-citizen.
3. Accept and adjust to the demands and stresses of parenthood, learning or relearning basics of child care, adjusting personal routines and needs to meet the child's needs, and trying to meet the spouse's needs as well.
4. Provide opportunities for the child to master competencies expected for each developmental stage, to allow the child to make mistakes and learn from them, to restrict the child reasonably and constantly for safety, and to attain the emotional developmental tasks described by Erikson (31).
5. Share responsibilities of parenthood and together make necessary adjustments in space, finances, housing, life-style, and daily routines that are healthy for the family (meals, sleep).
6. Maintain a satisfying relationship with spouse—emotionally, sexually, intellectually, spiritually, and recreationally—while maintaining a personal sense of autonomy and identity.
7. Feel satisfaction from being competent parents and the parenting experience but maintain contacts with relatives and the community.
8. Provide socialization experiences to help the child make the emotional shift from family to peers and society so that the child can become a functioning citizen.
9. Refine the communication system and relationships with spouse, children, and others and permit offspring to be autonomous after leaving home (5, 29, 65, 85).

Other authors also describe the reactions, roles, and responsibilities involved in parenting (1, 7, 8, 10, 41, 50, 52, 54, 56, 60, 62, 75, 81, 83).

As the children mature and leave home, the parents must rework their self-concepts as parents and people so they can assume new roles, responsibilities, and leisure activities to accomplish the last stage of parenthood, disengagement. You can assist the couple in meeting developmental tasks.

Disengagement or Contraction Stage

The **last,** or **disengagement or contraction, stage** occurs *when children leave and the partners must rework their separateness.* The middle-aged woman may return to work after the children leave home if she was not employed while childrearing; new roles evolve for each of the spouses. This is often a time for maximum contact between the partners, especially when retirement occurs. Retirement planning and preparation for the spouse's death must occur. Eventual bereavement, loneliness, and further role changes and losses will occur.

However, sometimes this stage does not last too long. The young adult who is unemployed, a college dropout, or divorced may return home to live. Sometimes teenage or young adult offspring return with children of his or her own because of divorce, economic problems, or other crises so that grandparents may become involved in raising the grandchildren. The aged parents or other relatives may be unable to continue to live independently and are included in the household of middle-aged offspring. Consequently, the tasks, functions, roles, and hierarchical relationships of the family must be reworked. Space and other resources must be reallocated. Time schedules for daily activities may be reworked. Privacy in communication, use of possessions, and emotional space must be ensured. Old parent-child conflicts and ideas about who is boss and how rules are set and discipline accomplished may resurface and should be discussed and worked through. These families can benefit from counseling; your guidance may be crucial. The middle-aged family is more fully discussed in Chapter 13.

Fox (33) offers the following suggestions to adult children and their parents to make living together more harmonious:

1. Remember what it was like when a new baby came home. No matter how beloved the child, disruptions are bound to occur. Realize that another relative's homecoming will be the same.
2. Everyone involved should remember whose house it is.
3. Realize that no matter how many years sons or daughters have been away, family procedures do not change. Mom may still be critical. Dad may be the constant advice-giver. Expect it.
4. Talk about resentments. Discuss problems if you think it will help.
5. Parents may say offspring are grown up. But that does not mean they believe it. Still, they cannot exert the same authority with a 30 or 40 year old as with a youngster.
6. Offspring and elderly parents must be flexible. It is unfair to expect the middle-agers who are the "hosts" to change their household and life routines too much.
7. Even if parents refuse money, adult offspring should insist on paying something, no matter how minimal. Otherwise the offspring are reinforcing the idea that parents are taking care of them. Elderly parents can also contribute financially most of the time.
8. When grandchildren are involved, set rules about who is in charge. To decrease dependency, babysitters should be hired when possible. Then family members do not feel obligated or constrained.
9. Determine length of the adult offspring's stay. It need not be a precise date, but future plans about leaving the home should be explicitly stated.
10. Both adult offspring and older relatives should share responsibilities if possible. But do not upstage mom or dad; for example, if mom loves cooking, do not make her feel useless by taking over in the kitchen.
11. Space permitting, privacy is important. The relative who has lived on his or her own is probably used to time and space alone.
12. Middle-agers should resist meddling in the affairs of either offspring or parents. They can advise. But grown offspring need to think for themselves, and older relatives expect to make their own decisions.
13. Realize that the living situation may be temporary. Living together may not be ideal for anyone. But some parents and offspring or middle-agers and their parents become closer during such periods.

FAMILY INTERACTION

Family interaction is a *unique form of social interaction based on a set of intimate and continuing relationships. It is the sum total of all the family roles being played within a family at a given time* (29). Families function and carry out their tasks and life-styles through this process.

Family therapists, psychiatrists, and nurses are giving increased attention to the emotional balance in family **dyads** or *paired role positions* such as husband and wife or mother and child. They have noted that a shift in the balance of one member of the pair (or of one pair) alters the balance of the other member (or pair). The birth of a child is the classic example (60). Dyads and emotional balance also shift in single-parent and step-parent families (50, 75, 80, 91, 92).

Interaction of the husband and wife or of the adult members living under one roof is basic to the mental, and sometimes physical, health of the adults and to the eventual health of the children. Two factors strongly influence this interaction: (1) the sense of self-esteem or self-love of each family member and (2) the different socialization processes for boys and girls (8).

Importance of Self-Esteem

The most important life task for each person—to feel a sense of self-esteem, to love and have a positive self-image—evolves through interaction with the parents from the time of birth onward and, in turn, affects how the person interacts in later life with others, including spouse and offspring.

The adult in the family who lacks self-acceptance and self-respect probably will not be a loving spouse or parent. Behavior will betray feelings about self and others because he or she will perceive no automatic acceptance and little love from others in the family. Because perception of an event is the person's reality, such a person in turn reacts in ways designed to defend self from the rejection that he or she *thinks* will be received: he or she may criticize, get angry, brag, demand perfection from others, or withdraw. In this way, he or she builds up self, the emotional reasoning being: "I may not be much, but others are worse." Such behavior is corrosive to any relationship but particularly one as intimate as the family's. Because of overt behavior, those intimate with him or her are not likely to appreciate or respond to the basic needs for love, acceptance, and respect. Indeed, the common responses to such behavior are counterattack or withdrawal, which, in turn, perpetuate the other's negative behavior. To remain open and giving in such situations is difficult for the mate but may be the only way to elevate the other's self-esteem. Perhaps only then can he or she reciprocate loving behavior. You can help family members realize the importance of respecting and loving one another and help them work through problems stemming from the low self-esteem of a family member (8).

Influence of Childhood Socialization

The second crucial influence on interaction between adults in the family is the difference in socialization processes for boys and girls. These differences are so embedded in the U.S. social matrix that until recently they had gone nearly unnoticed. There is a different social source for self-love in boys and girls. The girl is loved simply because she exists and can attract, as shown by the admiration pretty little girls receive. The girl is also taught to be subtle, for such behavior is part of her attraction. The boy is loved for what he can do and become; he must prove himself. Boys, especially from school age on, are given less recognition than girls for good looks and much recognition for what they can do. A boy learns to be direct, to brush aside distractions (sometimes including a woman's voice, for most disciplining will come from the mother and female schoolteachers and can be perceived as nagging after a while), and to get to the essence of things (8).

These concepts of what is appropriate boy and girl behavior are taught early and continue to affect heterosexual interactions throughout life. In traditional courtship, for example, the boy is expected to be in charge, to be dominant, to prove himself; the girl is expected to attract, to be passive. In marriage, however, these expectations cause problems, for the man is proving himself largely through his work, and this aspect of his earlier courtship behavior is now less visible to his wife. If the woman does not understand the dynamics of his behavior, she is likely to feel rejected and unloved, thinking she can no longer attract him. If the wife is also working, the husband may think of her as a competitor and work harder to keep his self-esteem. His physical self, including his involvement in lovemaking, is very much intertwined with his social, professional, and financial self, and failure in one is likely to cause feelings of failure in the total self, affecting his sense of masculinity, sexuality, and personhood (8).

All these facts are compounded by the shift in balance between the man and woman found in modern marriage, especially with the advent of the women's liberation movement. The husband often labors under the illusion that he enjoys the rights and responsibilities inherent in a patriarchal family system. Yet he must recognize the qualifications and drive for independence, the basic humanness, of his wife. You can help the couple to recognize the effect of their early socialization on their behavior and expectations and to work through misunderstandings. Help parents to overcome sexual stereotypes so that they do not inflict them on their children. Carmichael's book *Nonsexist Childrearing,* (20) may be helpful.

Variables Affecting Interaction Between the Child and Adult

Long before the child learns to speak, sensory, emotional, and intellectual exchanges are made between the child and other family members. Through such exchanges, and later with words, the child receives and tests instructions on how to consider the rights of others and how to respond to authority. The child also learns how to use language as a symbol, how to carry out certain routines necessary for health, how to compete, and what goals to seek. The games and toys purchased for and played with the child, the books selected and read, and the television programs allowed can provide key learning techniques.

The child's spontaneity can evoke in the adult fresh ways of looking at life long buried under habit and routine. The child says, "It's too loud, but my earlids won't stay down" or "I want one of those little red olives with the green around" or "Give me that eraser with the handle." The child can also recreate for the adult the difficulty of the learning process: "Is it today, tomorrow, or yesterday? You said when I woke up it would be tomorrow, but now you call it 'today.'"

Family interaction for the child and adult is also affected by the ordinal position and sex of the children and by the presence of an only child or of multiple births such as twins, of an adoptive child, or stepchild.

Parents tend to identify with their children and to treat them according to how they were treated as children. A parent can identify best with the child who matches his or her own sibling position. A man from a family of boys may not know how to interact with a daughter and may not empathize with her. In the process of identifying with the parent, the child picks up many of the parent's characteristics, especially if the child is the oldest or lone child. For example, the oldest boy may be dependent instead of independent if his father was the youngest sibling and retained his dependent behavior into adulthood. Using family constellation theory, Toman (90) describes features of each child in a family, based on sex and ordinal position, how the child feels about and interacts with people, and which ordinal position spouse he or she will most happily marry.

Ordinal Position of the Child

Birth order is important to development. Siblings, both same and opposite sex, have an important influence on each other as buddies, bullies, or heroes, and the early relationship often affects the adult relationship (44, 54, 57, 90). The firstborn, who is an only child until the second one comes along, may enjoy some advantages in achievement of intellectual superiority and perspective about life, including a greater sense of responsibility. He or she has more contact with adults and is the sole recipient of attention for a time. He or she becomes dominant over younger siblings. Secondborn boys with an older sister are more feminine than those with an older brother. The younger children benefit from the parents' experience with childraising and from having older siblings to imitate. Lastborns are also more sociable, possibly to ensure acceptance by older siblings or to gain parental attention. The lastborn may be more dependent. The middle child is likely to become caught between the jealousy of the older child and the envy of the younger, who may form a coalition against him or her. But he or she learns double or triple roles and is prepared for more kinds of relationships in adulthood. If two siblings are more than 6 years apart, they tend to grow up like only children (44, 90).

Only Child

The only child may feel more loneliness but develops more rapidly and may seem older and more serious than peers who have siblings. He or she lacks the opportunities siblings could provide. Thus he or she usually does not share feelings and experiences with someone close, cope with jealousy and envy from rivals in the home, or learn intimately about ways of the opposite- or same-sexed peers. The only child learns less about compromising with peers, sharing adult attention, and erecting strong defenses against the feelings displaced on him or her by adults and peers. He or she may prefer adults; the usual ways of relating and behavioral tactics do not work with peers.

Children are the logical targets for fulfilling many of the parents' frustrated ambitions and needs. In a large family these yearnings and aspirations can be parceled out among a number of children, but when there is only one child, this child can sense the parents' manipulation and expectations. Thus the only child usually is a peacemaker if he or she and the parents are the only household members. He or she is inadvertently brought into the parents' conflicts and is forced to help maintain harmony and preserve equilibrium in the household (57, 90).

In a family with only one child, there are few people to fulfill the many roles of a family; thus more is demanded of each member. The only child may be forced prematurely to assume roles for which he or she is ill equipped. The child may become deft at performing adult tasks and roles, but self-confidence in the capacity to do so may be uncertain (44, 57, 90).

The only child sometimes has special problems on becoming a parent, seeing in the child a longed-for brother or sister. The danger in the situation is that the child is also a rival for the spouse's attention. On reaching adolescence, the offspring may then pose a threat to the parent's own adult roles, and the parent may unconsciously become overly competitive (44, 57, 90). Yet the only child is now regarded as an answer for the parents who want the parenting experience but who also want time to fulfill their own careers.

Certainly the only child can develop into a wholesome, well-adjusted person. The qualities of being more serious, assertive, responsible, independent, curious, and able to entertain self and find satisfaction in personal pursuits frequently develop because of parental and home demands. These demands can enhance abilities to be a mature, capable adult. The greater opportunities available for adult contact, beginning at home, develop the only child's creativity, language skills, planning abilities, and intellectual potential. He or she has a high need to achieve and prefers the novel or complex. Firstborn and only children such as Cary Grant, Brooke Shields, Martha Collins, Ted Koppel, Joe Montana, John Updike, Isaac Newton, Franklin Roosevelt, Emile Zola, Herbert Spencer, Rainer Maria Rilke, and some of the American astronauts rank high on the roster of outstanding leaders, artists, and scientists.

As you counsel parents who plan for or have only one child, emphasize the need for peer activity and the danger of too much early responsibility and pressure.

Family With a Large Number of Children

The family with more than three or four children is less frequently seen now than in the past. The lastborn child may be less wanted than the first or middleborn, although parents feel more skilled and self-confident in rearing the younger children. Large families have advantages. Of necessity, the children learn thrift and conservation of resources and material goods. Members know the hot water supply is not unlimited, that food is not to be wasted, and that toys and clothing can be recycled. Children learn to share time, space, and possessions.

The children learn to do for themselves and each other; they learn responsibility. In a loving home, they have not only their parents' love but also that of siblings, a listening ear, respect, support, compassion, and help. If the parent does not have time to read to the 3 year old, the older sibling does. He or she gains more experience in reading, gains increased self-esteem from being helpful, and learns responsibility and caring. Each child learns cooperation, compromise, and tolerance and how to handle peer pressure. The effort, work, expense, and self-denial of having a large family can be offset by the rewards of watching children grow and develop and by a sense of contribution to the generations to come (54, 60, 87).

Your teaching and support can influence how well parents cope with responsibility of a large family.

Multiple Births

Twins or other multiple births have considerable impact on family interaction. If ovulation has been inhibited with contraceptive pills, multiple births are more likely once this method stops being used. Multiple fetuses in utero create many problems for the parents in relation to health of mother and babies, financial strain, ethical decisions if certain embryos may not live, and family relationships. The needs and tasks of these parents will differ from the parents who have a single birth.

Often these parents lack emotional and financial support and sufficient help with child care and household tasks. Your suggestions and support can influence how well the parents cope with their responsibility.

Because multiple births are often premature, the first 4 or 5 months are very demanding on the parents in terms of the amount of energy and time spent in child care; this means that the parents have less energy and time for each other or other children. The mother should have help for several months if possible—from the husband, a relative, friend, or neighbor. Financial worries and concern about space and material needs may also intrude on normal husband-wife relationships or on relationships with other children.

Although books discourage the mother of twins from breast-feeding or using alternate breast and bottle-feeding, the mother may be able to breast-feed both twins successfully by alternating breast- with bottle-feedings. The babies will not necessarily be poor breast-feeders with this arrangement.

You can suggest shortcuts in, or realities about, care that will not be detrimental to twin babies and that will give the parents more time to enjoy them. A diaper service, for example, is well worth the investment, for 1000 diapers may be used in a month's time. The parents should not be made to feel guilty if they are not as conscientious with two babies as they would be with one. Each can be given a total bath every other day instead of daily. Heating bottles before feeding is not necessary. The parents should try to avoid getting so wrapped up in meeting the babies' physical needs that resentment, anger, or excessive fatigue creep in. Multiple offspring should be fun as well as work.

Encourage the parents of twins (or multiple offspring) to perceive the babies as individuals and to consider the long-term consequences of giving them similar-sounding names, dressing them alike, having doubles of everything, and expecting them to behave alike. Tell parents about the U.S. national organization, Mothers of Twins, whose local branch can be a place to share feelings and ideas and gain practical suggestions. In the United Kingdom there is a Twins Clubs Association, a self-help organization with local chapters that provide educational and advocacy services.

Multiple-birth children usually are closer than ordinary siblings. These children have lived with each other from before birth on, so experiences are different from that of having various aged siblings. Parents often force one to be older and one to be younger in behavior; it is difficult for the one to play role of "older" because neither has the advantage of extra years of experience over the other, who is developmentally on the same level. With paternal twins, authority preference of parents tends to determine what age-ranks the girl and the boy will be ascribed. In contrast, identical twins meet the world as a pair; it is difficult to imagine life without each other. It takes longer to separate in adolescence and adulthood (they may not, emotionally or physically). Each tends to seek multiple birth persons as friends or mates.

They soon learn about the extra attention resulting from their birth status and may take advantage of the situation. Interaction between them is often complementary; for example, one twin may be dominant and the other submissive. Each learns from reinforcement of his or her experiences about the advantages of the particular role chosen. They learn to resist control by others and to manipulate others by acting alike and "in collusion." They do not have to manage conflicts with parents or others alone.

Siblings of a multiple birth usually are more detached from other siblings, even from parents, than each other. Twins may each receive less parental affection and communication because parents have less time to devote to each child. Thus twins are often slower to talk and many have a slower intellectual growth unless parents work to prevent it (60, 62). Yet the bond and sharing that occurs between twins or multiple birth individuals can have positive effects on development as well. The sense of severity and identity and the ability to share may be stronger, and these people have a unique empathy and ability to switch roles that enhances interpersonal relationships (2).

Gender of the Child

Gender also influences development within the family (54). In most cultures a higher value is placed on male than on female children. Actually, in some cultures only a boy's birth is welcomed or celebrated, and the family's status is partially measured by the number of sons. A family with several girls and no boys may perceive another baby girl as a disappointment. The girl may discover this attitude in later years from overhearing adult conversations, and she may try to compensate for her sex and gain parental affection and esteem by engaging in tomboy behavior and later assuming masculine roles.

If a boy arrives in a family that hoped for a girl, he may receive pressure to be feminine. He may even be dressed and socialized in a feminine manner. If the boy arrives after a family has two or three girls, he may receive much attention but also the jealousy of his sisters. Often he will grow up with three or four "mothering" figures (some may be unkind) and in a family more attuned to feminine than to masculine behavior. Developing a masculine identity may be more difficult for him, especially if there is no male nearby with whom to relate. In spite of being pampered, he may be expected by his family to be manly. The boy may feel envious of his sisters' position and their freedom from such expectations.

The girl who arrives in a family with a number of boys may also receive considerable attention, but she may have to become tomboyish to compete with her brothers and receive their esteem. Feminine identity may be difficult for her.

You can help parents understand how their attitude toward their own sexuality and their evaluation of boys and girls influence their relationship with their children. Emphasize the importance of encouraging the child's unique identity to develop.

Adopted Child

The adopted child may suffer some problems of the only child. In addition, the adopted child may have to work through feelings about rejection and abandonment by the biologic parents versus being wanted and loved by the adoptive parents. The child should be told that he or she is adopted as early as the idea can be comprehended. Usually by the preschool years he or she can incorporate the idea of being a wanted child.

Adopted children bring their own genes, birth experiences, biologic family ties, and often an extensive life history to their adoptive family. The adoptive family is not the same as a biologic family. Both adoptive parents and adopted children tend to feel they have less control over their situation than other families. Adoptive parents and adopted children are both likely to have experienced a sense of loss. It is not unusual for the adoptive child to seek his or her own biologic parents in late adolescence or young adulthood, especially if the child was old enough to remember both parents when adopted, even when the adoptive parents are truly considered the parents. This search may be a threat to adoptive parents, or they may feel secure enough to even assist the offspring in the search.

The adoptive parents' personal qualifications, their marital harmony, their love of the child, their acceptance of the child as is, and the child's having friends are major determinants of the child's adjustment and development. Factors not predictive of adjustment are socioeconomic status, occupational status, presence or absence of biologic siblings, age of parents, health of adopters, religion, or prior experience with children (4, 23, 72).

Definition of "suitable" adoptive parents has been liberalized. Adoption agency requirements of age, marital status, race, and mother's employment status are more flexible. The adoptive parent may be a man. Additionally, today's couples consider adoption even if they have their own children. Some believe they have a responsibility and enough love to provide a home for an existing child rather than add to the total population. Others are single persons who want to offer love and security to a child.

Social and legal changes have affected the kinds of children in need of adoption. Earlier adoption agencies served mainly Caucasian unmarried mothers who saw adoption as the only alternative for their babies. Today fewer infants are available because there is greater social acceptance of out-of-wedlock births; more unmarried mothers keep their babies. Contraceptives and abortions have also reduced the number of unwanted infants. A different category of adoptable children has grown in size, however. These children with "special needs" have at least one of the following characteristics: over age 5; black, biracial; or physically, emotionally, or cognitively handicapped. Increasingly, state legislatures terminate parental rights in cases of children in long-term foster care who have remained unvisited and ignored by their biologic parents and when the likelihood of the child's returning to his or her own home is minimal. New legislation has allowed abused children to become eligible for adoption (14–16, 28, 30, 39, 95).

Because of fewer available children in the United States, families are more likely to consider adopting a foreign child. Foreign adoption raises cultural, social, interracial, and emotional issues for the adoptive parents, their families and friends, and the specific community. Warren (95) discusses issues and concerns, qualifications, and the process.

Additional information is available from International Concerns Committee for Children, 911 Cypress Drive, Boulder, CO 80303 (95).

In spite of more liberal definitions of adoptability, the number of people applying to adopt a child, homes approved, placements made, and adoptions completed declined compared to the number of available children. Thus an increasing number of older or disabled children need permanent placement.

You may have an opportunity to educate adults about the opportunity for adopting an older child with special needs or to work with adoptive parents, who also have needs.

Adoption of a child with special needs involves four phases: (1) commitment of adults and child, (2) honeymoon or placement period, (3) storm period, and (4) adaptation and adjustment. The phases do not abruptly begin and end; each phase builds on the preceding phase and sometimes reversals occur. The phases, along with thoughts, emotions, and activities accompanying each phase, are summarized in Table 4–2. The adoptive process can terminate at any point. If termination is necessary, both sides—the family and child—need help to understand what happened and to understand that no *one person* is responsible. Future adoption procedures are enhanced if proper guidance is given with the first failure (14–16).

Stresses to adoptive families include the following:

1. Worry about child's heredity.
2. Parents choose to be parents; hence they are highly motivated to give parenting and thus will invest considerable expense and time.

3. The parents see themselves as chosen group because someone thought they should be good parents; the chosen group idea leads to problems such as difficulty in setting limits, increased stress in parenting role, and oversensitivity to problems in child.
4. Infertile couples may have feelings of hostility or inferiority that are projected on child; the child is a constant reminder of inability to conceive.
5. Adopted child or adolescent may project normal feelings of anger onto "adoptive" parents; parents may think normal developmental problems are a fact of adoption.
6. If one child is adopted and one is biologic, favoritism, insufficient rewards to adoptive child, or competition between children may result.
7. Sanctions and regards for role performance differ from biologic parents (e.g., the company may not have maternity leave for adoptive parents; there is little emotional support for adoptive parents in society).

TABLE 4-2. ADOPTIVE PROCESS

Phases	Thoughts and Emotions	Activities
Commitment of adult(s) and child(ren):	*Adult(s)* make general decision to adopt (stage 1), leading to decision to adopt specific child(ren) (stage 2).	*Adult(s)* prepare for adoption through dialogue with helpful people and agencies and sometimes attend sessions on adoption given by by adoption agency.
"Courting Stage"	*Child(ren)* express desire for adoption (stage 1), leading to decision on specific family (stage 2).	*Child(ren)* are counseled for potential adjustment by adoption agency staff. Visits are arranged and made between potential family and child(ren). All members involved (including existing children in family) get to know each other.
Placement:	*Parent(s)* are on an "emotional high"; excitement.	Household routines are altered to accommodate child(ren). Limit-setting is minimal. Parent(s) meet child(ren)'s whims.
"Honeymoon period" (child[ren] come to live with parent[s])	*Child(ren)* are excited but somewhat scared. "Can I trust these people?" "Will they send me away when I don't act my best?"	*Child(ren)* put on best behavior. Sometimes parent(s)' show of affection for child(ren) is not accepted because of child(ren)'s past negative parenting.
"Storm period"	*Parent(s)* are tired of permanent house guest(s), feel anger, disappointment, guilt and displace these feelings on each other and the child. They may wish the child would leave.	*Parent(s)* treat child(ren) or other family members with decreasing tolerance for behavior not in family norm.
	Child(ren) can no longer keep up good behavior but want to be loved and accepted.	*Child(ren)* may have tantrums, run away, try to reject parents before they reject him or her.
	Parent(s) may feel sense of failure. They may have expected too much of themselves and child(ren) and now may strike out at each other and other family members. Spouses may be jealous of time and energy mate gives to child(ren).	If the outcome is positive, the *parent(s)* will use problem solving, limit setting with flexibility, sense of humor, ongoing empathy and caring, supportive others, and community resources.
	Child(ren) may think, "They don't want me. What's going to happen to me?" and may live with anticipatory grief, fears of rejection, and insecurity, based on past hurts. Parent(s) and child(ren) test each other.	
Adaptation and adjustment phase (equilibrium occurs)	*All* believe they can live and work together; mutual trust is growing; family feels fused as a unit and able to handle frustrations and crisis.	Parent(s) are consistent with child(ren). *Parent(s)* and *child(ren)* can attend to outside interests without threatening family status.
	Child(ren) feel good about self, feel love and acceptance.	

8. Role autonomy is lacking. Adoptive parents need someone to agree that they will be good parents but need someone else to bear a child. These requirements inject dependence into a role considered independent, which may undermine parental confidence.

9. Community or school attitudes may be negative; one's "own" child is spoken of as biologic child. The child encounters these attitudes of distinguishing between "real" and "adoptive," which undermines the sense of belonging and can drive a wedge between parents and child (14, 16, 17, 39, 50, 51, 68, 94).

What was once viewed as a process that ended when the adoption decree was granted is now recognized as a condition that affects those involved throughout their lives. It is a permanent change in legal status. Adoption is a unique way of building families. These families are different from other families because of the circumstances that bring people to adoption and because of the way adoption continues to affect their lives (72, 82).

Adoptive parents, adoptive children, and adoptive family dynamics are different from birth parents, birth children, and birth family dynamics. Sometimes these differences generate problems within a family, and sometimes the adoption becomes the focus of other conflicts or unresolved family issues. Any time there are problems in an adoptive family, the significance of the adoption must be considered. Changes in the nature of adoptions have meant that more adoptive families have been seeking professional assistance and that professionals are having to consider the kinds of services the families may need and how to deliver them. Box 4–1 summarizes intervention guidelines for therapy with adoptive families (11, 14, 16, 17, 28, 39, 50, 51, 68).

Stepchild

The stepchild grieves and mourns the loss of a biologic parent from death or divorce and must also deal with problems associated with integration into a new family unit. The stepchild may have conflicting feelings of loyalty to the natural parent and to the stepparent, thinking that acceptance of the stepparent is rejection of the natural parent. The stepchild may also feel rejected by his or her remarried natural parent, seeing the stepparent as a rival for the parent's attention. Further, when there are stepsiblings, jealousy, conflict, and hate may be dominant feelings in the offspring. More on the stepparent family follows in the next section.

FAMILY LIFE-STYLES AND CHILDREARING PRACTICES

There is no single type of contemporary U.S. family, but the life-styles of many correspond to the factors dis-

---

■ **BOX 4-1.**
Intervention Guidelines for Adoptive Families

- Conventional treatment may not work well with adoptive families.
- Adoptive parents need validation as parents and of their decision to adopt.
- Adoptive parents must be included in therapeutic interventions to empower them further and to reinforce the adoptive commitment.
- In treating child-rooted problems, often the job will be to help parents modify their expectations.
- A child cannot successfully mourn the past and integrate it into the present circumstances if preoccupied with emotional survival. Developing a sense of safety and security is of paramount importance.
- Child-rooted barriers can come from unfinished emotional business, attachment disorders, or poor preparation for adoption.
- Adult-rooted barriers may stem from unfinished business, marital problems, or individual pathologies.
- Environmental barriers include lack of support or active disapproval from the extended family or the broader community.
- Any assessment is only useful if the assessed family accepts it as valid.
- In deciding to terminate an adoption that is not working, one must be committed to preserving the family's integrity, yet open to the removal of the child as a viable option.
- When an adoption is terminated, avoid judgment about reasons for its failure. Plans for adoption of another child should not be made until grief of the loss is resolved.

---

cussed in this section, including family structure, family cultural pattern, and the impact of the twentieth century. These factors, in addition to those already discussed, influence family interaction and so understanding will assist you in family care.

Family Structure

Childrearing and family relationships are influenced primarily by family structure. The biologic and reproductive unit considered typical in the United States is the mother-father-child group. Ordinarily the parents are married, have established a residence of their own, are viewed (along with their children) as an integral social unit, and live in an intimate, monogamous relationship. Emphasis in U.S. marriage is on pursuit of love in a romanticized way and on individual happiness rather than on family bonds as in many other cultures. Yet kinship ties are usually recognized on both sides of the family.

In many situations, however, a child may grow up in a family that differs from the typical one. An aunt, uncle, or grandparent may be a continuing member of the household unit; one or the other parent may be absent because of death, divorce, illegitimacy, military service, or occupation involving travel.

The single-parent family is increasingly common in numbers. *Families in which only one parent is living full time with offspring* are called single-parent families. Although death and illegitimacy may cause the family to have only one parent, divorce of the natural parents is the more common reason. In most cases these families have undergone a major change in life-style. A parent may have died either suddenly or after a long illness. If the parents are divorced, the family may have experienced considerable disruption before the breakup. Sometimes the single-parent family is a planned event. A woman, lacking a suitable partner but wanting to be a mother, will choose to have a child by artificial insemination; or a single man or woman may choose to adopt a child. Regardless of the reason for the situation, these families often encounter considerable stress, including financial strain—sometimes even poverty.

In many healthy persons emotional attachment to a dead or divorced spouse (or to the lost parent), with recurrent episodes of painful grief, may remain many years. Mourning in later life may be qualitatively different from that in earlier life; may be more prolonged and more difficult to complete; and may be related to less flexibility in aging, more rigid ego, and enormity of loss (spouse, identity, peer and family relations, sex companionship, style of living, routines and habits, economic security). The attachment for the spouse, lost either through divorce or death, which lasts for many years, may be unknown to even the closest friends or family of the survivor. Yet most mourners resolve their loss and become involved in life in new ways and with new people. The loss also offers an opportunity for personal development (23).

In the single-parent family the children may experience grief for the absent parent, guilt for their real or imagined part in the loss, shame for the change in their family structure, and fear about what changes the future may bring. Roles are changed. Each person may need to assume additional responsibilities and tasks. Parents may change their life-styles. Mother may go to work or school, for instance; father may move into an apartment; or both parents may begin dating. An adolescent may serve as a parent substitute to younger siblings, or other children may assume new household tasks. The initial task of this family is to accept its family structure as a workable option for family living.

Children living in this household often exhibit more adaptability, responsibility, and maturity than their peers. However, the child who lives with the parent of the opposite gender may have more difficulty with adjustment to the divorce or death of the other parent or to the remarriage of the parent than if the child lived with the same-gender parent. Inappropriate social behavior, difficulty with identity formation, depression, and poorer school performance may be manifested by the child. If there always was only one parent, the child may have evolved behavior and roles appropriate to the partner, regardless of the child's gender. This may also create later developmental problems (70).

Often an open discussion of the changed life-style, along with support from relatives, friends, and other single-parent families, enhances the problem-solving abilities of these persons. Family members may need professional help if they exhibit symptoms of more extreme dysfunction, grieving, or prolonged "acting-out" behaviors. The family may also need information about various community resources; a major concern for single-parent families is financial strain or poverty, especially for the woman, because of wage inequities, difficulty with divorce settlements and child support, or lack of preparation financially in case of parental death (70).

The stepfamily is also common. *The remarriage of a divorced or widowed parent with children may form a composite family unit known as the* **stepfamily.** The "wicked stepmother" myth pervades our culture; in addition, the common usage of the word *stepchild* denotes inferior status. These families may be formed in a variety of ways: a mother with children may remarry; a father whose children visit may remarry; either of the new parents may have an exspouse or children from a previous marriage (children and stepsiblings), and, to complicate this family even more, the remarried couple may decide to have children of its own. In-laws and several sets of grandparents complete the picture. This family is now a far cry from the typical nuclear family, and the interaction becomes increasingly complex. Because remarriages are fragile, the adults may divorce from the second marriage as well, creating more loss and devastation. If a third marriage or unmarried partnership occurs, there are more layers of relatives, many of whom hardly contact or know each other and who may not like each other at all. An unanswered question is whether the current generation of stepchildren will care for stepparents or other steprelatives in old age.

When a couple marries for the second or third time and either or both have children from a previous marriage, the new husband and/or wife becomes an instant stepparent. This addition of children to a couple's life differs from the situation of first-marriage couples, whose children are added at a slower pace. Additionally, the myth that familial love occurs via the marriage ceremony is common.

Adjustment to a new, unique family unit is the major task of the stepfamily. Stepfamilies go through stages of development:

1. Fantasy stage—the adults dream that past wrongs of the previous marriage will be fixed and everything will be fine; everyone will be made whole in the new marriage.

2. Reality stage—dreams of a unified family are destroyed, and the transition is seen as much more conflictual than anticipated. Everyone involved has lost something (92).

New members cannot be assimilated with an existing family; instead a new family unit is formed. New rules, customs, and activities must be developed. Conflictual values and family ghosts must be resolved. Table 4–3 summarizes stepfamily characteristics and tasks (91, 92).

All members of this new family bring a history of life experiences, relationships, and expectations to the stepfamily. Conflict often occurs when the values and rules of individuals or the former single-parent family differ from those of the second (92).

Conflicts about raising stepchildren can be the most explosive issue in remarriages. The partners must realize they cannot be "superparents' and they will not receive instant love from the stepchildren. In fact, the child may never be affectionate toward the stepparent; the divided loyalty between the birth parent and stepparent may be unresolvable. The adult may not really feel affection for the stepchild either, in spite of wanting to. Time must be spent between adult and child: it takes time and shared activity to build a trusting, caring relationship. Parents or children should not expect too much too fast. The stepparent should avoid criticism of or competition with the birth parent; a new niche must be fashioned. The stepparent should reach out to the child even if rejection is present, be fair and honest in interactions, and create time and space that is designated for only the stepchild. Discipline problems are best handled at first by the birth parent; later regulations and rules can be applied by either partner. Since most children are part of a single-parent home before they merge into a stepparent home, they are not likely to relinquish roles easily. Lastly, partners should focus on their marriage relationship and present an undivided front to the children (91, 92).

In time family members develop agreement about what is "right." Such agreement may include the "correct" church to attend, the "right" time for dinner, and how to celebrate birthdays. Open communication between members is essential to make decisions that are livable for all members.

In addition to adjusting in the family, stepfamilies must adjust to expectations of the outside world. Often differences in the reconstituted family are ignored because the family appears intact. Feelings of frustration, inadequacy, and isolation in family members stem from expectations that they feel as close to one another as blood relatives are expected to. The absent parent may still be an active influence in the original family. For instance, a divorced father may still contribute to his children's support and spend time with them on a regular basis, but they may be living with a stepfather. Even a deceased parent is remembered, not always accurately, and sometimes the stepparent is compared to the memory.

The child's ability to work through these feelings is influenced by age, sex, level of development, adaptive capabilities, and the understanding and support received from significant adults. He or she may need professional help to work through the difficulties of integration into a new family structure.

The stepfamily, like the single-parent family, needs to accept itself and be accepted as a combination of persons living together in a unique family unit. It is a potentially stressful situation that requires flexibility and adaptability of its members. Yet this family offers many opportunities for growth and friendship through the differing experiences of its members.

The number of stepfamilies continues to increase in the United States. Increasing numbers of children in America have at least one stepparent. In response to the growing number of these families, support groups such as the National Stepfamily Association operate to help them face their unique situations. In spite of the old adage that children are flexible and can "bounce back," the trauma of divorce is second only to death. Often the problems that arise in the second marriage are more devastating than earlier ones. The children know that the original parent will not return and they are faced with a new parent whom they often initially neither want nor accept emotionally. Counseling groups have

TABLE 4-3. COMPARISON OF STEPFAMILY CHARACTERISTICS AND TASKS

Stepfamily Characteristics	Stepfamily Tasks
Begins after many losses and changes	Dealing with losses and changes
Incongruent individual, marital, family life cycles and needs	Negotiating different developmental needs; synchronizing life cycles
Children and adults come with values and expectations from pervious families	Establishing new traditions and different expectations; clarify roles and values
Parent-child relationships predate the new couple	Developing a solid couple bond and forming new relationships
Biologic parent elsewhere in actuality or in memory	Creating a "parenting coalition"; the couple works on its union first
Children often members of two households	Accepting continual shifts in household composition: changing people, personal space, residence, responsibilities, roles
Legal relationship between stepparent and children is ambiguous or nonexistent	Risking involvement despite little societal support

Data from references 91 and 92.

started in schools, courts, and private practice to help these children (4, 36).

Another type of family structure has been termed *apartners*. Instead of getting married, a couple, who may have children by a previous marriage, chooses to maintain separate residences, take care of his or her own children, professional life, and everyday affairs but shares special times with each other on a regularly scheduled basis. Personal time and freedom, coupled with intimacy, are what the participants say they seek. Gay or lesbian couples may also have this arrangement, often because of social constraints rather than choice.

The single state (*never married, separated, divorced, widowed*) is another family structure. Today in the United States more individuals have chosen singlehood than in the past. Some would apply family developmental tasks to this person; however, it is no longer considered necessary to marry and bear children to be fulfilled and accomplished. The single state can promote development of creativity, object ties, and healthy narcissism through:

1. Privacy—being able to think and create in a peaceful atmosphere without interruption
2. Time—to travel, cultivate talents and interests, entertain and be entertained, follow intellectual pursuits
3. Freedom—being able to choose and make decisions, form friendships, use time as desired, depend on self, have a healthy narcissism
4. Opportunity—to extend borders of friendship, develop skills and knowledge, enjoy geographic moves or job mobility and success; the single person is often preferred for certain jobs or positions (5, 23)

Yet singlehood is not always happy for the never-married, separated, widowed, or divorced individual. It can be lonely. There can be too much unoccupied time and resulting depression. There can be too much space and freedom and the inability to make decisions. The silence of the home when entering from a day's work may be overwhelming. Talking and sharing both the joys and stresses and the daily routine events may be needed, but there is no one who really wants to be contacted or who responds other than in his or her own narcissistic way. There may be financial concerns or unwise use of money because of prior lack of opportunity with financial affairs. Others may expect the single person always to be available to help because he or she "has no family or obligations," but the single person may have difficulty receiving help in return—or even in asking for it. It is as if society expects the single person to manage everything alone. The person is a nonentity until someone needs something, and the single person is seen as available. In like manner, the single person

may be taken advantage of by home repairmen, by businesses, by acquaintances who pose as lovers, or by someone seeking an object interaction sexually. There may be places the single person cannot go because of cultural restrictions. Our society is couple oriented. Special holidays and anniversary dates can be especially painful. The person may be alone and forgotten by friends who are busy with their families; or even in a crowd of merrymakers, and in spite of a smiling face, the person may feel isolated and alone (23).

Your acceptance, support, validation, and teaching are crucial in promoting health in the single person.

Stepgeneration parents comprise a different kind of family *when the mother will not, does not, cannot, or should not care for her offspring*. Often it is the grandmother (occasionally only the grandfather) who comes to the rescue; this is an alternative to foster home placement. This phenomenon often is linked to drug and alcohol abuse or addiction or to physical, sexual, or emotional abuse of the child. In the process the grandparent(s) sacrifice personal needs and provide the love, security, and other needs for the child. The real concern is that the grandparent(s) may become ill or die before the child is reared. Most grandparents realize that the physical and emotional care and moral and spiritual guidance they give may prevent the grandchild from repeating the pattern the child was born into.

Family Size

Family size is related to distinctive patterns of family life and child development. Most children in the United States are members of a small family system—that is, one with three children or less. Some couples are choosing to have no children to pursue their own careers or professions or leisure interests, which become sublimation for children. Others make this choice because they believe the current world situation is not one into which to bring children.

The **small family system** has the following features: (1) emphasis is on planning (the number and the frequency of births, the objectives of childrearing, and educational possibilities); (2) parenthood is intensive rather than extensive (great concern is evidenced from pregnancy through every phase of childrearing for each child); (3) group actions are usually more democratic; and (4) greater freedom is allowed individual members. The child or children in the small family usually enjoy advantages beyond those available to children in large families of corresponding economic and social level, including more individual attention. On the other hand, these children may retain emotional dependence on their parents, grow up with extreme pressure for performance, and retain an exaggerated notion of self-importance.

The **large family,** generally thought of as one with

six or more children, is not a planned family as a rule. Parenthood is commonly extensive rather than intensive, not because of less love or concern but simply because parents must divide their attention more ways. In the very large family emphasis is on the group rather than on the individual member. Conformity and cooperation are valued above self-expression. Discipline in the form of numerous and stringent rules frequently is stressed, and there is a high degree of organization in the activities of daily living (23). If parents lack initiative and use their resources unwisely, disorganization may exist. For additional information see the section on The Family with a Large Number of Children, pp. 121–131.

Family Cultural Pattern

*The ways of living and thinking that constitute the intimate aspects of family group life comprise the **family cultural pattern*** (24). The family transmits the cultural pattern of its own ethnic background and class to the child, together with the parents' attitudes toward other classes.

Within the national cultural pattern of the United States, significant variations have been found in family cultural patterns and social systems (10). In Millstadt, Illinois, for instance, the German farm family provides a distinctive social system, with cultural features distinct from its Italian neighbors across the river in St. Louis. The Maine Yankee and the North Carolina rebel may speak the same language, but the meanings of the words used may be quite different because of regional variables. Thus how families rear their children depends on ethnic group and class, region, nation, and historical period.

Influence of Twentieth-Century Changes

Shift From an Agrarian to a Complex Technologic Society. This shift has produced dramatic changes for the U.S. family. A greater percentage of children now survives childhood than in 1900, and a higher percentage of mothers survives childbirth. Some marriages occur at an earlier age and some at a later age than in former generations. Fewer children are born to most parents, they are spaced closer together, and more first children are born to parents in their late thirties or early forties. Illegitimacy has lost its stigma, generally, and there is an increasing number of women who are single mothers by choice, whether they are teenagers or in their late thirties or early forties. Middle-aged couples now have more time together after their children are grown and leave home. Because of an increased life expectancy, families now have more living relatives than formerly, especially elderly relatives, for whom the family may have responsibility.

Other Trends Related to Living in a Complex Industrial Society. Families live primarily in urban or metropolitan areas. More women work outside the home. The U.S. woman who formerly stayed home and was the "homemaker" has also gone through several changes. Once homemaking took a good deal of time. Now modern conveniences make tasks easier. The woman who stays home today concentrates more on "mothering." Her outside activities may include volunteer work so she can control her hours and feel she has prime time at home yet is contributing outside the family unit. Family members are becoming better educated. Family incomes may be unstable; acquisition of personal housing and equipment sought early in the marriage is not always possible. Greater individual freedom exists. Sexual mores are changing, with trial and serial marriages. Value changes and different patterns of living apparently are the norm.

The emphasis on the family-kinship group has been replaced by acceptance of the nuclear or other types of family. Because Americans are so mobile and are increasingly living in smaller homes or in apartments, many ties with kin other than the immediate family are loosened or at least geographically extended. Sometimes close friends become "the family." Yet many Americans strengthen kinship ties through letters, telephone calls, and holiday and vacation visits. Religious influences affect family ties. Jews, with their many family traditions, are generally more embedded in a network of relatives than white Protestants are.

Rapid Change. Rapid change is a fact that families must acknowledge. Medical, pharmacologic, and scientific advances in birth technology and all areas of health, the increased number of single-parent families, the growing emphasis on the civil and economic rights of minority groups, and the women's liberation movement are only a part of the cultural expansion of this century. As people live longer, more older people will divorce, remarry, or cohabitate. Those who lack healthy emotional roots within their nuclear families, who have few or no kinship ties, who cannot adjust to rapid change, and who have little identity except as defined by job and income are more likely to become depressed, alcoholic, unfaithful to mate, or divorced (5, 40, 55, 57). Today's changing social environment makes it increasingly difficult for a parent to be certain of his or her identity. How, then, is he or she to provide emotional roots for the child?

U.S. Childrearing Practices. There is no one traditional national pattern, only the general concern that children develop "normally." Parents are encouraged through culture, education, and the mass media to use whatever the dominant childrearing theory is at the time. At the turn of the century, the dominant theory reflected the prevailing scientific belief in the primacy of heredity in determining behavior. In the early 1900s child care emphasized the importance of environment, and by the midthirties Freudian Psychoanalytic Theory had gained ascendency. Today Neo-Behavioristic theories are prominent. With each new wave of "knowledge," parents are bombarded by conflicting reports and condemnation of previous practices. Often the change in theory application occurs during the same parental generation so that parents do not trust their own judgment, and considerable inconsistency results. The inconsistency, rather than the theory, probably creates the main problems in childrearing. Sometimes parents strive to avoid rearing their children as they were reared but nevertheless do so unwittingly because of the permanency of enculturation. Children are often given approval and disapproval for their behavior and told they are "good" or "bad." This practice, along with inconsistency and other factors, contributes to competition and sibling rivalry.

Father's Role. The father's role is being reconsidered, and he is more active in child care (52, 54, 56). Still, the mother is primarily responsible for the crying baby and young child care. The infant is often unconsciously trained in privacy, individualism, and independence by being left alone in the crib or playpen much of the time. There is still, unfortunately, the fear of "spoiling" the infant if he or she is held too much or responded to spontaneously. Thus the infant may develop behavioral extremes to get needs met. He or she is being given the foundation to later stand out, push forward, to compete and achieve.

When the children are old enough to be out of the home, parents often strive to do things for their children and center their activities around their children's activities. Work responsibilities are not necessarily demanded, but there is subtle pressure for the children to repay by pleasing the parents through use of talents, organizational achievements, or honors won. Because of the small size of the nuclear family, the school-age child or adolescent may spend more time with peers than with family members. Because of the youth idealization of our culture, seniority does not invoke special respect for the older person (parent). The childrearing parent must offer more than age if he or she wants to maintain control.

A growing trend is for day-care centers or babysitters who are usually not relatives to care for children. What happens if the mother and parent-surrogate differ greatly about childrearing practices? The child generally acknowledges the authority of parents or at least the mother, but parent-surrogates affect him or her nevertheless. Any adult who is with the child reinforces behavior in the child that conforms to the adult's own standard of behavior. The child conforms to the adult's desires to gain approval. If the parent-surrogate acts in a way contrary to the values of the parents, both parents and child probably will be distressed.

Nursing Applications for Health Promotion

The family as the basic unit for the developing person cannot be taken for granted. Although family forms have changed and will continue to change, each person, to develop healthfully, needs some intimate surroundings of human concern. "No man is an island."

You will frequently encounter the entire family as your client in the health care system, regardless of the setting. You may be asked to do family-centered care, to nurse the client and the family or to do "family therapy." Yet you will not be able to carry out the nursing process with the family even minimally unless you understand the dynamics of family living presented in this chapter.

Rapid change, increasing demands on the person, technologic progress, and other trends mentioned seem to isolate people. Many families are not aware of the forces pulling them apart. More than ever, they need one place in their living where they can act without self-consciousness, where the pretenses and roles demanded in jobs, school, or social situations can be put aside. The living center should be a place where communication takes place with ease; where each knows what to expect from the other; where a cohesiveness exists that is based on nonverbal messages more than verbal; and where a person is accepted for what he or she is. The family may need your help in becoming aware of disruptive forces, of their maladaptive patterns, and of ways to promote an accepting home atmosphere.

In doing a family assessment, ask questions related to achieving the developmental tasks that were described earlier. Also, determine communication patterns and relationships, family health, access to health care, occupational demands and hazards, religious beliefs and practices, childrearing practices, participation in the community, and support systems. When you work with the family unit the information in Fig. 4–1 will help you assess the family's life-style and needs.

You can help families understand some processes and dynamics underlying interaction so that they, in turn, learn to respect the uniqueness of the self and of each other. Certainly members in the family need not always agree with each other. Instead they can learn to listen to the other person, about how he or she feels and why, accepting each person's impression as real for self. This attitude becomes the basis for mutual respect, honest communication, encouragement of individual fulfillment, and freedom to be. There is then no need to prove or defend the self.

Once the attitude "We are all important people in this family" is established, conflicts can be dealt with openly and constructively. Name calling and belittling are out of place. Families need to structure time together; otherwise individual schedules will allow them less and less time to meet. Parents need to send consis-

Meeting of Physical, Emotional, and Spiritual Needs of Members
Ability to provide food and shelter
 Space management as regards living, sleeping, recreation, privacy
 Crowding if over 1.5 persons per room
 Territoriality or control of each member over lifespace
 Access to laundry, grocery, recreation facilities
 Sanitation including disposal methods, source of water supply, control of rodents and insects
 Storage and refrigeration
 Available food supply
 Food preparation, including preserving and cooking methods, (stove, hotplate, oven)
 Use of food stamps and donated foods as well as eligibility for food stamps
 Education of each member as to food composition, balanced menus, special preparations or diets if required for a specific member
Access to health care
 Regularity of health care
 Continuity of caregivers
 Closeness of facility and means of access such as car, bus, cab
 Access to helpful neighbors
 Access to phone
Family health
 Longevity
 Major or chronic illnesses
 Familial or hereditary illnesses such as rheumatic fever, gout, allergy, tuberculosis, renal disease, diabetes mellitus, cancer, emotional illness, epilepsy, migraine, other nervous disorders, hypertension, blood diseases, obesity, frequent accidents, drug intake, pica
 Emotional or stress-related illnesses
 Pollutants that members are chronically exposed to such as air, water, soil, noise, or chemicals that are unsafe to health
Neighborhood pride and loyalty
Job access, energy output, shift changes
Sensitivity, warmth, understanding between family members
 Demonstration of emotion
 Enjoyment of sexual relations
  Male: Impotence, premature or retarded ejaculation, hypersexuality
  Female: Frigidity (inability to achieve orgasm), enjoyment of sexual relations, feelings of disgust, shame, self-devaluation; fear of injury, painful coitus
  Menstrual history, including onset, duration, flow, missed periods and life situation at the time, pain, euphoria, depression, other difficulties
Sharing of religious beliefs, values, doubts
 Formal membership in church and organizations
 Ethical framework and honesty
 Adaptability, response to reality

Satisfaction with life
Self-esteem

Childrearing Practices and Discipline
Mutual responsibility
 Joint parenting
 Mutual respect for decision making
 Means of discipline and consistency
Respect for individuality
Fostering of self-discipline
Attitudes toward education, reading, scholarly pursuit
Attitudes toward imaginative play
Attitudes toward involvement in sports
Promotion of gender stereotypes

Communication
Expression of a wide range of emotion and feeling
Expression of ideas, concepts, beliefs, values, interests
Openness
Verbal expression and sensitive listening
Consensual decision making

Support, Security, Encouragement
Balance in activity
Humor
Dependency and dominance patterns
Life support groups of each member
Social relationship of couple: go out together or separately; change since marriage mutually satisfying; effect of sociability patterns on children

Growth-Producing Relationships and Experiences Within and Without the Family
Creative play activities
Planned growth experiences
Focus of life and activity of each member
Friendships

Responsible Community Relationships
Organizations, including involvement, membership, active participation
Knowledge of and friendship with neighbors

Growing With and Through Children
Hopes and plans for children
Emulation of own parents and its influence on relationship with children
Relationship patterns: authoritarian, patriarchal, matriarchal
Necessity to relive (make up for) own childhood through children

Unity, Loyalty, and Cooperation
Positive interacting of members toward each other

Self-Help and Acceptance of Outside Help in Family Crisis

Figure 4-1. Family assessment tool.

tent messages to their children. To say "Don't smoke" while immediately lighting a cigarette is hardly effective.

Times of communication are especially necessary when children are feeling peer pressure; children, moreover, should be praised for what they do right rather than reprimanded for what they do wrong. Children need structure but should be told the reason for the structure if old enough to comprehend. As you help the

family achieve positive feelings toward and interaction with one another, you are also helping them to fulfill their tasks, roles, and functions. Review the adaptive mechanisms of families described in this chapter.

The person's health problems, especially emotional ones, may well be the result of the interaction patterns in childhood or in the present family. Knowledge of the variables influencing family interaction—parents' self-esteem and upbringing, number of siblings, the person's ordinal position in the family, cultural norms, family rituals—all will help you assist the person in talking through feelings related to past and present conflicts. Sometimes helping the person understand these variables in relation to the spouse's upbringing and behavior can be the first step in overcoming current marital problems.

You may help families explore and resolve ethical dilemmas related to their decisions whether their plans involve use of newer technology for getting pregnant or dealing with an adoptive child. Technology that allows infertile couples to become pregnant with in vitro fertilization may also cause parents to face major ethical dilemmas as they determine which of the fertilized embryos should be transplanted into the uterus and which should be frozen for future use. Exploration of feelings and implications is essential.

You may explore with the family the decision to use sperm donors for artificial insemination who are paid for their service. The donor should be carefully screened for a family history of inherited diseases and for current pathogens such as human immunodeficiency virus (HIV). Because some infections such as HIV, are present long before they may be detected (as long as 7 years), transmission of this disease via insemination may become known in the future. The donor is also screened in terms of race, intelligence quotient, physical characteristics, and health. Recipients may choose the baby's gender. Some women become pregnant after the first insemination; others require several inseminations (61).

Hiring a surrogate mother—a woman to become pregnant and bear the baby for the family—must also be carefully explored because of implications for the surrogate mother and her feelings, consequent feelings of the childrearing family, and legal issues (61).

Other decisions may not be as difficult but are key to future family development and relationships (e.g., helping adoptive parents relate with their child (4) or the homosexual family explain "coming out" to the children from an earlier marriage (35). These parents must be prepared to explain the child's origins when the child asks and to help the child understand that there are many kinds of families in the United States. We do not yet know the consequences, developmentally and emotionally, for children who are raised without guidance from the opposite gender or who are raised by only one parent. Your assessment, exploration, and teaching with such families are important.

More nursing research is needed in all of these areas. To help families explore values and ethical principles, you must *first* explore and resolve these issues within yourself. You cannot give another *the* answer; you can use therapeutic communication skills to enable clients to find their own answers.

You are a nurse, not a specialized family counselor, although with advanced preparation you could do

family therapy. But you can often sense lack of communication in a family. Through use of an empathic relationship and effective communication, teaching, and crisis therapy, you can encourage family members to talk about their feelings with one another and assist in the resolution of their conflicts. Help them become aware of the need to work for family cohesiveness just as they would work at a job or important project. Refer them to a family counseling service if the problems are beyond your scope. Your work with them should also help them better use other community resources such as private family or psychiatric counseling or family and children's services. Box 4–2 lists pertinent *nursing diagnoses*.

One family self-help resource can be the formation of a group of four or five complete family units (including stepfamily, single-parent, cohabitation, or the traditional unit) who contract to meet together over an extended period of time for shared educational experiences that concern relationships within their families. This setting provides a positive approach and affirms family members because a commitment is made for all persons—no matter what their age—to have both power and input into the group.

Your knowledge of the family life cycle, with developmental tasks to be performed at each stage, provides a foundation for learning the specifics of sequential development. This combined knowledge will help you in assessing the status of the family and the individual person in planning care, in intervention, and in objectively evaluating your effectiveness.

One liability in working with families of various economic levels and cultures may be *you*. For example, if you come from a middle-class U.S. background, that fact will affect your opinions about what constitutes family life. Your attitude toward nonconforming families or unconventional living arrangements may interfere with your objectivity and thus with your ability to assist some families. You will need to go through your own maturation process of learning that your way is not always the best or only way. The process is difficult. The book by Kramer (50) gives insights helpful to the person who is working with families.

Role of the Nurse in Well-Baby Care

You may care for well babies and mothers in a variety of settings—the clinic, hospital, home, or doctor's office. Your actions contribute significantly to their health.

Prenatal Care

Prenatal care to the mother and her partner may include physical assessment, teaching healthful practices for mother and baby, listening to mother vent frustrations or share fears, counseling her during periods of depression or uncertainty, and sharing her happy feelings about becoming a mother. You may conduct childbirth classes for mother and father so that they can better understand changes occurring in the mother and the nutrition and

■ **BOX 4-2.**
Selected Nursing Diagnoses Related to Family Nursing[a]

Pattern 2: Communicating

Impaired Verbal Communication

Pattern 3: Relating

Impaired Social Interaction
Social Isolation
Altered Role Performance
Altered Parenting
Potential Altered Parenting
Sexual Dysfunction
Altered Family Processes
Parental Role Conflict
Altered Sexuality Patterns

Pattern 4: Valuing

Spiritual Distress

Pattern 5: Choosing

Ineffective Individual Coping
Impaired Adjustment
Defensive Coping
Ineffective Denial
Ineffective Family Coping: Disabling
Ineffective Family Coping: Compromised
Family Coping: Potential for Growth
Decisional Conflict
Health Seeking Behaviors

Pattern 6: Moving

Diversional Activity Deficit
Impaired Home Maintenance Management
Altered Health Maintenance
Ineffective Breastfeeding
Altered Growth and Development

Pattern 7: Perceiving

Chronic Low Self-esteem
Situational Low Self esteem
Personal Identify Disturbance
Unilateral Neglect
Hopelessness
Powerlessness

Pattern 8: Knowing

Knowledge Deficit

Pattern 9: Feeling

Dysfunctional Grieving
Anticipatory Grieving
Potential for Violence: Self-Directed or Directed at Others
Post-Trauma Response
Anxiety
Fear

[a]Many of the NANDA nursing diagnoses are applicable to the ill individual in the family unit.
From North American Nursing Diagnosis Association, *NANDA Nursing Diagnosis Taxonomy I* (Rev.). St. Louis: North American Nursing Diagnosis Association, 1990.

hygiene necessary during pregnancy; know what to expect during labor, delivery, and postpartum; and prepare for an active role during birth. A maternity nursing book will give adequate detail to help you do prenatal assessment and care and intrapartal and postpartal assessment and intervention.

If the mother-to-be is unwed, you may also try to work with the father-to-be if both are willing. The father-to-be needs help in talking about his feelings and needs to support her, if they are compatible. He may also seek sex education.

To help the unwed parents and break the cycle for future generations, we must gain a better understanding of the unwed father. Do not perceive him as irresponsible or having taken advantage of an innocent girl. The relationship between the unwed mother and the father is not necessarily a hit-and-miss affair but often meaningful to both. If the parents-to-be are adolescents, they realize that a new life has been created as a result of their actions. They want to act in a responsible way.

They are concerned about the child's well-being (52, 56).

The unwed father can be encouraged to stand by the unmarried mother. Often he feels proud of fathering; he has proved his masculinity. The long-term consequences of having a child are such, however, that alternate solutions regarding the future of the child should be thoroughly explored with and by both partners. Alternatives include marriage, placing the child for adoption, or assumption by either parent or the grandparents of the responsibility for caring for and rearing the child. The man needs help in understanding how and why he became a father and the serious implications for the mother, the child, and himself.

Adolescents may admit that their sexual experiences were unsatisfactory, leaving them depressed, guilty, and scared. The good relationship with the girlfriend may have begun to deteriorate when sexual relations were started. Pregnancy comes as a shock to both. They know about contraceptives, but their use may have been sporadic, if at all, for some people believe that the spontaneity and sincerity of the sexual act are lessened when prepared for (52, 56).

Sex education must relate to the values of interpersonal relations and concern for others if it is to be successful. The implications and responsibilities of sexual behavior must be discussed with the teenagers. The difference between teenage love and a more mature relationship between people who are ready to meet the problems and responsibilities of adulthood should be discussed (52, 56).

Parents of the unwed father must be involved in helping their son; communication between the boy and parents should be reestablished. In addition, parents should assert themselves in helping the boy take responsibility for his actions and assist the boy in the case of marriage.

Efforts to prevent unwed pregnancies must be directed to improving and strengthening family life and developing a better respect for the father's role in the family. Many unwed fathers come from female-dominated homes or from homes in which the father is absent or inadequate in his role (52, 56).

Fathers can help adolescent sons by talking with and listening to them, by being slow to judge, by taking them to the job so the youth can see how the father earns a living, and by being a role model in relating maturely to the spouse and other women. Fathers can create an atmosphere in which the sons will want to talk about emerging sexual feelings and experiences (52, 56). If the adolescent son comes from a home where no father is present, the mother can work at listening to and discussing problems and feelings with the son. She may also be able to foster a bond between the son and another male member of the family.

Childbirth Education Classes

If you conduct childbirth education classes, try to interview each couple in their home early in the pregnancy, by the fourth month if possible, to observe their relationship and determine their response to pregnancy. Their response may be different and more honest in their own home than in class. During the classes include opportunities for both men and women to talk about the problems they feel are uniquely theirs, their feelings, or the commonality of the couvade syndrome. Provide anticipatory guidance about the couvade syndrome. Avoid pushing the father into participation and provide support for him. Focus childbirth education on the known benefits to the baby and parents and not on over-romanticized and dramatic statements about improved marital relationships. Educate both parents about family planning so that future pregnancies can be mutually planned. Refer either partner, or both, to psychologic counseling when necessary, especially if antisocial behavior is seen or if there has been fetal loss.

Labor

During labor you do necessary physical care, but you may also act as a coach for the mother, or you may support the father as he assists his wife. Flexibility in hospital routines for obstetric patients is usually possible and contributes to the parents' sense of control. In fact, negative feelings about traditional hospital deliveries have become so widespread that home delivers are increasing in many cities, often attended by a granny midwife instead of a professional doctor or nurse-midwife.

The physician and nurse or nurse-midwife can work as a team with the expectant couple. In some facilities the nurse-midwife assumes primary responsibility for the family unit. Whenever a mother delivers, she has the right to capable, safe care by qualified caretakers. Home deliveries can be carefully planned and safe. Hospital delivers can be more homelike. Maternity centers now provide families anticipating a normal childbearing experience with antepartum care that is educational in nature; labor and delivery in a homelike setting (but with adequate equipment) with discharge to home whenever it is safe for mother and baby, probably within 12 hours after delivery; and follow-up care by public health nurses in the home during the postpartum course. The labor-delivery rooms can be designed to accommodate the presence of the father or family during delivery and be less traumatic (cold, with intense lights) for the newborn. After the birth, the infant can remain with the mother, and the newborn's physical examination can be done in her presence with the father present. Childbirth should be a positive, maturing experience for the couple. Expectant parents have the right and responsibility to be involved in planning their care with the health team and to know what is happening. Cultural beliefs should be recognized, respected, and accommodated whenever possible. A positive childbearing experience contributes to a healthy family unit.

Delivery Methods

These methods are changing in some centers as doctors and midwives follow the trend set by Dr. Leboyer in France. The delivery room lights are dimmed; people speak softly or whisper; the infant is placed on the mother's abdomen to maintain body temperature and the prebirth curved position of the spine; the baby is massaged by mother and doctor; and the cord is not cut immediately. The baby is placed in warm water. Precautions are taken when necessary, but apparently delivery does not have to be so traumatic for the baby (53, 85).

Postpartum Period

In the early postpartum period assess mother and baby and give the mother physical care and assist her as necessary, even if she looks well and able. "Mother" the mother (18, 78, 79). Arrange the environment and hospital routines to enhance bonding between mother and baby. Listen to the mother's concerns; answer her questions; support her maternal behavior. In a nonthreatening way, teach the mother how to handle her baby. Help her begin to unlearn preconceived ideas about the baby and herself and to perceive herself and the baby positively. Give her special assistance if she is breast-feeding. After the initial "taking-in" period of having received special care and attention, the mother moves to the "taking hold" stage where she is able to care for the child (78, 79).

The interaction between the infant and primary caretaker is crucial. The mothering person helps the baby feel secure and loved, fosters a sense of trust, provides stimulation, reinforces certain behavior, acts as a model for language development, and trains the baby in basic learning strategies. In turn, maternal behavior is influenced by baby's cries, coos, smiles, activity, gazes, and by how well baby's behavior meets the mother's expectations.

Your significant contribution to the family unit is to promote attachment between parents and baby, encourage continuing contacts between the family and health professionals so that adequate health and illness care are received, and encourage parents to meet the baby's needs adequately. You can help the parents feel good about themselves and the baby.

You can be instrumental in continuing new trends in care to make the hospital or clinic environment more homelike while providing safe, modern care.

Continued Care in the Fourth Trimester

During the **fourth trimester,** the *6 or 8 weeks after delivery,* the mother needs assistance with child care and an opportunity to regain her former self physically and emotionally. Father also needs support as he becomes involved in child-care responsibilities (71). In the nuclear or single-parent family the parent(s) may struggle alone. Visits by a home health nurse may be useful. Some communities have a crisis line for new parents. You may be able to suggest services or help the parent(s) think of people who could be helpful.

As you assess the mother's functioning, consider her physical and emotional energy, support systems, and current level of parenting activity. If she apparently is not caring adequately for the child, assess for anemia, pain, bleeding, infections, lack of food or sleep, drug use, or other medical conditions that would interfere with her activity level and feelings of caring. Depression and postpartum blues are difficult to differentiate. In depression the mother is immobilized and forgets basic care, but with postpartum blues she may cry but care for the baby's physical needs.

The new mother usually has enough energy to do only top-priority tasks—eating, sleeping, baby care, and essentials for other family members. A house that is too clean is a danger signal that she is neglecting the baby, herself, or both (9).

The mother's support system is crucial for her energy maintenance, both physical and emotional. She needs direct support and assistance with daily tasks, plus moral support, a listener, a confidant. Support comes from personal and professional sources—the partner, parents, friends, other relatives, and the nurse, doctor, social worker, or pastor. Negative attitudes from others can drain emotional energy.

Bishop's (9) and Campbell and Smith's (19) guides to assess parenting feelings and adequate mothering may be helpful. Actual parenting skills can be manifested in various ways: touching, cuddling, a tender, soft voice tone, and loving gazes. Ability to obtain adequate medical care is typical of the caring parent; lack of use of medical services for the baby indicates a poor mother-child relationship. Additional information about parents' feelings and the parenting process are described in Chapter 7, pp. 207–215.

If the baby is progressing in normal fashion, focus on the mother's needs and concerns. Help her find nonprofessional support systems that can assist her when the professional is unavailable or that can help with child care. In addition to concern over child care, we must help the mother grow developmentally. Helping her stay in good physical and emotional health ensures better parenting.

A study of 117 women in early puerperium who had had vaginal deliveries and healthy newborns revealed that their teaching priorities may differ from what you believe is a teaching priority (26). Study results were analyzed with percentages in relation to all mothers, maternal age groups (teens, twenties, thirties), and parity groups (primiparas, multiparas). The maternal care topic of highest priority for all age and pariety groups was "Postpartum Complications." The infant care topic of highest priority for all age and pariety groups was "Infant Illnesses." The results suggest that these teaching topics are of most concern to mothers during the early postpartum period. The mothers' priorities assigned to other teaching topics varied by age and parity groups (26).

Care of Families Who Have a Child Born Prematurely or With Defect

Prematurity accounts for 50% of neonatal mortality, and premature infants who survive contribute significantly to the number of physically, intellectually, and emotionally handicapped children in the United States. Complications of prematurity include major and minor physical abnormalities, general motor incoordination, short attention span, distractibility and hyperactivity, difficulty separating from parents, preoccupation with the body, and scholastic underachievement (62, 85).

The last complications may be related more to an early disturbed mother-child relationship than to the prematurity, perinatal complications, or the child's birth defects. Typically the infant is rushed to the nursery after birth, thereby preventing physical or eye contact between mother and baby. The mother is often isolated from other mothers; professionals and family may avoid conversation about the baby. Mother often sees the baby in the premature or intensive care nursery at a distance and only indistinctly; or the baby may have been transported to a children's hospital at some distance so that visiting the baby after her discharge is difficult. The mother may have no opportunity to form any attachment feelings unless nursing staff foster the involvement in child care to the extent possible and keep her informed of baby's condition and progress. The baby who finally comes home to the parents may be a stranger for whom the mother has no maternal response or commitment. Additionally, the mother has developed little confidence in her mothering abilities and no caretaking regimen.

Behavior patterns in parents that strongly suggest a disturbed parent-child relationship and future problems in parenting the premature or defective child include the following behaviors:

1. Unable to talk about guilt feelings, fears, and their sense of responsibility for the child's early arrival with each other or others
2. Demonstrate no visible anxiety about the baby's condition, deny the reality, or displace anxiety onto less threatening matters
3. Make little effort to secure information about the baby's condition
4. Consistently misinterpret or exaggerate either positive or negative information about the baby and display no signs of hope as baby's condition improves
5. Receive no practical support or help from family or friends, and community resources are lacking
6. Unable to accept and use help offered

You may be instrumental in promoting certain procedures that can be used by hospital personnel to promote parent-child relationship:

1. Permit the mother to see and touch the baby as soon as possible, preferably in the delivery room; or transfer the baby to the mother's room in a portable incubator if the baby remains in the same hospital.
2. Permit the mother's involvement in baby's care as soon as possible. Take the mother to the premature care unit, teaching her to use the aseptic technique needed to touch, care for, and visit with the baby.
3. Provide an atmosphere that encourages questions.
4. Encourage parents to talk with each other, family members, and friends—using others for support.
5. Recognize that parent's excessive questions, demands, and criticisms are a reaction to stress and

not personal attacks on the professional worker or hospital.
6. Do not offer reassuring cliches or comforting statements too quickly. Encourage parents to cry, to face the reality of the situation.
7. Do not pressure parents to talk about their feelings all at once, but avoid using the excuse of "not wanting to probe" to avoid talking with them.
8. Encourage the mother to express breast milk if she wishes; the breast milk can be taken to a breast-milk bank and used for the infant. When the baby is sucking well, the mother can help bottle-feed the baby until the baby is strong enough to breast-feed.
9. Arrange for father to visit the baby before discharge, calling him about baby's progress at intervals when he is unable to visit.
10. Encourage the parents to handle the baby and do baby's care before discharge; teach about baby care as necessary while the parents are engaged in care of their baby.

Refer also to Chapter 7, pp. 245–248 for additional information. The book by Featherstone (32) is a useful reference. It was one of the first books written that focuses on family issues that occur when there is a developmentally disabled child, on the system as a whole, on the marital subsystem, and on the sibling subsystem. Because of the chronicity of developmental disability or some congenital defects, the article by Woods, Yates, and Primono (98) is a helpful reference.

Parent Education

To combat the problems associated with the high adolescent birthrate, some junior and senior high schools are establishing creative programs in parenthood education. Some hospitals and health clinics are initiating specialized prenatal and postnatal services for the adolescent mother and her at-risk infant. You can initiate nontraditional programs in your own community.

Some hospitals have established programs to help adolescent mothers become more effective parents. The adolescent mother who decides to keep her baby needs all the family and outside help she can get. She fears that whatever personal ambitions she has will be thwarted by the baby. Unmarried and unprepared for employment, she finds it almost impossible to make her own way in the world. Anger, frustration, and ignorance hamper her ability to attach to and appropriately care for the baby. Repeated pregnancies, child neglect and abuse, and welfare dependency often occur.

Formation of a mother's group, including women of various ethnic origins and income brackets, can provide parent education and support and foster talking about feelings. You should also educate parents about using community resources.

Your work with the mother may prevent maternal deprivation, insufficient interaction between mother and child, conditions under which the deprivation or even abuse develops, and negative effects on the child's development.

Working With Adoptive Families

You can help the adoptive parents in their adjustment. Assure them that attachment develops over time. Help them think through how and when to tell the child that he or she is adopted so that the child understands and is not traumatized. Help the parents anticipate how they will help the child cope when the child is taunted by peers about being adopted. Help them realize that the adopted child will probably seek answers to many questions when he or she gets older. Who were the parents? Their cultural, racial, or ethnic background? Their ages, occupations, interests, appearance? Why was he or she relinquished? What are the medical facts surrounding heredity and birth? Help parents realize that these questions do not mean that the child does not love them. Various articles supply information on adoption procedures, stresses encountered, and how to make adoption a success (14–17, 28, 30, 39, 48, 51, 68, 72, 82, 94, 95). Refer also to p. 248.

Working with Stepfamilies

The guidelines already discussed will be useful to you as you help the single-parent family or stepfamily adjust to its situation. The single-parent family can be referred to a local chapter of Parents Without Partners if the person seeks support from peers. Do not rush in with answers for these families until you have heard their unique problems. Acknowledge their strengths; help them formulate their own solutions. Often a few sessions of crisis therapy will be sufficient. Several references give further information (3, 36, 70, 74, 80, 91, 92, 96). Refer also to pp. 131–133.

Family Care Throughout the Life Cycle

You may be called on to assist families as they meet various developmental crises throughout the life cycle: school entry of the child, the adolescent period, children leaving home, divorce, retirement, death of a member. Your goal is health promotion and primary prevention. Your intervention early in the family life cycle may help establish a positive health trend in place of its negative counterpart. The care you give to young parents lays the foundation for their children's health. You may also find yourself becoming an advocate for families. The state or federal governments could support high-quality day care for the children of couples who want—or who are obliged—to pursue uninterrupted careers. Government dollars could be used in improving the schools in low-income neighborhoods (8, 10, 29, 54).

Another way to improve the family as an institution is from within. Parents should teach their children not just to get ahead but to serve, to cooperate, to be kind. The most disturbing force in America today is excessive competitiveness. People are obsessed with their jobs and with personal advancement and downgrade the family. We should be teaching our children to believe that family ties are the most rewarding values, that social, cultural and community activities can be deeply satisfying, and that the gratification from income and jobs is shallow by comparison (8, 10, 29, 54).

Our excessive competitiveness is being passed on to our children as parents try to produce "superkids." Misplaced educational pressure is likely to produce lopsided development and an aversion to schooling. To diminish the competitive atmosphere in schools, grades and examination should be dropped. Excessive competitiveness overlaps with excessive materialism. In most parts of the world materialism is balanced by spiritual values (e.g., dedication to God in Islamic countries, dedication to the nation in Israel, dedication to the family in Greece). By contrast, in America many children get their values—materialism, competitiveness, and brutality—from television. In turn, rates for violent crime are shockingly high. Parents should demand good programs from television producers and forbid their children's watching the violence and sordid sex. It is no wonder some youths panic at finding they have no supporting beliefs and turn to extremist cults and lifestyles and that the rate of teenage suicide has tripled in the past 20 years (8, 10, 29, 54).

Parents can make a profound difference by teaching spiritual values—helpfulness, cooperation, generosity, love—throughout childhood. Two-year-old children can be encouraged to help set the table and then be thanked and praised. Teenagers can be expected to work in hospitals and to tutor younger children. Such jobs should not be presented as distasteful. Children enjoy taking on adult jobs when they are presented as opportunities and efforts are appreciated (8).

Just as vital is a family atmosphere in which parents treat each other and their children with respect and affection and smile. The best forum is still meal time and the family meeting. When teenagers first give excuses why they cannot make it to a meal, parents should say very positively, "We like to have the whole family get together." Parents should avoid talking down to children and the attitude that being older makes them right but they can still be very clear about their beliefs and expectations (8, 10, 29, 54).

Parents must give careful attention to the topic of sex. We have done well to overcome the shame that used to surround sex; but in declaring sex more wholesome and natural, we have mistakenly ignored its tenderness, generosity, and intensely spiritual aspects. We have failed to instill that the impulse in idealistic youths to save intimacy for the ultimate partner has existed for centuries and has contributed to creativity in all the arts (59).

When parents are asked questions about sexual matters by 2-, 3-, and 4-year-old children, they should advance from anatomy and physiology to emphasize the loving and caring aspects of sex and marriage. An even greater influence on children is their parents' behavior toward and commitment to a partner and their admiration and respect for one another. Joking and disparaging remarks about marriage should be avoided. Parents can suggest that if young people want to claim the right to sexual freedom, they should be aware of the responsibilities. If a youthful marriage soon ends in divorce, parents can point out that no marriage succeeds by itself but must be continually cultivated, like a garden. It is wise to look for openings to discuss these topics when children are 9, 10, or 11 years of age. When they are 13 years old and beyond, they think their parents are hopelessly old-fashioned and consider peer opinions as the only truth (8, 54).

If we allow the strains of our society to worsen, then living here will be ever more painful. In our democracy we can control our society by guiding our children and using our political power. We need to move from an emphasis on ambitious individualism and self-centeredness into cooperation for the common good. We need leaders who have vision and courage, and we need mature parents who present a positive model for the future of the family and society.

REFERENCES

1. Ackerman, N., *Diagnosis and Treatment of Family Relations*. New York: Basic Books, 1972.
2. Anderson, M., The Mental Health Advantages of Twinship, *Perspectives of Psychiatric Care,* 23, no. 3 (1985), 114–116.
3. Andolfi, M., *Family Therapy: An Interactional Approach*. New York: Plenum Press, 1979.
4. Barth, R., and M. Berry, *Adoption and Disruption: Rates, Risks, and Responses*. Hawthorne, NY: Aldine de Gruyter, 1988.
5. Beavers, R., and R. Hampson, *Successful Families: Assessment and Intervention*. New York: W.W. Norton & Co., 1990.
6. Bell, A., M. Weinberg, and S. Hammersmith, *Sexual Preference: Its Development in Men and Women*. Bloomington, Ind: Indiana University Press, 1981.
7. Benedek, T., Parenthood During the Life Cycle. In Anthony, E. J., and T. Benedek, eds., *Parenthood: Its Psychology and Psychopathology*. Boston: Little, Brown, 1970, pp. 185–206.
8. Bettelheim, B., *A Good Enough Parent: A Book on Child-Rearing*. New York: Alfred A. Knopf, 1987.
9. Bishop, B., A Guide to Assessing Parenting Capabilities, *American Journal of Nursing,* 76, no. 11 (1976), 1784–1787.
10. Bossard, J., and E. Boll, *Sociology of Child Development* (4th ed.). New York: Harper & Row, 1960.
11. Bowlby, J., The Making and Breaking of Affectional Bonds, *British Journal of Psychiatry,* 130, (March, 1977), 201–210.
12. Bozett, F., ed., *Gay and Lesbian Parents*. New York: Preager Publishers, 1987.
13. ——, Social Control of Identity by Children of Gay Fathers, *Western Journal of Nursing Research,* 10, no. 5 (1988), 550–565.
14. Brockhaus, J., and R. Brockhaus, Adopting an Older Child—The Emotional Process, *American Journal of Nursing,* 82, no. 2 (1982), 288–291.
15. ——, Adopting a Child with Special Needs: The Legal Process, *American Journal of Nursing,* 82, no. 2 (1982), 291–294.
16. ——, Foster Care, Adoption, and the Grief Process, *Journal of Psychiatric Nursing and Mental Health Services,* 20, no. 9 (1982), 9–16.
17. Brodzinsky, D. M., et al. Psychological and Academic Adjustment of Adopted Children, *Journal of Consulting and Clinical Psychology,* 52 (1984), 869–878.
18. Brown, M., and J. Hurlock, Mothering the Mother, *American Journal of Nursing,* 77, no. 3 (1977), 439–441.
19. Campbell, S., and J. Smith, Postpartum: Assessment Guide, *American Journal of Nursing,* 77, no. 7 (1977), 1179.
20. Carmichael, C., *Nonsexist Childraising*. Boston: Beacon Press, 1977.
21. Cass, V., Homosexual Identity Formation: A Theoretical Model, *Journal of Homosexuality,* 4, no. 3 (1985), 219–235.
22. Clinton, J., Expectant Fathers at Risk for Couvade, *Nursing Research,* 35, no. 5 (1986), 290–294.
23. Colarusso, C., and R. Nemeroff, *Adult Development*. New York: Plenum Press, 1981.
24. Coleman, A., and L. Coleman, *Pregnancy: The Psychological Experience*. New York: Herder & Herder, 1972.
25. Coleman, P., *The Forgiving Marriage*. Chicago, Contemporary Books, 1989.
26. Davis, J., M. Brucker, and N. MacMullen, A Study of Mothers' Postpartum Teaching Priorities, *Maternal-Child Nursing Journal,* 17, no. 1 (1988), 41–50.
27. Dugan, A., Compadrazgo: A Caring Phenomenon Among Urban Latinos and Its Relationship to Health. In Leininger, M., ed., *Care: The Essence of Nursing and Health*. Detroit: Wayne State University Press, 1988, pp. 183–194.
28. Dunn, L., ed., *Adopting Children with Special Needs: A Sequel*. Washington, DC.: North American Council on Adoptable Children, 1983.
29. Duvall, E., and B. Miller, *Marriage and Family Development* (6th ed.). New York: Harper & Row, 1984.
30. Edwards, M.P., and F.E. Boyd, Adoption for Adolescents, *Child Welfare,* 54, no. 4 (1975), 298–299.
31. Erikson, E., *Childhood and Society* (2nd ed.). New York: W.W. Norton, 1963.
32. Featherstone, H., *A Difference in the Family*. New York: Penguin Books, 1981.
33. Fox, T., Tips on Making the Reunited Family Work, *St. Louis Globe-Democrat,* January 31, 1980. Reprinted in *LTC Notes:* The Catholic Health Association, 11, no. 2 (1981), 2–3.
34. Friedman, M., *Family Nursing: Theory and Assessment* (2nd ed.). Norwalk, Conn: Appleton-Century-Crofts, 1985.

35. Gantz, J., *Whose Child Cries: Children of Gay Parents Talk About Their Lives*. Rolling Hills Estates, Calif: View Press, 1983.

36. Gardner, R., *Psychotherapy With Children of Divorce*. New York: Jason Aronson, 1976.

37. Garrison, J., Part 7: Gay in America, A Special Report: Creating New Families. *San Francisco Examiner,* June 12, 1989, Sec. A, p 17.

38. Gieleghem, P., Discovery of the Couvade Phenomenon: Theory and Clinical Uses. In Leininger, M., ed., *Care: Discovery and Uses in Clinical and Community Nursing*. Detroit: Wayne State University Press, 1988.

39. Gil, O., and B. Jackson, *Adoption and Race: Black, Asian, and Mixed-Race Children in White Families*. New York: St. Martin's Press, 1983.

40. Goodrich, T., et al: *Feminist Family Therapy*. New York: W.W. Norton, 1988.

41. Gordon, T., *Parent Effectiveness Training*. New York: Peter H. Wyden, 1970.

42. Greenberg, M., and N. Morris, Engrossment: The Newborn's Impact Upon the Father, *American Journal of Orthopsychiatry,* 44, no. 4 (1974), 520–531.

43. Harris, M., and P. Turner, Gay and Lesbian Parents, *Journal of Homosexuality,* 12, no. 2 (1986), 101–113.

44. Hoopes, M., and J. Harper, *Birth Order Roles and Sibling Patterns in Individual and Family Therapy*. Rockville, Md: Aspen Publishers, 1987.

45. Hott, J., The Crisis of Expectant Fatherhood, *American Journal of Nursing,* 76, no. 9 (1976), 1436–1440.

46. Hrobsky, D., Transition to Parenthood: A Balancing of Needs, *Nursing Clinics of North America,* 12, no. 3 (1977), 457–468.

47. Hughes, C., An Eclectic Approach to Parent Group Education, *Nursing Clinics of North America,* 12, no. 3 (1977), 469–480.

48. Jewett, C.L., *Helping Children Cope With Separation and Loss*. Cambridge, Mass: The Harvard Common Press, 1982.

49. Kirkpatrick, M., C. Smith, and R. Roy, Lesbian Mothers and Their Children: A Comparative Survey, *Journal of Orthopsychiatry,* 51, no. 3 (1981), 545–557.

50. Kramer, J., *Family Interfaces: Transgenerational Patterns*. New York: Brunner/Mazel, 1987.

51. Krementz, J., *How It Feels to Be Adopted*. New York: Alfred Knopf, 1982.

52. Lamb, M., *The Father's Role*. New York: John Wiley, 1986.

53. LeBoyer's Babies, *Science News,* January 22, 1977.

54. Lidz, T., *The Person: His and Her Development Throughout the Life Cycle* (2nd ed.). New York: Basic Books, 1983.

55. Luepnitz, D., *The Family Interpreted: Feminist Theory in Clinical Practice*. New York: Basic Books, 1988.

56. Lynn, D., *The Father: His Role in Child Development*. Monterey, Calif: Brooks/Cole Publishing, 1974.

57. Messer, A., *The Individual in His Family: An Adaptational Study*. Springfield, Ill: Charles C Thomas, 1970.

58. Miller, B., Gay Fathers and Their Children, *The Family Coordinator* (October 1979), 544–556.

59. Miller, J., R. Jacobsen, and J. Bigner, The Child's Home Environment for Lesbian vs. Heterosexual Mothers: A Neglected Area of Research, *Journal of Homosexuality,* 7, no. 2 (1981), 49–56.

60. Minuchin, S., *Family Kaleidoscope*. Cambridge, Mass: Harvard University Press, 1984.

61. Montgomery, P., Should Surrogate Motherhood Be Banned? *Common Cause Magazine* (May/June 1988), 36–38.

62. Moshman, D., J. Glover, and R. Bruning, *Developmental Psychology*. Boston: Little, Brown, 1987.

63. Murphy, S., Family Study and Nursing Research, *Image,* 18, no. 4 (1986), 170–173.

64. Obrzut, L., Expectant Father's Perceptions of Fathering, *American Journal of Nursing,* 76, no. 9 (1976), 1440–1442.

65. Otto, H.A., Criteria for Assessing Family Strengths, *Canada's Mental Health,* 6 (1966), 257.

66. Perdue, B., J. Horowitz, and F. Herz, Mothering, *Nursing Clinics of North America,* 12, no. 3 (1977), 491–502.

67. Petze, C., Health Promotion for the Well Family, *Nursing Clinics of North America,* 19, no. 2 (1984), 229–237.

68. Plumey, J.H., *Successful Adoption*. New York: Harmony Books, 1982.

69. Public Health Problems Fuel Surge in Children in Foster Care, *The Nation's Health* (January 1990), 1, 11.

70. Reder, N., Single Parents/Dual Responsibilities, *The National Voter,* 39, no. 1 (1989), 9–11.

71. Rising, S., The Fourth Stage of Labor: Family Reintegration, *American Journal of Nursing,* 74, no. 5 (1974), 870 ff.

72. Ritchie, C., Adoption: An Option Often Overlooked, *American Journal of Nursing,* 89, no. 9 (1989), 1156–1157.

73. Robbins, M., and T. Schacht, Family Hierarchies, *American Journal of Nursing,* 82, no. 2 (1982), 284–286.

74. Roberts, C., and S. Feetham, Assessing Family Functioning Across Three Areas of Relationships, *Nursing Research,* 31, no. 4 (1982), 231–235.

75. Rosenthal, K., and H. Keshet, *Fathers Without Partners*. Totowa, NJ: Rowman & Littlefield, 1981.

76. Rossi, A., Transition to Parenthood, *Journal of Marriage and Family,* 30 (1968), 26–39.

77. ———, Transition to Parenthood. In Sze, W., ed., *Human Life Cycle*. New York: Jason Aronson, 1975, pp. 515–529.

78. Rubin, R., Attainment of the Maternal Role. Part 1: Processes, *Nursing Research,* 16, no. 3 (1967), 237–245.

79. ———, Attainment of the Maternal Role. Part II: Models and Referrants, *Nursing Research,* 16, no. 4 (1967), 342–346.

80. Sager, C., et al., *Treating the Remarried Family*. New York: Brunner/Mazel, 1983.

81. Satir, V., Love, Understanding, Communication Are Vital Elements of Family Health, *Parameters,* 4, no. 3 (1979), 8–10.

82. Schaffer, J., and C. Londstrum, *How to Raise an Adopted Child*. New York: Crown Publishers, 1989.

83. Schuller, A., The Family Comes First, *Possibilities* (May-June, 1987), 17–28.

84. Shavelson, E., et al., Lesbian Women's Perception of Their Parent-Child Relationships, *Journal of Homosexuality,* 5, no. 3 (1980), 205–215.

85. Sherwen, L., M. Scoloreno, and C. Wengerten, *Nursing Care of the Childbearing Family*. Norwalk, Conn: Appleton-Lange, 1991.

86. Skeen, P., and B. Robinson, Family Background of Gay

Fathers: A Descriptive Study, *Psychological Reports,* 59 (1984), 999–1005.

87. Smilkstein, G., The Cycle of Family Function: A Conceptual Model for Family Medicine, *Family Practitioner,* 11 (1980), 223.

88. Smith, S., Big Families Can Be Happy, Too, *Newsweek* (January 14, 1985), 12–13.

89. Terkelson, K., Toward a Theory of the Family Life Cycle. In Carter, E., and M. McGoldrich, eds., *The Family Life Cycle: A Framework for Family Therapy.* New York: Gardner Press, 1980, pp. 21–52.

90. Toman, W., *Family Constellation* (3rd ed.). New York: Springer, 1976.

91. Visher, E., and J. Visher, *Step Families: A Guide to Working With Step Parents and Step Children.* New York: Bruner/Mazel, 1979.

92. ——, *Old Loyalties, New Ties: Therapeutic Strategies with Stepfamilies.* New York: Brunner/Mazel, 1988.

93. Wachtel, E., and P. Wachtel, *Family Dynamics in Individual Psychotherapy: A Guide to Clinical Strategies.* New York: The Guilford Press, 1986.

94. Ward, M., Parental Bonding in Older Child Adoptions, *Child Welfare,* 40, no. 1 (1981), 24–34.

95. Warren, A., Adopting a Foreign Child, *Better Homes and Gardens,* 63, no. 10 (1985), 25–27.

96. Whall, A., *Family Therapy Theory for Nursing: Four Approaches.* Norwalk, Conn: Appleton-Century-Crofts, 1986.

97. Willie, C., *A New Look at the Black Family.* Bayside, NY: Bayside Press, 1976.

98. Woods, N., B. Yates, and J. Primomo, Supporting Families During Chronic Illness, *Image,* 21, no. 1 (1989), 46–50.

Chapter 5

Overview: Theories of Human Development

No theory explains everything about the person.
—Ruth Beckmann Murray

KEY TERMS

Psychology	Classical conditioning	Conscience	Anima/animus
Heterozygous	Behavior	Conscious	Personal unconscious
Homozygous	Learning	Preconscious	Collective unconscious
Polygenic inheritance	Operant conditioning	Unconscious materials	Mandala
Neurotransmitters	Transfer	Anxiety	Individuation
Ecology	Positive reinforcement	One Genus Postulate	Introversion
Anomie	Negative reinforcement	Prototaxic mode of experiencing	Extrovert
System	Behavior modification	Parataxic mode of experiencing	Modeling
Social system	Psychodynamic Theory	Syntaxic mode of experiencing	Maturational
Open system	Cognitive Theory	Concept of anxiety	Learning
Linkage	Id	Self-system	Equilibration
First Force	Instinctual forces	Consciousness	Assimilation
Second Force	Pleasure principle	Persona	Accommodation
Third Force	Ego	Shadow	Adaptation
Behaviorist	Reality principle		Schema
Neo-Behaviorist	Superego		Phenomenal field
Shaping	Ego ideal		Self-actualization

OBJECTIVES

Study of this chapter will enable you to:

1. Identify major theoretic perspectives for understanding the developing person.
2. Describe some physiologic theories about aspects of the developing person.
3. Identify major psychologic developmental theorists, according to their views about the developing person.
4. Compare major concepts of First, Second, and Third Force theorists.
5. Discuss ecologic theory as it applies to the developing person.
6. Apply concepts from at least three theories of development in care of the client.

In the past human development was considered something that just happened. Children at first were seen as little adults, only weaker and less capable. Gradually children were seen as different, not only in proportion, but in needs and characteristics. Until the twentieth century, the study of child development and advice on how to care for children was not based on the scientific method but on biases and folklore.

During the eighteenth century scientific, religious, economic, and social trends combined to foster the study of child development. The "nature versus nurture" argument began: The child was considered either the product of heredity or environment. With the rise of Protestantism, which emphasized self-reliance, independence, and responsibility for self and others, adults began to feel more responsible for how the child developed into an adult. With the Industrial Revolution, the family changed from a clanlike group to the nuclear family, and children became more visible and more important to their parents. In turn, parents concentrated more intensely on their offspring. Education was provided for children, and teachers became important in the child's development. As the spirit of democracy filtered into the home, parents became more uncomfortable about autocratic attitudes toward and discipline of children. Eventually the science of **psychology,** *the study of human behavior,* led people to understand themselves better by learning more about child behavior. By the nineteenth century all these forces had come together, and the study of the child was more common and systematic. Yet the study of child development was not based on the variety or sophistication of theory that was to evolve during the twentieth century (59).

The study of development, which began with study of the child, expanded in the beginning of the twentieth century to include adolescence as a transitional period of life. In the early twentieth century the study of the aged person began. By the mid-twentieth century, as more people were living longer, the study of aging and the aged person became popular. The study of young adulthood and middle age as developmental periods is a phenomenon of the past two or three decades. In the last quarter of the twentieth century, the focus is on the study of human development through the life span.

Persons continue to develop or undergo change—physically, emotionally, cognitively, spiritually, and socially—throughout the life span. Dying is seen as the last developmental phase, the final attempt to come to terms with self, others, and life in general. The study of the changes made by the individual and the family unit throughout the life span is the focus of this book. By learning more about ourselves and others, including how people respond to surrounding influences to meet basic needs, we hope to help people become better able to meet their individual potential and, in turn, create a better world.

Theories that are used to explain the developing person and the person's behavior use either a biologic, ecologic-social, or psychologic basis. Although we focus on the psychologic theories, a brief explanation of biologic and ecologic-social theories is given. The psychologic theories are divided according to their emphases—behaviorism, analytic, cognitive, and humanistic. Theorists who focus on these various psychologic theories have been grouped according to similarity of theories.

Keep in mind that any theory explains an aspect of the person. *The whole person is best understood when several theories are combined to explain the person's total development.* The theories have been developed by one or several methods for studying people.

CURRENT BIOLOGIC THEORIES

Basic to the person is his or her anatomic and physiologic structure and function. Various areas of the brain control certain functions and influence behavior. The huge quantity and vast range of sensory information that is transmitted to the cerebral cortex and the way in which the brain sorts, classifies, organizes, and interprets sensory information; handles input and output; considers expectations, past experiences, and other sources of information; and sends messages throughout the body are beyond the capability of any computer system. In many ways the human brain may be like that of other animals, but it differs in its capacity to think, make judgments, remember, use symbols, store maps of the body and the world, and create.

Research on the physiologic basis for behavior has gained sophistication with advancing technology in studying the brain and nervous system, endocrine functions, and physiologic responses in a variety of situations. These findings affect current beliefs about health, normality, and development. In the following discussion, theories related to genetic, biochemical, and neurophysiologic factors briefly are covered. For comprehensive study, refer to references listed at the end of the chapter (44, 51, 59). Also, Chapters 6 and 7 through 14 present physiologic factors that affect the person.

Genetic Factors

Understanding of the role of genetic factors has been derived historically from studies focusing on pedigree descriptions, incidence of abnormalities in generations of families, and more recently in direct visual examination of chromosomes and biochemical analyses of genetic material and enzymatic processes (51).

The Mendelian Law of Inheritance states that a dominant gene for a trait or characteristic in at least one parent will cause, on the average, one half of the children to inherit it. If both parents have the dominant gene, three fourths of their children will inherit the trait. When the trait is attributed to a recessive gene, the offspring does not inherit it unless the gene was received from both parents. If the gene was received from only one parent, the offspring is not affected but will probably pass on the gene to the child (the grandchild). If the spouses are **heterozygous** for a recessive gene (*both received the same gene type from only one of their parents*), one fourth of the children probably will be affected. If the spouses are **homozygous** for the recessive gene (the *same gene type was received from both of their parents*), all the children probably will inherit the trait or characteristic (44, 59).

The Mendelian law explains the occurrence of many physical traits such as eye color or height and may explain certain physiologic characteristics. However, the Mendelian law does not fully explain emotional or mental development and does not include social, moral, or spiritual development.

Deoxyribonucleic acid (DNA) is the genetic command center of every human cell. When DNA strands have defects, disease occurs. Some of the mutations may be inherited. Research is currently underway to develop a test to reveal risk for certain diseases based on genetic defects, which would enable us to determine ways to prevent illness related to risk factors.

Further, **polygenic inheritance,** the *combination of many genes acting together to produce a behavioral characteristic,* is believed to be a factor if certain characteristics or behavioral defects occur. Environmental effects contribute to the person's development of genetic potential from the moment of conception (39, 44, 59).

For example, three factors determine cholesterol levels: presence of a single gene, polygenetic inheritance, and environment. One gene plays a key role in determining serum cholesterol levels and subsequent risk for coronary artery disease. This gene causes blood cholesterol levels of 300 mg/dl and results in heart attacks between 30 and 39 years of age for men and in the sixties for women. However, it is found in only 3% of the population. Polygenetic inheritance determines blood cholesterol levels (120 to 300 mg/dl). Environmental factors that increase risk include cigarette smoking, inactivity, stress, and diet.

Cholesterol levels below 160 mg/dl are at a preventive level; 10% of the population fall in this category. These individuals need not worry about coronary artery disease, regardless of environmental factors or diet. People with levels above 180 mg/dl should have the ratio of high-density lipoproteins to low-density lipoproteins measured. Low-density lipoproteins carry most of the cholesterol in the blood, whereas high-density lipoproteins (the so-called "good lipoproteins") carry cholesterol to the liver for metabolizing or removal from the body (85).

Biochemical Factors

Research on the relationship between biochemical factors and behavior involves the areas of neurochemistry and hormones.

Neurochemistry is implicated in some behavioral development. The amount of biogenic amines, especially the **neurotransmitters,** *chemicals involved in transfer or modulation of nerve impulses from one cell to another,* apparently are related to mood. Catecholamines, including adrenalin, noradrenaline, dopamine, and serotonin, are important neurotransmitters in the brain and are involved in such emotional states as arousal, fear, rage, pleasure, motivation, exhilaration, sleep, and wakefulness (44). Such behavior, in turn, affects reactions of others, especially parents to the child, and the child's moods may affect child-rearing behavior.

Hormonal factors, based on changes in the endocrine system during stress or endocrine system disorders, may contribute to certain behavior. Steroid hormones are increased during stress behavior, which in turn may interfere with normal developmental processes physically and cognitively (51). Research findings indicate that higher thought processes influence both physiologic reactions and the subjective experience of emotional states (43, 51, 59).

Neurophysiologic factors mediate all physiologic processes and behavior via the nervous system; however, neurophysiologic factors in behavior and personality development are inconclusive. Some specific motor and speech functions and various sensations in different body parts can be traced to specific brain areas. For example, certain cells in the hypothalamus control temperature and emotional states but may also be related to sexual preference. There are also large areas of the cerebral cortex that do not have localized functions (44).

Children apparently are born with a predisposition to be outgoing or quiet, and there may be a chemical predisposition to seeking danger or high risk. Yet neurophysiology does not supply all the answers. A supportive environment may cause further development of certain neurophysiologic rudiments and promote further development of the neurophysiologic processes that are manifested: thus environment helps to produce a well-adjusted child. A hostile home environment, especially in early life, produces the opposite result.

Maturational Factors

The maturational view emphasizes the emergence of patterns of development of organic systems, physical structures, and motor capabilities under the influence of genetic and maturational forces. Because of an inherent predisposition of the neurologic, hormonal, and skele-tal-muscular systems to develop spontaneously, *physiologic and motor development occurs in an inevitable and sequential pattern in children throughout the world*. The growth of the nervous system is critical in this maturation unless the normal process is inhibited by severe environmental, physiologic, and emotional deprivation. Gesell, Ilg, and Ames (26) did extensive longitudinal studies in a large number of individuals from birth to 16 years of age from 1922 to 1946 that were instrumental in determining developmental sequences. Research by others since then has confirmed and added to their studies (27, 39, 44, 51, 59).

Gender differences may be inherent for some characteristics. For example, women generally have a greater response to the intuitive and analytic side of the brain, whereas men have a greater response to the spatial side of the brain. Yet many characteristics are the result of sociocultural influences; women from certain cultures may demonstrate characteristics common to men in other cultures. Gender differences are described in Chapters 10 to 14.

Biologic Deficiencies

Biologic stressors such as certain kinds of foods, lack of food, medications, or lack of sleep may change behavior and the course of development. These factors are discussed further in Chapters 6 and 12.

CURRENT ECOLOGIC THEORIES

Ecology is a *science that is concerned with the community and the total setting in which life and behavior occur*. A basic ecologic principle is that the continuity and survival of a person depends on a deliberate balance of factors influencing the interactions between the family or person and the environment.

Family is dependent on the resources and groups in the community to survive and continue its own development and to nurture adequately development of offspring. Further, climate, terrain, and natural resources affect family life-style and development and behavior of family members. The neighborhood may adversely affect development, especially if the person is reared in a family that lives in a deteriorating neighborhood or in an area with poor schools, inadequate housing, and high crime rate. Excessively crowded housing may create stresses within the family that contribute to sleep deprivation, bickering, incest, or other abuse, which, in turn, affects developmental progress in all spheres of the person. Job loss because of a changing community and the resultant financial problems may affect health-care practices and nutrition and, in turn, physical growth and emotional security.

Urbanization, rapid social changes, social stressors, discrimination, unemployment, poor housing, inadequate diet and health care, poverty, feelings of **anomie** (*not being part of society*), and negative self-image all contribute to stress and developmental difficulties in the vulnerable, immature person or in one without an adequate support system (59).

Sociologic variables, including family socioeconomic level and position in the community, and the prestige related to birth, race, age, cultural ties, and power roles affect development, behavior, and adaptation of the person and family. Certain behaviors may be expected from a person because of age, sex, race, religion, or occupation. The individual may experience role conflicts and developmental problems when there are discrepancies between norms and values and the demands of age, gender, occupation, or religion (51).

Cultures vary in their definitions of normal and abnormal behavior; cross-cultural comparisons of developmental norms are difficult. Theorists in each culture describe their research findings about normal child or adult characteristics or behavior based on norms of their culture and their cultural bias. For example, cognitive impairment in the elderly is rare in cultures that revere their elderly or in which people live only 20 or 30 years. What might be associated with homosexuality in our culture such as men embracing is considered normal man-to-man behavior in the Arab world.

Some authors believe that minorities must be evaluated by different psychologic criteria than those used for Caucasians. They cite adaptive personality traits that African-Americans have adopted to survive in American society (51).

Geographic moves may create many adjustments for the person as he or she attempts to meet norms of the new community. Developmental problems or dysfunctional behavior may occur among those who migrate (51). Persons who move often as children may never form chumships or close relationships later in adulthood. However, the mobile family and individual do learn coping skills that help them adjust to unfamiliar or stressful situations.

Some professionals and some lay people think abnormal behavior results from individual failure. In this view an individual's psychologic problems are the result of some personal circumstance such as deficient achievement of developmental tasks, immaturity, character defect, or maladjustment (51). An alternate view is to see the individual problems as stemming from social causes. The broad economic, political, cultural, and social patterns of the nation and particular subcultures can be viewed as determinants of individual developmental responses. Then the community is the place to begin making changes if individual dysfunction is to be decreased (51). Chapters 1, 2, and 4 discuss cultural, environmental, and family variables, and Chapters 7 through 14 present the interrelationship of these variables on the person.

Systems Perspective: General Systems Theory Applied to Behavior

First proposed by von Bertalanffy (88) the General Systems Theory presents a comprehensive, holistic, and interdisciplinary view. This theory proposes that the family, individual, various social groups, and cultures are systems. Nothing is determined by a single cause or explained by a single factor. Nothing can be studied as a lone entity, be it the environment; various sociocultural components, political-legal, religious, educational, and other social institutions or organizations; the person, family, group, or community; or the health-care delivery organization. All have interrelating parts, and all components interact with each other (3, 5).

A **system** is an *assemblage, unit, or organism of interrelated, interdependent parts, persons, or objects that are united by some form or order into a recognizable unit and that are in equilibrium* (1, 5, 52, 88).

People satisfy their needs within social systems. The **social system** is a *group of people joined cooperatively to achieve common goals, using an organized set of practices to regulate behavior* (5). The person occupies various positions and has defined roles in the social system. The person's development is shaped by the system; in turn, people create and change social systems (1, 52). The elements or components that are common to all systems are presented in Table 5–1. A given entity is not a system unless these characteristics are present (1, 5, 52, 88).

All living organisms (i.e., every person) comprise an open social system. An **open system** is *characterized by the ability to exchange energy, matter, and information with the environment to evolve into higher levels of heterogeneity, organization, order, and development* (1). Physically, there is a *hierarchy of components* such as cells and organ systems. Emotionally, there are levels of needs and feelings. Cognitively, a person has memories, knowledge, and cognitive strategies. Socially, the person is in a relative rank in a hierarchy of prestige roles such as boss, worker, adult, or child. Although internal stimuli are at work such as those governed by the nervous and endocrine systems outer stimuli also affect the person. The *boundaries or environment* such as one's skin, the limits set by others, social status, home, and community influence the person's *needs* and *goal achievement.* To remain healthy, the person must be able to *communicate* and must have *feedback:* the condition of the skin tells about temperature control; an emotional reaction signifies a sense of security, a job well done, or a failure; a pain signifies malfunction or injury. In turn, the person influences the external world through his or her developmental behavior. A constant *exchange of energy and information* must exist with the surrounding specified environment if the system is to be open, useful, and creative. If this information or energy exchange does not occur, the system becomes closed and ineffective.

TABLE 5-1. ELEMENTS AND CHARACTERISTICS OF A SYSTEM

Element	Definition/Example
Parts	The *system's components that are interdependent units.* None can operate without the other. Change in one part affects the entire unit.
	The person as a whole system is composed of physical, emotional, mental, spiritual, cultural, and social aspects. Physically, he or she is composed of the body systems—neurologic, cardiovascular, and so on. The health agency is one part of the health care system, and it, in turn, is composed of parts: the physical plant, employees, clients, departments that give services.
Attributes	*Characteristics of the parts* such as temperament, roles, education, age, or health of the person or family members.
Information/communication	*Sending of messages and feedback, the exchange of energy,* which varies with the system but is essential to achieve goals.
Boundary	A *barrier or area of demarcation that limits or keeps a system distinct from its environment* and within which information is exchanged.
	The skin of the person, home of the family, or walls of the health agency are boundaries. The boundary is not always rigid. Relatives outside the home are part of the family. The boundary may be an imaginary line such as the feeling that comes from belonging to a certain racial or ethnic group.
Organization	The *formal or informal arrangement of parts to form a whole entity so that the organism or institution has a working order that results in established hierarchy, rules, or customs.*
	The person is organized into a physical structure, basic needs, cognitive stages, and achievement of developmental tasks. Hierarchy in the family or health agency provides organization that is based on power (ability to control others) and responsibility. Nursing care may be organized into primary or team nursing, which is a way of differentiating services. The specialization of medical practice is also a way of organizing care. Organization in an institution is also maintained by norms, roles, and customs that each member must follow.
Goals	*Purposes of or reasons for the system to exist.* Goals may be long term or short term. Goals include survival, development, and socialization of the individual member of the family, or contributions to society.
Environment	The *social and physical world outside the system, boundaries, or the community in which the system exists.* The person's or family's environment may be a tribal enclave, farm, small town and surrounding area, or an urban neighborhood and surrounding city. Environment of a health-care system may be the city in which the agency is located or may extend to other states and countries for a major urban medical center.

Data from references 1, 5, 52, and 88.

Other social systems are the family; church; economic systems; politico-legal, educational institutions; and health care agencies.

Linkage *occurs when two systems exchange energy across their boundaries* (1). Industry, the church, or the health agency, for example, draws energy from its linkage to the family. In return, industry is willing to contribute to family welfare funds, United Fund, mental health campaigns, or ecologic improvements. The church maintains its role as prime defender of family stability. The health agency sets standards of health care.

Each person and family you care for is a system interacting with other systems in the community. Development and function are greatly affected by the interdependence and interrelationships of each component part and by all other surrounding systems.

CURRENT PSYCHOLOGIC THEORIES

A number of psychologic theories have been formulated to explain human development, behavior, and personality. This discussion is not exhaustive. A current model to help understand behavior and its underlying reasons and the approaches to working with people is to categorize the schools of thought (and the different theorists) under either First, Second, or Third Force theories. Differences between these *different theories or schools of thought* (**Force**) are significant in terms of their beliefs about human behavior and the perspectives from which their observations are made.

The **First Force** is *identified with the Behaviorist and Neo-Behaviorist schools of psychology,* whose focus is the stimulus-response link. Behaviorism views the person as an object or as a technical being. Technology is viewed as no different from the human and may be viewed as superior. The **Second Force** was *originally identified with Psychoanalytic Theory, both Freudian and Neo-Freudian (NeoAnalytic), but has been expanded to include cognitive and developmental theorists.* The **Third Force** was *first identified with humanistic psychology and now includes existential and phenomenologic theorists.*

Although the three Forces and families of theorists within each Force are discussed separately, a theorist who is considered in one of the families may disagree with another theorist from the same family. For example, some behaviorists would disagree with B.F. Skinner on some points. Further, no theorist or group of theorists has all the answers about human behavior. Yet the theorists within one Force hold certain ideas in common about development and behavior. This classification of theorists can assist you in synthesizing and using the main ideas of several theorists who hold similar views about the person and in realizing that often theorists who sound very different in their theory may be stating basically similar concepts.

Theorists that are mentioned in the following chapters are discussed under the First, Second, and Third Forces. The discussion about theorists is not comprehensive; no effort has been made to include all theorists that fall under any of the Forces.

FIRST FORCE THEORY

Overview

First Force theorists are **Behaviorists** who *adhere to stimulus-response conditioning theories.* This scientific approach to the study of the person generalizes results from animal experiments to people. The **Neo-Behaviorists**—*contemporary Behavioral theorists and the theorists in this school who have changed their ideas*—obtain data for laws of behavior by observing the human's behavioral response to stimuli. The person is considered in terms of component parts. The focus is on isolated, small units of behavior or parts of behavioral patterns that are objectively observed and analyzed from the perspective of nonmental, physiologic associations.

View of the Human

The person is seen as an object, a reactive organism responding mechanically, automatically, involuntarily, overtly, and quantitatively to past conditioning and present situations. The person is regarded as a product of learning. The person has sensory input and, in turn, acts to reduce a need; there is a natural tendency and drive to satisfaction. The person is acted on or reinforced by the environment, which causes learning and predictable behavior (7, 37).

Because the focus is on physiologic processes and identifiable aspects of the person, subjective, unobservable, unique, and inner aspects of the human are denied or dismissed as illusory. Undesirable behavior is removed from the person by **shaping,** *setting up the situation so that the person acts in a desired way and then is rewarded for the desired behavior* (7, 37, 59).

First Force Theorists

Early Theorists
Ivan Pavlov, a Russian physiologist, laid the foundations for the Behavioral School in the nineteenth century through his study of salivation and flow of digestive juices in dogs. His experiments established **classical conditioning,** whereby an *unconditioned or new stimulus is presented with a stimulus that is already known just before the response to the conditioned familiar stimulus. The organism learns to respond to a new stimulus in the same way it responded to a familiar stimulus.* Associations are shifted from one stimulus to another, with the same response being made to the substituted stimuli (36, 59).

John B. Watson is considered the founder of Behaviorism. His experiments showed that fears and phobias could result from classical conditioning in childhood and could, in turn, be unlearned in adulthood (39). He emphasized physiologic associations and connections in understanding physiologic processes.

Some present-day relaxation methods used by health-care providers are based on classical conditioning. The client is trained to respond to a therapist's direction by relaxing a muscle group; music is then played while the therapist gives directions for relaxing. Later the person is able to respond automatically by relaxing when music plays (37, 39). Classical conditioning is also used in the Lamaze preparation for childbirth or other kinds of childbirth education classes. Behaviorists believe emotions arise from body changes or are learned through classical conditioning. Emotions arise in the present situation based on past learning that is associated with the present event. For example, a person likes men with beards because he or she learned this response during childhood as a result of associating beards with a kindly bearded grandfather.

Skinner: Operant Conditioning Theory
Skinner is well known for his Operant Conditioning theory that used animal studies and built on the theories of Watson and Thorndike. According to Skinner, **behavior** is an *overt response that is externally caused and is primarily controlled by its consequences.* The environmental stimuli determine how a person alters behavior and responds to people or objects in the environment. Feelings or emotions are the accompaniments or result, not the cause of behavior. Innate or hereditary reflexes activate the internal glands and smooth muscles, but reflexive behavior accounts for little of human behavior (37, 79, 82).

Learning is a *change in the form or probability of response as a result of conditioning.* **Operant conditioning** is the *learning process whereby a response (operant) is shaped and is made more probable or frequent by reinforcement.* **Transfer** is an *increased probability of response in the future.* Responses or a set of acts are called operant because they operate on the environment and generate consequences. The important stimulus is the one immediately *following* the response, not the one preceding it. Operant conditioning occurs in most everyday activities, according to Skinner. People constantly cause others to modify their behavior by reinforcing certain behavior and ignoring other behavior. During development people learn to balance, walk, talk, play games, and handle instruments and tools because they are reinforced after performing a set of motions, thereby increasing the repetition of these motions. Social and ethical behaviors are learned as people are reinforced to continue them through their reinforcing of others for the same behaviors. Operant reinforcement improves the efficiency of behavior, whether the behavior is appropriate or inappropriate. Any attention, even if negative, reinforces response to a stimuli (37, 79, 81, 82).

Positive reinforcement occurs when the *presence of a stimulus strengthens a response;* **negative reinforcement** occurs when *withdrawal of a stimulus strengthens the tendency to behave in a certain way.* A positive reinforcer is food, water, or a smile. A negative reinforcer consists of removing painful stimuli. Skinner's theory emphasizes positive reinforcement (37, 82).

Application of Skinner's theory is threefold. His theory, when applied to clinical and classroom problems, is called *behavior modification.* When applied to courses of study, it is called *programmed learning.* When applied to correction of physiologic problems, it is called *biofeedback* (44, 82). As a nurse, you may use each of these applications in client care and teaching.

Behavior modification is the *deliberate application of learning theory and conditioning, thereby structuring different social environments to teach alternate behaviors and to help the person gain control over behavior and environment.* Shaping also achieves behavioral change. **Shaping** is the *gradual modification of behavior by breaking complex behavior into small steps and reinforcing each small step that is a closer approximation to the final desired behavior* (71, 76).

In behavior modification the behavior first must be reinforced each time it occurs. Reinforcement can be gradually tapered until the behavior is learned. Behavior that has been maintained by an intermittent schedule of reinforcement or partial reinforcement is highly resistant to extinction (71, 82, 94). For example, the child learns to talk not only through imitation of others but because of parental approval, love, and verbal responses that serve as rewards or reinforcement.

Sometimes aversive methods (e.g., seclusion) are used to change behavior. The purpose is not punishment but time out, as in allowing a tantrum to run its course without accidental reinforcement and without triggering similar behavior in other people. Strategies of punishment and deprivation, which are standard techniques in child rearing, are examples of using Skinner's principles of behavior modification. Some parents do not question sending a child to bed without a meal as punishment, and parents may even be criticized by other parents if they do not spank their children for naughty behavior.

Operant conditioning is used in many situations, including to:

1. Replace undesirable behaviors of normal or developmentally disabled children.
2. Reduce abnormal or self-destructive behavior.
3. Train parents, teachers, probation officers, and nurses to be more efficient in their roles.
4. Reduce specific maladaptive behaviors such as stuttering, tics, poor hygiene, or messy eating habits.
5. Control physical symptoms through biofeedback.

Figure 5–1 illustrates how development is viewed by First Force learning theorists. Table 5–2 presents key terms and definitions, with examples.

Cybernetic Principles. These principles take respondent and operant conditioning one step further to account for the continuous adjustment and modification necessary in learning complex, goal-directed behaviors. The learner becomes a control system between the stimulus and the response. The Cybernetic Theory of Learning suggests that learning results from the dynamic interaction between input (stimulus information), output (learner's response), and information feedback. Feedback modifies input, which in turn alters output.

Although each of the Behaviorists' theories sheds some light on learning complex motor skills, none accounts for the higher cognitive processes. Advocates of cognitive learning principles argue that the learner's ability to organize and process task-related information

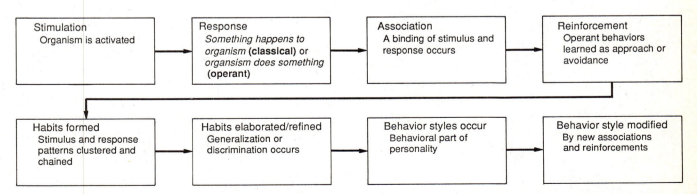

Figure 5-1. Development as viewed by learning theorists. Stimuli from inside or outside the organism are reinforced (positively or negatively) and on a particular schedule that determines their force and strength. Habits develop. The response processes of generalization and discrimination elaborate these habits and modify them. Effective habits are equated with effective development. This Force rarely speaks about the whole organism but rather about situationally determined behaviors.

TABLE 5-2. SELECTED TERMINOLOGY PERTAINING TO APPLICATION OF FIRST FORCE THEORY

Term	Definition	Example
Respondent conditioning	Pairing a neutral stimulus with a nonneutral stimulus until the person learns to respond to the neutral stimulus as to the nonneutral stimulus	Baby learns to "love" a sibling (nonneutral stimulus) because the sibling shakes a rattle and offers other toys (neutral stimulus) while cooing, touching, and smiling to baby.
Operant conditioning	Rewarding or punishing a response until the person learns to repeat or avoid that response in anticipation of positive or negative consequences	Preschooler returns toys to the toy box at the end of the day because he remembers the consequences: doing so is followed by 10 minutes of time with the parent; failure to do so results in sitting alone in his room for 5 minutes.
Positive reinforcement	Rewarding desired behavior to maintain that behavior	Parent buys a desired item for the child who earns an *A* in a course.
Negative reinforcement	Removing an aversive stimulus in response to behavior, which maintains that behavior	Parent allows the child to forgo household tasks if he complains when asked to do them, yet the child receives an allowance weekly.
Extinction	Suppressing a behavior by removing reinforcers that are maintaining the behavior	Parent does not give the child who complains about doing household tasks the allowance at the end of the week and explains why.
Punishment	Suppressing an undesirable behavior by using an aversive stimulus in response to the person's behavior	Parent spanks the child for running into the street.
Time out	Suppressing maladaptive behavior by removing the subject to a neutral environment, void of reinforcements, when the behavior is manifested	Parent makes the 4-year-old child sit facing a corner for 5 minutes after hitting a sibling.
Generalization	Transferring a conditioned response from the conditional stimuli to another stimuli	Child who is bitten by a dog fears all animals.
Systematic desensitization	Pairing an anxiety-causing stimulus with an induced state of relaxation to extinguish fearful behavior	Parent remains with the child who has been bitten by a dog when the child is in the vicinity of animals, gradually helps the child to relax, and eventually pet a very friendly dog.
Discrimination	Responding only to a specific stimuli	Toddler learns via punishing encounters with mother that playing in water in the bathtub is acceptable and playing in the water in the toilet is not.
Escape behavior	Initiating a response to escape an unpleasant or aversive stimulus	Adolescent brings the parents a gift when returning late from a weekend with a friend.
Avoidance learning	Arranging responses to avoid exposure to an aversive stimulus	Adolescent verbally refuses the offer and walks away from the person offering a marijuana joint after a bad experience with it.
Chaining	Developing complex behavior by focusing on the individual components of the behavior; this is done in a backward fashion	School child learns to clean his room with the parent instructing and assisting with each step of the task and then verbally repeating in reverse order the steps after the task is finished.
Shaping	Reinforcing successive approximations or small units of a desired response until that behavior is gradually achieved	Parent teaches the child to clean his room by praising him for doing every step of the process—vacuuming the rug, dusting each piece of furniture.
Fading	Removing gradually the reinforcement given to the person	Parent gives less and less verbal approval to the school child for doing assigned household tasks.

systematically is the critical variable in performing complex motor behaviors. It is this ability that enables the person to interact with a dynamic environment in carrying out decision-making skills.

To reconcile the objectivity of Behaviorism with the flexibility of cognitive principles, researchers are turning toward information-processing models of behavior. Such models address the concepts of information (in its technical sense), uncertainty, and redundancy. The amount of information that a given event generates or feeds back depends on how complex the event is and how likely or unlikely it is that the event will occur again. The amount of information that an event generates is directly proportional to its complexity and is inversely proportional to the probability of its occurrence. If an event is redundant, its uncertainty is reduced. Redundancy results in improvement because of practice. No single theory alone can account successfully for the many complicated processes involved in the acquisition and application of complex skills. Each theory offers some guiding principles about learning and teaching (59).

SECOND FORCE THEORY

Overview

Second Force theorists include those who adhere to **Psychoanalytic, Neo-Analytic,** and **Cognitive Learning** theories. These theorists generally believe data for study about the person come from within the developing person, observation of interpersonal relationships, and knowledge of the impact of social units, norms, and laws on the person. Data from early development are used to understand present behavior and goal direction. This group of theorists studies the person more comprehensively and as a social being, using experimentation, objective observation, and self-report methods. Second Force theorists give us a helpful view of causation and provide a way of dealing with developmental and behavioral problems (51).

View of the Human

Knowledge of genetics, developmental levels, effects of internal stimuli, unconscious processes, social relationships, and environmental context are all used to understand the person.

Reality is external and interpersonal—what people agree on. The person is a social organism with a developmental past on which to build and a level of readiness that influences or contributes to learning and behavior. The person has maturational and social needs that affect development, learning, and behavior; he or she seeks social role satisfaction and reacts to social values and symbolic processes. The person internalizes societal rules to gain approval, can understand cause-and-effect relationships and complex abstract issues, is capable of insight and emotions, and initiates action and makes choices. The goal of behavior is seen as reduction of symbolic or internal needs or tension (51).

The goal of developmental guidance and discipline is to help the person become an adaptive, effective social being, aware of and responsive to social reality and patterns. The person has to learn and follow socially prescribed values, customs, and norms to fit into society as an effective and well citizen. Development, learning, and behavior are also influenced strongly by the person's developmental level, personal history, cognitive processes and intellect, and intrapsychic processes (51).

Emphasis is on the person, even in the younger years, understanding self and his or her behavior. Increased insight promotes development and maturation.

If the person is not ready to learn or change behavior, the parent, teacher, or another acts as an external motivator or facilitator of readiness to change. Rewards are given through approval, affiliation, and various verbal and nonverbal methods. Learning and behavior change also are self-reinforcing to the person (51).

Second Force Theorists

Second Force theorists are numerous and can be divided into those with a psychodynamic perspective and those with a cognitive perspective. The **Psychodynamic Theory** or **perspective** *is then divided into two groups:* Psychoanalytic (Freud [15–20]) and Neo-Analytic (Jung [43], Adler [60], Rank [60], Horney [38, 68], Fromm [22], Sullivan [84], Erikson [11], and Berne [2, 4]). Freud is the Analytic theorist discussed in this section; Sullivan, Erikson, and Jung are the Neo-Analytic theorists presented. The Neo-Analytic theorists reinterpreted Freud's Psychoanalytic Theory in formulating their theories. Sullivan further developed new emphases in his Interpersonal Theory: (1) causation of behavior was seen as the result of dyad (mother-child) relationships and (2) development continued into adulthood. Erikson, in his Epigenetic Theory, expanded understanding of normal developmental stages and tasks through the life span, emphasized sociocultural influences to a greater degree, and saw the person as capable of emotional growth throughout life.

The **cognitive theory or perspective** includes theories about *mental or cognitive development*. Some have combined or modified concepts from behavioral and psychodynamic theories with an emphasis on cognitive processes to learn adaptive, satisfying behavior and to gain control over personal life. Such theorists are A. Bandura (Social Learning Theory) (3) and J. Piaget (Theory of Cognitive Development) (64–67).

In addition to the Second Force theorists who emphasize that people develop in sequential stages, other current "stage" theorists are George Vaillant (87), Roger Gould (32), Gail Sheehy (77), and Daniel Levinson (50). Their concepts and theories are referred to in Chapters 12 and 13 on young adulthood and middle age.

Moral development theories are also presented in this section. The focus is on *Kohlberg's Theory of Moral Development* (46–49) and Gilligan's Theory of Moral Development (28–30).

Psychodynamic Perspective

The **Psychodynamic perspective** is *concerned with the inner and unconscious processes of the person— drives, needs, motivations, feelings, and conflicts.* Past developmental experiences are important in the causation of behavior and for achieving present developmental tasks and maturity. Most of the Neo-Analytic theorists have paid little attention to biology. Because thoughts and feelings are not directly observable, these theorists infer them from overt behavior (51).

Freud: Psychoanalytic Theory.
Sigmund Freud, a Viennese neurologist, developed Psychoanalytic Theory, the first psychologic theory to include a fully developed explanation of abnormal behavior. He gave biologic factors little emphasis but used the medical model of emphasizing pathology and symptoms.

Freud's theory of personality seems complicated because it incorporates many interlocking factors. Major components are psychic determinism; psychic structures of id, ego, and superego; primary and secondary process thinking; the conscious-unconscious continuum; libido or psychic energy; behavior; anxiety and defense mechanisms; and psychosexual development. Some of his theory is discussed here and referred to in the chapters on childhood.

The psychic structures of the person are id, ego, and superego. **Id** is *the structure of personality that is an unorganized reservoir of psychic energy* and furnishes energy for the operation of the other two structures, the ego and superego. The id, present at birth, discharges tension and consists of **instinctual forces,** *biologic drives and impulses that must be satisfied for survival.* The id operates on the **pleasure principle,** *seeking immediate gratification and avoidance of discomfort* (18).

The **ego** is the *part of the personality that establishes relations with the environment through conscious perception, feeling, and action and serves to control impulses from id and demands of superego.* The ego operates on the **reality principle,** *whereby external conditions are considered and immediate gratification is delayed for future gains that can be realistically achieved.* Besides mediating between the demands of the id and superego, the ego controls access of ideas to the conscious, appraises the environment and external reality, uses various mechanisms to help the person feel safe emotionally, and guides the person to acceptable behavior. The ego also directs motor and cognitive functions (18).

Superego is the third personality structure to form, beginning in the preschool years. *It represents internalized moral code, rules, and norms of society, which restrain expression of instinctual drives in the person and prevent disruption of society.* The superego is not necessarily an accurate representation of cultural norms and parental prohibitions, but it is the child's interpretation of these norms and prohibitions. The superego, if well internalized, is active in directing the person's thoughts, feelings, and actions. The superego is composed of two systems: the ego ideal and the conscience. The **ego ideal** *corresponds to those aspects the parents believe are morally good and behavior or achievements to which the person aspires.* The **conscience** *corresponds to those aspects considered morally bad and is responsible for guilt feelings.* The superego can either reward or punish

the ego or the person's consciousness; the restrictions and fears stemming from the superego may be unrealistic and rigid (20, 51).

These three systems operate and interact as the structure of personality that Freud described in the conscious-unconscious continuum. Id is unconscious; ego and superego are both conscious and unconscious (20).

The **conscious** includes *all aspects of mental life that are currently in awareness or easily remembered.* The **preconscious** is the *element of mental life that can be remembered with help but is not currently at the level of awareness.* **Unconsciousness materials** are *those thoughts, feelings, actions, experiences, and dreams that are not remembered, are very difficult to bring into consciousness, and are not recognized if one is told of them.* The existence of the unconscious is inferred from behavior. Psychic energy is channeled by conscious and unconscious forces that are not always in harmony. The greater the degree of intrapsychic conflict, the greater the likelihood that mental events remain unconscious. The greater the unconscious conflict, the greater the vulnerability to anxiety (16, 20).

Anxiety is the *response of tension or dread to perceived or anticipated danger or stress and is the primary motivation for behavior.* There are two types of anxiety-provoking situations. Anxiety may be caused by excessive stimulation that the person cannot handle, of which birth is the prototype experience. Anxiety may also rise from intrapsychic or unconscious conflicts, unacceptable wishes, unknown or anticipated events, superego inhibitions and taboos, and threatened loss of self-image. If anxiety cannot be managed by direct action or coping strategies, the ego initiates unconscious defenses by warding off awareness of the conflict to keep the material unconscious, to lessen discomfort, and to maintain the self-image. Because everyone experiences psychologic danger, the use of defense mechanisms clearly is not a special characteristic of maladaptive behavior. Such mechanisms are used by all people, either singly or in combination, at one time or another, and are considered adaptive (15, 17, 19, 51). Commonly used ego adaptive (defense) mechanisms are described throughout the text in relation to the developmental era during which they arise.

Freud proposed five stages of psychosexual development and contended that personality was formed by age 5 years (16, 51). The stages in psychosexual development, each resolved in turn, are summarized in Table 5–3 and are referred to throughout the text.

Freud's ideas about psychosexual development are undoubtedly the most controversial aspects of his theory. Although many theorists agree that childhood experiences are very important in personality development, many reject Freud's assertions about childhood sexuality and the Victorian and stereotyped ideas about men and women (51).

Psychoanalytic Theory has been criticized for many

TABLE 5-3. FREUD'S STAGES OF PSYCHOSEXUAL DEVELOPMENT: LIBIDINAL EXTENSION

Stage	Major Body Zone	Activities	Extension to Others
Oral (0–1½ yr)	Mouth (major source of gratification and exploration)	Security—primary need Pleasure from eating and sucking Major conflict—weaning Incorporation (suck, consume, chew, bite, receive)	Sense of *We*—no differentiation or extension Sense of *I* and *Other*—minimum differentiation and total incorporation
Anal (1½–3 yr)	Bowel (anus) and bladder—source of sensual satisfaction, self-control and conflict (mouth continues in importance)	Expulsion and retention (differentiation, expelling, controlling, pushing away) (Incorporation still is used.)	Sense of *I* and *Other*—separation from other and increasing sense of *I*
Phallic (4–6 yr)	Genital region—penis, clitoris (mouth, bowel, and bladder sphincters continue in importance)	Masturbation Fantasy Play activities Experimentation with peers Questioning of adults about sexual topics Major conflict—Oedipus complex, which resolves when child identifies with parent of same sex (Mastery, incorporation, expulsion, retention continue.)	Sense of *I* and *Other*—fear of castration in boy Sense of *I* and *Other*—strengthened with identification process with parents Sense of *Other*—extends to other adults
Latency (6–10 yr)	None (penis, clitoris, mouth, anus)	Diffuse activity and relationships (Mastery, incorporation, expulsion, retention continue.)	Sense of *I* and *Other*—extends out of nuclear family and includes peers of same sex
Genital (puberty and thereafter)	Penis, vagina (mouth, anus, clitoris)	Full sexual maturity and function (Mastery, incorporation, expulsion, retention continue.) Addition of new assets with each stage for gratification Realistic heterosexual expression	Sense of *I* and *Other*—extends to other adults and peers of opposite sex

reasons (see an objective critique by Graves [33]). In contrast, Greenberg and Fisher (34) have reviewed the thousands of scientific studies done worldwide to check the validity of Freud's ideas and have found that Freud's model of personality development and behavior is supported by other studies. His theory continues to influence twentieth-century thought and research, especially in Western cultures, in relation to development and therapy of the ill person (35). Recently, feminist scholars have begun to reassess Freud's theory, recognizing the value of his ideas and their applicability to understanding men and women, boys and girls. (8)

You will find Freud's concepts pertinent to your understanding of the developing person and to nursing care.

Major Neo-Analytic Theorists. Neo-Freudians or Neo-Analysts follow Freud's theory in general but disagree with or have modified some of the original propositions. They maintain the medical model and share the view of intrapsychic determinism as the basis for external behavior. Some take into account the social and cultural context in which the person lives. Harry Stack Sullivan (84), Erik Erikson (11), and Carl Jung (41–43) are described briefly; Sullivan and Erikson are referred to throughout the text.

SULLIVAN: INTERPERSONAL THEORY OF PSYCHIATRY. Harry Stack Sullivan (84) formulated the Interpersonal Theory of Psychiatry. The theory focus is on relationships between and among people, in contrast to Freud's emphasis on intrapsychic sexual phenomena and Erikson's focus on social aspects. Experiences in major life events are the result of either positive or negative interpersonal relationships. Personality development is largely the result of the mother-child relationship, childhood experiences, and interpersonal encounters. There are two basic needs: satisfaction (biologic needs) and security (emotional and social needs). Biologic and interpersonal needs are interrelated. How biologic needs are met in the interpersonal situation determines sense of satisfaction and security and provides avoidance of anxiety.

Sullivan used the following biologic principles to understand the person's development:

1. *Principle of communal existence:* A living organism cannot be separated from the necessary environment to survive. For example, the embryo must have the correct intrauterine environment to live, and the baby must have love and human contact to become socialized or human.

2. *Principle of functional activity:* Functional or phys-

162 BASIC CONCEPTS RELATED TO THE DEVELOPING PERSON AND FAMILY UNIT

iological activities and processes affect the person's interaction with the environment.

3. *Principle of organization:* The person is systematically arranged physically and emotionally and within societies, and this organization enables function.

An important principle for the study and care of people is the **One Genus Postulate** that states *we are all more simply human than otherwise—hence more similar than different in basic needs, development, and in the meaning of our behavior.*

Sullivan postulated that people experience events in the following three modes. The differences between these modes are due to the crucial role of language in experience and development and are described further in Chapters 7, 9, and 10.

1. **Prototaxic mode of experiencing** refers to *experiences that occur in infancy before language symbols are acquired or to the first time a person experiences an event that is difficult to describe in words.*
2. **Parataxic mode of experiencing** refers to *experiences characterized by symbols used in a private (autistic) way and encompasses fantasy, magical thinking, and lack of cause-and-effect thinking that is seen in children and adults.*
3. **Syntaxic mode of experiencing** refers to *experiences of preadolescence, adolescence, and adulthood characterized by consensual validation, whereby persons communicate with each other using language or symbols that are mutually understood.* This mode of experiencing begins during the chum stage in the school-age child or thereafter.

Sullivan implied that the need to avoid anxiety and the need to gratify basic needs are the primary motivations for behavior. His **Concept of Anxiety** states that *anxiety has its origin in the prolonged dependency of infancy, urgency of biologic and emotional needs, and how the mothering person meets those needs. Anxiety is the result of uncomfortable interpersonal relationships, is the chief disruptive force in interpersonal relationships, is contagious through empathic feelings, and can be relieved by being in a secure interpersonal relationship.*

The **self-system** is the *internal organization of experiences that exists to defend against anxiety and to secure necessary security.* One aspect of the self-system is known as *good-me, bad-me, and not-me,* which refers to feelings about the self that begin to form in infancy.

Sullivan's developmental stages and concepts are described in Chapters 7 through 14 in relation to each developmental era and are pertinent to the understanding and care of the developing person and family unit.

ERIKSON: EPIGENETIC THEORY OF PERSONALITY DEVELOPMENT. Erik Erikson (11) formulated the Epigenetic The-

ory, based on the principle of the unfolding embryo: anything that grows has a ground plan out of which parts arise. Each part has its time of special ascendancy until all parts have arisen to form a functional whole. Thus each stage of development is the base for the next stage.

His theory explains step-by-step unfolding of emotional development and social characteristics during encounters with the environment. Erikson's psychosexual theory enlarges on Psychoanalytic Theory because it (1) is not limited to historical era, specific culture, or personality types, (2) encompasses development through the life span and is universal to all people, and (3) acknowledges that society, heredity, and childhood experiences all influence the person's development (11).

The following are basic principles of his theory, based on cross-cultural studies (11):

1. Each phase has a specific developmental task to achieve or solve. These tasks describe the order and sequence of human development and the conditions necessary to accomplish them, but actual accomplishment is done at an individual pace, tempo, and intensity.
2. Each psychosexual stage of development is a developmental crisis because there is a radical change in the person's perspective, a shift in energy, and an increased emotional vulnerability. During this peak time the potential in the personality comes in contact with the whole environment, and the person has some degree of success in solving the crucial developmental task of the specific era. How the person copes with the task and crisis depends on previous developmental strengths and weaknesses.
3. The potential inherent in each person evolves if given adequate chance to survive and grow. Anything that distorts the environment essential for development interferes with evolvement of the person. Society attempts to safeguard and encourage the proper rate and sequence of the unfolding of human potential so that humanity is maintained.
4. Each developmental task is redeveloped, reworked, and redefined in subsequent stages. Potential for further development always exists.
5. Internal organization is central to development. Maturity increases as the tasks of each era are accomplished, at least in part, in proper order.

Erikson proposed eight stages of development and described the developmental task of crisis for each stage. They are described in Chapters 7 through 14 in relation to each developmental era. His theory is widely accepted and used in understanding the developing person and in administering nursing care.

JUNG'S THEORY. Carl Jung (12, 43, 83), another Neo-Analytic theorist, proposed the following assumptions about personality structure:

Research Abstract

Drew, B., Differentiation of Hopelessness, Helplessness, and Powerlessness Using Erik Erikson's "Roots of Virtue," Archives of Psychiatric Nursing, *4, no. 5 (1990), 332–337.*

The North American Nursing Diagnosis Association has generated a diagnostic system for nursing practice that includes the diagnoses of hopelessness and powerlessness. The American Nurses' Association, through the Phenomena Task Force, states that hopelessness, helplessness, and powerlessness are phenomena of concern to nursing practice. These concepts have been discussed by a number of others.

This article differentiates between the phenomena of hopelessness, helplessness, and powerlessness, using Erik Erikson's conceptual framework, "Roots of Virtue." According to Erikson, hope is the earliest and most basic virtue, which develops with trust, and lies in the quality of the relationship between parents and child and in the consistency of the nurturing environment. The next virtue is will, or willpower, and self-control, which contrasts with helplessness, and is acquired as the child gains awareness of his or her personal impact on surrounding life events so that the child experiences control rather than helplessness. The next two developmental outcomes are purpose and skill, or competency, versus powerlessness. The rudiments of purpose are having a direction and focus to the striving, and in the young child purpose is attached to reality. Competency or skill promotes a strong ego, able to deal with the surrounding environment with confidence and with a realistic assessment of limits and controls of the person's world.

Three hypotheses may be developed from this framework: (1) hopelessness, helplessness, and powerlessness are relatively enduring traits; (2) stress is likely to elicit a particular state, depending on level of task frustration; and/or (3) type of response is dependent on type of stress. Depending on the individual and the stresses, each hypothesis may be appropriate. Research could be done to determine if there is a sequential relationship between the concepts. Has the most hopeless person previously experienced helplessness and powerlessness? Does one phenomenon predominate under stress? It appears that each phenomenon is qualitatively different and that each may be precipitated by current stresses but that the conflicts that emerge are often reminiscent of childhood issues. Knowledge of these issues can guide nursing assessment and intervention.

1. The **ego** or **consciousness** includes *awareness of self and the external world.*
2. The **persona** is the *image or mask presented to the outer world,* depending on the roles of the person.
3. The **shadow** consists of *traits and feelings that cannot be admitted to the self;* it is the opposite of ego or self-image.
4. The **anima** and **animus** in the personality refer to the *characteristics traditionally considered feminine and masculine.* Each person has both characteristics or is androgynous or bisexual with the feminine, nurturing, feeling side and the masculine, logical, assertive side. Socialization forces the person to overemphasize gender characteristics so that the opposite aspect of the person is not usually fully developed.
5. The unconscious is composed of two layers:
   a. The **personal unconscious** is unique, *contains all the repressed tendencies and feelings that build over the lifetime,* and *includes the shadow and some of the anima or animus.*
   b. The **collective unconscious** is *inherited and shared by all humankind and is composed of archetypes, or innate energy forces and organizing tendencies.* Archetype images are unknowable and are found in myths, art, dreams, and fantasies throughout the world and include the image of Earth Mother, Wise Old Man, death, the witch, rebirth, God. The archetypes influence the nature and growth of other parts of the personality. They are essentially unknowable, like instincts or innate perceptual tendencies.
6. **Self** is the most important archetype, our unconscious centeredness, wholeness, and meaning. It is an inner urge to balance and reconcile the opposing aspects of our personalities, represented in drawings of **mandalas,** *figures in which all sides are perfectly balanced around a center point.*
7. **Individuation** is the unattainable goal pursued by the self, which *involves finding the unique way, achieving a measure of psychic balance while separating self from societal conformity to goals and values.*
8. There are two basic personality types or tendencies:
   a. **Introversion** refers to being *inner-reflective, caught up in one's inner state, fears, hopes and feelings*. The introvert hesitates in relationships, is more secure in his or her inner world, and takes pleasure in activities that can be done alone.
   b. The **extrovert** confidently *engages in direct action and starts interactions with others.* The extrovert moves outward toward the world and prefers activities with people.

To Jung, life is a series of periods identified by different energy uses. Early childhood years were not emphasized in this developmental theory. The first period, until age 35 or 40 years, is a time of outward expansion. Maturational forces direct the growth of the ego and unfolding of capacities. After age 40, the person undergoes a transformation and looks for meaning in personal activities. With increasing age, there is increasing reflection. Late thirties and early forties were seen as important in life transition; this was seen as a time when energy from youthful interests was channeled to cultural and spiritual pursuits (43). Jung's theory is referred to again in the chapters on adulthood. His theory is gaining wider acceptance in the understanding of the developing adult.

Cognitive Perspective

Cognitive psychology deals with the person as an information processor and problem solver. The cognitive perspective is concerned with internal processes but emphasizes how people attempt to acquire, interpret, and use information to solve life's problems and to remain normal or healthy. It emphasizes conscious processes, present thoughts, and problem-solving strategies. The cognitive perspective has grown out of new directions in learning and psychodynamic theories. Some present-day learning theorists are becoming increasingly interested in what goes on within the person between the application of a stimulus and the response, and some current psychodynamic theorists are focusing on thinking and problem solving and on feelings and emotions. Relationships among emotions, motivations, and cognitive processes are being studied. Overlap between the cognitive perspective and other approaches is becoming more evident (44, 59).

Bandura: Social Learning Theory. Albert Bandura's Social Learning Theory (3) states that learning occurs without reinforcement, conditioning, or trial-and-error behavior since people can think and anticipate consequences of behavior and act accordingly. This theory emphasizes (1) the importance of vicarious, symbolic, and self-regulatory processes in psychologic functioning and (2) the capacity of the person to use symbols, represent events, analyze conscious experience, communicate with others at any distance in time and space, and plan, create, imagine, and engage in foresightful action. The person does not simply react to external forces: he or she selects, organizes, and transforms impinging stimuli and thus exercises some influence over personal behavior. There is a continuous, reciprocal interaction between cognitive, behavioral, and environmental determinants (3, 6).

Human nature is characterized as a vast potentiality that can be fashioned by direct and vicarious experience into a variety of forms of development and behavior within biologic limits. The level of psychologic and physiologic development restricts what can be acquired at any given time (3).

The person may be motivated by ideas or fantasies of future consequences or by personal goal-setting behavior. If the person wants to accomplish a certain goal and there are distractions from the task, the person visualizes how he or she will feel when the goal is attained. People respond evaluatively to their own behavior and tend to persist until the behavior or performance meets the goal (3).

Bandura (3) proposes that learning occurs through **modeling,** *imitation of another's behavior.* According to his theory, much of our daily behavior is learned by modeling. Imitation is one of the most effective forms of learning. Babies learn to speak by imitating the sounds of their parents; older children learn a number of behaviors by watching the teacher, parent, or peers. People learn how to be normal or abnormal. Maladaptive behavior arises from modeling when the child imitates abnormal parental behavior. Bandura's research also shows the power of watching television on people's behavior and that for some people the model of aggressive behavior will cause later acting-out behavior. This research is discussed further in Chapter 10.

Bandura's research combines aspects of First and Second Force theories and is pertinent to understanding certain aspects of the developing person. His theory is also pertinent to nursing case, especially the educational role.

Piaget: Theory of Cognitive Development. Jean Piaget (64–66) formulated the Theory of Cognitive Development. The bulk of his research was concerned with the child's thinking at particular periods of life and with studying differences among well children of a specific age. A great amount of empirical data was used in developing the theory. He believed that development is neither **maturational,** an unfolding of the innate growth process, nor **learning,** an accumulation of experiences. Rather, development is an active process resulting from **equilibration,** an *internal force that is set in motion to organize thinking when the child's belief system develops sufficiently to contain self-contradictions.*

Four factors interact within the person to stimulate mental development (66):

1. Maturation of the nervous and endocrine systems, which provides physical capabilities
2. Experience involving action, with a consequent discovery of properties of objects
3. Social interaction with opportunity to observe a wide variety of behaviors, gain direct instruction, and to receive feedback about individual performance
4. An internal self-regulation mechanism that responds to environmental stimuli

Intelligence is an adaptive process by which the person modifies and structures the environment to fit personal needs and also modifies self in response to environmental demands.

By interaction with the environment, the person constructs reality by assimilation, accommodation, and adaptation. **Assimilation** is *taking new and content experiences into the mind or cognitive structure.* **Accommodation** is the *revising, realigning, and readjusting of cognitive structure to take into account the new content.* **Adaptation** is the *change that results from the first two processes.* Piaget emphasizes the innate, inborn processes of the person as the essential force to start the process of equilibration or cognitive growth. Cognitive development proceeds from motor activity to interaction with the wider social world, and finally to abstract ideas. Development is seen as solidly rooted in what already exists, and it displays a continuity with the past. Adaptations do not develop in isolation; all form a coherent pattern so that the totality of biologic life is adapted to its environment. The theory focuses on development of intellectual capacities with little reference to emotional or social development (64–66, 89).

The thinking process is explained by schematic mental structures of pictures formed in response to stimuli. A **schema** is a *cognitive structure, a complex concept encompassing both motor behavior and internalized thought processes*. A schema *involves movement of the eyeballs, paying attention, and the mental picture that is formed as a result of the sensory process*. Thinking eventually involves using combinations of mental pictures, forming concepts, internalizing use of language or subvocal speech, drawing implications, and making judgments. When these internal actions become integrated into a coherent, logical system, they are considered logical operations. The schemata that are developed and the specific levels of function are unique to each person and in turn structure future learning. Learning is determined by (1) what is observed, (2) whether new information is fit into old schematic accurately or in a distorted way, and (3) how much increase in competence results from the encounter or experience (64–66).

Piaget divided human development into four periods: Sensorimotor, Preoperational, Concrete Operations, and Formal Operations. In each stage the person demonstrates interpretation and use of the environment through certain behavior patterns. He or she incorporates and restructures the previous stage and refines ability to perceive and understand. Suggested ages for each stage are indicated, but innate intellectual ability and environmental factors may cause variation. These periods are discussed with development of the infant, toddler, preschooler, schoolchild, and adolescent. You will find these stages pertinent to determining mental development of the person and corresponding educational approaches and activities.

Moral Perspective

Kohlberg: Theory of Moral Development. Lawrence Kohlberg (46, 48) formulated a Theory of Moral Development. Because moral development is related to cognitive and emotional development and to societal values and norms and is divided into stages by Kohlberg, he can be identified with Second Force theorists.

Moral reasoning focuses on 10 universal values: punishment, property, roles and concerns related to affection, roles and concerns related to authority, law, life, liberty, distribution of justice, truth, and sexual behavior. A conflict between two or more of these universal val-

ues necessitates a moral choice and its subsequent justification by the individual, requiring systematic problem solving and other cognitive capabilities (48, 49, 69).

Kohlberg theorized that a person's moral reasoning process and behavior develop through six stages over varying lengths of time. Each stage is derived from a prior stage and is the basis for the next stage. *Each moral stage is based or dependent on the reason for behavior and shows an organized system of thought by which the person is consistent in the level of moral judgment.* The person is considered in a specific stage when the same level of reason for action is given at least half the time. More advanced logical thinking is needed for each successive moral stage. One criterion of moral maturity, the ability to decide autonomously what is right and caring, is lacking in the Preconventional and Conventional Levels because in each level the person is following the commands of authority figures. If the person's cognitive stage is at Concrete Operations, according to Piaget, the person is limited to the Preconventional or Conventional Levels of moral reasoning. Even the person in Formal Operations may not be beyond the Conventional Level of moral maturity. Kohlberg found that 50% of late adolescents and adults are capable of Formal Operations thinking, but only 10% of these adults demonstrated the Post-Conventional Level in stages 5 and 6. Thus the person moves through stages, but few people progress through all six stages. Table 5–4 shows the three levels and six stages. Moral development is discussed in relation to each developmental era in Chapters 7 through 14.

Development of moral judgment is stimulated whenever (1) the educational process intentionally creates cognitive conflict and disequilibrium so that the person can work through inadequate modes of thinking, (2) when the person has opportunity for group discussion of values and can participate in group decision making about moral issues, and (3) the person has opportunity to assume responsibility for the consequences of behavior (49). Walker found that Kohlberg's moral stages were revealed over a 2-year interval in 233 subjects ages 5 to 63 years (90). Kohlberg's theory has application to nursing, education (49, 90, 91), and family counseling (93). Studies show that moral development continues as he describes through adulthood (53).

Gilligan: Theory of Moral Development. Gilligan's research on moral development has focused on women, in contrast to Kohlberg's focus on men. Gilligan found that moral development proceeds through three levels and two transitions, with each level representing a more complex understanding of the relationship of self and others and each transition resulting in a crucial reevaluation of the conflict between selfishness and responsibility. Women define the moral problem in context of human relationships, exercising care and avoiding hurt.

TABLE 5-4. PROGRESSION OF MORAL DEVELOPMENT

Level	Stage
Preconventional Person is responsive to cultural rules of labels of good and bad, right or wrong. Externally established rules determine right or wrong actions. Person reasons in terms of punishment, reward, or exchange of favors. Egocentric focus.	**I.** *Punishment and Obedient Orientation* Fear of punishment, not respect for authority, is the reason for decisions, behavior, and conformity. *Good* and *bad* are defined in terms of physical consequences to the self from parental, adult, or authority figures. The person defers to superior power or prestige of the person who dictates rules ("I'll do something because you tell me, and to avoid getting punished"). Average Age: toddler to 7 years
	II. *Instrumental Relativist Orientation* Conformity is based on egocentricity and narcissistic needs. The person's decisions and behavior are usually based on what provides satisfaction out of concern for self: something is done to get something in return. Occasionally the person does something to please another for pragmatic reasons. There is no feeling of justice, loyalty, or gratitude. These concepts are expressed physically ("I'll do something if I get something for it or because it pleases you"). Average age: preschooler through school age.
Conventional Person is concerned with maintaining expectations and rules of the family, group, nation, or society. A sense of guilt has developed and affects behavior. The person values conformity, loyalty, and active maintenance of social order and control. Conformity means good behavior or what pleases or helps another and is approved. Societal focus.	**III.** *Interpersonal Concordance Orientation* A. Decisions and behavior are based on concerns about others' reactions; the person wants others' approval or a reward. The person has moved from egocentricity to consideration of others as a basis for behavior. Behavior is judged by the person's intentions ("I'll do something because it will please you or because it is expected"). B. An empathic response, based on understanding of how another person feels, is a determinant for decisions and behavior ("I'll do something because I know how it feels to be without; I can put myself in your shoes"). Average age: school age through adulthood. Most American women are in this stage.
	IV. *Law-and-Order Orientation* The person wants established rules from authorities, and the reason for decisions and behavior is that social and sexual rules and traditions demand the response. The person obeys the law just because it is the law or out of respect for authority and underlying morality of the law. The law takes precedent over personal wishes, good intentions, and conformity to group stereotypes ("I'll do something because it's the law and my duty"). Average age: adolescence and adulthood. Most men are in this stage; 80% of adults do not move past this stage.
Postconventional The person lives autonomously and defines moral values and principles that are distinct from personal identification with group values. He or she lives according to principles that are universally agreed on and that the person considers appropriate for life. Universal focus	**V.** *Social Contract Legalistic Orientation* The social rules are not the sole basis for decisions and behavior because the person believes a higher moral principle applies such as equality, justice, or due process. The person defines right actions in terms of general individual rights and standards that have been agreed on by the whole society but is aware of relativistic nature of values and opinions. The person believes laws can be changed as people's needs change. The person uses freedom of choice in living up to higher principles but believes the way to make changes is through the system. Outside the legal realm, free agreement and contract are the binding elements of obligation ("I'll do something because it is morally and legally right, even if it isn't popular with the group"). Average age: middle-age or older adult. Only 20% or less of Americans achieve this stage.
	VI. *Universal Ethical Principle Orientation* Decisions and behavior are based on internalized rules, on conscience rather than on social laws, and on self-chosen ethical and abstract principles that are universal, comprehensive, and consistent. The rules are not concrete moral rules but instead encompass the Golden Rule, justice, reciprocity, and equality of human rights, and respect for the dignity of human beings as individual persons. Human life is inviolable. The person believes there is a higher order than social order, has a clear concept of civil disobedience, and will use self as an example to right a wrong. The person accepts injustice, pain, and death as an integral part of existence but works to minimize injustice and pain for others ("I'll do something because it is morally, ethically, and spiritually right, even if it is illegal and I get punished and even if no one else participates in the act"). Average age: middle-age or older adult. Few people attain or maintain this stage. Examples of this stage are seen in times of crisis or extreme situations.

Data from references 46–49.

In her studies women's moral judgment proceeded from (1) initial concern with survival, to (2) a focus on goodness, to (3) a principled understanding of others' need for care. Table 5–5 summarizes the three levels and two transitions of moral development proposed by Gilligan.

The focus on justice by Kohlberg is concerned with issues of inequality and oppression, and the theory values reciprocal rights and equal respect for individuals. The care focus proposed by Gilligan is concerned with issues of abandonment, and the theory values ideals of attention and response to need (28–30). Cooper (10) describes how the value of caring makes it pertinent to nursing.

Some people may combine both perspectives and incorporate them into their moral development—such values as honesty, courage, and community, which are implied in Kohlberg's Postconventional Level. More research in all age groups, men and women, and all races and ethnic groups is needed to understand moral development fully.

Friedman (21) tested Gilligan's claim that men and women differ in moral judgments. College students read four traditional moral dilemmas and rated the importance of 12 considerations for deciding how the protagonist should respond. There were no reliable sex differences on moral reasoning. Sex-typed personality measures also failed to predict individual differences in moral judgments.

THIRD FORCE THEORY

Overview

Third Force theorists include those who are proponents of **Humanistic Psychology, Existential Psychology,** and **Phenomenologic Psychology.** Humanistic and existential psychologies acknowledge the dynamic aspect of the person but emphasize the impact of environment to a greater degree.

Existentialism has its roots in philosophy, theology, literature, and psychology and addresses the person's existence in a hostile or indifferent world and within the context of history. It is phenomenologic in nature; the context, uniqueness, and everchanging aspects of events are considered. Existentialism regards human nature as unexplainable but emphasizes freedom of choice, responsibility, satisfaction of ideals, the burden of freedom, discovery of inner self, and consequences of action. Themes addressed include suffering, death, despair, meaninglessness, nothingness, vacuum, isolation, anxiety, hope, self-transcendence, and finding spiritual meaning. Transcendence of inevitable suffering, anxiety, and alienation is emphasized (13, 14). **Humanism** emphasizes self-actualization, satisfaction of needs, the individual as a rule unto himself or herself, the pleasure of freedom, and realization of innate goodness and creativity (86). Existentialists seek to answer the following questions: What are the possibilities of the person? From these possibilities, what is an optimum state for the person? Under what conditions is this state most likely to be reached? These disciplines strive to maximize the individuality and developmental potential of the person (9, 55, 57, 58, 86).

Because all behavior is considered a function of the person's perceptions, data for study of the person are subjective and come from self-reports, including (1) feelings at the moment about self and the experience, (2) meaning of the experience, and (3) personal values, needs, attitudes, beliefs, behavioral norms, and expectations. Perception is synonymous with reality and meaning. The person has many components—physical, physiologic, cognitive, emotional, spiritual, cultural, social, and familial—and cannot be adequately understood if studied by individual components. The person is also affected by many variables, both objective and subjec-

TABLE 5-5. GILLIGAN'S THEORY OF MORAL DEVELOPMENT

Level	Characteristics
I. Orientation of Individual Survival Transition	Concentrates on what is practical and best for self; selfish; dependent on others
1: From Selfishness to Responsibility	Realizes connection to others; thinks of responsible choice in terms of another as well as self
II. Goodness as Self-Sacrifice	Sacrifices personal wishes and needs to fulfill others' wants and to have others think well of her; feels responsible for others' actions; holds others responsible for her choices; dependent position; indirect efforts to control others often turns into manipulation through use of guilt; aware of connectedness with others
Transition 2: From Goodness to Truth	Makes decisions on personal intentions and consequences of actions rather than on how she thinks others will react; takes into account needs of self and others; wants to be good to others but also honest by being responsible to self; increased social participation; assumes more responsibilities
III. Morality of Nonviolence	Establishes moral equality between self and others; assumes responsibility for choice in moral dilemmas; follows injunction to hurt no one, including self, in all situations; conflict between selfishness and selflessness; judgment based on view of consequences and intentions instead of appearance in the eyes of others

Data from references 10, 28–30.

tive. All behavior is pertinent to and a product of the phenomenal or perceptual field of the person at the moment of action. The **phenomenal field** is the *frame of reference and the universe as experienced by the person at the specific moment (the existential condition)* (7, 9, 31, 56, 86).

View of the Human

The person is viewed as a significant and unique whole individual in dynamic interaction with the environment and in the process of becoming. In addition, the person is seen as holistic, with organizational complexity, more than the sum of the parts. The person is constantly growing, changing, expanding perceptual processes, learning, developing potential, and gaining insights. Every experience affects the person, depending on the perceptions. The person is never quite the same as he or she was even an hour or day earlier. The goals of the creative being are growth, feeling adequate, and reaching the potential. The person is active in pursuing these goals. Basic needs are the maintenance and enhancement of the self-concept and a sense of adequacy and self-actualization (7, 9, 31, 54, 56, 86).

Reality is internal; the person's reality is the perception of the event rather than the actual event itself. No two people will view a situation in exactly the same way. Various factors affect perception: (1) the sensory apparatus and central nervous system of the person; (2) time for observation; (3) opportunities available to experience events; (4) the external environment; (5) interpersonal relationships; and (6) self-concept. What is most important to the person is conscious experience, what is happening to the self at a given time. The person is aware of social values and norms but lives out those values and norms in a way that have been uniquely and personally defined (9, 56).

Perceptions are crucial in influencing behavior. Of all the perceptions that exist for the person, none is more important than those held about the self and the personal meaning and belief related to a situation. Self-concept is learned as a consequence of meaningful interactions with others and the world and has a high degree of stability at its core, changing only with time and opportunity to try new perceptions of self.

The truly adequate person sees self (and others) as having dignity, integrity, worth, and importance. Only with a positive view of self can the person risk trying the untried or accepting the undefined situation. The person can become self-actualized only through the experience of being treated as an adequate person by significant others. This person is open to all experiences, develops trust in self, and dares to recognize feelings, live life fully, and express uniqueness. The person feels a sense of oneness with other people, depending on the nature of previous contacts.

Third Force Theorists

The theorists of the Third Force include the humanists Abraham Maslow (Theory of Motivation and Hierarchy of Needs [54–56]) and Carl Rogers (Theory on Self-Concept and Client-Centered Therapy [45, 72–74]). Other humanistic theorists include Arthur Combs (9), Donald Snygg (9), Sidney Jourard (40), and Rollo May (57). Humanistic nursing as a framework has been developed by Josephine Paterson and Loretta Zderad (62). Although found as a thread in other nursing models, including Neuman's Health Care Systems Model (61), humanism is the basis for the views of Hildegard Peplau (63), Dorothy Johnson (70), and Martha Rogers (75). Only Maslow will be discussed in this chapter. References at the end of the chapter give information on other theorists who have contributed to nursing.

Maslow: Theory of Motivation and Hierarchy of Needs

Abraham Maslow originated the term *Third Force* to show the perspectives of creativity and potential for freedom in the person, aspects he believed were neglected in psychoanalytic and learning theories. Maslow studied normal people and mental health (31) in contrast to other developmental and personality theorists. One of his most important concepts is **self-actualization,** the *tendency to develop potentialities and become a better person,* and the need to help the person achieve the sense of self-direction implicit in self-actualization. Implicit in this concept is that people are not static but are always in the process of becoming different and better (31, 54–56).

The needs that motivate self-actualization can be represented in a hierarchy of relative order and predominance. The basic needs, always a consideration in client care, are as shown in Table 5–6.

Maslow's study of self-actualizing people refutes Freudian theory that the human unconscious, or id, is only bad or dangerous. In self-actualizing people the unconscious is creative, loving, and positive (31).

Although Maslow ranked these basic human needs from lowest to highest, they do not necessarily occur in a fixed order. The physiologic and safety needs (deficiency needs), however, are dominant and must be met before higher needs can be secured. Personal growth needs are those for love and belonging, self-esteem and recognition, and self-actualization. The highest needs of self-actualization, knowledge, and aesthetic expression may never be as fully gratified as those at lower levels. Individual growth and self-fulfillment are a continuing, lifelong process of becoming (31, 55).

To motivate the person toward self-actualization, there must be freedom to speak, to pursue creative potential, and to inquire; an atmosphere of justice, honesty, fairness, and order; and environmental stimulation and challenge (31). Many have trouble moving toward self-actualization because of the environment in which

TABLE 5-6. MASLOW'S THEORY OF HIERARCHY OF NEEDS

Needs*	Characteristics
Physiologic	Requirements for oxygen, water, food, temperature control, elimination, shelter, exercise, sleep, sensory stimulation, and sexual activity met
	Needs cease to exist as means of determining behavior when satisfied, re-emerging only if blocked or frustrated
Safety	Able to secure shelter
	Sense of security, dependency, consistency, stability
	Maintenance of predictable environment, structure, order, fairness, limits
	Protection from immediate or future danger to physical well-being
	Freedom from fear, anxiety, chaos, and certain amount of routine
Love and Belonging	Sense of affection, love, and acceptance from others
	Sense of companionship and affiliation with others
	Identification with significant others
	Recognition and approval from others
	Group interaction
	Not synonymous with sexual needs, but sexual needs may be motivated by this need
Esteem from Others	Awareness of own individuality, uniqueness
	Feelings of self-respect and worth and respect from others
	Sense of confidence, independence, dignity
	Sense of competence, achievement, success, prestige, status
	Recognition from others for accomplishments
Self-Actualization	Acceptance of self and others
	Empathetic with others
	Self-fulfillment
	Ongoing emotional and spiritual development
	Desire to attain standards of excellence and individual potential
	Use of talents, being productive and creative
	Experiencing fully, vividly, without self-consciousness
	Having peak experiences
Aesthetic	Desire for beauty, harmony, order, attractive surroundings
	Interest in art, music, literature, dance, creative forms
Knowledge and Understanding	Desire to understand, systematize, organize, analyze, look for relations and meanings
	Curiosity; desire to know as much as possible
	Attraction to the unknown or mysterious

*Needs are listed in ascending order. Physiologic needs are most basic; self-actualization is highest level of needs.
Data from references 31, 54–56.

they live. For example, socialization practices may hinder women in using fully their intellectual abilities. Men may be inhibited from expressing emotions of tenderness, love, or need of others by cultural norms. Deprivation of growth needs results in feelings of despair and depression and a sense that life is meaningless (31, 54–56).

REFERENCES

1. Anderson, R., and I. Carter, *Human Behavior in the Social Environment,* Chicago: Aldine, 1974.
2. Babcock, D., Transactional Analysis, *American Journal of Nursing,* 76, no. 7 (1976), 1152–1155.
3. Bandura, A., *Social Learning Theory.* Morristown, NJ: General Learning Press, 1977.
4. Berne, E., *Transactional Analysis in Psychotherapy: A Systematic Individual and Social Psychiatry.* New York: Grove Press, 1986.
5. Berrien, K., *General and Social Systems.* New Brunswick, NJ: Rutgers University Press, 1968.
6. Carruth, B., Modifying Behavior through Social Learning, *American Journal of Nursing,* 76, no. 11 (1976), 1084–1086.
7. Carter, S., The Nurse Educator: Humanist or Behaviorist? *Nursing Outlook,* 26, no. 9 (1978), 554–557.
8. Chodoran, N., *Feminism and Psychoanalytic Theory.* New Haven, Conn: Yale University Press, 1991.
9. Combs, A., and D. Snygg, *Individual Behavior: A Perceptual Approach to Behavior.* New York: Harper & Row, 1959.
10. Cooper, M., Gilligan's Different Voice: A Perspective for Nursing, *Journal of Professional Nursing,* 5, no. 1 (1989), 10–16.
11. Erikson, E., *Childhood and Society* (2nd ed.). New York: W.W. Norton, 1963.
12. Fordham, F., *An Introduction to Jung's Psychology.* Baltimore: Penguin Books, 1966.
13. Frankl, V., *Man's Search for Meaning.* New York: Washington Square Press, 1967.
14. ———, *The Unheard Cry for Meaning.* New York: Washington Square Press, 1978.
15. Freud, A., *The Ego and the Mechanisms of Defense.* London: Hogarth Press, 1937.
16. Freud, S., *A General Introduction to Psychoanalysis.* New York: Simon & Schuster, 1935.
17. ———, *The Problem of Anxiety.* New York: W.W. Norton, 1936.
18. ———, *Ego and the Id.* London: Hogarth Press, 1947.
19. ———, *Inhibitions, Symptoms, and Anxiety.* London: Hogarth Press, 1948.
20. ———, *Outline of Psychoanalysis.* New York: W.W. Norton, 1949.
21. Friedman, W., et al., Sex Differences in Moral Judgments: A Test of Gilligan's Theory, *Psychology of Women Quarterly,* 7, no. 1 (1987), 87.
22. Fromm, E., *The Art of Loving.* New York: Harper & Row, 1963.
23. Furth, H.G., and H. Wachs, *Thinking Goes to School:*

Piaget's Theory in Practice. New York: Oxford University Press, 1975.

24. Gesell, A., *The First Five Years of Life*. New York: Macmillan, 1940.

25. ——, and F. Ilg, *The Child From Five to Ten* (rev ed). New York: Harper, 1977.

26. ——, F. Ilg, and L. Ames, *Youth: The Years From 10 to 16*. New York: Harper & Brothers Publishers, 1956.

27. ——, et al., *Infant and Child in the Culture of Today: The Guidance of Development in Home and Nursery School*. New York: Harper Collins, 1974.

28. Gilligan, C., In A Different Voice: Women's Conceptualization of Self and of Mortality, *Harvard Educational Review*, 47, no. 4 (1977), 481–517.

29. ——, *In A Different Voice: Psychological Theory and Women's Development*. Cambridge, Mass: Harvard University Press, 1982.

30. ——, and D. Attanucci, Two Moral Orientations: Gender Differences and Similarities, *Merrill-Palmer Quarterly*, 34, no. 3 (1988), 332–333.

31. Goble, F., *The Third Force: The Psychology of Abraham Maslow*. New York: Grossman, 1970.

32. Gould, R., The Phases of Adult Life: A Study in Developmental Psychology, *American Journal of Psychiatry*, 129, no. 5 (1972), 521–531.

33. Graves, J., Psychoanalytic Theory. A Critique, *Perspectives in Psychiatric Care*, 11, no. 3 (1973), 114–120.

34. Greenberg, R., and S. Fisher, Testing Dr. Freud, *Human Behavior*, 7, no. 9 (1978), 28-33.

35. Hartmann, H., *Essays on Ego Psychology*. New York: International Universities Press, 1964.

36. Heidbreder, E., *Seven Psychologies*. Englewood Cliffs, NJ: Prentice-Hall, 1963.

37. Hilgard, E., and G. Bower, *Theories of Learning* (5th ed.). Englewood Cliffs, NJ: Prentice-Hall, 1981.

38. Horney, K., *The Neurotic Personality in Our Time*. New York: W.W. Norton, 1937.

39. Jones, F., K. Garrison, and R. Morgan, *The Psychology of Human Development* (2nd ed.). New York: Harper & Row, 1985.

40. Jourard, S., *Disclosing Man to Himself*. New York: D. Van Nostrand, 1968.

41. Jung, C., *Modern Man In Search of a Soul*. New York: Harcourt, Brace, & World, 1933.

42. ——, *The Undiscovered Self* (transl. by R.F.C. Hall). New York: Mentor Books, 1958.

43. ——, Psychological Types. In Adler, G., et al., eds. *Collected Works of Carl G. Jung*, Vol. 6. Princeton, NJ: Princeton University Press, 1971.

44. Kaluger, G., and M. Kaluger, *Human Development: The Span of Life* (3rd ed.). St. Louis: Times Mirror/Mosby, 1984.

45. Kirschenbaum, H., and V. Henderson, eds., *A Carl Roger's Reader*. Boston: Houghton Mifflin, 1989.

46. Kohlberg, L., ed., *Collected Papers on Moral Development and Moral Education*, Cambridge, Mass: Moral Educational Research Foundation, 1973.

47. ——, Moral Stages and Moralization: The Cognitive Developmental Approach. In T. Lickona, ed., *Moral Development and Behavior*. New York: Holt, Rinehart, & Winston, 1976, 31–53.

48. ——, *Recent Research in Moral Development*. New York: Holt, Rinehart & Winston, 1977.

49. ——, The Cognitive-Developmental Approach to Moral Education. In Scharf, P., ed., *Readings in Moral Education*. Minneapolis: Winston Press, 1978, pp. 36–51.

50. Levinson, D., *The Seasons of a Man's Life*. New York: Ballantine Books, 1978.

51. Lidz, T., *The Person: His and Her Development Throughout The Life Cycle* (2nd ed.). New York: Basic Books, 1983.

52. Loomis, C.P., *Social Systems*. New York: D. Van Nostrand, 1960.

53. Marchand, J.L., and J. Samson, Kohlberg's Theory Applied to the Moral and Sexual Development of Adults, *Journal of Moral Education*, 7, no. 4 (1982), 247–258.

54. Maslow, A., *Towards a Psychology of Being*, 2nd ed. New York: D. Van Nostrand, 1968.

55. ——, *Motivation and Personality*, 2nd ed. New York: Harper & Row, 1970.

56. ——, *The Farther Reaches of Human Nature*. New York: Viking Press, 1971.

57. May, R., *Psychology and the Human Dilemma*. New York: D. Van Nostrand, 1967.

58. Middleton, J., Existentialist as Helper? *Canadian Psychiatric Nursing*, 20, no. 3 (1979), 7–8.

59. Moshman, D., J. Glover, and R. Bruning, *Developmental Psychology: A Topical Approach*. Boston: Little, Brown, 1987.

60. Munroe, R., *Schools of Psychoanalytic Thought*. New York: Holt, Rinehart & Winston, 1955.

61. Neuman, B., The Betty Neuman Health-Care Systems Model: A Total Person Approach to Patient Problems. In Riehl, J.P., and C. Roy, eds. *Conceptual Models for Nursing Practice* (3rd ed.). New York: Appleton-Century-Crofts, 1988.

62. Paterson, J., and L. Zderad, *Humanistic Nursing*. New York: John Wiley, 1976.

63. Peplau, H., *Interpersonal Relations in Nursing*. New York: G.P. Putnam's Sons, 1952.

64. Piaget, J., *The Origins of Intelligence in Children*. New York: W.W. Norton, 1963.

65. ——, *Six Psychological Studies*. New York: Random House, 1967.

66. ——, and B. Inhelder, *The Psychology of the Child*. New York: Basic Books, 1969.

67. ——, and B. Inhelder. *Memory and Intelligence*. London: Routledge & Kegan Paul, 1973.

68. Quinn, S., *A Mind of Her Own: The Life of Karen Horney*. New York: Summit Books, 1987.

69. Rest, J., The Legacy of Lawrence Kohlberg, *Counseling and Values*, 32, no. 3 (1988), 156–162.

70. Riehl, J., and C. Roy, Theory and Models. In *Conceptual Models for Nursing Practice* (3rd ed.). New York: Appleton-Century-Crofts, 1988.

71. Rimm, R.C., and J.C. Masters, *Behavior Therapy Techniques and Empirical Findings*. New York: Academic Press, 1979.

72. Rogers, C., *Client-Centered Therapy*. Boston: Houghton-Mifflin, 1951.

73. ——, *On Becoming a Person*. Boston: Houghton-Mifflin, 1961.

74. ——, A Theory of Personality. In Millan, T., ed. *Theories of Psychopathology*. Philadelphia: W.B. Saunders, 1973.

75. Rogers, M., *An Introduction to the Theoretical Basis of Nursing*. Philadelphia: F.A. Davis, 1970.

76. Schwartz, M., *Biofeedback: A Practitioner's Guide*. New York: Guilford Press, 1987.

77. Sheehy, G., *Passages*. New York: Bantam Books, 1984.

78. Skinner, B.F., *The Behavior of Organisms*. New York: Appleton-Century-Crofts, 1938.

79. ——, *Walden Two*. New York: Macmillan, 1948.

80. ——, *Science and Human Behavior*. New York: Macmillan, 1953.

81. ——, *Beyond Freedom and Dignity*. New York: Alfred A. Knopf, 1971.

82. ——, *Cumulative Record* (3rd ed.). New York: Appleton-Century-Crofts, 1972.

83. Storr, A., *The Essential Jung*. Princeton, NJ: Princeton University Press, 1983.

84. Sullivan, H.S., *The Interpersonal Theory of Psychiatry*. New York: W.W. Norton, 1953.

85. Taylor, R., *Distinguishing Psychological From Organic Disorders*. New York: Springer, 1990.

86. Urban, H., Humanist, Phenomenological, and Existential Approaches. In Hersen, M., A. Kadzin, and A. Bellak, eds. *The Clinical Psychology Handbook* (2nd ed.). New York: Pergamon Press, 1991, pp. 200–219.

87. Vaillant, G., The "Normal Boy" in Later Life: How Adaptation Fosters Growth, *Harvard Magazine,* 6 (1977), 234–239.

88. Von Bertalanffy, L., *General System Theory*. New York: George Braziller, 1968.

89. Wadsworth, B., *Piaget's Theory of Cognitive and Affective Development* (4th ed.). New York: Longman, 1989.

90. Walker, L., A Longitudinal Study of Moral Reasoning, *Child Development,* 60, no. 1 (1989), 157–166.

91. Weinrich, H., Some Consequences of Replicating Kohlberg's Original Moral Development Study in a British Sample, *Journal of Moral Education,* 7, no. 1 (1977), 32–39.

92. West, J., and D. Burser, Gilligan and Kohlberg: Gender Issue in Moral Development, *Journal of Humanistic Education and Development,* 22, no. 4 (1984), 134–142.

93. Winsor, J., and F. Lower, *An Application of Kohlberg's Moral Reasoning Theory to Understanding Problems of Marital and Family Communication*. New York: Basic Books, 1992.

94. Wolpe, J., *Practice of Behavior Therapy* (3rd ed.). New York: Pergamon Press, 1991.

Chapter 6

The Developing Person: Principles of Growth and Development

Nothing has a stronger influence on their children than the unlived lives of their parents.
—Carl Gustav Jung

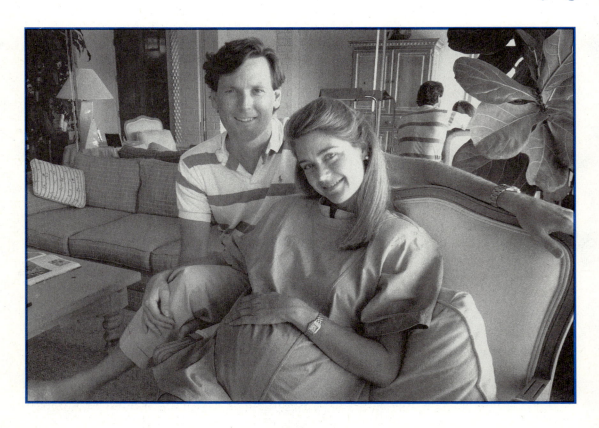

KEY TERMS

Social time	Cognitive competency	Gametes	Anoxia
Historical time	Emotional competency	Meiosis	Prematurity
Cohort	Social competency	Follicle	Low-birth-weight
Norms	Principle of Development	Ovulation	Hormone
Growth	Toward Self-Knowledge	Orgasm	Integration
Incremental growth	and Autonomy	Cervix	Regulation
Replacement growth	Principle of Differentiation	Fraternal twins	Morphogenesis
Hypertrophy	Cephalocaudal Principle	Identical twins	Socialization
Hyperplasia	Proximodistal Principle	Germinal stage	Resilient children
Development	Bilateral Principle	Embryonic stage	Child abuse
Developmental task	Principle of Asynchronous Growth	Fetal stage	Sexual molestation
Maturation	Principle of Discontinuity of Growth Rate	Conceptus	Emotional abuse
Biologic age	Chromosomes	Anemia	Neglect
Chronologic age	Genes	Pica	Maternal deprivation
Learning	Ovum	Teratogen	Failure to thrive
Critical periods	Zygote	Teratogenesis	Perceptual deprivation
Physical competency		Folklore	

OBJECTIVES

Study of this chapter will enable you to:

1. Define growth, development, and related terms.
2. Explore general insights into and principles of human behavior.
3. Discuss various influences that have an effect on the developing person: prenatal variables involving father, mother, and fetus; variables related to childbirth; early childhood variables, including child abuse; sociocultural experiences; and environmental factors.
4. Relate information in this chapter to yourself as a developing person.
5. Use information from this chapter when assessing the person through the life span.
6. Teach the person and family about factors that influence development of self or offspring, when appropriate.

Developmental theory, which discusses the person throughout the life span, centers around certain principles of and influences on the person's growth and development. Although growth and development are usually thought of as a forward movement or a kind of adding on such as increase in height and weight or the self-actualizing personality, the model can also apply to reversal, decay, deterioration, or death. Three kinds of reversals occur: (1) loss of some part such as occurs with catabolism (changing of living tissue into wastes or destructive metabolism), (2) purposefully changing behavior when it is no longer useful, and (3) death (83, 102).

Growth and development are generally characterized by the following: (1) direction, goal, or end state, (2) identifiable stage or era, (3) forward progression so that once a stage is worked through, the person does not return to the same position, (4) increasing specialization, (5) causal forces that are either genetic or environmental, and (6) potentialities and capabilities for various behaviors, and achievements (83, 102).

DIMENSIONS OF TIME

Lifetime or chronologic age is frequently used as an index of maturation and development but is only a rough indicator of the person's position on any one of the numerous physical or psychologic dimensions. Further, the society is a reference point for understanding the behavior; what is appropriate for a 14-year-old individual in one society is not in a different society (86).

Social time, or *social expectations of behavior for each age era,* is not necessarily synchronous with biologic timing. Neither chronologic age nor maturational stage is itself a determinant of aging status but only signifies the biologic potentiality on which a system of age norms and age grading can operate to shape the life cycle (86).

Historical time shapes the social system, and the social system creates a changing set of age norms and a changing age-grade system that shapes the person's life cycle. **Historical time** refers to a *series of economic, political, and social events that directly shape the life course of the person and long-term processes* such as industrialization and urbanization that create the social-cultural context and changing definitions of the phases of the life cycle (86).

A group of people born at a certain calendar time (**cohort**) has, as a group, a particular background and demographic composition so that most of the people of that specific age or generation will have similar experiences, level of education, fertility and childrearing patterns, sexual mores, work and labor force participation patterns, value systems, leisure patterns, religious behavior, consumer behavior, and ideas about life generally (86).

Social time is prescribed by each society in that all societies rationalize the passage of lifetime, divide life into socially relevant units, and transform calendar or biologic time into social time. Thus age grading occurs; the life cycle consists of a succession of formally age-graded, descriptive norms. Duties, rights, and rewards are differentially distributed to age groups. In societies in which division of labor is simple and social change is slow, a single age-grade system becomes formalized, and family, work, religious, and political roles are allocated. A modern, complex, rapidly changing society, which has several or overlapping systems of age status, has some tasks and roles that are tied to chronologic age and some that are more fluid or less defined. In every society there is a time to be a child and dependent, a time to be educated to whatever level is needed, a time to go to work, to marry, to have a family, to retire, and to die. The members of the society have a general consensus about these age expectations and norms, although perceptions may vary somewhat by age, sex, or social class. Thus there is some pressure to conform. If the person engages in the tasks earlier or later than others in the society, he or she is considered deviant. Patterns of timing can play an important role with respect to self-concept and self-esteem, depending on the person's level of awareness about his or her fit to social age norms and the rigidity in the culture. The young are more likely to deny that age is a valid criterion by which to judge behavior. The middle-aged and old adults, who see greater constraints in the age-norm system than do the young, have learned that to be off time involves negative consequences. Many of the major marks in the life cycle are ordered and sequential and are social rather than biologic, and their time is socially regulated (86).

The life course dimension is indexed by chronologic age, which serves as an indicator of the person's experience, including age-related organic changes affecting physical and mental functioning and including the probability of certain psychologic and social experiences (86).

This book is organized along chronologic lines, with the life cycle divided into different time periods rather than having content organized around a topical approach. The person's life is divided into the following chronologic stages: the prenatal period (from the moment of conception to birth); infancy (birth to 1 year); toddlerhood (1 to 3 years); preschool (3 to 6 years); school years (6 to 12 years); adolescence (12 to 20 or 25 years); young adulthood (20 or 25 to 45 years); middle age (45 or 50 to 65 or 70 years); and late maturity (65 or 70 years and over). These divisions are somewhat arbitrary because it is difficult to assign definite ages since individual lives are not marked off so precisely. In discussion of stage theories such as those of Freud, Erikson, and Piaget, we use the theorists' own age ranges, and the same reservations apply to them.

The study of development is not merely a search for facts about people at certain ages. The study involves finding *patterns* or *general principles* that apply to most people most of the time.

People are often at one level in one area of development and at another level in another area. For example, an 11-year-old girl may have begun to menstruate—an activity that marks her physical transition from childbirth to puberty—before she has outgrown many childish feelings and thoughts. A 48-year-old man who took several years to find his career direction, who married in his thirties, and who became a father in his forties may in many important psychologic ways be in the young adulthood period. On the other hand, his 49-year-old neighbor who settled early on a professional direction and into family life may already be a grandfather and may act and feel more like a middle-aged man. Furthermore, individual differences among people are so great that they enter and leave these age periods at different times of life. People are aware of their own timing and are quick to describe themselves as "early," "late," or "on time" regarding developmental tasks.

Ideal **norms,** *standards* or *expectancies,* for different behaviors vary among different groups of people. The entire life cycle is speeded up for the poor and working classes, who tend to finish their education earlier than middle- or upper-class people, to take their first jobs sooner, marry younger, have children earlier, reach the peak of their careers earlier, and become grandparents earlier. These differences are related to financial needs that make it imperative for poor and working-class people to get paying jobs earlier in life. People from more affluent backgrounds can pursue their educations for a longer time, can use young adulthood to explore options, and can delay becoming financially independent and beginning a family (34, 83, 102).

PRINCIPLES OF GROWTH AND DEVELOPMENT

Definitions

Certain words are basic to understanding the person and are used repeatedly. They are defined below for the purpose of this book.

Growth refers to *increase in body size or changes in structure, function, and complexity of body cell content and metabolic and biochemical processes up to some point of optimum maturity* (83, 102). Growth changes occur through incremental or replacement growth. **Incremental growth** refers to *maintaining an excess in growth over normal daily losses from catabolism, seen in urine, feces, perspiration, and oxidation in the lungs.* Incremental growth is observed as increases in weight or height as the child matures. **Replacement growth** refers to *normal refills of essential body components* necessary for survival (42). For example, once a red blood cell (erythrocyte) has entered the cardiovascular system, it circulates an average of 120 days before disintegrating when another red blood cells takes its place (42). Growth occurs through **hypertrophy,** *increase in the size of cellular structures* and **hyperplasia,** an *increase in the number of cells* (42). Growth during the fetal and infancy periods is achieved primarily through hyperplasia, which is gradually replaced by hypertrophic growth. Each body organ has its own optimum period of growth. Body tissues are most sensitive to permanent damage during periods of the most rapid hyperplastic growth.

Development is the *patterned, orderly, lifelong changes in structure, thought, or behavior that evolve as a result of maturation of physical and mental capacity, experiences, and learning and result in a new level of maturity and integration* (83, 116). Development should permit the person to adapt to the environment by either controlling the environment or controlling responses to the environment. Developmental processes involve interplay among the physiologic characteristics that define the person; the environmental forces, including culture, that act on him or her; and the psychologic mechanisms that mediate between them. Psychologic processes include the person's perception of self, others, and the environment, and the behaviors he or she acquires in coping with needs and the environment. Development combines growth, maturation, and learning and involves organizing behavior (28).

Developmental task is a *growth responsibility that arises at a certain time in the course of development, successful achievement of which leads to satisfaction and success with later tasks.* Failure leads to unhappiness, disapproval by society, and difficulty with later developmental tasks and functions (28).

Maturation refers to the *emergence of genetic potential for changes in form, structure, complexity, integration, organization, and function* (102).

Biologic age is the *level of physical growth and development.* **Chronologic age** is the *time since birth* and is not always identical to biologic age.

Learning is the *process of gaining specific knowledge or skill and acquiring habits and attitudes as a result of experience, training, and behavioral changes.* Maturation and learning are interrelated. No learning oc-

curs unless the person is mature enough to be able to understand and change his or her behavior (102).

GENERAL ASSUMPTIONS ABOUT BEHAVIOR

C. Buhler is a developmental theorist whose thinking in the early 1900s influenced a number of present well-known personality and developmental theorists.

Buhler (12) described the person's life course as having a definite basic structure and direction or goals. These structures and goals are evidence in the biologic life cycle and in psychologic development. The structure and phasic organization of the person's life, with its properties and potentials, determines the person's goals and is influenced by environmental circumstances, time limits, personal characteristics, and society's assignment of roles.

In Buhler's theory life is divided biologically into a nonreproductive phase (first 15 years, approximately), a reproductive phase from approximately 15 to 45 years, and then a decline and loss in the reproductive ability, first in the female and then in the male (after middle age for the woman and in old age for the man). Onset of reproductive ability, from puberty to 25 years, is followed by a peak period for reproductive ability and stationary growth (25 to 45 years). A period of gradual decline follows.

Psychologic development is not parallel to biologic development because (1) psychologic development is continuous, and (2) there is no exact parallel between the two aspects of life so far as tasks or goals are concerned. Psychologic and mental development may be behind biologic development, is generally independent of physical or biologic factors, and extends beyond reproductive abilities. The psychologic system develops in a maturational order and is influenced by learning and the impact of emotional experiences. Abilities, aptitudes, motives, and goals contribute to personality development (12).

The following statements have not been proved by strict scientific study, but they have been observed so regularly that they seem to be true.

The *person is a unified but open system* composed of the components of body, mind, feelings, and spirit, which are, in turn, continually influenced by the environment. The person, in turn, influences the environment (83, 102, 115).

All *persons are similar and have the same basic needs, but they are also unique* in following and expressing their own developmental patterns. The *One Genus Postulate* states that people are more similar than different simply because they are all Homo sapiens (115).

The *person is a unified whole.* Thus understanding the whole person is not possible through study of isolated components of the person (95).

The *person's life process evolves irreversibly;* the person cannot totally return to something he or she was developmentally (58, 95). Nevertheless, the past influences the person to some degree whether or not he or she is aware of the influence, and it sets the direction for present and future patterns of behavior (58, 115).

The *person responds as a total organism at any given moment to events, persons, or objects* in terms of personal perception, needs, and expectations (58).

Each person is a social being who has the capacity to communicate and react to other people and the environment. Thus the person can function in the social system and its various institutions such as family, school, and church (58).

The *person cannot understand the self without understanding others, and he or she cannot understand others without understanding the self.* Understanding the past and the parents helps to understand the self since developmental patterns of the parents are repeated in the child (115).

Culture and society determine guidelines for normal progression of development and behavior patterns. What is normal in one ethnic or racial group may be considered deviant or undesirable in another. Further, deviation from normal may occur in all or only certain areas of function. The child may show abnormally slow development in one area and unusually accelerated or a mature quality in another. Yet in spite of these differences, the child may be perceived generally by others as a normal person, depending on the degree of deviance.

Throughout life the person strives to reach optimum physical and emotional potential, barring great interferences. An inner drive or motivation propels him or her onward to meet the various developmental tasks. The person tries all types of adaptive behavior when interferences occurs. He or she may regress to work through unsolved problems from the past. Once a need is met or a goal is accomplished, the person is free to move on to new arenas of behavior (34, 115).

General Principles of Development

The following statements apply to the overall development of the person.

Childhood is the foundation period of life. Attitudes, habits, patterns of behavior and thinking, personality traits, and health status established during the early years (the first 5) determine to a large extent how successfully the person will continue to develop and adjust to life as he or she gets older. Early patterns of behavior persist throughout life, within the range of normalcy (34, 83, 102).

Development follows a definable, predictable, and sequential pattern and occurs continually through adulthood. All persons progress through similar stages, but the age for achievement varies since achievement depends on inherent maturational capacity interacting with the physical and social environment. The different areas of growth and development—physical, mental, emotional, social, and spiritual—are interrelated, proceed together, and affect each other; yet these areas mature at their own pace. The stages of development overlap, and the transition from one stage to another is gradual (34, 102, 115).

Growth and development are continuous, but they occur in spurts rather than in a straight upward direction. At times the person will appear to be at a standstill or even regress developmentally.

Growth is not necessarily accompanied by behavior change. As the child matures, he or she retains earlier ways of behaving, although there will be a developmental revision of habits. For example, the high-activity infant becomes a high-activity toddler or adult, but the object of the activity changes from diffuse interests to concentrated play to work. The young child's temperament is a precursor of later behavior, although the person is adaptable and changes throughout life.

Critical periods in human development *occur when specific organs and other aspects of a person's physical and psychosocial growth undergo marked rapid change and the capacity to adapt to stressors is underdeveloped. During these critical periods when tremendous demands are placed on the person, the individual has an increased susceptibility to adverse environmental factors* that may cause various types and degrees of negative effects. For example, implantation is a critical period, and at certain times during pregnancy certain substances are more likely to damage fetal structures (25). During adolescence the rapid physical growth may negatively affect social relationships or feelings about self. Middle or old age may be another critical period.

If appropriate stimuli and resources are not available at the critical time or when the person is ready to receive and use particular stimuli for the development of a specific psychomotor skill, the skill may be more difficult to learn later in the developmental sequence. However, learning of any psychomotor skill is also influenced by sociocultural factors; the extent to which any skill is influenced by genetics, environmental opportunity, cultural and family values and patterns, and emotional status is not fully known.

Mastering developmental tasks of one period is the basis for mastering the next developmental era, physically and emotionally. Certain times periods exist when the task can be best accomplished and the task should be mastered then; if the time is delayed, the person will have difficulty in accomplishing the task. Each phase of development has characteristic traits and a period of equilibrium when the person adjusts more easily to environmental demands and a period of disequilibrium when he or she experiences difficulty in adjustment. Developmental hazards exist in every era. Some are environmental and interfere with adjustment; others come from within the person (28, 34, 84, 103, 115).

Progressive differentiation of the self from the environment results from increasing self-knowledge and autonomy. The young child first separates as an object apart from mother. Gradually he or she becomes less dependent emotionally on the parents. As the child matures into adulthood, an increase in cognitive development enables more control over behavior. The person can think and act on his or her own and become more and more autonomous (102).

The *developing person acquires simultaneously competencies in four major areas:* physical, cognitive, emotional, and social. **Physical competency** includes *various motor and neurologic capacities* to attain mobility and manipulation and care for self physically. **Cognitive competency** includes *learning how to perceive, think, solve problems, and communicate thoughts and feelings* that, in turn, affect emotional and social skills. **Emotional competency** includes *developing an awareness and acceptance of self as a separate person, responding to other people and factors in the environment because others have been responsive to him or her, coping with inner and outer stresses, and becoming increasingly responsible for personal behavior.* **Social competency** includes *learning how to affiliate securely with the family first and then with various people in various situations.* These four competencies constantly influence one another. Health of one domain or the extent of competency affects the other domains or competencies. Lack of care or stimulation in any one area inhibits development of the other three areas. Repetition and practice are essential to learning. Rewarded behavior is usually repeated (83). The person optimally uses personal assets, inner resources, competencies, and abilities to keep energy expenditures at a minimum while focusing toward the achievement of a goal (102).

Readiness and motivation are essential for learning to occur. Hunger, fatigue, illness, pain, and the lack of emotional feedback or opportunity to explore inhibit readiness and lower motivation.

Many factors contribute to the formation of permanent characteristics and traits, including the child's genetic inheritance, undetermined prenatal environmental factors, family and society when he or she is an infant and young child, nutrition, the physical and emotional environment, and the degree of intellectual stimulation in the environment.

Progressive differentiation of the self from other people and the environment, the **Principle of Development toward Self-Knowledge and Autonomy,** is made apparent with the individual's increasing self-awareness and emergent self-concept. The young child achieves increasing ability to perceive himself or herself as an initiator of action on the environment and an increasing ability to regulate his or her own behavior, to think and act in an individual and unique way, and to become more autonomous. The ability to be autonomous and interdependent is reworked throughout life (83).

Principles of Growth

Several principles of growth are emphasized in the following pages, but the primary determinant of normal growth is the development of the central nervous system, which, in turn, governs or influences other body systems.

The **Principle of Differentiation** means that *development proceeds from (1) simple to the complex; (2) homogeneous to heterogeneous; and (3) general to specific* (83). For example, movement from *simple to complex* is seen in mitotic changes in fetal cell structures as they undergo cell division immediately following ovum fertilization by a sperm (42). All human embryos are anatomically female for the first 6 weeks of life; only through the action of specific hormones does the male embryo develop between the sixth and twelfth weeks of life (83). Differentiation from simple to complex motor skill is seen after birth as the baby first waves his or her arms and then later learns to control finger movements. The general body configuration of male and female at birth is much more similar than during late adolescence, thus indicating *movement from homogeneity to heterogeneity* (83). The mass of cells in the embryo is at first homogeneous, but the limbs of the 5-week-old embryo show considerable differentiation as the elbow and wrist regions become identifiable and finger ridge indentations outline the progressive protrusion of future fingers from the former paddle-shaped arm bud (42). *General to specific* development is observed in motor responses, which are diffuse and undifferentiated at birth and become more specific and controlled later. Baby first moves the whole body in response to a stimuli; later he or she reacts with a specific body part (102). The behavior of the child becomes more specific to the person or situation with increasing age.

The **Cephalocaudal, Proximodistal, and Bilateral Principles** all indicate that *major physical and motor changes invariably proceed in three bipolar directions.* **Cephalocaudal** (*head to tail*) means that the *upper end of the organism develops with greater rapidity than and before the lower end of the organism.* Increases in neuromuscular size and maturation of function begin in the head and proceed to hands and feet. For example, a comparison of pictures of a 5-week-old embryo during a period of several days clearly shows the extensive head growth, caused mainly by development of the brain, accompanied by further oblongation of the body structure from head to tail. Further, auditory, visual, and other sensory mechanisms in the head develop sooner than motor systems of the upper body. At the same time, the arm buds, first appearing paddle shaped, continue to change in shape and size more rapidly than do the lower limbs. After birth the infant will be able to hold the head erect before being able to sit or walk (102). **Proximodistal** (*near to far*) means that *growth progresses from the central axis of the body toward the periphery or extremities.* **Bilateral** (*side to side*) means that the *capacity for growth and development of structures is symmetric* (83); growth that occurs on one side of the body occurs simultaneously on the other.

The **Principle of Asynchronous Growth** *focuses on developmental shifts at successive periods in development.* A comparison of pictures of persons of different ages indicates that the young child is *not* a "small adult"; the proportional size of the head to the chest and of the torso to the limbs of younger and older persons is vastly different. Length of limbs in comparison to torso length is smaller in the infant than the schoolchild and greater in the aged than the adolescent because of the biologic changes of aging (83, 102).

The **Principle of Discontinuity of Growth Rate** refers to the *different rate of growth changes at different periods during the life span* (83). The *whole* body does not grow as a total unit simultaneously. Instead, various structures and organs of the body grow and develop at different rates, reaching their maximum at different times throughout the life cycle. For instance, in its rudimentary form the heart and circulatory system begin to function during the third week of embryonic life, continue to mature slowly compared to the rest of the body, and after the age of 25 years remains fairly constant in size (83, 102). Before birth the head is the fastest growing body party. The brain grows and develops according to a different pattern; this vital organ grows very rapidly during fetal life and infancy, reaching 80% of its maximum size at the age of 2 years. Full growth is seen at approximately 6 years of age (83, 102). Body growth is rapid in infancy and adolescence and relatively slow during school years.

All body systems normally continue to work in unity throughout the life span. Some physiologic characteristics such as oxygen concentration in the blood remain fairly stable throughout life. Others such as body temperature undergo minor changes, depending on age, hormonal balance, or time of day. Some characteristics change markedly during the life cycle such as pulse rate and fluid intake that are affected by changes in body surface, organ size, or maturity (102). Age-related changes occur at varying chronological periods. Structural deterioration usually precedes functional decline. Some organs and systems deteriorate more rapidly than others. In late life the capacity for adaptation changes and finally decreases. Before death, decline or deterioration usually affects most structural and many functional centers in the aged person (83).

The study of growth and development processes must focus on the complete continuum of the life cycle—from conception through death—to acquire a comprehensive understanding of the complexity of these processes and how these principles are activated throughout the life span.

DEVELOPING PERSON: PRENATAL STAGES AND INFLUENCES

The Beginning

The cell, the basis for human life, is a complex unit. Refer to the anatomy or physiology text for review of cell structure and function. This chapter presents a brief overview of the prenatal period as the beginning of life. For in-depth study of the biologic differences of the male and female, the reproductive process, including fertilization and development of the unborn child in utero, inheritance patterns, and the processes of labor and delivery, refer to an anatomy and physiology or developmental text and to a maternity nursing text (14, 25, 42, 83, 102, 103).

All body cells have 22 pairs of rod-shaped particles, nonsex **chromosomes** (*autosomes*), and a pair of sex chromosomes. The biologic female has two X chromosomes; the biologic male has one X and one Y chromosome. Each of the chromosomes contains approximately 20,000 *segments strung out like lengthwise beads* called **genes.** The genes, apparently located according to function, are made up of deoxyribonucleic acid (DNA), which processes the information that determines the makeup and specific function of every cell in the body. The genes play a major role in determining hereditary characteristics (25, 42, 102).

According to the Jacob-Monad (53) hypothesis, there are three different types of genes. Only one type is directly responsible for growth. The other two regulate genetic activity as a result of information from the rest of the reproductive cell. These synthesizing genes do not automatically perform the processes contained in their genetic code; their function is to be sensitive to environmental conditions within the cell. Thus gene expression is affected by the prevailing cellular environment of the fetus and the uterine environment, which are active in determining the structure and organization of each fetal system (53). Variation in the human results from common factors such as cross-over of genes in a variety of combinations, mutations, unusual sexual configurations, and other abnormalities in genetic process (42, 102). Many chromosomal defects can now be diagnosed (25).

The female reproductive cycle is more regular and is easier to observe and measure than is the male reproductive cycle (23). In contrast to the normal menstrual cycle, spermatogenesis normally occurs in cycles that continuously follow one another.

Approximately 14 days after the beginning of the menstrual period fertilization may occur in the outer third of the fallopian tube. The sperm cell from a male penetrates and unites with an **ovum** (*egg*) from a female to form a *single-cell* **zygote.** The sperm and ovum, known as **gametes** (*sex cells in half cells*), are produced in the reproductive system through **meiosis,** a *specialized process of cell division and chromosome reduction* (25, 42).

A newborn girl has approximately 400,000 immature ova in her ovaries; each is in a **follicle,** or *small sac.* **Ovulation,** *the expelling of an ovum from a mature follicle in one of the ovaries,* occurs approximately once every 28 days in a sexually mature female (42).

Spermatozoa, much smaller and more active than the ovum, are produced in the testes of the mature male at the rate of several hundred million a day and are ejaculated in his semen at *sexual climax* (**orgasm**). For fertilization to occur, at least 20 million sperm cells must enter a woman's body at one time. They enter the vagina and try to swim through the **cervix** (*opening to the uterus*) and into the fallopian tube. Only a tiny fraction of those millions of sperm cells makes it that far. More than one may penetrate the ovum, but only one can fertilize it to create a new human. The sex of the baby is determined by the pair of sex chromosomes; the sperm may carry either an X or Y chromosome, resulting in either a girl (XX zygote) or a boy (XY zygote). Thus the man determines the sex of the baby (25, 42).

Spermatozoa maintain their ability to fertilize an egg for a span of 24 to 72 to 90 hours; ova can be fertilized for approximately 24 hours. Thus there are approximately 72 to 90 hours during each menstrual cycle when conception can take place. If fertilization does not occur, the spermatozoa and ovum die. Sperm cells are devoured by white blood cells in the woman's body; the ovum passes through the uterus and vagina in the menstrual product (25, 42).

Multiple births may occur. Twins occur in approximately one of 86 births. Occasionally two ova are released within a short time of each other; if both are fertilized, **fraternal** (*dizygotic, or two-egg*) twins will be born. Created by different eggs and different sperm cells, the twins are no more alike in their genetic makeup than other siblings. They may be of the same or different sex. If the ovum divides in two after it has been fertilized, **identical** (*monozygotic, or one-egg*) twins will be born. At birth these twins share the same placenta. They are of the same sex and have exactly the same genetic heritage; any differences they will later exhibit are due to the influences of environment, either before or after birth. Other multiple births—triples, quadruplets, and so forth—result from either one or a combination of these two processes (25, 42).

Multiple births have become more frequent in recent years as a result of the administration of certain fertility drugs that spur ovulation and often cause the release of more than one egg. The tendency to bear twins apparently is inherited and more common in some families and ethnic groups than in others. Twins have a

limited intrauterine space and are more likely to be premature and of low-birthweight. They are therefore at greater risk for survival at birth (25).

After either single or multiple fertilization the zygote travels to the uterus for implantation or imbedding in the uterine wall. Progesterone secretion has prepared the uterus for the possible reception of the fertilized ovum. The continued secretion of ovarian estrogen and progesterone develops the uterus for the 9-month nurturance of the developing embryo and fetus in pregnancy. Continued secretion of estrogen during this period increases the growth of the uterine muscles and eventually enlarges the vagina for the delivery of a child. Continued secretion of progesterone during pregnancy serves to keep the uterus from prematurely contracting and expelling the developing embryo before the proper time. In addition, progesterone prepares the breast cells in late pregnancy for future milk production (25).

Stage of Prenatal Development

Life in utero is usually divided into three stages of development: germinal, embryonic, and fetal. The **germinal stage** *lasts approximately 10 days to 2 weeks after fertilization.* It is characterized by rapid cell division and subsequent increasing complexity of the organism and its implantation in the wall of the uterus. The **embryonic stage,** *from 2 to 8 weeks,* is the time of rapid growth and differentiation of major body systems and organs. The **fetal stage** *from 8 weeks until birth,* is characterized by rapid growth and changes in body form caused by different rates of growth of different parts of the body (25, 42).

The fetus is a very small but rapidly developing human being who is influenced by the maternal and external environment and to whom the mother responds, especially when fetal movement begins. Table 6–1 summarizes some major milestones in the sequential development of the **conceptus,** the *new life that has been conceived.* However, *being precise about the exact timing* is difficult (25, 42, 103, 116).

Prenatal Influences on Development

Heredity

Genetic information is transmitted from parents of offspring through a complex series of processes. Twenty-three pairs of chromosomes in the human germ cells divide into two gametes by meiosis, giving to each of these mature germ cells (female ovum and male spermatozoon) one half the genetic material necessary for producing a new individual. The specific hereditary information is carried on the chromosomes by thousands of genes, but the expression of gene characteristic is not a preprogrammed, unchangeable process (25, 42).

Further, hereditary factors do not by themselves fully determine what the person will become. Innate characteristics and environmental forces are closely re-

TABLE 6-1. SUMMARY OF THE SEQUENCE OF PRENATAL DEVELOPMENT

Time Period After Fertilization	Developmental Event
Germinal stage	
30 hr	First division or cleavage occurs.
40 hr	Four-cell stage occurs.
60 hr	**Morula,** *a solid mass of 12 to 16 cells;* total size of mass not changed because cells decrease in size with each cleavage to allow morula to pass through lumen of fallopian tube. Ectopic pregnancy within fallopian tube occurs if morula wedged in lumen.
3 days	Zygote has divided into 32 cells; travels through fallopian tube to uterus.
4 days	Zygote contains 70 cells. Morula reaches uterus; forms a **blastocyst,** *a fluid-filled sphere.*
4½ to 6 days	Blastocyst floats in utero. **Embryonic disk,** *thickened cell mass from which baby develops,* clusters on one edge of blastocyst. Mass of cells differentiates into two layers: (1) **ectoderm,** *outer layer of cells* that become the epidermis of skin, nails, hair, tooth enamel, sensory organs, brain and spinal cord, cranial nerves, peripheral nervous system, upper pharynx, nasal passages, urethra, and mammary glands; (2) **endoderm,** *lower layer of cells* that will develop into gastrointestinal system, liver, pancreas, salivary glands, respiratory system, urinary bladder, pharynx, thyroid, tonsils, lining of urethra, and ear.
6 to 7 days	**Nidation,** *implantation of zygote* into upper portion of uterine wall, occurs.
7 to 14 days	Remainder of blastocyst develops into the following: (1) **placenta,** *a multipurpose organ connected to the embryo by the umbilical cord* that delivers oxygen and nourishment from the mother's body and absorbs the embryo's body wastes, combats internal infection, confers immunity to the unborn child, and produces the hormones that (a) support pregnancy, (b) prepare breasts for lactating, and (c) stimulate uterine contractions for delivery of the baby. Placenta circulation evidenced by 11 to 12 days. (2) **Umbilical cord,** *a structure that contains two umbilical arteries and an umbilical vein and connects embryo to placenta.* Approximately 20 inches long and 1½ in diameter. Rapid cell differentiation occurs. (3) **Amniotic sac,** *a fluid-filled membrane that encases the developing baby,* protecting it and giving it room to move.
2 to 8 wk	Period during which embryo firmly establishes uterus as home and undergoes rapid cellular differentiation, growth, and development of body systems. This is a **critical period** *when embryo is most vulnerable to deleterious prenatal influences.* All developmental birth defects occur during **first trimester** *(3 months)* of pregnancy. If embryo is unable to survive, a **miscarriage** or **spontaneous abortion,** *expulsion of conceptus from the uterus,* occurs.
Embryonic stage	
15 days	Cranial end of elongated disk has begun to thicken.
16 days	**Mesoderm,** *the middle layer,* appears and develops into skin dermis, tooth dentin, connective tissue, cartilage, bones, muscles, spleen, blood, gonads, uterus, and excretory and circulatory systems. Yolk sac, which arises from ectoderm, assists transfer of nutrients from mother to embryo.
19 to 20 days	Neural fold and neural groove develop. Thyroid begins to develop.
21 days	Neural tube forms, becomes spinal cord and brain.
22 days	Heart, the first organ to function, initiates action. Eyes, ears, nose, cheeks, and upper jaw begin to form. Cleft palate may occur if defective development.
26 to 27 days	Cephalic portion (brain) of nervous system formed. Leg and arm buds appear. Stubby tail of spinal cord appears.
28 days	Crown to rump length, 4 to 5 mm.
30 days	Rudimentary body parts formed. Limb buds appear. Cardiovascular system functioning. Heartbeat 65 times per minute; blood flow through tiny arteries and veins. Lens vesicles, optic cups, and nasal pits forming. By end of first month, new life has grown more quickly than it will at any other time in life. Swelling in head where eyes, ears, mouth, and nose will be. Crown to rump length, 7 to 14 mm ($\frac{1}{4}$ to $\frac{1}{2}$ inches).
31 days	Eye and nasal pit developing. Primitive mouth present.
32 days	Paddle-shaped hands. Lens vesicles and optic cups formed.
34 days	Head is much larger relative to trunk. Digital rays present in hands. Feet are paddle shaped. Crown to rump length, 11 to 14 mm.
35 to 38 days	Olfactory pit, eye, maxillary process, oral cavity and mandibular process developing. Brain has divided into three parts. Limbs growing. Beginning of all major external and internal structures. Crown to rump length, 15 to 16 mm.
40 days	Elbows and knees apparent. Fingers and toes distinct but webbed. Yolk sac continues to (1) provide embryologic blood cells during third through sixth weeks until liver, spleen, and bone marrow assume function; (2) provide lining cells for respiratory and digestive tracts; (3) provide cells that migrate to gonads to become primordial germ cells.
42 days	Crown to rump length, 21 to 23 mm.
50 days	All internal and external structures present. External genitalia present but sex not discernible; yolk sac disappears, incorporated into embryo; limbs, hands, feet formed. Nerve cells in brain connected.
55 to 56 days	Eye, nostril, globular process, maxilla and mandible almost completely formed. Ear beginning to develop.
8 wk	Stubby end of spinal cord disappears. Distinct human characteristics. Head accounts for half of total embryo length. Brain impulses coordinate function of organ systems. Facial parts formed, with tongue and teeth buds. Stomach produces digestive juices. Liver produces blood cells. Kidney removes uric acid from blood. Some movement by limbs. Weight, 1 g. Length, 1–1½ inches (2.5–3.75 cm).

TABLE 6-1. SUMMARY OF THE SEQUENCE OF PRENATAL DEVELOPMENT (Continued)

Time Period After Fertilization	Developmental Event
Fetal Stage	
9 to 40 wk	Remainder of intrauterine period spent in growth and refinement of body tissues and organs.
9 to 12 wk	Eyelids fused. Nail beds formed. Teeth and bones begin to appear. Ribs and vertebrae are cartilage. Kidneys function. Urinates occasionally. Some respiratory-like movements exhibited. Begins to swallow amniotic fluid. Grasp, sucking, and withdrawal reflexes present. Sucks fingers and toes in utero. Makes specialized responses to touch. Moves easily but movement not felt by mother. Reproductive organs have primitive egg or sperm cells. Gender distinguishable. Head one third of body length. Weight, 30 g (1 oz). Length, 3 to $3\frac{1}{2}$ inches at 12 wk.
13 to 16 wk	Much spontaneous movement. Sex determination possible. **Quickening,** *fetal kicking or movement,* may be felt by mother. Moro reflex present. Rapid skeletal development. Meconium present. Uterine development in female fetus. **Lanugo,** *downy hair,* appears on body. Head one fourth of total length. Weight, 120 to 150 g (4 to 6 oz). Length, 8 to 10 inches. Fetus frowns, moves lips, turns head; hands grasp, feet kick. First hair appears. Ova formed in female.
17 to 20 wk	New cells exchanged for old, especially in skin. Quickening occurs by 17 wk. Vernix caseosa appears. Eyebrows, eyelashes, and head hair appear. Sweat and sebaceous glands begin to function. Skeleton begins to harden. Grasp reflex present and strong. Permanent teeth buds appear. Fetal heart sounds can be heard with stethoscope. Weight, 360 to 450 g (12 oz to 1 lb). Length, 12 inches.
21 to 24 wk	Extrauterine life, life outside uterus, is possible but difficult because of immature respiratory system. Fetus looks like miniature baby. Mother may note jarring but rhythmic movements of infant, indicative of hiccups. Body becomes straight at times. Fingernails present. Skin has wrinkled, red appearance. Alternate periods of sleep and activity. May respond to external sounds. Weight, 720 g ($1\frac{1}{2}$ lb). Length, 14 inches.
25 to 28 wk	Jumps in utero in synchrony with loud noise. Eyes open and close with waking and sleeping cycles. Able to hear. Respiratory-like movements. Respiratory and central nervous systems sufficiently developed; some babies survive with excellent and intensive care. Assumes head-down position in uterus. Weight, 1200 g ($2\frac{1}{2}$ lb).
29 to 32 wk	Begins to store fat and minerals. Testes descend into scrotal sac in male. Reflexes fully developed. Thumb sucking present. Mother may note irregular, jerky, crying-like movements. Lanugo begins to disappear from face. Head hair continues to grow. Skin begins to lose reddish color. Can be conditioned to environmental sounds. Weight, 1362 to 2270 g (3 to 5 lb). Length, 16 inches.
33 to 36 wk	Adipose tissue continues to be deposited over entire body. Body begins to round out. May become more or less active because of space constriction. Increased iron storage by liver. Increased lung development. Lanugo begins to disappear from body. Head lengthens. Brain cells number same as at birth. Weight, 2800 g (6 lb). Length, 18 to 20 inches.
37 to 40 wk	Organ systems operating more efficiently. Heart rate increases. More wastes expelled. Lanugo and vernix caseosa disappear. Skin smooth and plump. High absorption of maternal hormones. Cerebral cortex well-defined; brain wave patterns developed. Skull and other bones becoming more firm and mineralized. Continued storage of fat and minerals. Glands produce hormones that trigger labor. Ready for birth. Weight, 3200 to 3400 g (7 to $7\frac{1}{2}$ lb). Length, 20 to 21 inches. Baby stops growing approximately 1 wk before birth.

lated. Genetic endowment in respect to any trait may be compared to a rubber band. The rubber band may remain unstretched because of environmental influences, causing potential to remain dormant. Or the rubber band may be stretched fully, causing the person to excel beyond what seems his or her potential. The person in later maturity, for example, has had many years of changing environmental influences; what he or she has become is no doubt an expression of innate genetic potential and environmental supports and the wisdom to take advantage of both.

Embryologic development and principles of genetics affecting body structure and function are complex. A number of references provide additional information (14, 25, 42, 83, 84, 102, 103, 116).

Parental Age
Age of mother and number of previous pregnancies affect the health of the fetus (66). If the woman has had three or more pregnancies before the age of 20, the baby is less likely to be healthy. Pregnancy during the teen years is more frequently associated with prematurity and infant illness (103). Risk for the infant is least when the mother is in her twenties (25, 103,). The woman who becomes pregnant after age 35 may increase her risk of delivery complications and problems in the neonate. These problems include prematurity, low-birthweight, Down Syndrome, birth defects, and fraternal twinning (25, 103). The more pregnancies the woman has had, the greater the risk to the infant. Maternal physiology cannot support many pregnancies in rapid succession, and as age increases, the ability to cope with the stresses of pregnancy decreases (25, 103).

Age of the father can also adversely affect the health of the fetus. The risk of producing offspring with anomalies linked to autosomal-dominant mutations is higher when the father is age 40 or older (40).

Prenatal Endocrine and Metabolic Functions
Fetal growth and development are dependent on maternal endocrine and metabolic adjustments during pregnancy. The placenta helps to provide necessary estro-

gens, progesterone, and gonadotropin to sustain pregnancy and trigger other endocrine adjustments that involve primarily the pituitary, adrenal cortex, and thyroid. Fetal endocrine function is regulated independently from the mother, but endocrine drugs given to the mother may produce undesirable effects on the fetus (25, 42, 103).

Animal research indicates that later sexual characteristics and behavior may be affected by administration of or presence or absence of sex hormones during fetal development. This is the first critical period for sexual differentiation. Although the fetus has a chromosomal combination denoting male or female, the fetus must be exposed to corresponding hormones during pregnancy. If the male fetus is insensitive to androgen (a masculinizing hormone) and exposed to large amounts of estrogens (a feminizing hormone), the child may possess many female characteristics (25, 103). Testicular inductor substance causes production of fetal androgens that suppress anatomic precursors of the oviducts and ovaries and, in turn, cause the male genital tract to develop during the seventh to twelfth weeks. The male embryo's testosterone offsets the maternal hormone influences. Unless androgens are present, the external genitalia of the fetus will appear female regardless of chromosomal pattern. Estrogens are released in the genetically female embryo and are necessary for the fetus to develop female genitalia. Likewise, inspection of the external genitalia of a newborn female may show abnormal fusion of the labia and enlargement of the clitoris caused by an androgen agent taken by the mother early in her pregnancy (25).

The second critical period for sexual differentiation occurs just before or after birth, when sex typing of the brain may occur. Testosterone may influence the hypothalamus so that a noncyclic pattern for release of pituitary hormones, the gonadotropins, will occur in males and a cyclic pattern of gonadotropic release will occur in females (116).

Fetal and placental growth, nourishment, waste excretion, and total function are dependent on the adequacy of the mother's blood system. Inadequate hemoglobin or red blood cells interfere with fetal function (25, 42).

Maternal hyperglycemia helps promote transfer of excessive glucose across the placenta to the fetus, stimulating fetal insulin secretion—a potent growth factor (25, 37, 48, 78, 94). The diabetic mother is at high risk. The metabolic stress of fetal hyperinsulinism apparently contributes to increased anomalies (e.g., obesity of the newborn) (25, 37, 78). Many fetal metabolic defects can now be diagnosed (25, 116); congenital heart defects are the most common (94).

Maternal Nutrition

Nutrition is one of the most important variables for fetal health and prevention of prenatal and intrapartal complications. Scientists know that at least 60 nutrients are basic to the maintenance of healthy growth and development (25, 129). Lack of these nutrients over a period of time may depress appetite, encourage disease, and retard growth and development, including causing mental retardation. If the mother's nutritional state is not adequate, the fetus is deprived of nutrients (25, 64). During the first 2 months of pregnancy, the developing embryo consists mostly of water; later more solids in the form of fat, nitrogen, and certain minerals are added. Because of the small amount of yolk in the human ovum, growth depends on nutrients obtained from the mother (25).

Caloric and *protein* intake are of particular importance. Calories are implicated in cell multiplication, and protein is believed primarily related to enlargement of these cells. Therefore failure of the cells to receive sufficient protein and calories during critical periods of growth can lead to slowing down and ultimate cessation of the ability of these cells to enlarge, divide, and develop specialized functions. Lack of protein also affects later intellectual performance. Further, sufficient calories from fats and carbohydrates are needed so that protein is not used for energy. On the other hand, an excessive intake of protein and calories may produce excessive fat storage cells that do not disappear and may contribute to later obesity (85, 103).

Caloric requirements for the pregnant woman are approximately 300 calories higher than for the nonpregnant woman, contributing to a total weight gain of approximately 25 pounds (25). If the woman has not gained at least 10 pounds by 5 months' (20 weeks') gestation, she is at risk for delivery of an ill child. Low maternal weight at conception and little weight gain during pregnancy are associated with birth of a child who is underweight for gestational age and prone to developmental hazards (129). The overweight woman jeopardizes the fetus if she tries to lose weight during pregnancy; the effects of ketoacidosis, which results from calorie limitations, have been associated with neuropsychologic defects in the infant (45, 85, 103, 129).

Protein requirements are 1.5 g/kg daily for the pregnant woman, compared to the usual 1 g/kg daily (45). Nitrogen is the key element in protein that makes it different from fat or carbohydrate (130). More protein is needed for growth and repair of the fetus, placenta, uterus, and breasts and for increased maternal blood volume (25). High-protein diets have not demonstrated improvement in birth weight and are not recommended prenatally (110, 130).

Mineral intake, especially calcium and phosphorus, follows protein as the next most essential requirement. Calcium is mostly deposited in the infant during the last month of gestation; a good supply must be stored from the early months of pregnancy to meet this demand and minimize depletion of maternal reserves (92).

The recommended intake of phosphorous, sodium, zinc, iodine via iodized salt, magnesium, potassium, and fluoride remains essentially unchanged during pregnancy. Substantial decreases of minerals can predispose the offspring to debilitating conditions; for example, profound zinc deficiency can cause dwarfism, and severe iodine deficiency can lead to endemic cretinism characterized by multiple severe neurologic defects. Most diets that supply sufficient calories for appropriate weight gain also supply adequate minerals if iodized salt is used. The only exception is iron, which should be supplemented during pregnancy because the maternal blood volume may double as a result of increases in both plasma and erythrocytes. In addition, almost one fourth of the maternal iron is transferred to the placenta and fetus. These iron requirements are more prominent during the last two trimester periods of gestation (25, 103). Supplementation with 30 to 60 mg of ferrous iron during the last 3 to 4 months of pregnancy is beneficial in building and protecting maternal reserves and preventing iron deficiency anemia, which predisposes to being underweight and to congenital defects in the newborn. Salt should not be restricted unless edema develops.

Folic acid supplementation is used to prevent fetal malformations, especially neural tube defects and maternal anemia (25, 105). Additional iodine prevents inadequate physical and mental growth (45, 85). Further information on diet for the pregnant woman, including the vegetarian, is found in Chapter 12.

An adequate intake of vitamins acquired through foods affects normal metabolism. Although supplementary vitamins may be prescribed by the physician or purchased over the counter, natural foods are the best source of vitamins (45, 85). Vitamin and mineral preparations should not be substituted for food (25). This recommendation is supported by a 1986 study of vitamin C (ascorbic acid) and health practices and mortality (33). Vitamins B_{12} and B_6 contribute to the plasma demands during pregnancy. The requirement for vitamin C increases by one third; a reasonable diet can supply this amount. Large doses of vitamin C can interfere with vitamin B_{12} absorption and metabolism (25). As a vitamin C source, orange juice should be taken in moderation because of the emetic effect related to hyperacidity.

Maternal malnutrition, which usually is related to a lifetime of inadequate nutrition in the mother, has an adverse effect on her children and grandchildren. The fetal central nervous system is the structure most damaged; impaired intelligence performance results later in life (7).

Effects of inadequate nutrition are most severe for the pregnant adolescent who herself has growth requirements and for the mother with accumulated effects of several pregnancies, especially closely spaced ones. Nutritional deficiencies of the mother during her own fetal and childhood periods contribute to structural and physiologic difficulties in supporting a fetus. Improvement of the pregnant woman's diet when she has previously been poorly nourished does not appreciably benefit the fetus. The fetus apparently draws most of its raw materials for development from maternal body structure and lifetime reserves (45, 103). You have a significant role in teaching proper nutrition to children and adolescents.

Socioeconomic level significantly affects the mother's nutritional status. Regardless of ethnic or cultural background, families who are relatively affluent tend to choose foods from the traditional food groups and eat a better balanced meal. However, studies comparing mothers with deficient and adequate diet have not compared other variables often associated with dietary deficiency such as extreme stress, poverty, and deprived socioeconomic class (77, 85, 109).

In a study on Guatemala newborns it was found that the birth weight was significantly affected by the number of supplemental calories ingested by the mother during pregnancy but not by the supplemental protein intake (85). Stein and Klein (110) also failed to find any improvement in birth weight attributed specifically to a protein-enriched supplemental diet. Length of gestation was increased, with a corresponding increase in birth weight of infants born to mothers who were placed on a balanced protein-calorie supplementation; the same results were not found in the high-protein-only supplementation. In fact, some mild short-term psychologic adverse affects occurred in the latter group (99). The implications of these results are uncertain; further studies are needed.

In a Canadian study in which dietary needs for calories and protein were individually calculated for each woman based on body weight for height, with adjustments for protein deficiency and being underweight, the quality of maternal diets significantly improved and the incidence of low-birth-weight infants, stillbirths, neonatal mortality, and perinatal mortality were drastically reduced (129). Refer to Appendices I and II at the end of the book for the recommended daily allowances and major sources and functions of nutrients.

Anemia. The effects of maternal anemia on the fetus are less clear than those on the mother. **Anemia** *denotes a decrease in the oxygen-carrying capability of the blood,* which is directly related to a reduction in hemoglobin concentration. Anemia, regardless of its cause, has been associated with spontaneous abortion, prematurity, low-birth-weight, and fetal death—even in mild cases (hemoglobin level, 8 to 11 g) (25). A direct relationship between anemia and fetal distress has not been established unless the anemia of the mother is severe (hemoglobin less than 6 g).

The common association of anemia and inadequate maternal nutritional intake with lower educational levels and socioeconomic background is prominent in the literature (103, 129).

Iron Deficiency Anemia (IDA) accounts for 75% of all the anemias diagnosed during pregnancy (85). The iron requirements of pregnancy are considerable—close to 800 mg, of which 300 mg go to the fetus and placenta and 500 mg are used to expand the maternal hemoglobin mass (45). IDA (as well as underweight and congenital defects) develops unless adequate replacement of these and other natural maternal iron losses occur. The developing fetus may not suffer severe ill effects of the mother's decreased iron supply if its own hemoglobin production is maintained at a normal level (i.e., if the placental source of iron is of sufficient amounts for the fetus to establish and maintain normal hemoglobin levels) (25).

Sickle cell anemia in the mother, associated with sickle cell disease seen predominantly in the African-American population, may show a number of negative effects on the developing fetus. Changes in the mother's pathophysiologic state may lead to intrauterine growth retardation, premature labor, a reduction of 250 to 500 g in average birth weight, and even stillbirth related to the "sickling" or clumping of malshaped erythrocytes within the placental vascular system (25, 45, 103).

Pica. **Pica** is *eating nonfood substances* such as clay, unprocessed flour, cornstarch, coal, soap, toothpaste, mothballs, petrol, tar, paraffin, wood, plaster, soil, chalk, charcoal, cinders, baking powder, baking soda, powdered bricks, and refrigerator frost scrapes. Pica is common in children and women of all cultures who are hungry, poor, malnourished, and desire something to chew (103). Sometimes secrecy or superstitious beliefs accompany this habit. Some people such as African-Americans in the southern part of the United States and their descendants believe that eating red and white clay overcomes the chances of disfigured offspring. Pica is usually associated with iron deficiency; whether anemia is the cause or the effect is unknown. Certainly pica interferes with normal nutrition by reducing appetite (45, 103).

Environmental Hazards to the Fetus: Teratogenic Effects

Teratogens. A **teratogen** is an *agent that interrupts normal development and causes malformation.* **Teratogenesis** means *development of abnormal structures.*

Prominent environmental factors that have the potential of damaging the fetus include radiation, some food additives, various pollutants, chemical interactions, nicotine from smoking tobacco, pica, drugs, alcohol, maternal and paternal infections, and maternal stress. The timing of fetal contact with a specific teratogen is a crucial factor (Figs. 6–1 and 6–2). Susceptibility to teratogens, in general, decreases as organ formation advances (25). For instance, a teratogen introduced into the system of an embryo between 3 and 8 weeks of gestation when principal body systems are being established is likely to do much more harm than if it came in contact with the same conceptus during the third or eighth months. During the implantation period when the fertil-ized ovum lies free within the uterus and uses uterine secretions as its nutrition source, teratogens can kill the embryo (25, 42, 83, 93, 116). Even during the third trimester fetal cerebral vascular reaction to certain teratogens can be detrimental (18–20, 25).

There is no evidence that congenital malformations will always be produced when a teratogen is present, for the embryo has the inherent capacity to replace damaged cells with newly formed cells. Once implantation has occurred (7 or 8 days after fertilization), the embryo undergoes very rapid and important transformations for the next 4 weeks. The sequence of embryonic events shows that each organ (brain, heart, eye, limbs, and genitalia) undergoes a critical stage of differentiation at precise times. During these individual critical periods the embryo is highly vulnerable to teratogens, producing specific gross malformations. Each teratogen acts on a selected aspect of cellular metabolism (25).

In many malformations, a genetic predisposition combined with a teratogen is required to produce an abnormality (25). A substance can have adverse effects on the central nervous system but not on normal development of limbs. A teratogen may cause a variety of gross anomalies; a few show a preferential action on specific organs. For example, thalidomide anomalies are characterized by skeletal malformation; no other form of growth retardation is noted (25, 103, 116).

A complicated interplay exists among the father, mother, offspring, and teratogen. In addition to the critical period or developmental stage and genetic susceptibility, the degree to which a teratogen causes abnormalities depends on its dosage, absorption, distribution, metabolism, the physical state of the mother, and excretion by the separate body systems of mother and fetus. A teratogen that enters a mother's system also enters the system of her developing child, meaning that the so-called *placental barrier is practically nonexistent* (83, 103).

External Environmental Factors. Prenatally environmental factors such as high level of noise, radiation from multiple sources at work or from chest x-ray studies and pelvimetry, ultraviolet rays from the sun or sunlamp, and pollution of air, water, and food are increasingly shown as important for the newborn. Depending on dosage, radiation can be responsible for cell destruction that is linked to embryonic death, gross malformations, growth retardation, and an increased risk of malignancy in later life. Most of the commonly used diagnostic procedures cause only low level fetal x-ray exposure. If carefully performed and accurately interpreted, fetal ultrasonography can be used at no significant risk to the developing fetus (9, 25). Recent occupational research by Schorr et al. (100) shows no relationship between exposure to electromagnetic fields in video display terminals and an increased risk of spontaneous abortion via embryonic death. Certain trace metals and normal exposure to radi-

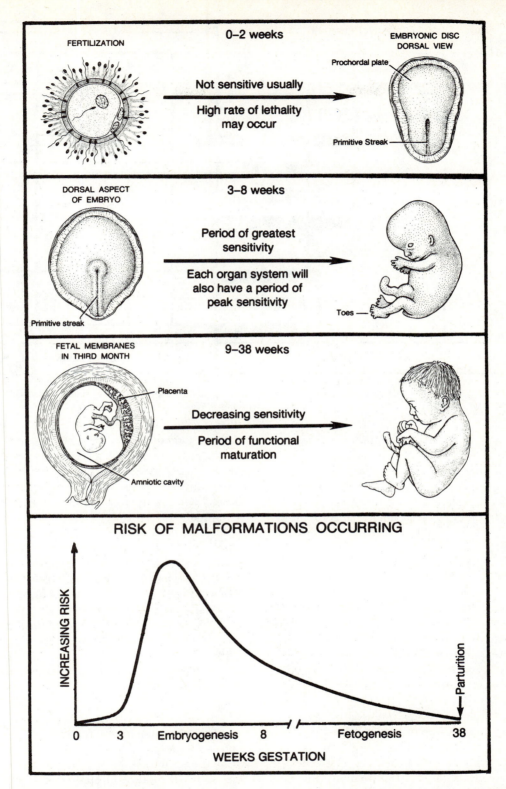

Figure 6-1. Periods of susceptibility to teratogens. (From Sadler, T.W., *Langman's Medical Embryology* [5th ed.]. Baltimore: Williams & Wilkins, 1985.)

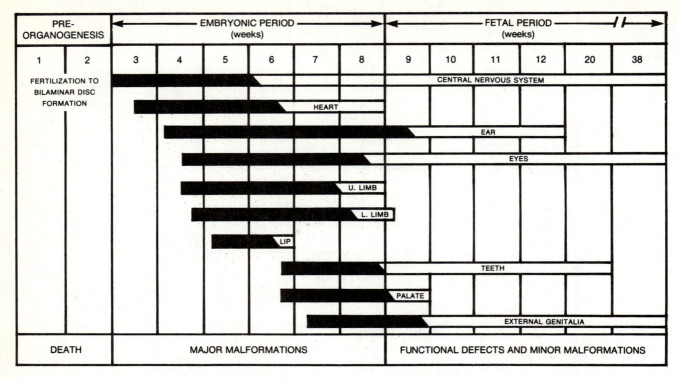

Figure 6-2.   Susceptibility of organ systems to teratogens. Solid bars denote highly sensitive periods. (From Sadler, T.W., *Langman's Medical Embryology* [5th ed.]. Baltimore: Williams & Wilkins, 1985.)

ation produce teratogenic effects, although they may be undetectable (25, 111, 116).

Occupational hazards include transfer of drugs and chemicals from the male to the female during intercourse—an action that later can negatively affect fertilization or implantation or, if the woman is already pregnant, can have teratogenic effects on the developing person. For example, decreased sperm count and infertility are related to paternal exposure to Diabromochloropapane (DBCP). Paternal exposure to toxic agents is most likely to result in male infertility or spontaneous abortions. Anesthetic gases, vinyl chloride exposure, chloroprene, or other hydrocarbons have all been connected to spontaneous abortions. Lead present in the environment directly increases sperm abnormalities, induces male infertility, and facilitates spontaneous abortion through either affected sperm or indirect contamination (22, 111).

Agent Orange, named for the orange strip wrapped around 11 million gallons shipped and sprayed in Vietnam, is composed of 2,4,5-T and other chemicals, including dioxin. Dioxin, a widely publicized, highly toxic substance is believed responsible for the many adverse effects of exposure to Agent Orange experienced by Vietnam veterans such as chloracne, latent extreme fatigue, liver damage, and joint pain in back, hips and fingers, plus increases in spontaneous abortions and congenital malformations—spina bifida, cleft lip, and neoplasms. A major study commissioned by the U.S. government was conducted to explain the linkage

of Agent Orange to reproductive problems encountered by veterans and the presence of abnormalities in their offspring (22, 87, 111, 118). However, no conclusive research investigations support a causal role between these chemicals and fetal anomalies. Continued research is warranted.

Smoking Tobacco. Smoking is associated with decreased maternal pulmonary function and with an increased incidence of abnormal bleeding during pregnancy (25, 110). Adverse effects of maternal smoking on the fetus extend to the categories of both morbidity and mortality (25, 43, 60, 120), including the risk of childhood cancer (54, 113). Although many of the hazards of smoking are well publicized, such as a higher percentage of stillbirths, spontaneous abortions and premature deliveries, it is estimated that nearly half the women who seek prenatal care classify themselves as "smokers" (25).

The prevalence of smoking has decreased more among Caucasian than African-American pregnant women and among those who are at least 20 years of age and are more educated. Unmarried mothers are much more likely to smoke than their counterparts. Smoking is perceived as a threat to normal growth and development patterns; one third of pregnant women can quit smoking during pregnancy, with another one third cutting down (64). Women who quit smoking during pregnancy are likely to resume the habit after delivery (60).

Low birth weight (less than 5½ pounds or 2.5 kg) increases as the number of cigarettes smoked daily increases. Nicotine, along with many other components of cigarette smoke such as cotinine, passes through the placenta and directly affects the fetus. Although it affects many systems of the developing person, the primary target is the cardiovascular system (103). Nicotine transferred to the fetus by the mother's smoking of one cigarette is enough to lower the pH and oxygen tension in its blood and decrease fetal oxygen (60). Furthermore, the carbon monoxide that crosses the placenta attacks the fetal hemoglobin, reducing the oxygen tension at the capillary level, which then induces hypoxia in the fetus (60).

Carbon monoxide is believed responsible for many cases of growth retardation later observed in offspring of smoking mothers (60, 103). Additionally, slight retardation in learning skills—reading and mathematics specifically—has been identified by researchers who conducted an extensive study on several thousand children between 7 and 11 years whose mothers had smoked during pregnancy (60).

Additionally, infants of smoking mothers may be more likely to develop Sudden Infant Death Syndrome (SIDS) and do have significantly more hospital admissions with the diagnosis of bronchitis or pneumonia in comparison to infants of nonsmoking mothers (43). Children of heavy smokers (10 or more cigarettes per day) have poorer physical and social development than offspring of light smokers or nonsmokers (38, 60). Deficiencies can be identified as early as age 3 years (38, 60).

The adverse effects of passive smoking present a new area of research. A 1991 Swedish study suggests that tobacco smoking exposure may be linked to preterm births (less than 37 weeks) but not to low birthweight (less than 2500 g) among full-term live births (1).

Based on the abundance of evidence pointing to the damaging effects of smoking to both mother and fetus, total avoidance of smoking during pregnancy is a primary objective of the National Cancer Institute and is a major medical recommendation (25, 127). Smoking cessation programs range from self-help to structured interventions. Maternal cigarette smoking and heavy caffeine use, both during and after pregnancy, are linked to increased rates of infantile apnea (120). For males, cigarette advertisements continue to link smoking with virility. However a growing body of research links smoking with reduced sperm count. Large doses of marijuana smoke produce the same effect (22).

Drug Hazards to the Fetus: Teratogenic Effects

The Food and Drug Administration (FDA) divides drugs into five categories that indicate a safety factor of maternal use during pregnancy. The question raised is: Do fetal risks outweigh benefits gained through use of a drug?

A drug that has a teratogenic effect in animals does not necessarily have the same effect in humans and vice versa. For instance, thalidomide caused very few malformations in animals but causes many in humans (25).

Drugs That Cross the Placenta. Many drugs cross the placenta to the fetus from the mother's blood. The placenta acts like a sieve, not a barrier. Thus no drug, whether obtained by prescription or over the counter, should be taken during pregnancy unless it is medically prescribed as necessary for the mother (25). Cunningham, MacDonald, and Gant (25) stress two basic points: (1) with rare exception, any drug that exerts a systemic effect in the mother will cross the placenta to reach the embryo or fetus, and (2) if an essential drug is administered during pregnancy, the advantages to be gained must clearly outweigh any risks inherent in its use. Physicians prescribe fewer drugs to pregnant women now than in the past; a drug is prescribed only if withholding it would cause a more serious consequence for the mother than its adverse effects on the fetus.

Aspirin (acetylsalicylic acid) and propoxyphene hydrochloride (Darvon) cross the placenta and should be avoided. Medications containing salicylates, including in combination with caffeine and phenacetin, are associated with an increased incidence of anemia, hemorrhage, prolonged gestation, perinatal mortality, and low-birthweight (91, 116). However, new research indicates that aspirin in low doses (60 mg/day) favorably influences the course of pregnancy for pregnancy-induced hypertension without exposing the fetus or newborn to hemorrhagic risks. Nonsteroidal anti-inflammatory drugs such as those containing ibuprofen may produce teratogenic effects during the last trimester (5).

Some antibiotics are teratogenic and should be given cautiously during pregnancy (91). Some women are plagued by urinary tract and other rather common types of bacterial infection during gestation. The question of safety of the embryo and fetus is raised when medications are prescribed to alleviate these medical problems. Penicillin has been used extensively during pregnancy and apparently is harmless to the embryo and fetus (8, 25, 93, 116). *Sulfonamides* are relatively safe but should be avoided during the last few weeks of pregnancy because of risk of neonatal hyperbilirubinemia. On the other hand, tetracycline therapy causes minor tooth defects, discoloration of the deciduous teeth, and distortion of bone growth (25). Streptomycin and other aminoglycosides are also excluded as drugs of choice because their use can result in deafness (25). Information pertaining to placental transmission of antimicrobial agents remains incomplete, although it is known that the period of maximum teratogenicity lasts until the ninth week of gestation (25).

Parental use of antiepileptic agents, particularly phenytoin and carbamazepine, increases the incidence of infant spina bifida, craniofacial defects, fingernail hypoplasia, and developmental delays (49). Some of the undesirable effects may be due to the epilepsy itself (27, 49). In the male, lowered sexual potency, decreased fertility, and sperm with decreased motility and abnormal structural changes have been identified (22).

Most cytotoxic drugs used in the treatment of maternal cancer are known to cross the placenta, as do many of the other drugs discussed here. These agents may cause abortion or fetal anomalies if taken during the first trimester. However, no ill effects on the fetus have been reported in cases in which the drugs were administered to the mother during the remainder of the pregnancy (25). Furthermore, the circulating cancerous cells of the mother appear not to invade or harm the developing embryo and fetus. The study of cytotoxic drugs and their potential effects on mother and infant continues.

Occupational hazards associated with pregnant nurses exposed to antineoplastic drugs during the first trimester include a significant increase in fetal loss (66). In the male research indicates that some cancer chemotherapy agents damage the sperm; sperm banking before therapy or perhaps artificial insemination of mates is an available option.

Hormones may also have a deleterious effect on the fetus. Taking sex hormones or oral contraceptives either just before or during pregnancy may harm the developing fetus (25, 91). Spontaneous abortion and cardiovascular defects in the newborn have been reported. A delayed consequence has been observed in adolescents or young women who develop vaginal or cervical cancer, which may be fatal. Adolescent and young adult female offspring of women who received diethylstilbestrol (DES) during the first trimester of pregnancy to prevent miscarriage are more likely to develop such cancers or show changes in vaginal tissue or vaginal and cervical structures. Daughters of women who were administered DES in the 1950s should have regular pelvic examinations. Sons of women who received DES may experience sterility and testicular abnormalities and cancer. Corticosteroids (e.g., prednisone) are other hormones that pass through the placenta barrier and may cause adverse effects to the fetus (25, 103, 111).

The diabetic mother should take the hormone insulin; oral antidiabetic drugs are not recommended because of the risk of neonatal jaundice and hypoglycemia (25). Large-for-gestational-age infants are generally born to women with insulin-dependent diabetes mellitus because of the influence of this growth factor on the fetus (25, 124).

Drug Abuse and Addiction. During pregnancy drug abuse and addiction continue to manifest themselves as major psychosocial and physical problems for both mother and child. Before 1968 only a few published reports documented this complication of pregnancy. Now substances commonly abused during pregnancy, taken individually or in combination, are known to have multiple effects on the developing person, on the outcome of pregnancy, and on neonatal neurobehavior (103). Infants exposed to addictive drugs in utero throughout pregnancy are at great risk for a higher rate of congenital malformations, obstetric complications, and perinatal mortality (22, 23, 25, 93, 111).

Effects of drug use on the fetus, neonate, and child depend on the type of drug ingested, dose, duration of drug use before and during pregnancy, and the state of maternal nutrition. There are fewer infant symptoms when the pregnant woman stops drug use in the first trimester of pregnancy than if drug use continues. Thus it is imperative to prevent drug use and to support the mother's efforts to stop drug use and to encourage adequate prenatal care and nutrition (132).

These drugs include amphetamines, barbiturates, cocaine (includes "crack" and "ice," potent and purified versions), ethchlorvynol (Placidyl), heroin, meperidine hydrochloride (Demerol), methadone, morphine, pentazocine hydrochloride (Talwin), propoxyphene hydrochloride, phencyclidine, known as "angel dust" (PCP), tetrahydrocannabinos (THC) or marijuana, and methamphetamine (25, 67, 91). Drugs that act on the central nervous system are often lipophilic and of relatively low-molecular weight characteristics, which facilitate crossing the so-called placental-fetal blood-brain barrier (25). Some drugs can be metabolized by the fetal liver and placenta; however these metabolites are water soluble (25). These drugs may interfere with blood flow to the placenta. A high incidence of maternal nutritional deficiency, anemia, and small pregnancy weight gain is also associated with drug use (45, 103).

Clinical assessment for substance abuse should include an evaluation of physical appearance, a nursing history, and a substance abuse interview. The client's demeanor, neatness, cleanliness, and affect may give subtle or overt clues. Urine samples of mothers are effective to screen for ingestion of illicit drugs; alcohol breath tests are appropriate to check maternal alcohol levels at periodic intervals. Interventions should address the habits of pregnant women comprehensively rather than focus on use of any one substance (131).

Low-birth-weight, short gestation, small size for gestational age, and major malformations occur more often among offspring of marijuana users (67). Numerous adverse effects of maternal drug addiction are reported in the literature, including prematurity, low birthweight and accelerated weight loss in the newborn period, depressed Apgar scores at birth, chromosomal abnormalities, and neuromotor abnormalities (18–20, 103, 132).

Addictive drugs such as heroin, codeine, and morphine in the mother's blood are related to a high incidence of obstetric complications: hypertension, toxemia, abruptio placenta, intrauterine growth retardation, spontaneous abortion, stillbirth, premature and breech delivery, and postpartum hemorrhage (resulting in part from poor prenatal care). Of the three drugs, cocaine in its various forms is the most devastating (18–20, 110, 132). Using urine samples to verify drug habits reveals maternal use of cocaine results in a greater reduction in fetal birthweight and body length, in addition to a smaller head circumference, than does marijuana (90, 132).

Chasnoff and associates (18–20) explain that cocaine acts peripherally to inhibit nerve conduction and prevent norepinephrine uptake at the nerve terminals, producing increased norepinephrine levels with subsequent vasoconstriction and a concomitant abrupt rise in blood pressure. Fetal cocaine exposure is linked to lowered birthweight, shorter gestation, smaller head circumference, and a higher incidence of cardiopulmonary pattern abnormalities (18, 75, 90).

Placental vasoconstriction also occurs, decreasing blood flow to the fetus with an increase in uterine contractibility. In the neonate tachycardia and hypertension are clearly associated with cerebrovascular hemorrhage. Computed tomographic (CT) scan of the neonate may confirm the presence of acute focal cerebral infarction.

A generation of children who were exposed to cocaine in the fetal state has an abnormally high incidence of "severe" physical and emotional problems. These children have a higher incidence of the following:

1. Learning difficulties
2. Impaired orientation
3. Growth retardation
4. Severe impairments in motor movements including simple movements like eating and dressing
5. Irritability
6. Tremors
7. Sensitivity to sounds
8. Various personality-social difficulties

Many of these children have been born to middle class and wealthy parents, a group increasingly using cocaine (18–20, 114).

The Brazelton Neonatal Behavioral Assessment Scale is recommended to evaluate normality of responses to environmental stimuli (103). Finnegan's Neonatal Narcotic Abstinence Syndrome (NAS) is useful for assessing neonatal withdrawal (114). The specific pattern of symptoms is dependent on (1) the type, amount, and combination of drugs used by the mother, (2) the length of time between drug exposure and delivery, and (3) the fetal ability to metabolize the drug. Box 6–1 presents the symptoms and signs that are typically observed in the neonate who has been addicted during pregnancy to cocaine, heroin, or another narcotic (18–20, 114, 132). Newborns may require up to 40 days of treatment during the withdrawal phase (20). The limited ability of the newborn to metabolize and eliminate these fat-soluble drugs may be responsible for postponement of withdrawal symptoms for 2 to 4 weeks in some infants (132).

The child of a cocaine-addicted mother is likely to demonstrate permanent physical and mental damage as a result of fetal anoxia and/or fetal or neonatal strokes (cerebrovascular hemorrhages) (20, 114). Long-term effects in the child of the cocaine or heroin-addicted

---

■ BOX 6-1.
Neonatal Narcotic Abstinence Syndrome: Manifestations of Narcotic Withdrawal

Central Nervous System (signs appear within first 24 hours)

- Hyperirritability
- Hyperactivity—hard to hold; failure to mold to mother's body
- Restlessness
- Incessant shrill cry
- Inability to sleep, disturbed rapid eye movements (REM) sleep
- Hypertonia of muscles
- Hyperactive reflexes
- Stretching
- Tremors
- Poor temperature regulation; fever
- Possible generalized convulsions

Respiratory System

- Rapid irregular breathing
- Yawning
- Sneezing
- Nasal stuffiness, congestion
- Excessive secretions
- Intermittent cyanosis
- Respiratory alkalosis
- Periods of apnea

Cardiovascular System

- Tachycardia

Gastrointestinal System

- Frantic sucking of hands; disorganized sucking behavior
- Difficulty sucking and feeding; poor closure of lips around nipple
- Appearance of being very hungry
- Sensitive gag reflex
- Regurgitation
- Vomiting
- Diarrhea
- Progressive weight loss

Skin

- Pallor
- Sweating
- Excoriation

Musculoskeletal System

- Small head size
- Short length

---

mother include the following characteristics: lower weight and shorter height than normal for age, smaller head circumference, and lower scores on perceptual and learning tests (114, 132).

Intrauterine growth retardation—an actual reduction in the number of cells in organs of the passively addicted fetus—probably is caused by the nutritional deficiencies associated with the maternal drug life-style (103). Observed chromosomal damage related to low Apgar readings requires more research. Neuromotor anomalies consist of decreased visual orientation: irregular sleep patterns—disorganized rapid eye movement (REM) periods and absence of "quiet sleep"; nonnutritive sucking; hyperactivity and impaired attention span; and a disturbed motor development with varying patterns (114). The decreased ability to orient to auditory and visual stimuli can have extensive effects on later character development and learning behaviors (103). Disrupted REM sleep patterns also directly affect the child's personality development (114).

Withdrawing the addicted woman before delivery causes the fetus to experience withdrawal distress caused by visceral vasoconstriction affecting circulation to the uterus. Intrauterine death may occur. The infant is born with drug addiction and experiences withdrawal symptoms in 2 to 4 days.

Fetal, maternal, paternal, and environmental factors all interact to produce neonatal withdrawal syndrome, which is actually a diverse collection of signs and symptoms demonstrated in the newborn (9, 114).

Mood Altering or Psychotropic Drugs. With the exception of phenothiazines used for major psychiatric conditions, these drugs, administered before and during pregnancy, should be avoided when possible because of their reported untoward effects on the developing person (9, 25). Such drugs ingested by the mother before conception or between conception and implantation are known to produce chromosomal anomalies in the embryo (9, 25). Minor tranquilizers and antidepressants can produce damaging effects, depending on the critical period of fetal development when the drug is circulated within the mother's system. For instance, thalidomide shows its teratogenic effects when ingested between days 28 and 42 of pregnancy (9). If psychotropic drugs are taken late in pregnancy, the neonate is likely to suffer drug toxicity, hypothermia, respiratory depression, hypotonia, convulsions, and withdrawal symptoms (25). Newborns of mothers who had taken lithium have been described as hypotonic, listless, and floppy (25). For treatment of stress-related illnesses in males, cimetidine (Tagamet) and sulfasalazine (Azulfidine) may temporarily suppress sperm production up to nearly 50% (22, 23).

Drug abuse in the father may also act as a teratogen. For example, marijuana abuse may cause chromosomal breaks in the father and contribute to fetal risk (112). Animal studies indicate that morphine-dependent and methadone-dependent males father offspring having decreased birth weight, increased stillbirth rates, and increased neonatal mortality rates (22).

Alcohol. Alcohol ingested before or during pregnancy serves as another common cause of abnormal changes in the fetus (21, 59, 70, 76, 110). Alcoholic beverages should be avoided; drinking as little as 3 ounces of liquor daily increases the chances of congenital defects (70), low-birth-weight, preterm delivery, stillbirth, abruptio placenta, or spontaneous abortion (110). In a study of 11,698 Danish women, alcohol consumption of 120 g/week or more was associated with a five times greater reduction in average birth weight in babies of smokers versus babies of nonsmokers. Alcoholism in the father may inhibit spermatogenesis and also act as a teratogen that contributes to chromosomal breaks or damaged genes, resulting in spontaneous abortion or birth defects. It is common for alcoholic men and women to marry, with each contributing to the development of Fetal Alcohol Syndrome (discussed below) to some degree (111). Even abstinence during the gestation period seems to be "too little too late" for infants born to mothers who have had a history of heavy alcoholic intake before conception (70). The affected newborn may suffer many of the signs and symptoms described in Neonatal Narcotic Abstinence Syndrome caused by maternal drug-related consumption. The term in this case is *Fetal Alcohol Syndrome (FAS)*. FAS, which results from excessive maternal ingestion of alcohol causes the following characteristics (21, 25, 55, 70, 71, 76, 110, 116):

1. Low-birth-weight
2. Small head
3. Flat facial profile or deformity
4. Ear and eye abnormalities
5. Poor motor coordination
6. Disturbed sleep patterns
7. Extra digits
8. Heart defects

Research conducted by Jones and Smith (55) indicates that perinatal mortality is abnormally high, impaired fine and gross motor development is continued as the surviving child matures, and the incidence of mental retardation is abnormally high when evaluated at age 7. Isouh et al. (52) add that the younger the mother at the onset of alcoholism, the higher is the incidence of speech and language problems in the offspring. These children who suffer the effects of maternal alcoholic intake via FAS are more prone than the average child to acquiring both classifications of bacterial infections—minor and life threatening (103). Lesser defects may occur in the offspring (10% risk of FAS) when the mother engages in moderate social drinking or when the woman drinks an average of 1 to 2 ounces of absolute alcohol daily in the months before pregnancy. Heavy paternal drinking may also be a factor in FAS (22, 76, 102). Growth is retarded throughout childhood, and mental and motor capabilities appear limited for life. FAS may rank second only to German measles as a cause of congenital disorders (70). New research suggests that continued, regular use of alcohol by the mother who breast-feeds can further impede motor development of the infant (71).

Effects of Folklore

Folklore can be defined as *strong beliefs about certain facets of or influences on basic aspects of life*. Most cultures, especially those that adhere less to scientific thinking, define certain desirable or forbidden activities for the pregnant woman. These superstitions, however, are often believed, feared, or unconsciously practiced even by well-educated or professional people, although they might not confess that they believe in them. The commonly experienced fear of giving birth to an abnormal infant causes the pregnant woman, or even the father-to-be, to act in ways that would otherwise be rejected or opposed. The more tightly the woman is bound by her culture, the more she follows the rules or taboos surrounding food, hygiene, activity, and contacts with other people. Many cultures emphasize that the woman should look at pleasant sights, think positive thoughts, eat certain foods, and pursue certain leisure activities to ensure a healthy, happy, talented child. Cultures usually emphasize that unhappy thoughts, aggressive actions, certain foods, unpleasant sights, or unusual or strenuous activity should be avoided to prevent bearing a sick, deformed, or dead baby. Often folklore practices do not interfere with scientific practices; therefore you should not ridicule or try to convince the mother to drop these practices since the resulting conflict she feels internally or from her culture may have adverse health effects. Further, folklore often evolves so that the pregnant woman is protected from hazards or given extra care that, in turn, meets her needs emotionally and physically.

Various references are available to give you further information about specific folklore that affects prenatal care (45, 103).

Maternal Infections: Hazardous Influence on the Fetus

The pregnant woman is more susceptible to infections. The placenta cannot screen out all infectious organisms; therefore infectious diseases in the vaginal region can travel up to the amniotic sac and penetrate its walls and infect the amniotic fluid. Diseases that have a mild effect on the mother may have a profound effect on the fetus, depending on gestational age (25).

Acquired Immune Deficiency Syndrome (**AIDS**) is transmitted from mother to fetus at some point near the actual birthing process; the exact mode of transmission is not clearly understood. In 1991 the majority of the 2500 cases of pediatric AIDS patients (less than age 5 years) acquired the infection directly from their mothers (81, 128). New research suggests that the fetal central nervous system can be infected in utero with neurodevelopmental deficiencies detected during infancy (73). Women who are infected with the human immunodeficiency virus (HIV) and women who are at risk for infection (intravenous [IV] drug users, Haitian-born, partners of IV drug users, partner of bisexual man) place the unborn fetus in serious jeopardy (89). The incuba-

tion period can range from 2 months to 5 years. To protect the health care provider, the Centers for Disease Control (CDC) emphasize the consistent use of blood and body fluid precautions for all patients (17).

The majority of AIDS cases in the pediatric age range (up to 13 years) result from acquiring HIV perinatally from infected mothers. Transmission of the virus through breast milk has also been reported. Other modes include transfusion, either prenatally or postnatally. Records indicate that the earliest year of birth for children with perinatally acquired AIDS was 1977; the earliest transfusion of blood known to have infected a child with HIV was 1978 (97).

Except for Kaposi's sarcoma, clinical manifestations of AIDS in newborns are different than those observed in adults. Newborns of HIV-seropositive mothers show no difference in birth weight, gestational age, head circumference, or Apgar score when compared to those born to seronegative mothers (81). These differences make the task of identifying and managing infected offspring just that more difficult. Conditions such as failure to thrive, *Candida* infections, generalized lymphadenopathy, brain involvement, diarrhea, and bacterial infections (bacteremia, pneumonia, otitis media) persist over time in AIDS-infected infants. Diagnosis of AIDS may take several months and includes intensive blood analysis with particular attention to significant changes in T-lymphocyte activity. Prognosis for infants of less than 1 year is bleak (101, 110). Some children have survived longer than expected with gamma globulin therapy, but AIDS-induced brain damage is ever a threat, along with devastation of other body systems (50, 82).

If the child-bearing-age women at high risk for HIV would stop bearing children, AIDS in children could be eliminated. It was predicted that 10,000 to 20,000 children under age 13 would be infected by 1991. Actually, only a little over 2000 cases were reported by 1990 in the United States (35, 50).

Adolescent AIDS cases are steadily rising, prompting CDC investigators to say that prevention efforts must go beyond providing information and must help adolescents develop motivation, attitudes, and skills to avoid behaviors that place them at risk for HIV infection (35, 50, 82). Information about HIV and AIDS is rapidly changing with new research. The journal *AIDS* is one source for current information.

Rubella (German measles) is another example of maternal infection that may occur during the first trimester with harmful effects. Rubella may go unnoticed by the mother, but it can cause fetal growth retardation and serious congenital anomalies in the eyes and ears, heart, or brain—and death. Approximately 1 in 600 children is born with congenital rubella (103, 121).

To minimize or prevent clinical features of the disease, large doses of gamma globulin are generally administered to nonimmunized pregnant women who have been exposed to rubella. Immunization of all female children before puberty can effectively retard the spread of rubella. The vaccine should never be administered to pregnant women; the rubella vaccine virus will cross the placenta just as the wild (community-acquired) rubella virus (25). The rubella vaccine is actually a live-virus vaccine containing a strain of rubella virus that has been somewhat altered. Therefore women who (1) are at risk, (2) are not aware of being pregnant, and (3) agree to prevent conception for a 3-month period should be vaccinated according to the U.S. Public Health Service Advisory Committee on Immunization Practices (121).

Small-for-date births are a fetal complication of maternal rubella. The fetus suffers an abnormal decrease in the absolute number of cells in most organs because of the viral interference with cell multiplication. The virus also causes adverse changes in the small blood vessels of the developing fetus and does profuse damage to the placental vascular system as well, thus interfering with the fetus' blood flow and oxygenation (25, 103).

Rubeola ("long measles") is also associated with congenital defects. Viruses causing mumps, smallpox, scarlet fever, and viral hepatitis may be related to formation of anomalies in utero, and during the last month of pregnancy they may cause a life-threatening fetal infection (8, 25).

Maternal syphilis causes severe adverse effects such as congenital syphilis, brain damage, spontaneous abortion (miscarriage), or stillbirth. Adequate treatment before the eighteenth week of pregnancy prevents syphilis in the fetus since the fetus appears relatively immune to syphilis, compared to other diseases, in early pregnancy.

Statistics show a drastic rise in congenital syphilis. Although necrosis of the umbilical cord (vein) is a clear indication that the newborn is infected, other symptoms may not appear until the fourteenth week of life (36). Symptoms include lesions of the skin and mucous membranes, coryza, anemia, and localized septicemia; or the child may appear healthy at birth with symptoms appearing in 2 to 6 weeks. Occasionally, symptoms may not appear for 2 years (6, 103). Treatment of the mother also ensures treatment of the ill fetus because penicillin readily crosses the placenta. Other antibiotics are available for those persons who are allergic to penicillin such as erythromycin (6, 103). Tetracycline is contraindicated during pregnancy (25). Newborns of mothers treated prenatally with erythromycin should be retreated (25).

Maternal gonorrhea and other less-known types of sexually transmitted disease (see the article by Benoit [6]) have varying degrees of negative effects on the mother and her offspring. These conditions are receptive to antibiotic treatments (6, 25).

Herpes simplex of the genital area is increasing in incidence. Thus the prevention and treatment of *perinatal herpes simplex* (type II) is of great public concern. Its primary source is maternal in nature in that genital herpes infections are sexually transmitted; consequently, affected women are mainly in the child-bearing age group (6, 11). The majority of genital infections are asymptomatic and difficult to recognize on clinical examination, thus making the identification of a mother whose fetus is in jeopardy very difficult (6, 24).

Unlike rubella, which readily crosses the placenta, the potential hazards of herpes simplex generally await the unsuspecting fetus in the maternal cervix or lower genital tract. The virus invades the uterus following the rupture of membranes or after contact is made with the fetus during the normal vaginal birth descent. Cesarean section is the delivery of choice if the infection has been diagnosed as a means of protecting the fetus from contamination (25).

Congenital and neonatal herpes simplex viral infections often prove lethal (6). A mortality rate of 60% and serious central nervous system and eye damages have been identified in half the survivors. Neonates may be asymptomatic. Because drug therapeutic measures taken thus far to cure the mother and newborn are ineffective, research in prevention and treatment of the infectious disease continues (6, 25).

Another dangerous infection is *Cytomegalic Inclusion Disease* (CID), which is caused by one of the herpes viruses and occurs in 1% to 2% of pregnant women and approximately half their babies. CID may go undetected in the mother and in the young child because the disease is asymptomatic, but laboratory analysis of infant cord blood detects the virus. The disease in the newborn is characterized by microcephaly, impaired growth, impaired intellectual ability, impaired hearing, enlarged liver and spleen, hemolytic anemia, and fracture of long bones (6, 25).

A *parasitic disease, toxoplasmosis,* is acquired by human contact with cat feces or eating inadequately cooked foods that contains the parasitic cysts. Transplacental transmission occurs during acute infection of the mother, but the disease causes congenital liver and brain damage and can result in convulsions, blindness, and mental retardation. The infected mother can be treated with medication, which probably reduces fetal damage. However, pregnant women who are not immune should be advised to not handle cats, cat feces, or litter boxes (25).

Fetal Infection

Intrauterine fetal infection caused by group B *Streptococcus* probably occurs with greater frequency than is clinically diagnosed (15). In the most serious of cases the clinical signs—apnea, respiratory distress, and shock—emerge at birth or within 48 hours (25). Immediate treatment is mandatory for survival. The death rate may be particularly high in preterm infants who show early signs and symptoms. Evidence points to the passage of this infectious agent during the birthing process via the maternal genital tract. Only penicillin is indicated for use as an antibiotic since no severe allergic reaction to the fetus or newborn has been reported (25).

Immunologic Factors

The fetus is immunologically foreign to the mother's immune system; yet the fetus is sustained. Selected antibodies of measles, chicken pox, hepatitis, poliomyelitis, whooping cough, and diphtheria are transferred to the fetus. The resulting immunity lasts several months after birth. Antibodies to dust, pollen, and common allergens do not transfer across the placenta (25).

The most commonly encountered interference with fetal development is incompatibility between maternal and infant blood factors, resulting in various degrees of circulatory difficulty for the baby. This problem is more complex than the commonly known Rh incompatibility. When a fetus' blood contains a protein substance, the Rh factor (Rh-positive blood), but the mother's blood does not (Rh-negative blood), antibodies in the mother's blood may attack the fetus and possibly cause jaundice, spontaneous abortion, stillbirth, anemia, heart defects, mental retardation, or death. Usually the first Rh-positive baby is not affected adversely, but with each succeeding pregnancy the risk becomes greater. A vaccine can be given to the Rh-negative mother within 3 days of childbirth or within 3 days of abortion that will prevent her body from making Rh antibodies. Babies affected by the Rh syndrome can be treated by repeated blood transfusions (25). In-depth information can be attained from a physiology or obstetrics text (14, 25, 42).

Maternal Emotions

The physical-psychologic interdependence between mother and fetus still is being studied; effects of the mother's elation, fear, and anxiety on the behavior and other developmental aspects of the baby are poorly understood. Anxiety, for instance, produces a variety of physiologic changes in the person because of activation of the hypothalamus and the sympathetic division response of the autonomic nervous system, which stimulates the adrenal medulla to produce adrenaline. Adrenaline, in turn, stimulates the anterior lobe of the pituitary to produce adrenocorticotropic hormone (ACTH), which activates the adrenal cortex to release cortisone. The results are increased heart rate, constriction of peripheral vessels, dilation of coronary vessels, decrease in gastrointestinal motility, and changed carbohydrate and protein metabolism, which also affects many body functions and changes in the adrenocortical hormonal system (25). These changes occurring in the pregnant woman contribute to hyperactivity of the fetus because increased maternal cortisone is secreted and enters the blood circulation, crossing the placenta to the fetus (25, 103). Because the fetus experiences only the consequences and not the cause of the emotion itself, the experience may mean nothing to the fetus (68). However, some studies indicate that maternal fear and anxiety induce the same sensations in the fetus (68). Animal studies indicate that stress-producing situations influence the fetus, causing changes in emotional states and also in learning activity after birth (29). Studies indicate that the human fetus responds with increased activity to loud noises in the environment (83). Maternal stress therefore may be considered a teratogen, resulting in physical and psychologic alterations of the developing person before and following birth.

A severe but not uncommon stressor for the pregnant woman is physical abuse or battering, which also involves fear, anxiety, and other feelings related to emotional abuse. Some men grow up rejecting their own needs for love and therefore find it difficult and threatening to meet the pregnant woman's emotional needs. Battering a pregnant woman may present a more extreme response of jealousy toward the unborn baby and anger at being displaced from the center of the woman's attention. Men also may fear and envy women's reproductive power ("womb envy," which is the other side of Freud's concept of women's penis envy). Such men deal with fear and envy by asserting physical power over the woman, often forcing himself sexually on the woman to the extent of manifesting sexual addiction or rape (51).

Maternal anxiety reactions are also related to physiologic responses of pregnancy such as nausea and vomiting, backaches, and headaches, which, in turn, affect the fetus.

The woman who begins pregnancy with inadequate psychic reserves is especially vulnerable to stresses and conflicting moods that accompany pregnancy (29). Do not assume harmony between the partners or happiness about the coming baby. The mother-to-be may have many feelings to resolve during pregnancy, as may the father-to-be. However, maternal emotionality during pregnancy has not been correlated with specific mother-child behavioral interaction.

Birth Defects Transmitted by the Father

Genes of both mother and father and the prenatal maternal environment may cause birth defects. Genetic mutations in sperm are being formed in a greater percent of the population. Mutations may be caused by exposure to irradiation, infection, drugs, and chemicals. These mutations occur more frequently as a man ages and may be responsible for various inborn disorders and congenital anomalies (Box 6–2) (25, 40, 87). For males this "cutoff" is 45 years of age; risks for chromosomal abnormalities may double when the male is 55 years or older (23, 40). The male may affect the unborn child in other ways as well. For example, recent research reveals the sperm of the man who uses cocaine may be affected by the substance and in turn adversely affect the ovum and developing child (130). Refer also to Chapter 2 for additional information on birth defects transmitted by the father, with a focus on Table 2–3.

VARIABLES RELATED TO CHILDBIRTH THAT AFFECT THE BABY

Medications

Analgesics and general anesthetics given during childbirth cross the placental barrier, affecting the newborn for days after delivery. Respiration after birth is negatively affected; artificial resuscitation may be needed for severe respiratory depression. Motor skills are also less adept, and more crying irritability is seen after birth. Local anesthetics also indirectly affect the fetus by reducing blood flow to the uterus thus affecting the fetal heart rate (9, 25).

Childbirth without drugs was first introduced in 1914 by Grantly Dick Read. He was followed by Dr. Fernand Lamaze. In recent times the natural childbirth method has become popular both to mother and father because they can both actively participate in the birth of their child. During natural childbirth classes parents learn about the physiology of pregnancy and childbirth, exercises that strengthen the mother's abdominal and perineal muscles, and techniques of breathing and relaxation during labor and delivery. The father acts as encourager and coach throughout the prenatal classes and during labor and delivery so that the birth experience is shared between the couple. Equally of benefit is the child who comes into the world without any ill effects from medication. Refer to literature from the American Society for Psychoprophylaxis in Obstetrics and obstetric nursing texts for more information on prepared childbirth.

Method of Delivery

In the early 1970s F. LeBoyer, a French obstetrician, developed a less traumatic method of delivering the baby by reducing intensity of new stimuli—light, gravity, and coolness. Lights are dim, only essential talking is allowed, and baby is placed on mother's abdomen until the cord stops pulsating (3 to 5 minutes). During this time the baby's back is gently massaged to simulate uterine contractions. Baby is wrapped in a warm blanket and placed to the mother's breast after the cord is cut. Baby is quieter and more alert as a result (103).

Inadequate Oxygenation

Anoxia, *decreased oxygen supply,* and increased carbon dioxide levels may result during delivery. Some degree almost routinely occurs from compression of the umbilical cord, reduced blood flow to the uterus, or placental separation. Fortunately, newborn babies are better able to withstand periods of low oxygen than are adults. Other causes of asphyxia, however, such as drug-induced respiratory depression or apnea, kinks in the umbilical cord, wrapping of the cord around the neck, very long labor, or malpresentation of the fetus during birth have more serious effects. Longitudinal studies over 7 years of anoxic newborns revealed lower performance scores on tests of sensorimotor and cognitive-intellectual skills and personality measures than for children with minimal anoxia at birth. Anoxia is also the principal cause of perinatal death and a common cause of mental retardation and cerebral palsy (25, 103).

Research Abstract

Gennaro, S., and M. Stringer, Stress and Health in Low Birthweight Infants: A Longitudinal Study, Nursing Research, *40, no. 5 (1991), 308–311.*

The emotional stress experienced by parents of preterm infants and the subsequent relationship between that stress and future infant outcomes have been an area of concern for several decades. This stress and two common stress responses, anxiety and depression, have been related to inappropriate use of acute care health facilities and to changes in parental perceptions of the low-birth-weight (<2500 g) infant. When family support is increased, lessening stress, a significant decrease in emergency room visits for low-birthweight infants has been documented. Parental stress also has a detrimental impact on subsequent infant growth and development. The mother's sense that the preterm infant is vulnerable ("vulnerable child syndrome") has been associated with childhood behavior problems. Maternal stress changes the quality of mother-infant interaction. Mothers with higher anxiety reported having less confidence in their parenting abilities and having infants with an increased incidence of feeding difficulties. Mothers of term and preterm infants who experienced increased negative life events and decreased social support were less satisfied with mothering and had a poorer quality of maternal-infant interaction. Depressed mothers were less responsive to their infants during the first 3 postpartum months.

The purpose of this study was to examine the association between maternal anxiety and depression, the use of health care services (infant acute care visits), and infant health outcomes (growth and development) in preterm low-birthweight infants.

The instruments used were the Multiple Affect Adjective Check List-Revised-State Form (MAACL-R), Bayley Scales of Infant Development, and the Neonatal Morbidity Scale (NMS). Maternal anxiety and depression were measured in the hospital during the first postnatal week and in the week following the infant's hospital discharge using the MAACL-R. Neonatal morbidity was determined by chart review throughout the infant's hospital stay using the NMS. Scores were assigned at days 3 and 7, and every 5 weeks thereafter until discharge. Data on the number of infant acute care visits were collected on each infant, beginning with hospital discharge and ending when the infant was 6 months adjusted age (chronologic age minus amount of prematurity). Infant growth and development were measured when the infant was 6 months adjusted age at a routine clinic visit.

The sample consisted of 63 mothers of low-birth-weight infants (36) and very-low-birth-weight infants (27) born over a $1\frac{1}{2}$ year period at an urban tertiary care center. The mean maternal age was 24 years (SD = 5.9). Most of the mothers in the study had vaginal deliveries, were multiparas, and were predominantly African-American. The mean infant birthweight was 1641 g, and the mean gestational age at birth was 31.4 weeks. Infants were hospitalized for an average of 31.7 days after birth.

Results indicated that the number of acute-care visits the infants experienced during the study period ranged from no visits to 17 visits. Mothers of infants with multiple acute care visits had significantly higher anxiety and more depression than the other two groups of mothers; the infants were not those who were the sickest during hospitalization. No significant relationships were found between maternal anxiety or depression experienced at birth and infant discharge, infant growth (weight, length, and head circumference), or development (motor or mental scale of Bayley Scales of Infant Development) at 6 months adjusted age.

Because of the smaller number of infants with inadequate growth at 6 months adjusted age ($N = 6$), the relationship between infant growth and maternal anxiety may not have been adequately tested.

Premature Birth and Low-Birth-Weight

Prematurity may have long-term consequences for the child. **Prematurity** is defined as the *infant born at gestational age of 37 weeks or earlier, combined with birth weight of less than 2500 g or $5\frac{1}{2}$ pounds.* Risk of death is greater to premature babies.

Later developmental and behavioral problems such as physical and mental retardation and hyperactivity may also be correlated with prematurity (29, 83). Treatment of the premature neonate in sterile, precisely controlled incubators causes the absence of environmental and sensory stimuli, which also contributes to retardation. Research shows 5 minutes of gentle rubbing hourly throughout the 24-hour day for 10 days showed positive effects immediately and later for infants in isolettes—they were more active and gained weight faster, and 7 months later they performed better on tests of motor development while appearing healthier and more active than control children (62, 63).

The small-for-gestational age or **low-birth-weight** (*less than $5\frac{1}{2}$ pounds or 2500 g*) infant may not be premature. Low birthweight is the major factor associated with death of the infant during the first 4 weeks of life. In one study 17.5% of battered women who delivered in private hospitals had low-birth-weight infants, compared to 4.2% of nonbattered women. The percentage for battered women was even higher in public hospitals (47). Being battered also doubles the chance of having a miscarriage. Battering may be one of the most frequent problems in pregnancy (13, 47).

The following maternal factors contribute to a higher risk of low-birth-weight babies (13, 25, 45, 103):

1. Underweight before pregnancy
2. Less than 21 pounds gained during pregnancy
3. Inadequate prenatal care
4. Age of 16 years or younger or 35 years or older
5. Low socioeconomic level

6. Poor nutrition during pregnancy
7. Smoking cigarettes during pregnancy
8. Use of addictive drugs or alcohol during pregnancy
9. History of prior abortions
10. Complications during pregnancy
11. High stress levels, including suffering physical battery or emotional abuse

A sixfold increase in the risk of low-birth-weight is associated with financial problems existing during the pregnancy, irrespective of the variables of race, poor health habits, and complications during pregnancy (7). A study of low-birth-weight children born to disadvantaged families showed that those who had received sensory stimulation in the nursery and additional sensorimotor stimulation from their mothers throughout the first year of life performed better on tests of intellectual and sensorimotor development at the end of the year than the children who had not received extra stimulation (102).

A study of 1000 infants for 3 years in eight U.S. cities indicated that the outcomes for premature and low-birth-weight infants can be significantly improved by intensive interventions for the first 3 years of the child's life. Children and families received the following services:

1. Weekly home visits in the first year of the child's life and biweekly thereafter
2. Attendance for the child at a special child development center after 12 months of age
3. Bimonthly group meetings for parents

Children who received these services showed higher intelligent quotient scores and fewer behavioral problems than did those who received no intervention (30).

Premature children differ from full-term infants in a number of ways, including sleep patterns, which are poorly organized with poorly differentiated sleep states. Shorter and less regular periods of each sleep state are exhibited and may persist beyond infancy. Because more growth hormone is released during sleep, disturbed sleep patterns in the premature may affect physical growth and size generally (25, 29).

EARLY CHILDHOOD VARIABLES THAT AFFECT THE PERSON

Nutrition

Nutrition can exert an important influence on growth and development, especially if nutritional deficiency diseases occur. Unfortunately, minimum, optimum, and toxic levels of nutrients are not well researched to date. However, inadequate nutrition may slow normal growth and apparently causes permanent effects of low intellec-

tual ability. As much as 30% of the brain's neurons may never be formed if protein intake is inadequate during the second trimester of pregnancy or the first 6 months of life. Children who suffer starvation do not catch up with growth norms for their group, although later in life adequate nutrition and socioemotional support help to offset the differences (29, 45).

Obesity in childhood more likely is related to eating patterns than to genetics, according to a study of weight differences between infants of obese and nonobese foster mothers. The babies weighed $4\frac{1}{2}$ pounds at birth and entered the foster homes at $3\frac{1}{2}$ weeks of age. Children cared for by obese foster parents also became obese. The mean weight of all children of obese mothers was heavier at all ages than for children of nonobese mothers. Children with excess cell mass from excessive caloric intake develop adult adipose cells early in life. Adipose stores continue to increase because of the increased number of adipose cells (2, 45, 103).

Even breast-feeding is not completely safe. Many drugs ingested by the mother are excreted in human milk (25,111). The newborn is susceptible to foreign substances because the body's principal detoxifying mechanisms are not functional, the enzyme system is immature, and kidney function is incompletely developed (25). Media reports indicate that pesticides in food and other environmental pollutants unknowingly ingested by the mother are excreted in human milk.

Stress

Stress related to emotional and sensory deprivation causes undesirable physical, emotional, and intellectual effects (29, 106–108). Some studies of the effects of mild physical stress on infants and rats reveal increased physical height, faster weight gain, and greater resistance to disease; however, variables for these studies appear poorly controlled, and the studies are primarily anecdotal. Other studies show that severe stress, discomfort, or pain cause the infant to perceive less external stimuli and to distort perceptions. Less tolerance for stress develops (83).

Effects of Practice on Neuromuscular Development

Effects of exercise or practice on developing early motor skills remain contradictory in reports. Apparently certain motor behavior appears when the body has the neuromuscular maturity for that behavior; practice of the behavior before its natural appearance does little to speed up long-term development, although it may appear that the child can do an activity earlier. Unpracticed children catch up, often doing the same activity in research studies only a few days later (83).

Endocrine Function

Mediation of hormones is crucial to the child and person throughout life. A **hormone** is a *chemical substance produced by an endocrine gland and carried by the bloodstream to another part of the body (the target organ) where it controls some function of the target organ.* The major functions of hormones include (1) integrative action, (2) regulation, and (3) morphogenesis. **Integration,** *permitting the body to act as a whole unit in response to stimuli,* results from hormones traveling throughout the body and reaching all cells of the body. For example, the response of the body to epinephrine during fright is generalized. Estrogen, although more specific in its action, affects overall body function. **Regulation,** *maintaining a constant internal environment or homeostasis,* results from all the hormones. The regulation of salt and water balance, metabolism, and growth are examples. In **morphogenesis,** the *rate and type of growth of the organism,* some hormones play an important part (42).

Growth hormone (*GH*) or *somatotropic hormone* (*STH*), secreted by the anterior pituitary gland and regulated by a substance called *growth-hormone-releasing-factor* (*GHF*), produced in the hypothalamus, affects morphogenesis by promoting the development and enlargement of all body tissues that are capable of growing. Growth hormone has three basic effects on the metabolic processes of the body: (1) protein synthesis is increased; (2) carbohydrate conservation is increased; and (3) use of fat stores for energy is increased (42).

Growth hormone is secreted in spurts instead of at a relatively constant rate. The lowest concentrations of plasma GH are found in the morning after arising; the highest concentrations occur between 60 and 90 minutes after falling asleep at night. The peak of GH is clearly related to sleep; thus the folk belief that sleep is necessary for growth and healing has been supported (42, 83).

SOCIOCULTURAL FACTORS THAT INFLUENCE THE DEVELOPING PERSON

Cultural and Demographic Variables

Culture, social class, race, and ethnicity of the parents—foods eaten by the pregnant woman, prenatal care and childbirth practices, child-rearing methods, expected patterns of behavior, language development and thought processes during childhood and adulthood, and health practices—variously affect the person from the moment of conception. However, the person will demonstrate some behaviors outside the cultural norm. If the child's parents are from a different ethnic or social background from most citizens of the area, the child may learn to talk, act, and think differently from most people. Conflict results between the person and the representatives (people and institutions) of the main culture, which, in turn, affects the child's ongoing development and care. Refer to Chapter 1 for in-depth discussion.

The health care given to the child by the parents is related to sociocultural status. For example, in urban areas parents of children who are adequately immunized are likely to have the following characteristics: (1) they perceive childhood diseases as serious; (2) they know about the effectiveness of vaccination; (3) they are older; (4) they are better educated; (5) they have smaller family size (number of children); (6) they read newspapers, listen to radio or television promotions of immunizations, and respond to these community educational efforts; and (7) they probably are Caucasian. Inadequately immunized children in urban areas are found in families in which the parents are young, poor, minimally educated, and non-White with a large number of children. The parents do not perceive childhood diseases as serious, do not know about the effectiveness of vaccines, or do not pay attention to health education in the mass media (83).

All the advantages of inheriting a good brain can be lost if the child does not have the right environment in which to develop it. Animal and human studies demonstrate that lack of physical or social stimulation has an effect on later behavior and development. For example, studies comparing rats raised in a stimulus-deprived environment and stimulus-rich environment showed that rats that had things to keep them interested, amused, and challenged had a greater number of neurons than the other rats and their brain cells were richer in biochemical content. Studies on rats also show that, although there cannot be an increase in the number of neurons after brain-cell division has stopped, the neurons that already exist can grow 15% larger and form more associations when the rat is given extra stimulation after being deprived. Thus the deprived rat can catch up in intellectual capacities.

The same apparently is true of humans, as demonstrated by Korean and Vietnamese children who were adopted by American parents. In a new, loving environment they improved in all spheres of behavior and intelligence (83).

Socialization Processes

Socialization is the *process by which the infant is transformed into a member of a particular society and learns the roles appropriate to sex, social class, and ethnic group or subculture* (86).

All humans experience socialization, the shaping of the person into a socially acceptable form, especially during the early year of life. Thus heritage and culture are perpetuated. The newborn is a biologic organism with physical needs and inherited characteristics, which will be socialized or shaped along a number of dimensions: emotional, social, cognitive, or intellectual, perceptual, behavioral, and expressive. During the period of socialization various skills, knowledge, attitudes, values, motives, habits, beliefs, needs, interests, and ideals are learned, demonstrated, and reinforced. Various people are key agents in the socialization process: parents, siblings, relatives, peers, teachers, and other adults. Certain forces will impinge on the person and interact with all the individual is and learns; these forces include culture, social class, religion, race or ethnicity, the community, the educational system, mass media, and various organizations. Certain factors may limit or enhance the socialization process: age, gender, rate and stage of development, general constitution, and innate intelligence. Integration of all the various individual and socializing forces will form the adult character, personality traits, role preferences, goals, and behavioral mode (86).

Socialization is a lifelong process of social learning or training through which the person acquires knowledge, skills, attitudes, values, needs, motivations, and cognitive, affective, and conative patterns that relate to the sociocultural setting. The success of the socialization process is measured by the person's ability to perform in the roles he or she attempts and to respond to rapid social change and a succession of life tasks (86).

The life cycle is seen as a succession of roles and changing role constellations. Certain order and predictability of behavior occur over time as the person moves through the given succession of roles. The person learns to think and behave in ways consonant with the roles to be played; performance in a succession of roles leads to predictable personality configurations (12, 28, 29, 86).

Community Support System

Community relationships influence primarily the parents, but they also influence the child. An emotional support system for the parents, physical and health-care resources in the community, and social and learning opportunities that exist outside the home promote the child's development and prepare him or her for later independence and citizenry roles. If the parents are unable to meet the child's needs adequately, other people or organizations in the community may make the difference between bare survival and eventual physical and emotional normalcy and well-being.

Cultures vary in the degree to which the new mother is given help. For example, in India the mother is assisted with child care and is allowed to do nothing except care for her baby for 40 days after delivery. Several decades ago mothers in the United States were hospitalized for 10 or 12 days, and the family helped at home for another couple weeks or so. Now the mother is sent home after 24 to 72 hours, often to assume total child care.

Physical health of the baby and emotional health of the mother in the months following delivery depend on whether or not she had assistance with infant care during the first month after delivery (103).

Family Factors

The family structure, developmental level and roles of family members, their health and financial status, their perception of baby, and community resources for the family influence the child's development and well-being. The child learns to behave differently and as an adult will have different values and expectations if he or she is reared in a single-parent, nuclear, extended, matrifocal, or patriarchal family or in a poor or wealthy family. The number of siblings, their sexes, and birth order influence how the child is treated and perceives self. The stresses on and crises within the family determine how well the child is cared for from birth, how and what is taught to the child, discipline measures, and how he or she looks at life. The family's presence or absence of work, leisure, travel, material comforts, habits of daily living, and the facade put on for society will affect the child's self-concept, learning, physical well-being, and eventual life-style. Refer to Chapter 4 for more information.

Spitz (106, 107) studied four different child-rearing situations to determine the effect on the young child. Children from professional, urban homes had the highest developmental quotient initially, and it stayed high. Children living in an isolated fishing village with poor nutrition, housing, hygiene, and medical care had a low developmental quotient in the first 4 months, and it remained low. Children born to delinquent women and reared in a penal institution by their mothers had a lower development quotient initially than children in the fishing village, but they gained slightly. Children from a Latin, urban background who were raised in a foundling home had an initial high development quotient, but the score was lowest of the groups studied at the end of the first year.

The children in the foundling home had been given minimum mothering by overworked nurses. The presence of the mother is sufficient to compensate for lack of material objects. The lack of development was related to lack of human stimulation since deterioration of the child was arrested if he or she were removed from the foundling home at 1 year of age.

The mother has traditionally been credited with having the most effect on the child, whether the outcome was good or bad. However, researchers now acknowledge the importance of the father and the effect of the father's presence or absence on the developing child (65, 74). The stability and strength of attachment between the child and family will largely determine the degree to which he or she will become a self-confident, productive citizen. The long-term emotional and physical environments are the most crucial variables in the child's measured performance at 10 years. A positive environment overcomes negative perinatal influences; a negative environment may have lasting effects (83).

Vulnerable and Resilient Children

Both vulnerable and resilient children develop within the same family system. Siblings brought up under chaotic situations, with alcoholic or drug-using parents, or in impoverished circumstances do not all develop the same personality traits. One becomes physically or emotionally ill, whereas the sibling thrives. There is no single set of qualities or circumstances that characterize such resilient children, but they are different from their vulnerable siblings from birth. **Resilient children** appear to be *endowed with innate characteristics that insulate them from the pain of their families and allow them to reach out to some adult who provides crucial emotional support.* These children typically have the ability to use some talent or personality traits to draw some adult to them as a substitute parent. Also these children seemed to recover quickly from stressors (119). Resilient children differ from their siblings. From birth these children are more alert to their surroundings. By 1 year of age, trust had been established with their mothers. There has been warm and secure relationships with the mother, regardless of other circumstances. By age 2, even when abused or neglected, these children are more independent, easy going, enthusiastic for activities, and able to tolerate frustration. By age $3\frac{1}{2}$, the resilient children are more cheerful, flexible, and persistent in the face of stress or failure. They show ability to seek help from adults (119).

The children closest emotionally to the distressed parent are most likely to show signs of distress. These children are more likely to be self-derogatory, anxious, depressed, and physically ill. However, hardships can leave even the resilient children with psychologic scars, although they tend not to become emotionally disabled. Even apparently well-adjusted, successful resilient children may pay a subtle psychologic cost. In adolescence they are more likely to cling to a moralistic outlook. In intimate relationships they are apt to be disagreeable and judgmental. They tend to be constricted and overcontrolled. If the disturbed parent is of the opposite gender, the resilient person is often emotionally distant in intimate relationships, breaking off relationships as they become more intimate. Some seek partners with problems, with the idea of rescuing or curing them (119).

Child Abuse

Child abuse is a negative influence on the developing person. It is currently an epidemic, and children are suffering more serious and brutal injuries. Parents who abuse their children are from every race, color, creed, ethnic origin, and economic level (15). As a nurse, you are crucial in preventing child abuse through your assistance to parents. **Child abuse** is a *pattern of abnormal parent-child interactions and attacks over a period of time that results in nonaccidental injuries to the child physically,*

emotionally, or sexually or from neglect. Other terms are *battered child* or *maltreatment syndrome.* Abused children range in age from neonate through adolescence.

You may be the first health worker to encounter such a child in the community. Be alert for signs of child abuse as you assess the injured or ill child. Nonaccidental physical injury includes multiple bruises or fractures from severe beatings; poisonings or overmedication; burns from immersion in hot water or from lighted cigarettes; excessive use of laxatives or enemas; and human bites. The trauma to the child is often great enough to cause permanent blindness, scars on the skin, neurologic damage, subdural hematoma, and permanent brain damage or death. **Sexual molestation,** *exploitation of the child for the adult's sexual gratification,* includes rape, incest, exhibitionism to the child, or fondling of the child's genitals. **Emotional abuse** includes *excessively aggressive or unreasonable parental behavior to the child,* placing unreasonable demands on the child to perform above his or her capacities, verbally attacking or constantly belittling or teasing the child, or withdrawing love, support, or guidance. **Neglect** includes *failure to provide the child with basic necessities of life* (food, shelter, clothing, hygiene, or medical care), *adequate mothering, or emotional, moral, or social care* (15, 31, 32, 44, 46, 72, 103). The parents' lack of concern is usually obvious. Abandonment may occur. In all forms of abuse the child frequently acts fearful of the parents or adults in general. The child is usually too fearful to tell how he or she was injured.

There are a number of characteristics of the potentially or actually abusive parent(s). Typically the abuser manifests the following characteristics:

1. Young in age
2. Emotionally unstable, unable to cope with the stress of life or even usual personal problems
3. Insufficiently mothered, rejected, or abused as a child
4. Lonely, few social contacts, isolated from people
5. Unable to ask for help, lack of friends or family who can help with child care
6. Does not understand the development or care needs of children
7. Living through a very stressful time such as unemployment, being abused by the spouse, or poverty
8. Personal emotional needs previously unmet; difficulty in trusting others
9. Angered easily; negative self-image and low self-esteem
10. No one from whom to receive emotional support, including partner
11. Expects the child to be perfect and to cause no inconvenience
12. May perceive the child as different, too active, or too passive, even if the child is normal or only mildly different.

Sometimes the child has mild neurologic dysfunction and is irritable, tense, and difficult to hold or cuddle. The child may have been the result of an unwanted pregnancy or premature or have a birth defect. Usually only one child in a family becomes the scapegoat for parental anger, tension, rejection, and hate. The child who does not react in a way to make the parent feel good about his or her parenting behavior will be the abused one (15, 31, 32, 44, 46, 72, 88, 102, 103).

Additional information about child and adolescent abuse is found in Chapters 7 through 11.

Prolonged Separation

Separation for more than 3 months from a mothering person leads to serious consequences because from approximately 3 to 15 months of age the presence of a consistently loving caretaker is essential. Physical and intellectual growth is impaired, and the baby will not learn to form and maintain trust or a significant relationship. He or she will either withdraw or seek precociously to adapt by getting attention from as many people as possible. Death may result even with the best possible physical care (83, 106–108).

Maternal Deprivation or Failure to Thrive

These are the terms used to describe infants who have insufficient contact with a mothering one and who do not grow as expected in the absence of an organic defect (83, 102, 106–108). These infants may be institutionalized or have a parent who does not exhibit affectionate maternal behavior. Deprivation during the second 6 months occurs when a previously warm relationship with the mother is interrupted. This deprivation is more detrimental to the child than the lack of a consistent relationship during the first 6 months. Another cause for failure to thrive is **perceptual deprivation,** *lack of tactile, vestibular, visual, or auditory stimuli,* resulting from either organic factors or the lack of mothering (102, 103). Touch and cuddling are essential for the infant; the skin is the primary way in which baby comes to know self and the environment.

Although damage to the child from maternal deprivation may be severe, not every deprived child becomes delinquent or a problem adult. Some infants who have lacked their mother's love appear to suffer little permanent damage. The age of the child when deprived or abused, the length of separation or duration of abuse, the parent-child relationship before separation or in later childhood, care of the child by other adults during separation from the parents, and the stress produced by the separation or abuse all affect the long-range outcome.

Spiritual Factors

Religious, philosophic, and moral insights and practices of the parents (and of the overall society) influence how the child is perceived, cared for, and taught. These early underpinnings—or their lack—will continue to affect the person's self-concept, behavior, and health as an adult, even when he or she purposefully tries to disregard these early teachings. Refer to Chapter 3 for more information.

Macroenvironmental Factors That Influence the Developing Person

The overall environment of the region in which the person lives and in the home affects development and health. The climate the person learns to tolerate, water and food availability, emphasis on cleanliness, demands for physical and motor competency, social relationships, opportunities for leisure, and inherent hazards depend on whether the child lives on a farm or in the city, on the seacoast or in a semiarid region, in the cold North or sunny South, in a mining town or a mountain resort area. Added to these effects are the hazards from environmental pollution that affect all societies, whether it is excrement from freely roaming cattle or particles from industrial smokestacks. No part of the world is any longer uncontaminated by pesticides; all parts have disease related to problems of waste control. On a more immediate level, the size, space, noise, cleanliness, and safety within the home will affect the person's behavior and health and the home environment he or she will eventually build.

Further discussion of effects of the macroenvironment on the person's health can be found in Chapter 2.

Nursing Applications

Your support, assistance, and teaching with the pregnant woman and her significant support system will contribute to more nurturing parenting. Refer to texts on obstetric and maternal-child nursing for additional information about nursing care of the woman during pregnancy, labor, delivery, and after delivery. Information is also given in Chapters 2, 7 through 11, and 17 that can be shared with the pregnant woman and parents for health promotion.

Consider the principles of growth and development as you assess people in different developmental eras. Carefully assess pregnant women to determine whether they are at risk because of any of the negative influencing factors. A helpful screening system for the woman prenatally and intrapartally and for the neonate has been devised (103). Help those who are at risk to get the care necessary to prevent fetal damage and maternal illness. Consider also the sociocultural and religious backgrounds and the life-style of the person you are caring for so that you do not overlook or misinterpret factors that are significant to the pregnant woman and her family.

Teach potential parents about the many factors discussed in this and following chapters that can influence the welfare of their offspring. Be aware of community services such as genetic screening and counseling, family planning, nutritional programs, prenatal classes, counseling for prevention of child abuse, and medical services. Join with other citizens in attempts to reverse environmental and child abuse hazards.

Your role with the child-abusing parent and the abused child is a significant one. To help parents and child, you must first cope with your own feelings as you give necessary physical care to the child or assist parents in getting proper care for the baby. Often parents who feel unable to cope with the stresses of childrearing will repeatedly bring the child to the emergency room for a variety of complaints or minor, vague illnesses or injuries. Be alert to the subtle message; talk with the parent(s) about himself or herself, the management of the child, feelings about parenting and the child, and who helps in times of stress. Establish rapport; act like a helpful friend; convey a feeling of respect for them as people (which may be difficult if you feel that the child abuser is a monster). Avoid asking probing questions too quickly; do not lecture or scold the parent about his or her childrearing methods. Help parents to feel confident and competent in any way possible. If possible, form a "cool mothering" relationship with the parent(s) (i.e., make yourself consistently available but do not push too close emotionally). Often the mother responds well to having a grandmotherly person (usually a volunteer) spend time with her in the home. In a sense the grandmotherly person is mothering the mother, but she is also assisting with a variety of household chores, giving the mother time to spend with her baby while unharried by demands of other children or household tasks. The grandmotherly person can also be a model on how to approach, cuddle, and discipline the child. Both you and the volunteer can share information about normal child behavior and developmental characteristics appropriate for age; the parent may expect the 6-month-old baby to obey commands. Convey that consistency of care is important. Realize that the parent will need long-term help in overcoming the abusive pattern. After a relationship has been formed, the abusing parent(s) may benefit from joining a group such as Parents Anonymous in which the problems of being a child abuser can be resolved and the information about normal development can be learned.

To avoid driving the parent away from potential help or becoming more abusive to the child, use the principles of therapeutic communication and crisis intervention discussed in Chapter 17. In your zeal to protect the child, intervene sensibly with the parents and the child to avoid further harm and to avoid disrupting any positive feelings that might exist between parents and child. Foster home care is not necessarily the answer; foster parents are sometimes abusive, too. Rapid court action may antagonize parents to the point of murdering the child or moving to a different geographic location where they cannot receive help. Refer the parents to

Parents Anonymous, a self-help parent's group that exists in some large cities, or to other local self-help crisis groups. For more information, refer to the "Symposium on Child Abuse and Neglect," *Nursing Clinics of North America,* 16, no. 1, March, 1981 (44, 63, 72, 102).

Further, cooperate with legal, medical, and social agencies to help the parent(s) and to prevent further child abuse—and possible death or permanent impairment of the child. Child abuse is against the law in every state, and every state has at least one statewide agency to receive and investigate suspected cases of child abuse. Any citizen or health worker can anonymously report a case of child abuse to authorities without fear of recrimination from the abuser. An investigation by designated authorities of the danger to the child is carried out shortly after reporting; the child may be placed in a foster home or institution by court order if the child's life is threatened. The goal of legal intervention is to help the parents and child, not to punish (63, 72).

Unless the problem of child abuse can be curbed, many of today's children will become the next generation of abusing parents.

Mothers and children constitute approximately two thirds of the population in any society. They are worth caring for physically and emotionally because of their worth to the future of the society.

REFERENCES

1. Ahlborg, G., and L. Bodin, Tobacco Smoke Exposure and Pregnancy Outcome Among Working Women: A Prospective Study at Prenatal Care Centers in Orebro County, Sweden, *Preventive Journal of Epidemiology,* 133, no. 4 (1991), 338–347.
2. American Academy of Pediatrics Committee on Nutrition, Toward a Prudent Diet for Children, *Pediatrics,* 73 (1984), 876.
3. American College of Obstetrics and Gynecologists, *Antepartum Fetal Surveillance, Technical Bulletin,* no. 107 (August 1987).
4. American Dietetic Association, Nutrition Management of Adolescent Pregnancy, *Journal of the American Dietetic Association,* 89 (1989), 104–109.
5. Benigni, A., et al., Effect of Low-Dose Aspirin on Fetal and Maternal Generation of Thromboxane by Platelets in Women at Risk for Pregnancy-Induced Hypertension, *New England Journal of Medicine,* 321, no. 6 (1989), 357–362.
6. Benoit, J., Sexually Transmitted Diseases in Pregnancy, *Nursing Clinics of North America,* 23, no. 4 (1988), 937–946.
7. Binsacca, D., Factors Associated With Low Birth Weight in an Inner-City Population: The Role of Financial Problems, *American Journal of Public Health,* 77, no. 4 (1987), 585–586.
8. Bobitt, J.R., Specific Bacterial Infections: Group B Streptococcus and Listeria. In Sciarra, J.J., ed., *Gynecology and Obstetrics.* Philadelphia: Harper & Row, 1982.

9. Briggs, G.G., R.K. Freeman, and S.J. Yaffe, *Drugs in Pregnancy and Lactation* (2nd ed.). Baltimore: William & Wilkins, 1986.

10. Brill, N., Emotional Abuse of Children, *American Journal of Psychiatry,* 1, no. 2 (1981), 41.

11. Brunell, P.A., Prevention and Treatment of Neonatal Herpes, *Pediatrics,* 66, no. 11 (1980), 5.

12. Buhler, C., The Developmental Structure of Goal Setting in Group and Individual Studies. In Buhler, C. and F. Massarik, eds., *The Course of Human Life.* NY: Springer-Verlag, 1968.

13. Bullock, B.L., and J. McFarlane, The Birth-Weight/Battering Connection, *American Journal of Nursing,* 89, no. 9 (1989), 1153–1155.

14. Bullock, B.L., and P.P. Rosendahl, *Pathophysiology: Adaptations and Alterations in Function* (2nd ed.). Glenview, Ill: Scott, Foresman, 1988.

15. Campbell, J.E., and J. Humphreys, *Nursing Care of Victims of Family Violence.* Reston, Va: Reston, 1984.

16. Castleman, M., Toxics and Male Infertility, *Sierra* 70, no. 2 (1985), 49–52.

17. Center for Disease Control, USDHHS, Recommendations for Assisting in the Prevention of Human T-Lymphotrophic Virus Type III/Lymphadenopathy-Associated Virus and Acquired Immunodeficiency Syndrome, *MMWR,* 34 (December 6, 1987), 721–726, 731–732.

18. Chasnoff, I.J., Prenatal Cocaine Exposure Is Associated With Respiratory Pattern Abnormalities, *American Journal of Disabled Children,* 144, no. 2 (1990), 583–587.

19. ———, and D. Griffith, Cocaine: Clinical Studies of Pregnancy and the Newborn, *Annals of the New York Academy of Sciences,* 562 (1989), 260–266.

20. ———, et al., Temporal Patterns of Cocaine Use in Pregnancy: Perinatal Outcomes, *Journal of the American Medical Association,* 261, no. 12 (1989), 1741–1744.

21. Clarren, S.K., and D.W. Smith, The Fetal Alcohol Syndrome, *New England Journal of Medicine,* 298, no. 19 (1978), 1063–1067.

22. Cohen, F.L., Paternal Contributions to Birth Defects, *Nursing Clinics of North America,* 21, no. 1 (March 1986), 51–66.

23. ———, *Clinical Genetics in Nursing Practice.* Philadelphia: J.B. Lippincott, 1984.

24. Committee on Infectious Diseases: Fetus and Newborn, Perinatal Herpes Simplex Virus Infections, *Pediatrics,* 66, no. 7 (1980), 1.

25. Cunningham, F., P. MacDonald, and N. Gant, *Williams Obstetrics* (18th ed.). Norwalk, Conn: Appleton-Lange, 1989.

26. Dorfman, D.H., and J.H. Glaser, Congenital Syphilis Presenting in Infants After the Newborn Period, *New England Journal of Medicine,* 323, no. 19 (1990), 1299–1302.

27. Dusitsin, N., et al., Development and Validation of a Simple Device to Estimate Birthweight and Screen for Low Birthweight in Developing Countries, *American Journal of Public Health,* 81, no. 9 (1991), 1201–1205.

28. Duvall, E., and B. Miller, *Marriage and Family Development* (6th ed.). New York: Harper & Row, 1984.

29. Dworetzky, J., and N. Davis, *Human Development: A Lifespan Approach.* St. Paul, Minnesota: West Publishing, 1989.

30. Early Intervention Improves the Developmental Outcome of Premature Infants, New Study Says, *Advances: Newsletter of The Robert Wood Johnson Foundation,* 3, no. 2 (1990), 3.

31. Elmer, E., *Children in Jeopardy: The Study of Abused Minors and Their Families.* Pittsburgh: University of Pittsburgh Press, 1962.

32. ———, Child Abuse: The Family's Cry for Help, *Journal of Psychiatric Nursing,* 5, no. 4 (1967), 338ff.

33. Enstrom, J.E., L.E. Kanim, and L. Breslow, The Relationship Between Vitamin C Intake, General Health Practices, and Mortality in Alameda County, California, *American Journal of Public Health,* 76, no. 9 (September 1986), 1124–1129.

34. Erikson, E., *Childhood and Society* (2nd ed.). New York: W.W. Norton, 1963.

35. Fairbanks, K.D., et al., AIDS Update, *Clinicians' Reviews,* 1, no. 6 (1990), 85–86.

36. Fojaco, R.M., G.T. Hensley, and L. Moskowitz, Congenital Syphilis and Necrotizing Funisitis, *Journal of American Medical Association,* 261, no. 12 (1989), 1788–1790.

37. Foster, D.W., Diabetes Mellitus. In Braunwald, E., et al., eds., *Harrison's Principles of Internal Medicine* (11th ed.). New York: McGraw-Hill, 1987.

38. Fox, N.L., M. Sexton, and J.R. Hebel, Prenatal Exposure to Tobacco: Effects on Physical Growth at Age Three, *International Journal of Epidemiology,* 19, no. 1 (1990), 66–71.

39. Fried, P.A., Marijuana Use by Pregnant Women and Effects on Offspring: An Update, *Neurobehavioral Toxicology and Teratology,* 4 (1982), 451–454.

40. Friedman, J.M., Genetic Diseases in the Offspring of Older Fathers, *Obstetrics and Gynecology,* 57, no. 6 (1981), 745–749.

41. Garn, S.M., et al., Effects of Maternal Cigarette Smoking on Apgar Score, *American Journal of Disabled Children,* 135, no. 6 (1981), 503–506.

42. Guyton, A., *Medical Physiology* (8th ed.). Philadelphia: W.B. Saunders, 1991.

43. Harlap, S., and A. Davis, Infant Admissions to Hospital and Maternal in First and Second Trimesters, *Lancet,* 2, no. 7 (1980), 1973.

44. Hayes, P., The Long-Term Treatment of Victims of Child Abuse, *Nursing Clinics of North America,* 16, no. 1 (1981), 139–147.

45. Hegarty, V., *Decisions in Nutrition.* St. Louis: Times Mirror/Mosby College Publishing, 1988.

46. Helberg, J., Documentation in Child Abuse, *American Journal of Nursing,* 83, no. 2 (1983), 236–239.

47. Helton, A., Battering During Pregnancy, *American Journal of Nursing,* 86, no. 8 (1986), 910–913.

48. Hill, J.D., and R.D. Milner, Insulin as a Growth Factor, *Pediatric Research,* 19 (1955), 879–886.

49. *HIV/AIDS Surveillance Report.* Atlanta: Center for Disease Control, USDHHS, April, 1991.

50. HIV and Children: A Growing Problem, *American Nurse* (November/December 1990), 21.

51. Hoff, L., *Battered Women as Survivors.* New York: Routledge, 1990.

52. Isouh, S., et al., Fetal Alcohol Syndrome Revisited, *Pediatrics,* 68, no. 10 (1981), 475.

53. Jacob, J., and J. Monad, Genetic Regulatory Mechanisms in the Synthesis of Proteins, *Journal of Molecular Biology,* 3 (1961), 318–356.

54. John, E.M., D.A. Savitz, and D.P. Sandler, Prenatal Exposure to Parents' Smoking and Childhood Cancer, *American Journal of Epidemiology,* 133, no. 2 (1991), 123–125.

55. Jones, K.L., and D.W. Smith, The Fetal Alcohol Syndrome, *Tetratology,* 12 (1975), 1.

56. Kaczmarek, R., et al., X-Ray Examinations During Pregnancy: National Natality Surveys 1963 and 1980, *American Journal of Public Health,* 79, no. 1 (1989), 75–77.

57. Kaiserman, M., and B. Rogers, Tobacco Consumption Declining Faster in Canada Than in the U.S., *American Journal of Public Health,* 81, no. 7 (1991), 902–904.

58. King, I., *Theory for Nursing: Systems, Concepts, Process.* New York: Delmar Publishing, 1981.

59. Klein, J., et al., Drinking During Pregnancy and Spontaneous Abortion, *Lancet,* 2, no. 7 (1980), 1976.

60. Kleinman, J.C., and A. Kopstein, Smoking During Pregnancy, *American Journal of Public Health,* 77, no. 7 (July 1987), 823–825.

61. Kramer, L., and M. Pierpont, Rocking Waterbeds and Auditory Stimuli to Enhance Growth of Preterm Infants, *Journal of Pediatrics,* 88 (February 1976), 297–299.

62. Kramer, M., et al., Extra Tactile Stimulation of the Premature Infant, *Nursing Research,* 24, no. 5 (September-October 1975), 324–334.

63. Kreitzer, M., Legal Aspects of Child Abuse: Guidelines for the Nurse, *Nursing Clinics of North America,* 16, no. 1 (1981), 149–161.

64. Kuzma, S.W., and D.G. Keeinger, Patterns of Alcohol and Cigarette Use in Pregnancy, *Neurobehavioral Toxicology and Teratology,* 3, no. 2 (1981), 211–221.

65. Lamb, M., *The Father's Role.* New York: John Wiley, 1986.

66. Lammer, E.J., et al., Classification and Analysis of Fetal Deaths in Massachusetts, *Journal of the American Medical Association,* 261, no. 12 (1989), 1757–1762.

67. Levin, S., et al., The Association of Marijuana Use With Pregnancy, *American Journal of Public Health,* 73, no. 10 (1983), 1161–1164.

68. Liley, A.W., The Fetus as a Personality, *Australia-New Zealand Journal of Psychiatry,* 6 (1972), 99ff.

69. Lindenberg, C., et al., A Review of the Literature on Cocaine Abuse in Pregnancy, *Nursing Research,* 40, no. 2 (1991), 69–75.

70. Little, R.E., et al., Decreased Birth Weight in Infants of Alcoholic Women Who Abstained During Pregnancy, *Journal of Pediatrics,* 96, no. 6 (1980), 974.

71. ———, et al., Maternal Alcohol Use During Breast-Feeding and Infant Mental and Motor Development at One Year, *New England Journal of Medicine,* 321, no. 7 (1989), 425–430.

72. Ludwig, S., A Multi-disciplinary Approach to Child Abuse, *Nursing Clinics of North America,* 16, no. 1 (1981), 161–165.

73. Lymon, W.D., et al., Detection of HIV in Fetal Control Nervous System Tissue, *AIDS,* no. 9 (1990), 917–920.

74. Lynn, D., *The Father: His Role in Child Development.* Monterey, Calif: Brooks/Cole Publishing, 1974.

75. MacGregor, S.N., et al., Cocaine Abuse During Pregnancy: Correlation Between Prenatal Care and Perinatal Outcome, *Obstetrics and Gynecology,* 74, no. 6 (1989), 882–885.

76. Marbury, M., et al., The Association of Alcohol Consumption with Outcome of Pregnancy, *American Journal of Public Health,* 73, no. 10 (1983), 1165–1168.

77. Mare, R., Socioeconomic Effects on Child Mortality in the United States, *American Journal of Public Health,* 72, no. 6 (1982), 539–547.

78. Menton, R.K., et al., Transplacental Passage of Insulin in Pregnant Women With Insulin-Dependent Diabetic Macrosomia, *New England Journal of Medicine,* 323, no. 5 (1990), 309–315.

79. Mercer, R., A Theoretical Framework for Studying Factors That Impact on Maternal Role, *Nursing Research,* 30, no. 2 (1981), 73–77.

80. Miller, G., A Theoretical Framework for Nursing Research in Child Abuse and Neglect, *Nursing Research,* 30, no. 2 (1981), 73–83.

81. Minoff, H.L., et al., Pregnancy Outcomes Among Mothers With Human Immunodeficiency Virus and Uninfected Control Subjects, *American Journal of Obstetrics and Gynecology,* 163, no. 5 (1990), 1598–1604.

82. Monamey, T., Kids with AIDS, *Newsweek* (September 1987), 51–57.

83. Moshman, D., J. Glover, and R. Bruning, *Developmental Psychology.* Boston: Little, Brown, 1987.

84. Mussen, P., et al., *Child Development and Personality* (7th ed.). New York: Harper & Row, 1990.

85. National Academy of Sciences Institute of Medicine, Subcommittee on Nutritional Status Weight Gain During Pregnancy, *Nutrition During Pregnancy.* Washington, DC: National Academy Press, 1990.

86. Neugarten, B., Adaptation and the Life Cycle, *Counseling Psychologist,* 6, no. 1 (1976), 16–20.

87. Olson, J., A. de Costa Pereira, and S. Olsen, Does Maternal Tobacco Smoking Modify the Effect of Alcohol on Fetal Growth? *American Journal of Public Health,* 81, no. 1 (1991), 69–73.

88. Olson, R., Index of Suspicion: Screening for Child Abuse, *American Journal of Nursing,* 76, no. 1 (January 1976), 108–110.

89. Parks, W.P., and G.B. Scott, An Overview of Pediatric AIDS: Approaches to Diagnosis and Outcome Assessment. In Broder, S. ed., *AIDS: Modern Concepts and Therapeutic Challenges.* New York: Marcel Dekker, 1987.

90. Petiti, D., and C. Coleman, Cocaine and the Risk of Low Birth Weight, *American Journal of Public Health,* 80, no. 1 (1990), 25–28.

91. *Physicians' Desk Reference.* Oradel, NJ: Medical Economics, 1991.

92. Pitkin, R.M., Calcium Metabolism in Pregnancy and the Perinatal Period, *American Journal of Obstetrics and Gynecology,* 151, no. 1 (1985), 99–109.

93. Porter, J.B., et al., Drugs and Stillbirth, *American Journal of Public Health,* 76, no. 12 (1986), 1428–1430.

94. Reece, E.A., and S.C. Hobbins, Diabetic Embryopathy: Pathogenesis, Prenatal Diagnosis and Prevention, *Obstetrics and Gynecology Survey,* 41, no. 6 (1986), 325–335.

95. Rogers, M., *The Theoretical Basis of Nursing.* Philadelphia: F.A. Davis, 1970.

96. Rogers, M.E., Health Hazards to Perinatal Handling of Antineoplastic Agents, *Occupational Medicine: State of the Art Review,* 2 (1987), 513–524.

97. Rogers, M.F., et al., Acquired Immunodeficiency Syndrome in Children: Report of the Center for Disease Control National Surveillance, 1982 for 1985, *Pediatrics,* 79, no. 6 (1987), 1008–1012.

98. Rose, F.W., Spina Bifida in Infants of Women Treated With Carbamazopine During Pregnancy, *New England Journal of Medicine,* 324, no. 10 (1991), 674–677.

99. Rush, D., Z. Stein, and M. Susser, A Randomized Controlled Trial of Prenatal Nutritional Supplementation in New York City, *Pediatrics,* 65, no. 4 (1980), 683.

100. Schnoor, T.M., et al., Video Display Terminals and the Risk of Spontaneous Abortion, *New England Journal of Medicine,* 324, no. 11 (1991), 727–733.

101. Scott, G.B., et al., Survival in Children With Perinatally Acquired Human Immunodeficiency Virus Type 1 Infection, *New England Journal of Medicine,* 321, no. 26 (1989), 1791–1796.

102. Schuster, C.S., and S.S. Ashburn, *The Process of Human Development: A Holistic Life-Span Approach* (2nd ed.). Boston: Little, Brown, 1986.

103. Sherwen, L., M. Scoleveno, and C. Weingarten, *Nursing Care of the Childbearing Family.* Norwalk, Conn: Appleton-Lange, 1991.

104. Smith, J., Care of the Hospitalized Abused Child and Family: A Framework for Nursing Intervention, *Nursing Clinics of North America,* 16, no. 1 (1981), 127–137.

105. Smithells, R.W., et al., Further Experience of Vitamin Supplementation for Prevention of Neural Tube Defect Recurrences, *Lancet,* 1, no. 8332 (1983), 1027–1031.

106. Spitz, R., Hospitalism. In *The Psychoanalytic Study of the Child,* Vol. 1. New York: International University Press, 1945.

107. ———, Hospitalism: The Genesis of Psychiatric Conditions in Early Childhood. In Sze, W., ed., *Human Life Cycle.* New York: Jason Aronson, 1975, pp. 29–43.

108. ———, and K.M. Wolf, Anaclitic Depression: An Inquiry into the Genesis of Psychiatric Conditions in Early Childhood. In *The Psychoanalytic Study of the Child,* Vol. 2. New York: International University Press, 1946, pp. 313–342.

109. Starfield, B., Child Health and Socioeconomic Status, *American Journal of Public Health,* 72, no. 6 (1982), 532–533.

110. Stein, Z., and J. Klein, Smoking, Alcohol and Reproduction, *American Journal of Public Health,* 73, no. 10 (1983), 1154–1156.

111. Stellman, J.M., The Effects of Toxic Agents on Reproduction, *Occupational Health and Safety,* April 1979, 36–43.

112. Stenchover, M., Fetal Risks from Paternal Medication, *Journal of American Medical Association,* 211 (February 23, 1970), 1382.

113. Stjernfeldt, M., et al., Maternal Smoking During Pregnancy and the Risk of Childhood Cancer, *Lancet,* 1, no. 8494 (1986), 1350–1352.

114. Strachan-Lindenberg, C., et al., A Review of the Literature on Cocaine Abuse in Pregnancy, *Nursing Research,* 40, no. 2 (1991), 69–75.

115. Sullivan, H.S., *Interpersonal Theory of Psychiatry.* New York: W.W. Norton, 1953.

116. Tanner, J.M., *Foetus into Man: Physical Growth from Conception to Maturity.* London: Open Books, 1978.

117. Taylor, P., et al., Polychlorinated Biphenyls: Influence on Birthweight Gestation, *American Journal of Public Health,* 74, no. 10 (1984), 1153–1154.

118. Theiler, P., A Vietnam Aftermath, *Common Cause Magazine* (November-December 1984), 29–34.

119. Thriving Despite Hardship: Key Childhood Traits Identified, *The New York Times,* October 13, 1987, Sec. I, 19.

120. Toubas, P., et al., Effects of Maternal Smoking and Caffeine Habits on Infantile Apnea: A Retrospective Study, *Pediatrics,* 78 (July 1986), 159–163.

121. United States Public Health Service Advisory Committee on Immunization Practices, Revised Recommendations on Rubella Vaccine, *Pediatrics,* 65, no. 6 (1980), 6.

122. Varney, H., *Nurse-Midwifery* (2nd ed.). Boston: Blackwell Scientific Publications, 1987.

123. Ward-Wimmer, D., Nursing Care of Children With HIV Infection, *Nursing Clinics of North America,* 23, no. 4 (1991), 719–729.

124. Whitley, R., et al., A Controlled Trial Comparing Vidarabine With Acyclovir in Neonatal Herpes Simplex Virus Infection, *New England Journal of Medicine,* 324, no. 7 (1991), 444–449.

125. Whitley, R., et al., Predictors of Morbidity and Mortality in Neonates With Herpes Simplex Virus Infections, *New England Journal of Medicine,* 324, no. 7 (1991), 450–454.

126. Windsor, R.A., and C.T. Orleans, Guidelines and Methodological Standards for Smoking Cessation Intervention Research Among Pregnant Women: Improving the Science and Art, *Health Education Quarterly,* 13, no. 2 (1986), 131–136.

127. ———, et al., Smoking Cessation and Pregnancy Intervention Trial: Preliminary Mid-Trial Results in Advances in Cancer Control: Screening and Prevention Research, *Progress in Clinical and Biological Research,* 339 (1990), 107–117.

128. Working Group on HIV Testing of Pregnant Women and Newborns, HIV Infection, Pregnant Women, and Newborns, *Journal of American Medical Association,* 264, no. 18 (1990), 2416–2420.

129. Worthington-Roberts, B., and S.R. Williams, *Nutrition in Pregnancy and Lactation* (4th ed.). St. Louis: Times Mirror/Mosby, 1989.

130. Yazigi, R., R. Odem, and K. Polakoski, Demonstration of Specific Binding of Cocaine to Human Spermatozoa, *Journal American Medical Association,* 266, no. 14 (1991), 1956–1959.

131. Zlatnik, F.J., and L.F. Burmeister, Dietary Protein in Pregnancy: Effect on Anthropometric Indices of the Newborn, *American Journal of Obstetrics and Gynecology,* 146, no. 2 (1983), 199–203.

132. Zuckerman, B., et al., Effect of Maternal Marijuana and Cocaine Use on Fetal Growth, *New England Journal of Medicine,* 320 (1989), 762–768.

Part III

The Developing Person and Family: Infancy Through Adolescence

Chapter 7

Assessment and Health Promotion for the Infant

A baby is God's opinion that the world should go on.
—Carl Sandberg

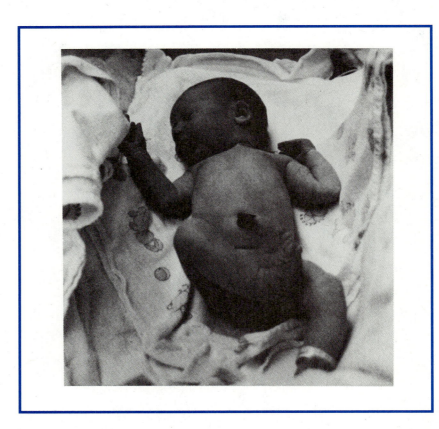

KEY TERMS

Neonate/newborn	Mongolian spots	Hernia	Cognitive behavior
Infant	Jaundice	Imperforate anus	Speech awareness
Mother (Parent[s])	Physiologic jaundice	Spina bifida	Speech
Crisis	Desquamation	Amblyopia	Language
Attachment	Umbilical cord	Colic	Undifferentiated cry
Bonding	Circumcision	Stools	Cooing
Engrossment	Phimosis	Colostrum	Babbling
Binding-in	Caput succedaneum	Burping	Lalling
Identification	Cephalohematoma	Weaning	Autistic
Claiming	Brown fat	Phenylketonuria (PKU)	Basic trust
Polarization	Surfactant	Immunizations	Mistrust
Psychologic abuse, battering, or maltreatment	Meconium	Herd immunity	Body image
	Reflex	Atopic dermatitis	Self-concept
Autistic behavior	Consummatory	Diaper dermatitis (rash)	Adaptive mechanisms
Anterior fontanel	Avoidant	Seborrheic dermatitis	Symbolization
Posterior fontanel	Exploratory	Oral candidiasis (thrush)	Condensation
Acrocyanosis	Social	Constipation	Incorporation
Lanugo	Attentional	Iron deficiency anemia	Displacement
Vernix caseosa	Micrograthia	Roseola infantum	Sexuality
Milia	Ptosis	Psychosocial development	Premature infant
Hemangiomas	Hydrocele	Intelligence	Congenital anomalies

OBJECTIVES

Study of this chapter will enable you to:

1. Define terms and give examples of basic developmental principles pertinent to the neonate and infant.
2. Discuss the crisis of birth for the family, factors that influence parental attachment and family response, and your role in assisting the family to adapt to this crisis and perform their developmental tasks.
3. Describe the adaptive physiologic changes that occur at birth.
4. Assess the neonate's physical characteristics and the manner in which psychosocial needs begin to be filled.
5. Contrast and assess the physiologic, motor, cognitive, linguistic, emotional, and social characteristics and adaptive mechanisms of the infant.
6. Discuss and assess the nutritional, sleep, movement, and play needs and patterns and sexuality development of the infant.
7. Interpret the immunization schedule and other safety and health promotion measures for a parent.
8. Discuss your role in assisting parents to foster the development of trust and a positive self-concept and to nurture the infant physically.
9. State the developmental tasks for the infant and behavior that indicates that these tasks are being met.
10. Compare parental behavior toward the infant who thrives with parental behavior toward the infant who fails to thrive.
11. Discuss your role in promoting parental attachment and preventing maternal deprivation and child abuse.
12. Begin to implement appropriate intervention measures with parents and baby after delivery and during the first year of life.

This chapter discusses the normal growth and development of the baby during the first year of life, baby's effect on the family, and the family's influence on baby. Measures to promote his or her welfare that are useful in nursing practice and that can be taught to parents are described throughout the chapter.

In this chapter the term **neonate,** or **newborn,** refers to the *first 4 weeks of life;* **infant** refers to the *first 12 months.* **Mother** or **parent(s)** are the terms used to *denote person(s) responsible for the child's care and long-term welfare.*

You can refer to an embryology and obstetric nursing book for detailed information on fetal development, prenatal changes, and the process of labor and delivery. This chapter builds on information presented in Chapters 4 and 6 and focuses on the developmental tasks of the infant and family after birth. The authors are aware that some characteristics and developmental tasks of the infant and family described here may vary in other countries. Certainly the infant will be slower to develop some characteristics and if he or she is born where there is famine, economic deprivation, political unrest or war, or devastation due to natural disaster. For example, for the child born in a refugee camp or between bombings, the parents have survival as the main task.

FAMILY DEVELOPMENT AND RELATIONSHIPS

The coming of the child is a **crisis,** a *turning point in the couple's life in which old patterns of living must be changed for new ways of living and new values* (59, 60, 77). The crisis may first be felt by the woman as she recognizes body changes and new emotional responses. The crisis may relate to losing the slim figure; determining how long she can work if she is in a career or profession and whether or not she can balance working and child rearing; making spatial changes in the home or moving to a new home to accommodate the baby; and balancing the budget to meet additional expenses. The crisis will be less if the baby is wanted than if the couple had planned on having no children. But having a baby is always a crisis—a change.

The crisis is greater when the baby is not planned for or wanted. Do not assume that either the woman or her partner is happy about the pregnancy. The woman may not deliberately seek an abortion, but she may not eat or may exercise vigorously in an effort to maintain a slim figure, not gain too much weight, or deny the pregnancy. Sometimes the man fears becoming a father and the consequent responsibility and loss of freedom. As the woman's pregnancy progresses and as she looks more pregnant and activity must be curtailed, the man may withdraw emotionally, be apathetic about the baby, spend more time with male friends, work associates, or other women, and avoid preparation for the baby's arrival. In turn, the woman spends more time alone and feels increasingly rejected, abandoned, depressed and angry. The woman may challenge the man's behavior, and more bickering, tension, resentment, and verbal (and sometimes physical) fighting occur in the martial relationship. The couple may separate unless both the man and woman are helped to admit and work through their feelings and recommit their love for each other. It is important that such assistance be given—for the future of both the baby and the parents (98).

"Your life will never be the same again." A starry-eyed expectant couple often hears this phrase. Being caught up in the romantic adventure of pregnancy, these words may fall on deaf ears. What do these words really imply?

With the advent of parenthood, a couple is embarking on a journey from which there is no return. To put it simply, parents cannot quit. Most losses in today's world are reversible. If the marriage partner is lost, the individ-ual can remarry; if a job is lost, a new position can be found. But an "I'll-try-it" attitude cannot be assumed toward parenthood. The child's birth brings a finality to many highly valued privileges and a permanence of responsibilities.

The young couple who has enjoyed an intense relationship suddenly finds a not-always-so-welcome onlooker and intruder. Gone for many years are sleeping late on Saturday mornings, last-minute social invitations or plans for a weekend trip, spontaneous sex, quiet meals by candlelight, an orderly house, and naps when desired. Of course, some of these activities can still be accomplished but never as freely as before. What was previously taken for granted now becomes a luxury. The "childhood" of parents comes to a screeching halt as the infant's needs take precedence.

Going to work, to visit friends, or even to shop is no easy task. Even a few hours away from home means making sure you have everything baby needs—bottle, food, pacifier, a few toys, a clothing change, and more than enough diapers. In addition to this armful, an infant seat or stroller must also be packed. By the time baby is dressed and everything is packed, Mom may want a nap more than anything else. Making sure baby is wearing a dry diaper before the final exit through the door becomes more important than the finishing touches of makeup or putting on the special jewelry for the outfit. If there are several small children to care for in addition to baby, the planning and effort are compounded, and older brothers and sisters can help with various tasks only to a certain point.

The intensity of the newcomer's demands may call for massive changes in life-style. Life changes have been correlated with illness susceptibility in the Social Readjustment Scale by Holmes and Rahe (60). When enough life changes occur within a year and add up to more than 300 points, trouble may lie ahead. Changes that may be connected with the addition of a family member total up to an ominous 397, as shown by the following list (59, 60). For some the score may be higher.

• Pregnancy	40
• Sex difficulties	39
• Gain of new family member	39
• Change in financial state	38
• Change in number of arguments with spouse	35
• Trouble with in-laws	29
• Wife begins or stops work	26
• Change in living conditions	25
• Revision of personal habits	24
• Change in recreation	19
• Change in church activities	19
• Change in social activities	18
• Change in sleeping habits	16
• Change in number of family get-togethers	15
• Change in eating habits	15
	397

Whether perceived as positive or negative, change always involves a sense of loss of the familiar, for the way it used to be. The vacuum created by the loss is a painful one and one for which parents are usually ill-prepared. The couple's life will never again be "normal" as they once knew it, but together the family now needs to find a "new normal."

If pregnancy and parenting create a crisis for a couple who want a baby, they are even more upheaving for the adolescent or for the woman who is the single-parent family—either unmarried or, if married, left by the husband or father to face pregnancy, birth, and child rearing alone. This adolescent/woman needs the support of and help from at least one other person during this period. A parent, relative, or friend can be a resource. Often the support and help of a number of people are needed. As a nurse, you may be the primary source of support. Your empathetic listening, acceptance, practical hints for better self-care and baby care, and general availability can make a real difference in the outcome of the pregnancy and in the mother's ability to parent—and in her ability to handle future crises. Referral to other resources and self-help groups such as Coping With Overall Parenting Experience (COPE) and Parents Without Partners or to a counselor may also be of great help to the mother.

Growth and Development of Parents

An increasing number of people are not prepared either intellectually or emotionally for family life because of the lack of nurturing or because of the difficult family life they experienced in childhood. Creating and maintaining a family unit are difficult in today's society. Many occupations demand travel, frequent change of residence, and working on Sundays and holidays, the traditional family days. The rapid pace of life and available opportunities interfere with family functions. The close-knit interdependence of the old family unit is being replaced with a group of individuals whose lives seem merely thrown together.

Expectations for self and others have increased. For example, the woman may be striving for success in several areas. No longer is being a wife and mother enough: many women seek a career as well. All these expectations conflict with a strong family life, for children demand parents become other-centered instead of self-centered.

In spite of today's difficulties in maintaining a family unit, the norm still exists to have children. Thus many couples wander rather naively into the developmental crisis of parenthood. In a culture in which adolescence may last until the mid-twenties, most young people are just getting used to being called Ma'am or Sir when suddenly they become Mom and Dad. Thus along with the developmental tasks of finding identity and intimacy may be superimposed the task of being generative as well.

"Pregnancy is preparation . . . birth is the event . . . parenting is a process" (34). Becoming a parent involves grieving the loss of one's own childhood and former life-style. The person must be in touch with and be able to express and work through feelings of loss before he or she can adapt and move on to a higher level of maturation. Being aware of the tremendous influence of parents on their children's development, parents may feel challenged to become the best persons they are capable of being. New parents may need to develop a confidence that they do not feel, an integrity that has been easy to let slide, and values that can tolerate being scrutinized. To grow and develop as a parent, the person needs to make peace with his or her past so that unresolved conflicts are not inflicted on the child.

After a baby joins the family, a number of problems must be worked through. The mother must deal with the separation from a symbiotic relationship with the baby. The reality of child care and managing a household may be a disillusionment after exposure to the American ideals inculcated by the mass media and advertising.

One of the potential problem areas that you can explore with parents is that of reestablishing a mutually satisfying sexual relationship, which is not a simple psychologic process but has intricate psychologic overtones for man and woman. You may also need to address the couple's desire for family planning (see Table 12–3 in Chapter 12 for information on contraceptive measures). Sexual relationships usually decrease during pregnancy, childbirth, and the postpartum period. By 6 weeks after birth the woman's pelvis is back to normal; lochia has ceased; involution is complete; and physically she is ready for an active sex life. But the mother may be so absorbed in and fatigued by the challenges and responsibilities of motherhood that the father is pushed into the background. Father may feel in competition with baby, resenting both the baby and his wife.

Either one may take initiative in renewing the role of lover, in being sexually attractive to the other. The woman can do this by getting a new hairdo or stylish clothes for the now slimmer outward figure. Inwardly, she can strengthen flabbly perineal muscles through prescribed exercise. Patience on the part of the husband is also necessary, for if an episiotomy was done before delivery, healing continues for some time, and the memory of pain in the area may cause the woman involuntarily to tense the perineal muscles and wish to forego intercourse. Happy couples who have a sound philosophy and communication system soon work out such problems, including the fact that the baby's needs will sometimes interrupt intimacy. For couples whose earlier sex life was unsatisfactory and who do not work together as a team, such problems may be hard to surmount. The woman may prolong nursing, complain of fatigue, ill health, or pain. The man may find other outlets (40).

Husband and wife must reestablish effective communication so that they can share feelings of pride, joy, anxiety, insecurity, and frustrations of early parenthood, avoid eclipsing their marriage by the new family roles, and understand the involvement of the multiple roles of mate, parents, and persons. Your support, suggestions, and assistance in helping the couple seek and accept help from family and friends fosters their ability to manage.

Given the whole realm of stresses and life changes associated with a baby's birth, it is understandable that at least initially parenting is at best a bittersweet experience. Parents feel strong ambivalences and what Angela Barron McBride (88) calls "normal crazy" thoughts and feelings toward this child whom they have together created.

The following stress factors may be used in your assessment to predict the likelihood of postpartum difficulties (49):

1. Primapara (woman having her first baby)
2. No relatives available for help with baby care
3. Complications of pregnancy in family history
4. Woman's mother dead
5. Woman ill apart from pregnancy
6. Woman ill during pregnancy
7. Woman's education higher than that of her parents
8. Male partner often away from home or not involved with pregnancy or child rearing
9. Woman with no previous experience with babies

Postpartum difficulties are also more likely if the parent is an adolescent or has suffered child abuse. The more past and present stresses, the more difficulty the woman has in coping with the postpartum experience (49).

Parenting is a risky process. It involves facing the unknown with faith because no one can predict the outcome when the intricacies of human relationships are involved. Parents grow and develop by taking themselves and their child one day at a time and by realizing the joy that can be part of those crazy, hectic early weeks and months. The feelings of joy and involvement increase as the parent-child attachment is cemented.

Because establishing this attachment is crucial to the long-term nurturing of the child and parental interest in the child, the process will be explored in depth to assist you in assessment and intervention.

Infant-Parent Attachment

Attachment is a *close and reciprocal relationship between two people that involves contact and close proximity and endures through time* (Fig. 7–1). **Bonding** usually refers to the *initial maternal feeling and attachment behavior immediately following delivery.* **Engrossment** is a term used to describe the *father's initial paternal response to the baby.* Table 7–1 outlines the

Figure 7-1.   Mother-infant attachment develops mutually over the first year of life. (From Sherwen, L.N., M.A. Scoloveno, and C.T. Weingarten, *Nursing Care of the Childbearing Family.* Norwalk, Conn: Appleton & Lange, 1991, p. 44.)

optimum behaviors of the infant, mother, and father in the typical order of progression in establishing this initial tie (8, 14–16, 32, 51, 62, 113, 115, 116, 135). The extent to which these behaviors are shown depend on how much contact is permitted by the hospital or staff between parents and baby.

Some research shows that all mothers do not initially follow the sequence of handling that is described in most of the literature and in Table 7–1. Some mothers initially use palms or arms to handle the infant and then their fingers to explore the infant. Often mothers simultaneously use fingers and palms and then arms and trunk to explore and hold the baby. These differences should be considered in assessment of maternal bonding and attachment (136, 137).

The state of the infant is a strong predictor of the relative frequency with which fathers display interactional behavior, affection, and comfort toward the infant. Very young crying infants are comforted or shown affectional behavior. Fathers are most likely to stimulate by touch those infants who are awake but not crying. Fathers are as likely to talk in a stimulating manner to crying as noncrying and to sleeping as awake infants. Perhaps fathers perceive talking as less soothing to crying infants than touch and less disturbing than touch to sleeping infants. Infant state behaviors are strongly related to affectional paternal responses, indicating that new fathers begin early to read and respond to infant cues (67).

Studies in bonding and attachment have been done primarily on middle-class, reasonably well-educated Caucasians. Bonding and attachment behaviors, especially for the male, could be different in other racial and cultural groups. Some cultures emphasize the mother as

TABLE 7-1. INFANT-PARENT ATTACHMENT BEHAVIORS

Infant	Mother	Father
Reflexly looks into mother's face, *establishes eye-to-eye contact* or *"face tie"*; molds body to mother's body when held	*Reaches* for baby; *holds high against breast-chest-shoulder area;* handles baby smoothly	Has great *interest in baby's face and notes eyes*
Vocalizes, cries, and *stretches out arms* in response to mother's voice; responds to mother's voice with *"dance"* or *rhythmic movements*	Talks softly in *high-pitched voice* and with intense interest to baby; puts baby face-to-face with her (*en face position);* eye contact gives baby sense of identity to mother	*Desires to touch, pick up, and hold baby;* cradles baby securely; shows more fingertip touching and smiling to male baby; has more eye contact with infant delivered by forceps or cesarean section
Roots, licks, then *sucks* mother's nipple if in contact with mother's breast; cries, smiles	*Touches* baby's extremities; examines, strokes, massages, and kisses baby shortly after delivery; puts baby to breast if permitted; oxytocin and prolactin released	*Looks for distinct features;* thinks newborn resembles self; perceives baby as beautiful in spite of newborn characteristics
Reflexly embraces, clambers, clings, using hands, feet, head, and mouth to maintain body contact	*Calls baby by name;* notes desirable traits; *expresses pleasure* toward baby; *attentive* to reflex actions of grunts and sneezes	*Feels elated,* bigger, proud after birth; has strong *desire to protect and care for child*
Odor of mother distinguished by breast-feeding baby by fifth day	*Recognizes odor* of own child by third or fourth day	

NOTE: Similar behaviors are seen with a premature baby but the timing will vary.

caretaker of the infant; the bond or attachment between father and child is less overt and may be emphasized later in childhood.

The first hour after birth apparently is a critical time for stimulating attachment feelings and bonding in the parents since then the baby tends to have eyes open, gazes around, has stronger sucking reflexes, cries more, and shows more physical activity than in subsequent hours (51).

In addition to causing an increased alertness in the baby, effective maternal-infant bonding can promote baby's physical health: transference of maternal nasal and respiratory flora to baby may prevent him from acquiring hospital strains of staphylococci; maternal body heat is a reliable source of heat for the newborn; and regular breast feedings can pass on the antibodies IgA and T and B lymphocytes to baby to protect against enteric pathogens (71, 106).

Binding-in is the term Rubin (115, 116, 118) uses to describe the *maternal-child relationship as a process that is active, intermittent, and accumulative over a period of 12 to 15 months*. Maternal identity is essential for the binding-in process, and both maternal identity and binding-in are either enhanced or inhibited by the infant's behavior and society. The process involves (1) identification of the infant by the mother as part of self and belonging to self; (2) claiming the child as her own emotionally and physically; and (3) polarization or separating the infant from the unity of self and fetus.

Maternal binding-in is stimulated by fetal movements and the physical needs of the newborn. After birth, fantasies about the child are replaced by an object to see, touch, hear, smell, and care for, which organizes maternal behavior and attitudes. Sex, size, and condition of the infant are critical to the maternal response. Complete **identification** occurs when the *mother knows by looking, touching, hearing, or smelling that the child is well or unwell, hungry or satisfied, comfortable or in distress.* **Claiming** *occurs with the mother's commitment to the child in labor and delivery and is seen in the pleasure with the birth of the child.* Claiming also occurs by association with significant others in the social environment who claim the infant and her. **Polarization,** *separating from the symbiotic relationship with the fetus, begins with labor and delivery.* Gradually the woman realizes the baby is not inside of her. The infant is held, nurtured, and compared to self and family members but is increasingly seen as a separate, unique individual and less as an extension of self and her own body image. Family life is reorganized; the baby is included in family activities. Over the period of the first year the mother can let go of the child as he or she gains motor, social, and emotional competence. The psychologic loosening allows the mother also to give the child more physical space (115, 116, 118).

Development of attachment between parent and baby continues through infancy. It involves emotional, cognitive, and socialization processes: loving through cuddling, touching, stroking, kissing, cooing and talking to, laughing, playing with, and reinforcing and teaching baby. Such contact should be consistent and done while caring physically for baby. The touching, cooing, talking and laughing can also be focused on baby while mother (or father) is preparing a meal, doing a household task, or waiting in a grocery line. The parent's voice across the room can also soothe and contributes to attachment. Further, just as the parent may need to learn to respond to the infant, sometimes the child needs prompting to be responsive to the parent and to signal needs and not just wait for every need to be automatically met.

Factors Influencing Maternal Attachment

Motherly feelings do not necessarily accompany biologic motherhood. Various factors affect the mother's attachment and care taking. Variables that are difficult or impossible to change include the woman's level of emotional maturity, how she was reared, what her culture encourages her to do, relationships with her family and partner, experience with previous pregnancies, and planning for and events during the course of this pregnancy (32, 62, 71, 106, 115, 117).

Deterrents to adequate mothering include the mother's own immaturity or lack of mothering, stress situations, fear of rejection from significant people, loss of a loved one, financial worries, lack of a supportive partner, and even the gender and appearance of the child. Separating mother and infant the first few days of life, depersonalized care by professionals, rigid hospital routines, and too early discharge from the hospital without adequate help also interfere with establishing attachment and maternal behaviors (16, 32, 52, 62, 71). Assess for these deterrents. Your nurturing of the mother and helping her seek additional help may offset the negative impact of these factors.

Parenting skills can be manifested in various ways. Although eye contact, touch, and cuddling are important, love can be shown by a tender, soft voice and loving gazes. Observe other indications of warm parenting feelings:

1. Calls the baby by name
2. Expresses enjoyment of the baby and indicates that the baby is attractive or has other positive characteristics
3. Looks at the baby and into baby's eyes
4. Talks to the baby in a loving voice
5. Takes safety precautions for the baby
6. Responds to the baby's cues for attention or physical care

Factors Influencing Paternal Attachment

Fatherly feelings do not necessarily accompany fatherhood. Bonding and attachment feelings in the father appear related to various factors: general level of education, participation in prenatal classes, gender of infant, role concept, attendance at delivery, type of delivery, early contact, and feeding method for baby (8, 14, 51, 135).

Support from the mother is most effective in reducing stress levels in expectant fathers; support from others is critical only if the expectant woman cannot be supportive. This may be because intimacy and self-disclosure for men is maintained primarily in the partner relationship. For the expectant woman, support from both the partner and others is critical in coping with stress, perhaps because women are socialized to value and depend on social relations to a greater extent than men (22).

Father is increasingly recognized as an important person to the infant and young child, not only as a bread-winner but also as a nurturer. Lack of a father figure can cause developmental difficulties for the child. Just as the mother is not necessarily endowed with nurturing feelings, the father is not necessarily lacking nurturing feelings. Some fathers seem to respond better to this role than their spouses.

The man who nurtures his children may meet some resistance in a society in which this role is sometimes considered unmanly, although social attitudes are changing. One father who was taking the basic child-raising responsibilities while his wife pursued the major family career was ostracized when he appeared at a meeting calling for "scout mothers." No women sat with him until he initiated conversation explaining why he was there. Occasionally the mother herself cannot understand when the father seems to cherish the nurturing role. She feels that her position is threatened, her husband is not acting "as a man," or he loves the children more than he loves her. Actually, the man who is allowed to express these feelings often simultaneously develops an even closer feeling for his wife.

Behavior Characteristic of Parental Difficulty in Establishing Attachment

Realize that parents tend to project their own feelings onto their child, turning the child into a figure from their own past. Negative feelings in the parent can create a dysfunctional relationship with the child.

Note the methods of relating to and holding the infant that would indicate the parent's *difficulty in establishing attachment:*

1. Maintains little or no eye contact with baby
2. Does not touch baby, or picks up baby at times to meet own needs
3. Does not support baby's head
4. Holds baby at a distance, at arm's length, loosely, or not at all
5. Appears disinterested in baby, preoccupied with something else when baby is present, and has a flat, fixed facial expression or unconvincing smile in response to your enthusiasm about baby
6. Perceives baby as unattractive or looking like someone who is disliked
7. Talks or coos to baby little or not at all
8. Has passive response to baby; allows baby to be placed in arms rather than reaching out to baby
9. Calls baby "it" rather than saying "my baby" or calling baby by name
10. Notes defects or undesirable traits in baby, even if baby is normal, or is convinced baby is abnormal
11. Avoids talking about baby, even when someone else initiates the topic
12. Expresses dissatisfaction with or revulsion about care of baby
13. Ignores baby's communications of cries, grunts, sneezes, and yawns

14. Gets upset when baby's secretions, feces, or urine touch body or clothes; perceives care of baby as revolting
15. Readily gives baby to someone else
16. Does not take adequate safety precautions with baby (e.g., in relation to diapering, feeding, covering baby, or baby's movements)
17. Handles the baby roughly, even after the baby has eaten or vomited
18. Gives inappropriate responses to baby's needs such as over- or underfeeding, over- or underhandling
19. Thinks baby does not love him or her
20. Expresses dislike of self, finds attribute in baby that is disliked in self
21. Complains of being too tired to take care of baby
22. Expresses fears that baby might die of a minor illness (10, 14, 31, 32, 115, 116)

You may not observe all these behaviors in the mother, initially or in the mother or father later, but a combination of several should alert you to actual or potential difficulty with being a parent.

Three components must be present before child abuse occurs: (1) the parents must have the potential for abuse; (2) there must be a special child; and (3) there must be a crisis or series of crises. The cycle of abuse can be prevented or treated by intervening with one of these components (90).

Parents Anonymous, a nationwide organization of and for adults with child abuse problems, recognizes six forms of child abuse: (1) physical abuse, (2) physical neglect, (3) emotional abuse, (4) emotional neglect, (5) verbal abuse, and (6) sexual abuse (90).

Be aware of the parent who has such *difficulty with attachment that maltreatment or abuse of the child results*. Types of abuse, signs and symptoms of the abused child, and characteristics of the child who suffers abuse, neglect, or material deprivation and characteristics of the abusing parent are presented in Chapter 6. Chapter 4 also describes characteristics and behaviors of the parent who has difficulty with parenting.

Garbarino, Guttmann, and Seeley (46) describe types of psychologic abuse, battering, or maltreatment. ***Psychologic abuse, battering or maltreatment*** is a *deliberate pattern of attack by a parent or an adult on a child's developmental status, sense of self, or social competence.*

Box 7–1 presents parental behaviors that are characteristic of psychologic abuse or maltreatment. As a result of maltreatment, the child becomes vulnerable to negative forces in the broader social environment, does not develop a sense of trust, and becomes emotionally, socially, and sometimes physically, ill (46).

Garbarino, Guttmann, and Seeley (46) discuss strategies and tools for identification and intervention with the family, individual child, and institutional network of social services.

BOX 7-1
Parental Behaviors Characteristic of Psychologic Maltreatment of the Infant

Rejecting
- Refuses to accept the child's attachment behavior or spontaneous overtures
- Refuses to return smiles and vocalizations

Isolating
- Denies child the experience of enduring patterns of interaction
- Leaves the child in its room unattended for long periods
- Denies access to the child by interested others

Terrorizing
- Exposes the child consistently and deliberately to intense stimuli or frequent change of routine
- Teases, scares, or gives extreme or unpredictable response to child's behavior

Ignoring
- Fails to respond to infant's spontaneous behavior that forms basis for attachment
- Does not respond to infant's smiles, vocalizations, or developing competence and changing skill

Corrupting
- Reinforces bizarre habits
- Creates alcohol or drug addictions
- Reinforces the child for oral sexual contact

From Garbarino, J., E. Guttmann, and J. Seeley, *The Psychologically Battered Child: Strategies for Identification, Assessment, and Intervention.* San Francisco: Jossey-Bass, 1987. Copyright 1986 by Jossey-Bass, Inc., Publishers.

Helberg (57) gives specific criteria for documentation of child abuse.

Switzer (134) describes legal definitions of child abuse in various states, who is required to report and reporting procedures, the legal effects of failure to report in various states, and confidentiality issues.

The article by Mittelman, Mittelman, and Wetu (95) shows pictures of both subtle and obvious abuse and gives detailed and specific description for clues that will assist you in assessing the child.

Personalizing Nursing Care to Promote Attachment

Call the child, mother, and father by their names during your care. Inquire about the mother's well-being; too often all the focus is on the baby. She is in a receptive state and must be emotionally and physically cared for. Father may also need nurturance before he can show caring and be helpful to mother and baby. Every minute of contact must be well used. Make favorable comments about the infant's progress. Compliment the mother on her intentions or ability to comfort, feed, or identify her baby's needs. Speak of the pleasure baby shows in response to the parent's ministrations. Reassure parents that positive changes in baby are a result of their care, and avoid judgmental attitudes or guilt statements. Encourage both parents to cuddle, look at, and talk to the baby; if necessary, demonstrate how to stroke, caress, and rock baby. Encourage parents to be prompt and consistent in answering the infant's cry. Encourage parents to rely on their own values and judgment, to trust their feelings, and to take action and responsibility for them. Parents will learn that the baby is tougher than he or she looks.

As you support, teach, and counsel, the following *interventions can promote mother-infant attachment and optimum infant stimulation:*

1. Assist mother soon after birth in gaining confidence in her ability to respond effectively to baby's cry through recognizing the meaning of the cry and using soothing measures such as rocking, redundant sounds, or swaddling.

2. Explain the infant's interactive abilities during the early puerperium and help the mother develop awareness of her own initial effective responses to the newborn's behavior.

3. Explain the basis of early infant learning as the discovery of associations, connections, and relationships between self and repeated occurrences. Explore how to provide variety and a gradually increasing level of stimuli complexity; sights, sounds, smells, movements, positions, temperatures, and pressure all provide learning opportunities and opportunities for emotional, perceptual, social, and physical development.

4. Call attention to baby and those behaviors that indicate developmental responsiveness such as reflex movements, visual following, smiling, raising chin off bed, rolling over, and sitting alone. Pupil dilation in the presence of another person or a valued object begins at approximately 4 weeks of age. During the first few weeks of life baby prefers the human face to other visual images.

5. Differentiate between contact stimulation and representative behaviors present in fetal life. Pressure and touch sensation are present a few months before birth; thus the newborn responds well to touch and gentle pressure. Rooting and hand-mouth activity occur in fetal life and is a major adaptive activity after birth.

6. Emphasize the importance of visual and auditory skills for developing social behaviors during the first 2 months of life.

7. Encourage mutual eye contact between mother and baby; all infant's efforts to vocalize should be reinforced. Eye contact between the dyad increases during the first 3 months of life and is soon accompa-

nied by other social responses—smiling and vocalization.

8. Encourage regular periods of affectionate play when the infant is alert and responsive. Mother may pick up and hold the baby close, encourage visual following and smiling, and talk to the infant, repeating sounds. Rhythm and repetition are enjoyed. Often baby is most alert after a daytime feeding.

9. Promote awareness in other family members of baby's competencies so that they can also respond to and reinforce the infant.

You can inform the nursing team about progress in the mother-infant interaction process to assist other members with assessment and intervention. Riesch and Munns (111) suggest that information about the infant's interactional potential and the maternal behaviors that support and enhance that potential should be included in all standard plans of maternal-neonatal nursing care.

Several tools are designed to help you assess baby, mother, and mother's attitude toward baby as you continue their care (10, 17, 27, 31). The *Neonatal Behavioral Assessment Scale* points out unique characteristics and strengths of the neonate (17). For example, you can demonstrate to the parents how the newborn can follow the direction of the mother's soft high-pitched voice as she moves from the line of baby's vision.

The *Neonatal Perception Inventory* gauges how the mother feels about the infant through how she feels about herself. Other inventories that question the mother about her perception of the baby are the *Average Perception Inventory and Your Baby*. They are completed at 1 and 2 days' postpartum, and two inventories are repeated again in 1 month, along with the *Degree of Bother Inventory*. If the infant is not perceived as better than average and if the degree of bother index is too high, psychiatric problems in the child may be predicted (21, 32). The *Blank Infant Tenderness Scale* can be used to measure mother's perceptions of infant tenderness needs and ability to give physical and emotional nurturance (12). The *Dyadic Interaction Code* is a tool for studying over time the interaction process between mother and newborn. There is rhythmicity in the mother-infant interaction, associated with synchronous interactions, heightened levels of positive affect, and extended periods of attention. The baby who is preterm, not healthy, or suffering from congenital anomalies may not be as responsive to the mother, thus interrupting rhythmicity and attachment (29).

Bishop (10) describes an extensive assessment tool that can be used to assess the mother's physical and emotional energy, support systems available to the mother, and the mother's current level of parenting activity. The tool is used for several visits, combining repeated observations and interviews, to obtain an accurate and comprehensive assessment. As you pinpoint problems by means of these inventories, you should be able to intervene or direct the parents to a helpful resource.

Incorporate the parents' cultural beliefs, values, and attitudes into your nursing care and modern health-care practices whenever possible. Maintaining important cultural traditions is one way to individualize care. Satz (121) gives specific examples of how she incorporated the values of the Navajo in promoting attachment. Specific traditions may extend to naming or bathing the baby, prenatal and postnatal care of mother, how to hold or dress baby, inclusion or exclusion of father from the delivery, and roles of various family members. Be sensitive to the preferences of clients who represent a culture different from your own. Listen to and observe carefully their requests. Listen to what is not said but is implied. Suggest rather than advise or direct when you teach.

Listen attentively for information and signs that give you clues to the parents' feelings about themselves, where they are in their own developmental growth, who they rely on for strength, their ideas about child discipline, and their expectations of the new child. As you see weaknesses or gaps in necessary information, you can instruct. If your approach is right, the parents will recognize you as a helpful friend. Mothers are receptive to your information and to your reinforcement of the mother's mothering skills.

While you are helping parents with discharge planning, remember that soon the complete focus on mother-father-new baby will be gone. Other roles will be reestablished: husband, wife, employer or employee, student, daughter, son, friend. The new parents will have to allow for all aspects of their personalities to function again. Baby will have to fit in.

While you are caring for baby, you will no doubt feel great satisfaction. However, remember that the child belongs to the parents; this is not *your* baby. Do not become so involved that through your actions you push aside the parents and cause them to feel ineffective.

Baby's Influence on Parents

Some babies have a high activity level and warm up easily to the parent; some are quiet, withdrawn, with a low activity level; and various other mixtures of activity level and temperament exist. The infant's dominant reaction pattern to new situations manifests an innate temperament, and the temperament affects the reactions of others, expecially the parents. They in turn will mold baby's reaction pattern (28, 106).

It is easy to love a lovable baby, but parents have to work harder with babies who are not highly responsive. You should assess the reactions between baby and parents since the style of child care that will develop has its basis here. A highly active mother who expects an intense reaction may have a hard time mothering a low-activity, quiet baby because she may misinterpret the baby's behavior, feel rejected, and in turn reject the child. Baby will be denied the stimulation necessary for development. If the mother is withdrawn, quiet, and unexpressive and has a high-activity baby, she may punish the baby for normal energetic or assertive behavior and ignore the bids for affection and stimulation. The child needs to feel his or her behavior will produce an effect or he or she will stop contacting the parents. Extreme parental rejection or lack of reaction causes the syndrome of neglect and deprivation, emotional illness, and **autistic behavior,** characterized by *self-absorption, isolation from the world, obsession with sameness, repetitive behavior, and lack of language communication with others* (7). An assertive child may become controlling with an indecisive mother and not learn that others also have needs and rights. If baby is controlled by mother, he or she cannot develop trust, independence, or ability to cope with persons on equal terms. If the mother overanticipates the child's needs, the child becomes passive and dependent.

Help parents understand the *mutual response* between baby and themselves, and help them learn to read the baby's signals and to give consistent signals to the baby. All parents feel incompetent and despairing at times when they are unable to understand the child's cues and meet needs, but if self-confidence is consistently lacking, the parent's despair may turn to anger, rejection, and abuse.

Expansion of Intrafamily Relationships

Grandparents-to-be and other relatives frequently become more involved with the parents-to-be, bringing gifts and advice, neither of which is necessarily desired. Yet their gifts and supportive presence can be a real help if the grandparents respect the independence of the couple, if the couple has resolved their earlier adolescent rebellion and dependency conflicts, and if the grandparents' advice does not conflict with the couple's philosophy or the doctor's advice. The couple and grandparents should collaborate rather than compete. Grandparents should be reminded not to take over the situation, and the couple's autonomy should be encouraged in that they can listen to the various pieces of advice, evaluate the statements, and then as a unit make their own decision. In addition, parents should refrain from expecting the grandparents to be built-in baby-sitters and to rescue them from every problem. Grandparents usually enjoy brief rather than prolonged contact with baby care. For the single parent, the grandparents or other relatives can be a major source of emotional and financial help and can provide help with child care.

You may assist the parent(s) in working with grandparents—resolving feelings of either being controlled or not adequately helped, understanding grandparents' feelings, accepting help, and avoiding excessive demands.

In some cultures the maternal grandmother has a major role in care of the pregnant and postpartum daughter and in care of the infant. The grandmother may give advice about nutrition, self-care, or baby care to the daughter; however, the advice may be contrary to scientific and medical knowledge and practices. Establish rapport with both the grandmother and the pregnant woman or the mother. Respect the role of the grandmother. Often the advice she gives is culturally based—the practices have maintained the group for centuries. The practices may be carried out along with modern-day health and medical practices. If the advice is truly harmful to the mother or baby, your rapport, nonjudgmental approach, and well-timed, low-key teaching to the grandmother may help her to accept the teaching you direct to the pregnant woman/mother. Indeed, if either or both grandparents are considered the head of the household, direct your attention initially to them and direct your teaching to them. Initial or exclusive focus on their daughter is likely to alienate them so that they discontinue coming for care or become resistive and not allow their daughter to carry out your teaching.

PHYSIOLOGIC CONCEPTS

Neonate—Physical Characteristics

The neonatal period of infancy includes the critical transition from parasitic fetal existence to physiologic independence. The normal newborn is described in the following pages; references 81, 106, 126, and 131 are used. Transition begins at birth with the first cry. Air is sucked in to inflate the lungs. Complex chemical changes are initiated in the cardiorespiratory system so that the baby's heart and lungs can assume the burden of oxygenating the body. The foramen ovale closes during the first 24 hours; the ductus arteriosus closes after several days. For the first time, baby experiences light, gravity, cold, and firm touch.

The newborn is relatively resistant to stress of anoxia and can survive longer in an oxygen-free atmosphere than an adult. The reason is unknown, as are the long-term effects of *mild* oxygen deprivation (106, 131).

General Appearance

The newborn does not match the baby ads and may be a shock to new parents. The mis-shapen head, flat nose, puffy eyelids and often undistinguished eye color, discolored skin, large tongue and undersized lower jaw, short neck and small sloping shoulders, short limbs and large rounded abdomen with protruding umbilical stump that remains to 3 weeks, and bowed skinny legs may prove very disappointing if the parents are unprepared for the sight of a newborn. The head, which accounts for one fourth of the total body size, appears large in relation to the body.

The **anterior fontanel,** a *diamond-shaped area at the top of the front of the head,* and the **posterior fontanel,** a *triangular-shaped area at the center back of the head,* are often called **soft spots.** These unossified areas of the skull bones, along with the suture lines of the bones, allow the bones to overlap during delivery and also allow for expansion of the brain as they gradually fill in with bone cells. The posterior fontanel closes by 2 or 3 months; the anterior fontanel closes between 8 and 18 months. These soft spots may add to the parents' impression that the newborn is too fragile to handle (82).

Reassure the parents that the newborn, although in need of tender, gentle care, is also resilient and adaptable. The head and fontanels can be gently touched without harm, although strong pressure or direct injury should be avoided. Reassure them also that the baby will soon take on the features of the family members and look more as they expected.

Apgar Scoring System

The physical status of the newborn is determined with the Apgar tool 1 minute after birth and then 5 minutes later. The newborn's respirations, heart rate, muscle tone, reflex activities, and color are observed. A maximum score of 2 is given to each sign, so that the score could range from 0 to 10, as indicated by Table 7–2. A score less than 7 means that the newborn is having difficulty adapting, needs even closer observation than usual, and may need life-saving intervention (125).

Gestational Age Assessment

In addition to using the Apgar score, assessment includes estimating gestational age to use parameters other than weight to assess an infant's level of maturity.

TABLE 7-2. ASSESSMENT OF THE NEWBORN: APGAR SCORING SYSTEM

Sign	0		1	2
Heart rate	Absent		Less than 100 beats per min	More than 100 beats per min
Respirations	Absent		Slow, irregular	Cry; regular rate
Muscle tone	Flaccid		Some flexion of extremities	Active movements
Reflex irritability	None		Grimace	Cry
Color	Body cyanotic or pale		Body pink; extremities cyanotic	Body completely pink

Modified from Sciarra, J.J., ed., *Gynecology and Obstetrics.* Philadelphia: Harper & Row, 1982.

By considering *both birth weight* and *gestational age,* you can categorize infants into one of several groupings. Problems can then be anticipated and, if present, be identified and treated early. Assessment can be done as early as the first day of life and should be done no later than the fifth day of life since external criteria such as hip abduction, square window, dorsiflexion of foot, and size of breast nodules change after 5 to 6 days of life. If the neonate is examined on the first day of life, he or she should be examined again before the fifth day to detect neurologic changes. The score can be affected by asphyxia or maternal anesthesia.

To assess gestational age several sources can be used: The *Dubowitz Guide to Gestational Age Assessment* includes an examination of 10 neurologic and 11 external signs (38). Ballard et al. (3) have modified the Dubowitz Scale. *Colorado Clinical Estimation of Gestational Age—A Guide* includes obstetric data and physical and neurologic criteria and defines when certain characteristics should be present. For best results, assess the infant according to the Dubowitz and Colorado scales. Add scores together; the sum of the scores will correlate with a certain gestational age in weeks. Plot the baby's weight and gestational age in weeks on the Colorado Growth Chart. This will place the infant in one of nine categories based on *age* and *weight*.

Skin

The skin is thin, delicate, and usually mottled, varies from pink to reddish, and becomes very ruddy when the baby cries. **Acrocyanosis,** *bluish color of the hands and feet,* is the result of sluggish peripheral circulation that occurs normally only a few days after birth. **Lanugo,** *downy hair of fetal life,* most evident on shoulders, back extremities, forehead, and temples, is lost after a few months and is replaced by other hair growth. The *cheesy skin covering,* **vernix caseosa,** is left on for protective reasons; it rubs off in a few days. **Milia,** *tiny white spots that are small collections of sebaceous secretions,* are sprinkled on the nose and forehead and should not be squeezed or picked; they will disappear. **Hemangiomas,** *pink spots* on the upper eyelids, between eyebrows, on the nose, upper lip, or back may or may not be permanent. **Mongolian spots,** *slate-colored areas* on buttocks or lower back in Black, Oriental, or Mediterranean babies, fade without treatment. If a birthmark is present, parents should be assured it is not their fault. **Jaundice,** *yellowish discoloration of skin,* should be noted. If it occurs during the first 24 hours of life, it is usually caused by blood incompatibility between mother's and baby's blood and requires medical investigation and possibly treatment. **Physiologic jaundice** normally appears on the third or fourth day of life because the excess number of red blood cells present in fetal life that are no longer needed are undergoing hemolysis, which in turn causes high levels of bilirubin (a bile pigment) in the bloodstream. The jaundice usually disappears in approximately 1 week when the baby's liver has developed the ability to metabolize the bilirubin. If bilirubin levels are excessively high, the neonate is placed under full-spectrum lights (phototherapy) to promote bilirubin breakdown. The baby's eyes must be covered during phototherapy.

Parents should be reassured about these and other conditions of the skin that normally occur. Foot or hand prints are made for identification since these lines remain permanently. **Desquamation,** *peeling of skin,* appears in 2 to 4 weeks.

Umbilical Cord

The *bluish-white, gelatinous structure that transports maternal blood from placenta to fetus* is the **umbilical cord.** It is cut 1½ to 3 inches from baby's abdominal wall. Because of the high water content, the stump of the cord dries and shrinks rapidly, losing its flexibility by 24 hours after birth. By the second day, it is a very hard yellow or black (blood) tab on the skin. Slight oozing where the cord joins the abdominal wall is common and offers an excellent medium for bacterial growth.

The area should be cleaned with cotton balls and alcohol several times daily until the cord has dropped off (6 to 14 days) and for 2 or 3 days after the cord falls off when the area is completely healed. Parents should be taught this procedure.

Circumcision

The *surgical removal of the foreskin,* **circumcision,** is done almost automatically on newborn males. In contrast to past belief, this is a painful procedure for the baby, as shown by the cry (103). The same reasons are given by people in different cultures either to do or not to do circumcision. These reasons include:

1. Sign of manhood
2. Cultural norms
3. Sexuality concerns
4. Hygienic, cosmetic, or comfort concerns
5. Biblical or religious mandate
6. Prevention of later genitourinary problems
7. Medical advice

The main difference among various cultural groups related to circumcision is the issue of pain. Some people believe the procedure is not harmful or even very painful to infants; others believe it is traumatic and dangerous (54). Although it is part of religious ritual for the Jewish male, most families have the boy circumcised to facilitate hygiene of the penis and to decrease the risk of penile cancer.

Although there are risks to circumcision, these complications occur infrequently. Irritation and infection can occur. Hemorrhage is the most common complication, requiring sutures or pressure dressings that can cause scarring, deformity, or **phimosis** *(tightening of the foreskin).* If the physician is not skilled, various surgical mishaps may occur. Although rare, septicemia with osteo-myelitis, pulmonary abscess, and death may occur. Physicians are now questioning the necessity of circumcision. Good hygiene provides the same medical benefits without the risk of surgery and the pain (103, 131). Parents may feel they have no choice about circumcision. Discuss the procedure with them so that their action is based on information. Further, you may share that the American Academy of Pediatrics states there are no medical indications for circumcision. However, urologists report that a small percentage of uncircumcized males develop genitourinary infections, inflammation of the glans, or phimosis (tightening of the foreskin) (131).

Weight, Length, and Head Circumference

In newborns these circumferences provide an index to the normality of development, and measurements should be accurate. The ***average birth weight*** of Caucasian male infants in America is $7\frac{1}{2}$ pounds (3400 g) and for girls is 7 pounds (3180 g). Newborn infants of African-American, Indian, and Oriental groups are smaller, on the average, at birth (102). The factors maternal age, parity, life-style, and the woman's previous state of nutrition and prenatal care also influence birth weight. In all instances female babies are somewhat smaller than males. Shortly after birth the newborn loses weight, up to 10% of birth weight, because of water loss, and parents should be told that this is normal before a steady weight gain, which begins in 1 or 2 weeks. Tissue turgor shows a sense of fullness because of hydrated subcutaneous tissue (82, 131).

In developing countries a large percentage of babies are born at home. Babies are not weighed at birth because scales are not available. However, measurements within 24 hours after birth of chest circumference (at nipple line) and mid-arm circumference (midway between acromium process and bend of elbow), when combined, were predictors of birthweight in one study. Based on accurate (92% to 97%) studies of 402 newborns in Thailand, The *Chulalongkorn University Birthweight Estimation Device,* a circular nomographic chart, has been developed. Estimation, if not precise measurement, of birthweight is important because low birthweight is the major factor associated with death of infants within the first 4 weeks of life (39).

Length is measured by having the child supine on a hard surface, extending the knees, placing the soles upright, and measuring from the soles of the feet to the votex (tip) of the head.

The ***average length*** of American infants at birth is just under 20 inches (50.8 cm). Boys range from 19 to 21 inches (48.2 to 53.3 cm); girls average slightly less. The bones are soft, consisting chiefly of cartilage. The back is straight and curves with sitting. The muscles feel hard and are slightly resistant to pressure (82, 131).

Measurement of **head circumference** is important in assessing the speed of head growth to determine if any abnormalities such as too rapid or too slow growth are present. The measurement is taken over the brow just above the eyes and across the posterior occipital protuberance. This standard measure of head size averages approximately 12.4–14.8 inches or 31–37 cm at birth, but variations of one half inch are common. Chest circumference is usually approximately an inch less than head size (131). Parents should be prepared for molding of the skull during vaginal delivery; **caput succedaneum,** *irregular edema of the scalp,* which disappears approximately the third day; or for **cephalohematoma,** *a collection of blood beneath the fibrous covering of the skull bones,* usually the parietal bones. Obstruction of the nasolacrymal duct is also common, and the excessive tearing and pus accumulation usually clears up when the duct opens spontaneously in a few months.

The baby's characteristic position during this period is one of flexion, closely imitating the fetal position, with fists tightly closed and arms and legs drawn up against the body. The baby is aware of disturbances in equilibrium and will change position, reacting with the Moro reflex.

Ethnic differences for weight, length, head circumference, and other measurements have been noted in Anglo and Mexican-American children ages 48 to 56 weeks. The Mexican-American child has shorter stature and greater weight for length than the Anglo child, with greater chest circumference, subscapular skinfolds, and estimated body fat, with no difference by gender. Head circumference is greater for males than females in both ethnic groups but is greater in Anglo than Mexican-American children. Thigh circumference is greater in Mexican-Americans than Anglos and in females than in males (75).

Despite widespread poverty and lack of access to medial care, Latinos in the United States, especially Mexican-Americans, have less risk of low-birth-weight babies and less infant mortality than do Caucasians or African-Americans. In Latin cultures the prevalence of traditional family values, better prenatal diets, fewer single mothers, strong extended families, and lower smoking rates may account for the difference. Health practices of Mexican-Americans deteriorate the longer they live in the United States as they become more likely to eat fast foods, smoke, and drink alcohol, activities that have serious health effects (73).

Other Characteristics

Several other characteristics are also normal and resolve themselves shortly after birth: swollen breasts that contain liquid in boys and girls; swollen genitalia with undescended testicles in the boy; and vaginal secretions in the girl, caused by maternal hormones. Genitalia size varies for boys and girls. Urine is present in the bladder, and the baby voids at birth.

Vital Signs

In the newborn vital signs are not stable.

Respiratory Efforts. Respiratory efforts at birth are critical, and immediate adaptations must occur to counter the decreasing oxygen level and increasing carbon dioxide level in the blood. Causes of respiratory initiations include cutting of the umbilical cord, which causes hypoxia, resulting in carbon dioxide accumulation; physical stimulation of the birth process; the sudden change in baby's environment at birth; the exposure to firm touch; and the cool air. If the mother were medicated during labor or if the baby is premature, the respiratory center of the brain is less operative, and baby will have more difficulty with breathing. *Respirations* range from 50 to 80 per minute during the first hour after birth and then decrease to 30 to 60 per minute. Respirations are irregular, quiet, and shallow and may be followed by an intermittent 5- to 10-second pause in breathing (125, 131).

Body Temperature. Body temperature ranges from 97° to 100° F (36.1° to 37.7° C) because (1) the heat-regulating mechanism in the hypothalamus is not fully developed; (2) shivering to produce heat does not occur; (3) there is less subcutaneous fat; and (4) heat is lost to the environment by evaporation, conduction, convection, and radiation. At birth amniotic fluid increases temperature loss by evaporation from the skin; thus diligent efforts to dry the skin are necessary. The wet newborn can lose up to 200 calories of heat per kilogram per minute (90 calories/min is the maximum the adult can lose). If the room is cool and the baby is placed in contact with cold objects, heat loss occurs by convection, radiation, and conduction. Excessive heat loss or cold stress may lead to apnea, respiratory depression, and hypoglycemia (131).

Thus baby should be placed next to mother's abdominal skin or breast initially and then wrapped well in blankets before being placed in a warm crib. Several mechanisms occur to help the newborn conserve heat: (1) vasoconstriction by which constricted blood vessels maintain heat in the inner body; (2) flexion of the body to reduce total amount of exposed skin (the premature baby does not assume a flexion of the extremities onto the body); (3) increased metabolic rate, which causes increased heat production; and (4) metabolism of adipose tissue that has been stored during the eighth month of gestation. This *adipose tissue* is called **brown fat** because it is *brown in color from a rich supply of blood vessels and nerves,* and it is unique in that it *aids adaptation to the stress of cooling.* Brown fat, located between the scapulae around the neck, behind the sternum, and around the kidneys and adrenal glands, accounts for 2% to 6% of the neonate's body weight and is metabolized quickly (125, 131).

Body temperature of the baby normally drops 1° to 2° F immediately after birth, but in a warm environment begins to rise slowly after 8 hours. Thus prevention of heat loss, especially during the first 15 minutes, is crucial to adaptation to extrauterine life (125, 131). Also, babies who have lost excessive amounts of heat cannot produce surfactant. **Surfactant** is a *thin lipo-protein film produced by the alveoli that reduces surface tension of the alveoli, allows them to expand and allows some air to remain in alveoli at end of expiration.* Thus it takes less effort to reexpand the lungs (125, 131).

Heart Rate. Heart rate ranges at birth from 100 to 160 beats per minute because of the immature cardiac regulatory mechanism in the medulla. The heart rate may increase to 170 to 180 beats per minute when the newborn cries and drop to 90 during sleep. The pulse rate gradually decreases during the first and subsequent years (125, 131).

Blood Pressure. Blood pressure may range from 40 to 50 mm of mercury (mm Hg) systolic, depending on cuff size or the instrument used for measurement. By the end of the first month, blood pressure averages 80/40 (125, 131).

Meconium

The *first fecal material* is sticky, odorless, and tarry. This **meconium** is passed from 8 to 24 hours after birth. Transitional stools for a week are loose, contain mucus, are greenish-yellow and pasty, and have a sour odor. There will be two to four stools daily. If the neonate takes cow's milk, the stools will become yellow and harder and average one to two daily.

Reflex Activity

Reflex activity is innate or built in through the process of evolution and develops while the baby is in utero. **Reflex** is an *involuntary, unlearned response elicited by certain stimuli,* and it indicates neurologic status or function (106, 125, 131). Individual differences in the newborn's responses to stimulation are apparent at birth. Some respond vigorously to the slightest stimulation; others respond slowly, and some are in between. Several types of reflexes exist in the neonate and young infant; consummatory, avoidant, exploratory, social, and attentional. **Consummatory reflexes** *such as rooting and sucking promote survival through feeding.* **Avoidant reflexes** are *elicited by potentially harmful stimuli* and include the Moro, withdrawing, knee jerk, sneezing, blinking, or coughing. **Exploratory reflexes** *occur when infants are wide awake and are held upright so that their arms move without restraint.* The visual object at eye level elicits both reaching and grasping reflexes. **Social reflexes** *such as smiling promote affectionate interactions between parents and infants* and thus have a survival value. Crying in response to painful stimuli, loud noise, food deprivation, or loss of support; quieting in response to touch, low soft tones, or food; and smiling in response to changes in brightness, comforting stimuli, or escape from uncomfortable stimuli are examples of innate reflexes that can be modified by experience and that persist throughout life. **Attentional reflexes,** including orienting and attending, *determine the nature of the baby's response to stimuli* and have continuing importance through development (106).

The nervous system of the newborn is both anatomically and physiologically immature, and reflexes should be observed for their presence and symmetry. These reflexes are described in Table 7–3.

Sensory Abilities

The newborn has more highly developed sensory abilities than was once supposed. Apparently a moderately enriched environment, one without stimulus bombardment or deprivation, is best suited for sensory motor development. Even premature babies placed in a stimulus-rich environment until discharged from the hospital learn more quickly and are healthier at 4 months than premature babies who lived in the traditional environment (74, 106).

The infant's use of the senses, innate abilities, and environment lay the ground work for intellectual development. Studies show that 20 minutes of extra handling a day will result in earlier exploring and grasping behavior by the infant. He or she is very sensitive to touch and vestibular (rocking, holding upright) stimulation; cutaneous and postural stimulation is necessary for development of the nervous system, skin sensitivity, and emotional health (18, 74). Moderate, gentle kinesthetic stimulation daily results in a baby who is quieter, gains weight faster, and shows improved socio-emotional function.

The first impressions of life, security, warmth, love, pleasure, or lack of them come to the infant through touch. Knowledge of the people around him or her, initially of mother, is gradually built from the manner in which baby is handled. He or she soon learns to sense mother's self-confidence and pleasure as well as her anxiety, lack of confidence, anger, or rejection. These early touch experiences and the infant's feelings through them apparently lay the foundation for feelings about people thoughout life.

Sensitivity to Pain, Pressure, and Temperature. Sensitivity to pain, pressure, and temperature extremes is present at birth; pain is shown by a distinct cry (45, 89). The baby is especially sensitive to touch around the mouth and on the palms and soles. Females are more responsive to touch and pain than males (82). The newborn reacts diffusely to pain since he or she has little ability to localize the discomfort because of incomplete myelinization of the spinal tracts and cerebral cortex (106, 126, 131). However, the baby's response to pain increases each day in the neonate period. Visceral sensations of discomfort such as hunger, overdistention of the stomach, passage of gas and stool, and extremes of temperature apparently account for much of the newborn's crying. At first the cry is simply a primitive

discharge mechanism that calls for help. He or she wails with equal force regardless of stimulus. In a few weeks baby acquires subtle modifications in the sound of the cry that provide clues to the attentive parent about the nature of the discomfort so response can be adjusted to the baby's need (45, 106).

Vision. Characteristics of newborn vision are:

1. Acuity—clarity of vision at a specific distance (8 to 20 inches)
2. Fixation—ability to direct eyes at same point in space for specific time (4 to 10 seconds)
3. Discrimination—demonstrated preference for particular sizes, shapes, colors, or pattern; discriminates large from small and intensity of color
4. Conjugation—ability of the eyes to move together; frequency of refixation is more frequent for newborn
5. Scanning—ability to move eyes over the visual field and focus on satisfying image
6. Accommodation—adjustment of eyes for distance; the preferred distance is 8 inches up to 1 month of age; at 4 months ability to adjust is on adult level (85)

The visual abilities of the newborn are apparent as he or she tracks or visually follows large moving objects beginning a day after birth; initial vision is blurred. Central vision is adequate for fixation and coordinated binocular eye movements. Infants prefer less complex stimuli and large pictures or objects. The eyes are as sensitive to changes in light intensity as adult eyes. Because eye movements are not yet fully coordinated and the neonate's eyeball is shorter than that of the adult, the newborn cannot focus on objects unless they are held approximately 8 to 20 inches from his or her face, until 2 months, when the lenses of the eyes become more flexible. The infant maintains contact with the environment through visual fixation, scanning, and tracking and pays more attention to stimuli from the face than to other stimuli (Fig. 7–2). The newborn looks at mother's face while feeding and while sitting upright, follows the path of an object, crying if it comes too close to his or her face. He or she apparently has innate depth perception, can define stripe and edge, and correlates touch with sight (81, 85, 106, 131). He or she apparently sees colors and prefers black and white to red, orange, or yellow. The newborn looks longer at colors of medium intensity (yellow, green, pink) than at bright (red, orange, blue) or dim (gray, beige) colors. The newborn focuses attention on patterned objects such as geometric shapes, large circles, dots, and squares in preference to solid colors. Babies also prefer real faces to mobiles. Pupils respond sluggishly to light, bright lights cause discomfort, and the newborn will blink and withdraw (131).

Parents should be reassured that the antibiotic ointment or solution correctly placed in baby's eyes at birth will not damage vision but prevents blindness if the

TABLE 7-3. ASSESSMENT OF INFANT REFLEXES

Reflex	Description	Appearance/Disappearance
Rooting	Touching baby's cheek causes head to turn toward the side touched.	Present in utero at 24 wk; disappears 3 to 4 mo; may persist in sleep 9 to 12 mo.
Sucking	Touching lips or placing something in baby's mouth causes baby to draw liquid into mouth by creating vacuum with lips, cheeks, and tongue.	Present in utero at 28 wk; persists through early childhood, especially during sleep.
Bite	Touching gums, teeth, or tongue causes baby to open and close mouth.	Disappears at 3 to 5 mo when biting is voluntary but seen throughout adult years in comatose person.
Babkin	Pressure applied to palm causes baby to open mouth, close eyes.	Present at birth; disappears in 2 or 4 mo.
Pupillary response	Flashing light across baby's eyes or face causes constriction of pupils.	Present at 32 wk of gestation; persists throughout life.
Blink	Baby closes both eyes.	Remains throughout life.
Moro or startle	Making a loud noise or changing baby's position causes baby to extend both arms outward with fingers spread, then bring them together in a tense, quivery embrace.	Present at 28 wk of gestation; disappears at 4 to 7 mo.
Withdrawing	Removes hand or foot from painful stimuli.	Present at birth; persists throughout life.
Colliding	Moves arms up and face to side when object is in collision course with face.	Present at birth or shortly after; persists in modified form throughout life.
Palmer grasp	Placing object or finger in baby's palm causes his or her fingers to close tightly around object.	Present at 32 wk of gestation; disappears at 3 to 4 mo, replaced by voluntary grasp at 4 to 5 mo.
Plantar grasp	Placing object or finger beneath toes causes curling of toes around object.	Present at 32 wk of gestation; disappears at 9 to 12 mo.
Tonic neck or fencing (TNR)	Postural reflex seen when infant lies on back with head turned to one side; arm and leg on the side toward which he or she is looking are extended while opposite limbs are flexed.	Present at birth; disappears at approximately 4 mo.
Stepping, walking, dancing	Holding baby upright with feet touching flat surface causes legs to prance up and down as if baby were walking or dancing.	Present at birth; disappears at approximately 2 to 4 mo; with daily practice of reflex, infant may walk alone at 10 mo.
Reaching	Hand closes as it reaches toward and grasps at object at eye level.	Present shortly after birth if baby is upright; comes under voluntary control in several months.
Orienting	Head and eyes turn toward stimulus of noise, accompanied by cessation of other activity, heartbeat change, and vascular constriction.	Present at birth; comes under voluntary control later; persists throughout life.
Attending	Eyes fix on a stimulus that changes brightness, movement, or shape.	Present shortly after birth; comes under voluntary control later; persists throughout life.
Swimming	Placing baby horizontally, supporting him under abdomen, causes baby to make crawling motions with his or her arms and legs while lifting head from surface as if he or she were swimming.	Present after 3 or 4 days; disappears at approximately 4 mo; may persist with practice.
Trunk incurvation	Stroking one side of spinal column while baby is on his or her abdomen causes crawling motions with legs, lifting head from surface, and incurvature of trunk on the side stroked.	Present in utero; then seen at approximately third or fourth day; persists 2 to 3 mo.
Babinski	Stroking bottom of foot causes big toe to raise while other toes fan out and curl downward.	Present at birth; disappears at approximately 9 or 10 mo; presence of reflex later may indicate disease.
Landau	Suspending infant in horizontal, prone position and flexing head against trunk cause legs to flex against trunk.	Appears at approximately 3 mo; disappears at approximately 12 to 24 mo.
Parachute	Sudden thrusting of infant downward from horizontal position causes hands and fingers to extend forward and spread as if to protect self from a fall.	Appears at approximately 7 to 9 mo; persists indefinitely.
Biceps	Tap on tendon of biceps causes biceps to contract quickly.	Brisk in first few days, then slightly diminished; permanent.
Knee jerk	Tap on tendon below patella or on patella causes leg to extend quickly.	More pronounced first 2 days; permanent.

Data from references 106, 125, 126, and 131.

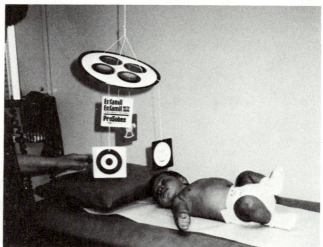

Figure 7-2. Infant has the ability to fix on the mother's face beginning at 1 day after birth and finds geometric objects interesting.
(From Sherwen, L.N., M.A. Scoloveno, and C.T. Weingarten, *Nursing
Care of the Childbearing Family*. Norwalk, Conn: Appleton & Lange,
1991, pp. 635, 847.)

mother should have an undetected gonorrheal infection.
Teach parents that baby needs eye contact and the opportunity to see the human face and a variety of changing scenes and colors. Providing a mirror or chrome
plate that reflects light and objects and rotating the bed
help the baby use both eyes, avoiding one-sided vision.
Hang cardboard black and white mobiles, especially
those that make sound, and have them within the reach
of baby's kicking feet. Later the infant enjoys other colors and designs that are within grasp. By age 2 months,
baby can see the ceiling and decorations on it. As baby
grows older the crib should be low enough that he or
she can see beyond the crib (81, 85).

Hearing.   Hearing is developed in utero when the fetus
is exposed to internal sounds of mother's body, such as
the heartbeat and abdominal rumbles (heard at 5 months),
and external sounds, such as voices, music, or a cymbal
clap (heard at 7 months). Hearing is blurred the first few
days of life because fluid is retained in the middle ear,
but hearing loss can be tested as early as the first day
(81). The neonate cannot hear whispers but can respond
to voice pitch changes. A low pitch quiets; a high pitch
increases alertness. Baby responds to sound direction—
left or right—but responds best to mother's voice, to
sounds directly in front of his or her face, and to sounds
experienced during gestation (131). Baby often sleeps
better with background songs or a tape recording of
mother's heartbeat (120). By 3 days of age, the newborn
discriminates between the voice of mother and another
female (137). Differentiation of sounds and perception
of their source take time to develop, but there are startle
reactions. The baby withdraws from loud noise (131).
    The presence of congenital (born deaf) hearing loss

is more common than ordinarily understood. It is believed that approximately $1\frac{1}{2}$% to 3% of infants born in the United States each year have a hearing loss severe enough to require special education or help. Box 7–2 is a guide for parents and health-care professionals to check for hearing ability in the neonate and infant (27).

Taste and Smell. Taste and smell are not highly developed at birth, but acid, bitter, salt, and sweet substances evoke a response. Taste buds for sweet are more abundant in early than late life. Breathing rhythm is altered in response to fragrance, showing some ability to smell (81, 106, 131).

Neonates differ in their appearance, size, function, and response. Girls are more developmentally advanced than boys and African-Americans more than Caucasians. The most accurate assessment is made by comparing the neonate against norms for the same sex and race (106, 131).

Special Considerations in Physical Assessment of the Neonate

When a newborn is examined, the primary concerns are neurologic status, congenital deformities, and metabolic disturbances. Any history of hereditary diseases and pregnancy and delivery information is essential. See Table 7–3 because reflex status indicates neurologic and some congenital deformities. The following are particular aspects to check when physically assessing the neonate (61, 106, 120, 130, 131).

A *small chin,* called **micrograthia,** may mean that the neonate will experience breathing difficulties since the tongue can fall back and obstruct the nasopharynx.

Ear position is important because there is a strong association between low-set ears and renal malformation or in a chromosomal aberration such as Down syndrome. The top of the ear should be in alignment with the inner and outer canthi of the eyes. The eustachian tube is shorter and wider than in the adult. To examine the neonate with an otoscope, the head should be stabilized and the pinna of the ear pulled back and up.

Discharges from the eye may be due to chemical irritation or to ophthalmic neonatorum from gonorrhea in the mother. A mongoloid slant in a Caucasian infant may suggest a chromosome abnormality.

Ptosis (*drooping*) of the eyelids should be a cause of concern. Drooping eyelids reduce the amount of light entering the retina and can decrease development of sight.

Conjunctival hemorrhage is usually of no significance. An infant lid retractor may be used to view the fundus if the muscles of the newborn keep the eyelids closed.

The **nose** should be patent. Flaring of the nostrils usually represents respiratory distress. A thick bloody discharge from the nose suggests congenital syphilis.

■ **BOX 7-2.**
Checklist to Detect Presence of Hearing In Infancy

From Birth to 2 Wk
Does Baby:

- Jump or blink when there is a sudden loud sound
- Stop crying when you start to talk
- Seem aware of your voice
- Stir in sleep when there is continuous noise close by
- Jump or blink when there is a sudden soft click such as a light switch or a camera click when the room is otherwise quiet
- Stop sucking momentarily when there is a noise or when you start to talk
- Look up from sucking or try to open eyes when there is a sudden noise

From 2 Wks to 10 Wks
Does Baby:

- Stop crying when you talk to him or her
- Stop movements when you enter the room
- Seem aware of your voice
- Sleep regardless of noises
- Waken when the crib or bassinet is touched
- Respond to comforting only when held against mother or familiar caretaker
- Cry at sudden loud noises
- Blink or jerk at sudden loud noises

From $2\frac{1}{2}$ Mo to 6 Mo
Does Baby:

- Always coo with pleasure when you start to talk
- Turn eyes to the speaker
- Know when father comes home and wriggle in welcome (if awake)
- Startle when you bend over the crib after awakening
- Seem to enjoy a soft musical toy (e.g., a crib musical toy)
- Cry when exposed to sudden, loud unexpected noise
- Stop movements when a new sound is introduced
- Try to turn in the direction of a new sound or a person who starts to talk
- Make many different babbling sounds when alone
- Try to "talk back" when you talk
- Start wriggling in anticipation of a bottle when you start preparing it (if the baby is awake and the preparation is out of sight, as the refrigerator door opening, and so on
- Know own name (smiles, turns, or otherwise gives an indication)

NOTE: If the child is hearing impaired or deaf, a source of information about treatment facilities and/or other educational materials for parents can be obtained from Galludet College, Washington, D.C.
Modified from *Can Your Baby Hear?* St. Louis: St. Louis Hearing and Speech Center, 1980.

The **mouth** should be inspected for cleft lip and cleft palate. Although spitting up is common in the newborn, projectile vomiting is not. The newborn should have very little saliva, and tonsillar tissue should not be present at birth.

The **chest** and **abdomen** are considered a unit in the newborn. The anteroposterior diameter is usually equal to the transverse diameter. Wide-set nipples may indicate Turner syndrome, a genetic disorder. Smaller breasts that contain liquid are not uncommon in both male and female. The breath sounds in the infant are bronchovesicular. If heart murmurs exist, they are usually best heard over the base of the heart rather than at the apex.

The **umbilical cord** should have two arteries and one vein. Auscultation of bowel sounds should precede palpating for masses, an extremely important procedure in the newborn.

The **genitalia** are examined for deformities. Only the external genitalia are examined in children. In uncircumcized males up to 3 months of age, the foreskin should not be retracted to avoid tearing the membrane. The testes should be palpated in the scrotum, although sometimes they are still undescended. A **hydrocele,** *a collection of watery fluid in the scrotum or along the spermatic cord,* and **hernia,** *a protrusion of part of the intestine through the abdominal muscles,* are common findings in males.

A bloody or mucous vaginal discharge may be present in girls. Fused labia are a serious anomaly, but simple adhesion may be due to inflammation.

Rectal temperatures will rule out **imperforate anus** *(lacking normal anal opening).*

The spine should be palpated for **spina bifida,** *a congenital neural tube defect characterized by anomaly in posterior vertebral arch.* Observation for symmetric bilateral muscle movements of the hips and knees is essential. The **hips** should be examined for dislocation by rotating the thighs with the knees flexed.

Extremities should be noted for the right number of fingers and toes and bilateral movements, and position of hands and feet should be checked.

Infant—Physical Characteristics

General Appearance

The growing infant changes in appearance as he or she changes size and proportion (106, 126, 131). The face grows rapidly; trunk and limbs lengthen; back and limb muscles develop; and coordination improves. By 1 month of age the baby can lift the head slightly when prone and hold the head up briefly when the back is supported. By 2 months the head is held erect, but it bobs when he or she is sitting unsupported.

Skull enlargement occurs almost as rapidly as total body growth during the first year and is determined mainly by the rate of brain expansion. From birth to 4 weeks, the head size increases to 14.75 inches (37.5 cm);

at 3 months to 15.75 inches (39.5 cm); at 20 weeks to 16.5 inches (41 cm); and at 30 weeks to 17 inches (43 cm). By the end of the first year the head will be two thirds of adult size (106, 126, 131).

Physical Growth and Emotional, Social, and Neuromuscular Learning

Physical growth and these areas of learning are concurrent, interrelated, and rapid in the first year. The first year of life is one of the two periods of rapid physical growth after birth. (The other period is prepuberty and postpuberty.) Baby gains $\frac{2}{3}$ ounce per day in the first 5 months and $\frac{1}{2}$ ounce per day for the next 7 months. Birth weight doubles by 5 to 6 months and triples by 12 months. Baby grows approximately 1 foot in the first year (82, 106, 131).

Physical and motor abilities are heavily influenced by genetic, biological, and cultural factors, nutrition, maturation of the central nervous system, skeletal formation, overall physical health status, environmental conditions, stimulation, and consistent loving care. African-American infants mature ahead of Caucasian infants in motor skills, bone ossification, and walking. This is apparently due to genetic factors and has evolutionary adaptive value (81, 82, 106). The skeletal system should be assessed for any orthopedic problems (83).

Table 7–4 divides further developmental sequence into 3-month periods for specific assessment (47, 82, 106, 126, 131). *It is only a guide,* not an absolute standard. Great individual differences occur among infants, depending on their physical growth and emotional, social, and neuromuscular responses. Girls usually develop more rapidly than boys, although the activity level is generally higher for boys. Even with these cautions, the table can be a useful tool if you observe overall behavior patterns rather than isolated characteristics.

Neurologic System

The neurologic system is immature, but it continues the fetal pattern of developing a functional capacity at a rapid rate. Consistent stimulus of the nervous system is necessary to maintain growth and development, or function is lost and cannot be regained.

Under 4 months of age baby does not look for an object hidden after seeing it, and when the same object reappears, it is as if the object were a new object. The infant has no knowledge that objects have a continuous existence: the object ceases to exist when it is not seen (21, 104, 105). The baby coordinates both eyes, and attends to and prefers novel stimuli. At 4 months he or she can focus for any distance and perceive shape constancy when the object is rotated at different angles (81, 131). Infants look longer at patterned stimuli of less complexity than at stimuli that have more complex designs or no lines or contours and can detect change of pattern (81). The infant is attracted by checkerboard designs, geometric shapes, and large pictures (circles, dots, and squares at least 3 inches high and with angles rather than con-

TABLE 7-4. ASSESSMENT OF PHYSICAL CHARACTERISTICS OF THE INFANT

1 to 3 Mo	3 to 6 Mo	6 to 9 Mo	9 to 12 Mo
Many characteristics of newborn, but more stable physiologically	Most neonatal reflexes gone. Temperature stabilizes at 99.4° F (37.5° C)		Temperature averages 99.7° F (37.7° C)
Heartbeat steadies at about 120 to 130 beats per min		Pulse about 115 per min	Pulse about 100 to 110 per min
Blood pressure about 80/40; gradually increases		Blood pressure about 90/60	Blood pressure 96/66
Respirations more regular at 30 to 40 per min; gradually decreases		Respirations about 32 per min	Respirations 20 to 30 per min
Appearance of salivation and tears			
Weight gain of 5 to 7 oz (141.75 to 198.45 g) per wk	Weight gain of 3 to 5 oz (85.05 to 141.75 g) per wk		Weight gain of 3 to 5 oz (85.05 to 141.75 g) per wk
Weight at 8 to 13 lb (3629 to 5897 g)	Weight at 15 to 16 lb by 6 mo (6.8 to 7.3 kg)	Birth weight doubled by 6 mo	Birth weight tripled; average 22 lb (10 kg)
Head circumference increases 1 inch up to 16 inches (40 cm)	Head size increases 1 inch (2.54 cm)	Head size 17.8 inches (43.21 cm)	Head size increases slightly more, about $\frac{1}{2}$ inch (18.3 inches or 45 to 46 cm)
Chest circumference 16 inches (40 cm)	Chest size increases over 1 inch (17.3 inches or 43 to 44 cm)	Chest circumference increases $\frac{1}{2}$ inch (17.8 inches or 44 to 45 cm)	Chest circumference increases about $\frac{1}{2}$ inch (18.3 inches or 45 to 46 cm)
Growth of 1 inch (2.54 cm) monthly	Growth of $\frac{1}{2}$ (1.27 cm) monthly	Growth of $\frac{1}{2}$ inch (1.27 cm) monthly	Growth of $\frac{1}{2}$ inch monthly; height 29 to 30 inches (72.5 to 75 cm), increased by 50% since birth
Tonic neck reflex and Moro reflexes rapidly diminishing	Most neonatal reflexes gone Palmar reflex diminishing		
Arms and legs found in bilaterally symmetric position			
Limbs used simultaneously, but not separately	Movements more symmetric		
Hands and fingers played with			
Clenched fists giving way to open hands that bat at objects			
Reaches for objects Plays with hands	Reaches for objects with accurate aim and flexed fingers	Palmar grasp developed Picks up objects with both hands; bangs toys	Throws objects
	Objects transferred from one hand to another by 6 mo	Bottle held with hands; holds own cookie	Puts toys in and out of container
	Bangs with objects held in one hand	Preference for the use of one hand	
	Scoops objects with hands		
	Begins to use fingers separately	Probes with index finger	Points with finger
		Thumb opposition to finger (prehension) by 7 mo	Brings hands and thumb and index finger together at will to pick up small objects
			Releases objects at will
Can follow moving objects with eyes when supine; begins to use both eyes together at about age 2 mo	Binocular depth perception by about 5 mo	Explores, feels, pulls, inspects, tastes, and tests objects	Makes mark on paper

(continued)

TABLE 7-4. ASSESSMENT OF PHYSICAL CHARACTERISTICS OF THE INFANT (Continued)

1 to 3 Mo	3 to 6 Mo	6 to 9 Mo	9 to 12 Mo
	Looks for objects when they are dropped		
	Improving eye-hand coordination	Hand-mouth coordination	
		Feeds self cracker and other finger foods	Eats with fingers; holds cup, spoon
	Eruption of one or two lower incisors	Begins weaning process	Has six teeth, central and lateral incisors; eruption of first molars at about 12 mo
Attends to voices	Binaural hearing present		
Raises chin while lying on stomach at 1 mo	Turns head to sound	Turns to sounds behind self	
Raises chest while lying on stomach at 2 mo; raises head and chest 45° to 50° off bed, supporting weight on arms			
Holds head in alignment when prone at 2 mo; holds head erect in prone position at 3 mo			
Supports self on forearms when on stomach at 3 mo	Rolls over completely by 6 mo		Rolls easily from back to stomach
Sits if supported.	Sits with support at 4 mo		
	Holds head steady while sitting		
	Pulls self to sitting position		
	Begins to sit alone for short periods	Sits erect unsupported by 7 mo	Sits alone steadily
			Pivots when seated
	Plays with feet		Puts feet in mouth
	Kicks vigorously		
	Begins to hitch (scoot) backward while sitting	Creeps or crawls by 8 or 9 mo	Hitches with backward locomotion while sitting
	Bears portion of own weight when held in standing position	Pulls self to stand by holding onto support	Sits from standing position without help
	Pushes feet against hard surface to move by 3 or 4 mo	Cruises (walking sideways while holding onto object with both hands) by 10 mo	Stands alone for a minute
			Walks when led by 11 mo
		Begins to walk with help	Walks with help by 12 to 14 mo
			Lumbar and dorsal curves developed while learning to walk
			Turning of feet and bowing of legs normal
			Beginning to show regular bladder and bowel patterns; has one or two stools per day; interval of dry diaper does not exceed 1 to 2 hr
			Not ready for toilet training
Smiles at comforting person reflexly	Smiles at person deliberately during interaction	Experiences separation anxiety about 7 to 9 mo	
			Begins to cooperate in dressing; puts arm through sleeve; takes off socks
Coos, chuckles; laughs	Babbles; plays with sounds		Improves previously acquired skills throughout this period

tours) (81). Full depth perception develops at approximately 9 months when the images received in the central nervous system from the macula of each eye are integrated. Visual stimulation of both eyes simultaneously is necessary for the baby to develop binocular vision. Otherwise **amblyopia** (*lazy eye*), *which is a gradual loss of the ability to see in one eye because of lack of stimulation of visual nerve pathways,* develops without damage to the retina or other eye structures. If visual stimulation is not lacking for too many weeks, the condition reverses itself. If one eye continues to do all the work for several months, blindness results in the other eye (106, 126, 131).

During infancy vital signs (temperature, pulse, respirations, and blood pressure) stabilize, as shown in Table 7–4.

Intersensory integration takes place in infancy; information from two sense modalities is interrelated. Four-month-old infants respond to relationships between visual and auditory stimuli that carry information about an object. Six-month-old infants look longer at television when both picture and sound are on than when only the picture is on. They look longer at patterns on television then other types of stimuli (81).

The haptic system is that body system pertaining to tactile stimulation. At birth all humans possess central nervous system ability to register and associate sensory impressions received through receptor organs in the skin and from kinesthetic stimuli that originate with neuromuscular stimulation from their contact with other humans. Sensory pathways subserving kinesthetic and tactile activities are the first to complete myelinization in infancy, followed by auditory and visual pathway myelinization.

Touching the infant from birth on provides the basis for higher-order operations in the neurologic, perceptual, muscular, skeletal, and cognitive systems. Each tactile act carries a physiologic impact with psychologic and sociocultural meaning. Much information is gained through discriminating one physical stimuli from another, with the form or quality of touch changing the perception of the tactile experience. Tactile stimulation is essential for both the beginning body image development and other learning (96, 143). Encourage parents to stroke, massage, and cuddle baby; to talk and sing to baby; and to provide toys that have primary colors, different textures, and movement.

Endocrine System

This system begins to develop primarily in infancy and childhood; it is limited in fetal life. Thus the child is very susceptible to stress, including fluid and electrolyte imbalance, during the first 18 months of life because the pituitary gland and adrenal cortex do not function well together and the adrenal gland is immature. The pituitary gland continues to secrete growth hormone and thyroid-stimulating hormone (begun in fetal life), which influence growth and metabolism (125, 131).

Respiratory System

The structures of the upper respiratory tract remain small and relatively delicate and provide inadequate protection against infectious agents. Close proximity of the middle ear, wide horizontal eustachian tube, throat, short and narrow trachea, and bronchi result in rapid spread of infection from one structure to the other. Mucous membranes are less able to produce mucus, causing less air humidification and warming, which also increases susceptibility to infection. The rounded thorax, limited alveolar surface for gas exchange, and amount of anatomical dead air space in the lungs or portion of the tracheobronchial tree where inspired air does not participate in gas exchange means that more air must be moved in and out per minute than later in childhood, causing increased respiratory rate. By age 1 year the lining of the airway resembles that of the adult. Respiratory rate at rest decreases gradually during the first year (106, 125, 131).

Gastrointestinal System

The gastrointestinal system matures somewhat after 2 to 3 months when the baby can voluntarily chew, hold, or spit out food. Saliva secretion increases and composition becomes more adultlike. Stomach capacity increases from 60 ml in the neonate to 250-300 ml in late infancy. The stomach's emptying time changes from $2\frac{1}{2}$ to 3 hours to 3 to 6 hours. Gastric hydrochloric acid is low; pepsinogen secretion nears adult levels at 3 months. Tooth eruption begins at approximately 6 months and stimulates saliva flow and chewing.

The small intestine is proportionally longer than it is in an adult; the large intestine is proportionally shorter. Peristaltic waves mature by slowing down and reversing less after approximately 8 months; then stools are more formed and baby spits up or vomits less. **Colic,** a term that indicates *daily periods of distress,* usually occurs between 2 to 3 weeks and 2 to 3 months and seems to have no remedy. X-ray films taken of such infants show unusually rapid and violent peristaltic waves throughout the intestinal tract. These movements are normally set off by a few sucking movements. Gas pressure in the rectum is also three times greater than in the average infant (106, 125, 131). Some physicians believe colic is caused by a deficiency of vitamin K, A, or E. Some mothers find that changing formula and giving plain, low-fat yogurt helps reduce the pains. When small yogurt feedings do not help, vitamin A and E supplements have been found effective. Apparently colic disappears as digestive enzymes become more complex, and normal bacterial flora accumulate as baby ingests a larger variety of food. By 2 months baby usually has two **stools** (*bowel movements*) daily. By 4 months there is a predictable interval of time between feeding and bowel movements. Breast-fed babies usually have soft, semiliquid stools that are light yellow in color. Breast-fed babies may vary more in the bowel movement pattern: the baby may have three or four watery stools a day or may go several days without a bowel movement. The stools of the formula-fed baby are more brown and formed.

The liver occupies a larger part of the abdominal cavity than an adult's liver does and remains functionally immature until age 1 year. Glycogen and vitamin storage is less effective than it is later in life.

As the autonomic nervous system and gastrointestinal tract mature, interconnections form between higher mental functions and the autonomic nervous system; the infant's gastrointestinal tract responds to emotional states in self or someone close to him or her (106, 125, 131).

Muscular Tissue

At birth muscular tissue is almost completely formed; growth results from increasing size of the already existing fibers under the influence of the growth hormone, thyroxin, and insulin. As muscle size increases, strength increases in childhood. Muscle fibers need continual stimulation to develop to full function and strength (106, 125, 131).

Skin

Structures typical of adult skin are present, but they are functionally immature; thus baby is more prone to skin disorders. The epidermal layers are very permeable, causing greater loss of fluid from the body. Dry, intact skin is the greatest deterrent to bacterial invasion. Sebaceous glands, which produce sebum, are very active in late fetal life and early infancy, causing milia and cradle cap, which go away at approximately 6 weeks. Production of sebum decreases during infancy and remains minimal during childhood until puberty, which accounts for the dry skin.

Eccrine (sweat) glands are not functional in response to heat and emotional stimuli until a few months after birth, and function remains minimal through childhood. The inability of the skin to contract and shiver in response to cold or perspire in response to heat causes ineffective thermal regulation (106, 125, 131).

Urinary System

Renal structural components are present at birth; by 5 months tubules have adultlike proportions in size and shape. The ureters are relatively short, and the bladder lies close to the abdominal wall. However, renal function is not mature until approximately 1 year of age; therefore the child is unable to handle increased intake of proteins, which are ingested if cow's milk is given too early (106, 125, 131).

Immune System

Components of the immune system are present or show beginning development. The phagocytosis process is mature, but the inflammatory response is inefficient and unable to localize infections. The ability to produce antibodies is limited; much of the antibody protection is acquired from the mother during fetal life. Development of immunologic function depends on the infant's gradual exposure to foreign bodies and infectious agents (106, 125, 131).

Red Blood Cell and Hemoglobin Levels

High at birth, these levels drop after 2 or 3 months and then gradually increase when erythropoiesis begins. Iron deficiency anemia becomes apparent around 6 months of age if the physiologic system does not function adequately to sustain red blood cell and hemoglobin levels. By the end of infancy white blood cells, high at birth, decline to reach adult levels. Red blood cell and hemoglobin levels reach adult norms in late childhood (106, 125, 131).

Increasingly, studies show that the health of the adult is influenced considerably by the person's health status in early life. Obesity, discussed in Chapters 10, 11, and 12, is an example. Blood pressure in adult years is apparently set by age 1 year; the mix of genetic and environmental influences such as diet, stress, and infections is unknown. One measure of childhood onset of a tendency toward hypertension (high blood pressure) and a possible screening method are being sought in the enzyme kallikrein, released by the kidney and found in the urine. Kallikrein causes the release of materials that dilate blood vessels and is lowest in people with hypertension; kallikrein is also lower in African-American children than in Caucasian children, even before a difference in their blood pressure is seen (102, 106, 125, 131).

Nutritional Needs

The feeding time is a crucial time for baby and mother: a time to strengthen attachment, for baby to feel love and security, a time for mother and baby to learn about self and each other, and a time for baby to learn about the environment. See Table 7–5 for a summary of the changing schedule and amount of food during the first year of life.

Breast-Feeding

Breast-feeding of infants has come in and out of fashion; however, the American Academy of Pediatrics recommends breast-feeding for the first 6 to 12 months of life. However, a large percent of infants are bottle-fed. Human milk is considered ideal because it is sterile, digestible, available, inexpensive, and contains the necessary nutrients except vitamins C and D and iron. Further, even in undernourished women, the composition of breast milk is adequate, although vitamin content depends on the mother's diet (55, 56, 76). Breast milk is all that baby needs the first 6 months of life. It contains higher levels of lactose, vitamin E, and cholesterol and less protein than cow's milk. The additional cholesterol may induce production of hormones required for cho-

TABLE 7-5. FEEDING SCHEDULES AND AMOUNTS DURING THE FIRST YEAR OF LIFE

Age of Infant	Schedule for Milk and Food	Amount of Milk Each Feeding
1 wk	Every 2–4 hr (six to eight feedings)	60–90 ml (2–3 ounces)
2–4 wk	Every 4 hr (six feedings)	90–120 ml (3–4 ounces)
1 mo	Every 4–5 hr (five or six feedings)	90–120 ml (3–4 ounces)
2–3 mo	Five feedings Sleeps through night May add rice cereal (fewest allergic reactions)	120–180 ml (4–6 ounces)
4–5 mo	Five to six feedings May add iron-fortified cereals, cooked, strained, pureed vegetables, and meat	150–210 ml (5–7 ounces) Average serving size for food—1–2 tablespoons
6–7 mo	Four to five feedings Enjoys finger foods May add foods with eggs, fruits, oven-dried toast, and soy or wheat flour Ready to eat solid foods, not just thickened feedings	210–240 ml (6–8 ounces) Serving size—2 tablespoons
8–9 mo	Three to four feedings Eats regular food, mashed or chopped; follows eating pattern of family Will accept variety of foods	240 ml (8 ounces) Needs additional fluids during days
9–12 mo	Three feedings May add juice by cup	Whole milk added at 12 mo

Data from references 56, 131, and 147.

lesterol breakdown in adulthood. Breast milk has a more efficient nutritional balance of iron, zinc, vitamin E, and unsaturated fatty acids (56, 147).

Because of the host-resistant factors in human milk, breast milk offers many advantages to the infant, including the premature infant. Immunoglobulins and antibodies to many types of microorganisms, especially those found in the intestinal tract, and enzymes that destroy bacteria are obtained from human milk. Living milk leukocytes, which further promote disease resistance, are also present in breast milk. Respiratory and gastrointestinal diseases, infantile obesity, and meningitis occur two to three times less frequently in breast-fed than in bottle-fed babies. Breast-fed babies are also less prone to allergies. Breast milk has growth-promoting substances not found in formula or cow's milk. Human milk kept refrigerated in a sterile container (not pasteurized and not frozen) can be given to premature infants to

prevent necrotizing enterocolitis, a frequently fatal bacterial invasion of the colon wall. *Even a brief period of breast-feeding gives immunologic and other benefits* (43, 56, 106, 147).

The mother's decision to either breast-feed or bottle-feed can be influenced by the obstetrician, pediatrician, hospital staff, husband, friends, and how her own mother fed her children, or there may be no decision making at all. It may be assumed from the start that the mother will feed either one way or the other. Recently in the United States more Anglo women, both of lower and higher economic status, are returning to breast-feeding.

In the study by Scrimshaw et al. (127) 82% of Mexican-American women planned to breast-feed for at least 1 month; 30% planned to breast-feed for more than 6 months. Mexican-American women who were more acculturated were less likely to breast-feed. Women who were married or planning to marry, rather than unmarried women, were more likely to breast-feed. Women who were less anxious prenatally and in postpartum were more likely to breast-feed. Bottle-feeding, on the other hand, seemed more often a decision made by the woman herself. Reasons for not breast-feeding included no milk, pain, husband against breast-feeding, and dislike for the procedure. Fewer women planned to breast-feed if they planned to return to work soon—a mandatory choice if the woman did not have economic support from the father or was not married.

The woman who works can be encouraged to breast-feed when at home, although in some work sites women could bring the baby so breast-feeding could be continued. The mother can be told of the benefits of breast-feeding to the baby and informed about community resources such as La Leche League.

Any woman is physiologically able to nurse her baby, with very rare exceptions (147). But childbirth, breast-feeding, and child rearing are sexual experiences for the woman. The woman's success in breast-feeding is related to other aspects of her psychosexual identity (20). She may choose not to breast-feed or to limit the lactation period because of personal preference, illness, or employment in a place where she cannot take baby with her. Further, in the United States feelings of embarrassment, shame, guilt, and disgust about breast-feeding are still apparent, in spite of today's openness about the subject; often medical personnel convey these feelings to woman who wish to breast-feed. In cultures in which breast-feeding is accepted, women breast-feed without difficulty. Mother keeps baby nearby day and night and feeds baby whenever he or she is hungry or needs comfort. Babies fed in this way seldom cry and are satisfied. In societies with a leisure class in which women are objects of amusement and pleasure and technology is king, women are less likely to breast-feed or to have success if they try. Breast-feeding is a learned social behavior. A positive social support system is essential for the woman who breast-feeds since fear of failure, embarrassment, anxiety, exhaustion, frustration, humiliation, anger, fear, or any stress-producing situation can prevent the effect of oxytocin and can block the flow of milk (20). The woman who really wants to breast-feed will develop the courage to do so as comfortably as possible when in public places. Rentscler (107) found that the pregnant woman's level of information and motivation for achievement were positively related to successful breast-feeding.

Preparation for breast-feeding begins during pregnancy. An adequate diet during pregnancy is an initial step toward successful lactation and breast-feeding. Teach the woman the importance and method of preparation. The woman may consult La Leche League literature for help.

During pregnancy the progesterone level is high, like just before menstruation. If a mother nurses after delivery, the pituitary gland secretes prolactin. The high levels of estrogen from the placenta that inhibited milk secretion during pregnancy are gone. As the baby sucks, the nipple is in the back of the mouth, and the jaws and tongue compress the milk sinuses. These tactile sensations trigger the release of the hormone oxytocin from the pituitary gland, which, in turn, causes the "let-down" response. The sinuses refill immediately, and milk flows with very little effort to the baby. This is the crucial time to learn breast-feeding. Oxytocin also causes a powerful contraction of the uterus, lessening the danger of hemorrhage (125).

Every effort should be directed toward making breast-feeding a comfortable, uninterrupted time (24). Effective techniques for mother getting into a comfortable position, holding the baby, and putting the baby to nipple are described in La Leche League literature, obstetric nursing and other child care books, and some booklets prepared by formula companies (24, 70, 106, 131). Mother needs an encouraging partner or family member, knowledgeable and supportive medical personnel to assist, acquaintance with other successful nursing mothers, and hospital routines that allow the baby to be with her for feeding when the baby is hungry and her breasts are full. The mother should not automatically receive medication to stop lactation, and the baby should not be fed in the nursery between breast-feedings. The mother whose milk does not let-down may need oxytocin, a period of relaxation, or perhaps a soothing liquid before feeding. She should, in any case, be encouraged to increase her fluid intake and meet the increased recommended dietary allowances for lactating women (131, 147).

The baby may be put to breast immediately after delivery and fed within 8 hours after birth to reduce hypoglycemia and hyperbilirubinemia (131). That is also a key time to promote bonding.

The first nourishment the baby receives after delivery from breast-feeding is **colostrum,** a *thin yellow secretion*. Colostrum is rich in carbohydrates, which the newborn needs, and serves as a laxative in cleaning out the gastrointestinal tract. Colostrum fed immediately after birth prevents against infection because it triggers antibody production. Depending on how soon and how often the mother nurses, true milk comes in the first few days (56, 131, 147).

The baby may nurse every hour or two at first or on demand, perhaps 15 to 30 minutes each time, but graduate to 3- to 4-hour intervals, by 4 months, obtaining more milk in shorter feeding sessions. If anxieties, excessive stimuli, and fatigue are dealt with appropriately, the mother's milk supply will increase or decrease to meet the demand. Alternating breasts with each feeding and emptying the breasts will prevent caking. The infant should grasp the areola completely to avoid excess pressure on the nipples. Generally breast-feeding babies get enough to eat; the child whose growth and weight are within the norm is being breast-fed adequately. The large or active infant may need supplemental feeding in addition to breast milk, even when mother's supply is not compromised. However, usually extra formula or baby food is not necessary before the fourth month. Food in addition to breast milk (or formula) should be introduced by the end of the sixth month. If mother received ample amounts of iron during pregnancy, her baby's iron stores should last 4 to 12 months, even on an iron-poor diet (43, 56, 147).

Premature infants can breast-feed earlier and with less effort than they can bottle-feed, but they need time to learn to suck. Physiologically, breast-feeding is an advantage; premature infants suck for approximately 25 minutes at one time, but the longer feeding fills the stomach more slowly. The infant controls the pace of breast-feeding and also avoids gastric distention, in contrast to bottle-feeding and the caregiver's controlling feeding pace, amount, and time (19).

Breast-feeding the premature infant is possible and desirable and can be a rewarding option for the mother and nutritionally and emotionally beneficial to the baby. Breast milk is more digestible, and milk from mothers with preterm babies has adequate protein, sodium, potassium, and chloride. It is not at that point adequate in calcium, phosphorus, iron, zinc, and copper. These substances can be provided in supplementary feedings designed for premature infants (43). Boggs and Rau (13) describe (1) the specific procedure for pumping the breasts; (2) how the mother can maintain a milk supply; (3) ways to enhance the experience for the mother, baby, and intensive care nursery staff; and (4) continuation of breast-feeding after discharge.

Alcohol, nicotine, many medications, including laxatives and barbiturates, and drugs and foreign substances such as chemical pollutants and pesticides pass into the milk and to the infant. Studies show that baby's exposure to the chemicals polybrominated biphenyl (PBB) and polychlorinated biphenyl (PCB) still present as residues can occur both through breast milk and in utero. PBB is used in fire-retardant materials and other products, and PCB is a semisynthetic, chlorinated, petroleum-derivative oil that is in so many products and pesticides that its contamination is now worldwide. The breast-feeding mother can easily ingest these or other chemicals in food or water, and the baby stores these chemicals in adipose and hepatic tissue since they are slowly excreted. Studies show that these chemicals (and perhaps others that are yet untested) produce a long-term effect of reduced scores on tests of attention, verbal ability, perceptual and perceptual-motor tasks, intelligence, and various other developmental abilities in the infant and young child. The immature and developing neurologic function of the infant (and fetus) more likely will be affected by such contamination than is the neurologic function of the adult. Infants exposed to such chemical contamination are more prone to a variety of symptoms and illnesses in childhood (79, 99, 114, 124, 128).

The mother should be informed of these hazards to her baby if she breast-feeds so that she can avoid harmful substances if possible. Foods without preservatives or dyes can be purchased; some food can be home-grown by families if they wish to exert the effort and use the space. All medications except essential ones should be avoided by the lactating woman; even prescribed medications should be taken with caution.

Weaning gradually, whether to a bottle or a cup, will lessen the discomfort of temporarily having a greater supply than demand. There are normal growth spurts during the first few months when the baby may demand more milk, or the mother may notice a lag as the infant's interests are directed more to the surroundings. She can assume that the infant is receiving enough milk if weight gain is normal, if he or she has six or more wet diapers a day, and if the urine is pale (131, 147).

Commercial Formulas

Commercial formulas are similar to each other and to human milk, but they are not exactly the same. Most have a slightly higher renal solute load than does breast milk. Special formulas have been developed to meet the needs of infants with phenylketonuria, fat malabsorption, and protein hypersensitivity. Modular formula, made by Ross Laboratories, consists of a core of proteins and vitamins and minerals to which different carbohydrates and fats can be added in increasing amounts. Normal growth and development are possible without breast-feeding. However, formula feeding causes greater deposits of subcutaneous fat (131).

Higher protein intake from formula produces a higher blood urea nitrogen level and serum or urine level of amino acids (except taurine). If soy protein isolate is used as a substitute for milk protein, it is supplemented with the amino acid methionine in the formula. Soy protein isolate formula supports growth similar to that of breast-fed babies except the preterm baby. Soy-based formulas are used for infants with lactose deficiency or galactosemia, for the baby in a vegetarian family, or for the baby who is allergic to cow's milk as regular formulas. Protein hydrolysate or meat-based formulas can be used for infants allergic to cow's milk or who have malabsorption problems. If the osmolality is too high, water is drawn from the tissue, causing dehydration. Necrotizing enterocolitis may also be more likely to result (147). Wink (148) compares human milk and formulas. This comparison is shown in Table 7-6.

Infants should receive supplemental iron by 4 months of age and preterm babies by 2 months. Iron-fortified formulas are the best source for formula-fed babies. Too high sodium level in the formula may cause transient elevation of blood pressure in neonates (147, 148).

Teach parents that care must be taken if the bottle is heated; it is not essential to heat it. Instruct the parents why baby bottles should preferably not be heated in the microwave. The bottle, nipple, and milk all become too hot and will cause oropharyngeal and esophageal burns. Further, the formula-filled disposable plastic liner of a commercial nurser may explode after removal of the heated bottle from the microwave, causing body burns.

Water intoxication is a growing concern with babies who are bottle-fed, especially in poor families when the mother receives Special Supplemental Food Program for Women, Infants, and Children (WIC) formula supplements. The formula allotment of one can per day is often consumed before the end of the month so that the baby is given either very diluted formula or only water to drink. The baby, receiving excess water and inadequate protein and other nutrients, retains water and suffers cerebral edema and electrolyte imbalance, and convulsions ensue. The condition can be life-threatening. Thus mothers in the lower socioeconomic levels are being encouraged to breast-feed.

Cow's Milk

Cow's milk is designed for another animal; thus it is not surprising that it varies considerably in composition from human milk. Cow's milk is unsuitable for the infant less than 6 months of age. Cow's milk contains from two to three times as much protein as does human milk, and a much greater percentage of the protein is casein, which produces a large, difficult-to-digest curd. It is higher in saturated fats and lower in cholesterol than is human milk, but the total fat content is comparable. However, the butterfat is poorly absorbed. Cow's milk contains half as much total sugar as human milk and

TABLE 7-6. COMPARISON OF HUMAN MILK AND FORMULA

Nutrient or Component	Human Milk	Formula (by National Standards)
Protein	1.6 g/100 kcal; whey: casein ratio of 60:40	1.8 to 4.5 g/100 kcal; average, 2.3 g/100 kcal; whey: casein ratio of 60:40
Carbohydrates	Lactose, 70 g/L (39% of calories)	Lactose, sucrose, corn syrup, corn syrup solids, maltodextrins, or tapioca starch (40% to 50% of calories)
Fats	50% of calories	3.3 to 6 g/100 kcal; at least 300 mg/100 kcal must be linoleic acid, polyunsaturated fat (30% to 54% of calories) Butterfat of cow's milk excreted; soy, coconut, corn, oleo, safflower, or medium-chain triglyceride oils added
Osmolality	300 mOsm/kg	400 mOsm/kg
Iron	1 mg/L	0.15 mg/100 kcal
Sodium		Higher than human milk
Potassium		Higher than human milk
Chloride		Same as human milk

Modified from Wink, D., Getting Through the Maze of Infant Formulas, *American Journal of Nursing,* 85, no. 4 (1985), 388–392.

also has galactose and glucose. Although it contains more sodium, potassium, magnesium, sulphur, and phosphorus than human milk, like human milk it is a relatively poor source of vitamins C and D and iron. One striking difference between cow's milk and human milk is the calcium content: cow's milk contains more than four times as much calcium, and babies fed cow's milk have larger and heavier skeletons. Whether or not this is normal or better is debatable. Two percent or skim milk should not be fed to infants because they will not gain weight (147, 148).

Water

The baby needs approximately 100 to 150 ml of water per kilogram of body weight daily to offset normal fluid losses. Some of this is obtained through the milk, but hot weather, fever, diarrhea, or vomiting quickly leads to dehydration. Infants become dehydrated more quickly than adults because they have a smaller total fluid volume in the body compared to body size (147). Water should be offered at least twice daily. Parents should know the *signs of dehydration*: dry, loose, warm skin; dry mucous membranes; sunken eyeballs and fontanels; slowed pulse; lower blood pressure and increased body temperature; concentrated, scanty urine; constipation or mucoid diarrhea; lethargy; a weak cry. Any combination of these symptoms implies the need for medical treatment.

Nutrient Requirements

After the initial period of adjustment (7 to 10 days after birth), the baby needs a daily average of 2.2 g of protein and 117 calories per kilogram (or 36 per pound) of body weight to grow and gain weight satisfactorily. Moderate protein intake is apparently well utilized and increases growth. No specific fat requirement is set, but some fats are necessary because they contain essential fat-soluble vitamins, furnish more energy per unit than carbohydrates and protein, promote development of the nervous system, and contribute to diet palatability. Adequate intake of vitamins and minerals, especially iron and fluoride, is essential. If the water supply is not fluorinated, supplementation should be given until 12 years of age to prevent dental caries. Recommendations for various ages can be found in Appendix I and in a nutrition text (56, 147).

Feeding Comfort

Mothers frequently need instruction about times and methods of **burping** (*bubbling, or gently patting baby's back*) the baby to reduce gaseous content of the stomach during feeding since the cardiac sphincter is not well developed (70). Young babies must be bubbled after every ounce and at the end of a feeding. Later they can be bubbled halfway through and again at the end. The infant should be moved from a semireclining to an upright position while the feeder gently pats the back. Because a new infant's gastrointestinal tract is unstable, milk may be eructated with gas bubbles. Adequate bubbling should occur before the infant is placed into the crib to prevent milk regurgitation and aspiration. The infant should be positioned prone (on abdomen) or laterally.

Solid Foods

There is no rigid sequence in adding solid foods to the infant's diet. (See Table 7–5 for guidelines.) Whatever solid food is offered first or at what time is largely a matter of individual preference of the mother or of the pediatrician. Ideally the infant's needs and developmental achievements such as eye-hand-mouth coordination and fine pincer grasp should be considered when introducing solids. A large, active baby may need cereal added to the diet at 2 months of age to satisfy hunger. A smaller, more lethargic baby may find it awkward to accept such supplements before 3 or 4 months.

The mother or nurse introducing the baby to solid foods should make it a pleasant experience. The foods offered should be smooth and well diluted with milk or formula. The infant should not be hurried, coaxed, or allowed to linger more than 30 minutes. New foods should be offered one at a time and early in the feeding while he or she is still hungry. Emphasize *not to add* salt or sugar to feedings to please the feeder's taste buds. Honey should *not* be added to feedings the first year because of the possibility of honey botulism (56).

Because fetal iron stores may last up to 6 to 12

months and because of an increasing incidence of allergies in infants introduced to a variety of solids before 3 months, many physicians now recommend later introduction of solids. Many pediatricians are also concerned about early feedings because of the possible relationship between overfeeding and infant and adult obesity (14% of overweight 6-month-old babies become overweight adults [43]). Some even encourage a total milk diet as a nutritionally adequate diet during the first 6 months.

Help the parents realize that when the baby is first fed puréed foods with a spoon, he or she expects and wants to suck. The protrusion of the tongue, which is needed in sucking, makes it appear as if baby is pushing food out of the mouth. Parents misinterpret this as a dislike for the food, but it really is the result of immature muscle coordination and possibly surprise at the taste and feel of the new items in the diet. This reflex gradually disappears by 7 to 8 months. The baby should not be punished for spitting out food. Further, baby begins to exercise some control over the environment by pacing the feeding.

When you or the physician suggests that the mother offer "table food" to the infant, ask what table food is in their home. Depending on the level of the household hygiene or the family food pattern, table food may or may not constitute an adequate or healthy diet. Family diet counseling may be necessary to ensure continued health of the family unit. Food supplies not only physical sustenance but also many personal and cultural needs. The introduction of foods characteristic of a culture provides the foundation for lifelong food habits and the basis for teaching a cultural pattern of eating.

Infant nutritional status can be assessed by measuring head circumference, height, and weight. The fat baby, with a differential of two or more percentiles between weight and length, more likely will become an overweight adult (44).

However, weight at birth or weight gain in infancy is not an accurate predictor of obesity in children. Small stature may indicate undernutrition unless there is a genetic influence from small-sized parents. Signs of nutritional deprivation include smaller-than-normal head size, pale skin color, poor skin turgor, and low hemoglobin and hematocrit levels (56).

Teach parents to avoid overfeeding—either milk or foods. Theories hold that babies who are fed more calories than they use daily develop additional fat cells to store unused energy sources. These fat cells proliferate in infancy and continue to replace themselves during childhood. Adults who were fat infants will have excess fat cells to fill through life and may have difficulty with weight control or may be obese. Another theory about the effect of infant feeding on adult weight is that eating patterns are difficult to change, especially if food symbolizes love, attention, or approval.

In addition to discussing the food quantities, quality, and nutrients needed by the baby, help parents to realize that food and mealtime are a learning experiences. The baby gains motor control and coordination in self-feeding; he or she learns to recognize color, shape, and texture. Use of mouth muscles stimulates the ability to make movements necessary for speech development. He or she continues to develop trust with the consistent, loving atmosphere of mealtime. Food should not be used as reward or punishment (by withholding food). The child should learn moderation in feeding quantity, and between-feeding snacks should be avoided or, if used, should be healthful, small in quantity, and given because the child is hungry in spite of eating at mealtime (56).

Unless you are an experienced mother, you may feel uncomfortable in teaching about feeding or other child care. Yet, you can share information gleaned from the literature, experiences of other mothers you have helped, and your own experiences if you have worked in the newborn nursery or helped a family member with a new baby. Do not tell the mother what method is best; give her the available information and then support her in her decision. Because feeding is one of the first tasks as a mother, she will need your guidance, assistance, and emotional support. You can offer suggestions such as the posture that will assure a comfortable position for her as she cradles the baby in her arms close to her body. Whether breast- or bottle-fed, the baby needs the emotional warmth and body contact. The bottle should never be propped because choking may result. Further, nursing-bottle mouth may develop; tooth decay is much higher in children when mothers use the bottle of milk, juice, or sugar water as a pacifier. The upper front teeth are most affected because liquids pool around these teeth when baby is drowsy or asleep (43, 56).

Mother-child contacts after birth are a continuation of the symbiotic prenatal relationship. The dependence of the baby on the mother and the reciprocal need of the mother for satisfaction from the child, proving her dependability and giving her confidence, are necessary to develop and continue the relationship. A successful feeding situation sets the foundation for the infant's personality and social development. It is the main means of establishing a relationship with another person and consequently the most basic opportunity to establish trust. Thus feeding is much more than a mechanical task. Your teaching attitude can convey its importance. If a father will be a primary nurturer, teach him the same way you would teach the mother.

Mercer (93) explored early psychophysiologic mother-infant interaction using the tenderness and anxiety theorems of Harry Stack Sullivan. Maternal anxiety and perception were assessed and related to changes in healthy infant satiety, anxiety, and bottle-feeding behavior. Blood samples were obtained from the infants just before and 60 minutes after feeding for determination of glucose and cortisol. Formula consumption was also noted. An empathetic linkage exists in healthy postpartum mother-infant couples. The interaction of both a mother's transitory anxiety around feeding time and overall anxiety is associated with changes in her infant's satiety and anxiety levels and feeding behavior. Relatively low maternal anxiety at feeding time is associated with both increased formula intake and decreased postfeed cortisol, the latter being indicative of a feeling of security. Extremely low maternal anxiety or apathy (which can result from anxiety) around feeding time is associated with both decreased formula intake and increased postfeed cortisol, the latter reflecting a feeling of insecurity. Thus maternal anxiety levels are a threat physically and emotionally to the infant. A mother's perception of the infant tenderness needs is related to her prefeed and feed anxiety level. Increased maternal tenderness is associated with low maternal anxiety before and during infant feeding.

Weaning

The *gradual elimination of breast-feeding or bottle-feeding in favor of cup and table feeding* (**weaning**) is usually completed by the end of the first year. Baby shows signs of making this transition: muscle coordination increases, teeth erupt, and he or she resists being held close while feeding. The two methods should overlap and allow baby to take some initiative and allow mother to guide the new method. Mother's consistency in meeting the new feeding schedule is important to development of a sense of trust.

The most difficult feeding to give up is usually the bedtime feeding because baby is tired and is more likely to want the "old method." After the maxillary central incisory teeth erupt, a night bottle should contain no carbohydrate to reduce decay in the deciduous teeth. During periods of stress the baby will often regress. Baby is also learning to wait longer for food and may object vigorously to this new condition.

The need to suck varies with different children. Some children, even after weaning, will suck a thumb or use a pacifier (if provided). The baby should not be shamed for either of these habits because they are not likely to cause problems with the teeth or mouth during the first 2 years.

Weaning coincides with a slower growth rate and will be accompanied by a decrease in appetite. Baby should not be forced to eat at the old rate during this period. Teach parents the meaning of the baby's behavior and how to adapt to this new period of development.

Asian infant-feeding patterns differ from those of many other countries, including the dominant culture in the United States, the United Kingdom, and Europe. Some Asian-born immigrants have traditionally breast-fed the baby for 1 to 3 years, after which the child is fed a plain diet of rice, lentils, some vegetables, occasionally eggs, fish or fruit, and rarely meat. The Moslem parent, a vegetarian, cannot use, for religious purposes, commercially prepared baby food that has any meat product in it. They may occasionally eat animals slaughtered according to Moslem religious laws and rituals (meat is then classed as *halal*), but such meat is difficult to find in non-Moslem countries. Thus eggs and milk are the primary sources of protein. If the diet for the weaned child is well planned, it can be adequate. Assess for steady weight gain; normal developmental behavior; healthy-appearing hair, skin, teeth, and eyes; energy; ability to play and sleep; and infrequent colds or other infections. The main difference between Western and Asian infant-feeding practices is lack of variety in diet and prolonged use of milk and certain baby foods (80).

Sleep Patterns

One of the most frequent concerns of a new mother is when, where, and how much baby sleeps. Awake, alert periods are altered by different types of feeding schedules.

The infant exhibits at least five states or levels of arousal: (1) regular or quiet sleep; (2) irregular, active, or rapid eye movement (REM) sleep; (3) quiet wakefulness; (4) active wakefulness; (5) crying; and (6) an indeterminate state of transition from one state of alertness to another (106, 131).

Every infant has a unique sleep pattern and no two babies—even if they are twins—have identical sleep habits. The following are some generalizations that can serve as a guide for the baby's first months. During regular or quiet sleep, eyes are closed, breathing is regular, and the only movements are sudden, generalized startle motions. Baby makes little sound. This is the low point of arousal; infant cannot be awakened with mild stimuli. During irregular, active REM sleep, baby's eyes are closed, breathing is irregular, muscles twitch slightly from time to time, and there are facial responses of smiles or pouts in response to sounds or lights. Baby may groan, make faces, or cry briefly. These are all normal patterns of an infant's sleep, and none of them requires attention. During quiet wakefulness, eyes are open, the body is more active, breathing is irregular, and there is varying spontaneous response to external stimuli. During active wakefulness, eyes are open; there is visual following of interesting sights and sounds, body movements, and vocalizations that elicit attention (106, 131).

The newborn and young infant spend more time in REM sleep than adults. In this state baby shows continual slow rolling eye movements on which are superimposed rapid eye movements. Additionally, respirations increase and are irregular, and small muscle twitchings are seen (106, 131).

As the infant's nervous system develops, baby will have longer periods of sleep and wakefulness that gradually become more regular. By 6 weeks, baby's biologic rhythms usually coincide with daytime and nighttime hours, and he or she will be sleeping through the night. Babies sleep an average of 16 to 20 hours a day for the first week. By 12 to 16 weeks these hours will be reduced to 14 or 15 a day. Usually this pattern will continue through the first year, with nap times getting shorter until the morning nap is eliminated. By 7 or 8 months, baby may sleep through the night without awakening. By the end of the first year, the baby may sleep 12 to 14 hours at night and nap 1 to 4 hours during the day (106, 126, 131).

Help parents understand that when a baby goes through the stage of separation anxiety about 8 months of age, bedtime becomes more difficult because he or she does not want to leave mother. Because the baby needs sleep, the parent should be firm about getting the child ready for bed. Prolonging bedtime adds to fatigue and separation fears. Caressing or singing softly while holding baby in a sleeping position in bed is calming; restraint is perceived as helpful rather than punitive. If the mother is available when the baby first awakes, he or she anticipates this pleasure, and sleep is associated with return of mother. If the baby awakes and cries during the night, the parent should wait briefly. Many times the crying will subside with the baby's growing ability to control personal anxiety feelings. Persistent crying indicates unmet needs and should be attended.

Frequently a mother becomes concerned if baby sleeps too long during the day, perhaps 6 or 7 hours without a feeding. If this happens frequently, it may help to awaken the baby during the day for regular feedings and attempt to establish a better routine with longer sleeping periods at night. Occasional oversleeping is little cause for concern. The physical preparations for sleep ideally include a room and a bed for the baby, especially after the first few weeks. Sharing the parents' bed or room may lead to later sleep problems for the infant and can be detrimental to the husband-wife relationship. The infant should at least have a consistent place for sleeping (be it box, drawer, or crib) and a clean area for supplies. Sometimes baby does not seem to sleep enough. Some babies sleep less and remain healthy. Other babies have chronic sleeplessness, which may be due to allergy to cow's milk; if so, a suitable milk substitute should be used (68).

A baby can sleep comfortably in an infant crib or bassinet during the first few weeks, but as soon as active arms and legs begin to hit the sides he or she should be moved to a full-sized crib. The crib slats should be no more than $2\frac{1}{2}$ inches apart. There should be no pillows used. The crib should have a crib border placed at the bottom of the slats to prevent catching the head between the bars. It should be fitted with a firm, waterproofed, easy-to-clean mattress and with warm light covers loosely tucked in. The sides of the crib should fit closely to the mattress so that the infant will not get caught and crushed if he or she should roll to the edge. Thin plastic sheeting can cause suffocation and should never be used on or around the baby's crib. Teach these safety measures to the parents.

Play Activity

The infant engages in play with self: with the hands or feet, by rolling, getting into various positions, and with the sounds he or she produces. Baby needs playful activity from both mother and father to stimulate development in all spheres. Share the following information with parents. You may need to teach the parents how to touch, cuddle, talk to, and play with the baby.

Certain toys are usually enjoyed at certain ages because of changing needs and developing skills. From birth to 3 months he or she needs colorful hanging toys that make sound—mobiles, rattles, bells, musical toys, even crinkling paper. From 3 to 6 months, baby needs toys to touch, grab, and mouth such as large wooden and nonsplintering plastic beads, clothespins, empty spools, and soft, stuffed toys to feel, squeeze, and hold. Baby enjoys splashing water during the bath and being read to during quiet time. From 6 to 9 months, motion toys and those that can be transferred from hand to hand are fun. Baby enjoys his or her image in the mirror, simple games with people such as peek-a-boo and pat-a-cake, and out-of-door excursions. From 9 to 12 months, baby enjoys toys that pull apart such as nesting, stack, or climbing blocks, boxes, mother's kitchen utensils, toys for bath and sand play to practice pouring, filling, and dumping, push-pull toys, music, nursery rhymes, and cuddle toys for bedtime. The baby can remain satisfied playing with self for increasing amounts of time but prefers to have people around. Baby enjoys being held briefly in various positions, being rocked, swinging for short periods, and being taken for walks.

Because much of baby's play involves putting objects into the mouth, a clean environment with lead-free paint is important. A small object that baby swallows such as a coin is passed through the digestive tract. However, small batteries used in cameras, calculators, and other electronic equipment may be hazardous if swallowed because they can rupture and release poisonous chemicals. Surgical removal may be necessary. Children gradually build an immunity to the germs encountered daily on various objects. However, health may be threatened by that which goes unnoticed. Sitting and playing in dirt or sand contaminated by dioxin, other pesticides or herbicides, or radiation is dangerous to the developing physiologic systems. Children's or parents' reading material, which can become play objects, may also be hazardous. The high lead content of the glossy color pages of magazines and newspaper inserts may account for some cases of lead poisoning in young children, who are eaters of the inedible. A study conducted by researchers at the Connecticut Agricultural Experiment Station revealed that the lead content of glossy paper printed in color—especially pages containing the color yellow—is so high that a child devouring a 4-inch square of it every day for 6 weeks could be at a critical stage of lead poisoning. Although black-and-white newsprint, the comics, and the black-and-white magazine stock are scarcely recommended for snacking, their lead content is dramatically lower than that of the shiny, colored pages, the research showed. Ideally, the child does not eat paper; yet most children have been observed sucking or chewing on corners of magazines or pieces of paper.

Toys need not be expensive, but they should be colorful (and without leaded paint), safe, sturdy, and easily handled and cleaned. They should be large enough to prevent aspiration or ingestion; they should be without rough or sharp edges or points, detachable parts, or loops to get around the neck, and some should make sounds and have moving parts.

Baby needs an unrestricted play area that is safe, although use of a playpen is necessary for short periods. Excess restriction or lack of stimulation inhibits curiosity, learning about self and the environment, and development of trust. Therefore baby should not wear clothing that is restraining, he or she should not be kept constantly in a playpen or crib, and he or she needs play objects and a loving parent who provides stimulating surroundings.

Verzemnieks (140) discusses ways to stimulate sensory development of the hospitalized child during routine care measures and common items in the hospital that can be used as toys such as medicine cups, souffle cups, empty tape cylinders, and various boxes. She also lists common household items that can be used in the home for toys that can provide fun and stimulate creativity—more so than some of the expensive toys on the market.

Parents should know the dangers of overstimulation and rough handling. Fatigue, inattention, and injury may result. The playful, vigorous activities that well-intentioned parents engage in such as tossing the baby forcefully into the air or jerking the baby in a whiplash manner may cause bone injuries or subdural hematomas and cerebrovascular lesions that later could cause mental retardation. Premature infants and male babies are twice as vulnerable as full-term girls, according to one study, because of the relative immaturity of their brains (106, 126).

Health Promotion and Health Protection

In addition to measures already discussed, including the safety measures in the previous section on play activity, the following measures also promote health.

At birth the neonate should have silver nitrate drops or ointment instilled in the eyes. Although less than 3% of mothers have gonorrhea, the possibility of blindness in the infant, along with the low cost and effectiveness of the treatment, makes this procedure mandatory (131).

Injecting 1 mg of vitamin K is effective in preventing hemorrhagic disease, which is caused in 1 of 2000 to 1 of 3000 live births by a transient deficiency of factor VIII production. Sickle cell screening can be obtained from in-cord blood (131).

During the first week of life the infant should be screened for **phenylketonuria** (*PKU*), *an inborn metabolic disorder characterized by abnormal presence of phenylketone and other metabolites of phenylalanine in the urine*. Hypothyroid screening is also recommended for all newborns. Refer to Appendices III and IV for a schedule of health screening measures for the infant.

Immunizations

Immunizations, *promoting disease resistance through injection of attenuated, weakened organisms or products produced by organisms,* are essential to every infant as a preventive measure. Before birth baby is protected from certain organisms by the placental barrier and mother's physical defense mechanisms. Birth propels baby into an environment filled with many microorganisms. Baby has protection against common pathogens for a time, but as he or she is gradually exposed to the outside world and the people in it, further protection is needed through routine immunizations, available from private physicians or public health clinics. Annually, millions of children in the developing world either are permanently disabled or die from childhood diseases that are preventable. The World Health Organization has as its goal to immunize every child against diphtheria, polio, measles, tetanus, and whooping cough and to protect against tuberculosis (131).

The infant needs the combination of diphtheria and tetanus toxoids and pertussis vaccine (DTP). The diphtheria bacillus is still prevalent, and the fully immunized person, protected against the disease, can acquire and transmit the disease as a carrier. Pertussis (whooping cough) is a serious disease for babies. Unimmunized children may have the disease, but the nonspecific manifestations often cause a delay in diagnosis. The infant needs oral polio vaccine, which carries a risk of one case of paralytic polio in 9 million doses, a risk far less than that of the disease. The infant should receive DTP at ages 2, 4, and 6 months and live oral polio vaccine (OPV) at 2 and 4 months, with an optional dose at 6 months (100, 129, 131, 138). At 1 year the infant should be given a tine test to detect possible tuberculosis (2). Nose drop influenza vaccine is available for infants 6 months or older. Vaccination is essential to provide **herd immunity,** *immunity to all susceptible persons,* especially pregnant women in the first trimester.

OPV should not be administered in households with immunodeficient individuals because OPV is excreted in the stool and could infect an immunodeficient person. Poliovirus vaccine inactivated (IPOL) is safe to give in these households. A primary series of IPOL for children and adults consists of three 0.5 ml doses administered subcutaneously at least 4 weeks, preferably 8 weeks, apart. (The first two doses can be given with the DTP immunizations at 2 and 4 months of age.) The third dose should follow at least 6 months, preferably 12 months, after the second dose. A booster of OPV should be given to the child before entering school unless the third dose was given on or after the fourth birthday. Use of IPOL is contraindicated in persons with a history of hypersensitivity to any component of the vaccine, including neomycin, streptomycin, and polymyxin B. If allergic reaction occurs within 24 hours of the first dose, no further doses should be given (64).

Parents should be told the importance of immunizations and should be helped to get them, for example, through flexible clinic hours or low-cost mass immunizations in a community. Parents should also keep a continuing record of the child's immunizations. Your teaching, encouragement, community efforts, and follow-up are vital.

One study showed that a mailed reminder about the date for immunization of the 6-month-old infant increased the chances that baby would receive the scheduled immunization, especially in families that had a record of not keeping clinic appointments. Other nurses have found that a telephone reminder works well in getting mothers to return for well-baby immunizations (151).

Safety Promotion and Injury Control

Safety promotion and injury control are based on the understanding of infant behavior. Accidents are a major cause of death to individuals less than 26 years of age. Risk factors that influence the occurrence of fatal childhood accidents include (1) host factors such as age and sex; (2) environmental factors such as hazardous play equipment, flammable clothing, and accessible poisons; and (3) parental characteristics such as socioeconomic status (146).

The risk of a fatal accident among infants during the first year of life is directly related to the level of the mother's schooling for both Caucasian and African-American children. Infants whose mothers completed 8 or fewer years of education had nearly double the rate of fatal accidents as infants whose mothers had some high school education in a study in North Carolina (145).

Epidemiologic studies report that the main causes of death for the infant are drowning; suffocation by inhalation and/or ingestion of food or by mechanical means (in bed or cradle, by plastic bag, or by polystyrene-filled pillows); transport accidents; and falls (23, 35, 107). Contrary to common belief, the baby is not immobile: he or she will not necessarily stay where placed. Baby rolls, crawls, creeps, walks, reaches, and explores.

Since he or she is helpless in water, the baby should never be left alone or with an unresponsible person while in water. The home and car have many often unnoticed hazards; thus the baby should never be left alone in either and should never roam freely in the car while it is in motion. Parents should use an approved car infant seat or harness (Fig. 7–3). Richi and Krzy (110) give a detailed description of various kinds of child car seats and restraints and the advantages of each. You can incorporate such information as you teach parents safety measures for their child. Baby's physical ability to move is developing, but he or she lacks reasoning ability, knowledge, experience, and self-control.

Falls can be avoided if the parents or nurse is responsible for doing the following: (1) keeping crib rails up; (2) maintaining a firm grasp of the baby while carrying or caring for him or her and supporting the head during the first few months; (3) using a sturdy high chair and car infant seat or harness with fasteners in place (this is law in many states); and (4) having a gate at the top of the stairs or in front of windows or doors that are above the first story (106).

Suffocation at home and in the health-care setting can be avoided by (1) removing any small objects that could be inhaled or ingested (safety pins, small beads, coins, toys, nuts, raisins, popcorn, balloons); (2) keeping plastic bags, venetian blind cords or other cords out of reach; and (3) avoiding the use of pillows in the crib or excessively tight clothing or bedcovers (35, 106, 107, 131).

Burns can be avoided by (1) placing the crib away from radiators or fireplaces; (2) using warm-air vaporizers with caution; (3) covering electric outlets; (4) avoid-

Figure 7-3. Infants should be transported in an approved automobile infant seat or harness. (From Sherwen, L.N., M.A. Scoloveno, and C.T. Weingarten, *Nursing Care of the Childbearing Family.* Norwalk, Conn: Appleton & Lange, 1991, p. 926.)

ing tablecloths that hang over the table's edge; (5) turning pot handles inward on the stove; (6) avoiding excessive sun exposure; and (7) avoiding smoking around the baby (106, 126).

Encourage parents to take a first-aid course (one directed to cardiopulmonary resuscitation, preventing airway obstruction, and other home and family concerns) that enables them to recognize hazards and take appropriate measures to avoid injury to loved ones. Teaching parents about the child's normal developmental patterns will also enable them to foresee potential accidents and take precautions.

Common Health Problems: Prevention and Treatment

Various conditions are common in the infant. Table 7–7 summarizes the problems, their signs or symptoms, and methods to prevent or treat them (61).

The incidence of *acute respiratory disease, bronchitis,* and *pneumonia* increases with the increasing number of cigarettes smoked by the mother or other family members, particularly in infants aged 6 to 9 months. In a prospective study of 10,672 infants for whom hospital admission during the first year of life was related to maternal smoking, findings supported the hypothesis that atmospheric pollution with tobacco smoke endangers

the health of nonsmokers. Infants of smoking mothers had significantly more admissions for bronchitis or pneumonia and more injuries (53). In households in which the mother smoked, the infant's urine cotinine levels were higher, especially in breast-fed babies during non-summer months. However, infants in a family in which any member smokes will suffer the effects of passive smoking from absorption of environmental tobacco smoke (30, 50).

The common health problems presented throughout these chapters reflect what are considered common today. Even in the last 25 years striking changes have occurred in patterns of disease caused by transmissible agents; thus, what was common in 1945 is not even seen in the 1990s. On the other hand, we have some diseases today that were not even named in 1945. For an overview of these changing patterns see the article by Lorber (84).

PSYCHOSOCIAL CONCEPTS

The *intellectual, emotional, social, and moral components can be combined into what is often referred to as* **psychosocial development.** The separation of these facets of growth is artificial for they are closely interre-

TABLE 7-7. COMMON HEALTH PROBLEMS IN INFANCY

Problem	Definition	Symptoms/Signs	Prevention/Treatment
Atopic dermatitis	Chronic inflammatory disease of skin, characterized by itching	Family history of allergic disease, especially asthma Onset: usually after 2 mo Rough, red, papular scaling areas, mainly on scalp, behind ears, on forearms and legs	Use warm water for baths. Apply lotions. Use soft cotton clothing. Keep fingernails short.
Diaper dermatitis	Inflammation of skin covered by diaper	Itching, irritability Redness on buttocks, genitalia papules, vesicles, and pustules	Keep area clean and dry. Allow air to circulate. Apply bland ointment or Burow's solution.
Seborrheic dermatitis ("cradle cap")	Oily, scaly condition occurring in areas with large numbers of sebaceous glands	Scaly eruption spreading to eyebrows, eyelids, nasolabial folds	Shampoo and massage scalp. More severe cases may require a selenium sulfide (e.g., Selsun) shampoo.
Oral candidiasis ("thrush")	Fungal infection found in mouth of infants	White, irregular plaques found in mouth	Administer oral medication (e.g., nystatin [Mycostatin]).
Constipation	Difficulty in passing stool; excessive firmness of stool; decreased frequency of defecation	Straining on defecation, lack of stool passage Sometimes anal tissue or perianal abscess	Give warm sitz bath. Apply petroleum jelly to anus. Give additional water to drink.
Iron deficiency anemia	Anemia associated with inadequate supply of iron for synthesis of hemoglobin	Hematocrit value less than 30 Pallor, lethargy Anorexia Poor weight gain Splenomegaly	Discontinue whole cow's milk and substitute commercial formula. Increase intake of foods high in iron content. Give ferrous sulfate.
Roseola infantum	Acute benign febrile illness; fever stops as rash appears	High sudden fever lasting for 3–4 days with few other symptoms Rash lasts 24–48 hr	Use antipyretic therapy.

Data from references 61, 84, and 130.

lated. Similarly, psychosocial, physical, and motor development greatly influence each other. Babies are born cognitively flexible rather than with preset instinctual behavior. A level of physiologic maturation of the nervous system must be present before environmental stimulation and learning opportunities can be effective in promoting emotional and cognitive development. In turn, without love and tactile, kinesthetic, verbal, and other environmental stimuli, some nervous system structures do not develop. Babies adapt and react to the environment with which they are confronted. Low-birth-weight and premature infants have neurologic deficits that predispose to an increased risk for developmental delays, and they are apt to have behavioral styles that are more difficult to handle, which reduces maternal involvement and the stimulation needed for development (92).

Cognitive Development

Intelligence is the *ability to learn or understand from experience, to acquire and retain knowledge, to respond to a new situation, and to solve problems.* It is a system of living and acting developed in a sequential pattern through relating to the environment. Each stage of operations serves as a foundation for the next (105). **Cognitive behavior** includes *thinking, perceiving, remembering, forming concepts, making judgments, generalizing, and abstracting.* Cognitive development is learning and depends on innate capacity, maturation, nutrition, gross and fine motor stimulation, touch, stimulation of all senses through various activities, language, and social interaction (82).

Sequence in Intellectual Development

The sequence described by Piaget corresponds rather roughly in time span to those described for emotional development. The infant is in the sensorimotor period of cognitive development (104, 105, 141).

The infant arrives in the world with great potential for intellectual development, but at birth intellectual capacities are completely undifferentiated.

Stage One, the Reflex Stage. This stage covers the neonatal period when behavior is entirely reflexive. Yet all stimuli are being assimilated into beginning mental images through reflexive behavior and from human contact.

Stage Two, Primary Circular Reactions. Primary circular reactions are response patterns where a stimulus creates a response and gratifying behavior is repeated. At 1 to 4 months, life is still a series of random events, but hand-mouth and ear-eye coordination is developing. The infant's eyes follow moving objects; eyes and ears follow sounds and novel stimuli. Responses to different objects vary. Baby does not look for objects removed from sight. He or she spends much time looking at objects in the environment and begins to separate self from them. Beginning intention of behavior is seen; he or she reproduces behavior previously done. For example, the 8-week-old infant can purposefully apply pressure to a pillow to make a mobile rotate, smile at familiar faces, and anticipate a routine such as diapering.

Stage Three, Secondary Circular Reactions. Stage three covers 4 to 8 months. Baby learns to initiate and recognize new experiences and repeat pleasurable ones. Intentional behavior is seen. Increasing mobility and hand control help him or her become more oriented to the environment. Reaching, grasping, listening, and laughing become better coordinated. Memory traces are apparently being established: baby anticipates familiar events or a moving object's position. The child repeats or prolongs interesting events. Activities that accidentally brought a new experience are repeated. Behavior becomes increasingly intentional. Habits developed in previous stages are incorporated with new actions. Baby will imitate another's behavior if it is familiar and not too complex.

Stage Four, Coordination of Secondary Schemata. In this stage, from 8 to 12 months, baby's behavior is showing clear acts of intelligence and experimentation. Baby uses certain activities to attain basic goals. He or she

---

CASE SITUATION: Infant Development

Michael, 8 months old, is sitting on the lap of his babysitter, Aunt Jennifer, who is reading a story to him. Aunt Jennifer smiles and chuckles as she reads. Michael responds by mimicking her mouth movements. She says "Ooooohh" with a widened O-shaped mouth, and Michael imitates the O-shape of her mouth while she speaks. Michael makes a long, loud "Ooooohh" sound. Aunt Jennifer responds with smiles and exclamations of enthusiasm, recognizing his achievement. Michael smiles and continues to repeat "Ooooohh."

Michael then attempts to imitate Aunt Jennifer's actions in reading the book. He reaches toward the book and makes babbling sounds as he swats at the book. Michael's coordination of vision, hearing, and tactile senses as he repeatedly imitates his aunt's facial expressions, reaches for the book, and engages in prespeech babbling demonstrates a common behavior of children in this age group. These behaviors demonstrate Piaget's Stage Three, Secondary Circular Reactions, of the Sensorimotor Stage of cognitive development.

realizes for the first time that someone other than self can cause activity, and activity of self is separate from movement of objects. He or she searches for and retrieves a toy that has disappeared from view. Shapes and sizes of familiar objects are recognized, regardless of the perspective from which they are viewed. Because of the baby's ability to differentiate objects and people from self and the increased sense of separateness, he or she experiences separation (eighth month) anxiety when the mothering figure leaves. Baby is more mobile; sitting, creeping, standing, or walking gives a new perception of the environment. Baby understands words that are said. Thus coordination of schema involves using one idea or mental image to attain a goal and a second idea or image to deal with the end result (47, 104, 105, 141). Baby systematically imitates another while observing another's behavior.

Reaffirm with parents that they can greatly influence the child's later intellectual abilities by the stimulation they provide for baby, the loving attention they give, and the freedom they allow for baby to explore and use his or her body in the environment (32). Many educational toys are on the market, but common household items can be made into educational toys. For example, a mobile of ribbons and colorful cutouts will attract as much attention as an expensive mobile from the store. Unbreakable salt and pepper shakers or small cardboard boxes partly filled with rice, sand, or pebbles makes a good rattle (1).

Communication, Speech, and Language Development

Communication between people involves facial expressions, body movements, other nonverbal behavior, vocalizations, speech, and use of language. A newborn is ready to communicate if parents and caretakers know how to read the messages. The first communications are through eye contact, crying, and body movements.

Speech awareness *begins before birth. In utero the fetus hears a melody of language,* equivalent to overhearing two people talk through the walls of a motel room. *This creates a sensitivity that after birth provides the child with clues about sounds that accompany each other.* If babies have been read to in utero, after birth they appear to prefer the sound of the stories they had heard in utero (101).

Speech is the *ability to utter sounds;* **language** refers to *the mother tongue of a group of people,* the *combination of sounds into a meaningful whole to communicate thoughts and feelings.* Speech development begins with the cry at birth, and the cry remains the basic form of communication for the infant. Baby's **cry** is **undifferentiated** for the first month; the *adult listener cannot distinguish between cries of hunger, pain, fear, and general unhappiness.* Parents learn to distin-

guish the meanings of different cries and grunts the baby makes in the first 2 or 3 months. At first baby responds to both soothing and distressing stimuli with similar sounds. Then other prespeech sounds are heard: (1) **cooing,** the *soft murmur or hum of contentment;* (2) *squealing* and *grunting;* (3) **babbling,** *incoherent sounds make by playing with sounds;* (4) **lalling,** the *movement of the tongue with crying and vocalization* such as "m-m-m"; (5) *sucking sounds;* and (6) *gestures.* Cooing and babbling begin at 2 or 3 months; squeals and grunts are heard by 6 months. The number of sounds produced by babbling gradually increases, reaches a peak at 8 months, and gives way for true speech and language development. Smiles, frowns, and other facial expressions often accompany the baby's vocalizations as do gestures of reaching or withdrawing to convey feelings (75, 131).

There is a biologic basis for speech; the brain has amazing ability to process and interpret verbal expressions over an infinite range. However, parent-child interaction is essential for the child to learn language and conversation. Further, there is a critical period during which young children need environmental stimuli, or they will not learn to speak even when the sensory stimulation is exchanged for sensory deprivation (101).

At first vocalizations are reflexive; no difference exists between the vocalizations of hearing babies and deaf babies before 6 months of age. Later, vocalizations are self-reinforcing, that is, the baby finds pleasure in making and hearing his or her own sounds, and responses from others provide further reinforcement. Reinforcement when desired sounds are made and when certain sounds are omitted is necessary for the infant to progress to language development. The child must also hear others speak to reinforce further the use of the sounds and language of the culture. Effective mothers speak to their children frequently, even while they are doing their housework (7, 82).

By 9 months baby will have made every sound basic to any human language. The sounds made in infancy are universal, but when he or she learns the native language, the potential to say all universal sounds is lost (82, 101).

At every age the child comprehends the meaning of what others say more readily than he or she can put thoughts and feelings into words. In speech comprehension, the child first associates certain words with visual, tactile, and other sensations aroused by objects in the environment. Between 9 and 12 months, baby learns to recognize his or her name and the names of several familiar objects, responds to "no," echoes and imitates sounds, repeats syllables, and may occasionally obey the parent (82).

Baby tries to articulate words from the sounds heard. Words are invented such as "didi" to mean a toy or food. Language is **autistic;** *he or she associates mean-*

ings with sounds made by the self, but the sounds are not meaningful to others, often even to the parents. By trial and error and by imitation and as a result of reinforcement from others, the baby makes the first recognizable words, such as "mama," "dada," "no," or "bye-bye" between 10 and 18 months of age. (If the correct sound is directed to the appropriate parent, the sound is reinforced, and the baby continues speech.) Words such as "mama" and "nana" are universal to babies in every culture because they result from the sounds the infant normally makes in babbling. By age 1 year baby has a vocabulary of approximately six words. Nouns typically are learned first. He or she learns to associate meaning with an object such as its name, size, shape, texture, use, and sound; then a word becomes a symbol or label for the object. Learning to speak involves pronouncing words, building a vocabulary, distinguishing between sounds such as "p*e*t" and "p*a*t" or "*h*ear" and "*n*ear" and then making a sentence. The baby's first sentence usually consists of one word and a gesture (82).

Teach parents that many factors influence speech and language development: innate intelligence, ability to hear, modification of the anatomic structures of the mouth and throat, sense of curiosity, parental verbal stimulation and interest, and encouragement to imitate others (82).

Emotional Development

Eight psychologic stages in the human life cycle are described by Erikson (41). He elaborates on the core problems or crisis with which each person struggles at each of these levels of development. In addition to these problems, the child has other tasks to accomplish that relate to the psychosocial crisis such as learning to walk. Emotional or personality development is a continuous process. No person succeeds or fails completely in attainment of the goal to reach at a particular point in personality development.

Developmental Crisis

According to Erikson (41), the psychosexual crisis for infancy is trust versus mistrust. **Basic trust** involves *confidence, optimism, acceptance of and reliance on self and others, faith that the world can satisfy needs, and a sense of hope or a belief in the attainability of wishes in spite of problems and without overestimation of results.* A sense of trust forms the basis for later identity formation, social responsiveness to others, and ability to care about and love others. The person accepts self, develops reachable goals, assumes life will be manageable, and expects people and situations to be positive. A sense of trust may be demonstrated in the newborn and infant by the ease of feeding, the depth of sleep, the relaxation of the bowels, and the overall appearance of contentment. **Mistrust** is a *sense of not feeling satisfied emotionally or physically, an inability to believe in or*

rely on others or self. It is characterized by lethargy, lack of weight gain, poor eating, excessive colic, lack of sleep, and failure to thrive. Later, predominant feelings and behaviors are pessimism, lack of self-confidence, suspicion and bitterness toward others, and antagonism. The person believes things will not turn out right; therefore he or she withdraws or may be dependent, clinging, and easily hurt, although he or she sets the self up to be hurt. Relationships and new experiences are avoided. Gratification cannot be delayed. Or, as the person gets older, he or she may bully others to be sure of coming out on top or behave in a controlling, sarcastic, aggressive manner. Sometimes mistrust is turned into pathologic optimism; the person gambles on everything turning out all right, thinking nothing can go wrong.

Security and trust are fostered by the prompt, loving and consistent response to the infant's distress and needs and by the positive response to happy, contented behavior. You can teach parents that they do not "spoil" a baby by promptly answering the distress signal—his or her cry. Rather, they are teaching trust by relieving tension. Parents should understand the meaning they convey through such care as changing diapers. Even if the techniques are not the best, baby will sense the positive attitude if it exists. If the parents repeatedly fail to meet primary needs, fear, anger, insecurity, and eventual mistrust result. If the most important people fail him or her, there is little foundation on which to build faith in others or self and little desire to be socialized into the culture. The world cannot be trusted. If the baby is abused, neglected, or deprived, he or she may suffer irreversible effects, as discussed in Chapter 6, pp. 199 to 200.

The infant who is in a nurturing, loving environment and who has developed trust is a happy baby most of the time. He or she is sociable and responsive to others. Attachment to the parent has been formed so that separation or stranger anxiety is experienced at approximately 7 to 9 months of age and may extend to 10 to 12 months. After a time the infant will again respond to strangers. One study found that sociable babies have sociable mothers and that sociable, friendly babies score higher on cognitive tests than less sociable or mistrusting infants (133).

The working mother may discuss her situation with you. Emotional development of the infant is not compromised by the working mother if she has time and energy to maintain consistent, loving, and stimulating responses when she is with baby. Quality of care rather than quantity of time is the essence of parenting and promoting emotional development. When work is not stressful and is a source of personal satisfaction for the mother, she is a more contented mother and gives the baby better care. The father's nurturance is also important, and often he is more involved in caring for the child when the mother works, which contributes to quality care. The lowest scores of adequate mothering are found in dissatisfied homemakers (82). Further, the effective mother does not devote the bulk of her day in the home to child rearing but instead designs an environment that is loving, adequately stimulating, and helpful to the child in gaining competency (82, 106).

Because so many mothers work today, an important subject to discuss is child-care arrangements or babysitting services. Even if the parent does not work, some time away from the baby is rejuvenating and enhances the quality of parenting. Each parent has different ideas about how often, if at all, to leave the baby with a sitter. Discuss characteristics to consider in a sitter. Point out that parents will probably be most satisfied with a sitter whose child-rearing philosophy and guidance techniques coincide with theirs and who has had some child-care training or experience.

The *sitter* should be physically and emotionally healthy, acquainted with the baby and the home, and like the baby. If possible, parents should keep the baby with the same sitter consistently, especially around 7 or 8 months when he or she is experiencing separation anxiety. The sitter should have exact instructions about where the parents can be reached; special aspects of care; telephone numbers of doctor, police, and fire department; name and telephone number of another family member; and the telephone number of a poison control center, if nearby. As more mothers return to work shortly after childbirth, there will probably be an increasing trend toward infant day-care centers. Factors to consider in choosing day care services are discussed in Chapter 9, pp. 287 to 288.

Development of Body Image

Body image, the *mental picture of one's body,* includes the external, internal, and postural picture of the body, although the mental image is not necessarily consistent with the actual body structure. Included also are attitudes, emotions, and personality reactions of the individual in relation to his or her body as an object in space, with a distinct boundary and apart from all others and the environment. The body image, gradually formulated over a period of years, is included in the **self-concept** *(awareness of self or me)* and *derives from reactions of others to his or her body, perceptions of how others react, experiences with his or her own and other bodies, constitutional factors, and physiologic and sensory stimuli* (122).

At birth the infant has diffuse feelings of hunger, pain, rage, and comfort but no body image. Pleasurable sensations come mainly from the lower face, the mouth-nose area, which has considerable nerve innervation. At first all the baby knows is self. Baby has the same attitude toward his or her body as toward other objects in the environment; the external world is an extension of self. Gradually, baby distinguishes his or her body from other animate and inanimate objects in the environment

as he or she bites a hand, bangs the head, grasps and mouths a toy, and experiences visceral, visual, auditory, kinesthetic, and motor sensations (122).

A primitive ego or self-development begins at approximately 3 months. Weaning, contact from others, and more exploration of the environment also heighten self-awareness. As the child approaches the first birthday, there is some coordination of these sensory experiences that are being internalized into the motor body image. He or she is aware that some body parts give greater pleasure than other parts and that there are differences in sensation when his or her body or another object is touched (122).

Without adequate somatosensory stimulation, body image and ego development are impaired as shown by studies of premature incubator infants who lacked rocking, stroking, and cuddling (11, 74). The infant's initial experiences with his or her body, determined largely by maternal care and attitudes, are the basis for a developing body image and how he or she later likes and handles the body and reacts to others.

Adaptive Mechanisms

Adaptive mechanisms are *learned behavioral responses that aid adjustment and emotional development.* At first the baby cries spontaneously. Soon baby learns that crying brings attention; therefore, he or she cries when uncomfortable, hungry, or bored. Other tools besides crying used in adaptation are experimentation, exploration, and manipulation. Baby uses the body in various ways to gain stimulation. He or she grabs and plays with whatever is within reach, whether it is father's nose or a toy. By the end of infancy, emotions of anger, fear, delight, and affection are expressed through vocalization, facial expression, and gestures.

The young infant does not understand waiting. But as baby meets with security and feels a sense of tenderness from caretakers, he or she begins to wait a short time between feeling hunger pains and demanding food. Instead of immediately screaming when a toy cannot be reached, baby will persist in repeating the action that will get him or her to the object. The baby is beginning to respond to the expectations of others and adapt to the family's cultural patterns.

If, however, care does not foster trust, the infant constantly feels threatened. At first he or she cries and shows increased motor activity, perhaps expressing rage, but may eventually feel powerless and become apathetic.

Adaptive mechanisms in infancy are called *primary process.* Some of these rudimentary methods of handling anxiety are symbolization, condensation, incorporation, and displacement. **Symbolization** *occurs when an object or idea comes to stand for something else because of associated characteristics.* For example, taking milk from mother's breast satisfies hunger. Soon the act also means pleasurable body contact, emotional response, and security. **Condensation** is the *reverse process. Several objects are fused into a single symbol.* The word *toy,* for example, comes to represent a variety of objects. **Incorporation** occurs when the *representation of mother or other objects is taken into the self and becomes a part of the understanding* and is the basis for the child's separation anxiety or attachment to parents. **Displacement** occurs when *emotions are transferred from an original object to another* such as from the mother to other family members or the babysitter (7, 82, 139).

Adaptive behavior is developed through structuring of the baby's potential. He or she needs both freedom to explore and exercise and consistent, pleasant restraints for personal safety, which together enable learning of self-restraint. Constantly saying "No" or confining the child to a walker or playpen does not help the learning of adaptive behavior.

One study compared the temperament of very-low-birth-weight (VLBW) infants to that of full-term infants at 6 and 12 months of age, assessed patterns of change in temperament from 6 to 12 months, and investigated effects of the neonatal experience on manifestations of temperament. The infants were free of congenital anomalies and appropriate for gestational age. At 6 months the VLBW infants were significantly less adaptable and more intense than full-term infants. There were significantly more "difficult" and fewer "easy" infants in the study group. However, although at 12 months the VLBW infants were less persistent than a full-term infant, the behavioral style clusters of the VLBW children did not differ significantly from full-term infants. The social environment of the VLBW infant plays an important role in the manifestation of childhood temperament as early as 6 months of age, but behavioral styles are modified during the first year of life with corrective nurturing (91).

Findings of another study confirm other researchers' findings that environmental factors can assist or sabotage developmental progress in a child who was originally at biologic risk. Developmental progress in very-low-birth-weight infants may be more sensitive to subsequent environmental influences than it is to past perinatal insults. The impact of the environment appears to become more powerful as the child matures (123).

There are two possible explanations for this finding. One explanation concerns the infant's natural self-righting tendencies. The infant may be temporarily deflected off course by premature birth, prolonged hospitalization, and illness around the time of birth, but once he or she is exposed to an even minimally appropriate environment, natural self-righting mechanisms have the potential to bring him or her back into the maturational trajectory characteristic of their species. A second explanation lies in the view of human development; the infant is changing and growing within the context of a transactional, organismic milieu. Negative past events become less important as the child, the parents, and the environment influence one another. The child elicits and reinforces parental responses, and parental behaviors and characteristics support developmental gains. The quality of the home environment and the passage of time significantly affect the outcome (123).

Sexuality Development

Sexuality may be defined as a *deep, pervasive aspect of the total person and the sum total of one's feelings and behavior as a male or female, the expression of which goes beyond genital response.* Sexuality includes the attitudes that are necessary to maintain a stable and intimate relationship with another person. Sexuality culminates in adulthood, but it begins to develop in infancy (139).

Gender is determined at the moment of fertilization. Chromosome combination and hormonal influences affect sexual development prenatally, as discussed in Chapter 6. Sometimes mothers respond to the fetus in a gender-differentiated way: an active fetus is interpreted as a boy, a quiet one as a girl. Prenatal position, according to folklore, relates to sex: boys are supposedly carried high, and girls are carried low.

Gender or sex assignment occurs at birth. The parents' first question is usually "Is it a boy or a girl?" The answer to this question often stimulates a set of adjectives to describe the newborn: soft, fine-featured, little, passive, weak girl; robust, big, strong, active boy, regardless of size or weight. The name given to baby also reflects the parents' attitudes toward the baby's gender and may reflect their ideas about the child's eventual role in life. Mothers, however, engage in less sex-typing stereotypes than fathers (82).

Occasionally external genitalia are ambiguous in appearance, neither distinctly male nor distinctly female. When this occurs, parents should be given as much support and information as possible to cope with the crisis; gender assignment based on chromosomal studies or appearance should be made as soon as possible (58).

The stereotypes about gender do have some basis in fact because at birth males usually are larger and have more muscle mass, are more active, and are more irritable than girls. Females are more sensitive to auditory, touch, and pain stimuli (6, 87). At 3 weeks of age males are still more irritable and are sleeping less than females.

Initially, mothers seem to respond more to male infants than to female infants (perhaps because male infants have traditionally been more highly valued). But by 3 months this reverses, and mothers are thought to have more touch and conversational contact with female infants, even when they are irritable. This reverse may occur because mothers are generally more successful in calming irritable daughters than irritable sons (97).

By 5 months baby responds differently to male and female voices, and by 6 months he or she distinguishes mother from father and as distinct people. At 6 months the female infant has a longer attention span for visual stimuli and better fixation to a human face, is more responsive to social stimuli, and prefers complex stimuli. The male infant has a better fixation response to a helix of light and is more attentive to an intermittent tone (4, 72, 87).

Also, when the babies are 6 months old, mothers imitate the verbal sounds of their daughters more than their sons, and mothers continue to touch, talk to, and handle their daughters more than their sons. Throughout infancy and childhood, female children talk to and touch their mothers more, whereas boys are encouraged to be more independent, exploratory, and vigorous in gross motor activity (82).

Fathers tend to treat the baby girl more softly and the baby boy more roughly during the last 6 months of infancy. At 9 months baby girl behaves differently with her mother than with her father. She will be rougher and more attention seeking with her father (72).

By 9 to 12 months, baby responds to his or her name, an important link to gender and role. Research indicates that girl babies are more dependent and less exploratory by 1 year than boys because of different parental behaviors to each sex. Parents appear to reinforce sex-coded behavior in infancy so that gender role behavior is learned on the basis of parental cues (72).

Infants receive stimulation of their erogenous zones during maternal care. The mouth and lower face are the main erogenous zones initially, providing pleasure, warmth, and satisfaction through sucking. Both sexes explore their genitalia during infancy. Erection in the male and lubrication in the female occur.

Explore sexuality development with parents. Help them be aware of the importance for sexuality development of their tone of voice, touch, behavior, and feelings toward the boy or girl. Help them develop ways to relate optimally to and promote trust and well-being in the child.

Developmental Tasks

Infancy is far from what some have assumed—a time for rigidly and mechanically handling the baby because he or she seems to have so little capability as an adapting human being. The following developmental tasks are to be accomplished in infancy (40):

1. Achieve equilibrium of physiologic organ systems after birth.
2. Establish self as a dependent person but separate from others.
3. Become aware of the alive versus inanimate and familiar versus unfamiliar and develop rudimentary social interaction.
4. Develop a feeling of and desire for affection and response from others.
5. Adjust somewhat to the expectations of others.
6. Begin to manage the changing body and learn new

motor skills, develop equilibrium, begin eye-hand coordination, and establish rest-activity rhythm.
7. Begin to understand and master the immediate environment through exploration.
8. Develop a beginning symbol or language system, conceptual abilities, and preverbal communication.
9. Direct emotional expression to indicate needs and wishes.

Explore these tasks with parents. Help them realize specific ways they enable their baby to achieve these tasks.

Nursing Applications

Your role with the infant and family has been discussed with each section throughout this chapter. See Box 7–3 for some *nursing diagnoses* that may apply to the infant.

BOX 7-3.
Selected Nursing Diagnoses Related to the Infant[a]

Pattern 1: Exchanging

Altered Nutrition: More than body requirements
Altered Nutrition: Less than body requirements
Altered Nutrition: Potential for more than body requirements
Constipation
Diarrhea
Impaired Gas Exchange
Potential for Infection
Potential for Injury
Potential for Suffocation
Potential for Poisoning
Potential for Trauma
Potential for Aspiration
Altered Protection
Potential Impaired Skin Integrity

Pattern 6: Moving

Impaired Physical Mobility
Sleep Pattern Disturbance
Ineffective Breastfeeding
Altered Growth and Development

Pattern 7: Perceiving

Sensory/Perceptual Alterations
Unilateral Neglect

Pattern 9: Feeling

Pain
Anxiety

[a]Other of the NANDA diagnoses are applicable to the ill infant.
From North American Nursing Diagnosis Association, *NANDA Nursing Diagnosis Taxonomy I* (Rev.). St. Louis: North American Nursing Diagnosis Association, 1990.

You can also be instrumental in establishing or working with community agencies that assist parents and infants. You may be called on to work with families who have adopted a child or with the single parent or with the reconstituted family who then has their own child (see also Chapter 4). You may work with a family whose child is not healthy or perfect or is born prematurely (see also Chapter 4), or you may work with a family who experiences sudden death of the infant.

Establishment and Use of Community Resources for Continuity of Care

Some sources of help that may be found in your community are summarized in Box 7–4.

In one large city two maternity nurses identified a need for a local organization that would offer courses in parenting. In addition to course offerings, the organization now hosts discussion groups for expectant and new mothers and for parents of toddlers. Recently a "postpartum hot line" was started. The despair of couples who experience postpartum problems is pointed out repeatedly. For example, "This is Julie. . . . We had our baby on the fourteenth. But (*tears*) you must have to be a pediatrician to be a mother. The baby is crying all the time; I don't know if I can continue to nurse her. . . . Everything is horrible!" (A home visit and a series of follow-up phone calls played a part in this mother's nursing her baby happily for 8 months [34].)

Instead of using referral to a community agency, a hospital may provide its own postpartal home-care services, especially for mothers and babies who are discharged from the hospital in 12 to 24 hours after delivery. Jones (66) describes how she set up such a service. Early discharge can have the advantages of treating mother and baby as well, not ill, reducing family separation time, and more directly involving father in care. Every woman or family, however, is not a candidate for early discharge. Prenatal preparation is necessary. Mother and baby must show no potential complications. Medical back-up care must be quickly available. Further, at times mother may get more rest and emotional support in the hospital than at home, depending on home and family conditions. In fact, visits by a nurse practitioner 1 hour daily for 3 days and then as needed for the first 2 weeks may *not* provide sufficient care (66). In contrast, the hospital may have a lay visitor program to assist the mother at home shortly after discharge (78).

Whenever visits are made in the home, assessment tools that can be used, if administered by a qualified person, are the *Denver II—Revision and Restandardization of the Denver Developmental Screening Test (DDST)* (see Fig. 9–2), a general scale that measures personal and social skills, language, and gross and fine motor abilities (44), the *Infant Temperament Questionnaire (ITQ),* which addresses various areas of temperament and behavior (28) and the *Home Observation for Measurement of the Environment (HOME)* in which the home-rearing situation is assessed (26).

■ BOX 7-4.
Community Resources for Parents

Classes on Parenting, Prenatal or Postnatal Care, Lamaze or Psychoprophylaxis Method of Childbirth
- Junior or senior college presenting nonacademic courses
- Hospital clinics
- Individual childbirth educators who are members of local and international Childbirth Education Association
- Crisis agencies such as Parent and Child, St. Louis
- Local Red Cross chapter
- Community health nursing services

Breast-Feeding Information
- La Leche League

Parent Support
- Voluntary self-help agencies such as Cesarean Support Group
- Mother's Center
- A Mother Experiencing Neo-Natal Death (A.M.E.N.D.)
- St. Louis Association for Retarded Citizens
- Parent and Child, St. Louis
- Association of Family Women
- Coping With Overall Parenting Experience (C.O.P.E.), Boston, Massachusetts
- Compassionate Friends, Box 1347, Oakbrook, IL 60521
- National Foundation for SIDS (Sudden Infant Death Syndrome), 1501 Broadway, New York, NY 10036
- National Sudden Infant Death Syndrome Foundation, 310 South Michigan Ave., Chicago, IL 60604

Crisis Attendance or Counseling
- Crisis hotlines such as Life Crisis Center or Parent and Child, St. Louis
- Family and Children's Services
- The clergy or other counselors

Care of the Premature Baby and the Baby With Congenital Anomalies

The principal threats to infant health are low birthweight and birth defects. The United States ranks eighteenth among industrialized nations for infant mortality, and the incidence for African-Americans is $2\frac{1}{2}$ times the average. The infant mortality rate is higher than the national average in areas where there is higher unemployment and, consequently, a lack of health insurance and lack of prenatal and obstetric care. Minority groups and adolescents are especially affected. Preterm and low-birthweight infants have higher rates of morbidity and mortality than normal weight infants. Preterm delivery accounts for approximately 10% of all births and 75% of

Research Abstract

Youngblut, J., C. Cherry, and M. Horan, Maternal Employment Effects on Family and Preterm Infants at Three Months, Nursing Research, *40, no. 5 (1991), 272–275.*

More than half (55%) of mothers with children less than 3 years of age are employed. For some of these women, employment is a necessity. The mother's employment places her in multiple roles and adds complexity to her life and the lives of her loved ones. A prime concern for these women is the effect that their employment will have on their children and on their families. When the child is born prematurely, concerns increase. A considerable body of research exists in which the effects of maternal employment on healthy children are reported; however, the results are conflicting. Research has been focused exclusively on the mother-child relationship, ignoring the context of the family.

The purpose of this study was to identify the effects of maternal employment status on family functioning and the developmental progress of the infant at 3 month of age who was born preterm. It was hypothesized that the mother's degree of choice and satisfaction with her employment status, rather than whether or not she was employed, would determine the employment's effects on the child and family. In addition, congruence between the mother's actual employment status and her attitudes about employment was hypothesized to have a positive impact on both family and child outcomes.

A convenience sample of 110 families was recruited from two neonatal intensive care units (NICUs). Criteria for inclusion in the study were that the infant was less than 37 weeks' gestation, size-appropriate for gestational age, hospitalized in the NICU for more than 1 week but less than 3 months, and free of anomalies that would preclude developmental progress and that the mother was living with a male partner acting as the father. Most parents were married, Caucasian, with at least a high school education, and with family incomes of $20,000 or more. Most of the fathers were employed, 40 mothers were employed outside the home. Fifty-nine of the preterm infants were male. Mean gestational age at birth was 32.6 weeks; mean birthweight was 1784.2 g. Average length of stay in the NICU was 31.6 days. At the time of interview, 98 infants were within 2 weeks of their 3-month birthday.

Data were collected in a $2\frac{1}{2}$ hour home visit. Hospital chart review by the research assistant at each site provided information about the infant's NICU stay. The mother's degree of choice about her employment status and her satisfaction with that choice were measured with a single Likert-type item. Beliefs and attitudes about maternal employment were measured with the Home/Employment Orientation (HEO) scale.

Three dimensions of family functioning—family cohesion, family adaptability, and family relationships—were measured. The FACES III questionnaire was used to measure cohesion and adaptability. Child outcome was measured with the Bayley Scales of Infant Development.

Findings of this study suggest that maternal employment does not adversely affect the preterm infant's development at 3 months of age. Having an infant whose development is more normal allows employment of the mother for more hours. Maternal employment may allow respite time for both the mother and the alternate caregiver so that the infant experiences responsive care more often. Exposure to additional caregivers may provide preterm infants with a wider range of stimuli that would enhance their motor development. Infants of employed mothers who reported having more choice about the employment decision had better motor development scores than infants whose mothers reported having less choice. It is likely that having a new baby in the house has a stronger influence on the family at 3 months' postpartum than do employment-related variables. Effects that could emerge when the child is older cannot be ruled out with the results of this study.

prenatal deaths. Of those who survive, 50% have neurologic defects requiring lifelong social and financial commitment. A preterm infant usually develops complications that necessitate neonatal intensive care at the cost of approximately $15,000 per day (132).

Birth defects are the leading cause of infant death in the United States. The most common defects are heart problems, central nervous system disorders, and defects of the respiratory system. The second leading cause of death is a combination of low birthweight, prematurity, and respiratory distress syndrome. These children also receive neonatal intensive care unit (NICU) treatment. The average total lifetime cost per survivor for NICU graduates has been estimated to range from $40,647 to $362,992, depending on infant birthweight and morbidity (9). The third major cause is Sudden Infant Death Syndrome (SIDS).

The United States is experiencing an epidemic of children born to mothers addicted to alcohol, cocaine, crack, and other such drugs. A generation of babies has already been affected and will present major problems to our society because of their developmental disabilities, uncontrollable behavior and rage, learning deficits, and lack of superego and remorse. There is an inadequate number of treatment centers and foster homes. Mothers or grandmothers are likely to bear the brunt of this crisis. For many parents and their families, birth of a baby will not bring joy but fear, grief, and depression—for a long time (36, 37, 69, 146).

However, there are times that the baby is preterm or premature or has a lasting problem for no known reason. Further, there are families who reach out to these babies with love and caring; as a result, the baby develops to the maximum potential. Supportive nursing care is a key factor for these families (6).

The major problem with the **premature infant** is that he or she is usually separated from the parents. Often the newborn is in an isolette on another hospital floor; sometimes he or she is transferred to another hospital. If the infant is in the same hospital, every possible opportunity for touch and eye contact should be given to the parents. (The parent can even hold the baby while the nurse gives a gavage feeding.) If the baby must stay in the premature nursery, arrange for the parents to view the baby at a time when he or she is most alert, for example, right before feeding time; help the parents feel welcome. A note similar to the following pinned to the crib can give parents much encouragement: "Hi Mom and Dad. I am so glad you could come to visit me. Signed, Patricia." Try to give as much information as possible to the parents about the baby's habits, strengths, and gains. This information could also be put in note form: "Dear Mom and Dad, I gained 2 whole ounces yesterday. This is a lot for my size. I'm also kicking my feet more. I think I will be a soccer player. I love you. Brian."

If the premature infant is in another hospital, father should be encouraged to visit the infant and to be the link between baby and the mother until she can visit. The father can explain the care the baby is getting, take photos of the baby to show his wife, and describe the daily gains. If you work in the premature nursery and if the parents cannot visit, you can take the initiative to call the parents to describe how the baby is changing, the baby's schedule, and environment. The parents, in turn, can express their feelings.

The guidelines presented earlier on teaching the mother ways to stimulate her infant can also be taught to the mother of the premature—for use whenever the baby's condition permits. Refer also to Chapter 4 for additional information.

Foster grandparents in the premature nursery can provide some of the nurturing, holding, and tactile stimulation that the premature needs for normal development if the parents and grandparents cannot visit the nursery and participate in care (106).

Cultures vary in the care of the premature. Premature babies in some countries are placed with their mothers 2 to 3 hours after birth and are sent home soon after birth because of economic status of the parents, problems with cross and nosocomial infections, and deep respect for natural processes. Anderson, Marks, and Wahlberg (2) describe a program in Bogota, Columbia, that is designed to give optimum care to premature baby and mother after early discharge from the hospital.

Parents of the **baby with congenital anomalies** (defects in physical structure or function) will need the same considerations as parents of the premature infant. They should be encouraged to see their infant as soon as possible to avoid fantasies that are often worse than the anomaly. Show them the normal parts and emphasize the baby's positive features. Above all, show your acceptance of the infant: hold, cuddle, and look at the infant as you talk to him or her. Give information about the anomaly and the possible prognosis. This is a difficult time for parents, and they will need ample time to express their grief, guilt, and worries. Your patience and support will be most helpful. Various references provide more in-depth information to share with parents pertinent to the specific disability (2, 25, 58, 131, 144). Refer to Chapter 4 for additional information on nursing practice with the family.

There are *ethical dilemmas* with care of the premature infant, especially if he or she is greatly preterm and very low birthweight, and with care of the infant that has a severe congenital anomaly. Infants who in 1960 would have had no chance for survival are today receiving care from health professionals armed with extensive knowledge and state-of-the-art technologies. In fact, among all babies born between the years 1970 and 1980, deaths during the neonatal period diminished by one half. Many infants with multiple and serious handicaps can now survive anywhere from weeks to years, which raises questions about the cost of their care and the quality of their lives (142).

The primary controversies of withholding treatment revolve around two questions: (1) should life-sustaining treatment be denied to any infant regardless of the infant's pathology, related handicaps, or suffering; and (2) if treatment is not considered appropriate in all cases, which infants should be denied it, on what grounds, and who should decide (142)?

Parents and members of the health-care and judicial systems continue to debate hotly the anticipated length and quality of many of those infants' lives. Some infants who are saved will continue as a financial and care burden for their parents the rest of the parents' and the child's lives.

The ethical, personal, and economic dilemmas posted by the use of life-sustaining technologies are considerable and have caused policymakers to consider withholding treatment from selected infants (142). Using high technology treatment methods may be experimentation and research, shrouded in the guise of treatment. The pivotal case of Baby Doe has come to exemplify just such an event. The case is discussed at length by Wakefield-Fisher (142).

It is suggested that nursing and medical associations establish joint committees to further clarify ethical issues and to suggest practices related to withholding life-sustaining treatment from infants. The associations could communicate recommendations to professionals, the Department of Health and Human Services, and hospital-based committees. Such action would align nurses and physicians, helping both groups understand and exchange information about the related issues. Direction from a joint committee could encourage providers to adopt a more uniform response to seriously ill infants in terms of standards of care (142).

Nurses increasingly have understanding of both the questions and legal and ethical responses related to withholding life-sustaining treatment from infants. Nurses must participate in the decision making over the next decade, based on adequate knowledge of the issue.

Care of the Family Experiencing Adoption and Infant Death

Mothers Who Adopt Out Their Newborns

These mothers are confronted with a crisis that involves bereavement. Ambivalence prevails during the prenatal period: love for baby, guilt about abandonment, and concern for his or her future. Therapeutic intervention begins prenatally by exploring with the mother the anticipatory grief, anger, depression, decisions about seeing the baby, and choice of postdelivery care. To promote bonding would be cruel, but the mother should have the opportunity—the reality—of holding and inspecting. Not to recognize the infant is to deny the pregnancy; seeing the infant gives concrete focus to the mother's grief. A maternity nurse-specialist should consult the relinquishing mother on a scheduled basis to promote the woman's personal growth, self-respect, and dignity. Refer also to Chapter 4 for more information on the adoptive process and family.

Parents Whose Infants Die

If the newborn dies, parents must work through the affectional-symbiotic bond developed within the mother in anticipation of the baby as perfect. Full expression of the grief, guilt, and anger is necessary. Many hospital practices tend to discourage these reactions by removing all evidence of the baby's existence. Nothing is left to confirm the reality of the baby's death. Parents should, if they desire, be permitted to view, touch, and hold their dead infant. Within the beliefs of the parents, some traditional bereavement service should be arranged to promote grieving and making the death real (71). Klaus and Kennell (71) suggest meeting with the parents three times after the death of the infant to assist them through normal mourning: right after birth, within the next 2 to 3 days before discharge, and in 3 to 6 months. During these visits you can effectively listen, encourage expression of feelings, and check for normalcy in the parents' feelings and reactions.

Although SIDS is at least as old as Biblical times, it did not become acceptable as a term for use on death certificates until the early 1970s. Formerly it was called *crib death*. This disease is a primary cause of death in infants after the first week of life (131). A typical case might be an apparently healthy infant, possibly with a slight cold, usually between the ages of 3 weeks and 7 months, who is put to bed and then found dead when the caretaker goes to check him or her. Usually the baby has not made a sound, and there is no evidence of struggle. Autopsy is the only means of making a diagnosis and may reveal widely diffuse petechiae across the pleura, minor inflammation of the upper respiratory tract, minor lung congestion and common viruses, or no unusual findings (106).

No one knows what causes SIDS but there are many theories: (1) the mild viral infection may affect nerves that affect lung activity; (2) inherent nerve deficit may affect the larynx, causing laryngospasm; (3) there may be decreased carbon dioxide sensitivity or sleep apnea, and (4) suffocation may result from rebreathing face down in polystyrene-filled cushions. Because there is no known cause, there is no known prevention (106), although close monitoring may aid prevention. Special monitoring devices for use in the home can be purchased.

The thrust for the nurse is in helping the parents or caretakers deal with their guilt, grief, and future psychologic balance. You should be able to direct these people to national or local help. National organizations are listed in Box 7–4. In some health departments there are nurses who are designated to make visits for as long as needed. Luscombe (86) describes a self-help group formed to assist parents with mourning and feelings of guilt, failure, and isolation after their infant's death. Information about the group can be obtained by writing P.R.I.D.E., P.O. Box 95, Neptune, NJ 07754.

No matter what birth takes place—normal or abnormal—the family is going through a type of *rebirth* in that their lives are forever changed by the event. Your guidance in this process may be felt for years.

REFERENCES

1. Alexander, M., Homemade Toys for Infants, *American Journal of Nursing,* 70, no. 12 (December 1970), 2557–2560.
2. Anderson, G., E. Marks, and V. Wahlberg, Kangaroo Care for Premature Babies, *American Journal of Nursing,* 84, no. 7 (1984), 807–809.
3. Ballard, J., et al., A Simplified Score for Assessment of Fetal Maturation in Newly Born Infants, *Journal of Pediatrics,* 95 (1979), 769–774.
4. Bardwich, J., *Psychology of Women: A Study of Biocultural Conflicts.* New York: Harper & Row, 1971.
5. Becerra, J., and J. Smith, Breastfeeding Patterns in Puerto Rico, *American Journal of Public Health,* 80, no. 6 (1990), 694–697.
6. Becker, P., et al., Outcomes of Developmentally Supportive Nursing Care for Very Low Birth Weight Infants, *Nursing Research,* 40, no. 3 (1991), 150–155.
7. Bettelheim, B., and A. Freedgood, *A Good Enough Parent: A Book on Child-Rearing.* New York: Random, 1988.
8. Bills, B., Enhancement of Paternal-Newborn Affectional Bonds, *Journal of Nurse-Midwifery,* 25, no. 5 (1980), 21–26.
9. Birth Defects Are Leading Cause of Infant Deaths, *MMWR,* 38, (1989), 633–635.
10. Bishop, B., A Guide to Assessing Parenting Capabilities, *American Journal of Nursing,* 76, no. 11 (November 1976), 1784–1787.
11. Blaesing, S., and J. Brockhaus, The Development of Body Image in the Child, *Nursing Clinics of North America,* 7, no. 4 (1972), 597–598.

12. Blank, D., Development of the Infant Tenderness Scale, *Nursing Research,* 34, no. 4, (1985), 211–215.

13. Boggs, K., and P. Rau, Breastfeeding the Premature Infant, *American Journal of Nursing,* 83, no. 10 (1983), 1437–1439.

14. Bowen, S., and B. Miller, Paternal Attachment Behavior as Related to Presence at Delivery and Preparenthood Classes: A Pilot Study, *Nursing Research,* 29, no. 5 (1980), 307.

15. Bowlby, J., *Attachment and Loss: Vol. 1.* New York: Basic Books, 1969.

16. ———, Disruption of Affectional Bonds and Its Effect on Behavior, *Canada's Mental Health Supplement,* no. 59 (January-February 1969), 2–12.

17. Brazelton, P.T., *The Neonatal Behavioral Assessment Scale* (2nd ed.). Philadelphia: J.B. Lippincott, 1984.

18. Brazelton, T., and B. Cramer, *The Earliest Relationship.* Addison-Wesley, 1990.

19. Breast Is Best—For Premies Too, *American Journal of Nursing,* 87, no. 11 (1987), 1403–1404.

20. Brock, D., Social Forces, Feminism, and Breast-feeding, *Nursing Outlook,* 23, no. 8 (September 1975), 556–561.

21. Broussard, E.R., and M. Sturgeon, Further Considerations Regarding Maternal Perception of the First Born. In Hellmuth, J., ed., *Exceptional Infant: Studies in Abnormalities,* Vol. 2. New York: Brunner/Mazel, 1971.

22. Brown, M., Social Support, Stress, and Health: A Comparison of Expectant Mothers and Fathers, *Nursing Research,* 36, no. 2 (1986), 74–76.

23. Budnick, L., and D. Ross, Bathtub Drownings in the United States, 1979–81, *American Journal of Public Health,* 75, no. 6 (1985), 630–633.

24. Burd, B., Encouragement Counts in Breast Feeding, *American Journal of Nursing,* 81, no. 8 (1981), 1491.

25. Butani, P., Reactions of Mothers to the Birth of an Anomalous Infant: A Review of Literature, *Maternal-Child Nursing Journal,* 3 (Spring 1974), 59–76.

26. Caldwell, B., *Home Inventory for Infants.* Fayetteville, Ark: Fayetteville Center for Development and Education, University of Arkansas, 1978.

27. *Can Your Baby Hear?* St. Louis: St. Louis Hearing and Speech Center, 1980.

28. Carey W.B., and S.C. McDevitt, A Review of the Infant Temperament Questionnaire, *Pediatrics,* 61 (1978), 735-738.

29. Censullo, M., B. Lester, and J. Hoffman, Rythmic Patterning in Mother-Newborn Interactions, *Nursing Research,* 34, no. 6 (1985), 342–348.

30. Chilmonczyk, B., et al., Environmental Tobacco Smoke Exposure During Infancy, *American Journal of Public Health,* 80, no. 10 (1990), 1205–1208.

31. Clark, A.L., Recognizing Discord Between Mother and Child and Changing it to Harmony, *American Journal of Maternal-Child Nursing,* 1, no. 2 (March-April 1976), 100–116.

32. ———, and Dyanne D. Affonso, Infant Behavior and Maternal Attachment: Two Sides of the Coin, *American Journal of Maternal-Child Nursing,* 1, no. 2 (March-April 1976), 94–99.

33. Committee of Infectious Diseases, American Academy of Pediatrics, *Report of the Committee of Infectious Diseases* (21st ed.). Elkgrove Village, Ill: American Academy of Pediatrics, 1988.

34. Cooksey, N., *What Is Parent and Child/St. Louis . . . ?* December, 1976.

35. Cushions May Cause Infant Death, *Washington University School of Medicine Outlook* (Fall 1991), 2–3.

36. Damrosch, S.P., and L.A. Perry, Self-Reported Adjustment, Chronic Sorrow, and Coping of Parents of Children with Down Syndrome, *Nursing Research,* 38 (1989), 25–30.

37. Dorris, M., *The Broken Cord.* New York: Harper Collins, 1991.

38. Dubowitz, L., and V. Dubowitz, *A Clinical Manual: Gestational Age of the Newborn.* New York: Addison-Wesley, 1977.

39. Dusitin, N., et al, Development and Validation of a Simple Device to Estimate Birthweight and Screen for Low Birthweight in Developing Countries, *American Journal of Public Health,* 81, no. 9 (1991), 1201–1205.

40. Duvall, E., and B. Miller, *Marriage and Family Development* (6th ed). New York: Harper & Row, 1984.

41. Erikson, E., *Childhood and Society* (2nd ed.). New York: W.W. Norton, 1963.

42. ———, *Toys and Reasons.* New York: W.W. Norton, 1977.

43. Feeding Your Child, *Parenting: Glennon Hospital for Children, St. Louis,* 1990, pp. 10–11.

44. Frankenburg, W.K., and J.B. Dodd, The Denver Developmental Screening Test, *Journal of Pediatrics,* 71 (1967), 181–191.

45. Fuller, B., Acoustic Discrimination of Three Types of Infant Cries, *Nursing Research,* 40, no. 3 (1991), 156–160.

46. Garbarino, J., E. Guttmann, and J. Steeley, *The Psychologically Battered Child: Strategies for Identification, Assessment, and Intervention.* San Francisco: Jossey-Bass, 1987.

47. Gesell, A., et al., *The First Five Years of Life.* New York: Harper Brothers, 1940.

48. Goldstein, J., A. Freud, and A.J. Solnit, *Beyond the Best Interests of the Child.* New York: The Free Press, Macmillan, 1973.

49. Gordon, R.E., E.E. Kapostins, and K.K. Gordon, Factors in Postpartum Adjustment, *Obstetrics and Gynecology,* 25, no. 2 (1965), 158–166.

50. Greenberg, R., et al., Passive Smoking During the First Year of Life, *American Journal of Public Health,* 81, no. 7 (1991), 850–858.

51. Greenburg, M., and N. Morris, Engrossment: The Newborn's Impact Upon the Father, *American Journal of Orthopsychiatry,* 44 (1974), 520–531.

52. Hall, L., Effect of Teaching on Primiparas' Perceptions of the Newborn, *Nursing Research,* 29, no. 5 (1980), 317–321.

53. Harlap, S., and A.M. Davies, Infant Admissions to Hospital and Maternal Smoking, *Lancet,* 1 (March 30, 1974), 529–532.

54. Harris, C., Cultural Values and the Decision to Circumcise, *Image,* 18, no. 3 (1986), 98–103.

55. Hartwick, N., Infant Formula: A Threat to Third-World Babies, *Graduate Woman,* 75, no. 6 (1981), 26–31.

56. Hegarty, V., *Decisions in Nutrition*. St. Louis: C.V. Mosby, 1988.

57. Helberg, J., Documentation of Child Abuse, *American Journal of Nursing,* 83, no. 2 (1983), 234–239.

58. Hill, S., The Child with Ambiguous Genitalia, *American Journal of Nursing,* 77, no. 5 (May 1977), 810–814.

59. Holmes, T.H., and M. Masuda, Life Change and Illness Susceptibility, *Separation and Depression AAAS* (1973), 161–186.

60. ——, and R.H. Rahe, The Social Readjustment Rating Scale, *Journal of Psychosomatic Research,* 2 (1967), 213–218.

61. Hoole, A., R. Greenberg, and C.G. Pickhard, *Patient Care Guidelines for Nurse Practitioners* (3rd ed.). Boston: Little, Brown, 1988.

62. Hurd, J.M.L., Assessing Maternal Attachment: First Step Toward the Prevention of Child Abuse, *Journal of Obstetric, Gynecologic, and Neonatal Nursing,* 4, no. 4 (July-August 1975), 25–30.

63. Infant Formula is not Microproof, *American Journal of Nursing,* 85, no. 4 (1985), 358.

64. IPOL (Poliovirus Vaccine Inactivated), *Nation's Health* (September 1991), 6.

65. Jackson, P., When a Baby Isn't Perfect, *American Journal of Nursing,* 85, no. 4 (1985), 396–399.

66. Jones, D., Home Early After Delivery, *American Journal of Nursing,* 78, no. 8 (1978), 1378–1380.

67. Jones, L.C., and E. Lenz, Father-Newborn Interaction: Effects of Social Competence and Infant State, *Nursing Research,* 35, no. 3 (1986), 149–153.

68. Kahn, A., et al., Insomnia and Cow's Milk Allergy in Infants, *Pediatrics,* 76 (December 1985), 880–884.

69. Kazak, A.E., and R. Marvin, Differences, Difficulties, and Adaptation: Stress and Social Networks in Families With a Handicapped Child, *Family Relations,* 33 (1981), 67–77.

70. Kelly, P., ed., *First Year Baby Care: An Illustrated Step-by-Step Guide for New Parents.* Deephaven, Minn: Meadowbrook Press, 1983.

71. Klaus, M., and J. Kennell, *Parent-Infant Bonding* (2nd ed). St. Louis: C.V. Mosby, 1982.

72. Kleeman, J., The Establishment of Core Gender Identity in Normal Girls, *Archives of Sexual Behavior,* 1 (1971), 103–116.

73. Kleimhuizen, J., Traditions Guard Hispanic Babies' Health, *USA Today,* February 4, 1991, Sec. D, p. 4.

74. Kramer, M., et al., Extra Tactile Stimulation of the Premature Infant, *Nursing Research,* 24, no. 5 (September-October 1975), 324–334.

75. Krantz, L., Comparison of Body Proportions of One-year Old Mexican American and Anglo Children, *American Journal of Public Health,* 71, no. 3 (1981), 280–282.

76. Lactation and Composition of Milk in Undernourished Women, *Nutrition Review,* 33, no. 2 (1975), 42–43.

77. Lamb, M., *The Father's Role.* New York: John Wiley, 1986.

78. Lay Visitor Program Helps New Parents, *American Journal of Nursing,* 79, no. 3 (1979), 421.

79. Lazieh, M., The Breast Feeding Worker—Risk or Benefit, *Occupational Health Nursing,* 30, no. 11 (1982), 34–37.

80. Lee, E., Asian Infant Feeding, *Nursing Mirror,* 160, no. 21 (May 22, 1985), 14–15.

81. Lerner, R., and D. Hultsch, *Human Development: A Life-Span Perspective.* New York: McGraw-Hill, 1983.

82. Lidz, T., *The Person: His and Her Development Throughout the Life Cycle* (2nd ed). New York: Basic Books, 1983.

83. Linley, J., Screening Children for Common Orthopoedic Problems, *American Journal of Nursing,* 87, no. 10 (1987), 1312–1316.

84. Lorber, B., Changing Patterns of Infectious Diseases, *American Journal of Medicine,* 84, no. 3 (1988), 569–578.

85. Lundington-Hoe, S., What Can Newborns Really See? *American Journal of Nursing,* 83, no. 9 (1983), 1286–1289.

86. Luscombe, K., P.R.I.D.E.—Parents Resolving Infant Death Experiences, *Free Association '85,* 12, no. 3 (1985) 1–7.

87. Macoby, R., Sex Differences in Intellectual Functioning, In Bardwich, J., ed., *Readings on the Psychology of Women.* New York: Harper & Row, 1972, pp. 34–44.

88. McBride, A.B., *The Growth and Development of Mothers.* New York: Harper & Row, 1973.

89. McDonald, B., Heeding the Baby's Cry, *Washington University School of Medicine Outlook,* 24, no. 1 (1987), 17–19.

90. McKeel, N., Child Abuse Can Be Prevented, *American Journal of Nursing,* 78, no. 9 (1978), 1478–1481.

91. Medoff-Cooper, B., Temperament in Very Low-Birth-Weight Infants, *Nursing Research,* 35, no. 3 (1986), 139–142.

92. ——, and B. Schraeder, Developmental Trends and Behavioral Styles in Very Low Birth-Weight Infants, *Nursing Research,* 31, no. 2 (1982), 68–72.

93. Mercer, D., Relating Mother's Anxiety and Perception to Infant Satiety, Anxiety, and Feeding Behaviors, *Nursing Research,* 35, no. 6 (1986), 347–361.

94. Mercer, R., Theoretical Models for Studying the Effect of Antepartum Stress in the Family, *Nursing Research,* 35, no. 6 (1986), 339–346.

95. Mittelman, R., H. Mittelman, and C. Wetu, What Child Abuse Really Looks Like, *American Journal of Nursing,* 87, no. 9 (1987), 1185–1188.

96. Montagu, A., *Touching: The Human Significance of the Skin* (3rd ed). New York: Columbia University Press, 1986.

97. Moss H., Sex, Age, and State as Determinants of Mother-Infant Interaction. In Bardwich, J., ed., *Readings on the Psychology of Women.* New York: Harper & Row, 1972, pp. 22–29.

98. My Husband Was Afraid to Be a Father, *Good Housekeeping* (September 1989), 34, 36–37.

99. Nebert, D., J. Elashoff, and K. Wilcox, Possible Effect of Neonatal Polybrominated Biphenyl Exposure on the Developmental Abilities of Children, *American Journal of Public Health,* 73, no. 3 (1983), 286–289.

100. O'Grady, R., and T. Dolan, Whooping Cough in Infancy, *American Journal of Nursing,* 76, no. 1 (1976), 114–117.

101. Out of The Mouths of Babes, *Newsweek* (December 15, 1986), 84–86.

102. Owen, G., and A. Lubin, Anthropometric Differences Between Black and White Preschool Children, *American Journal of Diseases of Children,* 126 (1973), 168–169.

103. Owens, M., A Crying Need, *American Journal of Nursing,* 86, no. 1 (1986), 73.

104. Piaget, J., *The Construction of Reality in the Child* (M. Cook, transl.). New York: Basic Books, 1954.

105. ———, *The Origins of Intelligence in Children.* New York: International University Press, 1952.

106. Pillitteri, A., *Child Health Nursing: Care of the Growing Family* (3rd ed.). Boston: Little, Brown, 1987.

107. Pitch the Polystyrene-Filled Pillows, *Washington University Magazine* (Fall 1991), 3.

108. Pridham, K., and M. Hansoen, Helping Children Deal with Procedures in a Clinical Setting: A Developmental Approach, *Journal of Pediatric Nursing,* 2, no. 2 (1987), 13–21.

109. Rentscler, D., Correlates of Successful Breast Feeding, *Image,* 23, no. 3 (1991), 151–154.

110. Richi, F., and R. Krzy, The Child In the Car: What Every Nurse Should Know About Safety, *American Journal of Nursing,* 83, no. 10 (1983), 1421–1424.

111. Riesch, S., and S. Munns, Promoting Awareness: The Mother and Her Baby, *Nursing Research,* 33, no. 5 (1984), 271–276.

112. Rising, S.S., The Fourth Stage of Labor: Family Integration, *American Journal of Nursing,* 74, no. 5 (1974), 870–874.

113. Robson, K., The Role of Eye-to-Eye Contact in Maternal-Infant Attachment, *Journal of Child Psychology and Psychiatry,* 8 (1976), 13–25.

114. Rogan, W., et al., Polychlorinated Biphenysl (PCBs) and Dichlorodiphenyl Dichloroethene (DDE) in Human Milk: Effects of Maternal Factors and Previous Lactation, *American Journal of Public Health,* 76, no. 2 (1986), 172–177.

115. Rubin, R., Attainment of the Maternal Role—Part I, *Nursing Research,* 16, no. 3 (1967), 237–245.

116. ———, Attainment of the Maternal Role—Part II, *Nursing Research,* 16, no. 4 (1967), 342–346.

117. ———, Cognitive Style in Pregnancy, *American Journal of Nursing,* 70, no. 3 (1970), 502–508.

118. ———, Binding-in in the Postpartum Period, *Maternal-Child Nursing Journal,* 6 (1977), 67–75.

119. Ruffing, M.A., Mothering and Early Infant Stimulation, *Nursing Forum,* 18, no. 1 (1979), 69–79.

120. Salk, L., The Role of the Heartbeat in the Relations Between Mother and Infant, *Scientific American,* 228, (May 1973), 24–29.

121. Satz, K., Integrating Navajo Tradition Into Maternal-Child Nursing, *Image,* 14, no. 3 (1982), 89–91.

122. Schilder, P., *The Image and Appearance of the Human Body.* New York: International University Press, 1951.

123. Schraeder, B., Developmental Progress in Very Low-Birth-Weight Infants During the First Year of Life, *Nursing Research,* 35, no.4 (1986), 237–242.

124. Schwartz, E., and W. Rae, Effect of Polybrominated Biphenyls (PBB) on Developmental Abilities in Young Children, *American Journal of Public Health,* 73, no. 3 (1983), 277–281.

125. Sciarra, J.J., ed., *Gynecology and Obstetrics.* Philadelphia: Harper & Row, 1982.

126. Scipien, G.M., et al., *Comprehensive Pediatric Nursing* (3rd ed.). New York: McGraw-Hill, 1986.

127. Scrimshaw, S., et al., Factors Affecting Breast-feeding Among Women of Mexican Origin or Descent in Los Angeles, *American Journal of Public Health,* 77, no. 4 (1987), 467–470.

128. Seagull, E., Developmental Abilities of Children Exposed to Polybrominated Biphenyls (PBB), *American Journal of Public Health,* 73, no. 3 (1983), 281–285.

129. Selekman, J., Immunization: What's It All About? *American Journal of Nursing,* 80, no. 8 (1980), 1440–1445.

130. Sherman, J.L., Jr., and S. Fields, *Guide to Patient Evaluation* (3rd ed.). Garden City, NY: Medical Examination Publishing, 1978.

131. Sherwen, L., M. Scoloveno, and C. Weingarten, *Nursing Care of the Childbearing Family.* Norwalk, Conn: Appleton & Lange, 1991.

132. Smith R., Infant Mortality and Prenatal Care, *Henry Ford Hospital Medical Journal,* 38, nos. 2 and 3 (1990), 137–139.

133. Stevenson, M., and M. Lamb, Effects of Infant Sociability and the Caretaking Environment on Infant Cognitive Performance, *Child Development,* 50, no. 2 (1979), 340–349.

134. Switzer, J., Reporting Child Abuse, *American Journal of Nursing,* 86, no. 6 (1986), 663–664, 668.

135. Toney, L., The Effects of Holding the Newborn at Delivery on Paternal Bonding, *Nursing Research,* 32, no. 1 (1983), 16–19.

136. Tulman, L., Mothers' and Unrelated Persons' Handling of Newborn Infants, *Nursing Research,* 34, no. 4 (1985), 205–210.

137. ———, Initial Handling of Newborn Infants by Vaginally and Cesarean Delivered Mothers, *Nursing Research,* 35, no. 5 (1986), 296–299.

138. Urdang, L., and H. Swallow, eds., *Mosby's Medical and Nursing Dictionary.* St. Louis: C.V. Mosby, 1983.

139. U.S. Department of Health and Human Service, New Recommended Schedule for Active Immunization of Normal Infants and Children, *Morbidity and Mortality Weekly Report,* 35, no. 37 (September 16, 1986), 577–579.

140. Verzemnieks, I., Developmental Stimulation for Infants and Toddlers, *American Journal of Nursing,* 84, no. 6 (1984), 749–752.

141. Wadsworth, B., *Piaget's Theory of Cognitive and Affective Development* (4th ed.). New York: Longman, 1989.

142. Wakefield-Fisher, M., Balancing Wishes with Wisdom: Sustaining Infant Life, *Nursing and Health Care,* no. 11 (1987), 517–520.

143. Weiss, S., The Language of Touch, *Nursing Research,* 28, no. 2 (1979), 76–80.

144. Whaley, L., and D. Wong, *Nursing Care of Infants and Children* (4th ed.). St. Louis: C.V. Mosby, 1991.

145. Wicklund, K., S. Moss, and F. Frost, Effects of Maternal Education, Age, and Parity in Fetal and and Infant Accident, *American Journal of Public Health,* 74, no. 10 (1984), 584.

146. Wikle, L., Chronic Stresses of Families of Mentally Retarded Children, *Family Relations,* 30 (1981), 281–288.
147. Williams, S.R., *Nutrition and Diet Therapy* (6th ed.). St. Louis: TimesMirror/Mosby, 1989.
148. Wink, D., Getting Through the Maze of Infant Formulas, *American Journal of Nursing,* 85, no. 4 (1985), 388–392.

149. ———, Better Breast Milk for Premies, *American Journal of Nursing,* 89, no. 1 (1989), 48–49.
150. Yotema, S., *Vegetarian Baby*. Ithaca, NY: Plenum, 1980.
151. Young, S., et al., Effectiveness of a Mailed Reminder on the Immunization Levels of Infants at High Risk of Failure to Complete Immunizations, *American Journal of Public Health,* 70, no. 4 (1980), 422–424.

Chapter 8

Assessment and Health Promotion for the Toddler

Train up a child in the way he should go, and when he is old, he will not depart from it.
—*Proverbs 22: 6*

KEY TERMS

Toddler stage	Astigmatism	Juvenile hypertension	Self-system
Separation anxiety	Strabismus	Parataxic mode	Good-me
Protest	Otitis media	Preoperational period	Bad-me
Despair	Dental caries	Egocentric	Not-me
Denial	Malabsorption syndrome	Syncretic speech	Primary identification
Myelinization	Impetigo	Telegraphic speech	Regression
Accommodate	Pharyngitis	Contraction	Suppression
Hyperopia	Acute nonspecific	Expansion	Denial
Spider nevi	gastroenteritis (diarrhea)	Autistic	Reaction formation
Mongolian spots	Varicella (chicken pox)	Autonomy	Projection
Cafe-au-lait spots	Reye's syndrome	Shame	Sublimation
Bruises	Rubella	Doubt	Discipline
Parallel play	Pinworms (*Enterobius*	Anal stage	
Myopia	*vermicularis*)	Self-concept	

OBJECTIVES

Study of this chapter will enable you to:

1. Discuss the effects of family and toddler on each other, the significance of attachment behavior and separation anxiety, and the family developmental tasks to be achieved.
2. Explore with parents ways to adapt to the toddler while they simultaneously socialize the child and meet their developmental tasks.
3. Assess a toddler's physical and motor characteristics and related needs, including nutrition, rest, exercise, play, safety, and health protection measures.
4. Assess a toddler's general cognitive, language, emotional, and sexuality development.
5. Describe specific guidance and discipline methods for the toddler and the significance of the family's philosophy about guidance and discipline.
6. Discuss with parents their role in contributing to the toddler's cognitive, language, emotional, self-concept, and moral development.
7. Discuss the commonly used adaptive mechanisms that promote autonomy and your role in assisting parents to foster the development of autonomy.
8. State the toddler's developmental tasks and ways to help him or her achieve them.
9. Work effectively with a toddler and the family in the nursing situation.

In this chapter development of the toddler and the family relationships are discussed. *Nursing responsibilities for health promotion of the child and family are discussed throughout the chapter.* The information in this chapter is the basis for care of the toddler and family in any setting.

Within the first year of life children make remarkable adaptation internally and externally to their environment. They sit, walk, remember, recognize others, begin to socialize, communicate more purposely with speech, and show more specific emotional responses.

The **toddler stage** *begins when the child takes the first steps alone at 12 to 15 months and continues until approximately 3 years of age.* The family is very important during this short span of the child's life as he or she acquires language skills, increases cognitive achievement, improves physical coordination, and achieves control over bladder and bowel sphincters. These factors lead to new and different perceptions of self and the environment, new incentives, and new ways of dealing with problems.

FAMILY DEVELOPMENT AND RELATIONSHIPS

Behaviorally, the toddler changes considerably between 15 months and 3 years, a change that in turn affects family relationships. Because of new skills, the child begins to develop a sense of independence, establishes physical boundaries between self and mother, and gains the sense of a separate, self-controlled being who can do things on his or her own. From the age of 2 years the child moves toward independence—from the protracted dependency of childhood toward adulthood independence, self-reliance, and object relations. The child attempts self-education through mastery and engaging parents and others in help when necessary. Without the myriad attempts to do things for himself or herself, the child would obtain no degree of autonomy in skills. The periods of practice that ensure reliable performance and skills are often periods of independent action. However, dependence on others and gratification of dependency needs are essential for optimum ego development. Dependency does not mean passivity, for the child is quite active in obtaining help by crying, screaming, taking an adult by the hand and pulling him or her to another area, or asking how to solve a problem. The toddler should neither be kept too dependent nor forced too quickly into independence (3).

The family of a toddler can be quiet and serene one minute and in total upheaval the next, resulting from the imbalance between the child's motor skills, lack of experience, and mental capacities. One quick look away from the toddler can result in a broken object, a spilled glass of milk, or overturned dish. The toddler's quickly changing moods from tears to laughter or anger to calm, combined with energy, sense of independence, and curiosity, also account for parents' labeling their toddler a *terrible two*.

Help parents realize this behavior is normal and necessary for maturation. Expecting, planning for, and trying to handle patiently each situation will reduce parent frustration.

The toddler is frequently jealous of younger siblings because of having to vie for the center of attention that was once his or her own: older siblings are resented because they are permitted to do things he or she cannot. Power struggles focusing on feeding and toilet training occur between parent and child. Family problems may also arise when the toddler's activities are limited because of parental anxieties concerning physical harm or because of their intolerance of the child's energetic behavior and unknowing infractions of societal rules.

You can inform parents that their social teaching likely will center on cleanliness and establishing reasonable controls over anger, impulsiveness, and unsafe exploration.

Influence of the Family

The chief molder of personality is the family unit, and home is the center of the toddler's world. Family life nurtures in the child a strong affectional bond, a social and biologic identity, intellectual development, attitudes, goals, and ways of coping and responding to situations of daily life. The family life process also imparts tools such as language and an ethical system in which the child learns to respect the needs and rights of others and provides a testing ground before he or she emerges from home. A loving, attentive, healthy, responsible family is essential for maximum physical, mental, emotional, social, and spiritual development in childhood (1).

Parents with high self-esteem provide the necessary conditions for the toddler to achieve trust, self-esteem, and autonomy (self-control) through allowing age-appropriate behavior. Parents with low self-esteem provoke feelings of shame, guilt, defensiveness, decreased self-worth, and "being bad" in the child by overestimat-

ing the child's ability to conform, inappropriately or forcefully punishing or restraining the child, denying him necessities, and withdrawing love (11).

Help parents work out their feelings about self in relation to the child. Changing parental attitudes are often evident. If the parent is delighted with a dependent baby and is a competent parent to an infant, the parent may be threatened by the independence of the toddler and become less competent. Some parents have difficulty caring for the dependent infant but are creative and loving with the older child. But if the parent's development was smooth and successful, if the inner child of the past is under control, and if he or she understands self, parental behavior can change to fit the maturing child.

Attachment Behavior

Attachment behavior is very evident during the toddler years. The symbiotic mother-child relationship is slowly being replaced by the larger family unit, but the toddler still needs mother close. Children need to be touched, cuddled, hugged, rocked. All young mammals need physical contact for normal brain tissue development and for the brain to develop receptors that inhibit secretion of adrenal hormones (glucocorticoids)—the stress hormones. Thus both the immune and neurologic systems are affected positively by touch and by emotional attachment (39, 55).

In a classic study in the 1950s two groups of young Ugandan children were compared—those reared in the traditional African way with much attention focused on the child and those reared in the emerging European or Western way with the child left with other caretakers. In the African model the mothers never left the child, carried the child on the back, and played with and stimulated the child. The European model was to bottle feed the child and leave it alone a great deal. The children raised in the African way were, at 2 years of age, more advanced in motor development, language, adaptivity, and personal-social relationships. Good health and the ability to relate are the result of loving relationships (1, 22). Other authors validate these results (7–9, 14, 27, 29, 33, 46, 55).

The toddler shows attachment behavior by maintaining proximity to the parent. Even when out walking, the child frequently returns part or all the way to the parent for reassurance of the parent's presence, to receive a smile, to establish visual, and sometimes touch, contact, and to speak before again moving away (9).

Although attachment is directed to several close people such as father, siblings, babysitter, and grandparents, it is usually greatest toward one person, mother. Attachment patterns do not differ significantly between children who stay home all day versus those who go to day-care centers since attachment is related to the intensity of emotional and social experience between child and adult rather than to physical care and more superficial contact. Attachment is as great or greater if the mother shows warm affection less frequently than if she is present all day but not affectionate. In comparing children raised in Israeli kibbutzim to American children, both groups are equally attached to their parents, although young children in the kibbutzim have a greater attachment to peers than do young American children because they depend more on peers for approval (7).

Separation anxiety, the *response to separation from mother,* intensifies at approximately 18 and 24 months. Anxiety can be as intense for the toddler as for the infant if the child has had a continuous warm attachment to a mother figure since he or she thinks an object ceases to exist when it is out of sight. The child who is more accustomed to strangers will suffer less from a brief separation. When separated, the child experiences feelings of anger, fear, grief, and revenge. An apathetic, resigned reaction at this age is a sign of abnormal development. The child who is separated from the parent for a period of time, as with hospitalization, goes through three phases of *grief and mourning*—protest, despair, and denial, which may merge somewhat—as a result of separation anxiety (9, 33).

During **protest,** *lasting a few hours or days and seen for short or long separations, the need for mother is conscious, persistent, and grief laden. The child cries continually, tries to find her, is terrified, fears he or she has been deserted, feels helpless and angry that mother left him or her, and clings to her on her return.* If he or she is also ill, additional uncomfortable body sensations assault the toddler (9, 33). The child needs mother at this time.

Despair *is a quiet stage, characterized by hopelessness, moaning, sadness, and less activity. The child does not cry continuously but is in deep mourning. He or she does not understand why mother has deserted him or her. The child makes no demands on the environment nor responds to overtures from others, including at times the mother. Yet the child clings to her if permitted.* Mother may feel guilty and want to leave to relieve her distress since she may feel her visits are disturbing to the child, especially when the child does not respond to her.

Mother needs help in understanding that the child's and her reactions are normal and that the child desperately needs her presence (9, 36). If she can be present, you can promote family-centered care through your explanations to the mother and child, by not being rigid about visiting hours, by attending to mother's (or father's) comfort and needs, and by letting the parent help care for the child. Protests, in the form of toddler's screams and crying, will thus be less intense. Be accepting if a parent cannot stay with the child. Parents may live great distances from the hospital or have occupational or family responsibilities that indeed prevent them from visiting the child as often as they desire. The parent may also be ill or injured. Be as nurturing to the toddler

as possible while the parent is away. Tell the toddler how much Mommy and Daddy love him or her and want to be present but cannot. If possible, have the parent leave an article with the child that is a familiar representation of the parent.

Denial, *which occurs after prolonged separation, defends against anxiety by repressing the image of and feelings for mother and may be misinterpreted for recovery.* The child now begins to take more interest in the environment, eats, plays, and accepts other adults. Anger and disappointment at mother are so deep that the child acts as if he or she does not need her and shows revenge by rejecting her, sometimes even rejecting gifts she brings. To prevent further estrangement, mother should understand that the child's need for her is more intense than ever (9, 36).

Continue the above interventions that promote family-centered care. Give mother (father) and child time together undisturbed by nursing or medical care procedures. Provide toys that help the child to act out the fears, anxiety, anger, and mistrust experienced during the hospitalization and separation. Encourage the parent to talk about and work through feelings related to the child's illness and absence from the family.

With prolonged hospitalization, the child may fail to discover a person to whom he or she can attach for any length of time. If the child finds a mother figure and then loses her, the pain of the original separation is reexperienced. If this happens repeatedly, the child will eventually avoid involvement with anyone but invest love in self and later value material possessions more highly than any exchange of affection with people.

Teach parents that immediate aftereffects of separation include changes in the child's behavior—regression, clinging, and seeking out extra attention and reassurance. If extra affection is given to the child, trust is gradually restored. If the separation has been prolonged, the child's behavior can be very changed and disturbed for months after return to the parents. The parent needs support in accepting the child's expressions of hostility and in meeting his or her demands. Counteraggression or withdrawal from the child will cause further loss in trust and regression.

Child abuse or maltreatment may begin or continue at this age. Even when parents seem concerned and loving, a child is not immune from abuse. Further, children today are exposed to a variety of potential abusers—babysitters, day-care workers, the parent's live-in lover or occasional friend, step-parents, extended family members, and neighbors. Be alert to signs and symptoms of child abuse, discussed in Chapters 4, 6, and 7.

Maltreatment of the young child is demonstrated by the parental behaviors described in Box 8–1. Box 8–2 lists physical signs of abuse, and Box 8–3 lists examples of parent-child interactions that indicate abuse. You often must be very patient and observant to detect child abuse because the child does not have the language

BOX 8-1.
Parental Behavior Characteristic of Psychologic Maltreatment of the Toddler

Rejecting

- Excludes actively from family activities
- Refuses to take child on family outings
- Refuses to hug or come close to child
- Places the child away from the family

Isolating

- Teaches the child to avoid social contact beyond the parent-child relationship
- Punishes social overtures to children and adults
- Rewards child for withdrawing from opportunities for social contact

Terrorizing

- Uses extreme gestures and verbal statements to threaten, intimidate, or punish the child
- Threatens extreme or mysterious harm (from monsters or ghosts or bad people)
- Gives alternately superficial warmth with ranting and raging at the child

Ignoring

- Is cool and apathetic with child
- Fails to engage child in daily activities or play
- Refuses to talk to child at mealtimes or other times
- Leaves child unsupervised for extended periods

Corrupting

- Gives inappropriate reinforcement for aggressive or sexually precocious behavior
- Rewards child for assaulting other children
- Involves the child sexually with adolescents or adults

From Garbarino, James, Edna Guttman, and James Seeley, *The Psychologically Battered Child: Strategies for Identification, Assessment, and Intervention.* San Francisco: Jossey-Bass, 1987. Copyright 1986 by Jossey-Bass, Inc., Publishers.

BOX 8-2.
Physical Signs of Abuse of a Child

- An injury for which there is no explanation or an implausible explanation.
- Injury is not consistent with the type of accident described (e.g., child would not suffer both feet burned by stepping into hot tub of water—he or she would step in with one foot at a time, or a child who tips a pot of hot coffee on his or her hand has a splash-effect burn, not a mitten appearance).
- Inconsistencies in the parents' stories about the reason for child's injuries.
- Parents quickly blame a babysitter or neighbor for an accidental injury.
- Child does not have total appearance of an accident—dirty clothes, face smudged, hair tousled.
- Large number of healed or partially healed injuries.
- Large bone fracture, multiple fractures, or tearing of periosteum caused by having limb forcibly twisted.
- Child flinches when your fingers move over an area not obviously injured, but it is tender due to abusive handling.
- Human bite marks.
- Fingernail indentations or scratches.
- Old or new cigarette burns.
- Loop marks from belt beating.
- Soft tissue swelling, hematomas.
- Clustered or multiple bruises on trunk or buttocks, in body hollows, on back of neck, or resembling hand prints or pinch marks.
- Bald spots.
- Retinal hemorrhage from being shaken or cuffed about the head.
- History of unusual number of accidents.

Data from references 29, 36, 42 and 54.

6. Determining whether or not they will have any more children
7. Rededicating themselves, among many dilemmas, to their decision to be a child-bearing family (13)

Help parents to be cognizant of these tasks. Encourage them to talk through concerns, feelings, and practical aspects related to fulfilling these tasks. Refer them to a counselor or community agency if help is desired.

PHYSIOLOGIC CONCEPTS

Physical Characteristics

General Appearance

The appearance of the toddler has matured from infancy. He or she has lost the roly-poly look of infancy by 12 to 15 months, with abdomen protruding, torso tilting forward, legs at stiff angles, and flat feet spaced apart. Limbs are growing faster than torso, giving a different proportion to the body. By 12 to 15 months, chest cir-

skills to tell you what has happened. The child's nonverbal behavior, play, and artwork may provide clues. Observation of the latter takes time and patience as well as the parent's presence (29, 36, 42, 54).

Family Developmental Tasks

The family with a toddler faces many new developmental tasks:

1. Meeting the spiraling costs of family living
2. Providing a home that is safe and comfortable and has adequate space
3. Maintaining a sexual involvement that meets both partners' needs
4. Developing a satisfactory division of labor
5. Promoting understanding between the toddler and the family

segment_naviASSESSMENT AND HEALTH PROMOTION FOR THE TODDLER **259**

BOX 8-3.
Interaction Signs of Parental Abuse of a Child

- Child flinches or glances about nervously when you touch him or her.
- Child seems afraid of parents or caregivers and is reluctant to return home.
- Parent issues threat to crying child such as "Just wait 'til I get you home."
- Parent remains indifferent to child's distress.
- Parent(s) blames child for his or her own injuries (e.g., "He's always getting hurt" or "He's always causing trouble").
- Parental behavior suggests role reversal; parent solicits help or protection from child by acting helpless (when child cannot meet parent's needs, abuse results).
- Parent repeatedly brings healthy child to emergency room and insists child is ill (parent feeling overwhelmed by parental responsibilities and may become abusive).
- Child has had numerous admissions to an emergency room, often at hospitals some distance from the child's home.

Data from references 29, 36, 42, and 54.

cumference is larger than head circumference. The child increasingly looks like a family member as face contours fill out with the set of deciduous teeth. By age 2, he or she has 16 teeth. Gradually the chubby appearance typical of the infant is lost; muscle tone becomes firmer as the fat-storing mechanisms change. Less weight is gained as fat; more weight is gained from muscle and bone (16, 29, 42, 54).

Rate of Growth

During toddlerhood, growth is slower than in infancy; but it is even, and development follows the cephalo-caudal, proximal-distal, and general-to-specific principles discussed in Chapter 6. Although the rate of growth slows, bone growth continues rapidly with the development of approximately 25 new ossification centers during the second year (55).

Between the first and second years the average height increase is 4 to 5 inches (10 to 12 cm). Average height increase the next year is $2\frac{1}{2}$ to $3\frac{1}{2}$ inches (6 to 8 cm). Weight gain averages 5 to 6 pounds (2.27 to 2.72 kg) between the first and second years. Birth weight is quadrupled by age 2 years. The 2-year-old child stands 32 to 33 inches (81 to 84 cm) and weighs 26 to 28 pounds (11 to 13 kg). At 30 months average height is 36 inches (91.5 cm), and weight is approximately 30 pounds (13.6 kg). By age 2 years, the girl has grown to 50% of final adult height, by age $2\frac{1}{2}$ the boy to 50% of adult height (16, 23, 33, 41, 48).

Neuromuscular Maturation

Neuromuscular maturation and repetition of movements help the child further develop skills. **Myelinization,**

covering of the neurons with the fatty sheath called myelin, is almost complete by 2 years. This enables the child to support most movement and increasing physical activity and to begin toilet training. Additional growth also occurs as a greater number of connections form among neurons, and the complexity of these connections increases. Lateralization or specialization of the two hemispheres of the brain has been occurring; evidence of signs of dominance of one hemisphere over the other can be seen. The left hemisphere matures more rapidly in girls than in boys; the right hemisphere develops more rapidly in boys. These differences may account for language ability in girls and spatial ability in boys. Handedness is demonstrated, and spatial perception is improving (16, 27, 41, 48). (Spatial ability will be complete approximately age 10). The limbic system is mature; sleep, wakefulness, and emotional responses become better regulated. The toddler responds to a wider range of stimuli and has greater control over behavior. The brain reaches 80% of adult size by age 2 (16, 27, 38). The growth of the glial cells accounts for most of the change (34, 38, 43).

Motor Coordination

Increasing gross motor coordination is shown by leg movement patterns and by hand-arm movements. Table 8–1 summarizes the increasing motor coordination skills manifested during the toddler years.

Vision

Visual acuity and the ability to **accommodate,** *to make adjustments to objects at varying distances from the eyes,* are slowly developing. Vision is **hyperopic,** *farsighted,* testing approximately 20/10 at 2 years. Visual perceptions are frequently similar to an adult's, even though the child is too young to have acquired the richness of symbolic associations. The child's eye-hand coordination also improves. At 15 months he or she reaches for attractive objects without superfluous movements (16, 27, 36).

Endocrine System

Endocrine function is not fully known. Production of glucagon and insulin is labile and limited, causing variations in blood sugar. Adrenocortical secretions are limited, but they are greater than in infancy. Growth hormone, thyroxin, and insulin remain important secretions for regulating growth (16, 27, 36).

Respiratory System

Respirations average 20 to 30 per minute. Lung volume is increased, and susceptibility to respiratory infections decreases as respiratory tract structures increase in size (36).

Cardiovascular System

The pulse decreases, averaging 105 beats per minute. Blood pressure increases, averaging 80 to 100 systolic and 64 diastolic. The size of the vascular bed increases, thus reducing resistance to flow. The capillary bed has

TABLE 8-1. MOTOR COORDINATION DURING THE TODDLER YEARS

Age (mo)	Characteristics
12–15	Walks alone; legs appear bowed Climbs steps with help; slides down stairs backward Stacks two blocks; scribbles spontaneously Grasps but rotates spoon; holds cup with both hands Takes off shoes and socks
15–18	Runs but still falls Walks backward and sideways (17 mo) Climbs to get to objects Falls from riding toys or in bathtub Hammers on pegboard Grasps with both hands Picks up small items off floor; investigates electric outlets; grabs cords and table cloths (15 mo) Clumsily throws ball Unzips large zipper Takes off easily removed garments Stacks three to four blocks (18 mo)
18–24	Falls from outdoor play equipment Walks stairs with help (20 mo) Walks up and down stairsteps alone, holding rail, both feet on step before ascending to next step Can reach farther than expected, including for hazardous objects Fingers food Brushes paint; finger paints Takes apart toys; puts together large puzzle pieces
24–30	Runs quickly; falls less Walks downstairs holding to rail; does not alternate feet Jumps off floor with both feet (28 mo) Throws ball overhand Puts on simple garments Stacks six blocks Turns door handles Plays with utensils and dishes at mealtimes; pours and stacks Turn book pages Uses spoon with little spilling; feeds self Brushes teeth with help
30–36	Walks with balance; runs well Balances on one foot; walks on tiptoes (30 mo) Jumps from chair (32 mo) Pedals tricycle (32 mo) Jumps 10–12 inches off floor (36 mo) Climbs and descends stairs, alternating feet (36 mo) Rides tricycle Sits in booster seat rather than high chair Stacks 8 to 10 blocks; builds with blocks Pours from pitcher Dresses self completely except tying shoes; does not know back from front Turns on faucet Assembles puzzles Draws; paints

Data from references 16, 23, 27, 33, 41.

increased ability to respond to hot and cold environmental temperatures, thus aiding thermoregulation. The body temperature averages 99° F (37.2° C) (27, 36).

Gastrointestinal System

Foods move through the gastrointestinal tract less rapidly, and digestive glands approach adult maturity. Acidity of gastric secretion increases gradually. Liver and pancreatic secretions are functionally mature (36, 54).

Skin

The skin becomes more protective against outer invasion from microorganisms, and it becomes tougher with more resilient epithelium and less water content. Less fluid is lost through the skin as a result. The skin remains dry because sebum secretion is limited. Eccrine sweat gland function remains limited. At this age eczema improves and the frequency of rashes declines (36).

Urinary System

By age 3, the bladder has descended into the pelvis, assuming adult position. Renal function is mature; except under stress, water is conserved, and urine is concentrated on an adult level (36, 54).

Immune System

Specific antibodies have been established to most commonly encountered organisms, although the toddler is prone to gastrointestinal and respiratory infections when he or she encounters new microorganisms. Despite environmental exposure, antibody IgC increases, IgM reaches an adult level, and IgA gradually increases. Lymphatic tissues of adenoids, tonsils, and peripheral lymph nodes undergo enlargement, partly because of infections and partly from growth. By age 3 years, the adenoid tissue reaches maximum size and then declines, whereas tonsils reach peak size around 7 years (20, 36, 54).

Blood Cell Components

Blood cell counts are approaching adult levels, although the hemoglobin and erythrocyte (red blood cell) count are lower. Sufficient iron intake is necessary to maintain an adequate erythrocyte level. Erythrocytes are formed in the bone marrow of the ribs, sternum, and vertebrae as in adulthood. During stress, the liver and spleen also form erythrocytes and granulocytes (42).

Development does not proceed equally or simultaneously in body parts and maturational skills. Sometimes a child concentrates so intently on one aspect of development (e.g., motor skills) that other abilities (e.g., toilet training) falter or regress. Illness or malnutrition may slow growth, but a catch-up growth period occurs later so that the person reaches the developmental norms. The brain is more vulnerable to permanent injury because destroyed cells are not replaced, although some brain cells may take over some functions of missing cells. Most children also show seasonal spurts in growth. Caucasians, for example, show more height increase in spring and more weight increase in fall (20). There are also cultural differences in growth and development. The African-American child develops motor skills at a greater pace than the Caucasian until age 3 years. The African-American child may be walking alone at 7 or 9 months, in contrast to 12 or 15 months. If all variables are controlled, the African-American child probably will be heavier and have more advanced skeletal development (27, 33).

Discuss physical characteristics of the toddler with the parents to help them adjust to his or her changing competencies.

Physical Assessment of the Young Child

The approach to the physical examination depends on the age of the individual. Adequate time should be spent in becoming acquainted with the child and the accompanying parent. A friendly manner, quiet voice, and relaxed approach help make the examination more fruitful. Hands should always be warmed before giving an examination but especially so in the case of the child.

No assessment is complete without knowing the antenatal, natal, and neonatal history. When the child is old enough, let him or her tell what conditions surround the visit even if the message is only "stomach hurt."

Many times you will be learning about the young child from the mother and will be learning about the mother's attitude. If other siblings are present, observe the interaction among the family members.

What are the mother's facial expressions? In what tone of voice does she talk? Does she look away or comfort the child if the child seems disturbed with a procedure?

What are the other siblings' reactions toward the toddler, the mother, and the health-care worker? What are the siblings' reactions in general?

Although the child may not talk much, general appearance can reveal much information. Does the child look ill or well? What is the activity level? Coordination? Gait, if walking? Reactions to parents, siblings, and examiner? Nature of cry, if present? Facial expressions (44, 45)?

Before 6 months of age the infant usually tolerates the examining table. Between 6 months and 3 to 5 years, most of the examination can be done from the mother's or caretaker's lap. After age 4 years much depends on the relationship established with the child.

The sequence of the examination with the young should be from least discomfort to most discomfort. Undressing can be a gradual procedure since children are often shy about this process. Some examiners prefer to go from toe to head or at least to start with auscultation, which is painless and sometimes fascinating to the child. It is best to leave the ears, nose, and mouth to the end because examination of these areas often initiates a negative response.

Generally the temperature should be taken rectally during the first years of life. Through the age of 2 years, the head circumference is measured at its greatest width and plotted on a growth curve scale that is compared to the norm (44, 45).

Blood pressure should be taken with the cuff that will snugly fit the arm. The first reading is recommended at age 3 years. The inflatable bladder should completely encircle the arm but not overlap. Artificially high blood pressure results if the cuff is too narrow or too short (44, 45). Because this is a procedure that causes some discomfort and it is important to get readings in a low-anxiety state, sensitive timing is needed to get desired results. It sometimes helps to make a game out of the procedure by allowing the toddler to help pump up the bulb or read the numbers on the gauge.

The skin can be examined for turgor by feeling the calf of the leg, which should be firm. **Spider nevi,** *pinhead-sized red dots from which blood vessels radiate,* are commonly found, as are **Mongolian spots,** *large, flat black or blue-and-black spots.* One or two *patches of light brown, nonelevated stains,* called **cafe-au-lait spots,** are within normal findings, but more may be indicative of fibromas or neurofibromas. **Bruises** (*ecchymoses*) are not abnormal in healthy active children, but their location is important. Bruises not on the extremities or on areas easily hit when falling may indicate child abuse, or excessive bruising may indicate blood dyscrasias (25, 44, 45).

Lymph nodes are palpable in almost all healthy young children. Small, mobile, nontender nodes often point to previous infection (44, 45).

When examining the head region, consider the following:

1. The auricles of the ears should be pulled back and down in young children and back and up in older children.
2. A complete hearing test with an audiometer should be done before a child enters school. Before that, the whisper technique or the use of a tuning fork is adequate.
3. A Snellen E chart can be used for testing visual acuity before the child knows the alphabet. Visual acuity at 3 years is 20/40 and at 4 to 5 years is 20/30.
4. Other aspects of the visual examination depend on the child's age and the suspected problem (e.g., after surgery for congenital cataracts).
5. Teeth should be examined for their sequence of eruption, number, character, and position (25, 46).

When examining the thorax and lungs, remember that breath sounds of young children are usually more intense and more bronchial and expiration is more pronounced than in adults. The heart should be examined with the child erect, recumbent, and turned to the left. Sinus arrhythmia and extrasystoles can be benign and are not uncommon (25, 46).

When standing, a child's abdomen may be protuberant; when lying down, it should disappear. The skilled examiner should be able to palpate both the liver and the spleen (46).

When examining the male genitalia, the testicles should be examined while the male is warm and in a sitting position, holding his knees with heels on the seat of the chair or examining table. Without warmth and abdominal pressure, the testes may not be in the scrotum (25).

Examination of the female genitalia is basically visual unless a specific problem in the area has developed.

When examining the extremities, the examiner may note bowlegs, which are common until 18 months. Knock-knees are common until approximately age 12 years. The toddler may appear flat-footed when first walking. All these characteristics are usually short term (25, 44, 45).

The neurologic examination is conducted throughout and is not much different from the sequence in the adult examination; however, the appropriate maturation level must be kept in mind.

Nutritional Needs

Nutritional needs of toddlers aged 12 to 24 months are listed in Box 8–4. Children less than age 2 should not receive low fat (2%) milk because they need the extra calories from fat for energy, for growth, and for brain development. Liver or another high-iron food should be served at least once a week. Toddlers like breads, sweets, mashed potatoes, milk, and snack foods; such a diet, if served exclusively, would impair health. Too much milk without adequate amounts of other foods is also undesirable because omission of meats and vegetables could lead to iron-deficiency anemia (17, 24, 37, 56).

The average serving size for the child of 2 to 3 years is as follows:

1. Milk, 6 ounces (three fourths glass); cheese, $\frac{1}{2}$ ounce or $\frac{1}{4}$ cup; yogurt, $\frac{1}{2}$ cup
2. Juice, 3 to 4 ounces ($\frac{1}{3}$ to $\frac{1}{2}$ cup)
3. Meat, $\frac{1}{6}$ pound
4. Egg, one medium size
5. Cereal, 3 tablespoons cooked; $\frac{1}{2}$ cup ready-to-eat
6. Bread, one half slice; cookies, 2; rice, $\frac{1}{2}$ cup; pasta, $\frac{1}{4}$ cup
7. Fruits and vegetables, one half of raw fruit, 2 to 4 tablespoons (up to $\frac{1}{4}$ cup) cooked (17, 24, 37, 56)

■ **BOX 8-4.**
Recommended Nutritional Intake for Toddlers (Ages 12–24 Mo)

- Meat or fish, an egg or cheese: two (1 ounce) servings
- Milk (whole): maximum of 4 cups (1 quart), preferably 3 cups
- Green and yellow vegetables: two or more ($\frac{1}{4}$ cup) servings
- Fruit: at least two servings
- Cereal, bread: at least two servings
- Fats and carbohydrates: to meet caloric needs

Each day offer the toddler three regular meals and three snacks; snacks may include fruits, vegetables, crackers, yogurt, small sandwich, or juice. Avoid high-sugar, fat, and high-salt snacks; they may be permitted for special occasions. Caloric needs are not high and increase slowly throughout the toddler period. The toddler's appetite typically declines at approximately 18 months. The child has finished a major growth spurt and needs fewer calories. Approximately 1000 calories per day are needed at age 1 year, and only 1300 to 1500 calories are required by age 3 (100 cal/kg/day) because the child is growing less rapidly than during infancy. Body tissues and muscles are growing; thus protein needs are not high, between 1 g of protein per pound or 1.8 g per kilogram of body weight daily. Vitamin supplements are rarely needed if food intake is balanced in nutrients. (Refer to Appendix I.) Fluoride supplements are helpful in areas without fluorinated water. Fluid requirements are approximately 115 to 125 ml/kg/day (17, 24, 37, 56).

Food intake, or its refusal, is one way for the toddler to show increasing independence. Decreased food intake may result from a (1) slower growth rate; (2) short attention span and distractibility by other stimuli; and (3) increased interest in the surroundings. However, how well the child eats is determined to a great extent by how parents manage mealtime, parental behavior toward food, and the atmosphere surrounding the meal.

Some suggestions to teach parents to avoid having mealtime be a battleground are to (1) serve food in small portions; (2) serve finger foods or cut food so that it can be eaten with the fingers; (3) let the child choose (it is not necessary for the toddler to sample every food served); (4) not include high-fat, high-salt, or carbohydrate foods such as soda, candy, or cake or empty nutrition snack foods in the choice; (5) offer a food again if has been rejected one time, without fussing about it; and (6) not insist that the child eat everything on the plate (17, 24, 37, 56).

The toddler is a great imitator; he or she eats the kind of foods eaten by the parents. Parental pressure or reprimands when the child does not eat a particular food conveys anxiety or anger and reinforces not eating, either because of the negative attention received or the stress response felt by the child. Toddlers can be fussy eaters or go on "food jags," preferring only a certain food. Advise parents to give the requested food for a few days until the child gets bored with it, while continuing to offer alternative foods. Or the toddler may overeat if parents overeat. If there is a high caloric intake, obesity may result. Excessive weight gain interferes with the physical mobility that is a part of being a normal toddler.

Teach parents about the nutritional needs and eating patterns of the toddler. Avoid serving too large a portion, which can be the beginning of overeating or cause refusal to eat all the food, with resultant conflict between parent and toddler.

Malnutrition may lead to slower growth, tooth decay, lowered resistance to disease, and even death. Signs of malnutrition include abdominal swelling, lethargy, lack of attention to stimuli, lack of energy, diminished muscle strength and coordination, changes in skin color, and hair loss. Females apparently are buffered better against effects of malnutrition or illness than males. Malnutrition delays growth, but children have great recuperative powers if malnutrition does not continue too long. When nutrition improves, growth takes place unusually fast until norms for weight, height, and skeletal development are reached. For example, Korean children who suffered early malnutrition but were adopted and raised by American parents in homes providing good nutrition performed as well on intellectual tests as their American-born peers (17, 37, 56).

A hospitalized toddler frequently regresses; refusing to feed self is one manifestation. The child needs a lot of emotional support and to feel some kind of control over his or her destiny and that he or she is not totally helpless and powerless. A way of assuring some area of control is by permitting the child to choose foods and encouraging him or her to feed self.

Play, Exercise, and Rest

Play and Exercise

Play is the business of the toddler. During play he or she exercises, learns to manage the body, improves muscular coordination and manual dexterity, increases awareness and organizes the surrounding world by scrutinizing objects, and develops beginning spatial and sensory perception. The child learns language and to pay attention and releases emotional tensions as he or she channels unacceptable urges such as aggression into acceptable activities; translates feelings, drives, and fantasies into action; and learns about self as a person. Through play the toddler becomes socialized and begins to learn right from wrong. The child learns to have fun and to master.

The child has little interest in other children except as a curious explorer. Play is solitary and **parallel;** *he or she plays next to but not with other children.* There is little overt exchange, but there is satisfaction in being close to other children. Toddler is unable to share toys and is distressed by demands of sharing since he or she has a poorly defined sense of ownership. Toddler will play cooperatively with guidance, however. By the end of 2 years, most children imitate adults in dramatic play by doing such things as setting the table and cooking. When selecting play materials for the toddler, remember likes and dislikes and choose a variety of activities because the attention span is short. (Safety and durability aspects of toys, as discussed in Chapter 7, must be considered.)

Table 8–2 presents suggested play activities and equipment for the child 18 months or 2 years of age.

Help parents understand the importance of play and safety. A relation exists between the quality of attachment between mother and baby and the quality of play and problem-solving behavior at 2 years of age. Toddlers who are securely attached at 18 months of age

CASE SITUATION: Toddler Development

The setting is an urban day-care center. The outdoor fenced, grassy play area, with a sandbox, a variety of climbing and swing play equipment, and wheeled toys, looks inviting. Indoors the wide hallways, a cubicle for each child's clothing and personal items, and a large room where the children play indicate that this is a busy center. The large room has several distinct play areas: a house corner, a large block corner, a music area with piano and other children's instruments, a reading corner with books, and an art area with large sheets of paper and crayons, pencils, chalk, and finger paints. Tables in the middle of the room are piled with toys. Large windows face the playground; potted plants and an aquarium add life to the bustling room.

Luis, 18 months of age, is a typical toddler: 24 pounds, 28 inches tall. He occasionally falls as he walks around the room but rises to his feet without help. He pulls a toy truck, then sits on a tractor and pushes himself with his feet. In a few minutes a pink ball on a shelf catches his attention, and he runs to it, grasping it with hands and forearms. He repeatedly sets the ball on the shelf to play with a nearby toy but returns again for the ball.

While Luis is holding the ball, another toddler approaches him to get the ball. Luis yanks away, displaying the typical toddler's egocentricism and inability to share. The other child hits Luis, who cries to get the teacher's attention and support. The teacher talks to each child, encourages both to hug and be friendly, and plays with the two children briefly as they share the ball. In a few minutes each child has been distracted to engage in another activity in the room.

Before lunch the teacher calls the group together for story time, which is limited to 10 minutes because of the toddler's short attention span. During this time the toddlers repeat a nursery rhyme that was part of the story and then sing the rhyme, demonstrating rote memory. Luis and the other toddlers enjoy music and rhyming play.

TABLE 8-2. SUGGESTED PLAY ACTIVITIES AND EQUIPMENT FOR TODDLERS

Age (mo)	Toy, Equipment or Activity
18	Push-pull toys (cars, trucks, farm tools)
	Empty and fill toys (plastic food containers, kitchen utensils, small boxes, and open-close toys)
	Big picture books—thick-paged, colorful, sturdy (child will turn two or three pages at a time, tear at thin pages)
	Stuffed animals with no detachable parts
	Baby dolls, large enough to hug, carry, cuddle, dress, feed
	Big pieces of plain paper or newspaper layers and crayons for scribbling
	Small blocks—builds a tower of two or three at a time
	Shape-sorting blocks or cube
	Small chair; small furniture to play "house"
	Rubber or soft ball
	Phonograph record, preferably sturdy plastic that child can manipulate by self; musical and sound toys; musical instruments simple to use
	Rocking horse; rocking chair
24	All of the above are enjoyed; child now turns book or magazine pages singly—still tears; builds tower of seven blocks and aligns cubes; makes circular strokes with crayon
	Puppets
	Pedal toys; dumping toys (dump trucks)
	Playdough and clay; mud; finger paints
	Jungle gym for climbing; sand box; small water pool for waterplay
	Pounding toys—hammer and pegs, drums, small boards
	Picture puzzles—two to four pieces (wooden or thick cardboard)
	Large, colored wooden beads to string
	Simple trains, cars, boats, planes to push-pull or sit on
	Kick ball

are more enthusiastic, persistent, cooperative, and able to share than if secure attachment has not developed. There is also more frequent and sophisticated interaction with peers at 3 years when secure attachment has formed in infancy (27). Discuss play patterns and toys with the parents.

Help parents realize the importance of offering playthings that can transform into any number of toys, depending on his or her mood and imagination at the time. The adult can be available or initially start a play activity with the child. However, the child should be encouraged to play independently, developing mastery, autonomy, and self-esteem in the process.

Verzemnieks (51) describes developmental stimulation, play activities, and toys for the hospitalized child. Box 8–5 summarizes how play can be used effectively with the ill child.

Rest

Rest is as essential as exercise and play, and although a child may be tired after a day full of exploration and exerting boundless energy, bedtime is often a difficult experience. Bedtime means loneliness and separation from fun, family, and, most important, the mother figure.

The toddler needs an average of 10 to 12 hours of sleep nightly plus a daytime nap.

Teach the following guidelines to parents for establishing a bedtime routine for the toddler:

1. Set a definite bedtime routine and adhere to it. If the child is overly tired, he or she becomes agitated and difficult to put to sleep.
2. Establish a bedtime ritual, including bath, a story, and a tucking-in routine. Begin approximately 30 minutes before bedtime. The tucking-in should be caring and brief.
3. If the child cries, which most children do briefly, go back in a few minutes to provide reassurance. Do not pick up the child or stay more than 30 seconds. If the crying continues, return in 5 minutes and repeat the procedure. Thus the parent can determine whether there is any real problem, and the child feels secure.
4. If extended crying continues, lengthen the time to return to the child to 10 minutes. Eventually fatigue will occur, the cry will turn to whimpers, and the child will fall asleep.
5. The child should remain in his or her bed rather than sleep for all or part of the night with parents. Bedtime routine becomes a precedent for other separations. However, if the parents make an occasional exception such as during a family crisis of major loss, trauma, or transition or if the child is ill, neither the marriage relationship nor the child's development will be hindered. It is important that the exception not become the routine.
6. As the child grows older, limit the number of times the child can get up, for any reason, after going to bed.

Sleep problems during hospitalization may show up through restlessness, insomnia, and nightmares. Increasingly, hospitals are permitting parents to spend the night in the child's room to lessen fears and separation anxiety. Cuddling is still important to a toddler, especially if hospitalized. If a parent cannot remain with a frightened child, you can hold and rock him or her while he or she holds a favorite object.

Health Promotion and Health Protection

Routine Immunizations

These immunizations remain a vital part of health care. The Center for Disease Control (CDC) estimates that only 65% of 2-year-olds in the United States are immunized (49). Measles remains one of the most common childhood diseases. The toddler should receive a rubeola (long measles), rubella, and mumps (MMR) combined vaccine at 15 months; at 18 months he or she should receive a combined vaccine of diphtheria, tetanus, and pertussis (DTP) along with oral polio virus vaccine (OPV) to complete the primary series (49). The tine test is repeated at 3 years of age. The young child should

---

■ **BOX 8-5.**
Techniques for Using Play While Caring for the Child

Physical Assessment

- Talk soothingly and calmly. Explain what you are doing as you do it.
- Blow on the stethoscope. Ask child to imitate.
- Have child listen to own heart beat with stethoscope.
- Name body parts and touch them. "Foot. Here is my foot." "Where are your eyes?" "There are your eyes!" "Where is your nose?" Guide the child's hands to touch.
- Use diversions—another toy, tickles (especially abdomen).
- Play peek-a-boo: cover your eyes, then child's. Hide your head with blanket, then child's head. When child covers own head, say, "Where's (name?)" Then delight in discovery.
- Use body movement, exercising child's arms and legs rhythmically while doing assessment.
- Sing a nonsense tune or talk animatedly.
- Talk about sensations: warm or cold, soft or rough as sensations are presented.
- Name body position: up or down, over.
- Encourage child to do examination of doll, teddy bear, toy animal.

Bathing

- Experiment with the properties of water in a small tub. Use items that float and sink—washcloth, plastic soap dish, paper cup, plastic lid, empty plastic cylinders, or toys at child's cribside. Talk about what happens.
- Identify body parts as you wash them. Give simple directions "Close your eyes." "Raise your arms." "Wash your hair.") Be sure to praise all help.
- Encourage child to "bathe" a doll, teddy bear, or toy animal.

Feeding

- Place the child in high chair or walker when he or she can sit unsupported. Tie toy or utensil to high chair to facilitate retrieval.
- Discuss the food: hot or cold, colors, textures, which utensils to use.
- Use an extra spoon and cup: one for you, one for baby.
- Experiment with food: fingerpaint with food on tray, make lines.

Diagnostic Procedures

- Explain to the child what you plan to do and are doing. Be honest but gentle.
- Tell the child it is all right to cry; comfort if child cries.
- Set up situation so child can do procedure on doll or toy animal. While child is imitating, talk about how much it hurts. Cuddle and comfort the child, cooing, singing softly, rocking after the procedure.
- Distract the child with empty dressing packages, encouraging crushing and listening to sounds.
- Make the sounds and touch different parts of child's body.
- Vocalize sounds related to procedure. Have child imitate you.

---

be vaccinated against life-threatening *Haemophilus influenzae* type B (Hb) or other influenza strains. The vaccine is recommended for all children who are 2 years of age or older and for children 18 months or older in high-risk groups, including children who attend day care (49). If the parent refuses to have the child immunized for religious reasons, emphasize the need to prevent exposure to these diseases, if possible, and the importance of continued good hygiene and nutrition. The age for MMR immunization was lowered to 12 months by the Los Angeles County Health Department as a way to reduce the number of children in the Latino community who were susceptible to measles (15).

Common health threats at this age are respiratory infections and home accidents. The causes for accidents are motor vehicles, burns, suffocation, drowning, poisoning, and falls. Accidents are the leading cause of death, and deaths from poisonings continue to increase. Areas outside the home—the yard, the street, the grocery cart—have greater hazard because today there is more contact with them. Communicable diseases are less a health threat than parasitic diseases.

Safety Promotion and Injury Control

Accidents are a major cause of death. Thus it is necessary to childproof the home. Teach parents they can prevent injury from furniture by:

1. Selecting furniture with rounded corners and a sturdy base
2. Packing away breakable objects and putting safety catches on doors

They can prevent falls by:

1. Avoiding hazardous waxing
2. Discarding throw rugs
3. Keeping traffic lanes clear
4. Placing gates at tops of stairways (Fig. 8–1) and screens on the windows
5. Placing toys and favorite objects on a low shelf

Burns are prevented by blocking access to electric outlets, heating equipment, matches, lighters, hot water, and appliances that heat and taking special care with fireworks. Placing tools and knives high on the wall or

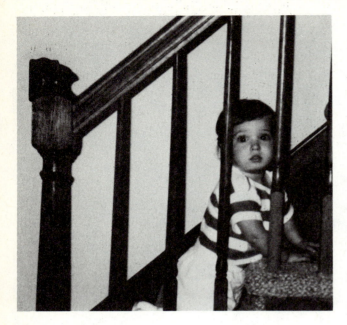

Figure 8-1. Toddlers should be prevented from climbing stairs, for example, by a portable gate. (From Sherwen, L.N., M.A. Scoloveno, and C.T. Weingarten, *Nursing Care of the Childbearing Family*. Norwalk, Conn: Appleton & Lange, 1991, p. 926.)

in a locked cabinet can prevent lacerations or more serious injury.

Parents may call you to help when their child has been injured or is ill. Know emergency care. A poison treatment chart is available from the National Poison Center Network, Children's Hospital, 125 DeSoto Street, Pittsburg, PA 15213. Many cities also have poison control centers to treat and give information to parents and professionals. The Red Cross is also a source of first-aid information. Teach parents to prevent poisoning through the steps outlined in Box 8–6.

■ **BOX 8-6.**
Parent Teaching to Prevent Poisoning

- Teach the child that medication and vitamins are not candy; keep them locked. Discard old medicine.
- Keep medicines, polishes, insecticides, drain cleaners, bleaches, household chemicals, garage products, and other potentially toxic substances in a locked cabinet out of the child's reach. Do not store them in containers previously used for food.
- Store nonfood substances in original containers with labels attached, not in food or beverage containers.
- If you are interrupted while pouring or using a product that is potentially harmful, take it with you. The toddler is curious and impulsive and moves quickly.
- Keep telephone numbers of the physician, poison control center, local hospital, and police and fire departments by the telephone.
- Teach the child not to eat berries, flowers, or plants; some are poisonous.

Thoroughly explore safety promotion with the parents since the following normal developmental characteristics make the toddler prone to accidents. He or she moves quickly and is impulsive. The inquisitive, assertive behavior helps him or her enjoy learning by touch, taste, and sight, but the curiosity can lead to hazards. The toddler enjoys playing with small objects that can be hazardous. He or she likes to attract attention; has a short attention span and unreliable memory; lacks judgment; has incomplete self-awareness; and imitates the actions of others.

Tell parents to teach the toddler to swim and always stay with the child when he or she is near water; not to allow boisterous play or sharp objects near a swimming pool, jungle gym, or sandbox; and to provide safety equipment and supervision.

Common Health Problems: Prevention and Treatment

The child must be carefully assessed for infections and other disease conditions because he or she lacks the cognitive, language, and self-awareness capacities to describe discomforts. Refer to Appendices III and IV for a schedule of health screening measures for the toddler. Table 8–3 summarizes common conditions, which are described more fully in the text.

Visual Defects

Visual defects may occur and may be difficult to detect. Squinting or holding objects very close or far from the face are clues that vision is faulty. **Myopia,** *nearsightedness,* and **astigmatism,** *unequal curvature in the refractive surfaces of the eye that interferes with clear focusing,* are two common refractive errors. **Strabismus** *(cross-eyes, wall eye) occurs because the eye muscles cannot move the eyes in parallel or coordinated movements.* Early assessment is essential.

Teach parents that prescribed eyeglasses correct myopia and astigmatism. Strabismus does not correct itself. The child will adjust by using only one eye; the other eye remains out of line and eventually loses visual function. The deviating eye can be brought back into binocular vision before age 6 years by having the child wear a patch over the better aligned eye to require the deviated eye to fixate or by surgery to alter attachment of extraocular muscles. Correcting strabismus and other visual problems is important for learning and for maintaining a positive self-concept. Because strabismus affects the child's appearance, it can be both psychologically and cognitively damaging. Further, no parent wants the child to grow up visually impaired in one eye, especially when the impairment could have been prevented (20, 36).

There is no accurate method available to tell the visual acuity of children less than age 3 years, but using Allen cards can provide useful data and will seem like play for the child. Familiar objects such as a birthday

TABLE 8-3. COMMON HEALTH PROBLEMS OF TODDLERS

Problem	Definition	Symptoms/Signs	Prevention/Treatment
Strabismus (crossed eyes, wall eyes)	Eyes are not straight or properly aligned	One or both eyes may turn in, turn out, turn up or down; may be constant or come and go	Glasses to correct related problem; patching; medication; surgery; eye exercises
Otitis media	Infection of middle ear, with accumulation of seropurulent fluid in middle ear cavity	Earache, fever, upper respiratory infection; decreased hearing; bulging tympanic membrane; disappearance of landmarks	Medication (antibiotic), sometimes decongestant; follow-up examination
Dental caries	Tooth decay	Obvious dark places or breakdown of teeth; pain	Supplemental fluoride; avoidance of sweets; directions to parents for cleaning teeth
Malabsorption syndrome	Lactose intolerance	Chronic vomiting, diarrhea, abdominal discomfort; flatulence; irritable	Trying other products beside milk (e.g., soybean formula)
Impetigo	Lesions caused by microorganism (usually *Streptococcus*)	Seropurulent vesicles on skin surrounded by erythematous base, with itching	Soaking and scrubbing lesions; cutting fingernails; oral or topical antibiotic
Pharyngitis (sore throat)	Inflammation of pharynx or tonsils or both; usually caused by a virus, sometimes by bacteria	Red throat, exudate, enlarged lymph nodes; fever; other upper respiratory infection symptoms	Antibiotic if appropriate; warm saline solution gargles; increased fluid intake; antipyretic if fever present
Acute, nonspecific gastroenteritis (simple diarrhea)	Inflammation of the gastrointestinal tract	Stools more frequent and liquid than usual	Discontinuing milk; giving clear liquid and an electrolyte solution, followed by simple foods
Varicella (chickenpox)	Acute, highly contagious disease caused by varicella-zoster virus	Rash occurring in crops of lesions beginning on trunk and spreading peripherally; itching; fever	Keeping fingernails short; using calamine lotion or prescription drug if itching intense; antipyretic if necessary
Rubella (3-day measles)	Viral disease characterized by rash and lymph node enlargement	Rash on face or neck, spreading to trunk and extremities; rash usually gone in 3 days	Prevention: immunization No specific treatment except symptomatic
Enterobius vermicularis (pinworms)	Parasitic infestation of the intestinal tract	Possibly asymptomatic; itching around anus; 1-inch white thready worms visible on perineum	Medication (treat all family members); personal hygiene; washing all laundry and bedclothes in hot water

Data from references 25, 44, and 45.

cake or horse are on each card. The child should first become familiar with the cards, and you should know that he or she does recognize the objects. Test each eye by covering the opposite eye and flashing the pictures one by one as the child identifies the objects. Gradually back away from the child and record the maximum distance at which the child can identify the objects. Thirty feet represents the maximum distance at which a child this age should identify the objects; if a toddler identifies them at 15 feet, his or her vision is 15/30 (44, 45).

Otitis Media
An infection in the middle ear is a common infection causing pain and fever. Sataloff and Colton (40) give detailed description of the types of otitis media, diagnosis, and treatment, as well as complications, including hearing loss.

Hearing Impairment
Mild *hearing loss* is frequently caused by middle-ear infections that accompany the common cold or ear trauma. Assessment of the child's auditory ability is cru-

cial to prevent language, social, and learning problems. Signs of impaired hearing include inability to speak by 2 years, failure to respond to noises that are out of sight, or tilting the head while listening (20, 36).

Encourage parents to obtain an early diagnosis. Educational treatment through lip reading and sign language during the toddler period prevents a later learning lag and psychologic problems.

Dental Caries
Dental caries occur infrequently in children less than 3 years old, but rampant *tooth decay* in very young children is almost always related to excessive intake of concentrated sweets or prolonged bottle feedings at nap and bedtime (bottle mouth syndrome).

The toddler should be weaned from the bottle or at least not allowed to fall asleep with it in his or her mouth (36). Teach parents that the adverse effects of bedtime feeding are greater than thumb sucking or the use of pacifiers. If deciduous teeth decay and disintegrate early, spacing of the permanent teeth is affected, and immature speech patterns develop. Discomfort is felt, emotional problems may result, and appearance is affected.

Encourage parents to take the child for the first dental visit between 18 and 24 months. Suggestions to help prepare the toddler or young child for the first dental visit are:

1. Explain what a dentist is in simple, positive terms.
2. Play dentist at home to prepare the child for the client role.
3. Prepare him or her for being alone in the dentist's office.
4. Describe dental instruments and how they are needed by the dentist.
5. Explain what x-ray machines are and how they take pictures of the teeth.
6. Never bribe the child to visit the dentist or use a dental visit as a form of punishment.
7. Avoid passing on parental or adult fears to the child (47).

Dental hygiene should be started when the first tooth erupts by cleansing the teeth with gauze or cotton moistened with hydrogen peroxide and flavored with a few drops of mouthwash. After 18 months the child's teeth can be brushed with a soft or medium toothbrush (36). Fluoride supplements are also believed to prevent caries.

A child with discolored teeth, pain, dental infection, or chipping of the front teeth should be referred to a dentist immediately. Irritability, restlessness, appetite disturbances, and behavioral changes may indicate dental caries (36).

Other Conditions

A child with *lactose deficiency* will have a **malabsorption syndrome** or *lactose intolerance*. Because there is not enough of the enzyme lactose to digest milk, the child has chronic vomiting and diarrhea, abdominal discomfort or pain, and flatulence and is irritable, often sleeping poorly. Milk is tolerated only in small amounts. Soybean formula is tried initially and may be digested.

One author described how she prepared in a blender a special formula that was a substitute for milk and milk products such as ice cream. After 5 weeks without symptoms, nonfat milk was introduced gradually in amount and number of feedings. The toddler was then able to tolerate some milk (18).

Another common problem usually caused by group A beta-hemolytic streptococci cause **impetigo,** in which the *upper layers of skin have honey-colored, fluid-filled vesicles that eventually crust, surrounded by a red base.* Impetigo is often a complication of insect bites, abrasions, or dermatitis that become infected with the organism. Some impetigo is contagious, and since acute glomerulonephritis may follow, proper identification of these lesions and appropriate antibiotic therapy is recommended (25).

Additionally, teach parents that fingernails should be trimmed to avoid spread of organisms via scratching. The toddler should have the lesions soaked and gently scrubbed three times a day to soften and remove crusts. Towels and clothing of the infected toddler should be kept and washed separately.

A problem that often begins in the toddler years is **pharyngitis,** *sore throat,* which involves *inflammation of the pharynx or tonsils or both.* Usually the cause is viral, but sometimes it is caused by group A beta-hemolytic streptococci and rarely by *Mycoplasma pneumoniae* and *Corynebacterium diphtheriae. It is not possible to determine the cause of pharyngitis by clinical features alone* (25).

A throat culture is needed to determine if the origin is due to group A beta-hemolytic streptococci. Because this organism has the potential to cause rheumatic fever, heart valvular disease, cervical lymphadenitis, otitis media, peritonsillar abscess, retropharyngeal abscess, sinusitis, and acute glomerulonephritis, proper identification and eradication of the organism with appropriate antibiotics are essential. For pharyngitis of any origin, antipyretic medication (if fever is present), warm saline solution gargles (if the older toddler can be taught this procedure), and increased fluid intake are in order (25). Other respiratory infections of a more severe nature may also occur. Consult a pediatric nursing text (36, 54).

Acute nonspecific gastroenteritis or **simple diarrhea** is often preceded by vomiting and is an *inflammation of the gastrointestinal tract during which stools are more liquid and frequent than usual.* The cause is unknown. (In contrast, some gastroenteritis can be traced to a bacterial infection, side effects of oral antibiotics, and food poisoning.) The toddler must be watched for signs of dehydration such as sunken eyes, dry mucous membranes, decreased skin turgor, and weight loss (25).

Treatment is varied, but generally the current diet, especially milk, should be discontinued. Small amounts of clear liquids such as cola (at room temperature and with the carbonation released) may decrease the vomiting tendency. These clear liquids should be alternated with an electrolyte solution such as Pedialyte. As diarrhea improves, easily absorbed foods such as flavored gelatin or bananas can be added. In a couple of days simple solid foods such as dry toast and plain baked potato should be tolerated. Cereal, if given, should be mixed with water. Milk, cheese, and eggs should not be added until the previously suggested foods are tolerated well (25).

Varicella (chicken pox) is an *acute, highly contagious disease* caused by the varicella zoster virus for which no vaccine is yet available. The main characteristic is a rash consisting of lesions that appear in crops and in rapid succession (6 to 8 hours), going from a flat macule to a fluid-filled vesicle that crusts.

You can determine that the lesion is chicken pox

because it begins on the trunk and spreads peripherally. Sometimes the lesions are in the mouth. Lesion formation and resolvement usually last for 3 to 5 days. Other symptoms, in addition to itching, are a fever that may cause headache, general malaise, and loss of appetite. Teach parents that treatment is symptomatic. Fingernails should be kept short to reduce scarring from scratching. Lotions such as calamine may help dry the skin and reduce itching. Occasionally a prescription drug will be used to reduce intense itching. Fever may be treated with an antipyretic drug other than aspirin, which may be associated with the development of Reye's syndrome. The child should be isolated as soon as possible and until the lesions have crusted. Complications are rare (25).

Reye's syndrome is a *rare but sometimes fatal disease of children who have been administered salicylates to treat respiratory or gastrointestinal illness or chicken pox.* In one multicenter study more than 90% of the children with Reye's syndrome had taken aspirin. During 1981 to 1985 1003 cases of Reye's syndrome, with 291 deaths, were reported to the CDC in Atlanta, whereas in 1985 only 91 cases were reported, probably because of decreased use of aspirin for children. Of those who survive Reye's syndrome, one third are likely to have permanent brain damage (25).

Teach parents to avoid use of aspirin with children and to substitute a nonsalicylate analgesic.

Rubella is a *viral disease characterized by a rash of 3-day duration, along with lymph node enlargement.* When acquired postnatally, it is mild. When acquired by a pregnant female, it is associated with a high degree of congenital malformations. To avoid the tragedy of malformation, *every 15-month-old should have the rubella vaccine.* Exceptions are only those toddlers who are receiving immunosuppressive therapy, who have immunodeficiency disorders, or who have malignant disease (25).

Pinworms (*Enterobius vermicularis*) *infest the intestinal tract and are the most common parasitic infestation in the United States.* Rare is the family with small children that escapes a bout with these slender, white, threadlike worms that average approximately 1 cm in length. Itching in the perianal region is the chief symptom. The cycle begins with oral ingestion of pinworm eggs. Eggs from the itching perianal region are picked up by the hands, especially of toddlers, and are put in their mouth, onto hands of other persons, and onto toys, rugs, and clothes. As hands touch these objects and go to the mouth, the infestation is multiplied. Once swallowed, the eggs pass through the intestinal tract in 15 to 28 days and hatch into larvae and then adult worms. At night when the child is still, the mature female worms migrate from the anus to the perineum where they deposit thousands of eggs, thus completing the cycle that will begin again with scratching (25).

Parents may be embarrassed to tell you about this infestation. Tell them that pinworms can be killed with a single dose of prescription medication. Usually all the symptomatic family members are treated at the same time. The real task, however, is stopping the cycle. Personal hygiene is extremely important, particularly handwashing before eating and after using the toilet. Careful washing of pajamas and bed sheets should be carried out after treatment. Favorite stuffed animals, chairs, and rugs often harbor the eggs and every effort should be made to cleanse these areas properly (25).

Juvenile hypertension has been defined as *sustained blood pressure levels above the 95th percentile on at least three measurements at different visits under circumstances where anxiety is minimized.* Another definition for children 3 to 12 years is a *diastolic pressure greater than 90 mm Hg* (32).

If hypertension is suspected, a complete investigation is warranted by a specialist interested in hypertension in children. Tell parents that many children will respond to an overall cardiovascular health program. If at all possible, drug therapy will be avoided (32).

Consult pediatric nursing texts for additional information on childhood illnesses and their assessment, care, and prevention (36, 54).

PSYCHOSOCIAL CONCEPTS

Cognitive Development

The intellectual capacity of the toddler is limited. The child has all the body equipment that allows for an assimilation of the environment, but he or she is just beginning intellectual maturity.

Learning occurs through several general modes: (1) natural unfolding of the innate physiologic capacity; (2) imitation of others; (3) reinforcement from others as the child engages in acceptable behavior; (4) insight, gaining understanding in increasing depth as he or she plays, experiments, or explores; and (5) identification, taking into self values and attitudes like those he or she is closely associated with through use of the other modes (23, 33, 41).

The toddler experiences the world in a **parataxic mode,** in that *wholeness of experience and cause-effect relationships do not exist.* He or she experiences parts of things in the present; they are not necessarily events connected with past and future (46). Repeating simple and honest explanations—for example, why a certain tool works or why he or she should not play in the street—will eventually lead to understanding of cause and effect.

The toddler's attention span lengthens. He or she likes songs, nursery rhymes, and stories, even though he or she does not fully understand simple explanations of them. He or she can name pictures on repeated exposure. The toddler plays alone sometimes but prefers being near people. He or she is aware of self and others in a new way.

Part of the toddler's learning is through imitation of the parents, helping them with simple tasks such as bringing an object, trying new activities on his or her own, ritualistic repetition of activity, experimenting with language, and expressing self emotionally. According to Piaget, the toddler finishes the fifth and sixth stages of the Sensorimotor Period and begins the Preoperational Period at approximately age 2 (41, 52).

In the *fifth stage* (12 to 18 months) the child consolidates previous activities involving body actions into *experiments* to discover new properties of objects and events and achieve new goals instead of applying habitual behavior. He or she no longer keeps repeating the same behavior to achieve a goal and performs familiar acts without random maneuvers. The child differentiates self from objects in the environment. Understanding of *object permanence, space perception,* and *time perception* can be observed in new ways. The child is aware that objects continue to exist even though they cannot be seen; he or she accounts for sequential displacements and searches for objects where they were *last* seen. Toddler manipulates objects in new and various ways to learn what they will do. For the first time, objects outside the self are understood as causes of action. Activities are now linked to internal representations or symbolic meaning of events or objects (memories, ideas, feelings about past event) (29, 52).

The *sixth stage of the Sensorimotor Period* (18 to 24 months) seems primarily a transitional phase to the preoperative period. Now the child does less trial-and-error thinking but uses memory of past experience and imitation to act as if he or she arrived at an answer. He or she imitates another who is out of sight. Toddler begins to solve problems, to foresee maneuvers that will succeed or fail, and to remember an object that is absent and search for it until it is found (29, 52).

In the *Preoperational Period* (2 to 7 years) thought is more symbolic; memory continues to form; and the child internalizes mental pictures of people, the environment, and ideas about rules and relationships. The child begins to arrive at answers mentally instead of through physical activity, exploration, and manipulation. Symbolic representation is seen in (1) the use of language to describe (symbolize) objects, events, and feelings, (2) the beginning of symbolic play (crossing two sticks to represent a plane), and (3) delayed imitation (repeating a parent's behavior hours later) (23). The toddler can understand simple abstractions, but thinking is basically concrete (related to tangible events) and literal. He or she is **egocentric** (*unable to take the viewpoint of another*); the ability to differentiate between subject and object, the real object and the word symbol, is not developed. He or she knows only one word for any object and cannot understand how the one word *chair* can refer to many different styles of chairs. If the flower is

called *flower* and *plant,* the child will not understand that more than one word can refer to the same object. Concept of time is *now* and concept of distance is whatever can be seen. The child imitates the thinking and behavior observed in another but lacks the past experience and broader knowledge that is essential for logical thought. This level of learning will continue through the preschool era (29, 52).

Pushing children to read and write at an early age has not been shown to produce long-lasting positive effects. It may cause the child to lose initiative, curiosity, desire to use ingenuity, and ability to cope with ordinary life stresses. The child knows inside what he or she can do. If the parents whom the child looks to for support and guidance are manipulating him or her to meet their needs, the child may come to mistrust parents and self. Before parents put the child in a preschool that emphasizes formal academics, they should consider what the child is not learning from missed playtime. Play that is parallel to and cooperative with peers helps the child develop language, motor, cognitive, nonverbal, and social skills; positive self-esteem; a sense of worth as an individual; and unique problem-solving skills in the face of stress (1, 34).

Teach parents about this aspect of development. This period can be trying and should be tempered by supportive guidance and discipline: parents' saying what is meant, providing environmental stimulation, showing interest in the child's activities and talking and working with the child, reinforcing intellectual attempts, and showing a willingness to teach with simple explanations. Much of the intellectual development now depends on the achievements of infancy, how parents used the baby's potential, and the *quality* of parent-child interaction rather than the *amount* of time, per se, that is spent with the child (29). The child learns to enjoy learning, which forms the basis for later school achievement.

Language Development

Learning to communicate in an understandable manner begins during this era. Through speech the toddler will gradually learn to control unacceptable behavior, exchange physical activity for words, and share the view of reality held by society.

The ability to speak words and sentences is not governed by the same higher center that controls understanding. The child understands words before they are used with meaning, and some children develop adequate comprehension but cannot speak (29).

Various theories explain language acquisition. Although First Force Theory, behaviorism or learning theory, explains some language learning through receiving reinforcement for imitation of language sounds, the number of specific stimulus-response connections that would be necessary to speak even one language could

Research Abstract

Free, T., et al., A Descriptive Study of Infants and Toddlers Exposed Prenatally to Substance Abuse, American Journal of Maternal-Child Nursing, *15, no. 4 (1990), 245–249.*

Children affected by prenatal abuse of alcohol and drugs are an increasing public health problem and a concern to nurses. Much of the literature describes maternal substance abuse and damage evident in neonates. The purposes of this pilot descriptive study were to determine characteristics of a sample of infants and toddlers who had been exposed as fetuses to substance abuse, to identify the health and developmental status of these children, and to determine who the caregivers were and the quality of care provided. Thus the interactive environment could be investigated.

The nonrandom, convenience sample consisted of 20 children and their caregivers from 15 families. These children had measurable amounts of alcohol or drugs in their urine or blood at birth, and prenatal substance abuse history was confirmed. Only 11 of the caregivers were biologic mothers; the other caregivers were grandmothers or aunts. Nineteen of the children were African-American; 13 families were from the lower socioeconomic level. Two children were 2 to 3 years old; five were 1 to 2 years old; and thirteen were less than 1 year of age. Mean maternal age was 29.6 years; mean educational level for caregivers was 11.6 years.

Data were collected using the Caldwell Home Scale, Home Observation for Measurement of the Environment, and Nursing Child Assessment Training. A health history, physical assessment, and developmental screening test were also performed to measure the children.

Results of the children's growth measures confirmed literature reports that many children exposed prenatally to alcohol or drugs fail to grow normally. In this sample three children born to alcoholic mothers had microencephaly. Six children were below the 5th percentile for weight and height; one was below the 5th percentile for weight; and one was below the 5th percentile for height. Of nine children born prematurely, five were below the 5th percentile for corrected height. The incidence of developmental delay was 35% (the delay in the general population is 3% to 5%). The greatest lags were in language and cognitive skills.

No statistically significant difference was found between mothers and other caregivers in the feeding of or interaction with the children, although caregivers were not substance abusers and the biologic mothers were. However, neither mothers nor caregivers provided a home environment conducive to promoting the child's cognitive development. The developmentally delayed children showed significantly lower scores on organization of the environment and had few opportunities for variety in daily stimulation.

The investigators concluded that the mothers' prenatal substance abuse and the quality of the home environment both affect the child's development. All of the families who participated in the study were motivated to obtain information about health and developmental interventions for their children, and nonsubstance-abusing caregivers requested information about how to help their family members who were abusing alcohol or drugs.

not be acquired in a lifetime. Nor does First Force Theory explain the sequence of language development, regardless of culture. However, learning principles can be used to modify acquired language deficits (27, 29).

Interactionist Theory (Second Force Theory) is used by most theorists to explain language development. Language develops through interaction between heredity, maturation, encounters with people and environmental stimuli, and life experiences. Humans are biologically prepared for language learning, but experience with the spoken word and with loving people who facilitate language acquisition is equally essential. Further, the child has an active role in learning language rather than a passive one. Adults modify their speech when talking to a child, and the child is more attentive to simplified speech. Mothers and fathers use different conversational techniques to talk with the child, who, in turn, teaches language in a broader way (27, 29).

Speech and language are major adaptive behaviors being developed during the second year. Speech enables the child to become more independent and to better make needs known. Speech is the mediation for thought processes. The greater the comprehension and vocabulary a child has, the further a child can go in cognitive processes. As the child and parents respond verbally and nonverbally to each other, the child learns attitudes and values and behaviors and ideas (27). The child first responds to patterns of sounds rather than to specific word sounds; if others speak indistinctly to the child, he or she will also speak indistinctly. The normal child will begin to speak by 14 months, although some children may make little effort to speak until after 2 years. By age 3, he or she may still mispronounce more than half the sounds (27, 54).

The toddler speaks in the present tense initially, using **syncretic speech,** in which *one word stands for a certain object, and has a limited range of sounds*. Single words represent entire sentences; for example, "go" means "I want to go." By 18 to 20 months he or she uses **telegraphic speech,** *two- to four-word expressions,* that contains a noun and verb and maintains word order such as "go play" and "go night-night." Variety on intonation also increases. A 2-year-old will introduce additional words and say "I go play" or "I go night-night." Conversation with parents involves contraction and expansion. The *child shortens into fewer words what the parent says but states the main message* (**contraction**); the *parent elaborates on, uses a full sentence, and interprets what the child says* (**expansion**). Expansion helps the child's language development (27). The toddler frequently says "no," perhaps in imitation of the parents and their discipline techniques, but may often do what is asked even while saying "no." Stuttering is common because ideas come faster than the ability to use vocabulary (27, 41).

Recognizable language develops sequentially. See

TABLE 8-4. ASSESSMENT OF LANGUAGE AND SPEECH DEVELOPMENT

Characteristic	1 Yr	1½ Yr	2 Yr	2½ Yr
Language understanding and basic communication	Understands "no-no" inhibition; knows "bye-bye" and pat-a-cake; says "mama," "dada" or some similar term for caretakers	Understands very simple verbal instructions accompanied by gesture and intonation; identifies three body parts; points to five simple pictures; points for wants	Identifies five body parts; finds 10 pictures; obeys simple commands	Points to 15 pictures; obeys two to three simple commands
Appearance of individual sounds	10 vowels, nine consonants in babbling and echoing	*p, b, m, h, w* in babbling		*t, d, n, k, g, ng* in words
Auditory memory imitation and repetition	Lalls; imitates sound; echoes or repeats syllables or some words (may not have meaning)		Meanings increasingly becoming associated with words	Repeats two digits; remembers one to two objects
Numerical size of vocabulary	One to two words	Adds 10-20 words a week	50–250–300 words if consistently spoken to	400–500 words
Word type	Nouns	Nouns, action verbs, some adjectives	Nouns, verbs, adjectives, adverbs	Pronouns, "I"
Sentence length	Single word	Single words expanding to three or four words, noun and verb	Two to five words; elemental sentence	
Description of vocalization and communication	Babbling, lalling, echolalia (repeating sounds)	Leading, pointing, jargon, some words, intonations, gestures	Words, phrases, simple sentences	Developmental language problems first seen
Purpose of vocalization and communication	Pleasure	Attention getting	Meaningful social control; wish requesting	
Speech content and style			Possessive "mine"; pronouns last grammar form learned; grammar depends on what is heard	
Percent intelligibility		20% to 25% for person unfamiliar with child	60% to 75%; poor articulation of some words	Vowel production—90%

Data from references 19, 23, 27, 33 and 41.

Table 8–4 for a summary of language and speech development.

The toddler's speech is **autistic** because *vocalizations have specific meaning only to the child*. He or she plays with sounds and incorrectly produces the majority of consonant sounds.

Apparently the child learns to speak in a highly methodical way, breaking down language into its simplest parts and developing rules to put the parts together. Children proceed from babbling to one-word and two-word sentences, use of word order and plurals, use of negative sentences, and the importance of phontics or a sound system (33). To communicate effectively, the child must learn not only the language and its rules, but also the use of social speech, which takes into account the knowledge and perspective of another person (23). This begins in toddlerhood and continues to develop through childhood as the child gains interpersonal and social experiences.

Teach parents that this is facilitated when they teach social language strategies to the child as they in-troduce him or her to life experiences. Through conversation with the family at mealtime and in other activities, vocabulary is enlarged, and the child learns family expressions that aid socialization. Mealtime provides a miniature society in which the toddler can feel secure in attempting to imitate speech. He or she gets positive reinforcement for speech efforts, especially for words that are selected, repeated frequently, and reinforced by eager parents. In addition, *being talked with, using adult words rather than baby talk, frequently throughout the day, being read to, and having an opportunity to explore the environment increase the child's comprehension of words and rules of grammar as well as organization and size of vocabulary and use of word inflections* (8).

Language development *requires a sense of security and verbal and nonverbal stimulation*. For a child to speak, he or she must have a loving, consistent relationship with a parent or caretaker. Unless the toddler feels that this person will respond to his or her words, toddler will not be motivated to speak. The toddler may not talk when separated from mother such as during hospitalization or the first day at day care. When being prepared for hospital procedures, the toddler needs simple and succinct explanations, with gestures pointing to the areas of the body being cared for, and verbal and physical displays of affection.

If a child is *delayed in speech,* carefully assess the child and family. Causes may include deafness or the inability to listen, mental retardation, emotional disturbance, maternal deprivation or separation from the parents, lack of verbal communication within the family and to the child, inconsistent or tangential responses to the child's speech, presence of twins, or parents' anticipating the needs of the child before he or she has a chance to communicate them.

Verbal interaction, an environment with a variety of objects and stimuli, and freedom to explore are crucial to help the young child use his or her senses and emerging motor skills and thereby are necessary to learn during the sensorimotor and preoperational states (53).

Emotional Development

The toddler is a self-loving, uninhibited, dominating, energetic little person absorbed in self-importance, always seeking attention, approval, and personal goals. Sometimes toddler is cuddly and loving. At other times, he or she bites or pinches and looks almost happy, feeling no sense of guilt or shame. There is little self-control over exploratory or sadistic impulses. The toddler only slowly realizes that he or she cannot have everything desired and that some behavior annoys others. He or she experiments with abandon in the quest for independence yet becomes easily frightened and runs to the parent for protection, security, reassurance, and approval.

Because the toddler still relies so much on the parents and wants their approval, he or she learns to curb the negativism without losing independent drives, to cooperate increasingly, and to develop socially approved behavior. Need for attention and approval is one of the main motivating forces in ego development and socialization.

The toddler often repeats performances and behavior that are given attention and laughed at; he or she likes to perform for adults and pleases self as much as the audience. He or she has a primitive sense of humor, laughs frequently, especially at surprise sounds and startling incongruities, and laughs with others who are laughing and at his or her own antics. Parents should give sufficient attention but not make the child show off for an audience, verbally or physically, and they should not overstimulate with laughter or games.

Developmental Crisis

The psychosexual crisis for the toddler is autonomy versus shame and doubt (14). **Autonomy** is *shown in the ability to gain self-control* over motor abilities and sphincters; to make and carry out decisions; to feel able to cope adequately with problems or get the necessary help; to wait with patience; to give generously or to hold on, as indicated; to distinguish between possessions or wishes of self and of others; and to have a feeling of good will and pride. Autonomy is characterized by the oft-heard statement, "Me do it." Mastery accomplished in infancy sets the basis for autonomy.

Using negativism, even displaying temper, dawdling, and rituals; exploring even when parents object; developing language skills, saying "no" although he or she may do as asked; and increasing control over his or her body or situations are some apparent ways the toddler is demonstrating developing autonomy and maintaining a sense of security and control. Ritualistic behavior is normal and at a peak at $2\frac{1}{2}$ years, especially at bedtime and during illness. Although autonomy is developing, emotions are still contagious. The toddler reflects others' behavior and feelings. For example, if someone laughs or cries, he or she will imitate for no apparent reason.

Shame and doubt are felt if autonomy and a positive self-concept are not achieved (14). **Shame** is *the feeling of being fooled, embarrassed, exposed, small, impotent, dirty, of wanting to hide, and rage against self.* **Doubt** is *fear, uncertainty, mistrust, lack of self-confidence, and feeling that nothing done is any good and that one is controlled by others rather than being in control of self* (14).

There is a limit to how exposed, dirty, mean, and vulnerable one can feel. If the child is pushed past the limit or disciplined or toilet trained too harshly, he or she can no longer discriminate about self, what he or she should be and can do. If everything is planned and done *for* and *to* the child, he or she cannot develop autonomy. The toddler's self-concept and behavior will try to measure up to the expectations of parents and others, but there is no close attachment to an adult. Apathy and withdrawal may occur, or he or she may become defiant, excessively negativistic, and physically overactive and develop behaviors opposite to expectations. A low frustration tolerance and difficulty with eating, digestion, elimination, and sleep may be seen. Too much shaming does not develop a sense of propriety but rather a secret determination to get away with things. As an adult, he or she may become either too compliant, letting self be controlled and manipulated in spite of being angry about it; or he or she may become impulsive, stubbornly assertive, obstinate, or negativistic, have little sense of responsibility, and want to get away with things. The person may give up easily in all efforts, withdraw, be compulsive in behavior, hoard objects, or be either messy or overmeticulous.

Discourage parents from creating an emotional climate of excessive expectations, criticism, blame, punishment, and overrestriction for the toddler because within the child's consciousness a sense of shame and doubt may develop that will be extremely harmful to further development. The child should not be given too much autonomy, or he or she will feel all-powerful. When a toddler fails to accomplish what he or she has been falsely led to believe could be achieved, the self-doubt and shame that result can be devastating. Aggressive behavior results if the child is severely punished or if parents are aggressive (3). With the proper balance of guidance and discipline, the toddler gains a sense of personal abilities and thus has the potential to deal with the next set of social adjustments.

Toilet Training

Toilet training is a major developmental accomplishment and relates directly to the crisis of autonomy versus shame and doubt or to what Freudian theory calls the **anal stage** (29). Independence and autonomy (self-control), not cleanliness, are the critical issues in teaching the child to use the toilet. For the process to work, the parents must do little more than arrange for the child to use the toilet easily. The parent supports rather than acts as a trainer and is interested in the child, not just the act (1). The toddler is interested in the products he excretes. The toddler gradually learns to control bowel and bladder. *Neuromuscular maturity,* which occurs from 1 to 3 years, with bowel before bladder control, *is necessary for regular, self-controlled evacuation* (16).

Many factors are involved besides biologic readiness since the toddler's fears, goals, and conflicting wishes also influence this learning experience. Psychologically, toilet training is complex. Mother gives approval not only for defecating properly but also for withholding feces. The sensations of giving and withholding feces, imitation of parents and siblings, approval from family, and pride in the accomplishments hasten toilet training. Being forced to do the parents' will may cause problems of negativism.

Bowel training is a less complex task than bladder training and should be attempted first. You can assist parents by alerting them to signs of readiness. The toddler shows physical readiness for bowel training when he or she defecates regularly and shows some signs of being aware of defecation such as grunting, straining, or tugging at the diaper. It also helps if the child can speak, understand directions, and manipulate the clothing somewhat. *Mental readiness* includes the child's wanting to watch people use the toilet (which should be allowed), wanting to flush the toilet, and asking questions about it. *Emotional readiness* includes feeling secure about using the toilet, pretending to use it, and asking to use it.

Some toddlers, after defecation, cry and indicate distress until they are changed. Others do not indicate discomfort and will play with and smear feces. They are curious, explore, and see nothing shameful about such behavior. They have not learned the aesthetic and cultural connotations of feces being "dirty" and "smelly" and not an object for play. But since play with feces must be restricted because it is unsanitary and non-

aesthetic, changing diapers immediately after defecation, using safety pins to keep the diaper on snugly, having well-fitted training pants, and showing parental disapproval are ways to prevent such play. In addition, encourage parents to provide opportunities for play and smearing with clay, sand, mud, paste, and finger paints to help the child develop natural potentials and divert instinctual urges into socially accepted behavior.

Parents may demonstrate inordinate interest in this aspect of development, producing anxiety over bowel training with possible harmful physical effects such as constipation or psychologic effects, which result from trying to meet excessive demands. Be aware of the development problems associated with toilet training, but remember that elimination is a natural process. Teach parents to approach toilet training in a matter-of-fact and relaxed way, to expect some resistance, and not to push the child or reflect anxiety. Every child by age 3 years can carry on this task with some help as to where and how. Culturally, American society seems to demand that mothers begin toilet training somewhere around 2 years of age, but $2\frac{1}{2}$ years would be soon enough (29). However, when younger parents follow the directions given in this chapter, grandma may defy them and secretly sit 1-year-old Suzie on the potty. Toilet training should not be started in turbulent periods such as hospitalization of the toddler, homecoming of a new baby, absence of the main caretaker from home, or a family crisis. Even when started in a calm period, some regression is natural.

Encourage the parents to have the child use a potty chair since it is mechanically easier than the family toilet, and the chair is his or her own. The potty chair should be in a place convenient for the child. Recommend that the child wear training pants and that training take place when disruptions in regular routine are at a minimum. The toddler should be praised for success. Parents should remain calm, reassuring, and supportive if the child has an accident.

Bladder training is more complex because the reflexes appropriate for bladder training are less explicit, neurologic maturation comes later, and urination is a reflex response to bladder tensions and must be inhibited. Bladder control demands more self-awareness and self-discipline from the toddler and is usually achieved between the ages of $2\frac{1}{2}$ and $3\frac{1}{2}$ years when physiologic development has progressed enough that the bladder can retain urine for approximately 2 hours. Waking hours and sleeping hours present two phases of control and differences in awareness of bladder function.

The series of events necessary for bladder training are that the toddler must first realize he or she is wet, then know he or she is wetting, next recognize impulses that tell that he or she is going to urinate, and finally control urinating until he or she is at the toilet (36). A physically ready child is able to stay dry for 2 or more hours during the day, and wake up dry from naps and may wake up dry in the morning.

You may help the parents by explaining the process of urination. Make it clear to the parents that both boys and girls can sit down while urinating and that both may try to stand like daddy. Sleeping control will be effective when the child responds to bladder reflexes and not before. Cutting down on fluids and other devices to reduce enuresis, or bed wetting, are not effective in gaining reflex control.

After waking control has been well established, sleeping control usually follows. Past 5 years of age, however, if nighttime control has not been achieved, there might be a physiologic or psychologic problem. Encourage medical attention if this problem persists, and consider possible emotional causes. Enuresis is discussed further in Chapter 9.

Body-Image and Self-Concept Development

Body Image

Body image development gradually evolves as a component of self-concept. The toddler has a dim self-awareness, but with a developing sense of autonomy, he or she becomes more correctly aware of the body as a physical entity and one with emotional capabilities. Toddler is increasingly aware of pleasurable sensations in the genital area and on the skin and mouth and is learning control of the body through locomotion, toilet training, speech, and socialization.

The toddler is not always aware of the whole body or the distal parts and might even consider distal parts such as the feet as something apart from self. Toddler does not always know when he or she is sick, tired, or too hot or when the pants are wet. The child also has difficulty realizing that body productions such as feces are separate from self; therefore he or she may resist flushing the toilet. Toddler is not aware of the influences on his or her body but is aware of general feelings and thoughts and increasingly of others' reactions to his or her body and behavior. For example, when the toddler is in control of the environment, the body feels good, wonderful, and strong. When things are not going well, if he or she cannot succeed or is punished excessively, the child feels bad and shameful.

Self-Concept

Self-concept is also made up of the feelings about self, adaptive and defensive mechanisms, reactions from others, and one's perceptions of these reactions, attitudes, values, and many of life's experiences.

As the child incorporates approval and disapproval, praise and punishment, gestures that are kind and forbidding, he or she forms an opinion about self as a person. How the person feels about self is determined to a great degree by the reactions of others and in turn later determines how he or she views others. The young child is very aware of the gradient of anxiety—mild, moderate, or severe. He or she watches for signs of approval and disapproval from others in relation to self. Increasingly there is recall about what caused discomfort or anxiety. Experiences of discomfort are first with

mother and then are generalized to other people, and much behavior becomes organized to avoid or minimize discomfort around others. Thus he or she gradually evolves adaptive and defensive behaviors and learns what to do to get along with others. The **self-system** gradually develops as an *organization of experiences that exists to defend against anxiety and to secure satisfaction* (46).

The various appraisals of others cause the child to form feelings of **good-me, bad-me,** or **not-me,** as the self-concept. The child is fully aware of reactions that convey approval, love, security, and because these make him or her feel good, a **concept of good-me** forms. *He or she likes self because others do, the basis of a positive self-concept.* Reactions of disapproval or punishment from significant adults increase the child's anxiety, and if this cycle continues, **bad-me,** a *negative self-concept,* results. If negative reaction is never-ending, the child may evolve defensive behaviors such as denial that prevent noticing the negative evaluations. Some appraisals from others evoke severe discomfort or panic; these *feelings and awareness of the situation are repressed and dissociated from the rest of the personality,* forming the **not-me part of the self.** *These are the ideas, feelings, or body parts that later seem foreign to the person.* For example, severe toilet training or punishing the child for masturbating or touching the genitals may be so traumatic and panic producing that he or she becomes almost unaware of the genital area. Later the person does not include the lower half of the body or the genital area in self-drawings or does not speak of sexual matters; he or she may be very inhibited about toileting, and a disturbed gender identity may be evident through behavior. The more feelings or life experiences that are dissociated, the more rigid the personality and the less aware of self he or she is in later life. Each person attempts to find ways to keep feelings of *good-me* and reduce the uncomfortable feelings elicited by the *bad-me* (46).

The direction of the self-concept and personality often follows the impetus given it in early childhood; the person remains fairly consistent in behavior and attitudes, although there are some changes throughout life as the person encounters new experiences and people. For example, if the young child internalizes feelings of being bad, unworthy, inadequate, perhaps because of race, color, or neighborhood, he or she will later have difficulty believing that he or she is good or competent, even when that is realistic. If the person has good, happy, adequate feelings about self because of childhood experiences, occasional failures will not dampen self-esteem or feelings of competence.

The child's major caretaker should have a positive self-concept and feel good about being a mother (father). If others in the family or if society debase the mothering one, there is injury to the child's self-esteem. Thus the issue of equality of women becomes critical. Equality as a person, the importance of the mother and homemaker role, and the importance of women to society and to the work world are all critical to successful child rearing. If the female caretaker doubts her own worth, is resentful of societal oppression, and has doubts about her own power and status, these negative feelings will be conveyed nonverbally to the child and will have a direct bearing on his or her sense of security and self-worth. This critical phase of development lies between 18 and 36 months (2).

Be mindful of body-image and self-concept formation as you care for toddlers, for it determines their reaction. Only through repetitious positive input can you change a negative self-concept to one that is positive. By stimulating a positive self-image, you are promoting emotional health. Teach parents to provide an environment in which the child can successfully exercise skills such as running, walking, and playing and feel acceptance of his or her body and behavior. Help them realize that as the child's autonomy develops, so too will a more appropriate mental picture of his or her body and emotions.

Adaptive Mechanisms

Before the child is 2 years old, he or she is learning the basic response patterns appropriate for the family and culture; a degree of trust and confidence, or lack of it, in the parents; how to express annoyance and impatience and love and joy; and how to communicate needs.

The toddler begins to adapt to the culture because of **primary identification.** He or she *imitates the parents* and responds to their encouragement and discouragement. With successful adaptation, the child moves toward independence. Other major adaptive mechanisms of this era include repression, suppression, denial, reaction formation, projection, and sublimation (29).

Repression *unconsciously removes from awareness the thoughts, impulses, fantasies, and memories of behavior that are unacceptable to the self.* The *not-me* discussed earlier is an example and may result from child abuse. **Suppression** *differs from repression in that it is a conscious act.* For example, the child forgets that he or she has been told not to handle certain articles. **Denial** is *not admitting, even when warned, that certain factors exist,* for example, that the stove is hot and will cause a burn. **Reaction formation** is *replacing the original idea and behavior with the opposite behavior characteristics.* For example, the child flushes the toilet and describes feces as dirty instead of playing in them, thus becoming appropriately tidy. **Projection** occurs when *he or she attributes personal feelings or behaviors to someone else.* For example, if the babysitter disciplines toddler, he or she projects dislike for her by saying, "You don't like me." **Sublimation** is *channeling impulses into socially acceptable behavior rather than expressing the original impulse.* For example, he or she plays with mud, finger paints, or shaving cream instead of feces, which is socially unacceptable.

Teach parents that the child's adaptive behavior is strengthened when he or she is taught to do something for self and permitted to make a decision *if that decision is truly his or hers to make.* If the decision is one that must be carried out regardless of the toddler's wish, it can best be accomplished by giving direction rather than by asking the child if he or she wants to do something.

Sexuality Development

Traditionally parents have handled sons and daughters differently during infancy, and the results became evident in toddlerhood.

Because parents encourage independent behavior in boys and more dependency in girls, by 13 months the boy ventures farther from mother, stays away longer, and looks at or talks to his mother less than does the girl. The girl at this age is encouraged to spend more time touching and staying near mother than is the boy. However, the separation process later seems less severe for girls. Perhaps boys should be touched and cuddled longer (29, 31).

Boys play more vigorously with toys than do girls, and they play more with nontoys such as doorknobs and light switches. Yet basically there is no sexual preference for toys, although parents may enforce a preference. A boy responds with more overt aggression to a barrier placed between him and his mother at 13 months of age than do girls. Boys show more exploratory and aggressive behavior than girls, and this behavior is encouraged by the father (29, 31). The female remains attentive to a wide variety of stimuli and complex visual and auditory stimuli. The female demonstrates earlier language development and seems more aware of contextual relationships, perhaps because of the more constant stimulation from the mother (6).

Society has traditionally been easy on girls in terms of achievement. If they excel, this is an added plus; if they do not, no one cares. Boys, however, are expected to achieve. As early as the toddler years this influence can be seen: girls are allowed to be more dependent, but boys are pushed to achieve. Attitudes, however, are changing about women's roles and abilities (4, 5).

Primary identification, *imitation and observation of the same-sexed parent,* contributes to gender identity. The child by 15 months is interested in his or her own and others' body parts. Both boys and girls achieve sexual pleasure through self-stimulation, although girls masturbate less than boys (possibly because of anatomic differences) (4).

By 21 months the child can refer to self by name, an important factor in the development of identity. By 2 years of age, the child can categorize people into boy and girl and has some awareness of anatomic differences if he or she has had an opportunity to view them (4).

By the end of toddlerhood, the child is more aware

of his or her body, the body's excretions, and his or her actions, and he and she can be more independent in the first steps of self-care. Ability to communicate verbally expands to the point that he or she can ask questions and talk about sexual topics with parents and peers.

Help parents to understand the developing sexuality of their child and to be comfortable with their own gender identification and sexuality so that they can cuddle the child and answer questions. Help them understand that a wide variety of play experiences will prepare the child for adult behavior and competence. They may talk through their concerns about a son's becoming a sissy if he plays with dolls or wears mother's high heels in dramatic play. Help parents realize that a daughter's playing with trucks does not mean she will become a truck driver.

Guidance and Discipline

Discipline is *guidance that helps the child learn to understand and care for self and to get along with others.* It is not just punishing, correcting, or controlling behavior, as is commonly assumed (29).

Everything in the toddler's world is new and exciting and meant to be explored, touched, eaten, or sat on, including porcelain figurines from Spain or boiling water. In moving away from complete dependency, the toddler demonstrates energy and drive and requires sufficient restrictions to ensure physical and psychologic protection and at the same time enough freedom to permit exploration and autonomy. Because mother must now set limits, a new dimension is added to the relationship established between mother and toddler. Before, mother met his or her basic needs immediately. With the toddler's increasing ability, freedom, and demands, the parent sometimes makes him or her wait or denies a wish if it will cause harm. The transition should be made in a loving, consistent, yet flexible manner so that the child maintains trust and moves in the quest for independence. Excessive limitations, overwhelming steady pressure, or hostile bullying behavior might cause an overly rebellious, negativistic, or passive child. Complete lack of limitations can cause accidents, poor health, and insecurity.

Mother is usually the main disciplinarian at this age, and her approach is important. When the mother is under high acute or chronic stress, support and help from others is the most significant factor in reducing a negative discipline approach to the child(ren), regardless of the mother's age, education, or marital status (10).

Through guidance and the parent's reaction, the child is being socialized, learning what is right and wrong. Because the child cannot adequately reason, he or she must depend on and trust the parents as a guide for all activities. He or she can obey simple commands. Later, the child will be capable of internalizing rules and

mores and will become self-disciplined as a result of having been patiently disciplined. Setting limits is not easy. Parents should not thwart the toddler's curiosity and enthusiasm, but they must protect him or her from harm. Parents who oppose the toddler's desire of the moment are likely to meet with anything from a simple "no" to a temper tantrum.

Teach parents the importance of constructive guidance and discipline. Temper tantrums result because the toddler hates being thwarted and feeling helpless. Once the feelings are discharged, the child regains composure quickly and without revenge. If temper tantrums, a form of negativism, occur, the best advice is to ignore the outburst; it will soon disappear. The child needs the parent's reaction for the behavior to continue. Belittling or beating the child does not help temper tantrums. If he or she is given more frustration than can be handled, fear, hostility, and anger mount, and the lack of verbal ability inhibits adequate outlet. Hence he or she strikes out, bites, or hits physically. Now toddler desperately needs mother's support, firm control, and mediation. The parent's calm voice, expressing understanding of feelings, and introduction of an activity to restore self-esteem are important to teaching self-control.

Because parents are sometimes confused about handling the toddler's behavior, you can assist them by teaching some simple rules:

1. Provide an environment in which the child feels respected.
2. Decide what is important and what is not worth a battle of will. For example, the child may not be wearing matched clothing but resists parental attempts to change. Avoid negativism and an angry scene by deciding that today it is all right for the child to wear an unmatched outfit.
3. Changing the mind, pursuing an alternate activity, or letting the child have his or her way is not giving in, losing face, being a poor parent, or letting the child be manipulative. When limits are consistent, changing a direction of behavior can be a positive learning experience for the child. The child is becoming aware of being a separate person, able to assert self and influence others.
4. Remove or avoid temptations such as breakable objects within reach or candy that should not be eaten to avoid having to repeatedly say "No."
5. Try not to ask open-ended questions for the child to decide about an activity when the decision is not really one the child can make.
6. Consider limits as more than restrictions but also as a distraction *from* one prohibited activity *to* another in which the child can freely participate. Distraction with alternatives or a substitute is effective with the toddler because attention span is short.
7. Reinforce appropriate behavior through approval and attention. The child will continue behavior that

gains attention, even if the attention is punitive, because negative attention is better than none to the child.

8. Set limits consistently so that the child can rely on the parent's judgment rather than testing the adult's endurance in each situation.

9. State limits clearly, concisely, simply, positively, and in a calm voice. For example, if the child cannot play with a treasured object, he or she should not be allowed to handle it. Say "Look with your hands behind your back" or "Look with your eyes, not your hands" rather than "Don't touch."

10. Set limits only when necessary. Some rules promote a sense of security, but too many confuse the child.

11. Provide a safe area where the child is free to do whatever he or she wants to do.

12. Do not overprotect the child; he or she should learn that some things have a price such as a bruise or a scratch.

13. Do not terminate the child's activity too quickly; tell him or her that the activity is ending (29, 41).

Each situation will determine the extent of firmness or leniency needed. The toddler needs grades of independence.

Moral-Spiritual Development

Birth through the toddler era might be termed the *pre-religious stage*. This label does not deny religious influences but simply points out that the toddler is absorbing basic intellectual and emotional patterns regardless of the religious conviction of the caretakers. The toddler may repeat some phrases from prayers while imitating a certain voice tone or body posture that accompanies those prayers. The child only knows that when he or she imitates or conforms to certain rituals, affection and approval come that add to the sense of identification and security. The "good" and "bad" are defined in terms of physical consequences to self.

Teach parents that the toddler can benefit from a nursery-school type of church program in which emphasis is on positive self-image and appropriate play and rest rather than on a lesson to learn. Toddler also needs to have others to imitate who follow the rules of society, and he or she needs rewards and reinforcement for good or desirable behavior.

Developmental Tasks

Development tasks for the toddler may be summarized as follows (13):

1. Settling into healthy daily routines
2. Mastering good eating habits
3. Mastering the basics of toilet training
4. Developing the physical skills appropriate to the stage of motor development
5. Becoming a family member

6. Learning to communicate efficiently with an increasing number of others

The constantly sensitive situation of the toddler, gaining autonomy and independence—at times overreaching and needing mother's help, at times needing the freedom from mother's protection—is one you can help parents understand. The child's future personality and health will depend partially on how these many opportunities are handled now. Your role in teaching and support is critical.

Nursing Applications

Your role with the toddler and family has been discussed with each section throughout this chapter. Box 8–7 lists some *nursing diagnoses* that may apply to the

 BOX 8-7.
Selected Nursing Diagnoses Related to the Toddler[a]

Pattern 1: Exchanging

Altered Nutrition: More than body requirements
Altered Nutrition: Less than body requirements
Altered Nutrition: Potential for more than body requirements
Potential for Infection
Potential for Injury
Potential for Suffocation
Potential for Poisoning
Potential for Trauma
Potential for Aspiration

Pattern 2: Communicating

Impaired Verbal Communication

Pattern 3: Relating

Impaired Social Interaction

Pattern 6: Moving

Impaired Physical Mobility
Altered Growth and Development

Pattern 7: Perceiving

Self-Esteem Disturbance
Sensory/Perceptual Alterations
Unilateral Neglect

Pattern 9: Feeling

Pain
Anxiety
Fear

[a]Other of the NANDA diagnoses are applicable to the ill toddler. From North American Nursing Diagnosis Association, *NANDA Nursing Diagnosis Taxonomy I* (Rev.). St. Louis: North American Nursing Diagnosis Association, 1990.

toddler, based on assessments that would be accomplished from knowledge presented in this chapter. Interventions include your role modeling of caring behavior to the toddler and family; parent and family education, support, and counseling; or direct care to meet the toddler's physical, emotional, cognitive, and social needs.

REFERENCES

1. Adams, D., *The Child Influencers*. Cuyahoga Fall, Ohio: Home Team Press, 1990.

2. Adams, P., What Women's Inequality Means to Children and Adolescents, *American Journal of Social Psychiatry,* 1, no. 1 (April 1981), 6–8.

3. Argyle, M., *The Psychology of Interpersonal Behavior*. Baltimore: Penguin Press, 1967.

4. Baker, S., and R. Henry, *Parents' Guide to Nutrition: Healthy Eating from Birth through Adolescence*. Reading, Mass: Addison-Wesley, 1986.

5. Bardwich, J., *Psychology of Women: A Study of Biocultural Conflicts*. New York: Harper & Row, 1971.

6. ———, and E. Douvan, Ambivalence: The Socialization of Women. In Bardwich, J., ed., *Readings on the Psychology of Women*. New York: Harper & Row, 1972, pp. 52–58.

7. Bettelheim, B., *A Good Enough Parent: A Book on Child-Rearing*. New York: Random, 1988.

8. Bossard, J.H.S., and E.S. Boll, *The Sociology of Child Development* (4th ed.). New York: Harper & Row, 1966.

9. Bowlby, J., *Attachment and Loss,* Vol. I. *Attachment*. New York: Basic Books, 1969.

10. Brandt, P., Stress-Buffering Effects of Social Support on Maternal Discipline, *Nursing Research,* 33, no. 4 (1984), 229–235.

11. Coopersmith, S., *The Antecedents of Self-Esteem*. San Francisco: W.H. Freeman, 1967.

12. DiLeo, J., *Children's Drawings as Diagnostic Aids*. New York: Brunner/Mazel, 1973.

13. Duvall, E., and B. Miller, *Marriage and Family Development* (6th ed). New York: Harper & Row, 1984.

14. Erikson, E.H., *Childhood and Society* (2nd ed.). New York: W.W. Norton, 1963.

15. Ewert, D., et al., Measles Vaccination Coverage Among Latino Children Aged 12 to 59 Months in Los Angeles County: A Household Survey, *American Journal of Public Health,* 81, no. 8 (1991), 1057–1059.

16. Falkner, F., and J.M. Tanner (eds.), *Human Growth* (2nd ed.). New York: Plenum Press, 1986.

17. Feeding Your Child, *Parenting:Glennon Hospital for Children,* 1990, pp 10–11.

18. Feigenberg, M., and J. Sotman, A Toddler with a Malabsorption Syndrome, *American Journal of Nursing,* 75, no. 6 (1975), 978–979.

19. Frankel, L., Warning Signals and Identification of Children With Learning Disabilities, *Health Values: Achieving High Level Wellness,* 9, no. 3 (1986), 3–7.

20. Freiberg, K., *Human Development: A Life Span Approach,* (4th ed). Boston: Jones and Bartlett, 1992.

21. Garbarino, J., E. Guttmann, and J. Seeley, *The Psychologically Battered Child: Strategies for Identification, Assessment, and Intervention*. San Francisco: Jossey-Bass, 1987.

22. Geber, M., The Psycho-Motor Development of African Children in the First Year and the Influence of Maternal Behavior, *The Journal of Social Psychology,* 47 (1958), 185–195.

23. Gesell, A., et al., *The First Five Years of Life*. New York: Harper & Brothers, 1940.

24. Hegarty, V., *Decisions in Nutrition*. St. Louis: Times Mirror/Mosby College Publishing, 1988.

25. Hoole, A., R. Greenberg, and C.G. Pickard, *Patient Care Guidelines for Nurse Practitioners* (3rd ed.). Boston: Little, Brown, 1988.

26. Jones, F., K. Garrison, and R. Morgan, *The Psychology of Human Development* (2nd ed.). New York: Harper & Row, 1985.

27. Kaluger, G., and M. Kaluger, *Human Development: The Span of Life* (3rd ed.). St. Louis: Times Mirror/Mosby, 1984.

28. Lamb, M., *The Father's Role*. New York: John Wiley, 1986.

29. Lidz, T., *The Person: His and Her Development Throughout the Life Cycle* (2nd ed.). New York: Basic Books, 1983.

30. Linley, J., Screening Children for Common Orthopedic Problems, *American Journal of Nursing,* 87, no. 10 (1987), 1312–1316.

31. Macoby, E., Sex Differences in Intellectual Functioning. In Bardwich, J., ed., *Readings on the Psychology of Women. I*. New York: Harper & Row, 1972, pp. 34–44.

32. Missouri Hypertension Control Program/Bureau of Chronic Diseases, Questions—Answers, Jefferson City, Mo. (n.d.).

33. Moshman, D., J. Glover, and R. Bruning, *Developmental Psychology*. Boston: Little, Brown, 1987.

34. Murphy, B., Pushing Up Baby, *Washington University School of Medicine Outlook,* 24, no. 3 (1987), 16.

35. New Evidence Links Reye's Syndrome and Aspirin, *The Nation's Health,* (May-June 1987), 20.

36. Pillitteri, A., *Child Health Nursing: Care of the Growing Family* (3rd ed.). Boston: Little, Brown, 1987.

37. Pipes, P., *Nutrition in Infancy and Childhood* (4th ed.). St. Louis: Times Mirror/Mosby, 1988.

38. Pridham, K., and M. Hansoen, Helping Children Deal With Procedures in a Clinic Setting: A Developmental Approach, *Journal of Pediatric Nursing,* 2, no. 2 (1987), 13–21.

39. Sagan, L., *The Health of Nations*. New York: Basic Books, 1987.

40. Sataloff, R., and C. Colton, Otitis Media: A Common Childhood Infection, *American Journal of Nursing,* 81, no. 8 (1981), 1480–1483.

41. Schuster, C.S., and S.S. Ashburn, *The Process of Human Development: A Holistic Life-Span Approach* (3rd ed.). Boston: Little, Brown, 1986.

42. Scipien, G.M., et al., *Comprehensive Pediatric Nursing* (3rd ed.). New York: McGraw-Hill, 1986.

43. Shapiro, L., et al., Obesity Prognosis: A Longitudinal Study of Children From Age 6 Months to 9 Years, *American Journal of Public Health,* 74, no. 9 (1984), 968–972.

44. Sherman, J.L., Jr., and S. Fields, *Guide to Patient Evaluation* (5th ed.). Garden City, NY: Medical Examination Publishing, 1987.

45. Silver, H. II, C.H. Kempe, and H. Bruyn, *Handbook of Pediatrics* (15th ed.). Los Altos, Calif.: Lange, 1987.

46. Sullivan, H.S., *Interpersonal Theory of Psychiatry.* New York: W.W. Norton, 1953.

47. Taking Care of Toddlers' Teeth, *Health Scene* (Fall 1987), 11.

48. Turner, J., and D. Helms, *Lifespan Development* (3rd ed.). New York: Holt, Rinehart & Winston, 1987.

49. U.S. Department of Health and Human Service, New Recommended Schedule for Active Immunization of Normal Infants and Children, *Morbidity and Mortality Weekly Report,* 35, no. 37 (September 19, 1986), 577–579.

50. Vaccinating Children Against *H. Influenzae, American Journal of Nursing,* 85, no. 6 (1985), 642.

51. Verzemnieks, I., Developmental Stimulation for Infants and Toddlers, *American Journal of Nursing,* 84, no. 6 (1984), 749–752.

52. Wadsworth, B., *Piaget's Theory of Cognitive and Affective Development* (4th ed.). New York: Longman, 1989.

53. Webb, P., Piaget: Implications for Teaching, *Theory Into Practice,* 19, no. 2 (1980), 93–97.

54. Whaley, L., and D. Wong, *Nursing Care of Infants and Children* (4th ed.). St. Louis: C.V. Mosby, 1991.

55. Why Children Need Their Parents' Time, *AFA Journal* (April 1991), 17–18.

56. Williams, S., *Nutritional and Diet Therapy* (6th ed.). St. Louis: C.V. Mosby, 1989.

Chapter 9

Assessment and Health Promotion for the Preschooler

The preschooler is constantly learning.
—*Ruth Beckmann Murray*

KEY TERMS

Preschool years	Second degree	Pressured sexuality	Peer group
Peers	Third degree	Ritualistic abuse	Physical activity
Oedipal or Electra stage	Encephalopathy	Neglect	Dramatic play
Identification	Strabismus	Concepts	Creative playthings
Day care	Diplopia	Concept formation	Quiet play
Family day care	Amblyopia	Action space	Permissive discipline
Nursery school	Acute purulent otitis media	Body space	Overpermissive discipline
Early school experiences	Conjunctivitis	Object space	Initiative
Montessori programs	Urinary tract infection	Map space	Guilt
Compensatory programs	Enuresis	Abstract space	Differentiation
Kindergarten	Nonspecific vulvovaginitis	Quantitative concepts	Articulate
Siblings	Measles	Concepts of causality	Integration
Dyads	Diarrhea	Animistic	Introjection
Active immunity	Postural problems	Egocentric	Secondary identification
Passive immunity	Juvenile hypertension	Transductive logic	Fantasy
Minor head injury	Child abuse	Absolute thought	Anthropomorphism
Minor lacerations	Physical abusive acts	Centering	Superego
Burns	Psychologic abuse	Reversibility	
First degree	Child sexual abuse	Peer	

OBJECTIVES

Study of this chapter will enable you to:

1. Compare the family relationships between the preschool and previous developmental eras and the influence of parents, siblings, and nonfamily members on the preschooler.
2. Explore with the family the expected developmental tasks and ways to meet them.
3. Visit several day-care centers and nursery schools, compare their values and services to parents and child, and discuss necessary adaptation by the preschooler in each setting.
4. Assess physical, motor, mental, language, play, and emotional characteristics of a 3-, 4-, and 5-year-old.
5. Describe the health needs of the preschooler, including nutrition, exercise, rest, safety, and immunization, and measures to meet these needs.
6. Explore with parents their role in contributing to the preschooler's cognitive, language, self-concept, sexuality, moral-religious, and emotional development and physical health.
7. Discuss measures to diminish the trauma of hospitalization for this age group.
8. Explore with parents effective ways for communication with and guidance and discipline of the preschooler to enhance his or her development.
9. Describe the developmental crisis of initiative versus guilt, the adaptive mechanisms commonly used that promote a sense of initiative, and the implications of this crisis for later maturity.
10. Discuss the developmental tasks and your role in promoting achievement of them.
11. Work effectively with a preschooler in the nursing situation.

In this chapter development of the preschool child and the family relationships are discussed. *Nursing responsibilities for health promotion for the child and family are discussed throughout the chapter. The information regarding normal development and needs serves as a basis for assessment.* Your role is to use information on assessment and health promotion in health education and counseling of families and in your care of the preschooler. You will find opportunity in many settings— the neighborhood, day-care center, church group, clinic, doctor's office, school, industrial setting, or hospital—to correct parents' misconceptions and validate their sound thinking about their child's development and the importance of the family's behavior for the child's emotional, physical, and social health. Principles of communication, health teaching, and crisis work also apply. Become active as a citizen to educate the public about needs of hospitalized children, promote needed legislation, or directly offset problems that affect children's health such as child abuse or lead poisoning. Promote quality day-care or preschool programs. The range of possible effective intervention is wide and will depend on your work setting and interest.

The **preschool years,** *age 3 through 5,* along with

infancy and the toddler years, form a crucial part of the person's life. The preschool child is emerging as a social being. He or she participates more fully as a family member but begins to grow slowly out of the family, spending more time in association with **peers,** *children of the same age.* Physical growth is slowing, but body control and coordination are increasing. Many body activities are becoming routine. Emotional and intellectual growth is progressively apparent in the ability to form mental images; express self in anger; become acquainted with the environment; have some perception of social relationships and the status of self as an individual compared with others; identify with the play group and follow rules; control primitive (*id*) impulses, and begin to be self-critical with references to a standard set by others (*superego formation*).

The parents, too, must learn to separate themselves from their growing child and revise decisions about how much free expression and initiative to permit the child while at the same time setting certain limits. The child's long step into the outside world is not always accomplished with ease for either the child or the parent. Thus gradually promoting more independence during the preschool years allows both the child and parents to be more comfortable about the separation that occurs when he or she goes to school.

FAMILY DEVELOPMENT AND RELATIONSHIPS

The family unit, regardless of the specific form, is important to the preschooler, and in turn the preschooler affects relationships within the family by his or her behavior. The close relationship of the baby to the mother and father gradually expands to include other significant adults living in the home, siblings, and other relatives, and they will have some effect on the child's personality.

In one study of the effect of parenting styles on preschoolers, children were divided into three groups: (1) friendly, self-controlled, and self-reliant; (2) discontented and withdrawn; and (3) low in self-reliance and self-control. Parents of the first group were significantly more controlling, demanding, and loving than parents of either of the other groups. Parents of the discontented and withdrawn children were also controlling, but they were detached instead of warm and loving. Parents of the children who were low in self-reliance and self-esteem were warm but highly permissive. This study is representative of a number of other studies that indicate that children of relatively demanding but loving parents usually are better adjusted, more independent, and more self-reliant (42, 51, 71). Other studies reveal that highly creative children have parents who are warm and loving and who expect more of them at an earlier age than do parents of less creative children (46). Parents who have a high need for achievement are more demanding that their children try new things and expect more of them at

an earlier age than do parents with less need for achievement. These ambitious parents emphasize independence, show an interest in their children's activities, give emotional rewards for competence, and set high goals for them. In turn, their children have a high need to achieve (51, 71).

Another study showed that the child's behavior affects parental reactions and is different toward each parent. When the child is more dependent in behavior, both parents interact more physically and verbally with the child and display more controlling behavior. In one study the girl child appeared to engage in specific tasks with father and in more personal interaction with mother. The father was more likely to help the child physically or become detached, whereas mother was more likely to encourage independence and to explain or question the child. More study must be done on the reciprocity of parent-child relationships and the effect of each on the other. For example, perhaps the parent who has been authoritarian and controlling over the child from birth on fosters dependent behavior in the child, which in turn stimulates more controlling behavior (42, 46).

Relationships with Parents

The preschooler's early emotional and physical closeness to the parents now leads to a different kind of relationship with them. This is the stage of the *family triangle, family romance,* or what Freud called the *Oedipal** or *Electra† Complex* (46).

Various authors say that knowledge of the Oedipal or Electra conflict as it exists in general western culture, the manner in which it is resolved, and the significance of it in the preschool era are essential for understanding the development of the adolescent and adult in American culture. Others feel that this theory has been overpublicized. The intensity of this situation appears related to family attitudes and culture (46).

During this **Oedipal** or **Electra stage** or *phase of pregenital sexuality, positive, possessive, or love feelings are directed mainly toward the parent of the opposite sex, and the parent of the same sex may receive competitive, aggressive, or hostile feelings.* The daughter becomes "Daddy's girl" and tries to imitate the mother's role; the father responds to her femininity. The son is "Mommy's boy" and imitates the father's role; the

---

*Oedipus, a hero of Greek mythology, was the son of King Laius and Queen Jocasta. At the time of Oedipus' birth, the oracle prophesied that Oedipus would kill his father and marry his mother. To avoid the prophecy, Laius ordered the infant abandoned so that he would die. Through a series of uncontrollable events, the infant survived, and the prophecy came true.
†Electra was a legendary Greek woman who was obsessed by an intense love for her murdered father and plotted with her brother to kill her mother and mother's lover, whom she blamed for the father's death.

mother responds to his masculinity. The parent of the same sex may be told, "I hate you. Go away." The child may declare to the opposite-sex parent that he or she will marry the parent someday. Help parents recognize these feelings as developmentally normal. During this phrase the child is establishing a basis for his or her own eventual mate relationship; the parents' positive handling of the Oedipal conflict is crucial.

Help the parents feel comfortable with the sexuality of the child and with their own sexuality so that they are neither threatened by nor ignore or punish the child's remarks and behavior.

As the parent of the opposite sex continues to show love to his or her mate and the child, and as the parents desexualize the relationship with the child, the erotic aspects gradually disappear. The child can them get on with one of the major preschool tasks—identification. **Identification** *occurs first through imitation of the same-sex parent's overt behavior and finally through introjection of attitudes, feelings, and values about sexual, moral, social, and occupational roles and behavior so that secondary identification results* (46).

In the one-parent or stepparent family (or in the abusive home), achieving identification may be more difficult. The little girl raised by a male may not fit in with other girls at school or be able to feel comfortable and relate to women later in life. The boy raised by a woman may relate to women but not to men.

Explore with parents the importance of identification with the same-gender parent or adult and ways to achieve this if the parent of the same gender as the child is not in the home. Divorced parents must understand that to the child divorce signifies rejection and that the missing parent no longer loves the child. The child feels at blame, and there may be guilt about the separation or about the relief felt after the separation if much discord preceded the divorce. Family discord may cause more distress than the absence of a parent, but the separation is still difficult. There are often practical problems such as financial or life-style changes and emotional trauma. After the divorce the child may manifest insomnia, grief and depression, digestive and elimination problems, irritability, anger, aggression, regressive behavior, fear, anxiety, and withdrawal. The child needs help in expressing feelings (through art, play, music, and talking) and in adapting to the change. The child needs loving interactions with an adult relative or friend who is of the same gender, and the mother or father should foster such a relationship. After divorce the child may have difficulty relating to or identifying with a stepparent. If possible, the child needs an ongoing involvement with the divorced parent who is no longer in the home. The child loves and needs both parents in most cases and needs to learn to live with and feel affection for and from the stepparent as well. The child needs help to develop a sense of history with the family of origin and the stepparent family, to maintain allegiance to the ab-

sent parent, and to develop new traditions. The effects of divorce on the child are considerable and long-term (59, 74).

These families benefit from (1) your empathy; (2) your listening ear; (3) your exploration of their own and the child's feelings; (4) your suggestions of practical ways of helping the child spend time with both biologic parents; (5) your discussion of ways to help the child mourn the loss he or she feels and adjust to the changed life situation; and (6) your counseling efforts and skills as the family works to resolve the crisis of separation, divorce, or remarriage.

Gender or Sexual Identity

Help parents realize that gender is reinforced through name, clothing, color of clothing and room, behavior toward, and expectations of the child. The innumerable contacts between the child and significant adults contribute to gender or sexual identification and should occur in this developmental period (42, 46, 51, 71). The sex of the child is a great determinant in personality development because each sex has different tasks and roles in every culture. Achieving a firm identity as a man or woman is basic to emotional stability and ego development.

In the United States most parents are less rigid about what clothing or colors are appropriate for boys and girls and are making an effort to teach both daughters and sons to talk about feelings, to do the same household tasks, and to engage in the same play activities. However, in some homes the daughter is reinforced for being cuddly, domestic, and emotional, and the son is reinforced for being physically aggressive or "tough." The 5-year-old son is not expected to set the table or help with dusting. Parents who have fixed ideas about gender-role behavior may not be responsive to your suggestions about the importance of both daughters and sons having the same play, learning, or social experiences or the appropriateness of pants and skirts for the daughters. Parental ideas frequently reflect their subcultural values and norms.

Explain parental reactions to and expectations of the child. Help them clarify their feelings and behavior and convey their respect to the child, regardless of gender. The gender assigned to the child by significant adults may be physically realistic or unrealistic. The feelings and needs of the parents strongly influence their reactions to the child so that gender assignment within the family can override biologic factors. The parent can "make" little boys out of infant girls or vice versa by the way they name, handle, dress, play with, touch, or talk to the child. Attitudes about activity and passivity and feelings of mastery or being mastered go into development of male and female traits in most cultures.

The Oepidal or Electra phase brings the development of sexuality to the foreground. The child is interested in the appearance and function of his or her own body, in variations of clothing and hairstyles (the child at first assigns gender on this basis) and in the bodies of others, especially in their sex organs (46). Children at this age feel a sense of excitement in seeing and feeling their own and others' nude bodies and of exposing themselves to other children or adults.

Although some body exposure goes on in the average American home, help parents realize that the child needs to learn clothing norms for the culture. Unless the parents live in a nudist camp, there are limits to undressing in public. Help the parents realize that their nudity may stimulate considerable fantasy in the child during this stage and that sexual feelings aroused in the child may be difficult for child or parents to handle.

The girl learns that she is equal to or surpasses boys in size, intelligence, and physical capacities and that there are obvious differences in their genital organs. The so-called *penis envy* of Freudian theory is not so much envy as fascination with the difference. It becomes envy if the parents convey the attitude that masculinity is superior to femininity. Questions about the boy's penis can be answered along with the information that she will later have breasts and be able to bear children.

The child has many questions about conception and childbirth and usually develops or expands a personal theory: babies come from a seed placed in the mother's mouth, from eating foods with seeds, from kissing, or from animals; babies are manufactured like household items; prenatally the baby sits on the mother's stomach, ingesting food as she eats; and babies come out of the anus or the navel.

Teaching Sexuality

Teaching sexuality to the child is enmeshed in the acquisition of gender identity and positive feelings about the self. The basis for sex education begins prenatally with the parents' attitudes about the coming child. Parents and other child educators or caretakers, including nurses, continue daily thereafter to form attitudes in the child and impart factual knowledge in response to questions. You can assist parents in acquiring information to answer the child's questions.

Because of the child's consuming curiosity, he or she asks many questions: Will the man in the television come out? How do I tie my shoes? Why is that lady's tummy so big? What is lightning? These questions are originally asked with equal curiosity. The adult's response will determine into what special category the child places questions about sex.

If parent-child communication has been open—if the child feels free to ask questions about sex and other topics, and if the parent gives satisfactory and correct answers without embarrassment—the basis for a healthy sexual attitude exists.

Although sex education must be tailored to the individual child's needs and interests and to the cultural, religious, and family values, the following suggestions are applicable to all children and can be shared with parents:

1. Recognize that education about the self as a sexual person is best given by example in family life through parents' showing respect and love for the self, mate, and the child.
2. Understand that the child who learns to trust others and to give and receive love has begun preparation for satisfactory adulthood, marriage, and parenthood.
3. Observe the child at play; listen carefully to statements of ideas, feelings, and questions and ask questions to understand better his or her needs.
4. Respond to the child's questions by giving information honestly, in a relaxed, accepting manner, and on the child's level of understanding. Avoid isolated facts, myths, or animal analogies. The question, "Where does baby come from?" could be answered, "Mommy carried you inside her body in a special place" rather than saying "The stork brought baby," "Baby was picked up at the hospital after a special order," or "God makes babies." Religious beliefs can be worked into the explanation while acknowledging human realities.
5. Teach the child anatomic names rather than other words for body parts and processes. Parents may hesitate to do this because they do not want the child to blurt out *penis* or *vagina* in public. Parents can teach the child that certain topics such as sexual and financial matters are discussed in the home, just as certain activities such as urinating are done in private.
6. Grabbing the genitals and some masturbation are normal. Children explore their bodies, especially body parts not easily seen and that give pleasurable sensations when touched. Masturbation should be accepted if it occurs in the home. The child should be taught that this is not normal behavior in public.
7. Playing doctor or examining each other's body parts is normal for preschool children. Parents should not overreact and should calmly affirm that they want the children to keep their clothes on while they play. Diversion from "playing doctor" is useful. If children seem to be using each other in a sexual way, they should be instructed that this is not acceptable.
8. Realize that sex education continues throughout the early years. The child's changing self motivates the same or different questions again and again. Remain open to his or her ongoing questions. Explanation about reproduction may begin with a simple statement, for example: "A man and a woman are required to be baby's father and mother. Baby is made from the sperm in the daddy's body and an

egg in the mother's body." A simple explanation of sperm and egg would be needed. Later the child can be given more detail.

Influence of Nonfamily Members

Help parents realize that other people may be significant to the child, depending on frequency and duration of contact, warmth of the relationship and how well the parents meet the child's needs (25, 46).

Other significant adults may include relatives, especially grandparents, aunts, uncles, and cousins who are peers; the teacher at the day-care center or nursery school; the babysitter; or neighbors. Servants, live-in help, the in-home caretaker, the babysitter, or the child's nurse-caretaker may provide positive or negative identification figures and should be chosen with care, especially those who live in the home. Relatives and friends also contribute to development of identity if contact is frequent.

Guests introduce the child to new facets of family life and parents' behavior, to different people with unfamiliar behavior, and to different ideas, religions, or occupations. Visits to others' homes aid socialization through comparison of the households, ability to separate from home, and interaction with people in new places.

Even domestic pets can be useful in meeting certain needs: loving and being loved; companionship; learning a sense of responsibility; and learning about sex in a natural way.

If the family uses day care, nursery school, or other early schooling for the child, the adults in the agency may exert a strong influence on the child.

Parents may ask you about each agency: the differences between them, their significance for the child, and the criteria for selection. Share the following information.

Day care is a *program to provide daily care away from home for any part of a 24-hour day, for compensation, or otherwise.* This program can be an important resource to many families: for example, when the single parent works and is the sole support of the family; when both parents work; when one parent is ill or a full-time student and the other parent works; or when the mother needs relief from child care for health or other urgent personal reasons.

Family day care is the *arrangement by a woman to care for mixed-aged children in the home.* Many home-care providers are former working women who want to remain in the home with their own children while continuing to contribute to the family budget by caring for several other children in the home. In most cases the number of children in the home is limited by law to six. The mixed ages of the children provide stimulation for each other, and the small number of children usually assures that each child gets the attention he or she needs.

Nursery school is usually a *half-day program that emphasizes an educational, socialization experience for the children to supplement home experiences.*

Early school experiences may include a *Montessori program, a compensatory program, or kindergarten,* which has now become the first step before school entry for most children in the United States. **Montessori programs** evolved from the Italian educator, Maria Montessori, who developed preschool education in Europe. They *emphasize: (1) self-discipline of the child; (2) intellectual development through training of the senses; (3) freedom for the child within a structure and schedule; and (4) meaningful individual cognitive experiences that are provided in a quiet, pleasant, educational environment.* **Compensatory programs,** which first began as Head Start and Follow Through Projects in the 1960s, *focus on making up for deprived conditions in the child's life, and include (1) giving physical care (good nutrition, dental care, immunizations); (2) fostering curiosity, exploring, creativity, and learning about the self and environment; (3) promoting emotional health through nurturing, positive self-concept, self-confidence, and self-discipline; and (4) teaching social skills and behaviors, how to interact with peers, teachers, and parents* (30, 42, 51, 71). **Kindergarten** is a *half- or whole-day educational program* for the 5-year-old child that may be an extension of either a nursery school or a part of the elementary school system. In some parts of the country, kindergarten attendance is mandatory for entry into first grade because the cognitive learning that is begun is a foundation for the cognitive program of the first grade. The social behaviors that are learned also prepare the child to be better disciplined in the school setting and to interact appropriately with teacher and peers. The half-day program also helps the child and parents to separate from each other for a period of time if that has not been done through nursery school or day care.

Criteria for selection of the day-center center or nursery school may be discussed with parents as they seek assistance with child care and education. Some of the same criteria are useful in selecting family day-care, Montessori, or compensatory program.

Criteria to observe for or ask about concern staff qualifications, approach to and care of the child, physical setup, and experiences or curriculum. The *day-care center* should be:

1. Operated by a reputable person or agency.
2. Licensed by a state authority.
3. Located conveniently close to the home.
4. Committed to philosophy of and beliefs about child rearing that are similar to those of the parents.
5. Able to provide a happy, comfortable, safe yet stimulating, living and play space for the child.
6. Staffed with certified teachers and other workers in an appropriate staff/child ratio.

7. Able to provide facilities for creative, dramatic, rough-and-tumble play; rest; meal service; bathroom; health services, and facilities for the child's clothing or other objects.
8. Able to provide supplies and equipment as required for the children.
9. Able to care for the sick child until the parent(s) can come for the child and willing to discuss with parents the child's illness or other behavior problems.
10. Operated at a cost comparable to other such facilities or on a sliding scale basis.

The above criteria also are applicable to *family day care,* although they would be applied to one adult in a home setting. The following questions should additionally be asked:

1. Is there backup help available to the adult if it is needed (e.g., in case she is ill or if her child or another child was injured or became ill)?
2. Does the adult take the children for trips in a vehicle? If so, are there child safety seats or belts appropriate to the child's age?
3. Is care provided on weekends, holidays, or in the evening?

The *nursery school* be operated by a reputable person or organization and provide the aforementioned except for a full noon meal. Usually only a midsession snack is served. In either center the parent should observe the program to learn about the philosophy of the staff regarding child rearing, care, and discipline; administrative policies; the use of professional consultants for educational, social, or medical concerns; and the educational qualifications of the staff. They should note the warmth, emotional characteristics, and competence of the staff as they and children work and play together. Cost of the program, when services are available, and the parents' obligations to the agency are other aspects to consider.

In *either agency* the child, under guidance of qualified staff, will get many experiences: socializing; investigating; imaginative experimenting; developing creative abilities; doing beginning problem solving; becoming more independent, secure, and self-confident in a variety of situations; handling emotions and broadening avenues of self-expression; learning basic hygiene and how to interact with others; and learning about the community in which he or she lives.

You can help parents be aware of these resources, answer their questions, and give suggestions regarding criteria for selection. As a nurse, you may also assist with primary prevention and health consulting to teachers, children, and parents in such an agency. For example, public health workers in Hennepin County, Minnesota, designed a program to promote optimum health and safety of children in day-care settings through health education to staff, technical assistance support, nurse-child

assessment, and evaluation of policies and procedures (37). The articles by Wenger et al. (76) and Johansen et al. (41) describe conditions of day care usually associated with disease.

There are no accurate predictors of later academic success for preschool children. Some studies show that when infants and young children in a ghetto were given a planned educational experience aimed at preventing retardation and promoting parental interaction, environmental stimulation, and experiential opportunity, the experimental group showed superior cognitive abilities at 5.5 years compared to children in a control group raised in the usual way. Other studies showed that 3-year-old children who were given special educational opportunities showed better intellectual performance at the end of second grade than did children in a control group (42, 51, 71). Other authors say that pushing the child to develop reading and mathematics skills too early will create problems: fatigue, stress-related illnesses, disciplinary problems, and parental burnout. (28).

If parents use a day-care center, family day care, nursery school, or early school program, help them understand that they remain the most important people to the child and that their love and involvement with the child are crucial for later learning and adjustment to life. The care or enrichment of a preschool center or program where children attend a few hours daily cannot undo deprivation or abuse that is present in a family. Help the working mother realize that her working does not necessarily deprive the child. Many career women tend to do better than full-time homemakers. They do not see the child as an end in itself; they allow the child to develop autonomy and initiative in creative ways because they have a sense of self-fulfillment in their own lives.

You can help the parents and child prepare for the separation if the child will be enrolled in a nursery school or day-care center. Help the parents realize, too, that the child's emotional and social adjustment and overall learning depend on many factors. Because each child interprets entrance into the agency on the basis of his or her own past experience, each differs in adjustment. Being with a number of children can be an upsetting experience. The child needs adequate preparation to avoid feeling abandoned or rejected. The mother must have confidence in the agency so that she can convey a feeling of pleasurable expectation to the child. The child should accompany the mother to see the building, observe the program, and meet the teachers and other children before enrollment. Ideally the child should begin attending when both mother and child feel secure about the ensuing separation, and the mother should be encouraged to stay with the child the whole first day or for a shorter period of time for several days until he or she feels secure without mother. If possible, the parent, rather than a neighbor or stranger, should take the child each day, assuring the child of the parent's return at the end of the day.

Relationships With Siblings

The discussion in Chapter 4 on the effect of the child's sex and ordinal position on family interaction is significant for understanding the preschooler.

Often the preschool child has **siblings,** *brothers or sisters,* either younger or older, so that family interaction is complex with many **dyads,** *groups of two people.* Siblings become increasingly important in directing and crystallizing the child's early development, partly because of their proximity but also because the parents change in their role with each additional child. Parents often are emotionally warmer after the firstborn, possible because they feel more experienced and relaxed. In the following discussion you should realize that the relationships described could occur at other developmental eras in childhood, but in the preschool years siblings begin to make a very definite impact (25, 46).

The sibling may be part of a multiple birth: twins, triplets, or more. Identical twins share traits, emotional bonds, and pain and communicate with each other in their own language in uncanny or mysterious ways, often when they are miles apart. Studies of identical twins who are reared separately in different environments can help to sort out the relative influence of heredity and environment. Twins seem to think about each other more than other siblings, so some of the ESP-like communication or experiences may be coincidence. Yet the extreme intimacy can be pathologic; there may be jealousy of each other or a symbiotic interdependence that interferes with identity formation of each individual. For the parents, raising twins creates a delicate balance.

You may give the following suggestions: (1) by the way parents talk to, dress, and handle twins (or other multiple births), help the children realize they are individuals first and twins second; (2) encourage each to develop separate interests, pursue different hobbies and subjects, or go to different schools to reduce competition and rivalry; (3) talk to the twins about different kinds of relationships, their own special closeness, the rewards of developing separate friendships, and the importance of separate intimate relationships, and (4) get help from the magazine *Twins* (Overland Park, Kansas), The National Organization of Mothers of Twins Clubs (Albuquerque, New Mexico), and the 300 chapters of TWINLINE (Berkeley, California), which can provide information to parents (2). Refer also to Chapter 4 for more information on multiple births.

Preschooler and New Baby

The arrival of a new baby changes life: the preschooler is no longer the center of attention but is expected by the parents to delight in the baby. It is important for parents to prepare the young child (toddler or preschooler) for a new arrival (Fig. 9–1). Although a space of 3 to 4 years is ideal, such ideal spacing does not always occur.

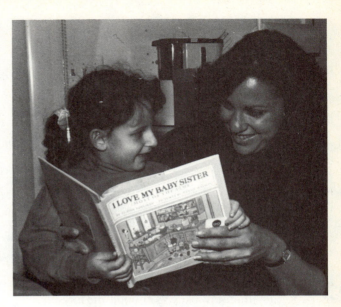

Figure 9-1. As birth approaches, parents can help prepare the preschooler for the arrival of the new sibling. (From Sherwen, L.N., M.A. Scoloveno, and C.T. Weingarten, *Nursing Care of the Childbearing Family.* Norwalk, Conn: Appleton & Lange, 1991, p. 537.)

When pregnancy is apparent, there are some ways for parents to prepare the older child:

1. Share the anticipation in discussions and planning. Let the child feel fetal movements. Show the child a picture of when he or she was a newborn. Talk about what he or she needed as a baby and the necessary responsibilities. Read books that explain reproduction and birth on his or her level.
2. Include the child as much as possible in activities such as shopping for furniture for the baby or decorating baby's room. The preschool child likes to feel important, and being a helper enhances this feeling.
3. Have the child visit mother and baby at the hospital, if rules permit, after delivery, or the older child can talk to mother by phone.
4. Encourage relatives and friends to bring a small surprise gift for the older child when they visit and bring a gift for baby. Have them spend time with the older child also rather than concentrating only on baby (70).

Accepting the family's affection toward the baby is difficult for the firstborn, and jealousy is likely to occur if more attention is focused on the baby than on him or her. As a result, the preschooler may regress, overtly displaying a need to be babied. He or she may ask for the bottle, soil self, have enuresis, lie in the baby's crib, or demand extra attention. The child may harm the baby, directly or indirectly, through play or handling baby roughly. He or she may appear to love the baby excessively, more than is normal. The child may show hostility toward the mother in different ways: direct physical or verbal attacks, ignoring or rejecting her, or displacing anger onto the day-care, nursery, or Sunday school teacher.

Teach parents that these outward behaviors and the underlying feelings should be accepted, for they are better handled with overt loving behavior than repressed through punishment. Jealousy can be handled by the parents in a variety of ways: tell the child about the pregnancy but not too far in advance because a young child has a poor concept of time. Convey that the child is loved as much as before, provide a time for him or her only, and give as much attention as possible. In addition, avoid ridicule; emphasize pleasure in having the child share in loving the new arrival and give increasing responsibility and status without overburdening him or her. Encourage the child to talk about the new situation or express hostility in play and involve him or her in preparing for the new baby. Although the preschooler may have to give up a crib, getting him or her a new big bed can seem like a promotion rather than a loss. Reading stories about feelings of children with new siblings can help the child express personal feelings. Other effective advice you can give about ways to handle jealous behavior are (1) do not leave the preschooler alone with the baby; (2) give him or her a pet or doll to care for as mother cares for the baby; (3) encourage the child to identify with the parents in helping to protect the baby since he or she is more grown up; and (4) avoid overemphasis of affection for the baby.

Older Child and Preschooler

The older sibling in the family who is given much attention for accomplishments may cause feelings of envy and frustration as the preschooler tries to engage in activity beyond his or her ability to get attention also. If the younger child can identify with the older sibling and take pride in the accomplishments while simultaneously getting recognition for his or her own self and abilities, the child will feel positive about self. If the younger child feels defeated and is not given realistic recognition, he or she may stop emulating the older sibling and regress instead. In turn, the older sibling can be helpful to the younger child if he or she does not feel deprived or is not reprimanded too much because of the preschooler.

Explore sibling relationships with parents and present suggestions for preventing conflicts. Often positive feelings exist between siblings. Quarrels are quickly forgotten if parents do not get overly involved. Because siblings have had a similar upbringing, they have considerable empathy for each other, similar values, similar superego development, and related perceptions about situations. Sibling values may be as important as the parents' values in the development of the child. Often recognition and other feelings of the sibling are of such importance to the child that he or she may conceal ability rather than move into an area in which the sibling has gained recognition, or he or she may engage in activity to keep the sibling from being unhappy. The children will learn to develop roles and regulate space among themselves to avoid conflicts unless conflictual behavior is given undue attention or the children are manipulated against each other by the significant adults.

Developmental Tasks of the Family

While the preschool child and siblings are achieving their developmental tasks, the parents are struggling with child rearing and their own personal developmental tasks. A discussion of parental developmental tasks while raising a preschooler follows:

1. Encourage and accept the child's evolving skills rather than elevating the parent's self-esteem by pushing the child beyond his or her capacity. Satisfaction is found through reducing assistance with physical care and giving more guidance in other respects.
2. Supply adequate housing, facilities, space, equipment, and other materials needed for life, comfort, health, and recreation.
3. Plan for predicted and unexpected costs of family life such as medical care, insurance, education, babysitter fees, food, clothing, and recreation.
4. Maintain some personal privacy and an outlet for tension of family members while including the child as a participant in the family.
5. Share household and child-care responsibility with other family members, including the child.
6. Strengthen the partnership with the mate and express affection in ways that keep the relationship from becoming humdrum.
7. Learn to accept failures, mistakes, and blunders without piling up feelings of guilt, blame, and recrimination.
8. Nourish common interests and friendships to strengthen self-respect and self-confidence and to remain interesting to the spouse.
9. Maintain a mutually satisfactory sexual relationship and plan whether or not to have more children.
10. Create and maintain effective communication within the family.
11. Cultivate relationships with the extended family.
12. Tap resources and serve others outside the family to prevent preoccupation with self and family.
13. Face life's dilemmas and rework moral codes, spiritual values, and a philosophy of life (25).

Explore with parents the challenges and practical ways of meeting these tasks within the specific family unit.

PHYSIOLOGIC CONCEPTS

Physical Characteristics

Growth

Growth during the preschool years is relatively slow, but changes occur that transform the chubby toddler into a sturdy child who appears taller and thinner. Trunk and limb growth is apparent. Although development does not proceed at a uniform rate in all areas or for all children, development follows a logical, precise pattern or sequence (33, 53, 77). The preschool child grows approximately 2 to 2½ inches (5 to 6 cm) and gains less than 5 pounds (2.2 kg.) *per year*. The child appears tall and thin because he or she grows proportionately more in height than in weight. The average height of the 3-year-old is 37 inches (94 cm); of the 4-year-old, 41 inches (104 cm) (or double the birth length); and of the 5-year-old, 43 to 52 inches (110 to 130 cm). At 3 the child weighs approximately 33 pounds (15 kg); at 4 years, 38 pounds (17 kg); and at 5 years, approximately 40 to 50 pounds (18 to 23 kg).

Vital Signs

The *temperature* is 98° to 99° F (36.7° to 37.2° C). The *pulse rate* is normally 80 to 110 and the *respiratory rate* approximately 30 per minute. Blood pressure is approximately 90/60 mm Hg, systolic and diastolic.

Other Characteristics

Vision in the preschooler is farsighted; the 5-year-old has 20/40 to 20/30 vision and is visually discriminative. By age 4, the cerebral cortex is fully connected to the cerebellum, permitting better control of fine muscle movements such as tying shoelaces, cutting with scissors, or holding a pencil or crayon. The child has 20 teeth, and by the end of the preschool period the child begins to lose deciduous teeth (42, 51, 71, 77). *Physical characteristics to assess* in this child are listed in Table 9–1. *Because each child is unique, the normative listings indicate only where most children of a given age are in the development of various characteristics.* Characteristics are listed by age in all following tables for reasons of understanding sequence and giving comparison. Consideration of only the chronologic age is misleading as a basis for assessment and care. The development of the whole and unique child and interrelationships among various aspects must be considered. Still, by using the norms for the child at a given age, you can assess how far the child deviates from the norm. *With more parental guidance, the child may reach norms ahead of age.*

Developmental Assessment

The Denver II—Revision and Restandardization of the Denver Developmental Screening Test (DDST) evaluates four major categories of development: gross motor, fine motor-adaptive, language, and personal-social (Fig. 9–2). It is used to determine whether a child is within the

normal range for various behaviors or is developmentally delayed. Like the original DDST, the Denver II is applicable to children from birth through 6 years of age. The age divisions are monthly until 24 months and then every 6 months until 6 years of age.

The Denver II differs from the DDST in items included in the test, test form, and interpretation. The previous total of 105 items has been increased to 125, including an increase from 21 DDST to 39 Denver II language items. A behavior rating scale has also been added. Items for which clinically significant differences exist (based on sex, ethnic group, maternal education, and place of residence) are discussed in a technical manual accompanying the test. If a child is delayed on one of these items, the examiner can look up norms for various subpopulations in the technical manual to consider whether the delay may be due to sociocultural or environmental differences.

Although it is not the purpose of this discussion to describe the administration and interpretation of the Denver II, the following points should be noted. First, to avoid errors in administration and interpretation, and hence invalid screening results, the examiner should carefully follow the protocol outlined by the test's authors. A manual-workbook, videotape, and proficiency test have been developed to ensure accurate administration and interpretation by examiners. Second, before administering the test, explanations should be given to both the child and parent(s). Parents should be advised that the Denver II is not an intelligence test but rather a means of helping the nurse observe what the child can do at a particular age.

Because the Denver II is nonthreatening, requires no painful or unfamiliar procedures, and relies on the child's natural activity of play, it is an excellent way to begin the health assessment (77). It provides a general assessment tool that can help guide treatment and teaching. The Denver II form and instruction manual can be obtained from Denver Developmental Materials, Inc., P.O. Box 6919, Denver, CO 80206–0919; (303) 355–4729.

It is important to consider genetics, family factors, nutrition, and social environment when you care for children who are developmentally delayed. Occasionally a child does not attain height within the norms for his or her age, although torso-leg proportions are normal, because the pituitary gland does not produce enough growth hormone (30, 53, 77). Growth hormone deficiency, which causes dwarfism in a preschool child, can now be treated with a synthetic growth hormone. The person still remains short in stature but is within a normal height range. The treatment is important because children who lag behind peers in growth are often teased, are kept from participating in certain play activities, and may have difficulty finding clothes or play equipment such as a bicycle that is of correct size. The child may be regarded by others as retarded in-

TABLE 9-1. ASSESSMENT OF PHYSICAL CHARACTERISTICS: MOTOR CONTROL

3 Years	4 Years	5 Years
Occasional accident in toileting when busy at play; responds to routine times; tells when going to bathroom	Independent toilet habits; manages clothes without difficulty	Takes complete charge of self; does not tell when going to bathroom
Verbalizes difference between how male and female urinate	Insists on having door shut for self but wants to be in bathroom with others	Self-conscious about exposing self
Needs help with back buttons and drying self	Asks many questions about defecation function	Boys and girls to separate bathrooms
Nighttime control of bowel and bladder most of time		Voids four to six times during waking hours; occasional nighttime accident
Runs more smoothly, turns sharp corners, suddenly stops	Runs easily with coordination	Runs with skill, speed, agility, and plays games simultaneously
	Skips clumsily	Increases strength and coordination in limbs
	Hops on one leg	
	Legs, trunk, shoulder, arms move in unison	
	Aggressive physical activity	
Walks backward	Heel-toe walk	May still be knock-kneed
Climbs stairs with alternate feet	Walks a plank	Jumps from three to four steps
Jumps from low step	Climbs stairs without holding onto rail	
	Climbs and jumps without difficulty	
Tries to dance but has inadequate balance, although sense of balance improving	Enjoys motor stunts and gross gesturing	Balances self on toes; dances with some rhythm
		Balances on one foot approximately 10 sec
Pedals tricycle	Enjoys new activities rather than repeating same ones	Jumps rope
Swings		Roller skates
		Hops and skips on alternate feet
		Enjoys jungle gym
Sitting equilibrium maintained but combined awkwardly with reaching activity	Sitting balance well maintained; leans forward with greater mobility and ease	Maintains balance easily
	Exaggerated use of arm extension and trunk twisting; touches end of nose with forefinger on direction	Combines reaching and placing object in one continuous movement
		Arm extension and trunk twisting coordinated
		Tummy protrudes, but some adult curve to spine
Undresses self; helps dress self	Dresses and undresses self except tying bows, closing zipper, putting on boots and snow suit	Dresses self without assistance; ties shoelaces
Undoes buttons on side or front of clothing	Does buttons	Requires less supervision of personal duties
Goes to toilet alone if clothes simple	Distinguishes front	Washes self without wetting clothes
Washes hands, feeds self	Brushes teeth alone	
May brush own teeth		
Catches ball with arms fully extended one out of two to three times	Greater flexion of elbow	Uses hands more than arms in catching ball
More refined hand movement	Catches ball thrown at 5 feet two to three times	Pours fluid from one container to another with few spills
Increasing coordination in vertical direction	Throws ball overhand	Uses hammer to hit nail on head
Pours fluid from pitcher, occasional spills	Judges where a ball will land	Interest and competence in dusting
Hits large pegs on board with hammer	Helps dust objects	Likes water play
	Likes water play	
Builds tower of 9 to 10 blocks; builds three-block gate from model	Builds complicated structure extending vertically and laterally; builds five-block gate from model	Builds things out of large boxes
Imitates a bridge	Notices missing parts or broken objects; requests parents to fix	Builds complicated three-dimensional structure and may build several separate units
		Able to disassemble and reassemble small object
Copies circle or cross; begins to use scissors; strings large beads	Copies a square	Copies triangle or diamond from model
Shows hand preference	Uses scissors without difficulty	Folds paper diagonally
Trial-and-error method with puzzle	Enjoys finer manipulation of play materials	Definite hand preference
	Surveys puzzle before placing pieces	Does simple puzzles quickly and smoothly
	Matches simple geometric forms	Prints some letters correctly; prints first name
	Prefers symmetry	
	Poor space perception	
Scribbles	Less scribbling	Draws clearly recognized lifelike representatives; differentiates parts of drawing
Tries to draw a picture and name it	Form and meaning in drawing apparent to adults	

Data from references 29, 42, 51, 53, 71, and 77.

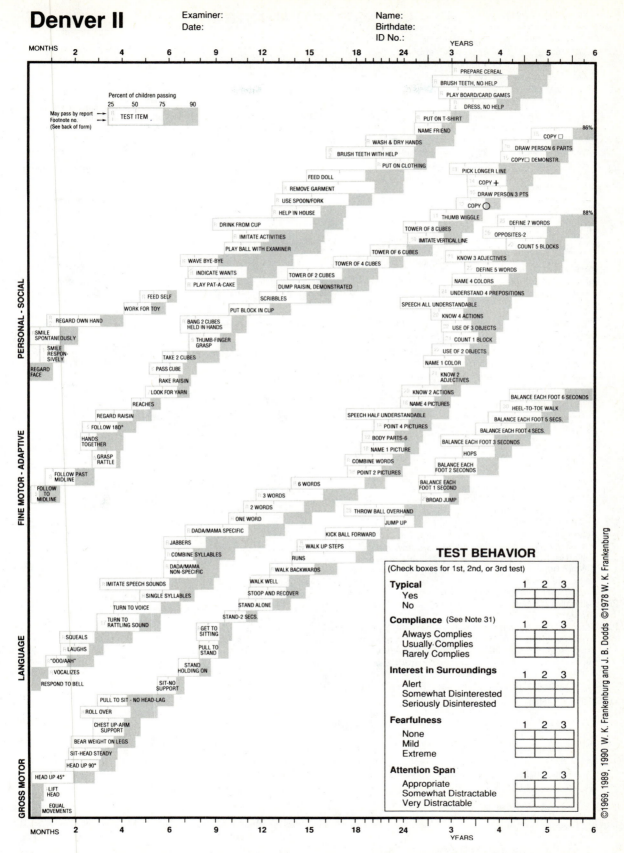

Figure 9-2. Denver II—Revision and Restandardization of the Denver Developmental Screening Test. (From W.K. Frankenberg and J.B. Dodds, 1990.)

(continued)

DIRECTIONS FOR ADMINISTRATION

1. Try to get child to smile by smiling, talking or waving. Do not touch him/her.
2. Child must stare at hand several seconds.
3. Parent may help guide toothbrush and put toothpaste on brush.
4. Child does not have to be able to tie shoes or button/zip in the back.
5. Move yarn slowly in an arc from one side to the other, about 8" above child's face.
6. Pass if child grasps rattle when it is touched to the backs or tips of fingers.
7. Pass if child tries to see where yarn went. Yarn should be dropped quickly from sight from tester's hand without arm movement.
8. Child must transfer cube from hand to hand without help of body, mouth, or table.
9. Pass if child picks up raisin with any part of thumb and finger.
10. Line can vary only 30 degrees or less from tester's line.
11. Make a fist with thumb pointing upward and wiggle only the thumb. Pass if child imitates and does not move any fingers other than the thumb.

12. Pass any enclosed form. Fail continuous round motions.
13. Which line is longer? (Not bigger.) Turn paper upside down and repeat. (pass 3 of 3 or 5 of 6)
14. Pass any lines crossing near midpoint.
15. Have child copy first. If failed, demonstrate.

When giving items 12, 14, and 15, do not name the forms. Do not demonstrate 12 and 14.

16. When scoring, each pair (2 arms, 2 legs, etc.) counts as one part.
17. Place one cube in cup and shake gently near child's ear, but out of sight. Repeat for other ear.
18. Point to picture and have child name it. (No credit is given for sounds only.)
   If less than 4 pictures are named correctly, have child point to picture as each is named by tester.

19. Using doll, tell child: Show me the nose, eyes, ears, mouth, hands, feet, tummy, hair. Pass 6 of 8.
20. Using pictures, ask child: Which one flies?... says meow?... talks?... barks?... gallops? Pass 2 of 5, 4 of 5.
21. Ask child: What do you do when you are cold?... tired?... hungry? Pass 2 of 3, 3 of 3.
22. Ask child: What do you do with a cup? What is a chair used for? What is a pencil used for? Action words must be included in answers.
23. Pass if child correctly places and says how many blocks are on paper. (1, 5).
24. Tell child: Put block on table; under table; in front of me, behind me. Pass 4 of 4. (Do not help child by pointing, moving head or eyes.)
25. Ask child: What is a ball?... lake?... desk?... house?... banana?... curtain?... fence?... ceiling? Pass if defined in terms of use, shape, what it is made of, or general category (such as banana is fruit, not just yellow). Pass 5 of 8, 7 of 8.
26. Ask child: If a horse is big, a mouse is __? If fire is hot, ice is __? If the sun shines during the day, the moon shines during the __? Pass 2 of 3.
27. Child may use wall or rail only, not person. May not crawl.
28. Child must throw ball overhand 3 feet to within arm's reach of tester.
29. Child must perform standing broad jump over width of test sheet (8 1/2 inches).
30. Tell child to walk forward, ⚬⚬⚬➝ heel within 1 inch of toe. Tester may demonstrate. Child must walk 4 consecutive steps.
31. In the second year, half of normal children are non-compliant.

OBSERVATIONS:

Figure 9-2. Continued

Nutritional Needs

tellectually. He or she may feel inferior, suffer a negative self-concept, lack initiative, and become withdrawn, depressed, or antisocial in later childhood or adult years.

The child needs the same food groups as the adult each day, but in smaller quantities. The child needs a gradual increase in caloric intake (1250 to 1600 calories per day or 90 to 100 kcal/kg/day). The slower growth rate and heightened interest in exploring the environment may lessen interest in eating. Box 9–1 outlines the daily nutritional needs of the preschool child. A rule of thumb for the size of servings is 1 tablespoon for each year of age: 3 tablespoons of fruit or vegetables for a 3-year-old; 5 tablespoons for a 5-year-old. Protein requirements remain high—30 to 36 g daily (or 3 g/kg/day). Without adequate fruits and vegetables, vitamins A and C usually are lacking. Calcium and iron (10 mg/day) are needed for storage and are assured through eating the foods de-

■ **BOX 9–1.**
**Recommended Nutritional Intake
for Preschoolers**

- Meat or meat substitutes: two to three ($1\frac{1}{2}$ to 2 ounce) servings
- Milk or equivalent milk servings: 1–$1\frac{1}{2}$ pints
- Vegetables and fruits: five or more servings
- Bread and cereals: four or more servings
- Fats, oils, sweets: use sparingly

scribed in Box 9–1 (54). (Refer to Appendix II.) Desserts should furnish protein, minerals, vitamins, and calories and should be a natural part of the meal, not used as a reward for finishing the meal or omitted as punishment.

Children who are reared in vegetarian families may be shorter in height and weigh less, but by the end of the preschool era, the child's growth velocity approaches the norm. In contrast, children reared in migrant families may be both inadequately nourished and below the norms for physical growth (67).

Midmorning, midafternoon, and evening snacks are necessary because of the child's high level of activity but should be wisely chosen: milk, juice, fruit wedges, vegetable strips, cereal without excess sugar, cheese cubes, peanut butter with crackers or bread, or plain cookies. Sweets (candy, raisins, sodas) should be offered only occasionally, not as a reward for behavior and not before a meal. This pattern will help prevent now and later the health problems associated with overeating sweet foods such as dental caries, malnutrition, or obesity and associating only pleasure with food. Lifetime food habits are being formed (54). Weight gain between 2 and 3 years for girls and 4 and 6 years for boys are the earliest times that are highly related to later obesity (65).

Teach parents about eating patterns, for they differ in each developmental era. Eating assumes increasing social significance for the preschooler and is still an emotional and physiologic experience. The child needs the right foods physically and a warm, happy atmosphere in which he or she is included in mealtime conversation. The family mealtime promotes socialization and sexual identification in relation to meal preparation, behavior during mealtimes, language skills, and understanding of family rituals and situation. The training is positive or negative, depending on the parents' example. Such learning is missed if there are no family mealtimes. Table manners need not be rigidly emphasized; accidents will happen, and parental example is the best teacher.

The preschooler's eating habits are simple. There may be periods of overeating or not wanting to eat certain foods, but they do not persist. The overall eating pattern from month to month is more pertinent to assess. Parenteral feeding practices, values related to food, preference for chubby children, and parental obesity were related to the preschooler's being obese in a study of Mexican-American children (1). Preschoolers who

follow their own appetite patterns are likely to maintain normal weight (1).

The sense of taste is keen; color, flavor, form, and texture are important. Foods should be attractively served, mildly flavored, whole, plain, separated and distinctly identifiable in flavor and appearance rather than mixed as in creamed foods, casseroles, and stews, except for spaghetti and pizza; and preferably lukewarm rather than too hot or too cold, including drinks. The preschooler likes to eat one thing at a time. Of all food groups, vegetables are least liked, whereas fruits are a favorite. He or she prefers vegetables and fruits crisp, raw, and cut into finger-sized pieces. Strong-tasting vegetables such as cabbage, onions, cauliflower, and broccoli and those with tough strings such as celery and green beans are usually disliked. Meats should be easily chewed and cut into bite-sized pieces. New foods can be gradually introduced; if a food is refused once, offer it again after several days.

If the child is eating insufficiently, the causes may include (1) eating too much between meals; (2) unhappy mealtime atmosphere; (3) attention seeking; (4) example of parental eating habits; (5) excessive parental expectations; (6) unavailability of adequate variety and quantity; (7) tooth decay, which may cause nausea or toothache with chewing; (8) sibling rivalry; (9) overfatigue; (10) physical illness; or (11) emotional disturbance. Parents should consider, too, the difference in eating pattern of the 3-, 4-, and 5-year-old, which can influence food intake. The 3-year-old either talks or eats, gets up from the table during meals but will return to eat more food, and rarely needs assistance to complete a meal. The 4-year-old normally combines talking and eating, rarely gets up from the table, and likes to serve self. The 5-year-old eats rapidly and is sociable during mealtime, so that family atmosphere is crucial (25, 46).

Measures to increase food intake include letting the child help plan the menu, set the table, wash dishes, or prepare foods such as stirring instant puddings or gelatin desserts, beating cake or cookie mix, or kneading dough. Other aids are serving meals in courses in a quiet environment in which there are few distractions; avoiding coaxing, bribing, or threatening; providing a premeal rest period; giving small, attractive servings; providing comfortable chair and table; allowing sufficient time for eating; and avoiding between-meal nibbling. Making food an issue and forcing the child to eat create eating problems, and the child is likely to win the battle. The child's appetite will improve as his or her growth rate increases nearer school age.

Hypochromic anemia, one of the most prevalent nutritional problems of young children, can be caused by inadequate intake of absorbable iron. Like other nutritional problems, hypochromic anemia is often associated with poor hygiene and chronic disease, but often it is a result of the slow transition from milk to solid foods. For reasons of convenience, economy, or ignorance, these children receive most of their calories from cow's milk—a very poor source of iron. Mothers of these children should be encouraged to gradually replace most of the milk with meats, eggs, and dark green, leafy vegetables in addition to fruits and cereal products. In severe cases iron supplements will be indicated (54).

Although vitamin-mineral supplements should not be a food substitute, many pediatricians recommend them, especially during these years when appetite fluctuates. Fluoride supplements should be continued if there is insufficient fluoride in the water.

Share information about nutritional needs and eating patterns and the psychologic aspects of food and mealtime with parents.

Exercise, Rest, and Sleep

This is the period when the child has a seeming surplus of energy and is on the move, sometimes to the point of fatigue. Thus the adult must initiate rest periods alternated with activity. Share the following information with parents.

The 3-year-old child does not always sleep at naptime but will rest or play quietly for 1 or 2 hours if undisturbed. The 4-year-old child resists naps but needs a quiet period. The 5-year-old child is unlikely to nap if he or she gets adequate sleep at night.

The preschooler may still take a favorite toy to bed; he or she likes to postpone bedtime and is ritualistic about bedtime routines such as prayers, a story, or music. Sleeping time decreases from 10 to 12 hours for the younger preschooler to 9 to 11 hours for the older preschooler. Dreams and nightmares may awaken the 3- or 4-year-old, causing fear and a move into bed with parents or older siblings. The 5-year-old sleeps quietly through the night without having to get up to urinate and has fewer nightmares.

If the parent responds with special attention to the child who awakens during the night, the sleep disturbance becomes worse. Parents should not become a sleep adjunct to the child (e.g., holding child in lap until he or she falls asleep again, picking up child as soon as he or she cries) because the child will not learn to fall asleep alone. The parent reinforces the waking behavior. Instead help the restless child develop sleep strategies such as cuddling a teddy bear or blanket or babbling to an imaginary friend. Parents should provide reassurance and set and stick to limits (28).

Dreams and nightmares occur during the light stages of sleep as a way to resolve emotional conflicts. During deep stages of sleep the child may sleepwalk or have night terrors. Often children do not awaken after they sleepwalk. In night terrors the child screams or cries, may thrash and squirm, is confused, does not respond to parents, behaves abnormally, and has tachycardia and tachypnea, dilated pupils, and sometimes facial contortions and diaphoresis.

Help the parents understand that calm reassurance is needed with night terrors. Wait out the attack without trying either to comfort or arouse the child. Further stimulation intensifies agitation. After 15 minutes or so, the child collapses back into sleep without memory of what happened. Sleep problems usually subside spontaneously, but the child and parents may need therapy if the problem persists several times weekly or over a period of time.

Health Promotion and Health Protection

Immunization Schedules

These schedules will be adjusted to the individual child; however, the 4-year-old should receive a DTP booster and a refeeding of oral polio virus vaccine (23, 64). Frequency of tuberculin testing depends on geographic region and personal environment. Inoculation for hepatitis B is also recommended (17).

Help parents realize that the state law of requiring immunizations before school entry is indeed a beneficial one since the organisms that cause childhood communicable diseases cannot be eliminated from the environment. The decrease in these diseases and their harmful effects has resulted only because of mass *inoculations of a disease antigen* (**active immunity**) or an *antibody* (**passive immunity**). The minimum reaction is far better than acquiring the disease.

Before giving an immunization, ask yourself the following questions:

1. Has the parent given consent? Members of some religious groups such as Church of Christ, Scientist (Christian Scientist) do not believe in immunizations. (The school district may allow these children to attend without immunization, based on parents' rights regarding their children.)
2. Is the vaccination (immunization) indicated based on the child's age and previous immunization record?
3. Are there any contraindications such as allergy to any of the constituents of the vaccine; presence of another infectious disease (febrile condition, dermatitis) or immunodeficiency disease; presence of malignancy or immunosuppressive therapy; or administration of gamma globulin, plasma, or blood transfusion in the previous 6 to 8 weeks that would have given passive antibodies?
4. Has the parent been informed of the method (route of administration) and benefits and risks involved in inoculation?
5. Has the parent informed you of any reactions or difficulties that occurred with or after previous immunizations? If the child has a minor reaction, remaining doses may be cut in half or thirds to decrease possibility of a systemic reaction. The child then returns an additional number of times to receive the full immunization series.

6. Has the parent been told that the antigens to the various diseases may be given separately but are usually combined for convenience of administration?

7. Has the vaccine been stored according to manufacturer's recommendations (usually refrigerated) and is there a date of expiration (53, 64, 77)?

Dental Care

Because caries frequently begin at this age and spread rapidly, dental care is equally important. Deciduous teeth guide in the permanent ones; they should be kept in good repair. Fluoride is important for preventing caries. If the child has teeth with deep grooves, a plastic coating can be applied to the teeth to prevent tooth decay and loss. If deciduous teeth are lost too early, permanent teeth grow in abnormally. Teeth should be brushed after eating, using a method recommended by the dentist, and intake of refined sugars limited to help prevent tooth decay.

Before entering school the child is usually required to have a physical examination (including urinalysis) and a dental examination. Refer to Appendices III and IV for a schedule of health screening measures for the preschool child.

Safety Promotion and Injury Control

The preschooler has more freedom, independence, initiative, and desire to imitate adults than the toddler but still has an immature understanding of danger and illness. This combination is likely to get him or her into hazardous situations.

A major responsibility of caretaking adults is safety promotion and injury control; the child needs watchfulness and a safe play area. The adult serves as a bodyguard while slowly teaching caution and keeping the environment as safe as possible. Other siblings can also take some, but not total, responsibility for the preschooler. Protecting the firstborn is simple since you can put dangerous objects away and there is likely to be more time and energy for supervision. When there are a number of children in a family, the activities of the older children may provide objects or situations that are dangerous to the younger ones.

Preschoolers need clear-cut safety rules, explained simply, repeatedly, and consistently; and you can help parents establish them. As the child learns to protect self, he or she should be allowed to take added responsibility for personal safety and should be given appropriate verbal recognition and praise that reinforce safe behavior. Constant threats, frequent physical punishment, and incessant "don'ts" should be avoided, for the child will learn to ignore them, feel angry or resentful, and purposefully rebel or defy adults, thus failing to learn about real danger. Also if the parent voices fear constantly, natural curiosity and the will to learn will be dulled; the child may fear every new situation.

Explore information in this section with parents so that they and you can use these safety suggestions.

1. Begin safety teaching early. Teaching done in the toddler years, for example, pays off later.

2. When you must forbid, use simple command words in a firm voice without anger to convey the impression that you expect the child to obey, for example, "stop," "no."

3. Phrase safety rules and their reasons in positive rather than negative terms when possible. For example, say: "Play in the yard, not the street, or you'll get hurt by cars"; "Sit quietly in the car to avoid hurt"; "Put tiny things (coins, beads) that you find in here (jar, bowl, box)."

4. Teach the child his or her full name, address, and telephone number (including zip code), and teach the child how to use the police or adults in service roles for help.

5. Teach the child not to give information over the phone about himself or herself or the family.

6. Encourage the child to share any "secrets"; emphasize that he or she does not have to be afraid to say anything.

7. Tell the child not to leave home alone or with a stranger. He or she should use a "buddy" system when going somewhere.

8. Never leave the child alone in public or unattended in a car.

9. Teach the child escape techniques, for example, how to unlock home doors or car doors.

10. Never leave the child home alone. Make sure that the babysitter is reliable.

11. Never allow play in or near a busy driveway or garage. Forbid street play if other play areas are available. Teach children to look carefully for and get away from cars. Drivers must take all possible precautions. A fenced yard or playground is ideal, although not always available.

12. Teach the child how safely to cross the street.

13. Teach the child to refuse gifts or rides from strangers, to avoid walking or playing alone on a deserted street, road, or similar area, and about the possibility of child molesters or abductors.

14. Keep matches in containers and out of reach.

15. Dispose of or store out of reach and in a locked cabinet as many poisons as possible: rat and roach killer, insecticides, weed killer, kerosene, cleaning agents, furniture polish, medicines. Sun tan lotion, shampoo, deodorants, nail polish, and cosmetics remain potential hazards; the child should be taught their *correct* use. The child is less likely to pull them out of cabinets or swallow them than when he or she was a toddler, but brightly colored containers or pills, powders, or liquids raise curiosity and experimentation. Bright-colored pills can be mistaken for candy.

16. Observe your child closely while he or she plays near water. Cover wells and cisterns. Fence ponds or swimming pools.

17. Keep stairways and nighttime play areas well lit.
18. Equip upstairs windows with sturdy screens and guards. Have hand rails for stairways.
19. Store knives, saws, and other sharp objects or lawn or power tools out of reach.
20. Remove doors from abandoned appliances or cars and campaign for legislation for appropriate disposal of them and for mandatory door removal.
21. Discourage playing with or in the area of appliances or power tools while they are in operation: a washing machine with a wringer, a lawn mower, a saw, or a clothes dryer.
22. Use safety glass in glass doors or shower stalls; place decals on sliding doors at child's eye level (and adult's eye level, too) to prevent walking or running through them.
23. Use adhesive strips in the bathtub.
24. Avoid scatter rugs, debris, or toys cluttered on the floor in areas of traffic.
25. Use seatbelts in the car that are appropriate for the weight of the child.

If the child continually fails to listen and obey, ask the following questions: Is the child able to hear? Is he or she intellectually able to understand? Are demands too many and expectations too great? Are statements too lengthy or abstract? Is anger expressed with teaching and discipline to the point that it interferes emotionally with the child's perception and judgment?

Accidents

Accidents are the most common cause of death. Approximately one third of the accidental deaths are caused by motor vehicles; the next most common causes are drowning, burns from fire or hot water, and poisonings (30). Running through sliding glass doors in homes, locking self in an abandoned refrigerator or freezer, and electric shocks from electric equipment also frequently cause severe injury or death. Falls can cause minor bumps, bruises, and lacerations. Animal bites are common.

Minor head injury is *any trauma to the head that does not alter normal cerebral functioning*. What appears a very minor head injury can result in a subdural or epidural hematoma—the preschooler bears very close monitoring. Parents or caretakers should be taught to check the preschooler every 2 hours in the first 24 hours after injury. If the preschooler cannot be awakened, is mentally confused, is unusually restless, disturbed, or agitated, starts vomiting, has a severe headache, has different sized pupils (unless previously that way), has weakness of arms or legs, has drainage from ears or nose, or has some sort of fit or convulsion, medical help must be sought (53, 66, 77).

Minor lacerations, *cuts,* should be examined for dirt and foreign objects even after they have been cleaned with warm water and soap. The laceration should be covered with a loose bandage that will keep out dirt and protect the wound from additional trauma. The parent or caretaker should watch for signs of infec-

tion: redness, heat, swelling, and drainage. The child should have updated tetanus prophylaxis (38, 51, 77).

Burns are *thermal injuries to the skin*. A **first-degree burn** usually *shows redness only;* a **second-degree burn** causes *blister formation,* sometimes with peeling and weeping. Scalds often produce this type of burn. A **third-degree burn** *chars the skin, causing a whitish appearance, and involves tissue under the skin*. It may cause anesthesia. Flame and hot metal often cause third-degree burns (39, 51, 53, 77).

For a first-degree burn the affected area should be plunged into cold water for a few minutes. Gentle washing with soap and water should be sufficient. A second-degree burn should have the same initial treatment. Blisters that form should be left intact, and the burned area should be covered with a nonadherent gauze and a bulky, dry, sterile dressing. Tetanus immunization should be up to date. A third-degree burn, any second-degree burn that covers an area greater than an adult's hand size, any facial burns, and any burn in which child abuse or neglect is suspected should be seen by the health care provider and physician (39, 51, 53, 77).

Accidental ingestions and poisonings occur under the age of 5 years, sometimes even when preventive measures as discussed in Chapter 8 are used. These ingestions can cause a great variety of symptoms and signs. The following guidelines should be taught to parents. The parent or caretaker should look for an empty container nearby if sudden unusual symptoms or abnormal odor to breath or clothes is observed. Try to determine what and how much was ingested and when. Call the poison control center for help. If there are no contraindications to vomiting (either from reading the side of the container or from getting directions at the poison control center), induce vomiting with syrup of ipecac. Mechanical stimulation of the posterior pharynx can be used to induce vomiting *except* with ingestion of corrosive agents such as lye, gasoline, or kerosene. The child should be taken to the nearest clinic that is set up to deal with these problems (39, 51, 53, 77).

The *bite of any animal* will probably have few symptoms other than pain at the site of puncture wounds or small lacerations. Dog bites are most common, although the child may have contact with other animals that bite or scratch. Bites from other children can also occur.

The chief concern is the possibility of rabies. It is essential to establish the vaccination status of the biting animal, if possible, for if the animal is properly vaccinated, there is little chance of acquiring and transmitting the disease to humans. Rabies prophylaxis will be determined by the physician. The wound should be washed with copious amounts of soap and water. After the soap is well removed, zephiran chloride or 40% to 70% alcohol or povidone-iodine solution should be applied. Tetanus prophylaxis should be up to date (5, 53).

Lead poisoning, especially in preschoolers, will produce **encephalopathy,** or *brain dysfunction.* The onset is insidious, with weakness, irritability, weight loss, and vomiting followed by personality changes and developmental regression. Convulsions and coma are late signs. Often history will reveal pica involving cracking paint in old homes, lead toys, old yellow and orange crayons, artist's paints, leaded gasoline, or fruit tree sprays (3).

A study investigated the average daily dietary lead intake of a cross-sectional sample of American children from birth to 5 years. Daily lead intake should not exceed 100 mg, and the study showed a daily average of 62 mg but a range from 15 mg to 234 mg. The higher levels may represent mouthing of objects and hands and the ingestion of some nonfood substances in addition to the lead content in food (3).

Prevention lies in keeping the preschooler in a leadfree environment as much as possible; someone should watch everything that goes in his or her mouth. You may call the housing inspector, with the family's permission, to test paint for lead. In many cities landlords are required to repaint the house interior when lead paint is found. Treatment for severe cases of lead poisoning involves hospitalization. General measures are to prevent reexposure to lead and to give the preschooler a high-calcium, high-phosphorus diet (milk) and large doses of vitamin D to help in removing lead from the blood by depositing it in the bones (3).

Common Health Problems: Prevention and Treatment

Teach parents that scheduled health maintenance visits to the doctor or nurse practitioner are important for early detection of problems.

Vision Problems

Vision is usually tested in the 4-year-old with an *E* chart, which is composed of capital *Es* with their legs pointing in various directions. You will point to the *Es* and ask the child to show you which direction each one is pointing. The child can use his or her fingers; verbalization is not necessary. First one eye and then the other should be tested. Visual fields can be tested much as with an adult. The parent or caretaker can hold the child, ensuring that his or her head remains straight forward. Using a small toy to place in the various visual fields is effective and can be made into a game. Vision can also be tested using Allen cards from the Denver eye screening test.

Colorblindness is more likely found in boys than in girls. Thus if a boy knows his colors, he can be asked to identify the basic colors in certain toys.

If an infant or toddler has had a "persistent deviating eye," he or she should have been referred to an ophthalmologist. **Strabismus** remains one of the most commonly seen abnormalities in preschool children. *Caused by the misalignment of each eye's optic axis, one or both of the child's eyes will turn in, out, up, or down.* **Double vision (diplopia)** next develops, followed by an *irreversible loss of vision in the suppressed eye* (**amblyopia**) if not treated early.

Functional amblyopia can be remedied through the use of corrective lenses, contact lenses, prisms, and vision training. Patching of one eye is often used. One test for detecting strabismus is to shine a penlight into the child's eyes. The light reflection should appear in the same position on each pupil if strabismus is not present (39, 51, 53, 57, 77).

Hearing Loss

Hearing loss should be suspected if the preschooler does not seem to hear as well as previously and has recurrent otitis media. Socialization and speech can become blocked if this occurs. Play techniques can be used with the preschooler to evaluate hearing. For example, earphones that will transmit various sounds can be placed on a child. He or she can be asked to put a peg in a pegboard every time a sound is heard. The result will be a variation of pure tone and audiometry (39, 51, 53, 57, 60, 77).

Acute purulent otitis media is usually a bacterial *infection of the middle ear with an accumulation of purulent fluid in the middle-ear cavity.* The preschooler will complain of earache, often have a fever, and have decreased hearing in the affected ear. Sometimes the tympanic membrane will perforate, and the purulent fluid will flow into the external canal. A nurse with physical assessment skills can make this diagnosis with an otoscope. Antibiotic treatment should be prescribed (39, 51, 53, 57, 60, 77).

As in toddlerhood, susceptibility to *upper respiratory infections* remains high. Because the lymphatic tissue known as tonsils and adenoids is more abundant at this time than in later life, these structures are often involved in the infectious process. Formerly it was nearly standard procedure for children to have tonsillectomies and adenoidectomies. However, with the evolving belief that the lymphatic tissue would later help with body defenses and realizing the risks involved and the fact that children still had upper respiratory infections after these surgeries, the trend went away from these procedures. "Large" tonsils, recurrent colds and sore throats, recurrent streptococcal pharyngitis, parental pressure, school absence, and "chronic tonsillitis" *are not* valid reasons for tonsillectomy and adenoidectomy. Valid reasons for surgery would include persistent nasal or oral obstruction, recurrent peritonsillar abscess, suspected tonsillar tumor, recurrent cervical lymph gland infection, and in some cases, recurrent ear problems (39, 51, 53, 57, 77).

Table 9–2 summarizes other common health problems.

Chronic health problems of the preschooler include glomerulonephritis (an *infection of the kidneys following infection elsewhere in the body*), leukemia, congenital heart defects, hemophilia, epilepsy, mental retardation, cerebral palsy, and emotional illness such as autism. For more information, consult a pediatric nursing book (38, 53, 77).

TABLE 9-2. COMMON HEALTH PROBLEMS OF PRESCHOOLERS

Problem	Definition	Symptoms/Signs	Prevention/Treatment
Conjunctivitis	Inflammation of the eyelids or conjunctivae or both; caused by bacteria or virus	Redness of conjunctivae; mild irritation; excessive lacrimation; normal vision	Cool compresses Appropriate eye drops
Urinary tract infection	Bacterial infection of part or all of the urinary tract, the collecting system of the kidneys, and the bladder	May be asymptomatic; urgency and frequency of urination; dysuria; flank and suprapubic pain; foul-smelling urine; fever	Appropriate antibiotic Increased water intake Personal hygiene
Enuresis	Involuntary passage of urine; occurs at night in 10% to 15% of 5-year-olds	Bedwetting	Reduction of liquid intake in the evening Maintaining appropriate attitude Signal device sometimes helpful Getting child up at specified times to urinate
Nonspecific vulvovaginitis	Inflammation of vulva and vagina; usually nonspecific organism responsible	Discharge; pruritus; erythema	Personal hygiene Wearing cotton underwear Avoidance of bubble baths and perfumed soaps Cold compresses to vulva
Measles	Highly contagious viral disease with severe complications	Rash (beginning at face and descending down body); 3 Cs—coryza, cough, conjunctivitis; Koplik's spots (red) on buccal mucosa; fever	Prevention: immunization If disease: isolation No specific therapy Symptomatic treatment
Diarrhea	Inflammation of gastrointestinal tract caused at this age by Giardia lambdia and Salmonella	Stools more frequent and liquid than usual	Sometimes antibiotics Personal hygiene Staying out of wading pools
Postural problems	Deviation of normal posture and normal spinal curves	Deviation seen as child bends anteriorly, laterally, posteriorly	Exercises prescribed by knowledgeable health care practitioner
Juvenile hypertension	Child more than age 3 years who has diastolic pressure greater that 90 mm Hg	Probably none other than blood pressure elevation	Referral for overall cardiovascular investigation

Data from references 39, 51, 53, 57, 60, and 77.

Abuse

An all-too-common health problem for the young child is *abuse, neglect,* or *maltreatment.* Garbarino, Guttmann, and Seeley (31) describe behaviors of the psychologically abusing parents (see Chapters 7 and 8) toward the young child.

Be aware that when you encounter children with some of the previous accidental occurrences or health problems, the origin of the problems may be the beatings, burns, shakings, handling, sexual abuse or incest, or neglect received at the hands of the parents, stepparents, day-care teacher, or other adult caretaker (47).

Role relationship of the child to the offender may be intrafamilial or extrafamilial (day-care worker, teacher, babysitter, family acquaintance). When the abuser is older, the age difference conveys that others will not believe the accusations of the child but the denial of the offender. Further, the role of the offender often also involves one of caretaker so that trust would be the normal feeling for the child (13).

The Federal Child Abuse Prevention and Treatment Act defines **child abuse** and **neglect** as the *"physical or mental injury, sexual abuse, negligent treatment, or maltreatment of a child under the age of 18 by a person*

who is responsible for the child's welfare under circumstances which indicate that the child's health or welfare is harmed" (79).

The three types of abuse (physical, psychologic, and sexual) may be present simultaneously, but frequently the child's symptoms and perceptions convey that one abuse experience is dominant (13).

Physical abusive acts *include being bit, punched, cut, burned, physically restrained, and tied up.* It is also considered abuse if the child witnesses this behavior between an adult and a child or between adults (13).

Psychologic abuse *is characterized by behaviors, activities, and words that intimidate, threaten, humiliate, shame, or degrade the child; blaming the child for the abuse; and threatening the child with harm* such as being locked in a box, removal of body parts, or death to self or family members if he or she tells about the abuse. (13)

Child sexual abuse is defined to *include immature children and adolescents engaged in sexual activities who do not fully comprehend the sexual act, who are unable to give informed consent, or who are forced to engage in activities that violate social taboos of family roles.* The child is victimized by the lack of choice in-

Research Abstract

Kelley, S., Parental Stress Response to Sexual Abuse and Ritualistic Abuse of Children in Day Care Centers, Nursing Research, *39, no. 1 (1990), 25–29.*

The sexual abuse of a child is a major crisis for the victim(s) and the parents. Evidence indicates that sexually abused children are affected negatively by the experience. Sexual victimization and subsequent disclosure are stressful events that alter the balance of the family and interfere with previous coping abilities. The sexually abused child incorporates the parents' reaction to the abuse, and increased behavioral symptoms appear in children who have encountered negative parental reactions.

The purpose of this study was to validate parental stress responses to extrafamilial sexual and ritualistic abuse. An increasing incidence of sexual abuse is occurring in day-care centers, and 13% of it has involved ritualistic abuse. It was hypothesized that parents of children sexually abused in day-care would demonstrate greater psychologic distress than parents of nonabused children and that parents of ritually abused children would demonstrate greater distress than parents of children sexually abused without rituals.

Ritualistic abuse practices often include ingestion of human excrement, semen, or blood; witnessing the mutilation of animals; threats with supernatural or magical powers; ingestion of drugs; and use of songs or chants. Child victims are threatened with the devil and physical harm to prevent disclosure of the ritualistic activities.

The sample consisted of a matched comparison group of 134 children: half had been abused in day-care centers; the other half had not been abused. The nonabused child group ranged in age from 4 to 11 years. The parents and the sexually abused children were divided into two groups based on whether or not there had been ritual sexual abuse. There were equal numbers of boys and girls.

The Symptom Checklist 90-R was completed by the parents to measure their psychologic distress. The Impact of Event Scale was administered to determine the conscious experience of the abuse on the parents. A Child Behavior Checklist and a demographic questionnaire were administered to the children.

Age of children when nonritualistic abuse began ranged from 1 to 4 years; mean duration of abuse was 13 months. Over one half (53%) were sexually abused more than 20 different times. Ages of the children when ritualistic abuse began was 1 to 7 years. Children in the ritualistic abuse group endured more extensive sexual abuse; each child was abused by 4.82 different offenders, with a range of 1 to 17 offenders for a duration of 16.5 months. Eighty percent were abused more than 20 times. Children in the ritualistic abuse group, in the context of cult worship, were abused physically, sexually, and psychologically and experienced more extensive sexual abuse.

The results indicated that parents of sexually abused children experienced clinically more psychologic distress than parents of nonabused children, including depression, interpersonal sensitivity, hostility, paranoia, and anxiety; and parents of ritually abused children had the most psychologic distress. Two years after disclosure, fathers were experiencing more distress than mothers. Parents continued to experience intrusive thoughts and images and conscious avoidance of ideas and emotions related to the child's abuse. Parental distress did decrease with distancing in time from the child's sexual victimization. Twenty-two percent of mothers of abused children had themselves been victimized as children.

To intervene efficiently, nurses must recognize sexual victimization as an acute and chronic stressor for parents. During the acute phase parents are dealing with feelings of shock, anger, denial, and guilt as well as entanglement in complex legal, mental health, and social service systems. Sexual abuse is also experienced by the parents as a chronic stressor because of long-term impact on the child, need for extended therapy, and legal proceedings, which may prevent closure on the event. Two years after the discovery of their child's sexual abuse, 52% of parents still had psychologic distress characteristic of PostTraumatic Stress Disorder and comparable to that found in studies of parents 2 years after their child had died from cancer. This distress was present despite therapy, although most received less than 6 months of treatment. Thus it appears that more treatment is needed, especially for women who have also been sexually victimized as a child. It has not yet been determined how long symptoms will last. More extensive research is needed on the effect of extrafamilial abuse on all family members.

volved. Sexual abuse is defined as pressured or ritualistic (44).

Pressured sexuality is an *adult's dominance used to ensure sexual control over the child so that there is loss of choice of consent and right to say no to the perpetrator; it often is accompanied by threats of violence to the child or family members* (12, 43).

Sexual activity that is child sexual abuse includes enforcing nudity or disrobing, genital exposure, observation of the child, photographing, kissing, fondling, masturbation, fellatio, cunnilingus, digital penetration of the anus or vagina, penile penetration of the vagina, and dry intercourse or forcing the child to perform sexual acts on other children or to watch sexual behavior between children and adults (67).

Ritualistic abuse refers to the *systematic and repetitive sexual, physical, and psychologic abuse of children by adults engaged in cult worship. The purpose of ritualistic abuse is to induce religious or mystical experiences for the adult participants.* Ritualistic behavior is linked with symbols of overriding power, authority, and purpose, often pseudoreligious or satanic in nature ("It is God's will that you be punished in this way for your sins"). There is the determined intent by the offender to convert the abused person to a victim role (13).

Indications of satanic ritual abuse include the following (43):

1. Use of special table or altar
2. Sex involving unusual practices
3. Imitations and reversals of the Catholic Mass
4. Ritual use of body fluids and excrement

5. Ritual use of a circle
6. Ritualized use of chants and songs, especially using names of demons
7. Use of animals and insects in ceremonies
8. Wearing of special masks and robes in ceremonies
9. Use of torches, candles, darkness, and body parts in ceremonies
10. Administration of drugs and potions
11. Dismemberment of infants and young children
12. Cannibalism of animals or humans; drinking of human or animal blood in ceremonies

The autonomic response to abuse is of two types: numbing and hyperarousal. Affective states may include passivity, anxiety, depression, anger, hostility, defiance, or rebellion. With hyperarousal, night terror, stomachache, startle reflexes, avoidance of people and places, crying, and enuresis may be noted. Alcohol and drug use may be a way to avoid the emotional pain. With numbing, there may be acting out of aggressive and sexualized behaviors and a lack of empathy for others (13). Federation (27) and Polk-Walker (55) also discuss feelings of the abused child and causes of abuse and treatment. More information about nursing assessment and intervention for the abused child is discussed in the section, "Nursing Applications" later in this chapter. Box 9–2 summarizes signs and symptoms of sexual abuse of the child.

A study of two groups of children attending day care who were sexually abused revealed differences using the TRIAD tool. One group (N = 32) was subjected to patterned sexual abuse. In this group the children's relationship with adult caretakers was sexual. Physical abuse and control of these children usually was opportunistic and aimed at immediate conquest of the child. The second group (N = 35) was subjected to sexual abuse within the context of ritual activities. Each form of abuse was scripted and aimed at performance of aggressive, erotic, and sadistic impulses of the abuser. Ritualistic abuse was more severe, and the child's fears continued longer after ritualistic abuse than after nonritualistic abuse. With ritualistic abuse there were significantly more physical abuse, more sexual acts, greater variation of sexual acts, and more offenders. The ritualistically abused children scored higher than the other abused children, although that group also had more symptoms than normal children. Of particular harmful impact were acts demanding sexual activity with other children, pornographic photography, and forced participation in rituals. Both groups had been highly stressed so that the children vacillated between great anxiety and numbness, for when the children reached a panic state, they went into dissociation (43).

Neglect

Not all abused children are battered. Some suffer just as cruelly from another type of abuse—parental neglect, either willful or unintentional. **Neglect** is a *lack of adequate food, clothing, shelter, love, concern, and attention*. Neglect can take many forms. A parent may neglect a child by simply "forgetting" about him or her (e.g., leaving him or her behind at a bus terminal after rounding up the other children), or a parent may sedate a rejected child to keep him or her quiet; belittle the child until he or she is convinced he or she is worthless; or hurt the child by physically abusing his or her pet or favorite toy.

Signs of a neglected child include the following (13):

1. Signs of malnutrition, including wasting of subcutaneous tissue, abdominal distention, thinness, pallor, dull eyes, sore gums
2. Inadequate clothing in cold weather
3. Apathy or hyperexcitability in the child
4. Behavior problems or emotional or developmental immaturity in the child
5. Parasitic infections
6. Depression or psychosomatic illness
7. Parental role-playing among siblings (when all the children in a family are neglected, older children will sometimes "mother" the younger ones)

Reactions to Illness and Hospitalization

During this stage, when the child has heightened feelings of sexuality, fears of dependency and separation, fantasies, feelings of narcissism, and rivalry with parents, he or she is particularly vulnerable to fears about body damage. The child perceives and fears dental, medical, and surgical procedures as mutilating, intrusive, punishing, or abandonment. The resulting conflicts, fears, guilt, anger, or excessive concern about the body can persist and influence personality development into adulthood.

Teach parents that many of these negative reactions can be averted by introducing the child to medical facilities and health workers when he or she is well. The best teaching is positive example. If the parent takes the child with him or her to the physician and dentist and if the child observes courteous professionals, a procedure that does not hurt (or an explanation of why it will hurt), and a positive response from the parent, a great deal of teaching is accomplished. These visits can be reinforced with honest answers to the many questions the preschooler will have.

Hospitalization should be avoided if possible. Preparation for hospitalization is important to reduce the separation anxiety and grief and mourning response described in Chapter 8. Most families have had some experience with a hospital and can give some explanation to the child.

Although children are forbidden in certain areas of a hospital, parents may arrange for a tour of the pediatric ward. The child should be told that special caring people work there and that if he or she is ever hospitalized, the parents will stay close by. The child can be further prepared through play, books, and appropriate films. Emphasize the importance of continued, ample contact with the child whenever either parent or child is

■ BOX 9-2.
Signs and Symptoms of Sexual Abuse of a Child

Disclosures

- States that someone removed child's clothes or handled or had contact with the genital area in some way
- Complains that an adult or older child touched or penetrated child's bottom, vagina, rectum, or mouth or that child touched an older child or adult's bottom, vagina, penis, or rectum
- Refers to blood or "white stuff" in genital area
- Describes detailed and age-inappropriate understanding of sexual behavior
- Hints about engaging in sexual activity

Physical Symptoms

- Somatic complaints: stomachaches, nausea, vomiting, headaches, leg aches
- Underwear excessively soiled due to reluctance to clean self or to a relaxed anal sphincter
- Semen or blood stains on child's underwear, skin, or hair or in mouth
- Bruises or abrasions in the genital or rectal area
- Vaginal or anal pain, burning when washed, pain when urinating or defecating
- Chronic constipation or urinary infections
- Constant fatigue, illness, flare-ups of allergies, vomiting
- On examination, relaxed anal sphincter, anal or rectal lacerations or scarring; child relaxes rather than tenses rectum when touched
- On examination, enlargement of vaginal opening and vaginal lacerations in girls, sore penis in boys; blood or trauma around genital area
- Presence of venereal disease, including infections such as trichimonas, herpes, or monilia

Behavior of Child

- Uncontrolled, hyperactive, wild
- Accident-prone or deliberately hurts self
- Negativistic; resistant to authority; mistrusts adults
- Overcompliant with authority; overly pleasing with adults
- Withdrawn; does not play; plays in lethargic, unfocused way
- Exhibits short attention span; has difficulty staying on task
- Does not learn readily
- Regressive, babyish, delayed, or disordered speech; significantly decreased speech production
- Sleep disorders: nightmares or night terrors, bed wetting, fear of going to bed
- Does not clean himself or herself after going to the bathroom
- Masturbates excessively; attempts to insert finger or other object in rectum or vagina
- Pulls down pants, lifts dress, or takes off clothes inappropriately
- Touches others sexually or asks for sexual activity
- Is sexually provocative or seductive in behavior
- Excessive bathing; preoccupation with cleanliness of self and surroundings
- Unusual reluctance to remove clothes (e.g., during visit to pediatrician, insistence on wearing underwear to bed)

Emotional Responses

- Low self-esteem, feeling of being "bad"; feels deserving of punishment
- Perceives self as dumb, ugly, unloved
- Is fearful and clingy; regresses to "baby" behavior
- Shows an unusual fear of people of a particular age group, gender, of policemen, doctors
- Is angry, aggressive, acts out
- Shows rapid mood changes inappropriate to the circumstances
- Sudden onset of anxiety or anxiety-related behavior (e.g., nail biting, grinding teeth, rocking)
- Is fearful of being touched; fears having genital area washed

---

hospitalized. Advise parents to (1) trust their intuition (they know the child best); (2) shop for a doctor and hospital; (3) prepare themselves so that they can prepare the child; (4) prepare the child a few days before hospitalization; and (5) be present at important times.

As a nurse, you will be in a position to offset the negative effects of hospitalization through planning individualized care, use of play or art therapy, and involvement in decision and policy making. The hospital personnel must make the ward as homelike as possible through gay decor and furnishings and provision for toys, a playroom, and central dining area. The staff can wear pastel uniforms or smocks and provide for the child to remain in his or her own clothes, keep a favorite toy, eat uninterrupted by procedures, and follow normal living routines when possible. Flexible visiting hours are es-

sential since the presence of the mother can dramatically revive a child's interest in getting well and improve eating, sleeping, and general behavior. Because a mother feels concern, partial helplessness, and perhaps guilt when her child is hospitalized, she may have an impaired relationship with her child and consequently the entire family. Family affection, concern, and questions should never be considered an interference. Instead, the family should be seen as collaborators in care. Answer questions and ask questions related to parents' questions to clarify further and inform or reinforce their ideas. Ideally, if the parent wishes, he or she should be allowed to stay with the child during care, procedures, tests, or treatments. If not feasible, one nurse should consistently care for the child while involving the parent as much as possible.

The parent needs to see the child receiving competent care and to feel that he or she is important to the child and capable as a parent, even if staying with the child is not possible. Encourage the parent to talk about feelings of fear, anxiety, guilt, shame, or sadness that may be present and related to the child's illness or hospitalization or children left at home. Avoid a critical attitude, voice tone, or disapproving nonverbal behavior that conveys to the parent that he or she is not managing well as a parent. Help parents to talk about the unique aspects of their child's or family life so that care can be truly individualized. For example, the child may prefer to wear his shorts instead of pajamas in bed. If an African-American child with an intricate hairstyle that was just arranged before admission is admitted, do not automatically do a routine admission shampoo. Realize that the Oriental or American Indian child may not talk as freely, at least initially, as the average Caucasian child, but this response reflects family and cultural child-rearing practices and does not mean that the child is retarded or does not understand you.

Obtain a developmental history from the mother on admission and use it to plan care to follow the child's usual living routine. Of great importance is the attitude of the staff caring for the child. The staff should be like the ideal parent: loving, honest, respectful, accepting, consistent. Cajoling, threatening, or rejection cannot help the child cope with problems. Acknowledge that children suffer great physical and emotional pain. Help the child get in touch with feelings and the pain. Do not tell him or her not to cry or that a procedure will not hurt when it will. Help the child displace aggression onto toys or staff rather than onto parents. Allow the child to be angry. Objective involvement is also important to avoid showing favoritism to only certain children. Several authors describe practical ways to help the child prepare for and cope with painful procedures (36).

PSYCHOSOCIAL CONCEPTS

Cognitive Development

The child in the Preoperational Stage is perceptually bound, unable to reason logically about concepts that are discrepant from visual cues. The child learns by being confronted with others' opinions and being actively involved with objects and processes (75). More important than the facts learned are the attitudes the child forms toward knowledge, learning, people, and the environment. Cognition and learning, at least partly a result of language learning and perceptual ability, can be studied through the child's handling of the physical environment and in connection with the concepts of number, casualty, and time, abstractions highly developed in western civilization (69).

By helping parents understand the cognitive development of their child, including concept formation, you will help them stimulate intellectual growth realistically, without expecting too much. **Concepts** *come about by giving precepts (events, things and experiences) a meaningful label; the name or label implies similarity to some other things having the same name and difference from things having a different name.* **Concept formation** *develops with perception progressing from diffuse to roughly differentiated and finally to sharply differentiated awareness of stable and coordinated objects.* The first concept is formed when a word comes to designate a crudely defined area of experience. As the late toddler and early preschooler acquire a number of words, each presenting a loosely defined notion or thing, the global meaning becomes a simple concrete concept. As perceived characteristics of things and events become distinguished from each other, the child becomes aware of differences among words, objects, and experiences such as dog and cat, baby and doll, men and daddy, approval and disapproval. However, the preschooler cannot yet define attributes and cannot make explicit comparisons of the objects. The attributes are an absolute part of the object such as bark and dog; hence the child is said to *think concretely.* What he or she sees or hears can be named, which is different from conceptual or abstract thinking about the object (69).

Concrete concepts become true concepts when the late preschooler can compare, combine, and describe them and think and talk about their attributes. At this point the child can deal with differences between concepts such as "dogs bark, people talk," but not until after the ages 6 or 7 will he or she be able to deal with opposites and similarities together (69). Box 9–3 summarizes categories of concepts that develop during this age period.

Some of the influences on concept development include the child's inability to distinguish between his or her own feelings and outside events; the ability to be impressed by the external, obvious features of a situation or thing rather than its essential features; his or her awareness of gaps in a situation; and emotional or contextual significance of words. The concreteness typical of a preschooler's concepts is found in the rambling, loosely jointed circumstantial descriptions. Everything is equally important and must be included. One must listen closely to get the central theme since young children learn things in bunches and not in a systematic, organized way. They can memorize and recite many things, but they cannot paraphrase or summarize their learning (46, 69).

Concepts of Relationships

These concepts involve time, space, number, and causation, are more abstract than those based on the immediately observable properties of things, and are greatly determined by culture (69).

Time Concept

For the preschooler, time is beginning to move; the past is measured in hours, and the future is a myth. At first

Categories of Concepts That Develop in the Preschool Years

Life: ascribes living qualities to inanimate objects
Death: associates death with separation, lack of movement; thinks dead people capable of doing what living people do
Body functions: has inaccurate ideas about body functions and birth process
Space: judges short distances accurately; aware of direction and distance in relation to body
Weight: estimates weight in terms of size; by age 5 can determine which of two objects feels heavier; notion of quantity—more than one, big, small
Numbers: understands up to 5
Time: has gradually increasing sense of time; present oriented; knows day of week, month, and year
Self: knows sex, full name, names of outer body parts by age 3; when begins to play with other children, self-concept begins to include facts about his or her abilities and race but not socioeconomic class
Sex roles: has general concept of gender, identity, and appropriate sex roles developed at age 5 or 6
Social awareness: is egocentric but forms definite opinions about others' behavior as "nice" or "mean"; intuitive; concept of causality is magical, illogical
Beauty: names major colors; prefers music with definite tune and rhythm
Comic: considers as comic funny faces made by self or others, socially inappropriate behavior, and antics of pets

space through play and exploration of his or her own body, up and down, front and back, sideways, next to, near and far, and later left and right. The child is not able until approximately age 6 to understand object space as a unified whole; he or she will first see a number of unrelated routes or spaces. He or she is generally aware of specific objects and habitual routes. The child does not see self and objects as part of a larger integrated space with multiple possibilities for movement. Map space and abstract space are not understood until later.

Quantitative Concepts

Notions of quantity are developed in the early preschool years such as one and more than one, bigger and smaller. Understanding of the quantity or amount represented by a number is not related to the child's ability to count to 10, 20, or higher, nor can he or she transfer numbers to notions of value of money, although he or she may imitate adults and play store, passing money back and forth. Ordinal numbers, indicating successions rather than totals, develop crudely in "me first" or "me last"; the concept of second or third develops later. The preschooler cannot simultaneously take account of different dimensions such as 1 quart equals 2 pints or equal volume in different-shaped containers (69). (See also Table 9–3.)

Concepts of Causality

The way of perceiving cause and effect is marginal. Things simply are. The child may be pleased or displeased with events but does not understand what brought them about. He or she does precausal thinking, confusing physical and mechanical causation or natural phenomena with psychologic, moral, or sequential causes. He or she frequently says "n' then," indicating causal sequence. When the child asks "why?" he or she is probably looking for justification rather than causation. Most things are taken for granted; the child assumes that people, including self, or some motivated inanimate being are the causes of events. Perception of the environment is **animistic,** *endowing all things with the qualities of life Westerners reserve for human beings.* There is little notion of accident or coincidence. It takes some time to learn that there are impersonal forces at work in the world. Thinking is also **egocentric:** *things and events are seen from a personal and narrow perspective and are happening because of self* (69).

The late preschooler fluctuates between reality and fantasy and a materialistic and animistic view of the world; most adults never completely leave behind the magical thinking typical of the preschooler. The child plays with the idea of a tree growing out of the head, what holes feel like to the ground, and growing up starting as an adult. The adult finds no meaning in music, art, literature, love, and possibly even science and mathematics without fantasy or magic.

formal time concepts have nothing to do with personal time. Adults are seen as changeless, and the child believes that he or she can mature in a hurry; thus the preschooler thinks he or she can grow up fast and marry his or her parent. Time concepts are further described in Table 9–3.

Spatial Concepts

These concepts differ markedly in children and adults. There are five major stages in the development of spatial concepts. First, there is **action space**, *consisting of the location or regions to which the child moves.* Second, **body space** *refers to the child's own awareness of directions and distances in relation to his or her own body.* Third, there is **object space,** *in which objects are located relative to each other and without reference to the child's body.* The fourth and fifth stages, **map space** and **abstract space,** are *interrelated and depend on knowing directions of east, west, south, and north; allocating space in visual images to nations, regions, towns, rooms; and the ability to deal with maps, geographic or astronomic ideas, and three-dimensional space* that use symbolic (verbal or mathematical) relationships (69).

The preschool child has action space and moves along familiar locations and explores new terrain. He or she is beginning to orient self to body space and object

Preoperational Stage

The Preoperational Stage is divided into the Pre-conceptual and Intuitive Phases. During the Pre-conceptual Phase, from 2 to 4 years of age, the child gathers facts as they are encountered but can neither separate reality from fantasy nor classify or define events in a systematic manner. Ability to define properties of an object or denote hierarchies or relationships among elements in a class is lacking. He or she is beginning to develop mental strategies from concept formation; concepts are constructed in a global way. He or she is capable of perceiving gross outward appearances but sees only one aspect of an object or situation at a time. For example, if you say, "Take the yellow pill," he or she will focus on either yellow or pill but cannot focus on both aspects at once. The child is unable to use time, space, equivalence, and class inclusion in concept formation. During the Intuitive Phase, lasting from approximately 4 to 7 years, the child gains increasing, but still limited, ability to develop concepts. He or she defines one property at a time, has difficulty stating the definition, but knows how to use the object. The child uses **transductive logic,** *going from general to specific in explanation,* rather than deductive or inductive logic. He or she begins to label, classify in ascending or descending order, do seriation, and note cause-effect relationships, even though true cause-effect understanding does not occur (56, 73).

The Preoperational Stage is characterized by the following: egocentric thought; literal thinking with absence of reference system; intermingling of fantasy, intuition, and reality; **absolute thought,** *seeing all or nothing without shades of gray or any relativity;* **centering,** *focusing on a single aspect of an object,* causing distorted reasoning; lack of concept of **reversibility,** *for every action, there is one that cancels it;* static thinking; difficulty remembering what he or she started talking about so that when the sentence is finished he or she is talking about something else; and inability to state cause-effect relationships, categories, or abstractions, believing that events that occur together belong together (46, 56, 73).

In general, the preschooler has a consuming curiosity. Learning is vigorous, aggressive, and intrusive. The imagination creates many situations he or she wishes to explore. Judgment is overshadowed by curiosity and excitement. The preschooler has begun to develop such concepts as friend, aunt, uncle; accepting responsibility; independence; passage of time, spatial relationships; use of abstract words, numbers, colors; and the meaning of cold, tired, and hungry. Attention span is lengthening.

The child's ability to grasp reality varies with individual intelligence and potential intelligence, the social milieu, and opportunities to explore the world, solve problems independently, ask questions, and get answers. (Table 9–3 summarizes major characteristics of mental development to help you in assessment [30, 33, 42, 51, 56, 69, 71, 73].)

An educational trend is underway to teach the preschooler more factual content and to provide some schooling from infancy on as seen in the large number of preschoolers in the United States who are enrolled in preprimary-school programs. Impetus for this trend stems from (1) the Head Start program in the 1960s, (2) women's liberation campaigns for day-care centers, (3) the growing realization by the middle class that competition for school achievement and college entrance will remain intense, (4) awareness that most of the brain is developed by age 4, and (5) the theory that at least half of all human intelligence is developed by age 4, possibly even earlier. Another theory states that by age 5 the intelligence quotient (IQ) is basically established, that attitudes toward learning and patterns of thinking will guide the child for the rest of his or her life (42, 51, 71). However, he or she needs informal learning opportunities, not facts.

Parents can enhance the child's growth by realizing the importance of the following approaches. Share this information with them. Refer to the article by Pontious (56) for ways to explain nursing procedures to a child.

The single most critical factor in the child's learning is a loving caretaker since that is whom the child imitates. How the mothering person speaks to, touches, and plays with the child governs the potential for socialization and cognitive development. This is true even for the child who had a low birth-weight and was at risk for developmental lag or disability (61). A child's problem-solving abilities are shaped by the parents' method for handling problems and by opportunities for problem solving. In families in which everyone gets a chance to speak out and jointly explore a problem, the child learns to express him or herself logically. Automatic obedience or acceptance of parental commands or decisions will interfere with reasoning (7). Important also are the opportunities provided for the child to learn, encouraging him or her to handle objects, explore, ask questions, and to play a variety of games. In the home the child learns how to learn or how not to learn. Teaching the child is more than telling him or her what to do. It involves demonstration, listening, and talking about the situation in direct and understandable terms and giving reasons. Cognitive development includes more than fluency with words, a good verbal memory, and information. It includes ability to use imagination, form mental pictures, and engage in fantasy appropriately, along with art, music, and other creative activities. It includes expanding skills in logical thinking. Most important, it involves increasing integration of many kinds of brain functions. Much integrated learning comes from the child's engaging in motor activity, play, and language games; talking with adults and peers; and paying attention to both trivial and important aspects of the environment (7, 46).

Creative methods of teaching for preschoolers is seen in educational programs such as *Sesame Street,* or *Mister Rogers' Neighborhood. Sesame Street,* presented

TABLE 9-3. ASSESSMENT OF MENTAL DEVELOPMENT

3 Years	4 Years	5 Years
Knows he or she is a person separate from another Knows own sex and some sex differences	Senses self one among many	Aware of cultural and other differences between people and the two sexes Mature enough to fit into simple type of culture Can tell full name and address Remains calm if lost away from home
Resists commands but distractible and responsive to suggestions Can ask for help Desire to please Friendly Sense of humor	States alibis because more aware of attitude and opinions of others Self-critical; appraises good and bad of self Does not like to admit inabilities; excuses own behavior Praises self; bosses or criticizes others Likes recognition for achievement Heeds others' thoughts and feelings; expresses own	Dependable Increasing independence Can direct own behavior; but fatigue, excessive demands, fantasy, and guilt interfere with assuming self-responsibility Admits when needs help Moves from direct to internalized action, from counting what he or she can touch to counting in thought; uses more clues
Uses language rather than physical activity to communicate	Active use of language Active learning Likes to make rhymes, to hear stories with exaggeration and humor, dramatic songs Knows nursery rhymes Tells action implied in picture books	Improves use of symbol system, concept formation Repeats long sentences accurately Can carry plot in story Defines objects in terms of use States relationship between two events
Imaginative Better able to organize thoughts Can bargain with him or her Sacrifices immediate pleasure for promise of future gain	Highly imaginative yet literal, concrete thinking Can organize his or her experience Increasing reasoning power and critical thinking capacity Makes crude comparisons	Less imaginative Asks details Can be reasoned with logically More accurate, relevant, practical, sensible than 4-year-old Asks to have words defined Seeks reality
Understands simple directions; follows normal routines of family life and does minor errands	Concept of 1, 2, 3; counts to five; does some home chores Generalizes	Begins to understand money Does more home chores with increasing competence Can determine which of two weights heavier Idea in head precedes drawing on paper or physical activity Interested in meaning of relatives
Knows age Meager comprehension of past and future Knows mostly today	Realizes birthday is one in a series and that birthday is measure of growth Knows when next birthday is Knows age Birthday and holidays significant because aware of units of time Loves parties related to holiday Conception of time Knows day of week	Understands week as a unit of time Knows day of week Sense of time and duration increasing Knows how old will be on next birthday Knows month and year Adults seen as changeless Memory surprisingly accurate
Has attention span of 10 to 15 min	Has attention span of 20 min	Has attention span of 30 min

as a lively, fast-moving, colorful program, emphasizes the alphabet, number concepts, similarities and differences, and positive body image. *Mister Rogers' Neighborhood* emphasizes positive body image, learning how things are done, and a personal one-to-one relationship between Mister Rogers and each child. It is difficult to assess the effect of these programs on the overall cognitive development of the child. Such programs appear to improve rote learning, although there is not much evidence that long-range concept formation is much different from what develops in children not exposed to these programs.

Because television is essentially a passive and solitary activity, more than occasional viewing may interfere with the purposes that more traditional play activities offer (see section on "Play Patterns," pp. 309 through 312). Thus television viewing can negatively affect self-concept and social skills, as well as motor, cognitive, and emotional learning (42, 51, 71).

Explore the use of television with parents. You can teach parents to see themselves as a parent educator rather than as "only a housewife" or "his pal, Dad." Parents can stimulate the intellectual development of their child by providing various practices: creating many and varied opportunities to learn about people and their environment; avoiding doing too much for the child; sharing activities with him or her; talking to him or her about situations the adult and child are in (shopping, cooking a meal, laundering); providing an interesting home; giving the child freedom to roam and follow natural curiosity within safe limits; giving daily individual attention to the child; obtaining information about child development and rearing from books, films, and other parents; experimenting with games and child-rearing practices and observing feedback from the child to determine which meet his or her needs; and avoiding the push to learn academic subjects too early, causing undue frustration and a negative attitude about learning and school later. The child will sense which activities provide interest and challenges without excess difficulty. Let him or her develop his or her own learning style and see you and other adults as sources of information and ideas.

Communication Patterns

People have three types of communication at their disposal: (1) somatic or physical symptoms such as flushed skin color on increased respirations; (2) action such as play or movement; and (3) verbal expression. The preschool child uses all of them.

Learning to use verbal expression—language—to communicate is an ongoing developmental process that is affected directly by the child's interaction with others. Language skills are enhanced, expanded, and refined as the child explores ideas with others and experiences a variety of social and educational environments. Language, cognition, and socialization are complex and interwoven. Verbal reasoning ability is dependent on the audible monologue of early toddler thinking, which then develops into inner speech and verbal thought (51, 71).

The child uses *language* for many reasons: to maintain social rapport, gain attention, get information, seek meaning about his or her experience, note how others' answers fit personal thoughts, play with words, and gain relief from anxiety. He or she asks why, what, when, where, how, repeatedly.

A child learns language from hearing it and using it. Words are at first empty shells until he or she has experiences to match. Parents should provide age-appropriate experiences so the child learns that words and actions go together. Equally important, parents should avoid saying one thing and doing another. Attaining trust in the utility and validity of verbal communication, learning that talking helps rather than hinders life, is crucial to transition from infancy to school years. If talking does not gain response from others or help the child solve problems and relate to those he or she needs or if the world is too troublesome, the child is likely to find refuge in fantasy and neglect social, communicative meanings of language.

Directing his or her own life depends on language and an understanding of the meaning of words and

logic with which they are used. When the child acquires language, he or she gradually becomes freed from tangible, concrete experiences and can internalize visual symbols, develop memory and recall, fragment the past, project the future, and differentiate fantasy from reality.

Language is also learned from being read to and having printed material available. Share the following suggestions with parents for choosing books for the preschooler. The book should be durable, have large print that does not fill the entire page, and be colorfully illustrated. The concepts should be expressed concretely in simple sentences and should tell a tale that fits the child's fantasy conception of the world such as a story with animals and objects who can talk and think like people; or the story should tell about the situations he or she ordinarily faces such as problems with playmates, discovery of the preschooler's world, nightmares, or the arrival of a new baby.

Follow and share with the significant adults in the child's life these *effective ways of talking with the preschooler:*

1. Try to maintain mutual respect as you talk with the child.
2. Do not discourage talking, questions, or the make-believe in the child's language; verbal explorations are essential to learn language. Answers to questions should meet needs and give him or her an awareness of adult attitudes and feelings about the topics discussed.
3. Tell the truth to the best of your ability and on the child's level of understanding. Admit if the answer is unknown, and seek the answer with the child. A lie is eventually found out and causes a loss of trust in that adult and in others.
4. Do not make a promise unless you can keep it.
5. Respond to the relationship or feelings in the child's experience rather than the actual object or event. Talk about the child's feelings instead of agreeing or disagreeing with what he or she says. Help the child understand what he or she feels rather than why he or she feels it.
6. Precede statements of advice and instruction with a statement of understanding of the child's feelings. When the child is feeling upset emotionally, he or she cannot listen to instructions, advice, consolation, or constructive criticism.
7. Do not give undue attention to slang or curse words, and do not punish the child for using them. The child uses these words for shock value, and attention or punishment emphasizes the importance of the words. Remain relaxed and give the child a more difficult or different word to say. If he or she persists in using the unacceptable word, the adult may say, "I'm tired of hearing that word, say _____ _____"; ask him or her not to say the word

again since it may hurt others, or use distraction. Children learn unacceptable words as they learn all others, and parents would be wise to listen to their own vocabulary.

8. Sit down if possible when participating or talking with children. You are more approachable when at their physical level.
9. Seek to have a warm, friendly relationship without thrusting yourself on the child. How you feel about the child is more important than what you say or do.
10. Through attentive listening and interested facial expression, convey a tell-me-more-about-it attitude to encourage the child to communicate.
11. Regard some speech difficulties as normal. Ignore stuttering or broken fluency that does not persist. Do not correct each speech error and do not punish. Often the child thinks faster than he or she can

articulate speech. Give the child time when he or she speaks.
12. Talk in a relaxed manner. Do not bombard the child with verbal information.

Table 9–4 is a guide for assessing language skills of the preschooler. During assessment keep in mind that how the child's parents and other family members speak and the language opportunities the child has influence considerably his or her language skills (32, 33, 42, 51, 71).

Play Patterns

Play is the work of the child. Play occupies most of the child's waking hours and serves to consolidate and enlarge his or her previous learning and promote adaptation. Play has elements of reality, and there is an earnestness about it. Piaget described play as assimilation;

TABLE 9-4. ASSESSMENT OF LANGUAGE DEVELOPMENT

3 Years	4 Years	5 Years
Appearance of individual sounds *y, f, v* in words	Appearance of individual sounds *sh, zh, th* in words	Appearance of individual sounds *s, z, th, r, ch, j* in words
Vocabulary of at least 900 words	Vocabulary of at least 1500 words	Vocabulary of at least 2100 words
Uses language understandably; uses some sounds experimentally	Uses language confidently	Uses language efficiently, correctly
Understands simple reasons	Concrete speech	No difficulty understanding others' spoken words
Uses some adjectives and adverbs	Increasing attention span	Meaningful sentences; uses future tense
	Uses "I" and other pronouns	Increasing skill with grammar
	Imitates and plays with words	Knows common opposites
	Defines a few simple words	
	Talks in sentences; uses past tense	
	Uses plurals frequently	
	Comprehends prepositions	
Talks in simple sentences about things	Talks incessantly while doing other activities	Talks constantly
Repeats sentence of six syllables	Asks many questions	No infantile articulation
Uses plurals in speech	Demands detailed explanations with "why"	Repeats sentences of 12 or more syllables
Collective monologue; does not appear to care whether another is listening	Carries on long involved conversation	Asks searching questions, meaning of words, how things work
Some random, inappropriate answers	Exaggerates; boasts; tattles; may use profanity for attention	Can tell a long story accurately, but may keep adding to reality to make story more fantastic
Intelligibility is 70% to 90%	Frequently uses "everything"	
Sings simple songs	Tells family faults outside of home without restraint	Intelligibility good; some distortion in articulation of *t, s*
	Tells story combining reality and fantasy; appears to be lying	Sings relatively well
	Intelligibility is 90%; articulation errors with *l, r, s, z, sh, ch, j, th*	
	Variation in volume from a yell to a whisper	
	Likes to sing	
Knows first and family name	Calls people names	Counts to 10 or further without help
Names figures in a picture	Names three objects he or she knows in succession	Repeats five digits
Repeats three digits	Counts to 5 without help	Names four colors, usually red, green, blue, yellow
Likes to name things	Repeats four digits	
	Knows which line is longer	
	Names one or more colors	
Talks to self or imaginary playmate	Talks with imaginary playmate of same sex and age	Sense of social standards and limits seen in language use
Expresses own desires and limits frequently	Seeks reassurance	
	Interested in things being funny	
	Likes puns	

── CASE SITUATION: Preschooler Development ──

Kalisha is an active, 38-month-old girl, who weighs 34 pounds (15.45 kg) and is 38 inches (95 cm) tall. She is playing on the sidewalk in front of her parents' home with her brother Marvin, 4 years old, and her next-door neighbor Lori, aged 5 years.

Kalisha is riding her small, two-wheeled bicycle, which has training wheels. Marvin and Lori are riding their small bicycles or scooters. Kalisha rides for a while, then stops to watch the others. Although involved in the same activity, she plays next to rather than with the older children. Several times Kalisha rides her bicycle into the path of her brother's approaching bicycle. The preschooler is typically intrusive in play, bombarding others by purposeful or accidental attack. Kalisha continues to ride and stop, always staying within her mother's view as she moves farther away and then nearer on her bicycle. She demonstrates the attachment behavior typical of this age by maintaining proximity to her mother.

When Marvin and Lori ride down the street, leaving Kalisha, she asks her mother to go with her to join them. She pulls her mother's hand insistently several times, and they walk together down the street. When she approaches the other children, Kalisha runs to them, laughing, and then gives Lori a hug. Lori chases Kalisha up the street, and Kalisha laughs and runs to her mother, seeking protection, security, assurance, and approval. Through this behavior she affirms that her mother is still the most important person in her life.

As the older children ride their bicycles on the sidewalk toward Kalisha, she laughs and shouts, then waves her arms, telling them, "I am the stop sign." She tells Lori to stop, but Lori rides by, laughing and saying, "You'll have to give me a ticket." On the return trip, Lori stops at Kalisha's command. Kalisha and Lori repeat this pattern several times, and each time Kalisha becomes more animated. She demonstrates autonomy and beginning initiative in these interactions, displaying the egocentrism typical of the preschooler as she commands events for her own needs and purposes and gains a sense of power through symbolic play.

---

play behavior involves taking in, molding, and using objects for pleasure and learning.

The preschooler is intrusive in play, bombarding others by purposeful or accidental physical attack. He or she is into people's ears and minds by loud, assertive talking; into space by vigorous gross motor activities; into objects through exploration; and into the unknown by consuming curiosity (26).

The preschool years are the pregang stage in which the child progresses from solitary and parallel play to cooperating for a longer time in a larger group. He or she identifies somewhat with a play group; follow rules; is aware of the status of self compared with others; develops perception of social relationships; begins the capacity for self-criticism; and states traits and characteristics of others that he or she likes or dislikes. At first the child spends brief, incidental periods of separation from the parents. The time away from them increases in length and frequency, and eventually the orientation shifts from family to peer group (25, 46, 48).

A **peer** is a *person with approximately equal status, a companion, often of the same sex and age,* with whom one can share mutual concerns. The **peer group** is a *relatively informal association of equals who share common play experiences with emphasis on common rules and understanding the limits that the group places on the individual.* The preschool play group differs from later ones in that it is loosely organized. The activity of the group may be continuous; but membership changes as the child joins or leaves the group at will, and the choice of playmates is relatively restricted in kind and number. This is the first introduction to a group that assesses him or her as a child from a child's point of view. The preschooler is learning about entering a new, different, very powerful world when he or she joins the group. Although social play is enjoyed, the child feels a need for solitary play at times.

The number and sex of siblings and the parent's handling of the child's play seems to influence behavior with the play group. If the family rejects the child, he or she may feel rejected by peers, even when the child is not rejected, causing self-isolation, inability to form close friendships, and ultimately real rejection.

Purposes of Play

The natural mode of expression for the child is play. Purposes of play include the following:

1. Develop and improve muscular strength, coordination, and balance
2. Work off excess physical energy
3. Communicate with others, establish friendships, learn about interpersonal relations, and develop concern for others
4. Learn cooperation, sharing, and healthy competition
5. Express imagination, creativity, and initiative
6. Imitate and learn about social activity, adult roles, and cultural norms

7. Test and deal with reality, gain mastery over unpleasant experiences
8. Explore, investigate, and manipulate features of the adult world
9. Learn about rules of chance and probability and rules of conduct and that at times one loses, but it is all right
10. Build self-esteem
11. Feel a sense of power, make things happen, explore and experiment
12. Provide for intellectual, sensory, and language development and dealing with concrete experiences in symbolic terms
13. Assemble novel aspects of the environment
14. Organize life's discrepancies privately and with others
15. Learn about self and how others see him or her
16. Practice leader and follower roles
17. Have fun, express joy, and feel the pleasure of mastery
18. Act out and symbolically work through a painful physical or emotional state by repetition in play so that it is more bearable and assimilated into the child's self-concept
19. Develop the capacity to gratify self and to delay gratification
20. Formulate a bridge between concrete experiences and abstract thought

Box 9–4 summarizes a classification of play according to its social characteristics (69, 77).

Play Materials

These materials should be simple, sturdy, durable, and free from unnecessary hazards. They need not be expensive. The child should have adequate space and equipment that is unstructured enough to allow for creativity and imagination to work unfettered. He or she will enjoy trips to parks and playgrounds. (The parents should be sure the child is not playing at dumps or at contaminated landfills.) Often creative, stimulating toys can be made from ordinary household articles: plastic pot cleaners, empty thread spools, a bell, yarn, or empty boxes covered with washable adhesive paper. The child may like the box more than the toy.

Increasing emphasis is being placed on high technology, interactive, and weaponry toys. These toys actually stifle imagination and discovery, and weaponry toys may cause fears, heighten aggressive fantasies, and cause injury and sometimes death. Young children need to direct their games to be in control of their play and their fantasies. They use play to work out problems, to practice skills, and to act out roles in preparation for later real life experiences. If the toy is too limiting, it will be cast aside by the child, regardless of how much the parent enjoys it. Some toys from infancy and toddlerhood are still enjoyed.

The play materials that are available will determine

■ BOX 9-4.
Types of Play Related to Social Characteristics

Onlooker play: Child watches others with no interactions or movement toward participation (e.g., use of television).
Parallel play: Child plays independently but next to other children; displays no group association.
Associative play: Children play together in similar or identical play without organization, division of labor, leadership, or mutual goals.
Cooperative play: Play is organized in group with others. There is planning and cooperation before play starts to form goals, division of labor, and leadership.
Solitary play: Child either by choice or because of lack of peers, entertains self in play. Play is often imaginative or studylike in nature.
Supplementary play: Play shifts from large group activities or games to focus on smaller group or board games.

Data from references 69 and 77.

---

the play activities. Play materials are enjoyed for different reasons. For example, **physical activity,** *which facilitates development of motor skills,* is provided through play with musical instruments and records for marching and rhythm, balls, shovel, broom, ladder, swing, trapeze, slide, boxes, climbing apparatus, boards, sled, wagon, tricycle, bicycle with training wheels, wheelbarrow, and blocks. Swimming, ice skating, roller skating, and skiing are being learned. **Dramatic play,** *which is related to the ability to classify objects correctly, take another's perspective, and do problem solving,* is afforded through large building blocks, sandbox and sand toys, dolls, housekeeping toys, nurse and doctor kits, farm or other occupational toys, cars and other vehicles, and worn out adult clothes for dress-up. This is a predominant form of play in childhood and also can include aspects of physical play. **Creative playthings,** *which promote constructive, nonsocial, cognitive, and emotional development,* include blank sheets of paper, crayons, finger or water paints, chalk, various art supplies, clay, plasticine, or other manipulative material, blunt scissors, paste, cartons, scraps of cloth, water-play equipment, and musical toys. **Quiet play,** *which promotes cognitive development and rest from physical exertion,* is achieved through books, puzzles, records, and table games (7, 46, 48). Children's songs, nursery rhymes, and fairy tales can absorb anxiety, entertain, soothe, reassure that life's problems can be solved, and support the child's superego.

The role of the adult in child's play is to provide opportunity, equipment, and safety and to avoid interference or structuring of play. (However, parents may need to restrict television watching, and children often want the structure of bedtime stories.) Allow the child to try things and enjoy personal activities. Assist only if he or she is in need of help. The child is not natural in play when he or she thinks adults are watching; avoid showing amusement or ridicule of play behavior or conversation. Allow playmates to work out their own differences. Distract, redirect, or substitute a different activity if the children cannot share and work out their problems. There are times to play with the child, but avoid overstimulation, teasing, hurry, talking about him or her as if he or she were not present, or doing the activity for the child. Let him or her take the lead. Try to enter the child's world. If he or she wants you to attend the teddy bear's 100th birthday party, go. A book that is creatively illustrated and gives many ideas for play activity for and with the preschooler is *Learning Through Play* by Jean Marzolla and Janice Lloyd (48).

Table 9–5 summarizes play characteristics as a further aid in assessment and teaching (32, 33, 48).

Share the above information with parents and explore their feelings about child's play and their role with the child.

Guidance and Discipline

The child learns how to behave by imitating adults and by using the opportunities to develop self-control. If the adult tells the child, "Tell him I'm not home" when the child answers the door, the child may at first be astonished, then accept the lie, and eventually use this behavior too.

The child needs consistent, fair, and kind limits to feel secure, to know that the parents care for and love him or her enough to provide protection—a security he or she does not have when allowed to do anything, regardless of ability. Limits should be set in a way that

TABLE 9-5. ASSESSMENT OF PLAY CHARACTERISTICS

3 Years	4 Years	5 Years
Enjoys active and sedentary play	Increasing physical and social play	More varied activity More graceful in play
Likes toys in orderly form Puts away toys with supervision	Puts away toys when reminded	Puts away toys by self
Fantasy not yielding too much to reality Likes fairy tales	Much imaginative and dramatic play Has complex ideas but unable to carry out because of lack of skill and time	More realistic in play Less interested in fairy tales More serious and ready to know reality Restrained but creative
Likes solitary and parallel play with increasing social play in shifting groups of two or three	Plays in groups of two or three, often companions of own sex Imaginary playmates Projects feelings and deeds onto peers or imaginary playmates May run away from home	Plays in groups of five or six Friendships stronger and continue over longer time Chooses friends of like interests Spurred on in activity by rivalry
Cooperates briefly Willing to wait turn and share with suggestion	Suggests and accepts turns but often bossy in directing others	Generous with toys Sympathetic, cooperative, but quarrels and threatens by word or gesture Acts out feelings Wants rules to do things right; but beginning to realize peers cheat, so develops mild deceptions and fabrications
Some dramatic play-house or family games Frequently changes activity Likes to arrange, combine, transfer, sort, and spread objects and toys	Dramatic and creative play at a peak Likes to dress up and help with household tasks Does not sustain role in dramatic play; moves from one role to another incongruous role No carry over in play from day to day Silly in play	Dramatic play about most life events, but more realistic Play continues from day to day Interested in finishing what started, even if it takes several days More awareness of yesterday and tomorrow Enjoys using tools and equipment of adults
Able to listen longer to nursery rhymes Dramatizes nursery rhymes and stories Can match simple forms Enjoys cutting, pasting, block building Enjoys sand and water play Enjoys dumping and hauling toys Rides tricycle	Concentration span longer Sometimes so busy at play forgets to go to toilet Reenacts stories and trips Enjoys simple puzzles with trial-and-error method Poor space perception Uses constructive and manipulative play material increasingly Enjoys sand and water play	Perceptive to order, form, and detail Better eye-hand coordination Rhythmic motion to music Likes excursions Interested in world outside immediate environment Enjoys cutting out pictures, pasting, working on special projects Likes to run and jump, play with bicycle, wagon, and sled

Data from references 32, 33, and 48.

preserves the self-respect of the child and parent and should not be applied angrily, violently, arbitrarily, or capriciously, but rather with the intent to educate and build character. Only when the child can predict the behavior of others can he or she accept the need to inhibit or change some of his or her behavior and work toward predictable and rational behavior. The parent should be an ally to the child as he or she struggles for control over inner impulses and convey to the child that he or she need not fear impulses.

The preschooler needs discipline that is permissive with limits. However, *permissive discipline* must be distinguished from *overpermissive* discipline. **Permissive discipline** *accepts the childish behavior of the child as normal and recognizes that the child is a person with a right to have all kinds of feelings and wishes that may be expressed directly or symbolically.* It sets realistic limits but is not harsh or demanding of perfection. The adult should distinguish between the wish and act and set limits on the act, not on the wish. Feelings and wishes must be identified and expressed verbally or through other outlets; it may be necessary to limit or redirect actions since destructive behavior cannot be tolerated.

Overpermissive discipline *permits undesirable behavior that can become harmful or destructive.* It causes the child to feel insecure and anxious; he or she perceives others' disapproval and believes that the parents do not care. Further, the child is unable to accomplish what he or she is ready to do because of lack of external or self-control; and he or she does not learn to like self. In turn, fantasies will increase, and the child will demand more privileges than should be granted. The vicious circle is uncomfortable for adult and child alike.

Share the above information and explore with parents the importance of their guidance to the child. *Techniques for guidance and limit setting* that would be helpful to you personally in working with children and should be shared with parents when indicated are as follows:

1. Convey authority without anger or threat to avoid feelings of resentment, fear, or guilt.
2. Be positive, clear, and consistent; let the child know what is acceptable behavior.
3. Place specific limits on special actions when the occasion arises, maintaining some flexibility in rules.
4. Recognize the child's wish, and put it into words, "You *wish* you could have that but . . . "; point out ways the wish can be partially fulfilled when possible.
5. Help the child express some resentment likely to arise when restrictions are imposed. "I realize you don't like the rules but. . . . "
6. Enforce discipline by adhering to the stated rules kindly but firmly. Do not argue about them nor initiate a battle of wills. Spanking is one way to discipline, but it may show the child an undesirable way of handling frustration. Spanking may interfere with superego development by relieving guilt too easily; the child feels he or she has paid for the misbehavior and is free to return to mischievous activity.
7. Positive suggestions rather than commands and "don'ts" help the child to learn how to get what he or she wants at the time and how to form happy relationships with others.
8. If the child has no choice about a situation, give direction that conveys what he or she has to do, for example, "It is time now to. . . . "
9. Convey that adults are present to help the child solve problems that cannot be solved alone.
10. Control the situation if the child has temporarily lost self-control; remove him or her from the stimulating event; stay with the child; talk quietly; use distraction or diversion if necessary; encourage thinking through the problem and finding a fair solution after he or she has become calm. Convey that you feel the child can regain self-control and handle the situation and can rejoin the group or continue the former activity when he or she feels ready (46).

A behavior modification technique that can be used to discipline an aggressively acting out child is *time-out*. Time-out involves immediately placing the child after a mean act in a quiet, uninteresting place (hall, small room, or corner of a room) for 5 to 15 minutes to remove the child from positive reinforcement. Time-out stops the misbehavior and is unpleasant enough to increase the possibility that the child will not repeat the undesirable act. The child learns accountability for behavior when time-out is linked to rules, limits, and extreme behavior. The child as part of the family unit should have input into formulating the rules and limits and the discipline method of time-out. This method should not be viewed by the child as a way to get out of cleanup or other tasks. During time-out the child may be requested to write sentences—positive and no longer than five words ("I will be polite"). Time-out is a method to help parents avoid nagging, spanking, screaming, lecturing, or being abusive and yet help parents feel in control and handle misbehavior so the child's behavior can improve. *The child should be helped to realize time-out means his or her behavior, not him or her, is rejected; thus use of rewards to reinforce desired behavior is necessary* in conjunction with this time-out method.

Emotional Development

If the child has developed reasonably well and if he or she has mastered earlier developmental tasks, the preschooler is a source of pleasure to adults. He or she is more a companion than someone to care for. The various behaviors discussed under development of physical, mental, language, play, body image, and moral-religious aspects contribute to his or her emotional status and development. The beginning motor self-control, high-energy level, use of language, ability to delay somewhat immediate gratification, ability to tolerate separation from mother, curiosity, strong imagination, and desire to move, all propel him or her to plan; attack problems; start tasks; consider alternatives; learn aggressively; direct behavior with some thought, logic and judgment; and appear more self-confident and relaxed. Tolerance of frustration is still limited, but flares of temper and frustrations over failure pass quickly. As the child is learning to master things and handle independence and dependence, so is he or she increasing mastery of self and others and learning to get along with more people, both children and adults. The preschooler attempts to behave like an adult in realistic activity and play and is beginning to learn social roles, moral responsibility, and cooperation, although he or she still grabs, hits, and quarrels for short bursts of time.

If the child has the opportunity to resolve the Oedipal triangle, to establish a sense of gender, and to identify with mature adults, if the attitude about self is sound and positive, and if he or she has learned to trust and have some self-control, he or she is ready to take on the culture. The preschooler begins to decide what kind of person he or she is, and self-concept, ego strength, and superego will continue to mature. Self is still very important, but he or she does not feel omnipotent.

Developmental Crisis

The psychosexual crisis for this era is initiative versus guilt, and all the aforementioned behaviors are part of achieving initiative (26). **Initiative** is *enjoyment of energy displayed in action, assertiveness, learning, increasing dependability, and ability to plan.* Natural initiative is desirable; however, it is important for parents not to expect too much or to push the child excessively. Studies indicate that teachers can identify Type A behaviors in young children (competitiveness, impatience, hostility, pseudoleadership) and that these children have a cardiovascular responsivity similar to adults with Type A behavior. Some of the Type A behavior may be the result of innate temperament, but parental practices or behavior may also have an influence (10, 11).

If the child does not achieve the developmental task of initiative, there is an overriding sense of guilt from the tension between the demands of the superego, or expectations, and actual performance.

Guilt is a *sense of defeatism, anger, feeling responsible for things that he or she is not really responsible for, feeling easily frightened from what he or she wants to do, feeling bad, shameful, and deserving of punishment.* A sense of guilt can develop from sibling rivalry, lack of opportunity to try things, or restriction on or lack of guidance in response to fantasy or when parents interfere with the child's activity. They stifle initiative by doing things for the child or by frequently asking, "Why didn't you do it better?" If the guilt feelings are too strong, the child is anxious and easily frightened, and he or she cannot organize activity and cannot do what he or she is neuromuscularly, mentally, and socially ready to do. Such a child develops a rigid superego that exercises strong control over behavior but at the same time feels resentment and bitterness toward the restrictive adult. Excessive guilt and lack of initiative development may be shown in a variety of behaviors: poor motor coordination, stammering speech, fears, nightmares, eating and elimination problems, irritability, regressed behavior, inability to separate from mother without panic, fear of strangers, temper tantrums, or lack of interest in peers or childhood activities.

You can help parents understand that if the child is to develop a sense of initiative and a healthy personality, they and other significant adults must encourage use of imagination, creativity, activity, and plans. Punishment must be limited to those acts that are truly dangerous, morally wrong, socially unacceptable, or with a harmful or unfortunate consequence for self or others. Parents should encourage the child's efforts to cooperate and share in the decisions and responsibilities of family life. The child develops best when he or she is commended and recognized for accomplishments. Appropriate behavior should be reinforced so that it will continue. Affirming a child's emotional experience is as important as affirming his or her physical development. Parents should set aside a time each day, perhaps near bedtime, for the child to review emotional experiences. If there has been joy, pride, or anger, it can be recounted to the parents. In talking, the child conjures up the feelings once again and integrates these feelings with the event. This promotes emotional growth. The preschooler needs to learn what feelings of love, hate, joy, and antagonism are and how to cope with and express them in ways other than physically. He or she needs guidance toward mature behavior.

Self-Concept: Body-Image and Sexuality Development

Self-concept, including body image, is gradually developing in these years. Positive self-concept develops from parental love, effective relations with peers and others, success in play and other activities, and gaining skills and self-control in activities of daily living. Body boundaries and sense of self become more definite to the preschooler because of developing sexual curiosity and awareness of how he or she differs from others, increased motor skills with precision of movement and maturing sense of balance, improved spatial orientation, maturing cognitive and language abilities, ongoing play activities, and relationship identification with his or her parents.

The pleasurable feelings associated with touching the body and genitals and with masturbation and play involving rocking or riding toys heighten self-awareness but also anxiety and anticipation of punishment. If the child is threatened or punished because of sexual curiosity, he or she may repress feelings about and awareness of the genitals or other body parts and develop a distorted body image. Of course, he or she must be taught that society does not condone handling of genitals in public. The preschooler must be able to stroke the body with affection; he or she needs adult caresses as well.

Learning about the body, where it begins and ends, what it looks like, and what it can do, is basic to the child's identity formation. Included in the growing self-awareness is discovery of feelings and learning names for them. The child is beginning to learn how he or she affects others and others' responses, and he or she is learning the rudiments of control over feelings and behavior. The concept of body is reflected in the way the child talks, draws pictures, and plays. The child with no frame of reference in relation to self has increased anxiety and misperception of self and others. Fantasies about self affect later behavior.

Parental and cultural attitudes about sex-appropriate behavior for boys and girls may heighten anxiety and body-image confusion, especially if the child's behavior and appearance do not match the expectations of others.

The artistic productions of the preschooler tell us about self-perceptions. The 3-year-old draws a man consisting of one circle, sometimes with an appendage, a crude representation of the face, and no differentiation of parts. The 4-year-old draws a man consisting of a circle for a face and head, facial features of two eyes and perhaps a mouth, two appendages, and occasionally wisps of hair or feet. Often the 4-year-old has not really formulated a mental representation of the lower part of the body. The 5-year-old draws an unmistakable person. There is a circle face with nose, mouth, eyes, and hair; there is a body with arms and legs. Articles of clothing, fingers, and feet may be added. The width of the person is usually approximately one half the length (22, 32, 33). The child may think of the body as a house (46). For example, while eating, he or she may name the various bites as fantasy characters who will go down and play in his or her house. The child may create an elaborate play area for them. (You can take advantage of this fantasy if eating problems arise.)

When the 3-year-old is asked his or her gender, the child is likely to give his or her name; the 4-year-old can state gender, thus showing a differentiation of self.

Discuss with the parents the concept of body image and how they can help the child's formulation of self. The child needs opportunities to learn the correct names and basic functions of body parts and to discover his or her body with joy and pride. Mirrors, photographs of the child, weighing, and measuring height enhance the formation of his or her mental picture. The child needs

physical and mental activity to learn body mastery and self-protection and to express feelings of helplessness, doubt, or pain when the body does not accomplish what he or she would like or during illness. The preschooler needs to manipulate the tools of his or her culture to learn the difference between self and machines, equipment, or tools. The child needs to be encouraged to "listen" to the body—the aches of stretched muscles, tummy rumblings, stubbed toes—and to understand what he or she feels. To deny, misinterpret, misname, or push aside physical or emotional activities and feelings promotes an unrealistic self-understanding and eventually a negative self-concept and unwhole body image. Specific nursing measures after illness or injury help the child reintegrate body image (8, 22, 51, 53, 56, 77).

Adaptive Mechanisms

Development proceeds toward increasing differentiation, articulation, and integration. **Differentiation** *involves a progressive separation of feeling, thinking, and acting and an increased polarity between self and others.* Differentiation is seen in the child's ability to **articulate** or *talk about the perceived experience of the world and the experience of self as a being.* **Integration** is seen in the *development of structured controls and adaptive or defensive mechanisms* (42, 51, 71).

With increasing differentiation, articulation of language, perceptions, and experience, and integration of experience and adaptive mechanisms into self, the child is better able to talk about fears and other feelings. The infant demonstrates behaviorally and through crying that he or she fears sudden movements, loud noises, loss of support, flashing lights, pain, strange people, objects, or situations, and separation from familiar people. The toddler's fears of being alone, the draining bathtub, the vacuum cleaner, the dark, dogs or other animals, high places, insecure footing, and separation from familiar people are expressed behaviorally and vocally, although the adult may have difficulty determining which fear is being expressed because of imprecise language skills. The preschooler has gained both language and conceptual ability, greater experience, and a greater imagination. Now he or she can talk about and play out the fears of being alone, ghosts, masks, the dark, strange noises, strangers, dogs, tigers, spiders, bears, and snakes, closed places, thunderstorms, and separation from loved ones. These fears decline by age 5 but may persist until age 7 or 8.

What the preschool child sees through the media or hears in stories (including traditional fairy tales) may produce great fear. The child has no way of knowing, unless explanations are given, that the big bad wolf will not eat him or her, or that the Indians attacking wagon trains will not attack his or her home next. Fears of ghosts, monsters, robbers, kidnappers, and other fantasized characters last through the preschool years until age 7 or 8, especially if parents do not talk about them and help the child differentiate between reality and imagination. Help parents realize that to instill realistic fear is adaptive: viewing and reading experiences that do not emphasize violence, bad people, or fearsome objects or animals, but rather gentle and calm experiences, are helpful for the child to gain a sense of self-control over fears.

The child encounters a variety of frustrations as he or she engages in new activities, expects more of self, and others expect more of the child. Disappointments arise. The child must learn to cope with frustrations just as he or she learns to handle and overcome fears. Teach parents that they can help by (1) showing concern and acceptance of the child's feelings; (2) helping the child talk about the feelings; (3) exploring with the child possible causes for the feelings; (4) helping the child realize that emotions have reasons and that they can discover causes for personal feelings; (5) emphasizing that the child is neither expected to be perfect nor should expect that everything will always go as desired; and (6) helping the child make a decision about handling the frustrating situation, thus learning problem-solving strategies. How the parent handles frustrations and problems sets an example for the child.

During the preschool years certain adaptive mechanisms are at a peak. They include introjection, primary and secondary identification, fantasy, and repression. These mechanisms may be used in other developmental eras to aid or hinder adjustment. Mechanisms previously discussed are also used in response to situations.

Introjection, *taking attitudes, information, and actions into the self through empathy and learning,* along with primary identification (imitation) are essential for secondary identification to occur. Through **secondary identification** the *child internalizes standards, moral codes, attitudes, and role behavior, including gender, as his or her own, and in his or her own unique way.*

Through **fantasy,** or *imagination,* the child handles tension and anxiety related to the problems of becoming socialized into the culture, family, and peer group. As the child mentally restructures reality to meet personal needs, he or she is gradually learning how to master the environment realistically. Because the child has difficulty distinguishing between wish and reality, parents must be gently realistic when necessary without shattering fantasies when they are needed or cause no problem. Parents must realize that an active imagination is normal at this age and provides tension release.

The child has fantasies about many things, shown in fondness for fairy tales and in the fears expressed. Some cultures allow magic, symbols, and fantasy to play a significant part in life; all cultures retain some. If the child is forced to distinguish reality too early or too quickly, if imaginings are not accepted, and if creativity is not encouraged, he or she is likely to lose the attri-

butes that contribute to the creative adult—a personal and social loss to be avoided.

Repression occurs as the culture and parents continue to insist firmly on reality and following the rules. Excessive repression is related to guilt feelings, harsh punishment, or perceived strong disapproval and will later interfere with memories of this period and result in constricted creativity and restricted behavior. Some repression such as that related to the Oedipal conflict is necessary to free the child's energies for new tasks to be learned.

You can help parents understand the processes of differentiation, articulation, and integration as related to emotional development, ways to help the child learn coping skills, and the normality and importance of these adaptive mechanisms.

Moral-Spiritual Development

A great influence on the child during these early years is the parents' attitude toward moral codes, the human as creative being, spirituality, religion, nature, love of country, the economic system, and education. They convey to the child what is considered good and bad, worthy of respect or unworthy. With the developing superego and imitation of and identification with adults, the child is absorbing a great deal of others' attitudes and will retain many of them throughout life. He or she is also beginning to consider how his or her actions affect others.

There are some general considerations you may find helpful pertaining to moral and religious education. The child cannot be kept spiritually neutral. He or she hears about morals and religion from other people and will raise detailed questions about the basic issues of life: Where did I come from? Why am I here? Why did the bird (or Grandpa) die? Why is it wrong to do . . . ? Why can't I play with Joey? How come Billy goes to church on Saturday and we go to church on Sunday? What is God? What is heaven? Mommy, who do you like best: Santa Claus, the Easter Bunny, the tooth fairy, or Jesus? These questions, often considered inappropriate from the adult viewpoint, should not be lightly brushed aside, for how they are answered is more important than the information given.

Example is the chief teacher for the child; if adult actions do not match the words, he or she quickly notices and learns the action. For the child, the parent is like God, omnipotent. Parents would be wise to remember this and try to live up to the high ideals of the child while at the same time introducing him or her to the reality of the world, for example, that parents do make mistakes. Talking with the child about such a mistake and asking forgiveness (if the child was wronged) will help him or her understand the redeeming power of a moral code, religion, or an ideal philosophy.

There are two major methods of religious education: indoctrination or letting the child follow the religion of his choice. Help parents realize that neither meets the real issues. The preschooler does not follow any religion because he or she understands it but because it encompasses daily life, offers concomitant pleasure, and is expected of him or her. The preschooler accepts the religion of the parents because to the child they are all-powerful. He or she is trusting and literal in the interpretation of religion. The first religious responses are social in nature; bowing the head and saying a simple prayer is imitated but is like brushing teeth to the young preschooler. The child likes prayers before meals and bedtime, and the 3-year-old may repeat them like nursery rhymes. The 4-year-old elaborates on prayer forms, and the 5-year-old makes up prayers.

Interpretation of religious forms and practices, influenced by the child's mental capacity and experiential contact, is marked by mental processes normal for the age: (1) egocentricism; (2) **anthropomorphism,** *in which the child relates God to human beings he or she knows;* (3) fantasy rather than causal or logical thinking; and (4) animism. The child thinks either God or human beings are responsible for all events. God pushes clouds when they move; wind is God blowing; thunder is God hammering; the sun is God lighting a match in the sky.

Thus the child needs consistent, simple explanations matched with the daily practices and religious ceremonies, rituals, or pictures. Encourage parents to discuss religion and related practices with the child. The preschool child is old enough to go to Sunday school, vacation Bible school, or classes in religious education that are on an appropriate level for the child. Religious holidays raise questions, and the spirit of the holiday and ceremonies surrounding it should be explained. In America where Christmas and Easter have become secularized and surrounded with the myths of Santa Claus and Easter Bunny, the child's fantasy and love of parties are likely to minimize the religious significance of the days. There is no harm to moral-religious development in telling the child about these myths so long as they are used to convey the religious spirit of the days rather than used as an end in themselves. The child thinks concretely, and embodiments of ideas such as the material objects used in any religion convey abstract meanings that words alone do not. When he or she expresses doubt about the myths, a more sophisticated explanation may be presented.

Conscience, or Superego, Development

This development is related to moral-religious training, discipline, conditioning of behavior (smiles, loving words), modeling of parents and others for correct behavior, being given reasons for behavior, and other areas of learning. The **superego,** *that part of the psyche that is critical to the self and enforces moral standards,* forms as a result of identification with parents and an introjection of their standards and values, which at first are questioned (46). At this point the child is in the Pre-

conventional Period, Stage 2, of moral development (see Chapter 5, Table 5–4). The preschooler usually behaves even if there is no external authority standing around to avoid disapproval, although he or she will slip at times. The superego can be cruel, primitive, and uncompromising. The child can be overobedient or resentful because parents do not live up to what the child's superego demands. The child is likely to overreact to punishment. This all-or-nothing quality of the superego is normally tempered later; a strict superego does not necessarily mean that the child has strict parents, but rather that he or she perceives them as strict. It is the result of the child's interpretation of events, teaching, admonitions, demands of the environment, discipline, punishment, fears, and guilt and anxiety about fantasized and real deeds.

Superego development will continue through contact with teachers and other significant adults through the years. If the superego remains too strict, self-righteous, or intolerant of others, the person in adulthood will develop a reaction formation of moralistic behavior so that prohibition rather than initiative will be a dominant pattern of behavior.

If the superego does not develop and if no or few social values are internalized, the child will be increasingly regarded as mischievous or bad in his or her behavior. Eventually he or she may have no guilt feelings and no qualms about not following the rules. The child is then on the way to truancy, delinquency, or becoming mentally ill, emotionally inadequate and unable to form mature relationships or follow social or ethical standards.

The child continues the moral development previously begun—learning a greater sense of responsibility, empathy, mercy, compassion, and fairness. The parents are the major teachers as they relate to the child fairly with compassion and gentleness. They teach also by being reliable and responsive. Further, they teach when they point out to the child the consequences of his or her behavior to others. If the child hurts another child physically or emotionally, the child needs to know that. Then the child learns an appropriate sense of guilt. That does *not* mean that the parent abuses the child or uses brute force to teach pain. Rather, discussion and reasoning, along with asserting authority (restraining and calming an angry, aggressive child) when necessary, are ways to influence positively the child's moral outlook. Withdrawal of love and physical punishment are not effective ways to teach moral behavior. In response to physical punishment, the child acts out even more physically or verbally from the consequent anger. Withdrawal of love results in a terrified, withdrawn, passive child who cannot respond to messages to be caring to others (63). If the child feels valued and values self, he or she will in turn treat other people, animals, the environment, and things as if they are valuable.

Discuss with parents the importance of superego

development and beginning moral development during this period. Share the preceding information.

Developmental Tasks

In summary, the developmental tasks for the pre-schooler are the following:

1. Settle into a healthful daily routine of adequately eating, exercising, and resting.
2. Master physical skills of large- and small-muscle co-ordination and movement.
3. Become a participating member in the family.
4. Conform to other's expectations.
5. Express emotions healthfully and for a wide variety of experiences.
6. Learn to communicate effectively with an increasing number of others.
7. Learn to use initiative tempered by a conscience.
8. Develop ability to handle potentially dangerous sit-uations.
9. Lay foundations for understanding the meaning of life, self, the world, and ethical, religious, and phil-osophical ideas (25).

Discuss with parents how these tasks may be achieved and encourage them to talk about their concerns or problems as they help the child mature in these skills.

When the preschool child becomes more realistic, relinquishes some fantasies, substitutes identity for rivalry with the parent of the same sex while seeking admiration of the parent of the opposite sex, and feels a sense of initiative rather than excessive guilt, he or she is ready to enter the period of latency.

If maladaptive behavior such as failure in language development, destructiveness, or excessive bedwetting persists, the parents and child need special guidance. You can obtain information on causes, associated behavior, and care for these and other special problems from a pediatric nursing book.

Nursing Applications

Your role with the preschooler and family has been discussed in each section throughout this chapter. Box 9–5 lists some *nursing diagnoses* that may apply to the preschooler based on assessments that would result from knowledge presented in this chapter. Interventions include your role modeling of caring behavior to the preschooler and family; child, parent, and family education, support, and counseling; or direct care to meet the preschooler's physical, emotional, cognitive, social, or spiritual and moral needs.

Because child abuse, especially sexual abuse, is epidemic in this country, some detail about the nurse's role is described. It is critical that the nurse and other health team members intervene to protect the child and work

---

■ BOX 9-5.
Selected Nursing Diagnoses Related to the Preschooler[a]

Pattern 1: Exchanging

Altered Nutrition: More than body requirements
Altered Nutrition: Less than body requirements
Altered Nutrition: Potential for more than body requirements
Potential for Infection
Potential for Injury
Potential for Poisoning
Potential Impaired Skin Integrity

Pattern 2: Communicating

Impaired Verbal Communication

Pattern 3: Relating

Impaired Social Interaction

Pattern 5: Choosing

Impaired Adjustment

Pattern 6: Moving

Sleep Pattern Disturbance
Feeding Self-care Deficit
Toileting Self-care Deficit
Altered Growth and Development

Pattern 7: Perceiving

Body Image Disturbance
Self-esteem Disturbance
Sensory/Perceptual Alterations
Unilateral Neglect
Hopelessness

Pattern 8: Knowing

Knowledge Deficit

Pattern 9: Feeling

Pain
Anxiety
Fear

[a]Other NANDA diagnoses are applicable to the ill preschooler. From North American Nursing Diagnosis Association, *NANDA Nursing Diagnosis Taxonomy I* (Rev.). St. Louis: North American Nursing Diagnosis Association, 1990.

---

with the family to improve parenting. Neither the child who is being abused nor the abusive family can develop and mature normally. The same is true for the family in which the child has been abused by someone from outside the family.

Assessment must be done carefully. The TRIADS checklist assesses the dimensions of child abuse. This acronym represents the assessment areas of:

Type of abuse (physical, psychologic, sexual)

Role relationship of victim to offender (intrafamilial or extrafamilial)

Intensity of abuse (way abuse began and ended, number of times abuse occurred, and number of offenders involved)

Autonomic response of the child

Duration of abuse (length of time over which abuse occurred, ranging from days to years)

Style of offender or abuse

Style of abuse relates to the offender's techniques and access to the child (13): (1) whether it occurs spontaneously and explosively and without anticipation on the part of the child; (2) if there are antecedent cues that alert the child to a series of acts; or (3) if acts are repetitively patterned, ritualistic, or ceremonial to control how the child can act.

If you suspect abuse, establish rapport and talk with the child alone. However, do not pry. If the child finds it difficult to talk, gently offer to draw some pictures or play with the child to gain information as follows:

1. What has happened to you? The child may not answer because he or she (a) thinks abuse is normal, (b) is terrified that parents will be more abusive if they knew he or she told, (c) feels loyalty to the parents and fears desertion, or (d) believes abuse is deserved.
2. Tell me everything that happened just before that.
3. Has anyone ever told you to take off your panties?
4. Has anyone ever put his or her finger (or another object) between your legs?
5. Does anyone ever get in bed with you at night?

Obtain information related to the points on the TRIADS checklist. Such information must also be obtained if incest is the issue.

When you talk with the parents about the subject of child abuse, do not give the impression that you are criticizing them, trying to impart your own values, or acting as their judge. Putting them on the defensive will not make them cooperate, and it may keep them from accepting help from other health care professionals. Do your best to be tolerant and understanding. Try to determine how realistically they perceive the child, how they cope with the stresses of parenting, and to whom they turn for support. As you talk, attempt to get the parents' answers to the following questions (13, 27, 79):

1. What do you do when he or she cries too much? If that does not work, what do you do?
2. Does the child sleep well? What do you do when he or she does not sleep?
3. How do you discipline him or her?
4. How do you feel after you have disciplined the child?
5. Are you ever angry because the child takes up so much of your time?

6. Does he or she take up more time than your other children or require more disciplining? If yes, why?
7. Do you think he or she misbehaves on purpose?
8. Whom do you usually talk to when your child upsets you? Is that person available now?
9. Was this child planned? (Do not assume that every woman who wanted an abortion or could have gotten one did so.)
10. Did both you and your partner want this child?
11. Does the child remind you of a relative or former spouse that is disliked? (Explore this possibility with gentle questions: "It must be really upsetting for you when he acts like his father. What goes through your mind then?" "In what ways is she like your mother? Do those characteristics irritate you?").

As you discuss things, try to determine what the situation is at home. Does one or both of the parents seem unduly distressed? Perhaps they are facing other stresses with which they cannot cope such as a job loss, loneliness, illness, or alcoholism.

Explain your suspicions to the parents, obtain necessary information, and indicate you want to help. The parents may be relieved that someone recognized the problem. However, they may also object strenuously and try to take the child home. The doctor may have to get an order from the police or other legal authorities to retain the child.

If you suspect sexual abuse, find out the following from the parents;

1. What words or names does the child use to describe various body parts?
2. What are the names of family members and frequent visitors?
3. Who babysits for the child?
4. What are the family's sleeping arrangements?
5. Does the child have behavioral problems such as excessive masturbation?
6. Does the child have any phobias or excessive fears of any person or place? Any nightmares?

Parents may not be involved in the sexual abuse and may be unaware of its occurrence. Work up gradually to the subject of their child's being abused. Inform them of your suspicions in private and without judgment. Do not bombard the parents with questions they will interpret as accusatory. Offer your support, telling them of your concern for the child. Suggest counselors who would be helpful for the child and parents. Give them ideas on how to help the child work through feelings about the trauma. Advise parents not to punish or scold the child when he or she works through emotions through masturbation or by playing with dolls (13, 79).

A pelvic examination is necessary if the child has been sexually abused; however, this procedure should be done carefully after explanation is given to the child, questions are answered, rapport is established, and the child feels some sense of security. A visual examination of the whole body, including the genital and rectal regions, should be done before a pelvic examination. Allow plenty of time for every step of the examination. The prepubescent vagina is extremely sensitive, and the doctor may want to sedate or anesthetize the child before the examination. A sterile plastic medicine dropper lubricated with sterile water should be used to obtain specimens. A nasal speculum or infant-sized vaginoscope, lubricated with water and warmed, can be used with the young child. Test the child for venereal disease (girls who are past menarche should be tested for pregnancy) (13, 79).

You are a key factor in *intervention*. However, do not engage in rescue fantasies. You are limited in what you can do, although reporting to the appropriate professionals is necessary action for intervention.

Interventions for the abused child include the following (12, 13, 27, 47, 55):

1. Relaxation techniques and psychopharmacology to reduce hyperactivity, nightmares, enuresis, and startle responses—sensory disruption
2. Thought stopping, clarification, and reframing of beliefs and linking distress directly to the trauma experience to reduce perceptual-cognitive disruptions
3. Desensitizing the child to fearful involvement with others, focused role playing to discriminate threatening exploitative behavior from safe behavior, and empathy training to reduce interpersonal disruption

Treatment objectives for the sexually abused child include the following, using play therapy:

1. Child will express feelings about being sexually abused.
2. Child will reenact incidents of sexual trauma; anatomic dolls will be used for the child to show where she or he has been touched by the adult and to allow the child to vent anger felt for the adult.
3. In an appropriate but satisfying way, child will diffuse anger, shame, humiliation, tension from secrecy, fear, and guilt and work through feelings of being damaged.
4. Child will learn to respect her or his body and the right to have physical and psychologic boundaries.
5. Child will learn to improve judgment process with adults and strangers and to handle sexual confrontations.
6. Child will demonstrate less acting out at school or home.
7. Child will discuss bad dreams and nightmares to be reassured of safety.

Crayons, paints, chalkboards, punching bags, bean bags, and dolls are media to use in treatment. Simple teaching tools, basic vocabulary, and keen observation are essential. Repetition of stories, re-creation of tele-

phone conversations with the perpetrator, and drawing and painting are essential for beginning resolution (27, 55).

If you are in a health care facility and suspect child abuse, report it to the doctor and appropriate health team members. Also report your suspicions to the proper agency—the police, the district attorney's office, a child-protective service, or a social service group. *Carefully document all evidence of abuse,* your interview of and actions with parents and child, any agencies or persons contacted about the abuse, and any agencies to which the parents were referred. All 50 states and the District of Columbia provide immunity to professionals who report suspected or actual abuse. In some states failure to report abuse is a crime (79).

List the names of children who are repeatedly brought to the hospital with injuries. Make sure the notes on the chart include what the parents said, how they reacted, and how they explained the accident. Provide other hospitals in the area with the names on file. Urge them to do the same with their files. Take the time to check with other hospitals when you have a case you question (79).

A neglected child needs help as much as one who has been abused. Careful assessment and interviewing of child and parents are essential. Notify your community's child protection service and document thoroughly your findings and interventions. Many of the guidelines described above are applicable.

REFERENCES

1. Alexander, M., and J. Blank, Factors Related to Obesity in Mexican-American Preschool Children, *Image,* 20, no. 2 (1988), 79–81.
2. Anderson, M., The Mental Health Advantages of Twinship, *Perspectives in Psychiatric Care,* 23, no. 3 (1985), 114–116.
3. Bander, L.K., et al., Dietary Lead Intake of Preschool Children, *American Journal of Public Health,* 73, no. 7 (1983), 789.
4. Bartlett, A., et al., Controlled Trial of *Giardia lamblia:* Control Strategies in Day Care Centers, *American Journal of Public Health,* 81, no. 6 (1991), 1001–1006.
5. Bates, B., *A Guide to Physical Examination and History Taking* (4th ed.). Philadelphia: J.B. Lippincott, 1987.
6. Bell, D., et al., Illness Associated with Child Day Care: A Study of Incidence and Cost, *American Journal of Public Health,* 78, no. 4 (1988), 479–484.
7. Bettelheim, B., *A Good Enough Parent: A Book on Child-Rearing.* New York: Alfred A. Knopf, 1987.
8. Blaesing, S., and J. Brockhaus, The Development of Body Image in the Child, *Nursing Clinics of North America,* 7 no. 4 (1972), 601–607.
9. Bonner, A., and R. Dale, *Giardia lamblia:* Day Care Diarrhea, *American Journal of Nursing,* 86, no. 9 (1986), 918–920.
10. Brown, M., and C. Tanner, Type A Behavior and Cardio-

vascular Responsivity in Preschoolers, *Nursing Research,* 37, no. 3 (1988), 152–155.

11. ——, and C. Tanner, Measurement of Type A Behavior in Preschoolers, *Nursing Research,* 39, no. 4 (1990), 207–211.

12. Burgess, A., Intra-Familial Sexual Abuse. In Campbell J., and I. Humphreys, eds., *Nursing Care of Victims of Family Violence.* Reston, Va: Reston Publishing, 1984.

13. ——, C. Hartman, and S. Kelley, Assessing Child Abuse: The TRIADS Checklist, *Journal of Psychosocial Nursing and Mental Health Services,* 28, no. 4 (1990), 6–14.

14. ——, M. McCausland, and W. Wolbert, Children's Drawings as Indicators of Sexual Trauma, *Perspectives in Psychiatric Care,* 19, no. 2 (1981), 50–58.

15. ——, et al., Child Molestation: Assessing Impact in Multiple Victims (Part I), *Archives of Psychiatric Nursing,* 1, no. 1 (1987), 33–39.

16. Cadman, D., et al., The Usefulness of the Denver Developmental Screening Test to Predict Kindergarten Problems in a General Community Population, *American Journal of Public Health,* 74, no. 110 (1984), 1093–1097.

17. CDC Endorses Plan to Inoculate All US Children for Hepatitis B, *Nation's Health* (July 1987), 12–13.

18. Chorba, T., et al., Control of a Non-Foodborne Outbreak of Salmonellosis: Day Care in Isolation, *American Journal of Public Health,* 77, no. 8 (1987), 979–981.

19. Critchley, D., Therapeutic Group Work With Abused Preschool Children, *Perspectives in Psychiatric Care,* 20, no. 2 (1982), 79–85.

20. De Santis, V., Nursery Rhymes: A Developmental Perspective. In Solnit, A., and P. Neubauer, eds., *The Psychoanalytic Study of the Child,* Vol. 41. New Haven, Conn: Yale University Press, 1986, pp. 601–626.

21. Dewey, K., et al., Height and Weight of Southeast Asian Preschool Children in Northern California, *American Journal of Public Health,* 76, no. 7 (1986), 806–808.

22. DiLeo, J.H., *Young Children and Their Drawings.* Springfield, Ill: Springer, 1971.

23. Doster, S., et al., Measles and Rubella: Our Remaining Responsibilities, *American Journal of Nursing,* 83, no. 5 (1983), 490–491.

24. Dreskin, W., and W. Dreskin, *The Day Care Decision: What's Best for You and Your Child.* New York: M. Evans, 1983.

25. Duvall, E., and B. Miller. *Marriage and Family Development* (6th ed.). New York: Harper & Row, 1984.

26. Erikson, E.H., *Childhood and Society* (2nd ed.). New York: W.W. Norton, 1963.

27. Federation, S., Sexual Abuse: Treatment Modalities for the Younger Child, *Journal of Psychosocial Nursing,* 24, no. 7 (1986), 21–24.

28. Foster, R., M. Hunsberger, and J. Anderson, *Family-Centered Nursing Care of Children.* Philadelphia: W.B. Saunders, 1989.

29. Frankenburg, W., et al., *Denver II—Revision and Restandardization of the Denver Developmental Screening Test.* Denver: Denver Developmental Materials, 1980.

30. Freiberg, K., *Human Development: A Life Span Approach* (4th ed.). Boston: Jones & Bartlett, 1991.

31. Garbarino, J., E. Guttmann, and J. Seeley, *The Psychologically Battered Child: Strategies for Identification, Assessment, and Intervention.* San Francisco: Jossey-Bass, 1987.

32. Gessel, A., and F. Ilg, *The Child From Five to Ten.* (rev. ed.) New York: Harper & Collins, 1977.

33. ——, et al., *The First Five Years of Life,* New York: Harper & Brothers, 1940.

34. *Health United States, 1982.* Washington, DC. U.S. Government Printing Office (1982), Publication No. PHS 83–1232.

35. Hegarty, V., *Decisions in Nutrition.* St. Louis: Times Mirror/Mosby College, 1988.

36. Heiney, S., Helping Children Through Painful Procedures, *American Journal of Nursing,* 91, no. 11 (1991), 20–24.

37. The Hennepin County Child Care Consultation Program, *American Journal of Public Health,* 76, no. 11 (1986), 1357–1358.

38. Holmes, J., and L. Magiera, *Maternity Nursing.* New York: Macmillan, 1987.

39. Hoole, A., R. Greenberg, and C.G. Pickard, *Patient Care Guidelines for Nurse Practitioners* (3rd ed.). Boston: Little, Brown, 1988.

40. Immunizations Still Important for Children, *Health Scene* (Fall 1987), 11.

41. Johansen, A., A. Leibowitz, and L. Waite, Child Care and Children's Illness, *American Journal of Public Health,* 78, no. 9 (1988), 1175–1177.

42. Kaluger, G., and M. Kaluger, *Human Development: The Span of Life* (3rd ed.). St. Louis: Times Mirror/Mosby, 1984.

43. Kelley, S., Parental Stress Response to Sexual Abuse and Ritualistic Abuse of Children in Day Care Centers, *Nursing Research,* 39, no. 1 (1990), 25–29.

44. Kempe, C., Sexual Abuse: Another Hidden Pediatric Problem, *Pediatrics,* 62 (1978), 582.

45. Lamb, M., *The Father's Role.* New York: John Wiley, 1986.

46. Lidz, T., *The Person: His and Her Development Throughout the Life Cycle* (2nd ed.). New York: Basic Books, 1983.

47. Lieske, A., Incest: An Overview, *Perspectives in Psychiatric Care,* 19, no. 2 (1981), 59–62.

48. Marzolla, J., and J. Lloyd, *Learning Through Play.* New York: Harper & Row, 1972.

49. Messer, A., *The Individual in His Family, An Adaptational Study,* Springfield, Ill: Charles C. Thomas, 1970.

50. Miller, S., *The Psychology of Play.* Harmonds-Worth, England: Penguin Books, 1974.

51. Moshman, D., J. Glover, and R. Bruning, *Developmental Psychology.* Boston: Little, Brown, 1987.

52. Piaget, J., *Origins of Intelligence in Childhood* (2nd ed.). New York: International Universities Press, 1953.

53. Pillitteri, A., *Child Health Nursing: Care of the Growing Family* (3rd ed.). Boston: Little, Brown, 1987.

54. Pipes, P., *Nutrition in Infancy and Childhood* (4th ed.). St. Louis: Times Mirror/Mosby, 1989.

55. Polk-Walker, G., What Really Happened? Incidence and Factor Assessment of Abused Children and Adolescents, *Journal of Psychosocial Nursing,* 28, no. 11 (1990), 17–22.

56. Pontious, S., Practical Piaget: Helping Children Understand, *American Journal of Nursing,* 82, no. 1 (1982), 114–117.

57. Potter, D., ed., *Assessment,* Springhouse, Penn: Intermed Communications, 1982.

58. Pridham, K., and M. Hansoen, Helping Children Deal with Procedures in a Clinic Setting: A Developmental Ap-

proach, *Journal of Pediatric Nursing,* 2, no. 2 (1987), 13–21.

59. Runyon, N., and P. Jackson, Divorce: The Impact on Children, *Perspectives in Psychiatric Care,* 24, nos. 3 and 4 (1987/1988), 101–105.

60. Sataloff, R., and C. Colten, Otitis Media: A Common Childhood Infection, *American Journal of Nursing,* 81, no. 8 (1981), 1480–1483.

61. Schilder, P., *The Image and Appearance of the Human Body.* New York: International Universities Press, 1951.

62. Schraeder, B., J. Rappaport, and L. Courtwright, Preschool Development of Very Low Birthweight Infants, *Image,* 19, no. 4 (1987), 174–178.

63. Schulman, M., *Moral Development Training: Strategies for Parents, Teachers, and Clinicians.* Menlo Park, Calif: Addison-Wesley, 1985.

64. Selekman, J., Immunization: What It's All About? *American Journal of Nursing,* 80, no. 8 (1980), 1440–1445.

65. Shapiro, L., et al., Obesity Prognosis: A Longitudinal Study of Children From Age 6 Months to 9 Years, *American Journal of Public Health,* 74, no. 9 (1984), 968–972.

66. Sherman, J., Jr., and S. Fields, *Guide to Patient Evaluation* (5th ed.). Garden City, NY: Medical Examination Publishing, 1989.

67. Shull, M.W., et al., Velocities of Growth in Vegetarian Preschool Children, *Pediatrics,* 60, no. 10 (1977), 410–417.

68. Sigroi, S., *Handbook of Clinical Intervention in Child Sexual Abuse.* Lexington, Mass: Lexington Books, 1982.

69. Stone, J., and J. Church, *Childhood and Adolescence: Psy-chology of the Growing Person* (5th ed.). New York: Random House, 1984.

70. Troy, P., et al., Sibling Visiting in the NICU, *American Journal of Nursing,* 88, no. 1 (1988) 68–69.

71. Turner, J., and D. Helms, *Lifespan Development* (4th ed.). New York: Harcourt & Brace, 1991.

72. U.S. Department of Health and Human Service, New Recommended Schedule for Active Immunization of Normal Infants and Children, *Morbidity and Mortality Weekly Report,* 35, no. 37 (September 19, 1986), 577–579.

73. Wadsworth, B., *Piaget's Theory of Cognitive and Affective Development* (4th ed.). New York: Longman, 1989.

74. Wallerstein, J., Children After Divorce: Wounds That Don't Heal, *Perspectives in Psychiatric Care,* 24, nos. 3 and 4 (1987/1988), 107–113.

75. Webb, P., Piaget: Implications for Teaching, *Theory Into Practice,* 19, no. 2 (1980), 93–97.

76. Wenger, J., et al., Day Care Characteristics Associated With *Haemophilus influenza Disease, American Journal of Public Health,* 80, no. 12 (1990), 1455–1458.

77. Whaley, L., and D. Wong, *Nursing Care of Infants and Children* (4th ed.). St. Louis: C.V. Mosby, 1990.

78. Williams, P., The Metro-Manila Developmental Screening Test: A Normative Study, *Nursing Research,* 33, no. 4 (1984), 208–212.

79. Yorker, B., The Prosecution of Child Sexual Abuse Cases, *Journal of Child Psychiatric Nursing,* 1, no. 2 (1988), 50–57.

Chapter 10

Assessment and Health Promotion for the Schoolchild

If you are concerned about yourself, plant rice. If you are concerned about your family, plant trees. If you are concerned about your nation, educate your children
—*Chinese Proverb*

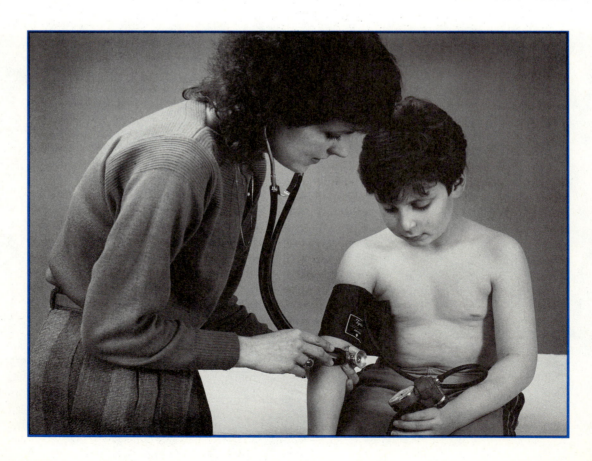

KEY TERMS

School-age years	Herpes simplex	Conservation	Collaboration
Middle childhood	Contact dermatitis	Decentering	Industry
Late childhood	Tinea corporis	Cognitive conflict	Inferiority
Juvenile period	Tinea capitis	School-phobic child	Sexuality education
Preadolescence/pre-pubescence	Warts	Gifted child	Sex education
Power-assertive discipline	Pediculosis humanus capitis	Syntaxic, consensual communication	Ritualistic behavior
Love-withdrawal discipline	Mumps	Gang	Reaction formation
Inductive discipline	Diabetes mellitus	Chum stage	Undoing
Latch key child	Rabies	Chum	Isolation
Fluoride mottling	Concrete operations	Altruism	Fantasy
Accommodative esophoria	Classification	Homosexuality	Regression
Scoliosis	Seriation	Competition	Malingering
Obesity	Nesting	Morality of constraint	Rationalization
Otitis externa	Multiplication	Compromise	Sublimation
Serous otitis media	Reversibility	Cooperation	
Allergic rhinitis	Transformation	Morality of cooperation	

OBJECTIVES

Study of this chapter will enable you to:

1. Discuss the family relationships of the schoolchild and the influence of peers and other adults on him or her.
2. Explore with the family members their developmental tasks and ways to achieve them.
3. Compare and assess the physical changes and needs, including nutrition, rest, exercise, safety, and health protection, for the juvenile and preadolescent.
4. Assess intellectual, communication, play, emotional, self-concept, sexuality, and moral-spiritual development in the juvenile and preadolescent and influences on these areas of development.
5. Discuss the crisis of school entry and ways to help the child adapt to the experience of formal education, including latch key care.
6. Discuss the physical and emotional adaptive mechanisms of the schoolchild and how they contribute to his or her total development, including meeting the developmental crisis of industry versus inferiority.
7. Discuss the significance of peers and the chum relationship to the psychosocial development of the child.
8. Explore with parents their role in communication with and guidance of the child to foster healthy development in all spheres of personality.
9. Discuss influence of media on behavior.
10. State the developmental tasks of the schoolchild and discuss your role in helping him or her to achieve them.
11. Work effectively with the schoolchild in the nursing setting.

As growth and development continue and the child leaves the confines of the home, he or she emerges into a world of new experiences and responsibilities. If previous developmental tasks have been met and the child has developed a healthy personality, he or she will continue to acquire new knowledge and skills steadily. If previous developmental tasks have not been met and the child's personality development is immature or warped, the child may experience difficulties mastering the developmental tasks of the school-age child. Peers, parents, and other adults can have a positive, maturing influence if the child is adequately prepared for leaving home, if individual needs are considered, and if he or she has some successful experiences.

The **school-age years** can be divided into **middle childhood** (*6 to 8 years of age*) and **late childhood** (*8 to 12 years of age*) (43, 126). The school-age years can also be divided into the juvenile and preadolescent periods. *At approximately age 6, the* **juvenile period** *begins, marked by a need for peer associations.* **Preadolescence** *usually begins at 9 or 10 years of age and is marked by a new capacity to love, when the satisfaction and security of another person of the same sex is as important to the child as personal satisfaction and security. Preadolescence ends at approximately 12 years with the onset of puberty. Preadolescence is also called* **prepubescence** *and is characterized by an increase in hormone production in both sexes,* which is preparatory to eventual physiologic maturity. Psychologic and social changes also occur as the child slowly moves away from the family. *This chapter discusses characteristics to assess and measure for you to use in relation to health care for the child and family* (186).

FAMILY DEVELOPMENT AND RELATIONSHIPS

Relationships With Parents

Although parents remain a vital part of the schoolchild's life, the child's position within the family is altered with his or her entry into school. Parents play a major role in socializing the child to the adult world. They contribute to the socialization process in at least five ways: (1) by assuming the role of love providers and caretakers; (2) by serving as identification figures; (3) by acting as active socialization agents; (4) by determining the sort of experiences the child will have; and (5) by participating in the development of the child's self-concept (43, 70, 98).

The schoolchild now channels energy into intellectual pursuits, widens social horizons, and becomes familiar with the adult world. He or she has identified with the parent of the same sex and through imitation and education continues to learn a social role. The family atmosphere has much impact on the child's emotional development and future response within the family when he or she becomes an adolescent. Research indicates that children can become positive in their behavior whether they are reared in either authoritarian or permissive homes if parents are consistent in their approach. The permissive child-rearing style does not necessarily produce a child with undisciplined behavior, and the authoritarian style does not necessarily produce aggressive or inhibited children (10, 101). Nevertheless the disciplinary style and parenting practices used in the home are important influences on the child, and several different disciplinary styles are used by parents. In **power-assertive discipline,** the *parent uses threats, commands, spankings, and withdrawal of privileges.* The parent controls the behavior of the child because the parent is in a position of power. With **love-withdrawal discipline,** the *parent relies on the child's fear that he or she will lose the emotional support, affection, and/or approval of the parent. The parent may also appeal to the child's reason, pride, or desire to be grown up;* this is **inductive discipline,** the form of discipline that apparently is the most effective in establishing self-regulation (70).

Although parental support is needed, the schoolchild pulls away from overt signs of parental affection. Yet during illness or when threatened by his or her new status, he or she turns to parents for affection and protection. Parents get frustrated with behavioral changes, antics, and infractions of household rules.

The romantic notion of the "typical American two-parent family with a male wage earner and a mother who stays home to care for two children" has been prevalent in the United States. This stereotype represents few American families (only 7% of school-age children) (117). It ignores the following (171):

1. Families of the millions of children whose mothers work outside home (73% of mothers with school-age children)
2. Millions of single-parent families who are more likely to be poor (25% of all children less than 18 years live with a single parent)
3. Millions of families that have at least one child with a physical, mental, or emotional handicap
4. Hundreds of thousands of children who do not have homes of their own—who live with relatives or doubled up or in shelters, which may serve as home and school
5. Millions of teenage parents, themselves merely children, struggling to raise another generation

The media report that children constitute the poorest age group in the United States, for at least 20% of all children are below the poverty line. One half of African-American children and more than one third of Latino children live in poverty. Being poor affects all dimensions of development.

However, not only poor, minority, or single-parent families need help. Many middle-class or upper-class families do not feel confident about raising their children. They may have all the help that professionals and housekeepers and nursemaids can give and may not be able to exercise effective control over what their children see on television or eat (44, 101).

Although the poor child frequently shares the helplessness of an unemployed parent, the higher-income child often feels the relentless pressure on the parent who is a high-powered corporate executive, lawyer, professor, or government official preoccupied with his or her own survival. Too often the demands of the workplace encroach on the needs and happiness of the family (44, 101).

In some families abuse, neglect, or maltreatment occur. Refer to Chapters 4, 6, 7, and 9 for background information about precipitating factors, characteristics of abusing parents, and signs, symptoms, and treatment of abuse. The research of Garbarino, Guttmann, and Seeley (54) shows that psychologic abuse or maltreatment of the school child is demonstrated by the behavior described in Box 10–1. Refer also to references 17, 18, 20, 47, 65, 103, 152, 187, 189, 216.

The **latch key child,** the *child who has the door key because no one is home when the child returns from school,* is seen increasingly since more than 70% of women with children under 18 work. Children voice different feelings about the working mother and having no one home to meet them after school. Some like it. They

BOX 10-1.
Parental Behavior Characteristic of Psychologic Maltreatment of the Schoolchild

Rejecting

- Communicates negative definitions of self to the child
- Creates a sense of "bad-me" or negative self-concept by consistently calling child negative names such as stupid, dummy, monster
- Belittles child's accomplishments regularly
- Scapegoats child in the family system

Isolating

- Removes child from normal social relations with peers
- Prohibits child from playing with or inviting children into the home
- Withdraws child from school

Terrorizing

- Places child in double bind
- Demands opposite or conflicting behavior or emotions simultaneously from the child
- Forces child to choose one of the two parents
- Changes rules of the house or of relationship with parents frequently
- Criticizes constantly so that child has no prospect of meeting expectations

Ignoring

- Fails to protect child from threats or intervene on behalf of the child
- Does not protect child from assault from siblings or other family members
- Does not respond to child's request for help or feedback

Corrupting

- Rewards child for stealing, substance abuse, assaulting other children, and sexual precocity
- Goads child into attacking other children
- Exposes child to pornography
- Encourages drug use
- Reinforces sexually aggressive behavior
- Involves child sexually with adolescents or adults

From Garbarino J., E. Guttman, and J. Seeley, *The Psychologically Battered Child: Strategies for Identification, Assessment and Intervention.* San Francisco: Jossey-Bass, 1987. Copyright 1986 by Jossey-Bass, Inc., Publishers.

sons that are usually the basis for mother working (73). Some girls say they want to work as a result, and some want to be homemakers when they grow up. More programs such as YWCA Latch Key Programs and day-care centers that provide longer hours of care are being established to accommodate the child after school. Safety measures are critical. If the child is to return home before the parent arrives, the child should be taught the following measures:

1. Teach children not to display keys and always to lock doors. Keep a spare key at a neighbor's house.
2. Tell children not to go into the house after school if the door is ajar, a window is open, or if anything looks unusual. Teach children not to open the door to anyone unless the person has been approved by the parent.
3. Teach children not to get in cars with strangers.
4. Teach children first-aid procedures and prepare a safety kit.
5. Teach safety rules to children who are expected to cook. Microwave ovens are the safest. Parents should not expect too much from the child.
6. Emphasize such fire safety rules as (a) leaving the house and not returning to it if a fire starts and practicing fire drills and evacuation at home, including determining a safe place to meet outside the home.
7. Teach children about weather-related safety: (a) stay in the house in an electric storm; (b) stay in the storm cellar or in the safest part of the house during a tornado warning (practice tornado drills with children); and (c) keep a flashlight handy in case of power failures.
8. Prevent drowning by (a) instructing children that they should never swim without adult supervision and (b) teaching older children caring for infants and toddlers about safe bathing methods.
9. Use locked storage for firearms. Instruct children that only adults may handle the firearms.
10. Teach children to tell callers that their parents are busy rather than saying "They're not here."
11. Keep police, fire department, and other important telephone numbers by the phone. Be sure children know how to report emergencies.
12. Investigate the neighborhood for families who will be at home and available for help with emergencies.
13. Establish clear rules about what may or may not be done until parent gets home.
14. Offer children a choice of activities.
15. Discuss with children what to do after school. Recommend specific activities other than television.

The child must be given time—physically, emotionally, mentally, and socially—to be a child and to learn about the world around him or her at an individual pace. Too often parents want to hurry the child into adulthood. The result will be a chronologic adult who

enjoy the solitude, privacy, responsibility, and closeness of each other at day's end. Some hate it for the same reasons. Some tolerate it out of necessity, disliking the separation and lack of time together. Some are afraid for themselves and their mothers. Some are proud of mother and how they are managing together. Some become discipline problems. All understand the financial reasons and sometimes the career and emotional reastill acts and feels like a child. Television, firms, advertisements, peers, and neighbors all exert pressure to wear adult clothes, to be sexually precocious, to manipulate parents into fewer limits and less guidance, to take technology, materialism, and money for granted, and often to participate in a multitude of after- (or before-) school activities (15). Parents believe their child must be the "early maturer." The pressures and hurry, especially in the middle-class and lower-upper-class urban family, are contributing to a growing number of troubled children who are emotionally distressed or ill or who are antisocial. The child abuses self and others with alcohol, drugs, and sexual activity. He or she also may search for peace among various cults or even through suicide. If the child must be *hurried* through childhood and if the child cannot be accepted for who he or she is, feelings of being unloved, rejected, and inferior grow ever deeper and bigger.

If we are committed to the family remaining the basic child-rearing institution—and we have not invented anything better for children than parents—our attitudes and policies must catch up with the fact that millions of Americans families need help at different times for various reasons to raise their children well. As a nurse, you care for the family and the individual. Help parents clarify and act on their values. As a school nurse, your assessment may be the key to a child's receiving necessary care since many children do not have a family doctor. You can conduct many health promotion activities described throughout this chapter. You can counsel and teach both parents and children (12, 163, 164, 180, 182). Be aware of cultural beliefs and practices as you work with children and families. A family who has lived in this country for several generations may follow the same cultural patterns as the family who is a new immigrant (151). Finally, as a citizen, your vote on action to pass health-related legislation is important and may be as crucial to health promotion as immunizations (70).

Relationships With Siblings

Although parental influence is of primary importance, the child's relationship with siblings affects personality formation. The influence of siblings on the development of the school-age child depends on a number of factors, including the age and gender of the siblings, number of children in the family, proximity of their ages and the type of parent-child interaction (125).

Relationships between the school-age child and siblings vary from jealousy, rivalry, and competition to protectiveness and deep affection. Siblings tend to get along more harmoniously when they are the same sex, but boys usually are more physically aggressive at all ages. School-age children need privacy and personal space. Quarrels and conflicts erupt when this need is violated (70, 98, 126, 129, 193). Although sibling jealousy is less acute in school-age children than in preschool children,

it still exists. An older child may be jealous of the attention given to younger siblings and may resent having to help with their care. The younger school-age child may feel jealous of the freedom given to older siblings. School-age children may feel the need to compete for parental attention and academic excellence. Parental comparisons of siblings' scholastic and artistic abilities or behavior should be avoided since they add to jealousy and resentment.

Adjustment outside the home is generally regarded as easier for the child with siblings than for the only child, who may develop a very close, intense relationship with the parents. The only child may cling to the notion of being the center of the family and may expect to be the center of attention in other groups as well. As a result, he or she may find the give and take of social living difficult (169). The differences in socialization between small and large families and for the only child is discussed in Chapter 4.

Family Development Tasks

Family activities with the school-age child revolve around expanding the child's world. Family development tasks include the following:

1. Take on parenting roles.
2. Adjust the marital system and the life-style to allow physical, emotional, and social space for the child(ren).
3. Keep lines of communication open among family members.
4. Work together to achieve common goals.
5. Plan a life-style within economic means.
6. Find creative ways to continue a mutually satisfactory married life or satisfactory single parenthood.
7. Maintain close ties with relatives.
8. Realign relationships with the extended family to include parenting and grandparenting roles.
9. Expand family life into the community through various activities.
10. Validate the family philosophy of life. The philosophy is tested when the child brings home new ideas and talks about different life-styles he or she encountered, forcing the family to reexamine patterns of living (42).

These tasks are manifested differently by families from various cultural backgrounds; those who are homeless, live in poverty, or are migrants; or those who live in war-torn or Third World countries. As you care for families and assist them to meet these tasks, consider the uniqueness of the family situation.

Adoptive families have the same developmental tasks as other families. An issue for adoptive parents, however, is how to help their adopted child(ren) feel a part of the family, especially if adoption occurs at an age when the child remembers the process.

Table 10–1 describes the adopted child's perception of adoption during the school years and how adoptive parents may respond.

The adopted child especially struggles with identity issues because of uncertainties about the past, especially when the child is of different racial or ethnic origin than parents. The adolescent may become especially rebellious, saying, for example, "I don't have to obey you—you're not my real mom." Parents must remain open to the youth's questions, sustain an accepting and open atmosphere, expect turbulence, and help him or her find other supportive adults. Parents should not smother with concern, give into unreasonable demands, or hold a grudge against the child who is acting ungratefully. (Most adolescents do.) Adoption is not a constant issue, but parents cannot ever completely retreat from it (117, 164).

Relationships Outside the Family

As the child's social environment widens, other individuals begin to function as role models and to influence the child. The child strives for independence and establishes meaningful relationships with peers, teachers, and other significant adults. These relationships provide the child with new ideas, attitudes, perspectives, and modes of behavior. Although the parents remain role models, the influence of the family and the time spent with family diminish. Parents may feel a loss of control and may actually experience ambivalent feelings toward the child's peers and new adult role models. Influences outside the family may cause the child to verbalize less love and respect for parents, to resent limits imposed by the family, and to question ideas, attitudes, and beliefs held by the family. Through contacts with the peer group, the child acquires a basis for judging the parents as individuals and learns that parents can make mistakes (43, 51, 70, 131, 169).

The schoolchild has a growing sense of community that changes with increased mobility and independence and added responsibility. His or her understanding broadens to include a sense of boundaries, distance, location, and spatial relationships of resources and organizations, demographic characteristics, and group identity (169).

As a nurse, you are in a key position to listen to and explore with families their concerns about being parents, achieving the expected developmental tasks, and adjusting to the growing and changing child as he or she interacts with parents, siblings, other relatives, peers, and other adults outside the home. At times you may validate their approach to a given situation. At other times you may help them clarify their values so they can, in turn, better guide the child. Such practical suggestions as how to plan more economically a nutritious meal or handle sibling rivalry can help a distraught parent feel and become more effective.

In the United States a large number of children live not in their own home but in facilities ranging from individual foster family and group homes to large institutions. Too many of these children are unnecessarily or prematurely removed from their homes before anyone has tried to work with or provide services to their families, who may be in poverty or unable to provide needed care but who love their children and are doing the best they can. If a poor rural family has no privy and no water, the answer is not to take away the children. Rather, your ability to maneuver the welfare system to provide a privy and a well may be the beginning of improved health for the entire family. Tens of thousands of children have been placed in inappropriate facilities for long periods of time, often away from their communities and even out of their states. They are shunted around frequently and denied a sense of permanence, loving attachments, and the chance to trust and be continuously nurtured by caring adults. They languish in twilight, often neither returned home nor provided a permanent new family through adoption (44).

Most parents try to do right by their children, but they may lack access, confidence, information, and power to deal alone with the people and institutions who could give help. Your ability to see beyond the obvious and to help the family use community resources effectively to meet basic needs is often the first step in promotion of both physical and emotional health. Your

TABLE 10-1. ADOPTED CHILD'S PERCEPTIONS AND SUGGESTED PARENTAL RESPONSES

Age (Yr)	Child's Perception	Suggested Parental Response
5–7	Begins to grasp full notion of adoption, that parents are not blood relatives, and that most children live with biologic parent(s) Feels sense of loss	Emphasize that child is important to them and was chosen. Answer questions comfortably and naturally. Explain it is normal for child to have mixed emotions about adoption.
8–11	Fantasizes and wonders about birth parents Realizes is different from nonadopted children Wants to question parents about adoption but fears appearing disloyal or ungrateful Feels grief and goes through mourning process Frequently asks questions about why birth parents relinquished him or her, parents' appearance and whether there are siblings	Discuss the adoption openly, when appropriate, to help the child vent curiosity and feelings. Help child accept fact he or she is different and emphasize other differences as well. Answer questions truthfully. Do not criticize or overpraise birth parents. Adjust depth of answer to age of child. Realize children who are not adopted also fantasize they are.

help may involve much effort over a period of time as you deal with a bureaucratic system and gain increasing empathy for the struggling family.

PHYSIOLOGIC CONCEPTS

Physical Characteristics

The child between 6 and 12 years old exhibits considerable change in physical appearance (43, 125, 126, 138, 169, 193, 206). Growth during this stage of development is hypertrophic (cells increase in size) instead of hyperplastic (cells increase in number). The growth rate is usually slow and steady, characterized by periods of accelerations in the spring and fall and by rapid growth during preadolescence (169).

Weight, Height, and Girth

These measurements vary considerably among children and depend on genetic, environmental, and cultural influences. African-American children and Caucasian children from lower socioeconomic groups usually are smaller in weight and height (166). An earlier study comparing 4167 Spanish-surnamed and 2322 non-Spanish surnamed children also suggested that growth retardation is more reflective of socioeconomic than ethnic-genetic factors. (41).

Changes in the height, weight, body mass index, triceps skinfold, and arm and estimated midarm muscle circumferences in lower socioeconomic Mexican-American children 6 through 17 years of age, from Texas, were documented on the basis of surveys done in 1972 and 1983. With the exception of height in youths aged 14 to 17, all parameters showed gains at most ages and in particular an increase in adipose tissue. These trends confirm the large proportion of relatively short but heavy children among Mexican-Americans (110).

The average schoolchild grows 2 to $2\frac{1}{2}$ inches (5 to 6 cm) per year to gain 1 to 2 feet (30 to 60 cm) in height by age 12. A weight gain of 4 to 7 pounds (2 to 3.5 kg) occurs per year. The average weight for a 6-year-old boy is 48 pounds (21.5 kg), and the average height is 46 inches (117 cm). By age 12 the average child weighs approximately 88 pounds (40 kg) and is more than 59 inches tall (150 cm). During the *juvenile* or *middle childhood period* girls and boys may differ little in size; their bodies are usually lean, with narrow hips and shoulders. There is a gradual decrease in the amount of baby fat with an increase in muscle mass and strength. Although the amount of muscle mass and adipose tissue is influenced by muscle use, diet, and activity, males usually have more muscle cells, and females have more adipose tissue. Muscle growth is occurring at a rapid rate. The muscles are changing in composition and are becoming more firmly attached to the bones. Muscles may be immature in regard to function, resulting in children's vulnerability to injury stemming from overuse, awkwardness, and inefficient movement. Muscle aches may

accompany skeletal growth spurts as developing muscles attempt to keep pace with the enlarging skeletal structure. As the skeletal bones lengthen, they become harder. Ossification, the formation of bone, continues at a steady pace. The schoolchild loses the pot-bellied, swayback appearance of early childhood. Abdominal muscles become stronger; the pelvis tips backwards and posture becomes straighter (16, 126, 169, 193, 206).

Vital Signs

Vital signs of the schoolchild are affected by size, gender, and activity. Temperature, pulse, and respiration gradually approach adult norms with an average *temperature* of 98° to 98.6° F (36.7° to 37° C), *pulse rate* of 70 to 80 per minute, resting pulse rate of 60 to 76 per minute, and *respiratory rate* of 18 to 21 per minute. The average *systolic blood pressure* is 94 to 112, and average *diastolic blood pressure* is 56 to 60 millimeters of mercury. As respiratory tissues achieve adult maturity, *lung capacity* becomes proportional to body size. Between the ages of 5 and 10, the respiratory rate slows as the amount of air exchanged with each breath doubles. Breathing becomes deeper and slower. By the end of middle childhood, the lung weight will have increased almost 10 times. The ribs shift from a horizontal position to a more oblique one; the chest broadens and flattens to allow for this increased lung size and capacity. (61, 126, 138).

Cardiovascular System

The *heart* grows slowly during this age period; the left ventricle of the heart enlarges. After 7 years of age, the apex of the heart lies at the interspace of the fifth rib at the midclavicle line. Before this age, the apex is palpated at the fourth interspace just to the left of the midclavicle line. By the age of 9, the heart weighs six times its birth weight. By puberty, it weighs ten times its birth weight. Even though cardiac growth does occur, the heart remains small in relation to the rest of the body. Because the heart is smaller proportionately to the body size, the child may tire easily. Sustained physical activity is not desirable. The schoolchild should not be pushed to run, jog, or engage in excessively competitive sports such as football, hockey, or racquetball (126, 138, 169, 193).

Hemoglobin levels are higher for Caucasians than African-Americans for 10- to 15-year-olds. In all likelihood racial differences in hemoglobin levels during childhood exist independent of nutritional values. Racial differences are consistent with those for infants, preschool children, teen-agers, pregnant women, and athletes, unrelated to nutritional variables (132).

Head

The growth of the *head* is nearly complete; head size measures approximately 21 inches (53 cm) and attains 95% of its adult size by the age of 8 or 9 years. The sinuses strengthen the structured formation of the face, reduce the weight of the head, and add resonance to the voice. The child loses the childish look as the face takes on features that will characterize him or her as an adult. Jaw bones grow longer and more prominent as the mandible extends forward, providing more chin and a place into which *permanent teeth* can erupt. Girls lose teeth earlier than boys; deciduous or baby teeth are lost and replaced at a rate of four teeth per year until approximately age 11 or 12. The "toothless" appearance may produce embarrassment for the child. The first permanent teeth are 6-year molars that erupt by age 7 and are the keystone for the permanent dental arch. Evaluation for braces should not be completed until all four 6-year molars have appeared. The second permanent molars erupt by age 14, and the third molars (wisdom teeth) come in as late as age 30. Some persons' wisdom teeth never erupt (Fig. 10–1). When the first permanent central incisors emerge, they appear too large for the mouth and face. Generally the teeth of boys are larger than those of girls (126, 169 193). Children who live in areas with high fluoride content in the drinking water may demonstrate **fluoride mottling** (*brownish permanent discoloration*) of the teeth in late childhood and adolescence (23).

Gastrointestinal System

Secretion, digestion, absorption, and excretion become more efficient. The stomach shape changes and its capacity increases. Maturity of the gastrointestinal system is reflected in fewer stomach upsets, better maintenance of blood sugar levels and an increased stomach capacity (193).

Urinary System

This system becomes functionally mature during the school years. Between the ages of 5 and 10, the kidneys double in size to accommodate increased metabolic functions. Fluid and electrolyte balance becomes stabilized, and bladder capacity is increased, especially in girls. Urinary constituents and specific gravity become similar to those of an adult. However, 5% to 20% of school-age children have small amounts of albuminuria (126, 169).

Vision

The shape of the eye changes during growth, and the normal farsightedness of the preschool child is gradually converted to 20/20 vision by age 8. By age 10 the eyes have acquired adult size and shape. Binocular vision is well developed in most children at 6 years of age; peripheral vision is fully developed. Girls tend to have poorer visual acuity than boys, but their color discrimination is superior (169). Large print is recommended for reading matter and regular vision testing should be part of the school health program.

Immune System

Lymphoid tissues reach the height of development by age 7, exceeding the amount found in adults. The body's ability to localize infection improves. Enlargement of adenoidal and tonsillar lymphoid tissue is normal, as are sore throats, upper respiratory infections, and ear infections, which are caused by the excessive tissue growth and increased vulnerability of the mucous

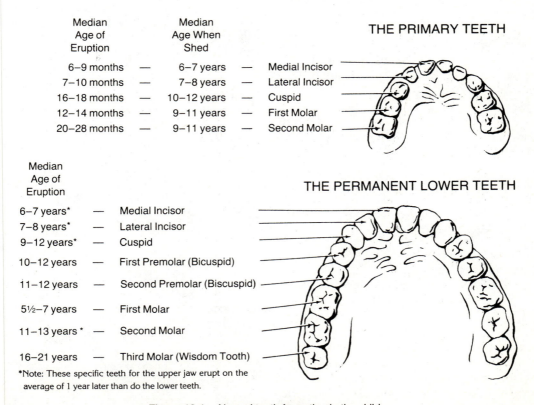

Median Age of Eruption		Median Age When Shed		
6–9 months	—	6–7 years	—	Medial Incisor
7–10 months	—	7–8 years	—	Lateral Incisor
16–18 months	—	10–12 years	—	Cuspid
12–14 months	—	9–11 years	—	First Molar
20–28 months	—	9–11 years	—	Second Molar

THE PRIMARY TEETH

Median Age of Eruption		
6–7 years*	—	Medial Incisor
7–8 years*	—	Lateral Incisor
9–12 years*	—	Cuspid
10–12 years	—	First Premolar (Bicuspid)
11–12 years	—	Second Premolar (Biscuspid)
5½–7 years	—	First Molar
11–13 years *	—	Second Molar
16–21 years	—	Third Molar (Wisdom Tooth)

*Note: These specific teeth for the upper jaw erupt on the average of 1 year later than do the lower teeth.

THE PERMANENT LOWER TEETH

Figure 10-1. Normal tooth formation in the child.

membranes to congestion and inflammation. The frontal sinuses are developed near age 6. Thereafter all sinuses are potential sites for infection. The immunoglobulins IgG and IgA reach adult levels by age 9, and the child's immunologic system becomes functionally mature by preadolescence (126, 169).

Neuromuscular Development

By age 7 the brain has reached 90% of adult size. The growth rate of the brain is greatly slowed after age 7, but by age 12 the brain has virtually reached adult size. Myelinization is complete; memory has improved. The child can listen better and make associations with incoming stimuli. Neuromuscular changes are occurring along with skeletal development. Neuromuscular coordination is sufficient to permit the schoolchild to learn most skills he or she wishes (169).

The transformation of the "clumsy" 6-year-old into the coordinated 12-year-old is due in part to maturation of the *central nervous system* and improved transmission of nerve impulses. The 6-year-old moves constantly—hopping, running, roller skating. The child walks a chalk mark with balance. Hands are used as tools in manipulative skills of hammering, cutting, pasting, tying shoes, and fastening clothes. Large letters or figures are made as he or she awkwardly grasps a pencil or crayon (169, 206).

Children of 7 have a lower *activity level* and enjoy active and quiet games. The child sees small print without difficulty, reverses letters less frequently while printing, and prints sentences. The 8-year-old moves energetically but with grace and balance, even in more active sports. Increased myelinization improves the child's reaction time and coordination. Longer arms permit more skillful throwing. He or she grasps objects better and writes rather than prints because the hands are larger and he or she has better small-muscle coordination. The 9-year-old moves with less restlessness, is skillful in manual activities because of refined hand-eye coordination, and uses both hands independently. This child strives to improve coordination and to perfect physical skills, strength, and endurance. The preadolescent, aged 10 to 12, has energetic, active, restless movements with tension releases through finger drumming or foot tapping. Skillful manipulative movements nearly equal those of the adult, and physical changes preceding pubescence begin to appear (126, 169, 206).

Prepubertal Sexual Development

During the *preadolescent* or *prepuberty period,* both males and females develop preliminary characteristics of sexual maturity. This period is characterized by the growth of body hair, a spurt of physical growth, changes in body proportion, and the beginning of primary and secondary sex characteristics (126). They demonstrate some of the same physical changes such as increased weight and height, vasomotor instability, increased perspiration, and active sebaceous glands. There is an increase in fat deposition approximately 1 year before the height spurt. These fat deposits last approximately 2 years or until skeletal growth and muscle mass increase. Females have more subcutaneous fat deposits, and the fat is lost at a slower rate, accounting for the fuller appearance of the female figure (126, 193, 206).

The girl's growth spurt begins as early as 8 years; the average is 10, and maximum height velocity· is reached around 12 years. The boy's growth spurt begins near 12 years; maximum height velocity is reached by approximately 14 years. The male grows approximately 4 inches (10 cm) per year for $2\frac{1}{2}$ years and then begins a slower rate of growth. The female grows an average of 3 inches (7.5 cm) per year until menarche begins. For both males and females, the growth spurt begins in the hands and feet and progresses to the calves, forearms, hips, chest, and shoulders; the trunk is the last to grow appreciably (126, 206).

As sebaceous glands of the face, back, and chest become active, acne (pimples) may develop. These skin blemishes are caused by the trapping of collected sebaceous material under the skin in small pores. The preadolescent and later the adolescent are concerned with their appearance; these blemishes cause considerable embarrassment. The young person and the family may resort to use of numerous techniques such as skin specialists, sun lamps, diets, makeup, lotions, and creams to alleviate this problem. Basically, the skin should be kept clean. If the problem persists, a dermatologist should be seen. To prevent the youth's withdrawal from social contact, the parents and youth should be encouraged to seek medical attention as early as possible after acne occurs. Acne is further discussed in Chapter 11.

Vasomotor instability with rapid vasodilation causes excessive and uncontrollable blushing. This condition usually disappears when physical growth is completed.

Boxes 10–2 and 10–3 list physical changes that occur in girls and boys during prepuberty or preadolescence.

■ BOX 10-2.
Physical Changes in Girls During Preadolescence

- Increase in transverse diameter of the pelvis
- Broadening of hips
- Tenderness in developing breast tissue and enlargement of areolar diameter
- Axillary sweating
- Change in vaginal secretions from alkaline to acid pH
- Change in vaginal layer to thick, gray, mucoid lining
- Change in vaginal flora from mixed to Döderlein's lactic-acid–producing bacilli
- Appearance of pubic hair from 8 to 14 years (hair first appears on labia and then spreads to mons; adult triangular distribution does not occur for approximately 2 years after initial appearance of pubic hair)

These physical changes for females are listed in the approximate sequence of their occurrence (125, 126, 138, 169, 193, 206).

BOX 10-3.
Physical Changes in Boys
During Preadolescence

- Axillary sweating
- Increased testicular sensitivity to pressure
- Increase in size of testes
- Changes in color of scrotum
- Temporary enlargement of breasts
- Increase in height and shoulder breadth
- Appearance of lightly pigmented hair at base of penis
- Increase in length and width of penis

These physical changes for males are listed in the approximate sequence of their occurrence (125, 126, 138, 169, 193, 206).

Teach parents about the physical and growth characteristics of the school-age child and the importance of nutrition, rest, immunizations, healthful activity, and regular medical and dental care. The rest of the chapter refers to variables that influence physical health.

Physical Assessment of the School-Age Child

Information will be gained from the child, the parents or caretakers, or both when assessing the child.

A child may be better at drawing than at explaining what is wrong. For example, when asked to draw a big circle where it hurts, the child can normally identify the part if given a simple outline drawing of a child.

The child over age 10 may wish to talk to the health care provider without the parent present. Being alert to the child's chronologic and developmental stage and his or her relationship with parents or caretakers will guide you in interviewing. Remember that the child is not there in isolation. Where the child lives (house or apartment, rural or urban area), how much personal space he or she has (own room, own bed), parents' marital situation, presence or absence of siblings, what is usually eaten, how much exercise and rest in 24 hours, who cares for the child after school if parents are working, and how he or she spends free time are all important in assessing the health status.

When doing a review of systems, remember to use words the child understands. For example, instead of asking if the child has ever experienced any otitis problems, simply ask as follows: Do your ears ever ache? Can you always hear when people talk to you?

In assessing skin, remember that the school-age child is subject to allergic contact dermatitis, warts, herpes type 1, ringworm, and lice. When seeing any rash, a thorough history is in order to determine the diagnosis and necessary treatment.

A considerable number of children who appear normal in a vision screening test may suffer from accommodation and convergence difficulty. Close work becomes exhausting and almost overwhelming and may be the basis for poor achievement in school. One fairly common problem, **accommodative esophoria,** *in which the eyes converge excessively in response to accommodation,* can be corrected by the use of eyeglasses for near work (49, 155).

Understanding that visual function is more than reading the 20/20 line on a Snellen chart will help you suggest a more comprehensive visual examination when a child is experiencing difficulty with school work.

Children and their parents do not always react predictably when there is a need for corrective lenses. Some children may feel self-conscious with their peers when wearing glasses. Parents may react as if the child's visual problem were a flaw and will deny it, stating that they are sure the child will outgrow the problem, ignore the information, or even go from doctor to doctor in search of reassurance.

If you are able to provide accurate information, using the principles of therapeutic communication, it will be exceedingly valuable to a child and family who are having difficulty adjusting to the need for therapy for a visual impairment. (This also holds true when therapy or a corrective device is needed on another body area.)

When assessing a child's hearing and ears, remember that hearing should be fully developed by age 5. By age 7, most children should speak clearly enough to be understood by adults. If either of these factors seems deficient, a thorough investigation into congenital or inherited disorders and how this deficiency affects daily activities and communication is in order (155).

In the young child, because the ear canal slants up, pull the auricle down, but not back as you would in an adult, when using the otoscope. Also, the ear canal is short in the young child, so take care not to insert the ear tip too far. The otoscope should be controlled so that if the young child moves suddenly, you can protect against the otoscope's hitting the ear drum. The cone of light is more indistinct in a child than in an adult (155).

Keep in mind the following as you continue assessment of the child's body systems: (1) if you think you hear fluid in the lungs, check the child's nose because sounds caused by nose fluid can be transmitted to the lungs; (2) a S_3 sound and sinus arrhythmia are fairly common in children's heart sounds; (3) a child's liver and spleen usually will enlarge more quickly than an adult's in response to disease; (4) the bladder is normally found much higher in a child than in an adult, and the kidneys can more often be palpated; (5) the genitalia should be inspected for congenital abnormalities that may have been overlooked and for irritation, inflammation, or swelling; and (6) developmental guidelines must be used to assess the nervous system, specifically language development, motor and sensory functions, and cerebral function (9, 155).

In the last 10 years musculoskeletal and posture problems, especially scoliosis detection, have gained wide attention. **Scoliosis,** *lateral curvature of the spine,* is more common in girls than in boys and is of two types, functional and structural. Ask the child to bend over and touch the toes without bending the knees and keeping the palms of the hands together. If the child has functional scoliosis, the external curve will disappear with this exercise; if it is structural, the curve will remain and sometimes become more pronounced. Early diagnosis is extremely important to arrest this problem (49, 155). Refer the child and family to an orthopedic specialist. If scoliosis is not corrected early in life, it can result in mobility problems, obstructive pulmonary disease, and problems with body image later in life.

Nutritional Needs

Although caloric requirements per unit of body weight continue to decrease for the schoolchild, nutritional requirements remain relatively greater than for the adult. (See Appendix I.) The young schoolchild requires approximately 80 calories per kilogram daily or 35 calories per pound. By age 10 there is a decrease in the calories per kilogram for both boys (45 calories/kg) and girls (38 calories/kg). An individual child may require more or fewer calories than the Recommended Dietary Allowances (RDA), depending on size, activity, and growth rate (151, 208). Therefore the total caloric range is approximately 1600 to 2200 daily. Daily caloric needs can be approximated for the child by the following formula: 1000 calories the first year plus 100 calories for each additional year (151, 208).

Protein requirement for growth is 1 g per pound or 36 to 40 g of protein daily. Vitamin and mineral requirements are similar to those for the preschool child. Because of enlargement of ossification centers in the bone, vitamin D (400 units) and a large intake of calcium (800 to 1200 mg) are needed daily. Vitamin C needs are not met as easily as other nutritional requirements (151, 208). Many of the fruit-flavored juices supply significant amounts of ascorbic acid.

Water intake may be overlooked; the schoolchild needs $1\frac{1}{2}$ to 3 quarts daily, depending on the size of the child.

Nutritional needs for the schoolchild include one or more servings daily of the foods listed in Box 10–4 (126, 151, 208).

Lunch for schoolchildren is often a cola, bag of potato chips, brownies, and ice cream. They do not eat the food provided by the school lunch program because they "do not like it." Because junk food and fast foods have also permeated the home, the child may get little else to eat. Further, schools have vending machines with junk food readily available. Thus American children eat too much salt, sugar, fat, and cholesterol, and 25% have a cholesterol level greater than 170, which is extremely high for children. By adolescence these same children will show signs of clogged arteries (176).

The school lunch program offers the child the best

> ■ **BOX 10-4.**
> **Recommended Nutritional Intake for Schoolchildren**
>
> • Meats and eggs (alternates: dry beans, dry peas, and lentils): two or more of a 2 or 3 oz serving
> • Milk (whole, skim, or powdered): 2–4 cups
> • Fruits and vegetables (including a dark green or deep yellow vegetable for vitamin A and a fruit or vegetable that contains high vitamin C): five or more servings
> • Breads and cereals: four or more servings to meet caloric needs
> • Fats and carbohydrates: use sparingly

chance for a nutritious meal. Since 1946 a federally subsidized lunch has included meat or another protein, two servings of fruit and/or vegetables, a grain, and milk for low cost or at no charge if the student is from a low-income family. However, the lunch can be high in fat (40% of total calories for the meal). Thus foods in this program should be baked, not fried (176).

Anyone over the age of 2 years should daily consume no more than 30% of their total calories in fat; however, the average person aged 6 to 19 years consumes 37% of his or her calories in fat (208).

Children eat what their parents eat. More fruits and vegetables must be eaten in the home so that children develop a taste for them, and school lunch programs must persist in serving them.

Discuss with parents the importance of a balanced diet and foods that supply specific nutrients.

Nutritional assessment is determined by obtaining a history of the child's food intake; looking at the general appearance and skin color and turgor; correlating height and weight; measuring subcutaneous tissue; checking for dental caries, allergies, and chronic illness; testing hemoglobin and hematocrit levels, and determining physical, cognitive, emotional, and social well-being (151, 208).

Eating Patterns

It is important to discuss the child's eating needs and patterns with parents so that they can provide a diet with adequate caloric intake and nutrients. By age 8 years children have increased appetites; by age 10 their appetites are similar to those of adults. Despite increasing appetites, children seldom voluntarily interrupt activities for meals. Television, sports, and other activities compete with meal times. Parents should be encouraged to establish a consistent schedule for meals and to allow their school-age child to participate in the meal planning. The schoolchild of 6 or 7 is capable of learning about healthful eating and of helping plan and prepare meals. Such activities develop a healthy sense of industry and independence in the child if they are not overdone.

Mealtime continues to cause dissension within most families. Parents are often upset by their child's terrible table manners. The young child stuffs food in his or her hands, spills it, and incessantly chatters throughout the meal. The time the family spends together eating can be much more pleasant if manners are not over-emphasized. If discipline during meals is necessary, it should be kept to a minimum. When mealtime becomes a time of stress, digestive problems, poor eating habits, or a temporary aversion to food may occur. Making a fuss over eating certain foods may cause the child to reject them more strongly. Experience and time will improve eating patterns, as shown in Table 10–2 (56, 57, 125, 193).

Food preferences and dislikes become strongly established during the school years. However, by age 8 the child will try new or previously disliked foods. Food likes and dislikes are often carried over from the eating experiences of the toddler and preschooler. In addition, it is easy for the schoolchild, influenced by peers, television commercials and other forms of advertisement, and the availability of junk food, to avoid nutritious foods and to fill up on empty calories.

The child mimics family attitudes toward food and eating. In many families food is equated with love and affection, an attitude that may result in the child's becoming overweight. Companionship and conversation at the child's level are essential during mealtime, for the child wants to talk and participate in a group. He or she especially likes picnics and eating with peers. Because food and eating are such vital social and cultural concerns, the source of a nutritional problem may be as much a psychosocial problem as a physiologic one.

Diet is also influenced by a child's activities. If the child has been active all day, he or she will be hungry and ready to eat. On the other hand, if the child has had limited activity or emotional frustrations during the day, he or she may have no appetite. The schoolchild has more freedom to move without parental supervision and often has small amounts of money to spend on candy, soft drinks, and other treats. In addition, the schoolchild is eating on his or her own for the first time. Peer influence will frequently determine the child's lunch. Schools have attempted to satisfy current eating preferences of this age group by offering a la carte selections such as french fries, hot dogs, pizza, and salads as well as balanced meals. Total and saturated fat and sodium content should be reduced in both school lunches and home meals.

Share the following suggestions with parents to improve nutrition and meal-time:

1. Make food attractive and manageable.
2. See that food intake is sufficient.
3. Provide a rest period before meals.
4. Have a firm understanding with the child that play and television do not take precedence over eating properly.
5. Between-meal snacks are necessary and enjoyed and do not interfere with food intake at meals if eaten an hour or longer before mealtime. Milk, cheese, fresh fruits and vegetables, peanut butter, and fruit juices are desirable snacks for both general nutritional needs and dental health.
6. Breakfast is crucial for providing the child with sufficient calories to start the day. The child who attends school without breakfast frequently exhibits fatigue and poor attention (169).

Undernutrition in children can be manifested in retarded growth, underweight, fatigue, lassitude, restless-

TABLE 10-2. SUMMARY OF EATING PATTERNS OF SCHOOLCHILDREN

6 Years	7 Years	8 Years	9 Years	10 Years	11 Years	12 Years
Has large appetite	Has extremes of appetite	Has large appetite	Has controlled appetite	Goes on eating sprees	Has controlled appetite	Has large appetite
Likes between-meal and bed-time snacks	Improves table manners	Enjoys trying new foods	Eats approximately an adult meal	Likes sweet foods	Improves table manners when eating in a restaurant	Enjoys most foods
Is awkward at table	Is quieter at table	Handles eating utensils skillfully	Acts more adult-like	Criticizes parents' table manners	Enjoys cooking	Has adultlike table manners
Likes to eat with fingers	Is interested in table conversation	Has better table manners away from home	Becomes absorbed in listening or talking	Has lapses in control of table manners at times		Participates in table discussions in adult-like manner
Swings legs under table, often kicking people and things	Leaves table with distraction			Enjoys cooking		
Dawdles						
Criticizes family members						
Eats with better manners away from family						

ness, irritability, and poor school performance and work output. Anorexia and digestive disturbances such as diarrhea and constipation signal improper utilization of nutrients. Poor muscular development may be evidenced by a child's posture—rounded shoulders, flat chest, and protuberant abdomen. Prolonged undernutrition may cause irregularities in dentition and may delay epiphyseal development and puberty (151, 169, 208).

Undernutrition and overnutrition may have the same causative factors: the child may be reflecting food habits of other family members; the parents and child may displace unrelated anxieties on food and mealtime; or eating may serve as a reward or punishment by both parents and child. *Overnutrition* and overweight are rarely caused by metabolic disturbances. **Obesity** is sometimes defined as an *individual who is 20% or more above ideal weight*. Obesity is the most frequent nutritional disorder of children in developed countries (208). In addition, childhood obesity can have serious social and emotional effects that may carry into adulthood (124). Prevention of childhood obesity through early nutrition education and established exercise habits is important. Forty percent of overweight 7-year-olds and 70% of overweight 10-year-olds become overweight adults. (91).

Parents should be encouraged to promote food to their children as nourishment for their bodies, not as a reward or punishment. They should promote food as necessary and enjoyable. A healthy child's appetite corresponds to physiological needs and should be a valuable index in determining intake. Too often parents expect young children to eat as much as the parents do. The child should neither be forced to eat everything on his/her plate nor made to feel guilty if second portions of mother's special dish are not eaten.

You can help parents learn about adequate nutrition for their child as well as what behavior to expect at each age. You can also aid teachers as they plan lessons on nutrition. For example, learning activities for the schoolchild could include visiting grocery stores, dairies, or farms as well as taking part in tasting parties and playing store. They could plan menus, cook various foods, and taste them. Such activities are unlimited.

Increasingly, dietary intake of excess sugar, food coloring, and other additives is being related to the child's behavior, especially hyperactivity. The whole family can benefit from natural foods, foods that have a minimum of preservatives or additives, and foods that are cooked properly (115, 168).

Rest and Exercise

There is no rule of thumb for the amount of rest a child should have. Hours of sleep needed depend on variables such as age, health status, and the day's activities. Schoolchildren usually do not need a nap. They are not using up as much energy in growth as they were earlier.

A 6-year-old usually requires approximately 11 hours of sleep nightly, but an 11-year-old may need only 9 hours (206). The schoolchild does not consciously fight sleep but may need firm discipline to go to bed at the prescribed hour. Sleep may be disturbed with dreams and nightmares, especially if he or she has considerable emotional stimulation before bedtime.

Exercise is essential for muscular development, refinement of coordination and balance, gaining strength, and enhancing other body functions such as circulation, aeration, and waste elimination. The schoolchild should have a safe place to play and simple pieces of equipment. Because there are times when bad weather will keep a child from going outside, supplies should be available that will facilitate exercise indoors.

Parents should play actively with their children sometimes. Children benefit from their parents' knowledge of various activities and are encouraged by the attention. Exercise then becomes fun, not work. In America where the child can be constantly entertained by television, parents must sometimes encourage exercise.

Review the child's rest and exercise needs with parents. At the same time, you may have an opportunity to discuss with parents how they are meeting their own needs for rest and exercise and how the parents and child can engage in activities that are mutually interesting and healthful.

Health Promotion and Health Protection

Immunizations

Immunization against measles, mumps, rubella, and polio should be given to the schoolchild if it has not been previously given. Diphtheria and tetanus toxoids combined with pertussis vaccine (DTP) and oral poliovirus vaccine (OPV) must be given as indicated in previous chapters. Booster doses of DTP should be given by 6 years of age; pertussis vaccine is not necessary for children over this age. Live measles, mumps, and rubella viruses vaccine (MMR) should be given between the ages of 11 and 12. Girls should receive rubella vaccine before they enter puberty to prevent congenital defects in the baby should they be exposed to rubella during pregnancy. Boys should be immunized against mumps before the age of 12; mumps contracted during or after puberty can cause sterility. The need for tuberculin tests depends on the prevalence of tuberculosis and the risk of exposure (2, 3, 195, 196, 206). The influenza virus vaccine, pneumococcal vaccine, and hepatitis B vaccine are recommended for children in certain high-risk groups (2, 3, 193, 206).

In the United States 20 million children under 13—almost 40% of all children—are not immunized against one or more preventable major childhood diseases. (In the developing world 95% of the children are not immunized against common contagious diseases) (195, 196, 197, 206).

Emphasize to parents the importance of immunization and record keeping. Supply parents with information about free immunization programs and school requirements for immunization. Inform them of an appropriate immunization schedule. They should know, for example, that if 7-year-old Tommy steps on a rusty nail, he is protected from tetanus because of DTP immunization at age 5. Before a child receives an immunization, he or she should be told why and where it will be given. Such explanations will elicit cooperation and help the child to understand that neither the illness nor treatment is being imposed because he or she is bad.

Safety Promotion and Injury Control

Accidents are of major concern for this age group and for younger children. Accidents are the single largest cause of deaths among schoolchildren; they are fatal nearly four times more often than cancer, the next leading cause of death. Motor vehicle accidents account for half of the accidental deaths in this age group. Other accidents that threaten children are fires, falls, drownings, and poisonings (5, 78, 130, 190, 197, 211). Even though school-age children have developed more refined muscular coordination and control, their use of bicycles, skateboards, roller skates, and sports increases their risk for injury. They are susceptible to cuts, abrasions, fractures, strains, sprains, and bruises. The incidence of injury is significantly higher in school-age boys than girls, and the death rate of boys is twice that of girls (206). Some of the injuries sustained during sporting activities may cause permanent disability because of damage to the epiphyseal cartilage or the neuromuscular system.

There is a group of children who apparently are *accident-prone*. They suffer more accidental injuries than the overall childhood population. Although the causative factors have not been completely determined, children who are overreactive, restless, impulsive, hostile, and immature are frequently found in this group (206).

Parents should be encouraged to provide more supervision and attention to these children and to repeat, even to children who are not accident-prone, cautions as necessary. The child forgets when involved in play; conceptual thinking and judgment are not well developed so that the child does not foresee dangers.

Accident prevention should be taught and enforced in school and at home. You must promote safety by helping parents and children identify and avoid hazards. The school-age child has increasing cognitive maturity, including improved ability to remember past experiences and anticipate probable outcomes of his or her actions. This makes the child a good candidate for safety instructions (206).

Safety education should include information about the hazards of risk taking and improper use of equipment. Injury prevention should address motor vehicle injuries, drownings, burns, poisonings, falls, and sports-related injuries. The child should be taught the proper use of seatbelts in motor vehicles. Safe pedestrian behavior should be emphasized by teaching the child the proper way to cross streets, how to read traffic signals, and the dangers of street play. You should stress the safety and maintenance of two-wheeled vehicles (such as bicycles) and encourage the use of safety apparel where applicable (82). Water safety and survival skills should be taught with basic swimming skills at an early age. Families who go boating must teach related safety measures to their children.

Farm children are at risk for accidental injury or death when they accompany or assist parents with farm work. Teach farm parents the following rules to reduce hazards:

1. Do not allow children as extra riders on equipment.
2. Do not allow children to play with idle machinery.
3. Leave any equipment that might fall such as front-end loaders in the down position.
4. When self-propelled machinery is parked, brakes should be locked and keys removed from the ignition.
5. Always leave a tractor power-take-off unit in neutral.
6. When starting machinery—and especially when reversing it—know where the children are.
7. Maintain machinery in good repair, particularly protective shields, and seat belts.
8. Do not permit children to operate machinery until they have completed safety training.
9. Fence farm ponds and manure pits.
10. Place fixed ladders out of reach, or fit with a special barrier; store portable ladders away from danger areas.
11. Shield dangerous machinery components and electric boxes and wiring and place out of easy reach or fit with locking devices.
12. Place warning decals on all grain bins, wagons, and trucks.
13. Maintain lights and reflectors for all equipment used on roads.
14. Do not expect children to work with farm animals or with machinery that is beyond their maturity physically or mentally (5, 201).

Children are killed not only as a result of accidents. Death by homicide has increased markedly in the United States and perhaps throughout the world. Child homicides are more common if the mother is unmarried, teenage, or a high-school dropout, and homicide rates are higher for African-Americans (210).

Meal preparation can be fun for the school-age child, but the hazards of sharp knives, hot stoves, microwave ovens (the health effect of microwave radiation leakage is still unknown [217]), and hot liquids must be kept in mind. Supervise the use of matches or flammable chemicals, and teach the child the proper behavior if clothing becomes ignited. A family-designed fire escape plan should be initiated and practiced monthly.

Most boys and girls love to climb trees; adults should teach them how to climb in the safest possible way. Explain the dangers involved in climbing electric poles, water towers, and other dangerous structures. Instruct the child in the proper use of playground equipment and in the need to pick up toys from the floor to prevent falls.

Instruct parents to keep potentially dangerous products in properly labeled receptacles. Educate the child about the dangers of taking nonprescription drugs and chemicals. Gun accidents are common during the school-age period (98). Parents who have a gun should keep it under lock and place the key in a child-proof location. Children of this age should be taught safety rules concerning guns.

You can advise parents of the hazards associated with organized contact sports; stress the use of protective head, elbow, and knee gear. Instruct the child in the proper use of sporting equipment, especially the more hazardous devices—skis, trampolines, skateboards, mopeds, and all-terrain vehicles.

You can reinforce any teaching that takes place in the home. Books, films, and creation of a mock situation can all supplement your verbal instruction. You and the parents will repeat the same cautions endlessly. Yet, caution and concern can be overdone. When a child is overly anxious about his or her welfare, tension can lead not only to accident-proneness but to being hurt worse when he or she does encounter danger. In the face of danger, panic prevents clear thinking and skillful action. In addition, overcaution stifles independence, initiative, and maturing. It is important to realize the necessity of shifting responsibility to the child with increasing age.

Responsibility for the child's health rests with the parents, but you can emphasize to parents the importance of regular examinations at a clinic or from a family physician and dentist. Every child should have a thorough preschool examination, including visual and auditory screening and posture and general health examination. Correction of health problems is essential since they may be a cause for injuries, illness, or difficulties with school work or peers. Realize that in the United States millions of children get basically no health care.

As a nurse you have a responsibility to strengthen the school health program in your community through direct services; teaching the board of education, teachers, parents, and students about the value and use of such a program in spite of costs; and working for legislation to finance and implement programs that do more than first-aid care. A school health program should supervise not only the child's physical but also emotional, mental, and social health. Instruction in personal hygiene, disease prevention, nutrition, safety, family life, and group living are of interest to the schoolchild and should be under the direction of the school nurse.

If there are chronically ill or disabled students in school, special preparation should be given to the teachers, the students, and the parents. You can promote understanding of the child and his or her condition, of the child's need to use individual potential, and of a total rehabilitation program. Several references will be helpful (16, 107, 126, 175, 181, 188, 206).

Common Health Problems: Prevention and Treatment

Although the child should now remain basically healthy, health problems do exist.

Inform parents of the need to treat both acute and chronic conditions. *Respiratory conditions* (colds, sore throats, and earaches) account for more than 50% of the reported acute illnesses among children in this age group. *Infective and parasitic diseases* (scabies, impetigo, ringworm, and head lice) are of concern because of their health threat to the child and to others. *Diseases of the digestive tract* (stomachaches, peptic ulcers, colitis, diarrhea, and vomiting) may have a psychosocial and a physiologic cause. Visual and hearing impairment, sickle cell anemia, asthma, hyperactivity, epilepsy, migraine headaches, hypertension, diabetes mellitus, and obesity are *chronic health problems* that may affect the school-age child (160, 215). The child may have been born with a congenital anomaly that can be only partially corrected or a disease such as hemophilia that needs continuing treatment. A considerable number of schoolchildren have risk factors that in adults are predictive of coronary heart disease: hypertension, increased serum cholesterol and triglycerides, and obesity. The elementary school population may also be the main reservoir of infectious hepatitis type A, for schoolchildren often have a mild undiagnosed disease that is spread person to person (72).

Because of the short urethra, girls are prone to *urinary infection;* this may be diagnosed by reddened genitals, a feeling of burning on urination, and an abnormal appearance and chemical analysis of the urine. Normal urinary output from 6 to 12 years is from 500 ml to the adult output of 1500 ml daily. Pinworms accompany urinary tract infections in approximately 50% of the cases (72).

The 7-year-old has fewer illnesses but may complain of *fatigue* or *muscular pain*. It is common to call these "growing pains"; however, this is not accurate since growing is not painful. Tension, overactivity or exertion, bruising, or injury may cause the leg pains. Pains in the knees with no exertional signs are also common in school-age children. Such pains usually occur late in the day or night and disappear in the morning (49).

Children with persistent leg pains should be referred to a physician. The 8- and 9-year-olds are generally healthy but may complain of minor aches to get out of disagreeable tasks. Such behavior should not be reinforced by undue attention.

Visual impairments that occur in the younger child may be undetected and untreated until the child attends school. Visual acuity may not develop normally. Box 10–5 lists signs and symptoms to assess when defective vision is present (49, 72). It is essential that visual problems be corrected.

Table 10–3 summarizes other common health problems, their definitions, symptoms and signs, and prevention or treatment measures (49, 72, 155).

■ **BOX 10-5.**
Signs and Symptoms Indicating Defective Vision in Schoolchildren

Behavior

- Attempts to brush away blur; rubs eyes frequently; frowns, squints
- Stumbles frequently or trips over small objects
- Blinks more than usual; cries often or is irritable when doing close work
- Holds books or small playthings close to eyes
- Shuts or covers one eye, tilting or thrusting head forward when looking at objects
- Has difficulty in reading or in other schoolwork requiring close use of the eyes; omits words or confuses similar words
- Exhibits poor performance in activities requiring visual concentration within arm's length (e.g., reading, coloring, drawing); unusually short attention span; persistent word reversals after second grade
- Disinterested in distant objects or fails to participate in games such as playing ball
- Engages in outdoor activity mostly (e.g., running, bicycling), avoiding activities requiring visual concentration within arm's length.
- Sensitive to light
- Unable to distinguish colors
- Steps carefully over sidewalk cracks or around light or dark sections of block linoleum floors
- Trips at curbs or stairs
- Poor eye-hand coordination for age, excessively hard-to-read handwriting, difficulty with tying shoelaces or buttoning and unbuttoning

Appearance

- Crossed eyes (iris of one eye turned in or out and not symmetric with other eye)
- Red-rimmed, encrusted, or swollen eyelids
- Repeated styes
- Watery or red eyes

Complaints

- Cannot see blackboard from back of room
- Blurred or double vision after close eye work
- Dizziness, headaches, or nausea after close eye work
- Itching, burning, or scratchy feeling eyes

Data from references 49 and 72.

There is increasing concern about the schoolchild's risks for cardiovascular disease. Study of 71 monozygotic and 34 same-sex dizygotic twin pairs ages 6- to 11-years-old in the Philadelphia area revealed that children with characteristics of type A behavior and its subcomponents—triglycerides, systolic blood pressure, and obesity—have a genetic predisposition to cardiovascular disease, but that some people have a greater response to environmental factors, which also influence these characteristics.

Type A behavior apparently is an outcome of an interaction between physiologic factors based on (1) sympathetic reactivity, which may be due to genetics or early conditioning; (2) cognitive reactions to certain situations; and (3) psychologic traits. Because weight, lipid profiles, and blood pressure have both substantial environmental and genetic origins, nurses should encourage reduction of fat in the diet, increased physical exercise, and smoking cessation (120).

Rabies, an *acute infectious disease characterized by involvement of the central nervous system, resulting in paralysis and finally death,* is fortunately not a common disease but comes from a common problem: the biting of a human by a mammal (48). Refer to Chapter 9 for treatment.

If a diagnosis of rabies is considered, it must be reported to the local health department and Centers for Disease Control (CDC) in Atlanta. The CDC staff will act as consultants for the use of antirabies vaccine and all other factors surrounding the case. The latest CDC recommendations are found in the *Morbidity and Mortality Weekly Report* (195). Prevention is in keeping the child away from unfamiliar animals, particularly ones that act agitated, in seeing that all pets are properly vaccinated, and in taking steps to get preexposure immunization for high-risk children—those living or visiting in countries where rabies is a constant threat (48).

Increasingly, the ill effects of *smoking and drug and alcohol abuse* are emerging as a regular health problem among adolescents. These habits are influenced by the habits of parents, siblings, and peers. In one study over 50% of the boys were given their first cigarette by parents. The boys did not enjoy smoking but felt a need to do it to show off; knowledge of the effects of cigarette smoking was not a deterrent (59).

In addition to the ill effects caused by actual smoking, children in families with cigarette smokers have an increased rate of respiratory conditions and cancer. These small children have an increased number of days per year when their activities are restricted because of illness (215). Teach parents that smoking may be interfering with the normal growth and development of schoolchildren and that parental and other adult example is important. For example, in the West and Southwest United States, adult Hispanics have tended to smoke fewer cigarettes than non-Hispanic Whites. One study showed that Hispanic children also smoked less

TABLE 10–3. COMMON HEALTH PROBLEMS OF SCHOOLCHILDREN

Problem	Definition	Symptoms/Signs	Prevention/Treatment
Otitis externa	Inflammation of the external auditory canal and auricle	Pain in ear aggravated by moving the auricle; exudate in ear canal	Prevention: keep instruments out of ears. Keep dirty water out of ear. Use acetic acid (2%) solution in ear after swimming. After the fact, use antibiotic and/or steroid drops.
Serous otitis	Accumulation of non-purulent fluid in middle ear	Fullness and crackling in ear; decreased hearing	Administer decongestants (questionable help).
Allergic rhinitis	Allergic reaction affecting nasal mucosa (and sometimes conjunctiva)	Clear, thin nasal discharge; breathes through mouth; often does "allergic salute" (rubs nose upward)	Find offending irritant or antigen and try to eliminate. Take antihistamines. Obtain work-up by allergist if problem persists.
Herpes type I	Vesicular eruption of skin and mucous membranes above the umbilicus (usually mouth)	Soreness of mouth from eruption of mucosa; inflammation and swelling; sometimes fever and enlarged lymph glands (submandibular)	Apply Zovirax ointment to slow down severity. Drink adequate fluid. Use saline solution mouthwash. Administer antipyretic. Isolate from susceptible persons.
Contact dermatitis	Vesicular formation on skin, usually from poison ivy or poison oak	Itching and formation of vesicles, sometimes on most body parts	Apply cold compresses and drying lotion. Sometimes administer cortisone-based oral medicine or injections. Learn how to avoid plants.
Tinea corporis (ringworm of nonhairy skin)	Superficial fungal infection involving face, trunk, or limbs	Red, patch areas that scale and are oval in shape; usually asymptomatic or mildly itchy; no systemic signs	Apply a topical antifungal daily for 2 or 3 wk.
Tinea capitis (ringworm of the head)	Fungal infection involving scalp	Same as tinea coporis	Apply fungal cream persistently. Sometimes it is necessary to shave hair.
Warts	Intradermal papillomas	Usually appear as common (on hands or fingers) or plantar (on feet)	Dichloroacetic acid will often dissolve them. Other removal methods are available from dermatologist.
Pediculus humanus capitus (headlice)	Infestation of head, hair, scalp with stated organism	Itching scalp; see nits or ova as little dots attached to base hairs	Shampoo with approved medication. Apply antihistamine for itching. Comb out any remaining ova-nits. Boil all head care items.
Mumps	Viral disease characterized by acute swelling of salivary gland, especially the parotid	Anterior ear pain; headache; lethargy; anorexia; vomiting; complication orchitis (*inflammation of one or both testes*)	Prevention: obtain vaccine. Use only supportive treatment such as antipyretics (not aspirin-products) and encouraging fluid intake.
Diabetes mellitus type I (formally called juvenile diabetes)	Inherited disease with metabolic component that causes elevated blood sugar and vascular component that causes effects on eyes and kidneys	Increased urination; increased thirst and hunger; weight loss and fatigue	Obtain work-up by appropriate health care practitioner. Follow diabetic diet and exercise recommendations. Administer insulin.

than non-Hispanic White children. Interestingly, to date Hispanics have had fewer respiratory diseases associated with cigarette smoking—lung cancer, emphysema, and chronic obstructive pulmonary disease, presumably because of lower tobacco consumption (49, 60, 79, 184).

The school nurse and teacher can do considerable health teaching, giving students an introduction to positive health habits. Some programs emphasize that the body is a beautiful system, that no one should abuse the system by doing or using anything damaging, and to "just say no." The program should emphasize that people can be happy and active when they avoid the use of alcohol, drugs, or cigarettes to offset the preponderance of advertising that links youth, beauty, and excitement with these activities (49, 59, 163, 164, 180). Emphasize to adults that more effective than organized educational attempts is the influence of significant adults, those who take a personal interest in the child and who set an example: parents who neither smoke, drink, or use drugs nor give cigarettes, alcohol, or drugs to their children; the teacher who not only teaches content but also lives the teaching; parents and health care providers who have quit smoking; the athletic coach who is committed to no smoking; nurses and obstetricians who can help young women change habits; and the nurse or pediatrician who counsels children and adolescents. Equally important, or more so, is the peer group; leaders of the peer group who have positive health habits should be used as models (10). Peer communication is also effective for initiating hygienic habits. You may have a role in working with the peer group.

PSYCHOSOCIAL CONCEPTS

Cognitive Development

The schoolchild has a strong curiosity to learn, especially when motivation is strengthened by interested parents and opportunities for varied experiences in the home and school.

Learning, behavior, and personality are complex and are not easily explained by one theory. This section uses information from a number of theorists. Refer to Chapter 5 for a review of how the three major schools of theorists explain the development of learning, behavior, and personality (80).

Pattern of Intellectual Development

This pattern can be traced through the school years (56, 57, 141, 143, 145, 200). In American culture the 6-year-old is supposed to be ready for formal education. The child in first grade is frequently still in the Preoperational Stage. Thinking is concrete and animistic; he or she is only beginning to understand semiabstract symbols. Thus the basis for formal study is lacking and depends on the direction and guidance of adult authority. The child still defines objects in terms of their use and effect on self. He or she reads and knows numbers, but this ability depends on previous help. Learning occurs frequently through imitation and incidental suggestion. Because of centering, the child may not be able to consider parts and wholes in words at the same time. The child who cannot accurately do reversals may confuse *was* and *saw*. The child who cannot follow transformations may not be able to sound out words; individual sounds of *c, a,* and *p* may not be recognized as *cap*. Apparently there is a high correlation between ability to converse and beginning reading achievement (202).

At approximately age 7 the child enters the stage of

Concrete Operations, *which involves systematic reasoning about tangible or familiar situations and the ability to use logical thought to analyze relationships and structure the environment into meaningful categories.* The child must have interactions with concrete materials to build understanding that is basic for the next stage (144, 202). He or she uses visible props to form mental images and learn about many aspects of a concept or one aspect of a broad concept. For example, a car (broad concept) can be identified as a Ford or a Chevrolet (one aspect). This identification is based on instruction or experience and the use of memory. During this period the child becomes less egocentric, less animistic, and better able to do cause-effect and logical reasoning. A number of mental strategies or operations are learned (200).

Operations characteristic of this stage include classification, seriation, nesting, multiplication, reversibility, transformation, conservation, and decentering (52, 141, 148, 200, 202).

1. **Classification** involves *sorting objects in groups according to specific and multiple attributes* such as length, size, shape, color, class of animals, or trademark. School children can identify which kind of Ford is approaching on the highway.
2. **Seriation** involves *ordering objects according to decreasing or increasing measure* such as height, weight or strength. The child knows A is longer than B, B longer than C, and A longer than C.
3. **Nesting** involves *understanding how a subconcept fits into a larger concept.* For example, a German shepherd is one kind of dog; a reclining chair and a dining room chair are both chairs.
4. **Multiplication** involves *simultaneously classifying and seriating,* using two numbers together to come out with a greater amount.
5. **Reversibility** involves *returning to the starting point or performing opposite operations or actions with the same problem or situation.* The child can add and subtract, multiply and divide the same problems. A longer row of clips can be squeezed together to form a shorter row and vice versa; the child realizes the number of clips has not changed.
6. **Transformation** involves the *ability to see the shift from a dynamic to static or constant state, to understand the process of change, and to focus on the continuity and sequence, on the original and final states.* For example, the child realizes or anticipates how a shorter row of pennies was shifted to become a longer row or the gradual shift in level of fluid in a container as it is poured into another container and the increasing level of fluid in the second container.
7. **Conservation** involves *understanding transformation conceptually and that a situation has not changed, to see the sameness of a situation or object*

CASE SITUATION: Schoolchild Development

Sarah, age 10 years, and Joshua, her 6-year-old brother, are visiting their grandmother, aunt, uncle, and cousins for the day. Sarah is thin, with narrow shoulders and hips and little adipose tissue, although she has considerable muscle mass.

A luncheon is being held for her grandmother's birthday, and Sarah is eager to help her aunt and cousins prepare the food, set the table, and make party favors. Sarah and Megan, her 9-year-old cousin, divide the nuts and candies into party cups to set at each person's plate. They do this systematically and logically, using the concepts of seriation and classification, so that each person receives an identical number of candies and nuts. This is typical of the Concrete Operations stage of cognitive development.

Sarah and Megan go to play school in Megan's room where there is a toy chest, dolls, bookshelves,

and chalkboard. Sarah plays the teacher, writing multiplication tables on the board and talking to Megan and to pretend students. She demonstrates concrete transformations as she solves multiplication problems. Sarah pretends the class is being bad and reprimands them as a teacher would. In this behavior she demonstrates understanding of relationships between various steps in a situation. It is apparent that Sarah's teacher is a role model for her; this is common among school-age children.

Sarah asks Megan for advice on solving the problems and on reprimanding the pretend class. This exchange of information is typical of the syntaxic mode of communication and consensual validation that is observed in the schoolchild. By incorporating Megan's ideas and answers, she shows that she cares about Megan's thoughts.

---

in spite of a change in some aspect, and that mass or quantity is the same even if it changes shape or position. For example, six paper clips moved from a 6-inch line to an 8-inch line remain six paper clips. Water in boiled form is vapor, which can return to water and freeze. It is still the same amount of water; nothing is lost in the process.

8. **Decentering** involves *coordination of two or more dimensions,* or the ability to focus on several characteristics simultaneously. For example, space and length dimensions can be considered; the youngest child would consider only one or the other. When 12 paperclips are spread from 6 inches to 12 inches, the child realizes the clips are spread and there are not more clips.

These operations increase in complexity as the child matures from an empirical to logical orientation. The child can look at a situation, analyze it, and come up with an answer without purposefully going through each step. For example, if two rows of coins have been spread out, the child does not have to count the coins. He or she realizes that nothing was added or subtracted to the rows, so each row still has the same number.

The child learns and can recall associations between sequences and groupings of events. At first he or she makes associations within a certain context or environment; later memory is used to transfer these associations to different contexts or environments. The child also rehearses; in the time between a learning experience and a memory test or application of learning he or she goes over mentally what has been learned (125, 200).

Thus by age 7 the child is more reflective and has a

deeper understanding of meanings and feelings. He or she is interested in conclusions and logical endings. Now language is used freely, not only to establish rapport but to inquire and give a running commentary on the matters at hand. Attention span has lengthened enough that the child may work several hours alone on an interesting activity. He or she is more aware of the environment and the people in it. Although still interested in fairies, Superman, and magic, the child is beginning to have a scientific interest in causes and conditions. He or she is serious about such concepts as government and civilization and enjoys inventing with household odds and ends or using a chemistry or carpentry set. The child can seriate by length and understands area or mass (56, 125).

The 8-year-old's thinking is less animistic and more aware of the impersonal forces of nature. The child does not grasp complex rules and instead improvises simple ones. He or she is intellectually expansive, inquiring about the past and future, the insides of earth and people, primitive people or people of other cultures, and his or her own race and nationality. This is a favorable time to strengthen sensible attitudes against racial prejudice and reinforce natural tolerance and sympathy for others. The child begins to understand logical reasoning, conclusions, contexts, and implications. He or she is less self-centered in thinking and understands more than a personal perspective. He or she learns by experience as well as from others (56, 125).

The 9-year-old is realistic, reasonable, self-motivated, and intellectually energetic and curious. The child has a growing capacity to put mind and energies to tasks on his or her own initiative and with minimal direction. The child is so busy and involved that he or she does not like to be interrupted and may work for 2 to 3 hours without anyone's reinforcement. The child likes to compete with self so that he or she repeatedly tries an activity until the activity is mastered to satisfaction. At this age the child is an excellent pupil and a perfector of skills. He or she likes to plan in advance. If a task is complicated, he or she asks to have successive steps explained. If unsuccessful in doing the task, he or she is realistic in self-appraisal. He or she likes to classify, identify, and make inventories or lists. The child is likely to know all the facts and figures about a baseball team, flags of different countries, or distinctions among different cars or airplanes. He or she can seriate by weight. The focus is on details. He or she does not like magic and believes in law (and that rules can be flexible) as much as luck or chance (56, 125).

The 10-year-old's thinking is concrete and matter of fact. He or she likes to reason and to participate in elementary discussions about social problems. A reasonable amount of homework is accepted without resentment because learning is enjoyable. The child wants to measure up to a challenge, defined in the social norms of the group. He or she likes to memorize, identify facts, locate cites on a map, or list serially familiar items. There is still difficulty in seeing relationships, but he or she likes to think in terms of cause and effect. Attention span may be short and choppy. Frequently planned shifts in activity and a friendly classroom are helpful to intellectual activity. He or she ranges out into a wide sphere of interests and yet concentrates on each for the moment (56, 125).

The 11-year-old has boundless curiosity but is not reflective. Thinking is concrete and specific. The child likes action in learning, to move about the classroom freely or try experiments. He or she concentrates well when working competitively with one group against another. The child prefers a certain amount of routine, wants school to be related to reality, and is better at rote memorization than at generalization. By now he or she can understand relational terms such as weight and size (56, 125).

The child at 12 years likes to learn and consider all sides of a situation. He or she is more independent in doing homework, entering a self-chosen task with zeal and initiative. Motivation comes by an inner drive rather than by competition, but he or she likes group work. The child is better able to classify, arrange, and generalize, understands conservation of volume, and likes to discuss and debate. He or she is beginning abstract thinking. Verbal, formal reasoning is possible. Now the moral of a story is understood (56, 125).

Discuss the child's changing cognitive abilities with parents and ways they can contribute to the cognitive achievement. If parents do not understand that certain cognitive behavior is age appropriate, their interactions with and guidance of the child may be less effective.

Cognitive development and an increasing under-standing of implications and consequences and of cause-effect relations may be a factor in the changing fearfulness of the child. By age 7 or 8 most fears that are typical of preschoolers (darkness, spooks) have been resolved. The young schoolchild is fearful of natural hazards, unsafe conditions, loss of parents, war (when the country is involved in war), school problems, disease, body injury, separation, excess punishment, death, breaking the moral code, and hell. Ten- and 11-year-olds report fears of dangerous animals, people, machines, weapons, vehicles, natural hazards, war, the bomb, disease, separation from or death of loved ones, personal death, breaking the moral code, and hell. Some of these fears (e.g., fear of vehicles or dangerous people) are realistic as the child increasingly moves out into the community alone. Adults also express some of these same fears (123, 213).

As a nurse, remember that the school-age child has great fear of body injury, disease, separation from loved ones, death, excess punishment (some diagnostic and treatment procedures seem like punishment), and doing wrong actions. Miller (123) gives specific suggestions for nursing practice that help offset the child's fears.

Concept of Time

Concept of time evolves during the early school period (56, 57). The time sense of the 6-year-old is as much in the past as the present. The child likes to hear about his or her babyhood. The future concerns the child primarily in relation to significant holidays. Duration of an episode has little time meaning. Time is counted by the hours; minutes are disregarded.

The 7-year-old is interested in the present. Sense of time is practical, sequential, and detailed. The child likes a personal watch since he or she can read a clock and knows the sequence of months, seasons, and years. Passage of time from one event to another and a specific time with a specific task are understood; thus he or she plans the day (56).

The 8-year-old is more responsible in relation to time and is extremely aware of punctuality. The 9-year-old can tell time without difficulty, plans the day, and generally tries to pack in more than possible. He or she likes to know how long a task will take when asked to do it. The child is especially interested in ancient times (56).

The 10-year-old is less driven by time than the 9-year-old. He or she is interested in the present; the best time is now. The child is able to get places on time with his or her own initiative. The 11-year-old child feels the relentless passing of time and is more adept at handling time. He or she feels the difference between time dragging and flying by and defines time as a distance from one event to another (57).

The 12-year-old defines time as duration, a measurement, and plans ahead so he or she feels life is under personal control. He or she is well rooted in the present but is excited about what will happen in the future (57).

You can help parents understand that their school-age children do not have adult concepts of time. The mother who is distraught because her 6- or 7-year-old constantly dawdles in getting ready for school can be helped by understanding the child's concept of time. The mother must still be firm in direction but not expect the impossible. She can look forward to improvement in the 8-year-old.

Understanding maturing time concepts will also aid you as you explain the sequence of a procedure to the schoolchild in the doctor's office, school, clinic, or hospital.

Spatial Concepts

These concepts also change with more experience (56, 57). The 6-year-old is interested in specific places and in relationships between home, neighborhood, and an expanding community. He or she knows some streets and major points of interest. By the age of 7 the sense of space is becoming more realistic. The child wants some space of his or her own such as a room or portion of it. The heavens and various objects in space and in the earth are of keen interest (56).

For the 8-year-old personal space is expanding as the child goes more places alone. He or she knows the neighborhood well and likes maps, geography, and trips. He or she understands the compass points and can distinguish right and left on others as well as one self (56).

Space for the 9-year-old includes the whole earth. He or she enjoys pen pals from different lands, geography, and history. For the 10-year-old space is rather specific, the place things such as buildings are. The 11-year-old perceives space as nothingness that goes on forever, a distance between things. He or she is in good control of getting around in the personal space (56, 57).

The 12-year-old understands that space is abstract and has difficulty defining it. Space is nothing, air. He or she can travel alone to more distant areas and understands how specific points relate to each other (57).

Encourage the parents to discuss spatial concepts with the child to facilitate abstract reasoning. Pontious (153) and Webb (202) give practical suggestions for using Piaget's concepts in care and teaching of children.

Box 10–6 summarizes other concepts that the school child formulates.

Entering School

School entry is a crisis for the child and family, for behavior must be adapted to meet new situations. The school experience has considerable influence on the child because he or she is in formative years and spends much time in school. School, society's institution to help the child develop the fullest intellectual potential and a sense of industry, should help the child learn to think critically; make judgments based on reason; accept criti-

---

■ **BOX 10-6.**
Categories of Concepts Developed During the School Years

Life: is aware that movement is not sole criterion of life.
Death: accepts death as final and not like life; thinks of death as an angel or bogeyman; thinks personal death can be avoided if one hides, runs fast, or is good. Traumatic situations arouse fear of death. By age 10 or 11, realizes death is final, inevitable, and results from internal processes. Belief in life after death depends on religious teachings.
Body functions: has many inaccurate ideas about body functions until taught health class; needs repetitive sex education; becomes more modest for self but interested in seeing bodies of adults. Performs complete self-care by 9 years.
Money: begins to understand value of coins and bills.
Self: clarifies ideas of self when sees self through eyes of teachers and peers and compares self with peers; by 11 or 12 years considers self to be in brain, head, face, heart, and then total body.
Sex roles: has clear concept of culturally defined sex role and that male role is considered more prestigious.
Social roles: is aware of peers' social, religious, and socioeconomic status, accepts cultural stereotypes and adult attitudes toward status; group conscious.
Beauty: judges beauty according to group standards rather than own aesthetic sensibilities.
Comedy: has concept of comedy or what is funny influenced by perception of what others think is funny.

---

cism; develop social skills; cooperate with others; accept other adult authority; and be a leader and follower. The child who attends a school with children from various ethnic or racial backgrounds or with children who have immigrated will also learn about cultures, and possibly several languages, first hand (Fig. 10–2). The course of instruction should be such that every child has a sense of successful accomplishment in some area. However, not only school promotes these cognitive and social skills. The home and other groups (e.g., peer or organized clubs) are important in their own way for intellectual and social development and for promoting a sense of achievement and industry.

Regular attendance at school starts early for some children, perhaps at $2\frac{1}{2}$ to 3 years in nursery school. But not all children are emotionally ready for school, even at age 6 or 7. If the child is unprepared for school, separation anxiety may be intense. The demands of a strange adult and the peer group may be overwhelming.

Various actions such as teaching the child his or her address and full name, independence in self-care, and basic safety rules help prepare the child for school. The preschool physical and dental examination and an orientation to the school and teacher promote a sense of anticipation and readiness. Parents should examine their

Figure 10-2.   Exposure to a variety of peers is important for the school-age child. (Copyright © T. Rosenthal, Super-stock, Inc.)

attitudes about the child's entering school. Some parents seem eager to rid themselves of a portion of responsibility. Others are worried about the new influences and fear loss of control. Because the parents' attitudes so strongly affect the child, they should verbalize the positive aspects.

The parent or classroom teacher (and the nurse in the health care setting) can stimulate the child's learning in the following ways:

1. Let each child's success be measured in terms of improved performance.
2. Structure for individuation, not for convergence. Avoid having all learning activities structured so that there is only one right answer.
3. Provide activities that are challenging, not overwhelming.
4. Arrange for the child to accomplish individual activities in company of peers, when appropriate, since peer interaction provides encouragement and assistance.
5. Demonstrate problem solving and thinking behavior to serve as a model for the child (202).
6. Use a multisensory teaching approach (199).

There is increasing societal pressure to accelerate the child in the educational process. Piaget contends that optimum comprehension results from numerous experiences over a period of time. Studies of schoolchildren show that a child can quickly learn a specific and advanced task but often with limited retention and transfer. Further, apparent shifts from Concrete to For-mal Operations may result from experiences unrelated to education. Direct verbal instruction and use of **cognitive conflict** (*getting the child to question perceptions*) can result in acquisition of conservation abilities, but transfer apparently is limited. Success at learning tasks of increasing complexity depends on levels and interactions of subskills already possessed by the learner. Rather than concentrating on learning of specific tasks, the home or classroom setting should encourage thinking in the child. A variety of experiences and teaching methods increases comprehension, learning, and transfer, which promote acceleration to the next cognitive level. Piecemeal acceleration often results in distorted or incomplete conceptual development that may hamper future thinking (125, 202).

The *teacher-pupil relationship* is important, for it is somewhat similar to the parent-child relationship. Often, however, the classes are so large that the teacher is unable to give much individualized time and attention to each child or to become acquainted with his or her uniqueness. Although the teacher sometimes represents a greater authority figure than the parents, the emotional bond between parent and child is ordinarily stronger than that between teacher and child, and the wise teacher does not act like a substitute parent. The child needs from the teacher a wholesome friendliness, consideration, fairness, sense of humor, and a philosophy that encourages his or her maturity. The teacher should be emotionally and physically healthy and have a thorough understanding of child development.

Problems of the family and child are brought into

sharp focus when the child enters school. The teacher sees many difficulties: the loneliness of an only child; the pain of the child with divorce or death in the family; the negative self-image of the child who is not as physically coordinated or intellectually sharp as his or her peers; the child with dyslexia or learning difficulties; the **school-phobic child** *who is fearful about or refuses to attend school*. Several theories have developed about the school-phobic child, one of which describes an overprotective mother, a sense of insecurity and uncertainty, and a sense that mother does not want the child to leave home and gain independence. Very little has been written about the father's role, but he has been viewed by some as passive and by some as firm and controlling. School phobia or separation anxiety can be an indicator of underlying schizophrenia, or it can be nothing more than a normal child with a temporary conflict (49, 133).

School experiences are vivid in the child's memory. The child needs someone to listen to and talk about these experiences when he or she arrives home. This strengthens language skills, self-concept, and self-respect. If the child is put off or no one is there to listen, he or she will increasingly turn inward and may refuse to talk when the adult is ready. The parents' taking a few minutes from supper preparation can be very important to the child.

Help parents realize that the child's ability to learn and achieve in school is affected by factors other than intellectual ability. The educational level of the parents is one of the strongest predictors of a child's academic performance and measured intelligence. Failure to achieve may be the child's reaction to a hostile home environment, poor nutrition, physical illness, a troubled classroom, or a teacher's personal problem. Even the design of the school or physical attributes and appearance of the classroom may contribute to poor achievement. If the child cannot see or hear well, is uncomfortable or bothered by distractions and noise, feels unsafe, or has insufficient space, attention, interest, and learning are reduced. Further, some classrooms are built to foster rigid teacher behavior; some children need more flexibility in the program (25, 171). Parents may project their inferiority feelings onto the child, and he or she believes that it is useless to try. The child may be punishing self out of guilt about past misdeeds, real or imagined, or may be asking for attention; or he or she may have been placed in the wrong learning group, either above or below personal abilities. Occasionally these negative factors cause a child to try harder, to sublimate and overcompensate, and to achieve well if ability is present.

Too much pushing by parents for the child to be a success, perfect in physical skills, the most intellectual, or a hard worker can backfire. The pressure that is generated may be so intense that the child eventually does not succeed at anything. Perfectionistic, highly successful, career- or professionally focused parents are apt to push the child too much. If a parent cannot admit mistakes, he or she is unlikely to tolerate mistakes made by the child, and all of us—parents and children—*do* make mistakes. The child may become a perfectionist from parental example and behavior. Certain signs and symptoms are clues. The *perfectionistic child* manifests:

1. Extreme concern about appearance.
2. Avoidance of tasks, play, or school because of fear of failure.
3. Dawdling or procrastinating on easy tasks to avoid harder ones or working so slowly on projects that creativity is lost.
4. Jealousy and envy of the apparent success and perfection of others.
5. Wanting to do something for which the child has no ability or talent.
6. Low tolerance for mistakes (e.g., the boy who wins the race may feel he was not successful because he did not set any records) (10, 15, 34, 101).

If these behaviors are present teach the parents to work on relaxing themselves and the child and developing a sense of tolerance and humor. They can join the child in new activities—done for fun and without competition. They and the child can set realistic goals. They can praise the child's efforts, not focus on the outcome. You may be their counselor, or you may refer them to counseling (15, 34).

School difficulty may arise from the misuse of intelligence quotient (IQ) testing. IQ scores are not the same as intelligence; IQ scores tell what the child has learned at school. An IQ score can go up or down many points in 1 year. The child with a low IQ score may be placed in the class for slow learners; 1 year in such a group may damage the child for the rest of the school years, even if he or she is later placed with a brighter group. Teachers are likely to respond to this child differently, expecting little and offering little. Attention is usually directed to the child who scored high, which further improves the score. IQ scores can predict academic success generally, but they say nothing about a child's curiosity, motivation, inner thoughts, creativity, ability to get along with people, or ability to be a productive citizen (113). Group standardized aptitude, achievement, and vocational tests used in schools (and the business world) cost more than they are worth (125). Certainly children should not be separated into gifted or retarded classes only on the basis of IQ scores.

Standardized achievement tests should be given less weight in educational decisions; they do not screen even for mental retardation with any real-life validity. Of adults who scored below 79 on individually administered IQ tests (and who would have been labeled mentally retarded had they been in school), 84% had completed 8 or more years of school, 83% had a job, 80% were financially independent, and almost 100% could do their shopping or travel alone. The ability to handle school-related content declines after leaving school; ability to handle the real world increases (125).

IQ test scores are affected by ethnic, racial, cultural, and language biases, the testing environment, and gender (113, 125). For example, many African-Americans score lower than Caucasians on IQ tests; but when the test is given by a African-American person, they score higher than if it is given by a Caucasian, possibly because they turn hostile feelings inward when under the direction of Caucasians. Stress and low self-expectations also adversely affect scores. African-American children score lower than Caucasian children on tests involving abstraction but higher on rote-memory tests (43, 125). Male-female differences are also striking. In the early school years boys and girls have equal scholastic standing, although girls may be superior. Later, males surpass females on tests of speed and coordination of gross motor acts, spatial-quantitative problems, mechanical tasks, types of quantitative reasoning, and in the subjects of mathematics, science, social studies, and citizenship. Females surpass males in fine motor skills, perceptual skills, memory, numerical computations, verbal skills, and in the subjects of writing, music, reading, and literature. The test scores are the result of stereotyped social training and value systems. Girls are rewarded for acting "feminine"; they may drop behind to gain approval. Yet females are as capable as males in all avenues of educational attainment if society allows, expects, or demands it (125).

The child from a minority group sometimes fares considerably worse in school than does the average child because of being handicapped with fewer verbal skills, the middle-class orientation of school programs and examinations, inadequately trained teachers and inferior school facilities in deprived areas, low motivation to achieve or compete, and the effect of the parents' and teacher's expectations on the child. Research shows that children tend to achieve what adults expect of them (125, 149). Research also indicates that early childhood enrichment programs for disadvantaged children improve performance in the school years, but those enrichment programs should continue in the school years (64, 101).

Research results show a low correlation between IQ scores, cognitive ability, and personality in the preschool years. However, teachers perceive students who show initiative or plunge into a new activity as the brightest and those who participate little or not at all as the least intelligent. Apparently the self-fulfilling prophecy occurs because of differential teacher expectations and differences in teacher interactions with various students—by the seventh grade a high correlation between personality characteristics and IQ scores exists (101, 122, 125, 202).

A classroom with diversity in the children's intellectual ability, skills, and personality is helpful to the child; he or she learns about the real world. A low percentage of disabled, retarded, or maladjusted children in a classroom will not adversely affect the normal child. However, putting the exceptional child in a normal classroom does not make him or her feel normal; he or she still is perceived and perceives self as different. The exceptional child may need special classes to get the help needed; teachers cannot be expected to specialize in all areas of education, and large classrooms prevent teachers from spending the necessary time with the child who has learning disabilities (125, 173). Legislation has forced "mainstreaming" or inclusion of the special students back into the regular classrooms.

The **gifted child** is *characterized by superior educability and consumption of information and by ability to produce information, concepts, and new forms.* The gifted child demonstrates to a greater extent than other children the seven types of intelligence: logical-mathematical, linguistic, musical, spatial, body-kinesthetic, interpersonal, and intrapersonal (122). The child is adept at problem solving and problem finding. The gifted child is considered educationally exceptional, and the child's full intellectual, creative, and leadership potential may be neglected if (1) parents are not attuned to the child's abilities and needs; (2) parents or teachers are threatened by the gifted child who grasps concepts more quickly than they; (3) parents do not value cognitive, creative, or leadership abilities; (4) the child is not given freedom to explore and be different; or (5) the school system does not have a program suited for his or her abilities (37, 67, 81, 122, 135, 140, 159, 170).

The articles by Miller (122) and Schwartz (170) detail the identification of and the emotional, social, and mental characteristics of gifted children and explain how the classroom teacher can help such children find their place in the world. Often the gifted child is misunderstood. Research indicates, however, that the gifted have higher self-esteem than others and that gifted students are more popular with their peers than other children (122, 135, 170).

You can encourage parents to respect the individual interests and talents of their child. If parents are not intimidated by the child's unusual interests and behavior, they will not fear deviations from neighborhood patterns and thereby not crush budding interests or creativity. That is perhaps the essence of raising a gifted child—to facilitate, provide opportunity, let alone, not hold back, or insist that something be done a certain way. Likewise, the wise parent will be able to await the sprouting of interests that do not come quickly to the surface, even if the child is behind other children or group norms. It takes courage and patience to let the child develop at his or her pace. You can be supportive to parents as they let the child assert his or her own initiative in a situation, even if the child is not at first successful. The impulse toward growth and development must first come from the individual's budding inclinations, not from a desire to conform to another's expectations.

Some parents believe the present public school system is inadequate to teach their children the needed skills. They are usually well-educated professionals and wish to teach their own children at home. References by several authors (33, 157, 161) explore various facets of this movement.

The *ill child* poses unique problems for the school and parents. An issue of mounting emotional intensity in many communities is whether children who have the human immunodeficiency virus (HIV) or acquired immunodeficiency syndrome (AIDS), regardless of cause, can attend school with other children. Although not a common health problem, the child with AIDS has a unique problem in school, at home, or when hospitalized. Although no spread by casual contact has been reported, the dilemma of how to handle these children is overwhelming (9).

Currently, these children are being treated with gamma globulin or with the drug AZT in a few selected hospital or clinic settings. School systems are handling the child in a variety of ways. In some systems no one except a small panel knows which child, if any, has AIDS, which prevents the child from stigma but does not protect him or her from asserting self too much or getting into situations in which an already low resistance might be compromised even further. Other school districts mandate that the child be taught at home. The lack of financial aid is a problem at all levels of living and treatment. Most of the children with AIDS do not have a family financial or insurance support system (1, 69, 86).

Klug (86) has detailed information on AIDS in the child from birth on and its effects and complications. She states that children with AIDS can remain in school except when viral infections in others threaten the infected child's immune system and health. The school nurse is in a key role to work with parents, teachers, school administrators, members of the school board, and the schoolchildren to help them understand the disease; to reduce fear, myths, and irrationality; and to ensure health and welfare of all the people in the school building. Your communication and negotiation skills and knowledge place you in a special role to be listened to by others, to be an advocate for the child and family, and to facilitate sensible decisions.

In working with parents, you may describe parenting as analogous to growing a garden. The gardener is successful because he or she does not thrust impossible patterns on the plants, respects and even nurtures their peculiarities, tries to provide suitable conditions, protects them from serious threats to life, does not continually poke or probe to make plants sprout more quickly, does not seize the new sprouts to pull open the leaves, and does not trim them all to look alike. As with plants, so it is with children. *They* must do the growing and developing and only through their own motivation (Fig. 10–3).

You, the teachers, and administrators must work together for the health and safety of the child. Guns and

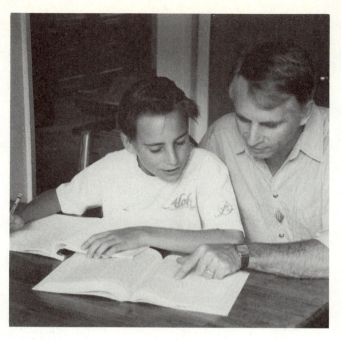

Figure 10-3. Parents nurture their children by providing support and encouraging their efforts and activities. (From Berger, K.J., and M.B. Williams, *Fundamentals of Nursing: Collaborating for Optimal Health.* Norwalk, Conn: Appleton & Lange, 1992, p. 313.)

other weapons do not belong in school, and the school must be kept safe from gunmen and snipers. All adults must know how to protect the children and themselves (50). The teacher can pass his or her observations about the child and environment on to you. You can work with the child, parents, teachers, and administrators as a consultant or counselor. Treating difficulties early is likely to prevent major and long-term problems. You must help the parents understand that they are ultimately responsible for their child's behavior and learning. Box 10–7 summarizes how parents can assist the child. Their understanding of growth and development through your teaching and their knowledge of the school and its functions through attending parent-teacher association meetings will help them in this demanding job. Parents with little education may need to learn the same subjects their children are learning to be able to help their children. Special classes could be arranged.

Intellectual Needs of the Hospitalized Child

You can help meet the hospitalized child's needs. A hospital tour, if it can be prearranged, helps the child feel acclimated during illness when his or her energy reserve is low. Because the child is beginning logical thought, he or she needs simple information about the illness to decrease the fear of the unknown and promote cooperation in the treatment plan. He or she needs to handle and become familiar with the equipment used. Heiney (66) describes practical ways to help the child deal with painful procedures.

■ **BOX 10-7.**
Suggestions for Parents About Children's Homework

Do's

- Let your children know you believe they can do well. Encourage self-evaluation.
- Minimize time spent watching television.
- Help your children organize. Encourage them to do the most difficult task first.
- Talk and read to your children.
- Go to your children's school and volunteer.
- Encourage outside activities and having friends at home.
- Work with your children's teachers and let the teachers know you understand and are supportive.
- Insist on good eating habits.
- Plan activities with your children.
- Be a good example.

Don'ts

- Dwell on the negative by criticizing.
- Allow the television to be your babysitter.
- Do it for the children.
- Leave them to their own devices.
- Forget to encourage verbal exchange.
- Push them to have every minute scheduled or send them off to play.
- Criticize and interfere with everything you do not understand.
- Allow constant eating.
- Send them off without you to family functions (e.g. school plays, pot-luck dinners).
- Say, "Do as I say and not as I do."

The child who must spend long periods in the hospital needs to learn about the outside world. Some hospitals take chronically ill children to the circus, athletic events, and restaurants. Teachers are also employed so that the child can continue with formal education.

Use of Nonschool Time

Help parents realize the importance of the use of time by the child when he or she is not in school. One study of more than 200 children in grades 3, 6, 7, 9, and 11 gave interesting results, although results may have been influenced by the fact that these children lived in an affluent community in the East (183). These results may help you talk with parents about their awareness of the child's activity and the importance of how the child uses time. In this study children preferred activities with parents such as going to museums or theaters or working on hobbies or projects to watching television. These children spent little time on "learning-related" activities, such as model building, stamp collecting, visits to muse-

ums and art exhibits. In fact, they expressed a strong desire for "more interesting after school activities." Homework and reading received little time, from a daily weekday average of 45 minutes for third graders to 75 minutes for ninth graders. One half as much time was spent on homework on weekends. Almost one half of the students enjoyed reading "often," but most stated that they opposed more homework. Students at all grade levels were not involved in attending church and community events or in volunteering in community service activities. Yet they expressed a strong desire to participate in such programs at all ages.

If parents cannot initiate attendance at learning-related activities with their children, for whatever reasons, perhaps school and other education-related agencies should offer learning-related activities held at convenient, accessible locations throughout the community. A number of school districts have developed school-business partnerships, internship programs, and other work-related projects designed to help students better understand the realities of the world of work. In a Midwest school district one seventh grade science teacher has held, for over a decade, well-attended weekend family field trips to interesting places, related to classwork, for parents and seventh graders. The teacher believes the extra time and effort are well spent; the school system is supportive. Parents endeavor to get their children into his class, partly for the field trip experiences.

Parents, teachers, and school administrators may wish to examine "the seventh grade slump." Seventh graders watch more television than do all other groups, participate less in learning-related activities, and dislike school more than do other groups. A reexamination of the seventh grade academic programs, extracurricular activities, and out-of-school opportunities for growth would be useful (183).

At all grade levels studied, parents seem to spend little time with children. Children want more time with parents. *Talk with parents to help them examine the role they now play in their children's lives, their various commitments, their priorities, and their importance to the child.* This is difficult when children come from homes with working mothers or from one-parent homes. Nevertheless, this issue is worth raising. Perhaps other caring adults are available also to spend time with the children. Human interaction is an important need for children—in fact, for people of all ages (117, 183).

Communication Patterns

Many factors influence the child's communication pattern, vocabulary, and diction. Some of these factors have been referred to in previous chapters. Influences include (1) speech and verbal and nonverbal communication pattern of parent(s), siblings, other adults such as teacher, and peers; (2) attitudes of others toward the child's efforts to speak and communicate; (3) general environmental stimulation; (4) opportunity to communicate with a variety of people in a variety of situations; (5) intellectual development; (6) ability to hear and articulate; (7) vocabulary skills; and (8) contact with television or other technology (101, 125).

The 6-year-old has command of nearly every form of sentence structure. The child experiments less with language, using it more as a tool and less for the mere pleasure of talking than during the preschool period. Now language is used to share in others' experiences. He or she also swears and uses slang to test others' reactions. The child enjoys printing words in large letters (56, 57, 101, 125).

At 7, the child can print several sentences, and at 8 he or she is writing instead of printing. By 9, the child participates in family discussions, showing interest in family activities and indicating an individuality. Verbal fluency has improved, and common objects are described in detail. Writing skill has improved; he or she usually writes with small, even letters. By 10, he or she can write for a relatively long time with speed. The preadolescent may seem less talkative, withdrawing when frustrated instead of voicing anger. Sharing feelings with a best friend is a healthy outlet (56, 57, 101, 125).

As the child shares ideas and feelings, he or she learns how someone else thinks and feels about similar matters. The child expresses self in a way that has meaning to others, at first to a chum and then to others. Thus he or she is validating vocabulary, ideas, and feelings. The child learns that a friend's family has similar life patterns, demands of the child, and frustrations. He or she learns about self in the process of learning more about another. The child recalls what has happened in the past, realizes how this has affected the present, and considers what effect present acts will have on future events. The child uses **syntaxic, or consensual, communication** *when he or she sees these cause-and-effect relationships in an objective, logical way and can validate them with others* (186).

Convey love and caring, not rejection, when you talk with children. Love is communicated through nonverbal behavior such as getting down to the child's eye level and through words that value feelings and indicate respect. Children understand language directed at their feelings better than at their intellect and the overt action. Do not overreact to normal behavior. Avoid talking about touchy areas, if possible, or the child's babyhood. He or she is struggling to be grownup; any reminder of younger behavior creates anxiety about potential regression (101). The principles of communicating with the preschooler discussed in Chapter 9 are also applicable to the schoolchild.

Effects of Television on the Child

Television and movies have a powerful influence on a child's communication and behavior patterns. Children watch an average of 4 hours of television daily—more time than is spent on school homework (102). The average child will have viewed from 15,000 to 22,000 hours or more of television by high school graduation; he or she will have spent fewer hours in formal classroom study (102, 125, 183).

If watching television is controlled by responsible parents, cognitive and social learning can be enhanced. Educational programs can model prosocial behaviors and present and reinforce techniques associated with various sports (102). For the person unable to attend church, the religious programs can be a substitute. Scenic programs have an esthetic value. Geographic, science, historical, or dramatic presentations are educational and/or relaxing. Television has the potential to educate, socialize, and teach content and communication skills. However, even viewing ordinary programs has serious limitations, including the following (58, 125, 127, 165, 178, 179):

1. Promotes passive rather than active learning
2. Increases passivity from continual overstimulation
3. Encourages low-level, nonconceptual thinking
4. Takes time away or distracts from more creative and stimulating activity; reduces creativity of the child
5. Encourages short attention span and hyperactivity through its use of snappy attention-getting techniques
6. Causes lack of understanding or comprehension of what is seen because of fast pace of programming
7. Causes loss of interest in less exciting but necessary classroom or home activities
8. Creates a desire for the superficial rather than depth of information
9. Creates uncertainty about what is real and unreal in life and family
10. Promotes a desire for unhealthy products such as high-sugar or high-salt snacks, other products not normally used by the family, or toys or other products that may be unhealthy or dangerous
11. Creates a confusion of values

Heavy television viewing is associated with lower school achievement. School teachers report that more children are entering school with decreased imaginative play and creativity and increased aimless movement, low frustration level, poor persistence and concentration span, and confusion about reality and fantasy. Rapid speech and constantly changing visuals on television prevent reflection. The child does not learn correct sentence structure, use of tenses, or the ability to express thought or feeling effectively. The result may be a child who is unable to enunciate or use correct grammar and who is vague in the sense of time and history, and cause-and-effect relationships (112, 125, 194, 212, 214).

Understanding television can involve active mental work for the young child, but often the child does not understand content, motives, or feelings; integrate events shown; or infer conditions not shown (135, 178).

Those are the mental processes that are stimulated by adult and peer interactions and reading literature. Often television is used in the home to the extent that it stifles family interaction and bombards with noise, excitement, speed, and misdirected humor. The stereotypic, simplistic, and often romanticized view of family life shown by most programs is unrealistic and probably not attainable. False expectations about things and people are raised; most advertising is sexist, ageist, and racist, showing women as uninterested in or incapable of anything except putting on diapers and using detergents. Most advertisements are directed to middle-class young Caucasians.

Science fiction conveys that life in the future may be scary and difficult at best. The child may have nightmares. A steady diet of science fiction may influence the child's present and future value systems (125, 194).

Some television programming is frankly pornographic; the values depicted are lack of loyalty or commitment to relationships, the beautiful and young body, immediate gratification, and narcissism. Movies and daytime dramas depict "jumping into bed and from bed to bed." Consequences of such behavior and relationships are not shown (129). Often such programming is at prime viewing time. The child who has unsupervised television watching cannot miss programs about family life that teach unhealthy values (102).

The violence in television programming is graphic, explicit, realistic, and intensely involving and affects both children and adults but the children more so because they have less ego control. Children act out more directly what they see and hear. Many programs directly or indirectly teach violent behavior, showing specifically how to carry out violent acts. It is not unusual when a rape, hostage-taking, suicide, or homicide is described on the evening news on television to have, either locally or nationally, a number of such incidents repeated within a few days (102). The live and explicit portrayals of violence suggests that violence is normal and justified. Realistic or punitive consequences of violent behavior are not shown; the viewer gets the idea and forms an attitude over time that it is courageous to be violent, that violence is rewarded or socially acceptable, and that the violent person is the hero with whom to identify. Further, continual viewing of violence desensitizes the person to violence in general; it is no longer a noteworthy act in the home or society. Even worse, television violence shows inequality and domination; the most frequent victims are women, the old, and children. Research results on the effects of violence over a 15-year period in the United States have not shown a decrease in the television violence portrayed (119, 139, 178, 179).

Teach parents that, increasingly, research indicates that seeing violent, sexually seductive programs or pornographic material on television or on films has the following *long-term negative effects* on children (87, 94, 102, 112, 119, 125, 165, 178, 179, 212):

1. Gives an unrealistic, irreverent view of life
2. Teaches values of violence and materialism; teaches lack of respect for life and dignity of person; teaches justification of violence
3. Presents sexual stimulation that the child cannot handle
4. Confuses values
5. Shows an unquestioning acceptance of dishonest, aggressive, violent, exploitative, or manipulative behavior toward others
6. Presents gender and racial stereotypes (e.g., the man is typically portrayed as more important, competent, authoritative, assertive, and aggressive than the woman; the minority person may be shown as incompetent; the American Indian often is stereotyped as a violent killer)
7. Stimulates fear and anxiety
8. Stimulates and causes acting out of or identification with aggressive and sexual impulses, anger, and hostile feelings
9. Promotes excessive fears about war and the bomb, about walking in one's own neighborhood, about the "violent" world, and about the police who only use force
10. Increases aggressive behavior (in some children behavioral changes may last 10 years)
11. Increases emotional problems

Children who have grown up in stable families, who feel secure and loved, and who have a variety of interests and relationships will not be adversely affected by the aggression, violence, and sex of television. They can separate fantasy from fact and all of their fantasy is not based on television. Children growing up without positive identification models, who are already shaky in their self-concept and identity formation, are affected very negatively. Likewise, children from troubled or dysfunctional homes lack the supervision or guidance to help them handle and sort through what they see and hear (119).

Discuss with parents the need to limit the amount of television viewing (2 hours a day); do alternative activities with their children; screen what their children are viewing; and work to reduce the trend to more violent and pornographic programming. Parents can be more vigilant about programs their children watch. Television programming can be improved. Networks and advertisers, of course, hope that parents will disregard research findings that make-believe violence makes for real violence in many settings. As long as violence on television is profitable, programming will contain violence. Parents can rebel: writing letters to stations, writing letters to advertisers, and refusing to buy the products advertised. This is a significant area of life that affects the child's and the family's physical, emotional, cognitive, social, and spiritual health.

Organizations such as the American Medical Association, National Education Association, and Parent-Teacher Association have united in opposition against programming containing violent and sexual excesses. Many parent, school, community, health care, and religious leaders are joining efforts to gain more educational and less destructive programming, including the National Coalition on Television Violence, which is directed by a psychiatrist. Opposition against video games is mounting in the belief that they foster some of the same problems as excess television (102).

In essence, interaction with parents and others and real experiences, not passive observations, help the child learn to work through conflicts of development and to solve problems.

Play Patterns

Peer Groups

Peer groups, including the gang and the close chum, provide companionship with a widening circle of persons outside the home and are extremely important to the school-age child. Between the ages of 7 and 9, children usually form close friendships with peers of the same sex and age. Later in this age group, peers are not necessarily of the same age. Children must earn their membership in the peer group, and being accepted by one's peers and belonging to a peer group are major concerns for this age group. Many factors determine a child's acceptance, including attractiveness and friendliness. Peer groups provide companionship and a chance for children to compete and to compare themselves with others their own age. Peer groups develop their own sets of values and goals, and each group member will have a specific status or role. These groups provide the child an opportunity to test mastery in a world parallel to adult society, with rules, organization, and purposes (43, 70, 126, 206).

Play Activities

Play activities change with the child's development. From 6 to 8 years he or she is interested chiefly in the present and in the immediate surroundings. Because he or she knows more about family life than any other kind of living, the child plays house or takes the role of various occupational groups with which there is contact: mailcarrier, nurse, storekeeper, teacher. Although the child is more interested in playing with peers than parents, the 6- or 7-year old will occasionally enjoy having the parent as a "child" or "student." This allows the child to have imaginary control over the parent and also allows the parent to understand how the child is interpreting the parent or how the child perceives the teacher.

Both sexes enjoy some activities in common such as painting, cutting, pasting, reading, collecting items such as baseball cards or stamps, simple table games, television, digging, riding a bicycle, running games, skating, and swimming. Again, the parent can sometimes enjoy these activities with the child, especially if the parent has a special talent the child wishes to learn. The child imitates the roles of his or her own sex and becomes increasingly realistic in play. By age 8, collections are a favorite pastime, and loosely formed, short-lived clubs with fluctuating rules are formed (88).

The schoolchild, usually near 8 or 9 years of age, enjoys computerized and electronic games, which give a sense of control and power; of being a peer with, or even superior to, the adult; of challenge and inventiveness; and an enjoyment of complexity and expandability. The computer can be a tool for robot thinking or for development of thought; for passivity or releasing aggressive impulses or creativity; for play or for learning. Computer toys can help the schoolchild understand the nature of systems and control of information—skills needed in the adult world. However, let the child take the lead in when to move into computer games. There is no need to rush the child. He or she can pick up the skills and the enjoyment at any age. Further, some schoolchildren will prefer reading, painting, playing an instrument, doing crafts, camping, or playing sports to working with computers. These skills and what these activities teach are as essential to the workplace as the ability to operate a computer (87).

From 9 to 12 years the child becomes more interested in active sports but continues to enjoy quieter activity. He or she wants to improve motor skills. The child may enjoy carpenter or mechanics tools, advanced models, or puzzles, or camera and film. Adult-organized games of softball, football, or soccer lose their fun when parents place excessive emphasis on winning. The hug from a teammate after hitting a home run means more than just winning. Further, adults' taking over the games robs the child of independence (193).

Creative talents appear; the child may be interested in more complicated arts and crafts, science projects, music, or dance. At approximately age 10, sex differences in play become pronounced. Each sex is developing through play the skills it will later need in society; this is manifested through the dramatizing of real-life situations. The child's interest in faraway places is enhanced through a foreign pen pal and through travel (57).

Gang Stage

In preadolescence the gang becomes important. A **gang** is a *group whose membership is earned on the basis of skilled performance of some activity, frequently physical in nature. Its stability is expressed through formal symbols such as passwords or uniforms.* Gang codes take precedence over almost everything. They may range from agreement to protect a member who smoked in the boys' restroom at school to boycotting a school dance. Generally, gang codes are characterized by collective action against the mores of the adult world. In the gang children discharge hostility and aggression against peers rather than adults and begin to work out their own social patterns without adult interference. Unfortunately, some gangs do turn their hostility against other youths or adults. When this occurs, the pattern is laid for delinquent behaviors (126, 193, 206). However, these groups are not necessarily offenders against the law. Gang formation is loosely structured at first, with a transient membership that cuts across all social classes. Early gangs may consist of both boys and girls in the same groups. Later, separate gangs for each sex occur (206).

Chum Stage

The chum stage occurs around 9 or 10 years of age and sometimes later when affection moves from the peer group and gang to a **chum,** a *special friend of the same sex and age.* This is an important relationship because it is the child's first love attachment outside the family, when someone becomes as important to him or her as self. Initially, a person of the same sex and age is easier than someone of the opposite sex to feel concern for and to understand. The friend becomes an extension of the child's own self. As he or she shares ideas and feelings, the child learns a great deal about both self and the chum. The child discovers that he or she is more similar to than different from others and learns to accept self for what he or she is. Self-acceptance of uniqueness increases acceptance of others so that the child of this age is very sociable, generous, and sympathetic, enjoys differences in people, and is liberal in ideas about the welfare of others. He or she learns that others can do things differently but that they are still all right as people. It is also through the chum relationship that the child learns the syntaxic mode of communication described earlier, for he or she learns to validate word meanings in talking with the chum. Thus ideas about the world become more realistic. Loyalty to the chum at this age may be greater than loyalty to the family (186). **Altruism,** a *concern for others in various situations,* and an ability to respond to others' happiness and distress, to develop intimate associations, including with individuals of the opposite gender, and a sensitivity and concern for all humanity result from high-level chumship (186).

The chum stage has homosexual elements, but it is not an indication of homosexuality. It provides the foundation for later intimacy with an individual of the opposite sex and close friends of both sexes. If the child does not have a chum relationship, he or she has little capacity for adolescent heterosexuality or adult intimacy. According to Sullivan, fixation at this level results in homosexuality (186). Other theories regarding causation of homosexuality also have been proposed (see Chapter 12).

Help parents understand the importance of the gang and chum stages.

Tools of Socialization

Competition, compromise, cooperation, and beginning collaboration are progressive tools the schoolchild uses in accomplishing satisfying relationships with peers. **Competition** is *comprised of all activities that are involved in getting to a goal first, of seeking affection or status above others.* When the child is competing, he or she has rigid standards about many situations, including praise and punishment. For example, regardless of the circumstance, the child believes that the same punishment should be given for the same wrongdoing. He or she cannot understand why a 3-year-old sibling and he or she should not be punished similarly for spilling milk on the kitchen floor. Similarly, the child thinks he or she should be praised for dressing self as is the 3-year-old. *The child accepts adult rules as compulsory and rigid; he or she experiences a* **morality of constraint** (142).

Compromise, a *give-and-take agreement,* is gradually learned from peers, teachers, and family. The child becomes less rigid in standards of behavior. **Cooperation,** an *exchange between equals by adjusting to the wishes of others,* results from the chum relationship with its syntaxic mode of communication (186). Through the **morality of cooperation** the *child begins to understand the social implications of acts.* He or she learns judgment through helping make and carry out rules (142). **Collaboration,** *deriving satisfaction from group accomplishment rather than personal success,* is a step forward from cooperation and enables experimentation with tasks and exploration of situations (101, 186).

If a child does not learn how to get along with others, future socialization will be inhibited. For example, if a person is fixated at the competition level and does not learn how to compromise or cooperate, he or she is hard on self and is a hard person with whom to live. Eventually the person derives satisfaction only from competing but fails to enjoy the accomplishment, the end product. If a child is not relating well with peers, a group assertiveness training program can effectively increase social and assertive behavior through reinforcement procedures, relaxation techniques, guided imagery, and behavior contracts (97).

Guidance and Discipline

In guidance, parents should invite confidence of the child as a parent, not as a buddy or pal. The child will find pals among peers. In the adult he or she needs a parent! The atmosphere should be open and inviting for the child to talk with the parents, but the child's privacy should not be invaded. The parents should see the child as he or she is, not as an idealized extension of themselves.

The schoolchild has a rather strict superego and also uses many rituals to maintain self-control. He or she prefers to initiate self-control rather than be given commands or overt discipline, and stability and routine in his or her life provide this opportunity. You can talk with parents about methods of guidance and the importance of not interfering with behavior too forcefully or too often. The child needs some alternatives from which to choose so that he or she can learn different ways of behaving and coping and be better able to express self later. If development has been normal during the preschool years, the child is now well on the way to absorbing and accepting the standards, codes, and attitudes of society. He or she needs ongoing guidance rather than an emphasis on disciplinary measures. Parents that are too controlled or punitive contribute to fearfulness in the child. If the parent is perceived as supportive and encouraging of autonomy, the child is less likely to be fearful. Research indicates that preadolescent girls perceive their mothers as more supportive but also more punitive than their fathers. Upper-middle-class parents are perceived by their daughters as less punitive and more autonomy granting than are lower-middle-class parents, and lower-class parents are perceived as even more punitive and less autonomy granting by their daughters (213). Boys who are less warmly treated by their parents are more responsive to social or peer influences than girls, which has implications for later antisocial behavior (101).

For some parents, guiding a child can be a problem. They will ask, "When, what kind, and how much should you punish a child?" "How do you handle guilt or hostile feelings that often accompany discipline?" You are in a position to help parents learn the value of positive guidance techniques (10, 32, 93, 101, 108, 126, 193).

When expressing anger to children, describe what you see, feel, and expect. Do not lower the child's self-esteem by humiliating him or her, especially in front of others. The child's dignity can be protected by using "I" messages: "I am angry. I am frustrated." Such statements are honest and are safer than "What's your problem? You are stupid!" If repeated frequently, the child may believe that he or she is stupid and carry that self-image for years. Although shouting is not recommended, the parent who shouts displeasure at the danger or inconvenience *only* is probably harming the child much less than the parent who quietly and continually verbalizes personal assaults against the child. Ideally, the limit should be set with firm conviction and should only deal with one incident at a time. More than one message can confuse the child.

Our grandparents are reputed to have disciplined their children with authority and certainty. By contrast, some of today's parents seem afraid of their children. The child needs an understanding authority and a good example. He or she needs to know what constitutes unacceptable behavior and what substitute will be accepted. For instance, say, "Food is not for throwing; your baseball is." He or she will not obey rules if parents do not. Inconsistent discipline, or the "Do as I say, not as I do" approach, will lead to maladjustment, conflict, and aggression. The suggestions about guidance listed in Chapter 9 are applicable to the schoolchild as well.

Guidance at this age takes many other and less dramatic forms. A mother can turn the often harried "getting back to school clothes" experience into a pleasant lesson in guidance. She can accompany the child on a special shopping trip in which he or she examines different textures of material, learns about color coordination, understands what constitutes a good fit, and appreciates how much money must be spent for certain items. This principle can be carried into any parent-schoolchild guidance relationship such as learning responsibility for some household task or earning, handling, and saving money.

Emotional Development

The schoolchild consolidates earlier psychosocial development and simultaneously reaches out to a number of identification figures, expands interests, and associates with more people. Behavioral characteristics change from year to year. Table 10–4 summarizes and compares basic behavior patterns, although individual children will show a considerable range of behavior. Cultural, health, and social conditions may also influence behavior (43, 56, 57, 101, 125).

Developmental Crisis

The psychosexual crisis for this period is industry versus inferiority. **Industry** is *an interest in doing the work of the world, the child's feeling that he or she can learn and solve problems, the formation of responsible work habits and attitudes, and the mastery of age-appropriate tasks* (46). The child has greater body competence and applies self to skills and tasks that go beyond playful expression. The child gets tired of play, wants to participate in the real world, and seeks attention and recognition for efforts and concentrations on a task. He or she feels pride in doing something well whether a physical or cognitive task. A sense of industry involves self-confidence, perseverance, diligence, self-control, cooperation, and compromise rather than only competition. There is a sense of loyalty, relating self to something positive beyond the moment and outside the self. Parents, teachers, and nurses may see this industry at times as restlessness, irritability, rebellion toward authority, and lack of obedience.

The danger of this period is that the child may develop a sense of **inferiority,** *feeling inadequate, defeated, unable to learn or do tasks, lazy, unable to compete, compromise, or cooperate,* regardless of his or her actual competence (46). The child, and later the adult if this stage is not resolved, will not like to work or try new tasks; he or she will be moody, anxious, oversensitive to and isolated from others, excessively meek, and lacking in perseverance. Regressive behavior, excess fear of body injury or illness, or psychosomatic disorders may be observed. The child may try to prove self by various acting-out behavior such as lying or stealing. If the child feels excessively ashamed, self-doubting, guilty, and inferior from not having achieved the developmental tasks

TABLE 10-4. ASSESSMENT OF CHANGING BEHAVIORAL CHARACTERISTICS IN THE SCHOOLCHILD

6 Years	7 Years	8 Years
Self-centered	Self-care managed	Expansive personality but fluctuating behavior
Body movement, temper outbursts release tension	Quiet, less impulsive but assertive	Curious, robust, energetic
Behavioral extremes; impulsive or dawdles, loving or antagonistic	Fewer mood swings	Rapid movements and response; impatient
Difficulty making decisions; needs reminders	Self-absorbed without excluding others; may appear shy, sad, brooding	Affectionate to parents
Verbally aggressive but easily insulted	Attentive, sensitive listener	Hero worship of adult
Intense concentration short time, then abruptly stops activity	Companionable; likes to do tasks for others	Suggestions followed better than commands
Security of routines and rituals essential; periodic separation anxiety	Good and bad behavior in self and others noted	Adult responsibilities and characteristics imitated; wants to be considered important by adults
Series of three commands followed, but response depending on mood	High standards for self but minor infractions of rules; tattles, alibis, takes small objects from others	Approval and reconciliation sought; feelings easily hurt
Self-control and initiative in activity encouraged when adult uses counting to give child time ("I'll give you until the count of 10 to pick up those papers")	Concern about own behavior; tries to win over others' approval	Sense of property; enjoys collections
Praise and recognition needed	Angry over others' failure to follow rules	Beginning sense of justice but makes alibis for own transgressions
		Demanding and critical of others
		Gradually accepts inhibitions and limits

9 Years	10 Years
More independent and self-controlled	More adultlike and poised, especially girls
Dependable, responsible	Mores self-directive, independent
Adult trust and more freedom without adult supervision sought	Organized and rapid in work; budgets time and energy
Loyal to home and parents; seeks their help at times	Suggestions followed better than requests, but obedient
More self rather than environmentally motivated; not dependent on but benefits from praise	Family activities and care of younger siblings, especially below school age, enjoyed
More involved with peers	Aware of individual differences among people, but does not like to be singled out in a group
Own interests subordinated to group demands and adult authority	Hero worship of adult
Critical of own and others' behavior	Loyal to group; chum important
Concerned about fairness and willing to take own share of blame	Some idea of own assets and limits
More aware of society	Preoccupied with right and wrong
	Better able to live by rules
	Critical sense of justice; accepts immediate punishment for wrongdoing
	Liberal ideas of social justice and welfare
	Strong desire to help animals and people
	Future career choices match parents' careers because of identification with parents
	Sense of leadership

11 Years	12 Years
Spontaneous, self-assertive, restless, curious, sociable	Considerable personality integration; self-contained, self-competent, tactful, kind, reasonable, less self-centered
Short outbursts of anger and arguing	Outgoing, eager to please, enthusiastic
Mood swings	Sense of humor; improved communication skills
Challenges enjoyed	More companionable than at 11; mutual understanding between parents and child
On best behavior away from home	Increasingly sensitive to feelings of others; wishes good things for family and friends; caught between the two
Quarrelsome with siblings; rebellious to parents	Others' approval sought
Critical of parents, although affectionate with them	Childish lapses, but wishes to be treated like adult
Chum and same-sex peers important; warm reconciliation follows quarrels	Aware of assets and shortcomings
Secrets freely shared with chum; secret language with peers	Tolerant of self and others
Unaware of effect of self on others	Peer group and chum important in shaping attitudes and interests
Strict superego; zeal for fairness	Ethical sense more realistic than idealistic
Future career choices fantasized on basis of possible fame	Decisions about ethical questions based on consequences
Modest with parents	Less tempted to do wrong; basically truthful
	Self-disciplined; accepts just discipline
	Enthusiastic about community projects

Research Abstract

Meininger, J., E. Stashinko, and L. Hayman, Type A Behavior in Children: Psychometric Properties of the Matthews Youth Test for Health, Nursing Research, *40, no. 4 (1991), 221–226.*

Type A children have been reported to exhibit more impatience and aggression, under-report fatigue, and make greater efforts to excel when performance criteria are ambiguous. There is evidence that type A and type B children are different in responsiveness. However, rating type A behavior in children may be as problematic as is rating such behavior in adults since type A individuals comprise a diverse group.

Anger and hostility components of type A behavior may stem from a profound sense of insecurity. Children who are insecurely attached develop an anger-oriented appraisal and coping style similar to the type A behavior described for adults. Attachment difficulties during sensitive periods of development can create low self-esteem and inferiority. The sense of personal inadequacy leaves type A individuals vulnerable to personal threats. The overt manifestations of type A behavior are viewed as defensive mechanisms in response to perceived threats.

A study of 216 twins (dizygotic and monozygotic) between 6 and 11 years of age revealed lower type A scores in this sample, and a consistent gender effect was not found. There was no evidence to conclude that type A behavior, as it is conceptualized for children, is linked with clinically evident coronary heart disease in adulthood.

all along, emotional and behavioral problems may occur. Withdrawal, depression, speech difficulties, fire-setting or other extreme antisocial behavior, or self-destructive or aggressive acts may be displayed. Sometimes opposite behavior may occur as the person tries to cope with feelings of being no good, inferior, or inadequate. Instead, the person might immerse self in tasks to prove personal worth and gain attention, become aggressive, bossy, and overcompetitive. He or she will want his or her own way regularly. There is no time for play or camaraderie. The child who is the "teacher's pet" because he or she is such a "good little worker" may well suffer a sense of inferiority. If work is all the child can do at home and school, he or she will miss out on a lot of friendships and opportunities in life, now and later, and eventually become the adult who is a slave to technology: he or she cannot stop working.

There are sharp differences in how children bear up under stress such as abuse or divorce. Some children become nervous, withdrawn and feel inferior; some are illness-prone and slow to develop. Other children are resilient, shrug off the stressors, thrive, and go on to be industrious, have high self-esteem, and as adults lead highly productive lives. Still other children have protective factors that buffer against risks. True, some children are born with an innately easy-going temperament that handles stressors better than do children with a nervous, overreactive disposition, but even highly reactive children can acquire resilience if they have a stabilizing, attentive parent or mentor (55).

Studies with monkeys show that when vulnerable monkeys are placed with attentive foster mothers, they go from the usual timid behavior to being assertive and socially outgoing. At puberty they are able to leave the native troop, and the monkeys then move to the top of the hierarchy and become leaders.

Vulnerable children, if placed in the right environment, also become productive and competent adults. Children who have robust, sunny personalities are lovable and readily win affection, which further builds self-esteem and an identity. Robust children are flexible but persistent and will continue to look for a solid relationship—neighbor, teacher, relative—until they find at least one such adult. Then they distance self from the conflictual or abusive home, at least emotionally (4, 55, 204, 205).

Resilient children are likely to have personality characteristics similar to those of both traditional male and female characteristics—outgoing and autonomous, nurturant and emotionally sensitive. Resilient children are likely to have a number of protective factors, but the key is a basic, consistent, lasting, trusting relationship with an adult who is supportive and who is a beacon presence from infancy on. Then the child's ability to cope improves naturally as he or she develops and gains experience.

When the child's environment is overwhelmingly stressful, extra support and love are especially important. If the child is facing multiple stressors, it is more difficult for outside intervention to help the child. The more the risk factors, the worse is the outcome for the child, regardless of the intervention. However, basic health, social, and educational programs must be provided to assist the child to adapt to the extent possible—now and in future adult life (4, 55, 204, 205).

Teach parents that they can contribute to a sense of industry and avoid inferiority feelings by not having unrealistic expectations of the child and by using the suggested guidance and discipline approaches. They can encourage peer activities and home responsibilities, help the child meet developmental crises, and give recognition to his or her accomplishments and unique talents. They must remember that part of the time their child may regress to jumping on the couch, drumming nervously on the table with fingernails, and insisting that keeping clean is only for parents. At other times they will marvel at the poised, contented child who is visiting so nicely with their guests.

Self-Concept, Body-Image, and Sexuality Development

Until the child goes to school, self-perception is derived primarily from the parents' attitudes and reactions toward him or her. The child who is loved for what he or she is learns to love and accept self. If parental reactions have been rejecting, if he or she has been made to feel ugly, ashamed, or guilty about self or his or her behavior, the child enters school feeling bad, inadequate, or inferior. A positive self-concept is imperative for happiness and personality unity.

The child with a positive self-concept likes self and others; believes that what he or she thinks, says, and does makes a difference; believes he or she can be successful and can solve problems; has a realistic estimate of personal abilities and limitations; and expresses feelings of pleasure and enjoyment (26).

A negative self-image causes the child to feel defensive toward others and self and hinders adjustment to school and academic progress. Low self-concept children show more social withdrawal, academic difficulties, and inappropriate attention seeking than high self-concept children (214).

At school the child compares self with and is compared by peers in appearance, motor, cognitive, language, and social skills. If he or she cannot perform as well as other children, peers will perceive the child negatively, and eventually he or she will perceive self as incompetent or inferior because self-image is more dependent on peers than earlier. Schoolchildren are frequently cruel in their honesty as they make derogatory remarks about peers with limitations or disabilities.

Unattractive children may receive discriminatory treatment from parents, teachers, and babysitters because adults have learned the social value of beauty. Unattractive children are judged more antisocial and less honest than attractive children. Thus if an unattractive child expresses innocence, he or she is less likely to be believed. Attractive children are better liked by peers and adults and are judged to have a higher IQ and to be more likely to attend college. Because people tend to act as others expect them to, the prophecy is likely to become true (12). It is important for you to avoid this kind of reaction.

Cultural attitudes also affect self-concept. In studies with African-American and Caucasian children, both races of children indicated a distinct preference for dolls of their own color, but in the 1960s African-American children preferred white dolls instead of black dolls. The awakening of Black political consciousness in the 1960s was a forerunner of a more positive self-image in the African-American person (101, 125).

Self-concept and body image are also affected by gender and grade level of the child, father's education, history of illness, and type of illness, if any. Williams (207) found that American and Filipino boys did not score significantly different in body image, whereas Filipino girls scored lower than American girls. Third-grade American children had a better understanding of the body than Filipino third graders, but fifth graders in both cultures did not score significantly different from each other. American and Filipino children whose fathers had a college education did not score significantly differently; however, Filipino children whose fathers had less education scored lower in body organ knowledge than American children whose fathers were not college educated. Regardless of these variables, ill Filipino children did not score significantly lower in body image and concept of illness than American children. More research is needed on the child's concept of self, body, and illness, both in this and other cultures.

Biracial children are increasing in number, and their special racial status affects racial identification, self-concept, self-esteem, and school adjustment. They must deal with overt racism affecting children of color, cope with outsiders who view their families as abnormal, and sometimes cope with the loyalty issues and negative feelings from the extended family of each parent. Positive parental feelings about racial identification and positive extended family relationships are critical to sound emotional adjustment of the child and a positive self-concept. The child may have difficulty identifying with either parent because of racism, and these feelings and issues must be discussed (24).

Parents, teachers, and health-care professionals can contribute to a positive self-esteem and competence in performance by emphasizing the child's positive, healthy characteristics and reinforcing the child's potential. You can be instrumental in fostering a healthy relationship. Then the child, especially a girl who is competent in many activities, retains this competence in the teen years. Studies show girls can be as excellent as boys in a wide variety of activities (62).

The perception and reaction of the teacher, nurse, and parent are extremely important. The parent and nurse should listen carefully to the child's own estimate of self, school progress, and relationship with peers. The teacher should be informed if the child questions his or her adequacy. The nurse can assess and help correct physical or emotional problems.

The teacher (or nurse) can intervene when derogatory remarks are made among classmates. Teacher may move a child into another work or play group appropriate for his or her ability or explain to peers in simple language the importance of accepting another who is at a different developmental level. Meanwhile, teacher should encourage the child who has the difficulty. In turn, the nurse supports the teacher in such action. Thus the school experience may either reinforce or weaken the child's feeling about self as a unique, important person, with specific talents or abilities. If he or she is one of 30 children in a classroom and receives little attention from the teacher, self-concept may be threatened.

The child's body image and self-concept are very fluid. Schoolchildren are more aware of the internal body and external differences. They can label major organs with increasing accuracy; heart, brain, and bones are most frequently mentioned, along with cardiovascular, gastrointestinal, and musculoskeletal systems. The younger child thinks that organs change position, and organ function, size, and position are poorly understood. Organs such as the stomach are frequently drawn at the wrong place (this may reflect the influence of television ads). Children generally believe that they must have all body parts to remain alive and that the skin holds in body contents; consider the impact of injury or surgery on the child. This is an excellent age to teach about any of these inaccuracies (54, 154).

The child is changing physically, emotionally, and socially. Physique is changing. Sexual identity is strengthening. He or she is learning how to get along with more people, both peers and adults, and is developing academic skills. Table 10–5 shows how aspects of the child's view of self change through the school years (10, 12, 32, 54, 56, 57, 154).

Self-concept, body image, and sexuality development are interrelated and are influenced by parental and societal expectations of and reactions to each sex. You can assist parents in promoting a positive self-concept and body image. During latency boys and girls are similar in many ways, but differences are taught. Girls reportedly are less physically active, but they have greater verbal, perceptual, and cognitive skills than boys. Girls supposedly respond to stimuli—interpersonal and physical, including pain—more quickly and accurately than boys. They seem better at analyzing and anticipating environmental demands; thus their behavior conforms more to adult expectations, and they are better at staying out of trouble. Girls are encouraged to depend on and to rely on others' appraisals for self-esteem more than boys. Girls are not usually forced to develop internal controls and a sense of independent self in the way that boys are because of the difference in adult reactions

TABLE 10-5. ASSESSMENT OF CHANGING BODY-IMAGE DEVELOPMENT IN THE SCHOOLCHILD

6 Years	7 Years	8 Years
Is self-centered	Is more modest and aware of self	Redefines sense of status with others
Likes to be in control of self, situations, and possessions	Wants own place at table, in car, and own room or part of room	Subtle changes in physical proportion; movements smoother
Gains physical and motor skills	Has lower level physical activity than earlier	Assumes many roles consecutively
Knows right from left hand	Does not like to be touched	Is ready for physical contact in play and to be taught self-defense mechanisms
Regresses occasionally to baby talk or earlier behavior	Protects self by withdrawing from unpleasant situation	Is more aware of differences between the sexes
Plays at being someone else to clarify sense of self and others	Dislikes physical combat	Is curious about another's body
Is interested in marriage and reproduction	Engages less in sex play	Asks questions about marriage and reproduction; strong interest in babies, especially for girls
Distinguishes organs of each sex but wonders about them	Understands pregnancy generally; excited about new baby in family	Plays more with own sex
May indulge in sex play	Concerned he or she does not really belong to parents	
Draws a man with hands, neck, clothing, and six identifiable parts	Tells parts missing from picture of incomplete man	
Distinguishes between attractive and ugly pictures of faces		

9 Years	10 Years
Has well-developed eye-hand coordination	Is relatively content with and confident of self
Enjoys displaying motor skills and strength	Has perfected most basic small motor movements
Cares completely for body needs	Wants privacy for self but peeks at other sex
Has more interest in own body and its functions than in other sexual matters	Asks some questions about sexual matters again
Asks fewer questions about sexual matters if earlier questions answered satisfactorily	Investigates own sexual organs
Is self-conscious about exposing body, including to younger siblings and opposite sex parents	Shows beginning prepubertal changes physically, especially girls

11 Years	12 Years
States self is in heart, head, face, or body part most actively expressing him or her	Growth spurt; changes in appearance
Feels more self-conscious with physical changes occurring	Muscular control almost equal to that of adult
Mimics adults; deepening self-understanding	Identifies self as being in total body or brain
Masturbates sometimes; erection occurs in boys	May feel like no part of body is his or hers alone but like someone else's because of close identity with group
Discusses sexual matters with parents with reticence	Begins to accept and find self as unique person
Likes movies on reproduction	Feels joy of life with more mature understanding

to each sex. Innate physiologic differences become magnified as they are reinforced by cultural norms and specific parental behaviors (7).

Stereotypes are changing, however. Girls can cope with aggression and competition just as boys can. Title IX of the Education Amendments of 1972 prohibited persons from being excluded from educational programs and activities because of sex; females may now legally participate in school sports programs and qualify for competitive athletics against boys. (Postpubescent girls should not engage in heavy collision sports against boys, however, because of potential injury resulting from the girls' lesser muscle mass per unit of body weight [125].)

Research shows that fears about the girl's harming her childbearing functions or her feminine appearance as a result of normal rigorous activity are unfounded. Traditionally, girls and women in rural areas have worked very hard physically with no ill effects. In addition, primarily the male hormones, not vigorous exercise, produce big bones, muscle mass, and a masculine appearance (125). Early physical education activities teach general coordination, eye-hand coordination, and balance—basic movements that carry over into all movement and sports. Rigorous conditioning activities such as gymnastics are suggested for achieving high levels of physical fitness for prepubertal girls and will improve agility, appearance, endurance, strength, feelings of well-being, and self-concept.

Sexuality Education

Sexuality education, *learning about the self as a person who is a sexual being,* has begun by the school years. The child can learn that both sexes have similar feelings and behavior potential, which can instill attitudes about maleness and femaleness for adulthood. The traditional stereotypes of the aggressive, competitive, intelligent, clumsy, brave, and athletic man and the passive, demure, gentle, graceful, domestic, fearful, and emotional woman must be discarded by parents, teachers, and other adults so that they will not be learned by the schoolchild. At this age both sexes are dependent and independent, active and passive, emotional and controlled, gentle and aggressive. Keeping such a range of behavior will contribute to a more flexible adult who can be expressive, spontaneous, and accepting of self and others.

You will have to work through your own stereotypes to help the parents, child, and child's peers avoid sex typing.

Sex education, *factual information about anatomy, physiology, and birth control methods,* should begin now for both sexes. By 7 or 8, children usually know that both sexes are required for childbirth to occur, but they are not sure how.

Almost all parents will experience at least some anxiety and embarrassment when they discuss sex with their children. Remember that these parents have come from a generation taught that the discussion of sex was at least partially taboo. Ideas about sexual behavior and what should be taught varies with socioeconomic level and age group.

Following are some guidelines for parents, teachers, or yourself when handling this subject:

1. Know the facts.
2. Do not lecture or preach.
3. Do not skip anything because the youngster says, "I already know." Chances are the child has some twisted facts.
4. Answer all questions as honestly as possible.
5. Do not force too much at one sitting. Aim the information at the child's immediate interest. Do not pry into the child's feelings and fantasies. Try to make the conversation as relaxed as possible.

Many elementary schools introduce basic sex education at the fourth grade level. Usually parents are asked to preview the film or presentation and give permission for their child to participate. Ideally this procedure will stimulate a bond among parents, child, and teacher so that all focus on accurate and positive education. In planning a sex education program, realize that there probably will be parents both in favor of and opposed to sex education classes. It is important to explore and clarify the attitudes of parents and teachers during the early planning phases.

Self-concept and sexuality can be traumatized by sexual advances from adults, sometimes family members. Burgess and her colleagues (17–20) and other authors (65, 103, 189) provide useful references for gaining additional information.

Burgess and Holmstrom (17) describe a study of school-age children who were sexually molested, feelings about the traumatic event, stages of resolution, defense mechanisms used by the children and parents, the issues, feelings of and difficulties for the parents in the community who joined together to prosecute the offender (a busdriver), other community issues, and the therapists' role with the children and parents over a period of time. Swanson and Braggio (187) discuss the dynamics of and consequent problems of father-daughter incest. Other references discuss factors that contribute to sexual abuse, the trauma to the child and family members, treatment, and legal implications; refer also to Chapter 9 (17–21, 47, 152, 216).

Adaptive Mechanisms

The schoolchild is losing the protective mantle of home and early childhood and needs order and consistency in life to help cope with doubts, fears, unacceptable impulses, and unfamiliar experiences. Commonly used adaptive mechanisms include ritualistic behavior, reaction formation, undoing, isolation, fantasy, identification, regressing, malingering, rationalization, projection, and sublimation (101).

Ritualistic behavior, *consistently repeating an act in a situation,* wards off imagined harm and anxiety and provides a feeling of control. Examples include stepping on cracks in the sidewalk while chanting certain words, always putting the left leg through trousers before the right, having a certain place for an object, or doing homework at a specific time.

Reaction formation, undoing, and isolation are related to obsessive, ritualistic behavior.

Reaction formation is used frequently in dealing with feelings of hostility. The child may unconsciously hate a younger brother because he infringes on the schoolchild's freedom, but such impulses are unacceptable to the strict superego. To counter such unwanted feelings, the child may become the classic example of a caring, loving sibling.

Undoing is *unconsciously removing an idea, feeling, or act by performing certain ritualistic behavior.* For example, the gang has certain chants and movements to follow before a member who broke a secret code can return. **Isolation** is a *mechanism of unconsciously separating emotion from an idea because the emotion would be unacceptable to the self.* The idea remains in the conscious, but its component feeling remains in the unconscious. A child uses isolation when he or she seems to talk very objectively about the puppy who has just been run over by a truck.

Fantasy *compensates for feelings of inadequacy, inferiority, and lack of success* encountered in school, the peer group, or home. Fantasy is necessary for eventual creativity and should not be discouraged if it is not used excessively to prevent realistic participation in the world. Fantasy saves the ego temporarily, but it also provides another way for the child to view self, thus helping him or her aspire to new heights of behavior.

Identification is seen in the hero worship of teacher, scoutmaster, neighbor, or family friend, someone whom the child respects and who has the qualities the child fantasizes as his or her own.

Regression, *returning to a less sophisticated pattern of behavior,* is a defense against anxiety and helps the child avoid potentially painful situations. For example, he or she may revert to using the language or behavior of a younger sibling if the child feels that the sibling is getting undue attention.

Malingering, *feigning illness to avoid unpleasant tasks,* is seen when the child stays home from school for a day or says he or she is unable to do a home task because he or she does not feel well.

Rationalization, *giving excuses when the child is unable to achieve wishes,* is frequently seen in relation to schoolwork. For example, after a low test grade, the response is, "Oh well, grades don't make any difference anyway."

Projection is seen as the child says about a teacher, "She doesn't like me," when really the teacher is disliked for having reprimanded him or her.

Sublimation is a major mechanism used during the school years. The child increasingly *channels sexual and aggressive impulses into socially acceptable tasks* at school and home. In the process, if all goes well, he or she develops the sense of industry.

Use of any and all of these mechanisms in various situations is normal, but overuse of any one can result in a constricted, immature personality. If constricted, the child will be unable to develop relationships outside the home, to succeed at home or school, or to balance work and play. Achieving a sense of identity and adult developmental tasks will be impaired.

Help parents understand the adaptive mechanisms used by the child and how to help the child use healthy coping mechanisms.

Child in Transition

American families are on the move. Moving from one part of the country to another, or even from one community and school system to another, brings a special set of tasks that should be acknowledged and worked through. Some families, because of the military or other career or as part of an exchange program, may live in another country for a number of years or move from country to country. This poses another kind of adjustment and set of tasks. Children who were born in a foreign country and then return with their parents to the United States undergo culture shock. They feel like citizens of another country and visitors in the land of which they are a citizen. Lykins (106) describes the feelings of children of the "Third Culture" who have seen much of the world, know more than one language, who are cognizant of and accepting of various life-styles, and who speak, dress, eat, and behave as if they were still in another land. He also describes family and employment dynamics. Educational considerations that must be made in school are also discussed. These students usually want to return to the country in which they had lived for some time, although they feel patriotism for the United States.

The school-age child is especially affected by a geographic move if he or she is just entering or is well settled into the chum stage. The child cannot understand why he or she cannot fit into the new group right away. Because routines are so important to the schoolchild, he or she is sometimes confused by the new and different ways of doing things. The parents will need to consult with the new school leaders about their child's adjustment.

If a family can include the schoolchild in the decision about where to move, the transition will be easier. If not, then the following ideas can still be used. Share them with parents. Ideally, the whole family should make at least one advance trip to the new community. If possible, the new home and town should be explored, and the child should visit the new school so that he or she can establish mentally where he or she is going. Writing to one of the new classmates before the actual move can enhance a feeling of friendship and belonging. If the child has a special interest such as gymnastics or dancing, a contact with the new program can form another transitional step.

When parents are packing, they are tempted to dispose of as many of the child's belongings as possible, especially if they seem babyish or worn. *Do not do this.* These items are part of the child, and they will help him or her feel comfortable and at home during adjustment to a new home and community.

Sometimes parents in the new community are reticent about letting their children go to the new child's house. The new parents should make every attempt to introduce themselves to the new playmates' parents, assuring them that the environment will be safe for play; or parents can have a get-acquainted party for the few children who are especially desired as playmates or chums.

Just as the family initiated some ties before they moved, so should they keep some ties from the previous neighborhood. If possible, let the child play with old friends at times. If the move has been too far for frequent visits, allow the child to call old friends occasionally. If possible, plan a trip back so that some old traditions can be reviewed and friends can be visited. The trip to the old neighborhood will cement in the child's mind that "home" is no longer there but in the new location.

The parents must accept as natural some grieving for what is gone. Letting the child express his or her feelings, accepting these feelings, and continuing to work with the above suggestions will foster the adjustment.

The nurse can foster the above through noticing the new child, watching his behavior, working with the teacher and peers, and contacting parents if necessary.

Moral-Spiritual Development

You can assist parents in understanding the importance of their role and that of peers, school, and even literature and the media in moral and spiritual development (128, 129, 167). If you care for a child over a period of time, you will also contribute to this development.

In the school years the child usually moves from the fairy tale stage of God's being like a giant to the realistic or concrete state of God's being like a human figure. For the Christian child, Jesus is an angelic boy growing into a perfect man.

The child is learning many particulars about his or her religion such as Allah, God, Jesus, prayer, rites, ancestor worship, life after death, reincarnation, heaven, or hell, all of which are developed into a religious philoso-phy and used in interpretation of the world. These ideas are taught by family, friends, teachers, church, books, radio, and television.

The child of 6 can understand God as creator, expects prayers to be answered, and feels the forces of good and evil with the connotation of reward and punishment. The 6-year-old believes in a creative being, a father figure who is responsible for many things such as thunder and lightning. The adult usually introjects the natural or scientific explanation. Somehow the child seems to hold this dual thinking without contradiction. The adult's ability to weave the supernatural with the natural will affect the child's later ability to do so. Coles (30) discusses his studies of spiritual development in children. Most children, even those from an atheistic background, develop a concept of God and are likely to believe in God. However, children may not discuss their views if they fear ridicule or rejection from a secular society (30).

The developing schoolchild has a great capacity for reverence and awe, continues to ask more appropriate questions about religious teaching and God, and can be taught through stories that emphasize moral traits. The child operates from a simple framework of ideas and will earnestly pray for recovery and protection from danger for self and others. The child believes that a Supreme Being loves him or her, gives the earth and a house, and is always near. He or she may say, however, "How does God take care of me when I can't see Him?" "Allah's here, but where?" "I don't know how to love God like I love you, Mommy, because I've never touched Him."

In prepuberty the child begins to comprehend disappointments more fully and realize that his or her answer to problems or desires to change the world quickly are not always possible (171). He or she realizes that self-centered prayers are not always answered and that no magic is involved. The child can now accept totally the scientific explanation for thunder and lightning. He or she may drop religion at this point; or because of strong dependence on parents, the child may continue to accept the family preference. Yet the blind faith that previously existed is gradually replaced by reason.

The schoolchild can be in the Conventional Stage of moral development, according to Kohlberg (89). (See Chapter 5, Table 5–4.) Beliefs about right and wrong have less to do with the child's actual behavior than with the likelihood of getting caught for transgression and the gains to derive from the transgression. Other factors that influence moral development include the child's intelligence, ability to delay gratification, and sense of self-esteem. The child with a high sense of self-esteem and a favorable self-concept is less likely to engage in immoral behavior, possibly because he or she will feel more guilty with wrongdoing. Thus moral behavior may be more a matter of strength of will or ego strength than of strength of conscience or superego. Morality is not a fixed behavioral trait but rather a decision-making capacity. The child progresses from an initial premoral stage, in which he or she responds primarily to reward and punishment and believes rules can be broken to meet personal needs, through a rule-based highly conventional morality, and finally to the stage of self-accepted principles (89).

Part of moral development is the ability to follow rules. Unlike the preschooler who initiates rules without understanding them, the 7-year-old or the 8-year-old begins to play in a genuinely social manner. Rules are mutually accepted by all players and are rigidly followed. Rules come from some external force such as God and are believed timeless. Not until the age of 11 or 12, when the formal operations level of cognition is reached, does the child understand the true nature of rules—that they exist to make the game possible and can be altered by mutual agreement (142).

Piaget (142) also identified stages of moral development as he studied the child's pattern of reasoning to think about moral issues. These stages are:

1. Premoral—the child has no regard for rules.
2. Heteronomous—the child obeys rules because of fear of authority or powerful figures.
3. Autonomous—the child follows rules freely, expressing mutual rights and obligations. The person is increasingly able to distinguish between principles and rules, and at more advanced stages the person applies principles to guide behavior in specific situations instead of automatically following established rules.

Moral development is related to self-discipline and empathy, and how this is taught varies with the culture. For example, a study showed that Japanese and American mothers approach the task of discipline and moral development differently. For instance, reactions of Japanese mothers to the child's public misbehavior is to ask, "How do you think this makes the storekeeper feel when you run around the store? How do you think it makes me feel?" From an early age the Japanese child is taught to consider the feelings of others, to think out the consequences of his or her behavior and not just obey rules, which fosters discipline and thoughtfulness that facilitates academic performance later. In contrast, the Western child is told what to do and often is spoken to with an anger level that arouses rebellion rather than self-restraint and a selfishness rather than a spirit of cooperation (10).

A study of children ages 10 to 14 in seven cultures, including the United States, Europe, and Asia, revealed that this era is a crucial time for learning moral views and to obey rules. Almost all children in all cultures realized that laws and rules are norms that guide behavior and require obedience from all, and they realized that chaos would result without them (102, 167). In five of the seven cultures children accepted that rule breaking might be permissible for higher moral reasons. In six of the seven cultures parents were seen as most able to make children follow rules. Only in Japan did the teacher rank higher than the parents. Police ranked at least fourth in all cultures except India. Thus affiliative, nurturant strategies rather than punitive ones were seen as most effective in inducing compliance and assuring the stability of systems (102, 167).

Developmental Tasks

Although the schoolchild continues working on past developmental tasks, he or she is confronted with a series of new ones (42):

1. Decreasing dependence on family and gaining some satisfaction from peers and other adults
2. Increasing neuromuscular skills so that he or she can participate in games and work with others
3. Learning basic adult concepts and knowledge to be able to reason and engage in tasks of everyday living
4. Learning ways to communicate with others realistically
5. Becoming a more active and cooperative family participant
6. Giving and receiving affection among family and friends without immediately seeking something in return
7. Learning socially acceptable ways of getting money and saving it for later satisfactions
8. Learning how to handle strong feelings and impulses appropriately
9. Adjusting the changing body image and self-concept to come to terms with the masculine or feminine social role
10. Discovering healthy ways of becoming acceptable as a person
11. Developing a positive attitude toward his or her own and other social, racial, economic, and religious groups

The accomplishment of these tasks gives the schoolchild a foundation for entering adolescence, an era filled with dramatic growth and changing attitudes. Your support, teaching, and guidance can assist the child in this progression.

Nursing Applications

Your role in caring for the school-age child and family has been described in each section of the chapter. Assessment, using knowledge about this era that is presented in this chapter, is the basis for *nursing diagnosis*. Nursing diagnoses that may be applicable to the school child are listed in Box 10–8. Interventions may involve measures that promote health (e.g., immunization or control of hazards); teaching, support, counseling, or

---

■ **BOX 10-8.**
Selected Nursing Diagnoses Related to the School-Age Child[a]

Pattern 1: Exchanging

Altered Nutrition: More than body requirements
Altered Nutrition: Less than body requirements
Altered Nutrition: Potential for more than body require-
ments
Potential for Infection
Potential for Injury
Potential for Trauma
Potential Impaired Skin Integrity

Pattern 2: Communicating

Impaired Verbal Communication

Pattern 3: Relating

Impaired Social Interaction
Social Isolation

Pattern 4: Valuing

Spiritual Distress

Pattern 5: Choosing

Ineffective Individual Coping
Impaired Adjustment
Health Seeking Behaviors

Pattern 6: Moving

Impaired Physical Mobility
Fatigue
Sleep Pattern Disturbance
Diversional Activity Deficit
Bathing/Hygiene Self Care Deficit
Dressing/Grooming Self Care Deficit
Altered Growth and Development

Pattern 7: Perceiving

Body Image Disturbance
Self-esteem Disturbance
Sensory/Perceptual Alterations
Hopelessness
Powerlessness

Pattern 8: Knowing

Knowledge Deficit

Pattern 9: Feeling

Pain
Dysfunctional Grieving
Anticipatory Grieving
Anxiety
Fear

[a]Other NANDA diagnoses are applicable to the ill school-age child.
From North American Nursing Diagnosis Association, *NANDA Nursing Diagnosis Taxonomy I* (Rev.). St. Louis: North American Nursing Diagnosis Association, 1990.

---

spiritual care with the child or family; or direct care measures to the ill child. Your understanding of the child developmentally will enable you to give holistic care—care that includes physiologic, emotional, cognitive, social, and spiritual aspects of the person.

REFERENCES

1. Allard, R., Beliefs About AIDS as Determinants of Preventive Practices and of Support for Coercive Measures, *American Journal of Public Health,* 78, no. 4 (1988), 448–452.
2. American Academy of Pediatrics, Committee on Infectious Diseases: Prevention of Hepatitis B Virus Infections, *Pediatrics,* 75, no. 2 (1985), 362–364.
3. ———, Committee on Infectious Diseases: Recommendations for Using Pneumococcal Vaccine in Children, *Pediatrics,* 75, no. 6 (1985), 1153–1158.
4. Anthony, E.J., and B. Cohler, *The Invulnerable Child.* New York: Guilford, 1987.
5. Attitudes of Safety Preserve Young Lives, *Farm Week* (April 1, 1991), p. 7.
6. Baker, S., and R. Henry, *Parents' Guide to Nutrition: Healthy Eating From Birth through Adolescence.* Reading, Mass: Addison-Wesley, 1987.
7. Bardwick, J., and E. Douvan, Ambivalence: The Socialization of Women. In Bardwick, J., ed., *Readings on the Psychology of Women.* New York: Harper & Row, 1972, 52–58.
8. Barker, P., and D. Lewis, The Management of Lead Exposure in Pediatric Populations, *Nurse Practitioner: American Journal of Primary Health Care,* 15, no. 12 (1990), 8–10.
9. Bates, B., *A Guide to Physical Examination and History Taking* (4th ed.). Philadelphia: J.B. Lippincott, 1987.
10. Bettelheim, B., and A. Freedgood, *A Good Enough Parent: A Book on Child-Rearing.* New York: Random, 1988.
11. Black, J., AIDS: Preschool and School Issues, *Journal of School Health,* 56, no. 3 (1986), 93–95.
12. Blaesing, S., and J. Brockhaus, The Development of Body Image in the Child, *Nursing Clinics of North America,* 7, no. 4 (1972), 601–607.
13. Boyce, W.T., et al., Playground Equipment Injuries in Large, Urban School District, *American Journal of Public Health,* 74, no. 9 (1984), 984–986.
14. Brazelton, T., What Parents Need to Say (Children's Fears of War), *Newsweek* (February 26, 1991), 52.

15. Brinley, M., How Much Is Too Much?, *W D Specials* (March 1988), p. 28 ff.

16. Bullough, B., and V. Bullough, *Nursing in the Community*. St. Louis: C.V. Mosby, 1990.

17. Burgess, A., and L. Holmstrom, Sexual Trauma of Children and Adults, *Nursing Clinics of North America,* 10, no. 3 (September 1975), 551–563.

18. ———, C. Hartman, and S. Kelley, Assessing Child Abuse: The TRIADS Checklist, *Journal of Psychosocial Nursing and Mental Health Services,* 28, no. 4 (1990), 6–14.

19. ———, M. McCausland, and W. Wolbert, Children's Drawings as Indicators of Sexual Trauma, *Perspectives in Psychiatric Care,* 19, no. 2 (1981), 50–58.

20. ———, et al., Child Molestation: Assessing Impact in Multiple Victims (Part I), *Archives of Psychiatric Nursing,* 1, no. 1 (1987), 33–39.

21. Burgess, E., Sexually Abused Children and Their Drawings, *Archives of Psychiatric Nursing,* 2, no. 2 (1988), 65–73.

22. Burgess, J., *Children, Adolescents and Nutrition*. New York: Grollier, 1988.

23. Butler, W., V. Segreto, and E. Collins, Prevalence of Dental Mottling in School-Aged Lifetime Residents of 16 Texas Communities, *American Journal of Public Health,* 75, (1985), 1408–1412.

24. Buttery, T., Biracial Children: Racial Identification, Self-Esteem, and School Adjustment, *Kappa Delta Pi Record,* 23, no. 2 (Winter 1987), 50–53.

25. Cacha, F., How Safe Are Students in School?, *Kappa Delta Pi Record,* 18, no. 3 (Spring 1982), 72–73.

26. Children Really Want Guidance in the Evolving Process of Self-Discovery, *Possibilities* (January–February 1989), 12–13.

27. Clore, E., Dispelling the Common Myths About Pediculosis, *Journal of Pediatric Health Care,* 3, no. 1 (1989), 28–33.

28. ———, Pediculosis Screening and Treatment, *School Nurse,* 6, no. 3 (1990), 14–18.

29. Coleman, D., Thriving Despite Hardship: Key Childhood Traits Identified, *New York Times,* October 13, 1987, p. 19 ff.

30. Coles, R., *The Spiritual Life of Children*. Boston: Houghton Mifflin, 1990.

31. ———, Children of Crisis, *The Privileged Ones, The Well Off, and the Rich in America,* Vol. 5. Boston: Little, Brown, 1978.

32. Comer, J., and A. Pouissant, *Black Child Care*. New York: Simon & Schuster, 1975.

33. Common, R., and M. MacMullen, Home Schooling—A Growing Movement, *Kappa Delta Pi Record,* 23, no. 4 (Summer 1987), 114–117.

34. Conroy, M., Is Perfectionism Killing Your Kid? *Better Homes and Gardens* (November 1987), 79–80.

35. Cookfair, J., *Nursing Process and Practice in the Community*. St. Louis: Mosby–Year Book, 1991.

36. Coopersmith, S., *The Antecedents of Self-Esteem*. San Francisco: W.H. Freeman, 1967.

37. Dagenais, R., and R. Morris, A Gifted Program That Is Making a Difference, *Kappa Delta Pi Record,* 25, no. 1 (Fall 1988), 24–27.

38. Daley, S., Little Girls Lose Their Self-Esteem on Way to Adolescence, Study Finds, *New York Times,* January 8, 1991.

39. Davidson, D.M., et al., School-Based Blood Cholesterol Screening, *Journal of Pediatric Health Care,* 3, no. 1 (1989), 3–8.

40. Diseker, R., et al., A Comparison of Height, Weight, and Triceps Skinfold Thickness of Children Ages 5–12 in Michigan (1978), Forsyth County, North Carolina (1978), and Hanes, Part I (1971–1974), *American Journal of Public Health,* 72, no. 7 (1982), 730–733.

41. Duncan, B., A. Smith, and F. Briese, A Comparison of Growth: Spanish-Surnamed With Non-Spanish Surnamed Children, *American Journal of Public Health,* 69, no. 9 (1979), 903–907.

42. Duvall, E., and B. Miller, *Marriage and Family Development* (6th ed). New Yorker: Harper & Row, 1984.

43. Dworetzky, J., and N. Davis, *Human Development: A Lifespan Approach*. St. Paul, Minn: West Publishing, 1989.

44. Edelman, M., Justice for Children Everywhere, *Today's Education* (February–March 1979), 41–45.

45. Edelson, E., *Food & Your Child*. New York: Time-Life Books, 1988.

46. Erikson, E., *Childhood and Society* (2nd ed.). New York: W.W. Norton, 1963.

47. Federation, S., Sexual Abuse: Treatment Modalities for the Younger Child, *Journal of Psychosocial Nursing,* 24, no. 7 (1986), 21–24.

48. Fergusen, C., and L. Roll, Human Rabies, *American Journal of Nursing,* 81, no. 6 (1981), 1175–1179.

49. Foster, R., M. Hunsberger, and J. Anderson, *Family-Centered Nursing Care of Children*. Philadelphia: W.B. Saunders, 1989.

50. Frederick, S., Ready for the Battle, *Believers' Voice of Victory,* 17, no. 6 (June 1989), 6–7.

51. Friar, L., and P. Grenoble, *Teaching Your Child to Handle Peer Pressure*. Chicago: Contemporary Books, 1988.

52. Furth, H., and H. Wachs, *Thinking Goes to School: Piaget's Theory in Practice*. New York: Oxford University Press, 1975.

53. Garbarino, J., E. Guttmann, and J. Seeley, *The Psychologically Battered Child: Strategies for Identification, Assessment and Intervention*. San Francisco: Jossey-Bass, 1987.

54. Gelbert, E., Children's Conceptions of the Content and Functions of The Human Body, *Genetic-Psychologic Monographs,* 65 (1962), 293–411.

55. Gelman, D., The Miracle of Resiliency, *Newsweek Special Issue* (Summer 1991), 44–47.

56. Gesell, A., and F. Ilg, *The Child From Five to Ten* (rev. ed.). New York: Harper Collins, 1977.

57. ———, F. Ilg, and L. Ames, *Youth: The Years from Ten to Sixteen*. New York: Harper & Brothers, 1956.

58. Goldman, J., The Taming of the Tube, *Health* (July–August 1990), 42–47.

59. Gordon, L., and D. Haynes, Smoking-Related Attitudes and Behaviors of Parents of Fourth-Grade Students, *Journal of School Health,* 51, no. 6 (1981), 408–412.

60. Greenberg, M., et al., Cigarette Use Among Hispanic and Non-Hispanic White School Children, Albuquerque, New Mexico, *American Journal of Public Health,* 77, no. 5 (1987), 621–622.

61. Grossman, D.S., Circadian Rhythms in Blood Pressure in School Age Children of Normotensive and Hypertensive Parents, *Nursing Research,* 40, no. 1 (1991), 28–34.

62. Hancock, E., *The Girl Within.* New York: Ballantine, 1990.

63. Haugaard, J., and N. Reppucci, *The Sexual Abuse of Children.* San Francisco: Jossey-Bass Publishers, 1989.

64. A Head Start Does Not Last, *Newsweek* (January 27, 1992), 44–45.

65. Heindle, M.C., Symposium on Child Abuse and Neglect: Foreword, *Nursing Clinics of North America,* 16, no. 1 (1981), 101–102.

66. Heiney, S., Helping Children Through Painful Procedures, *American Journal of Nursing,* 91, no. 11 (1991), 20–24.

67. Hickie, K., School's Just Too Boring for Many of Our Gifted Children, *Sydney Morning Herald,* December 18, 1991, p. 3.

68. Hirschmann, J., and L. Zaphiropoulos, *Solving Your Child's Eating Problems.* New York: Fawcett Columbine, 1985.

69. HIV and Children: A Growing Problem, *American Nurse* (November/December 1990), 21.

70. Hoffman, L., et al., *Developmental Psychology Today* (5th ed.). New York: Random House, 1988.

71. Hoier, T., Child Sexual Abuse: Clinical Interventions and New Directions, *Child and Adolescent Psychotherapy,* 4, no. 3 (1987), 179–185.

72. Hoole, A., R. Greenberg, and C.G. Pickard, *Patient Care Guidelines for Nurse Practitioners* (3rd ed.). Boston: Little, Brown, 1988.

73. How Kids Rate Their Working Moms, *Women's Day* (June 16, 1987), 6–7.

74. Hubbard, G., Perceived Life Changes for Children and Adolescents Following Disclosure of Father-Daughter Incest, *Journal of Child and Adolescent Psychiatric and Mental Health Nursing,* 2, no. 2 (1989), 78–82.

75. Human Nutrition Information Service, *Making Bag Lunches, Snacks, and Desserts Using the Dietary Guidelines.* Washington, DC: U.S. Government Printing Office, 1988.

76. Igoe, J.B., Beyond Green Beans and Oat Bran: A Health Agenda for the 1990s for School Age Youth, *Pediatric Nursing,* 16, no. 3 (1990), 289–292.

77. Immunizations Still Important for Children, *Health Scene* (Fall 1987), 11.

78. Injury-Proofing the School-Age Child, *Patient Care,* 23, no. 15 (1989), 178.

79. John, E., D. Savitz, and D. Sandler, Prenatal Exposure to Parents' Smoking and Childhood Cancer, *American Journal of Epidemiology,* 133, no. 2 (1991), 123–125.

80. Kantrowitz, B., and P. Wingert, How Kids Learn, *Newsweek* (April 17, 1989), 50–56.

81. Karamessinis, N., Personality and Perceptions of the Gifted, *G/C/T,* 1, no. 1 (May–June 1980), 11–13.

82. Karp, S., A 10-point Program for Bicycle Safety, *Contemporary Pediatrics,* 4, no. 6 (1987), 16–21, 24, 26–27.

83. Katz, L., Telling Children About Divorce, *Parents* (July 1986), 152.

84. Kempe, C., Sexual Abuse: Another Hidden Pediatric Problem, *Pediatrics,* 62 (1978), 582.

85. Kleinsasser, A.M., Equity in Education for Gifted Rural Girls, *Rural Special Education Quarterly,* 8, no. 4 (1988), 27–30.

86. Klug, R., Children with AIDS, *American Journal of Nursing,* 86, no. 10 (1986), 26–31.

87. Kohl, H., Should I Buy My Child a Computer? *Graduate Woman,* 76, no. 6 (1982), 20–23.

88. Kohlberg, L., Development of Moral Character and Moral Ideology. In Hoffman, M.L., (ed.), *Review of Child Development Research,* Vol. 1. New York: Russell Sage, 1964, pp. 383–432.

89. ———, *Recent Research in Moral Development.* New York: Holt, Rinehart & Winston, 1971.

90. ———, "Stages of Moral Development as a Basis for Moral Education." In Beck, C.M., B.S. Crittenden, and E.V. Sullivan, eds., *Moral Education: Interdisciplinary Approaches.* New York: Paulist Press, 1972, pp. 23ff.

91. Kolata, C., Obese Children: A Growing Problem, *Research News,* 232, no. 4 (1986), 20–21.

92. Kozinetz, C., Two Noninvasive Methods to Measure Female Maturation, *Journal of School Health,* 56, no. 10 (1986), 440–442.

93. Lamb, M., *The Father's Role.* New York: John Wiley, 1986.

94. Lambo, A., Children's Ability to Evaluate Television Commercial Messages for Sugared Products, *American Journal of Public Health,* 71, no. 9 (1981), 1060–1062.

95. Lamon, S., The British Primary School, *Kappa Delta Pi Record* (Spring 1985), 71–73.

96. Laskin, D., Safety at Home: An Ounce of Prevention is Worth a Pound of Cure, *Parents,* 65, no. 9 (1990), 111–112.

97. Leone, S., and J. Gumaer, Group Assertiveness Training of Shy Children, *School Counselor,* 27, no. 2 (1979), 134–141.

98. Leshan, E., *When Grownups Drive You Crazy.* New York: Macmillan, 1988.

99. Lesser, G. Education and the Mass Media. In Talbot, N., ed., *Raising Children in Modern America.* Boston: Little, Brown, 1976, pp. 319–331.

100. Levine, C., The DPT Dilemma, *Parents,* 62, no. 4 (1987), 228–231.

101. Lidz, T., *The Person: His and Her Development Throughout the Life Cycle* (2nd ed.) New York: Basic Books, 1983.

102. Liebert, R., and J. Spraskin, *The Early Window: Effects of Television on Children and Youths* (3rd ed.). New York: Pergamon Press, 1989.

103. Lieske, A., Incest: An Overview, *Perspectives in Psychiatric Care,* 19, no. 2 (1982), 59–63.

104. Louv, R., *Childhood's Future.* Boston: Houghton Mifflin, 1990.

105. Lutz, M., The Effects of Family Structure and Regular Places of Care on Preventive Health Care for Children, *Health Values: Achieving High Level Wellness,* 14, no. 1 (1990), 38–45.

106. Lykins, R., Children of the Third Culture, *Kappa Delta Pi Record* (Winter 1986), 39–43.

107. Lynds, B., S. Seyler, and B. Morgan, The Relationship Between Elevated Blood Pressure and Obesity in Black Children, *American Journal of Public Health,* 70, no. 2 (1980), 171–173.

108. Mackey, W., *Fathering Behaviors: The Dynamics of the Man-Child Bond*. New York: Plenum Press, 1985.

109. Maddocks, G., Growing to Independence, *Nursing Mirror,* 152, no. 21 (1981), viii–xiv.

110. Malina, R., A. Zuvaleta, and B. Little, Body Size, Fatness, and Leanness of Mexican-American Children in Brownsville, Texas: Changes Between 1972 and 1983, *American Journal of Public Health,* 77, no. 5 (1987), 573–577.

111. Manning, M., Disappearing Childhood: 6 Going on 16, *Kappa Delta Pi Record* (Fall 1985), 14–18.

112. Markham, L., and J. Smith, Nickelodeon: An Alternative to Usual Television Fare? *Kappa Delta Pi Record,* 19, no. 4 (Summer 1983), 125–128.

113. Marten, D., Cognitive Assessment of Diverse Populations, *Kappa Delta Pi Record* (Winter 1986), 35–38.

114. Mason, J.O., Forging Working Partnerships for School Health Education, *Journal of School Health,* 59, no. 1 (1989), 18–20.

115. Matthews, P., Fast Food, *Nursing Times,* 82, no. 11 (1986), 47–49.

116. Mayer, S., and C. Jenicks, Growing Up in Poor Neighborhoods: How Much Does It Matter? *Science,* 243 (March 1989), 1441–1445.

117. McCormick, J., and P. Wingert, Whose Child Am I Anyway? *Newsweek Special Issue* (Summer 1991), 58–60.

118. McKee, A., *The AAUW Report: How Schools Short-Change Girls*. New York: American Association of University Women, 1992.

119. Media, Violence May Be Linked, *University News* (September 21, 1990), 1, 8.

120. Mennger, J., et al. Genetics or Environment? Type A Behavior and Cardiovascular Risk Factors in Twin Children, *Nursing Research,* 37, no. 8 (1988), 341–348.

121. Micozzi, M., Childhood Hypertension and Academic Standing in the Philippines, *American Journal of Public Health,* 70, no. 5 (1980), 530–532.

122. Miller, D., Who is Gifted? A Quick Grasp of Concepts is One Clue, *Independent School,* 39, no. 4 (1980), 12–16.

123. Miller, S., Children's Fears: A Review of the Literature With Implications for Nursing Research and Practice, *Nursing Research,* 29, no. 4 (1979), 217–223.

124. Morgan, J., Prevention of Childhood Obesity, *Comprehensive Pediatric Nursing,* 9 (1986), 33–38.

125. Moshman, D., J. Glover, and R. Bruning, *Developmental Psychology*. Boston: Little, Brown, 1987.

126. Mott, S., S. James, and A. Sperhac, *Nursing Care of Children and Families* (2nd ed.). Redwood City, Calif: Addison-Wesley, 1990.

127. Murphy, E., *God Cares When I Don't Feel Good*. Elgin, Ill: David C. Cook, 1987.

128. Murphy, E., *God, You Fill Us Up With Joy: Psalm 100 For Children*. Elgin, Ill: David C. Cook, 1987.

129. Murphy, S., *The Early Development of Sibling Relationships in Childbearing Families*. San Francisco: University of California, 1989.

130. National Center for Health Statistics, *Health,* No. PHS 84-1232. Washington, DC: U.S. Government Printing Office, 1987.

131. Newman, B., and P. Newman, *Development Through Life: A Psychosocial Approach* (5th ed.). Pacific Grove, Calif: Brooks/Cole, 1991.

132. Nicklas, T., et al., Racial Contrasts in Hemoglobin Levels and Dietary Patterns Related to Hematopoiesis in Children: The Bogalusa Heart Study, *American Journal of Public Health,* 77, no. 10 (1987), 1320–1323.

133. Oakley, M., School Phobia, *Res Medica,* 3, no. 2 (1986), 11–14.

134. Oda, D., A Viewpoint on School Nursing, *American Journal of Nursing,* 81, no. 9 (1981), 1677–1678.

135. Oh, To Be Young and Gifted, *Newsweek* (February 23, 1987), 63–65.

136. Orbach, I., *Children Who Don't Want to Live: Understanding and Treating the Suicidal Child*. San Francisco: Jossey-Bass, 1988.

137. Ornstean, A., A Difference Teachers Make: How Much, *Educational Forum,* 49, no. 1 (Fall 1984), 109–117.

138. Papalia, D., and S. Olds, *Human Development* (4th ed.). New York: McGraw-Hill, 1989.

139. Parke, R., and R. Slaby, The Development of Aggression. In Hetherton, E., and P. Mussen, eds., *Handbook of Child Psychology, Vol. 4: Socialization, Personality, and Social Development*. New York: Wiley, 1983.

140. Paul, J., Educating the Gifted, *American Educator,* 4 (Summer 1980), 6–7.

141. Piaget, J., *Judgment and Reasoning in the Child*. New York: Humanities Press, 1928.

142. ——, *The Moral Judgment of the Child*. New York: Harcourt, Brace, 1932; The Free Press, 1965.

143. ——, *The Growth of Logical Thinking From Childhood to Adolescence*. New York: Basic Books, 1958.

144. ——, *The Origins of Intelligence in Children*. New York: W.W. Norton, 1963.

145. ——, *The Child's Conception of Numbers*. New York: W.W. Norton, 1965.

146. ——, and B. Inhelder, *The Psychology of the Child*. New York: Basic Books, 1969.

147. ——, and Barbel Inhelder, *Memory and Intelligence*. New York: Basic Books, 1973.

148. ——, Introduction. In Schwebel, M., ed., *Piaget in the Classroom*. New York: Basic Books, 1973.

149. Piersel, W., G. Brody, and T. Kratochwill, A Further Examination of Motivational Influences on Disadvantaged Minority Group Children's Intelligence Test Performance, *Child Development,* 48 (1978), 142–145.

150. Pink, W., Creating Effective Schools, *Educational Forum,* 49, no. 1 (Fall 1984), 91–107.

151. Pipes, P.L., *Nutrition in Infancy and Childhood* (4th ed.). St. Louis: C.V. Mosby, 1989.

152. Polk-Walker, G., What Really Happened? Incidence and Factor Assessment of Abused Children and Adolescents, *Journal of Psychosocial Nursing,* 28, no. 11 (1990), 17–22.

153. Pontious, S., Practical Piaget: Helping Children Understand, *American Journal of Nursing,* 82, no. 1 (1982), 115–117.

154. Porter, C., Grade School Children's Perceptions of Their Internal Body Parts, *Nursing Research,* 23, no. 5 (September–October 1974), 384–391.

155. Potter, D., ed., *Assessment*. Springhouse, Penn: Intermed Communications, 1982.

156. Price, J., et al., School Nurses' Perceptions of Childhood Obesity, *Journal of School Health,* 57, no. 8 (1987), 332–336.

157. Rakestraw, J., and D. Rakestraw, Home Schooling: A

Question of Quality, an Issue of Rights, *The Educational Forum,* 55, no. 1 (1990), 67–77.

158. Reek, J. van, M. Drop, and J. Joosten, The Influence of Peers and Parents on the Smoking Behavior of Schoolchildren, *Journal of School Health,* 57, no. 1 (1987), 30.

159. Rice, B., Going for the Gifted Gold, *Psychology Today,* 13 (February 1980), 55–58+.

160. Richards, W., Allergy, Asthma, and School Problems, *Journal of School Health,* 56, no. 4 (1986), 151–152.

161. Richoux, D., A Look at Home Schooling, *Kappa Delta Pi Record,* 23, no. 4 (Summer 1987), 118–121.

162. Robbins, K., D. Branding-Bennett, and A. Hinman, Low Measles Incidence: Association with Enforcement of School Immunization Laws, *American Journal of Public Health,* 71, no. 3 (1981), 270–274.

163. Robinson, T., School Nurse Practitioners on the Job, *American Journal of Nursing,* 81, no. 9 (1981), 1674–1676.

164. Rosenberg, M., *Growing Up Adopted.* New York: Bradbury Press, 1989.

165. Rubenstein, E., Television and Behavior: Research Conclusions of the 1982 NIMH Report and Their Policy Implications, *American Psychologist,* 38, (1983), 820–825.

166. Scholl, T., et al., Ethnic Differences in Growth and Nutritional Status: a Status of Poor Schoolchildren in Southern New Jersey, *Public Health Reports,* 102, no. 3 (1987), 278–283.

167. Schulman, M., *Moral Development Training: Strategies for Parents, Teachers, and Clinicians.* Menlo Park, Calif: Addison-Wesley, 1985.

168. Schultz, C., Sulfite Sensitivity, *American Journal of Nursing,* 86, no. 8 (1986), 914.

169. Schuster, C.S., and S.S. Ashburn, *The Process of Human Development: A Holistic Approach* (3rd ed.). Boston: Little, Brown, 1986.

170. Schwartz, J., Early Identification of Gifted, Talented, and Creative Children, *Kappa Delta Pi Record,* 20, no. 1 (Fall 1983), 24–28.

171. Schwartz, J., Portrait of a Generation, *Newsweek Special Supplement* (Summer 1991), 6–9.

172. Schwebel, M., and J. Raph, eds., *Piaget in the Classroom.* New York: Basic Books, 1973.

173. Scott, M., The Real Issue of Mainstreaming: The Education of the Nonhandicapped, *Kappa Delta Pi Record,* 19, no. 1 (Fall 1982), 17–20.

174. Selekman, J., Immunization: What's It All About? *American Journal of Nursing,* 80, no. 8 (1980), 1440–1445.

175. Shapiro, L., et al., Obesity Prognosis: A Longitudinal Study of Children From Age 6 Months to 9 Years, *American Journal of Public Health,* 74, no. 9 (1984), 968–972.

176. Sherman, J.B., and M.A. Alexander, Obesity in Children: A Research Update, *Journal of Pediatric Nursing: Nursing Care of Children and Families,* 5, no. 3 (1990), 161–167.

177. Sieving, R.E., and S.T. Zirbel-Donisch, Development and Enhancement of Self-Esteem in Children, *Journal of Pediatric Health Care,* 4, no. 6 (1990), 290–296.

178. Singer, D.C., A Time to Re-Examine the Role of Television in Our Lives, *American Psychologist,* 38 (1983), 815–816.

179. Singer, J.L., and D.E. Singer, Implications of Childhood Television Viewing for Cognition, Imagination, and Emotion. In Bryant, J., and D. Anderson, eds., *Children's Understanding of Television: Research on Attention and Comprehension.* New York: Academic Press, 1983.

180. Southall, C., Innovative School Nursing in Harlem: Family Life and Sex Education, *American Journal of Nursing,* 77, no. 9 (1977), 1473–1476.

181. Spradley, B.W., *Community Health Nursing: Concepts and Practice* (3rd ed.). Glenview, Ill: Scott, Foresman/Little, Brown, 1990.

182. Spratlen, L.P., Nurse-Role Dimensions of a School-Based Hypertension Screening, Education, and Follow-up Program, *Journal of School Health,* 52, no. 3 (1982), 174–178.

183. Stedwitz, U., C. Lariviere, and V. Rogers, What Do Kids Do When They're Not in School? *Kappa Delta Pi Record* (Winter 1988), 44–47.

184. Stjernfeldt, M., et al., Maternal Smoking During Pregnancy and the Risk of Childhood Cancer, *Lancet,* 1, no. 8494 (1986), 1350–1352.

185. Strickland, D., Friendship Patterns and Altruistic Behavior in Preadolescent Males and Females, *Nursing Research,* 30, no. 4 (1981), 222, 228, 235.

186. Sullivan, H.S., *The Interpersonal Theory of Psychiatry.* New York: W.W. Norton, 1953.

187. Swanson, L., and M.K. Biaggio, Therapeutic Perspectives in Father-Daughter Incest, *American Journal of Psychiatry,* 142, no. 6 (1985), 667–674.

188. Tesler, M., and M. Savedra, Coping With Hospitalization: A Study of School-Age Children, *Pediatric Nursing,* 7, no. 2 (1981), 35–40.

189. Thomas, J., and C. Rogers, Sexual Abuse of Children: Case Finding and Clinical Assessment, *Nursing Clinics of North America,* 18, no. 1 (1981), 179–188.

190. Thompson, D., et al., A Case-Control Study of the Effectiveness of Bicycle Safety Helmets in Preventing Facial Injury, *American Journal of Public Health,* 80, no. 12 (1990), 1471–1474.

191. Thompson, S., Summertime and Ticks, *American Journal of Nursing,* 83, no. 5 (1983), 768–769.

192. Tripp-Reimer, T., Retention of a Folk-Healing Practice (Matiasma) Among Four Generations of Urban Greek Immigrants, *Nursing Research,* 32, no. 2 (1983), 97–101.

193. Turner, J., and D. Helms, *Lifespan Development* (3rd ed.). New York: Harcourt & Brace, 1991.

194. U.S. Department of Health and Human Services, *Television and Behavior: Ten Years of Scientific Progress and Implications for the Eighties.* Washington, DC: The Department, 1982.

195. ——, New Recommended Schedule for Active Immunization of Normal Infants and Children, *Morbidity and Mortality Weekly Report,* 35, no. 37 (September 19, 1986), 577–579.

196. ——, *Public Health Service: Parents' Guide to Childhood Immunizations.* Atlanta: Centers for Disease Control, 1988.

197. ——, *Office of Maternal and Child Health USA '89,* No. HRS-MCH 8915. Washington, DC: Bureau of Maternal and Child Health Resources Development, 1989.

198. Vasquez, J., Context of Learning for Minority Students, *Educational Forum,* 52, no. 3 (1988), 243–253.

199. Vessey, J., Comparison of Two Teaching Methods on

Children's Knowledge of Their Internal Bodies, *Nursing Research,* 37, no. 5 (1988), 262–267.

200. Wadsworth, B., *Piaget's Theory of Cognitive and Affective Development* (4th ed.). New York: Longman, 1989.

201. We Kill Too Many Farm Kids, *Successful Farming* (February 1989), 18A–18P.

202. Webb, P., Piaget: Implications for Teaching, *Theory Into Practice,* 19, no. 2 (1980), 93–97.

203. Weinberg, A., et al., A Pilot Study on Cholesterol Screening in the School Environment, *Journal of School Health,* 58, no. 8 (1988), 62.

204. Werner, E., *Vulnerable but Invincible.* New York: Adams-Bannister-Cox, 1989.

205. Werner, E., *Against the Odds.* New York: Adams-Bannister-Cox, 1990.

206. Whaley, L., and D. Wong, *Nursing Care of Infants and Children* (4th ed.). St. Louis: C.V. Mosby, 1990.

207. Williams, P., A Comparison of Philippine and American Children's Concepts of Body Organs and Illness in Relation to Five Variables, *International Journal of Nursing Studies,* 15 (1978), 193–203.

208. Williams, S.R., *Nutrition and Diet Therapy* (6th ed.). St. Louis: Times Mirror/Mosby, 1989.

209. Winkelstein, M.L., Fostering Positive Self-Concept in the School Age Child, *Pediatric Nursing,* 15, no. 3 (1989), 229–233.

210. Winpisinger, K., et al., Risk Factors for Child Homicides in Ohio: A Birth Certificate-Based Case-Control Study, *American Journal of Public Health,* 81, no. 8 (1991), 1052–1054.

211. Wintemute, G., et al., Drowning in Childhood and Adolescence: A Population-Based Study, *American Journal of Public Health,* 77, no. 7 (1987), 830–832.

212. Wolfe, H., Television—Reflector or Creator of Values? *Graduate Woman,* (May–June 1979), 14–16.

213. Yanni, M., Perception of Parents' Behavior and Children's General Fearfulness, *Nursing Research,* 31, no. 2 (1982), 79–82.

214. Yeger, T., and S. Miezitis, Self-Concept and Classroom Behavior of Preadolescent Pupils, *Journal of Classroom Interaction,* 15, no. 2 (1980), 31–37.

215. Yoos, L., Chronic Childhood Illnesses: Developmental Issues, *Pediatric Nursing,* 13, no. 1 (1987), 25–28.

216. Yorker, B., The Prosecution of Child Sexual Abuse Cases, *Journal of Child Psychiatric Nursing,* 1, no. 2 (1988), 50–57.

217. The Zap Generation, *Newsweek* (February 26, 1990), 56–57.

Chapter 11

Assessment and Health Promotion for the Adolescent and Youth

For some, adolescence is short; for others, adolescence extends many years.
——*Ruth Beckmann Murray*

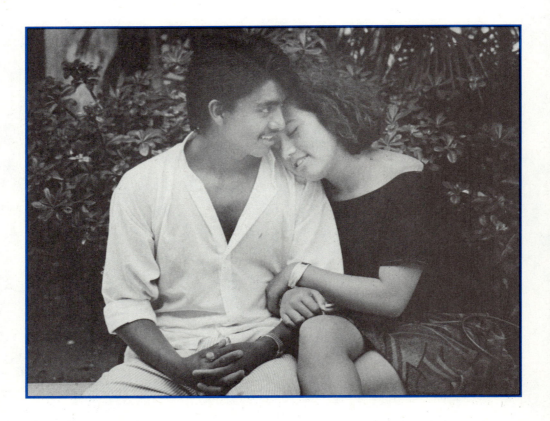

KEY TERMS

Puberty	Anorexia nervosa	Musculoskeletal chest pain	Candidal
Spermatogenesis	Bulimia	Strain or sprain	Trichomonal
Menstruation	Obesity	Minor ankle sprain	Nonspecific
Pubarche	Peer group	Hordeolum or stye	Chlamydia trachomatis
Menarche	Peer-group dialect	Epistaxis	Phthirus pubis
Adolescence	Identity	Acne vulgaris	Contraception
Preadolescence	Identity formation	Dental caries	Abortion
Early adolescence	Personal or real identity	Gingivitis	Incest
Middle adolescence	Ideal identity	Tinea pedis or athlete's foot	Drug abuse
Late adolescence	Claimed identity	Infectious mononucleosis	Drug
Sperm production	Identity diffusion	Hepatitis	Drug dependence
Nocturnal emissions	Sexuality	Rocky Mountain spotted fever	Addiction
Sex hormones	Masturbation	Lyme disease	Tolerance
Androgens	Ego	Sexually transmitted diseases	Cocaine
Estrogens	Frustration	Vaginitis	Kindling effect
Progesterones	Conversion		Crack or rock
Ovulation	Teen walkaway		
Primary dysmenorrhea	Teen runaway		

OBJECTIVES

Study of this chapter will enable you to:

1. Discuss the impact of the crisis of adolescence on family life and the influence of the family on the adolescent.
2. Explore with the family its developmental tasks and ways to achieve them while giving positive guidance to the adolescent.
3. Correlate the physiologic changes and needs, including nutrition, exercise, and rest, of early, middle, and late adolescence to those that occurred in preadolescence.
4. Discuss with parents the cognitive, self-concept, sexuality, emotional, and moral-spiritual aspects of development of the adolescent and ways in which the family can foster their healthy progress.
5. Identify examples of adolescent peer-group dialect and use of leisure time in your region, and discuss how knowledge of them can be used in your health-promotion activities and teaching.
6. Explore the developmental crisis of identity formation with the adolescent and the parents, the significance of achieving this crisis for ongoing maturity, and how to counteract influences that interfere with identity formation.
7. Describe the developmental tasks of adolescence and how the adaptive mechanisms commonly used assist the adolescent in achieving them.
8. Assess and work effectively with an adolescent with instructor supervision.
9. Discuss the challenges of the transitional period to young adulthood and your role in assisting the late adolescent into young adulthood.
10. Discuss common health problems of the adolescent, factors that contribute to them, and your role in contributing to the adolescent's health.

How can I best describe my son? He is 13 years old but could pass for 16 physically and mentally. He has the physique of a football player and appears to grow taller each day. His general knowledge is superior because he watches television for at least 2 hours a day, scans the morning and evening papers, and listens to the radio periodically during the day. He is full of contradictions; for example, he talks about love, but a hug or sign of affection from his mother will send him running to his room.

HISTORICAL AND CULTURAL PERSPECTIVES

Adolescence has long been considered a critical period in human development, and the search for an understanding of the adolescent can be traced historically. Early writers such as Rousseau, Francke, and Froebel directed their interest toward the education of the adolescent and his or her characteristics. In the late nineteenth century psychologists molded the Darwinian concepts into psychologic terms and firmly established adolescence as an inevitable stage in human development. Before the twentieth century, however, most people thought of themselves as young adults after puberty.

Adolescence is a long developmental stage, and because it differs cross-culturally, it is the most difficult to define. It is like old age in the United States, for each population is considered something of a burden and unable to contribute much to society. In the United States children are physiologically maturing at an earlier age. The increase in adult height and the change in age at which physical maturation occurs are called a secular growth trend. This trend is attributed to improved nutrition and health practices. Along with early maturation, the developmental era is being extended because of social, economic, employment, industrial, and family changes. For some people adolescence ends in the teens, but for most the period ends in the mid- twenties (55, 93, 135, 143, 144, 152). However, adolescence is not so prolonged in all countries or cultures. Certainly in some cultures when puberty occurs, rites of passage signal adulthood.

DEFINITIONS

In the past many people equated puberty and adolescence; they are now considered separate components. Puberty is preceded by prepuberty (discussed in Chapter 10).

Puberty is the *state of physical development between 10 and 14 years for females and 12 to 16 years for males when sexual reproduction first becomes possible with the onset of* **spermatogenesis** (*production of spermatozoa*) *and* **menstruation** (*onset of menses.*) Common law usually fixes puberty at 12 years for females and 14 years for males. **Pubarche** refers to the *beginning development of certain secondary sex characteristics that precedes the actual onset of physiologic puberty.* Some define puberty as a process involving a number of physical changes over a period of time that culminates in menstruation and spermatogenesis. The female may be unable to conceive for 1 to 2 years after **menarche,** the *first menstrual period,* and the male is usually sterile for a year or more after ejaculation first occurs. Some studies have shown, however, that some males become fertile at the onset of pubertal development (48, 55, 93, 135, 151, 206).

Adolescence is the *period in life that begins with puberty and extends for 8 to 10 years or longer until the person is physically and psychologically mature, ready to assume adult responsibilities and be self-sufficient because of changes in intellect, attitudes, and interests* (116, 220). Exceptions occur; some people never become psychologically mature. This definition does not reflect the individuality of the adolescent. Generalizations should be avoided as much as possible to prevent unjustified expectations from the adolescent.

Keniston (107) has delineated this period further between puberty and young adulthood by calling the period from 20 to 25 years *youth.* He believes that the affluent culture, especially in urban areas, has often created additional time before adult responsibilities must be assumed. For the purpose of this chapter, however, the adolescent period is divided into the subperiods of preadolescence, early, middle, and late adolescence. (The term *youth* is used interchangeably with adolescence.) Although age ranges are assigned to each subperiod, they are approximate; each adolescent may vary as to when and how he or she proceeds through the various stages.

Preadolescence, the *stage of prepuberty,* is discussed in Chapter 10 since these children are a part of the school-age population in America.

Early adolescence *begins with puberty and lasts for several years* (11 or 12 to 13 or 14 for females and 12 or 14 to 16 for males). The growth spurt focuses attention on self and the task of becoming comfortable with body changes and appearance. The teen tries to separate from parents; the dependency-independency struggle is shown by less involvement in family activities (and chores, if possible), being critical of the parents, and rebellion against parental and other adult discipline and authority. Conformity to and acceptance of peer-group standards and peer friendships are gaining in importance. The peer group usually consists of same-sexed friends; however, the adolescent has an increased interest in the opposite sex. Group activities with peers are popular (93, 143, 144).

Middle adolescence *begins when physical growth is completed and usually extends from age 13 or 14 to 16 for females and 14 or 16 to 18 or 20 for males.* The major tasks during this period are achievement of ego identity, attainment of greater independence, interest in the future and career planning, and establishment of heterosexual relationship. Peer-group allegiance, at a peak in 15- to 16-year-olds, is manifested by clothing, food, and other fads, preferred music, and common jargon. Experimentation with adultlike behavior and risk taking is common in an attempt to prove self to peers. Sexual experimentation often begins now (or earlier) as a result of social exploration and physical maturation. Changes in cognitive functioning may first be evident in that the person moves to more abstract thinking, returning to more concrete operations during times of stress (134).

Some teens are expected to move into the tasks of young adulthood at this point. Although they may be employed or independent in other ways, developmentally the person probably is in late adolescence.

Late adolescence *may occur from approximately 20 to 25 years of age.* The person has usually finished adolescent rebellion, formed his or her views, and established a stable sense of self. The youth is not fully committed to one occupation and questions relationships to existing social, vocational, and emotional roles and lifestyles. He or she may be a student or an apprentice (93, 107, 143, 144). Lack of economic freedom may be a concern and prolong dependence on parents. The value system is being clarified; issues of philosophy, religion, life and death, and ethical decisions are being analyzed. The peer group has lost its primary importance, and the youth may take the final step in establishing independence from parents by moving away from home. More adultlike friendships begin between late adolescents and their parents as the earlier family turbulence subsides. At the same time there is more individual dating and fewer group activities with friends; often the first emotionally intimate relationship develops with a member of the opposite sex. At that point the person is developmentally a young adult, having made the transition from adolescence. He or she is more realistically aware of strengths and limits in self and others (134).

FAMILY DEVELOPMENT AND RELATIONSHIPS

Developmental Tasks

The overall family goal at this time is to allow the adolescent increasing freedom and responsibility to prepare him or her for young adulthood.

Although each family member has personal developmental tasks, the family unit as a whole also has developmental tasks. They include the following (54):

1. Provide facilities for individual differences and needs of family members.
2. Work out a system of financial responsibility with the family.
3. Establish a sharing of responsibilities.
4. Reestablish a mutually satisfying marriage relationship.
5. Strengthen communication within the family.
6. Rework relationships with relatives, friends, and associates.
7. Broaden horizons of the adolescent and parents.
8. Formulate a workable philosophy of life as a family.

Discuss the developmental tasks and how to achieve them with the family. Generally speaking, the developmental tasks for a family at this time involve maintaining a grasp on these facets of life that continue to have meaning while striving for a deeper awareness and understanding of the present situation.

Family Relationships

During early adolescence the teen remains involved in family activities and functions. Gradually family relationships change, and the adolescent develops social ties and close relationships outside the family. The family's beliefs, life-styles, values, and patterns of interaction influence the development of these relationships, as can socioeconomic level of the parents. The media report that one of every five children less than 17 years old live in poverty. Poverty affects all spheres of family and individual development (135, 139, 144).

It is during middle and late adolescence that the most severe changes occur in the parent-child relationship. The relationship must evolve from a dependency status to mutual affection, equality, and autonomy. This process of achieving independence usually creates family turmoil, conflict, and ambivalence as both parents and adolescent learn new roles. The emancipation process must be gradual. Parents should gradually increase the teenager's responsibilities and allow privileges formerly denied. The adolescent wants to make independent decisions and to have increased freedom of movement. At the same time, he or she wants financial support, food, and safe sanctuary. Parents must resist granting instant adult status when the child reaches teen years and instead remember that the adolescent needs to be independent yet dependent. Although he or she protests, the teen values parental restraints if the restraints are reasonable. The adolescent feels more self-confident in exploring the environment if reasonable limits are imposed. Parents should listen to their adolescent's viewpoints concerning restrictions. Views may offer hints about the readiness for more independence and freedom (135, 143, 144, 154, 220).

Most ambivalence and negative behavior in the adolescent stems from self-perceived external restrictions. Teenagers may fight for grownup privileges that they never use—the actual battle is more important than the privilege. Disagreements and conflicts about sexual behavior, dress, drugs, school performance, homework, friendship, family car and telephone privileges, manners, chores and duties, money, and disrespectful behavior frequently disrupt family harmony (93, 118, 220).

In addition to other conflicts, the youth must also work through feelings for the parent of the opposite sex and unravel the ambivalence toward the parent of the same sex. He or she reworks some of the gender identity and family triangle problems that remain from the preschool era. In an attempt to resolve this ambivalence, the adolescent may strive to be as different as possible from the parent of the same sex. Frequently affection is turned to an adult outside the family—teacher, relative, family friend, neighbor, mentor, clergy person, or someone in public life. "Crushes" of this nature are very common; they are usually brief and may occur once, twice, or on numerous occasions. Idolizing another adult person causes the adolescent to want to please that person; therefore the adolescent's actions and language may change when the idolized person is present. Frequently the adolescent identifies so completely with this person that he or she absorbs some of the person's adult characteristics into the personality. These relationships are not harmful to the adolescent unless the person who is chronologically an adult still feels confused and rebellious toward society and fosters immaturity. On the contrary, an adult outside the family usually will be more objective than the parent and can help the adolescent grow toward psychologic maturity. Parents are experiencing sexuality changes at the same time. They are facing midlife and menopause and are concerned with self-perceived decreased sexual attractiveness and potency.

During this period parents may believe they are not as important to the adolescent as before. The adolescent complains that parents are old-fashioned and "out of it." He or she may appear hostile and resent parental authority and guidance. The teen seeks to find flaws in parental behavior and may try to build barriers between self and the parents to prove independence. The adolescent is critical, argumentative, and generally remote with both parents; a previously close and confiding relationship with the parents is lost. In their presence the adolescent may ridicule parents. This rejection is not consistent; response to parents varies with mood changes. At times the relationship can be close and positive; the adolescent may actually support the parents in the presence of peers (93, 143, 144, 206).

In addition to dealing with a loss of authority, parents are faced with other stresses. They are forced to redefine past child-parent relations and rethink their own values. Parents may also be forced to evaluate their own career choices as their adolescent begins vocational pursuits. Competition between parents and the teen may exist; parents may actually admit to not liking the adolescent. They may be anxious to relinquish financial, physical, and emotional child-rearing responsibilities to increase their own freedom (2, 116, 206).

Stresses that frequently produce family discord grow out of conflicting value systems between the old and new generations. Parents are confused by the change from the firm, strict discipline that they experienced to the apparent lack of discipline or permissiveness. Even a balance between the two extremes serves as a threat to some parents. Many of today's parents lived as adolescents in a world restricted to a certain geographic area. The authority of their parents often went unquestioned; questions were not tolerated by the parents. Today's adolescents are a generation born with television, an instrument that has brought remote corners of the world into their homes and minds and has fostered the asking of questions instead of relying on authority.

Parents need help to see that the adolescent is a product of his or her time and the teen is reflecting what is happening socially.

Youngs' book (229) is a practical reference for parents and professionals on the teenager's behavior, factors that contribute to stress response, signs and symptoms that the youth and the family are having problems, and how to manage tense situations and teenage behavioral problems.

Parental and adolescent response to the ambivalence and conflicts of this period varies. Parents may adhere to rules and the status quo to bolster their own security or cultural traditions rather than change for the offspring's benefit. Some parents cannot change as quickly as the child during puberty. Parents may overprotect. Others may be reluctant to admit that their child is establishing

an independent life-style; they may dread facing the empty-nest stage (2, 154). If the adolescent has come from a family that has provided past opportunities to learn responsibility, self-reliance, skills, and self-respect, he or she will make a smoother transition from childhood dependency to adulthood independence. If parents have been too liberal, overly permissive, or uninterested, the adolescent will have more difficulty adjusting because the past lacked structure and a system of standards or values. He or she has no point of reference to determine if the behavior is suitable and decisions appropriate (69, 154).

Fortunately some parents trust their offspring to live the basic values they taught, although at times behavior may appear differently. They realize that today's adolescent is growing up in a different historical era than when they were young, and they can accept the changes that result. They work at being communicative and flexible, yet supportive. They encourage but do not push or probe. They question the offspring to encourage thinking. They give reasons for rules and are firm when necessary. They accept that the adolescent may be as large as an adult but still behave childishly at times. The parents' behavior is adultlike so that they are a model for their offspring. They feel enough self-confidence that they do not have to belittle the adolescent. They are not threatened by his or her sexuality, and they maintain a balance of closeness and distance so that the adolescent can rework gender identity. If the parent-child relationship has been close in the past, it can remain close now in spite of superficial problems and responses.

Adolescence is not a period of conflict between parents and offspring in all cultures. For example, in Oriental and Indian cultures, some African groups, the Arabian countries, and certain European countries, behavior norms and role expectations provide the basis for a smoother transition from child to adult than is expected in the United States. Nontechnologic societies have less adolescent-parent conflict because there is less choice in occupations and life-styles and less variance between generational behavior (64).

Discuss the above information with parents. Help them understand the interaction between parents and offspring. Encourage the parents to maintain open lines of communication. Adolescents must feel free to seek help from parents; they respond to honesty, fairness, and sincere interest. In essence, the adolescent must be understood and accepted as a person while being allowed as much independence as can be handled. The home should provide an accepting and emotionally stable environment for the adolescent since the home situation affects later marital adjustments and the type of parent that he or she will become.

A factor that may affect parent-adolescent communication and relationships is the stepfamily or adoptive family structure. Often adopted adolescents struggle with whether they really belong to the family. (Refer also to Chapter 4). The National Council for Adoption estimates that 60,000 adoptions take place annually in the United States, including the adoption of 10,000 children from other countries. Because of the proliferation of divorce, single-parenting, and stepfamilies, adoptive children have plenty of company; parents can assure the adolescent he or she is not alone in feeling different. Parents and the adopted adolescent may wish to attend group sessions organized by Minnesota-based Adoptive Families of America, which has 260 chapters nationwide. The organization plans activities by nationality. Adoptive parents learn about the child's native culture, and adopted children are with others who share their heritage, ethnicity, and appearance. Thus identity and self-esteem can be strengthened. Adopted children statistically fare better than would have been predicted from their socioeconomic roots.

Abuse, Neglect, and Maltreatment

Abuse, neglect, and maltreatment occur to millions of adolescents, although health care professionals may not be alert to physical or psychologic cues. The adolescent who is physically abused may be present in the emergency room with some of the same kinds of injuries that are seen in the younger child (see Chapters 4, 6, 7, and 9). Sometimes bruises and lacerations are concealed from peers, teachers, and health care providers by cosmetics and clothes. Careful screening and astute communication skills are essential. You must establish a relationship and interview the adolescent alone. Then you are more likely to learn of physical, sexual, and psychologic abuse (maltreatment) or neglect.

Maltreatment of the adolescent is demonstrated by the behaviors described in Box 11–1. Other references that describe physical, psychologic, and sexual abuse are 21, 22, 24, 71, 80, 93, 102, 164).

PHYSIOLOGIC CONCEPTS

Influences on Physical Growth

The precise physiologic cause for the physical changes characteristic of this period is unknown. It appears that the hypothalamus, probably in some way related to brain maturation, initiates the pubertal process through secretion of neurohumoral releasing factors. These neurohumors stimulate the anterior pituitary gland to release gonadotrophic hormones, somatotropic hormone (STH) or growth hormone (GH), thyroid-stimulating hormone (TSH), and adrenocorticotropic hormone (ACTH). The amygdala in the limbic system also apparently changes function and promotes hormonal production (93, 135, 220).

Gonadotrophic hormones (follicle-stimulating hormone [FSH] and luteinizing hormone [LH]) stimulate the gonads to mature and produce sex hormones. FSH stimulates the ovaries in females to produce estrogen and the development of seminiferous tubules in males; LH stimulates the Leydig cells in the testes to produce tes-

---

■ BOX 11-1.
Parental Behavior Characteristics of Psychologic Maltreatment of the Adolescent

Rejecting

- Refuses to acknowledge changing social roles and to move to autonomy and independence
- Treats adolescent like a young child
- Subjects adolescent to verbal humiliation and excess criticism
- Expels youth from family

Isolating

- Tries to prevent youth from participating in organized and informal activities outside the home
- Prohibits adolescent from joining clubs or after-school activities
- Withdraws youth from school to work or perform household tasks
- Punishes youth for engaging in normal social activity such as dating

Terrorizing

- Threatens to expose youth to public humiliation such as undressing youth, forcing encounter with police or stay in jail
- Threatens to reveal intensely embarrassing characteristics (real or fantasized) to peers or adults
- Ridicules youth in public regularly

Ignoring

- Abdicates parental role
- Shows no interest in youth as person or in activities; refuses to discuss adolescent's activities, plans, interests
- Concentrates on activities or relationships that displace adolescent from affections

Corrupting

- Involves youth in more intense or socially unacceptable forms of sexual, aggressive, or substance abuse behavior; forces youth into prostitution
- Rewards aggressive or scapegoating behavior to siblings, peers, or adults
- Encourages trafficking in illicit drug use or alcohol use or in sex rings

From Garbarino, J., E. Guttmann, and J. Seeley, *The Psychologically Battered Child: Strategies for Identification, Assessment, and Intervention.* San Francisco: Jossey-Bass, 1987. Copyright 1986 by Jossey-Bass, Inc., Publishers.

---

tosterone. Growth and development of the adrenal cortex and stimulation of the secretion of androgens are promoted by ACTH. These androgens are responsible for producing secondary sex characteristics. Stimulation of deoxyribonucleic acid (DNA) synthesis and hyperplastic cell growth, particularly of the bones and cartilage, is produced by STH. Under the influence of TSH, thyroxin secretion is slightly increased during the pubertal period. Thyroxin levels increase to meet body metabolic need (93, 135, 220).

Both male and female hormones are produced in varying amounts in both sexes throughout life. During the prepubescent years, the adrenal cortex secretes a small amount of sex hormones. However, it is the sex hormone production that accompanies maturation of the ovaries and testes that is responsible for the physiologic changes observed in puberty. Physiologic changes in the male are produced by androgens, whereas large amounts of estrogens produce the changes in the female. Both forms of gonadal hormones stimulate epiphyseal fusion by repression of the pituitary growth hormone, thus slowing physical growth at the end of puberty.

Physical Characteristics

Growth

Adolescence is the second major period of accelerated growth (infancy was the first). The adolescent growth spurt occurs approximately 2 years earlier in the female than in the male. During the years of the growth spurt, females grow $2\frac{1}{2}$ to 5 inches (6 to 12.5 cm) and gain 8 to 10 pounds (3.5 to 4.5 kg); males average 3 to 6 inches (7.5 to 15 cm) and gain 12 to 14 pounds (5.5 to 6.5 kg). In the initial phase of the growth spurt, the increase in height is due to lengthening of the legs; later, most of the increase is in the trunk length. The total process of change takes approximately 3 years in females and 4 years in males (55, 69, 134, 135, 220).

Every system of the body is growing rapidly, but physiologic changes occur unevenly within the person. Variation exists in age of onset of puberty and rapidity of growth between different groups of people as well. For example, Chinese show an earlier height spurt and menarche and more advanced skeletal maturity than Europeans (134).

Sexual Development

Four physical characteristics define puberty for most adolescents as they observe themselves and each other (65, 93, 135, 220).

Females
- Height spurt: ages 8 to 17 years; peak age, 12
- Menarche: 10 to 16 years; average age, 12.5
- Breast development: 8 to 18 years
- Pubic hair: 11 to 14 years

Males
- Height spurt: 10 to 20 years; peak age, 14
- Penile development: 10 to 16 years
- Testicular development: 9 to 17 years
- Pubic hair: 12 to 16 years

Menarche is the indicator of puberty and sexual maturity in the female. Ovulation usually occurs 12 to 24 months after menarche. The onset of menarche varies

among population groups and is influenced by heredity, nutrition, health care, and other environmental factors. In the United States the average age of onset is 12.3 to 12.6 years. Research on the onset of menarche has revealed conflicting results. Some researchers have shown a relationship between the height and weight of a girl and menarche (69). Onset of menarche also varies from country to country: in Sweden, 12.9 years; in Italy, 12.5 years; in Africa, 13.4 to 14.1 years (134).

Secondary sex characteristics in the female begin to develop in prepuberty (see Chapter 10) and may take 2 to 8 years for completion. Breast enlargement and elevation occur; areola and papillae project to form a secondary mound. Axillary and pubic hair grows thicker, becomes darker, and spreads over the pubic area (55, 135).

Spermatogenesis (**sperm production**) and seminal emissions mark puberty and sexual maturity in the male. The first ejaculate of seminal fluid occurs approximately 1 year after the penis has begun its adolescent growth, and **nocturnal emissions,** *loss of seminal fluid during sleep,* occur at approximately age 14 (69).

Secondary sex characteristics in the male also begin in prepuberty (see Chapter 10) and may take 2 to 5 years for completion. Changes in body shape, growth of body hair, and muscle development may continue until 19 or 20 or even until the late twenties. North American males complete growth in stature by 18 or 19 years, with an additional $\frac{1}{2}$ to 1 inch (1 to 2 cm) in height occurring during the twenties because of continued vertebral column growth. The penis, scrotum, and testes enlarge; the scrotum reddens, and scrotal skin changes texture. Hair grows at the axilla and base of the penis and spreads over the pubis. Body hair generally increases, especially facial hair. The voice deepens (55, 135, 220).

Sex hormones are biochemical agents that primarily *influence the structure and function of the sex organs and appearance of specific sexual characteristics.* **Androgens** are *hormones that produce male-type physical characteristics and behaviors.* **Estrogens** are *hormones that produce feminine characteristics.* **Progesterones** are *female hormones that prepare the uterus to accept a fetus and maintain the pregnancy.* All three sex hormones are in both sexes. Androgens are in greater amounts in males; the other two hormones are in greater amounts in females (69). More information about the function of sex hormones can be obtained in any physiology text.

The 28-day menstrual or reproductive cycle is controlled by an intricate feedback system involving (1) the hypothalamus, which audits the level of the hormones in the bloodsteam; (2) the anterior lobe of the pituitary and its hormones, FSH and LH; (3) the ovaries and their hormones, estrogen and progesterone; and (4) the interplay between the ovarian hormones and FSH and LH (69).

At the onset of the cycle, when the estrogen level is lowest, the shedding of the endometrium (lining of the uterus) occurs. The hypothalamus, because of the low estrogen level, stimulates the pituitary gland to release FSH, which causes the maturation of one of the ova-containing ovarian or graafian follicles and increased production of estrogen. This is the time of the highest level of estrogen in the bloodstream. In response to estrogen, the endometrium begins to thicken to prepare to receive the zygote if fertilization occurs (69).

In response to the high level of estrogen, the anterior pituitary releases LH. The sudden increase of LH triggers **ovulation,** *release of the mature ovum,* from the follicle, which happens approximately 14 days after the onset of the cycle. The LH moves to the ruptured follicle, which causes the development of the glandular corpus luteum. This produces both estrogen and progesterone, which, when acting together, cause the glands of the endometrium to prepare further for the nourishment of a possible zygote (69).

If fertilization of the ovum by a sperm cell does not occur, the ovum deteriorates. The pituitary stops production of both FSH and LH, and the corpus luteum becomes dormant and atrophies. The resulting drop in estrogen and progesterone levels stimulates the shedding of the endometrial lining, which consists of blood, mucus, and tissues, or the menstrual discharge. Menstruation lasts 3 to 5 days. The cycle then begins anew (69). **Primary dysmenorrhea,** *painful menstruation occurring without any evidence of abnormality in the pelvic organs,* may occur. The cause is unknown, but endocrine factors, natural pain processes, and psychologic factors have all been considered. Various analgesics have been used for this condition through the years. More recently the nonsteriod, anti-inflammatory agents have been used with some success. Some women find that adherence to a certain diet such as one with decreased caffeine and sugar and increased protein intake and exercise habits may decrease symptoms. Heat to the painful area may be palliative. (94).

In the male the hormonal system for reproductive behavior is much simpler because there is no cyclical pattern. The male gonads, the testes, serve to produce sperm continuously and to secrete androgens. The major androgen is testosterone (69).

Just as FSH promotes the development of the ovum in the female, FSH promotes the development of sperm in the male. A continuous level of sperm production takes place in the seminiferous tubules inside the testes. The secretion of LH (also called interstitial cell-stimulating hormone [ISCH]) stimulates the Leydig cells lying in between these tubules to secrete the androgen (69).

Musculoskeletal System

Structural changes—growth in skeletal size, muscle mass, adipose tissue, and skin—are significant in adolescence. The skeletal system grows faster than the supporting muscles; hands and feet grow out of proportion to the body; and large muscles develop faster than small muscles. Poor posture and decreased coordination re-

sult. Males and females differ in skeletal growth patterns; males have greater length in arms and legs relative to trunk size, in part because of a prolonged prepubertal growth period in boys. (Males are also more clumsy than females.) Males also have a greater shoulder width, a difference that begins in prepuberty. Ossification of the skeletal system occurs later for boys than girls. In girls, estrogen influences ossification and early unity of the epiphyses with shafts of the long bones, resulting in shorter stature (69, 134, 220). Muscle growth continues in males during late adolescence because of androgen production. Muscle growth in females is proportionate to growth of other tissue. Adipose tissue distribution over thighs, buttocks, and breasts occurs predominantly in females and is related to estrogen production (69).

Skin

Skin texture changes. Sebaceous glands become extremely active and increase in size. Eccrine sweat glands are fully developed, are especially responsive to emotional stimuli, and are more active in males. Apocrine sweat glands also begin to secrete in response to emotional stimuli (69).

Cardiovascular System

The heart grows slowly at first compared to the rest of the body, resulting in inadequate oxygenation and fatigue. The heart continues to enlarge until age 17 or 18. Systolic blood pressure and pulse pressure increase; blood pressure averages 100 to 120/50 to 70. Pulse rate averages 60 to 68 beats per minute. Females have a slightly higher pulse rate and basal body temperature and lower systolic pressure than males. Hypertension is increasing in adolescents, both Caucasian and African-American, in males, in the obese, and in those with a family history of hypertension. Higher systolic pressure occurs in urban dwellers; higher diastolic pressure has been seen in those who smoked and lacked regular exercise. Routine hypertension screening should be done. The upper limit for normal blood pressure in individuals from 11 to 17 years old is 130/90 (69, 134, 202).

Respiratory System

The respiratory system also grows slowly relative to the rest of the body, contributing to inadequate oxygenation. Respiratory rate averages 16 to 20 per minute. Males have a greater shoulder width and chest size, resulting in greater respiratory volume, greater vital capacity, and increased respiration. The male's lung capacity matures later than that of the female, which is mature at 17 or 18 years (220).

Blood Components

Red blood cell mass and hemoglobin concentration increase in both sexes because of increased hormone production. Hematocrit levels are higher in males; platelet count and sedimentation rate are increased in females, and white blood cell count is decreased in both sexes. Blood volume increases more rapidly in males. By late adolescence, males average 5000 ml and females 4200 ml of blood (220).

Gastrointestinal System

This system matures rapidly from 10 to 20 years. By age 21 all 32 *teeth* have usually appeared. *Stomach capacity* increases to approximately 1 quart (more than 900 ml), which correlates with increased appetite as the stomach becomes longer and less tubular; increased gastric acidity occurs to facilitate digestion of the increased food intake. *Intestines* grow in length and circumference. Muscles in the stomach and intestinal wall become thicker and stronger. Elimination patterns are well established and are related to food and fluid intake. The *liver* attains adult size, location, and function (69, 135).

Fluid and electrolyte balance changes reflect changes in body composition in terms of bones, muscle, and adipose tissue. Percentage of body water decreases, reaching adult levels. Approximately 60% of the male's total body weight is fluid, compared to 50% in the female; the difference is caused by the greater percentage of muscle mass in the male. Exchangeable sodium and chloride decline; intracellular fluid and body potassium levels rise with the onset of puberty. Again, because of their greater muscle mass, males have a 15% higher potassium concentration (69, 134).

Urinary System

Urinary bladder capacity increases; the adolescent voids up to $1\frac{1}{2}$ quarts (1500 ml) daily. Renal function is like that of the adult (69).

Special Sense Organs

The eyeball lengthens, increasing the incidence of myopia in early adolescence. Auditory acuity peaks at 13, and from that age on, hearing acuity gradually decreases. Sensitivity to odors develops at puberty; the female's increased sensitivity to musklike fragrances may be related to estrogen levels (69, 220).

Unique Differences

Racial differences in physical development occur, although adult statures are approximately the same. For example, African-American boys and girls attain a greater proportion of their adult stature earlier. Skeletal mass is greater in the African-American person; using Caucasian norms means that bone loss could go undetected. The normal value for hemoglobin concentration is 1 g less for African-American. Thus a low hemoglobin reading for African-Americans has a different nutritional implication; the person may not be iron deficient (89, 224). Continued research is necessary to determine other differences that may exist.

Because of the changing body, the adolescent needs information about the normality of anatomic and physiologic changes in addition to sex education. Adults should be cautioned not to pass on superstitions and taboos (e.g., that girls must rest and not participate in social or sport activities or that they should not take

showers during menstruation). The adolescent male must be told that the release of spermatic fluid through nocturnal emissions is *not* the result of disease or punishment for masturbation or sexual daydreaming.

If the parents are knowledgeable about pubertal growth changes, they can predict coming physical changes based on how the teen presently looks, which can be reassuring to the child whose onset of puberty is delayed. This may be more difficult in one-parent families since the man or woman is less equipped to understand and help the opposite-sexed child.

You can be very helpful in teaching the adolescent and in helping parents understand what they should teach their children. They both need realistic information about these subjects and an opportunity for discussion. Additional information can be obtained from the local library or health association, doctor, religious leader, counselor, or personal product companies. Having this knowledge can eliminate much fear and guilt and will help the adolescent understand his or her normal development.

Physical Assessment of the Adolescent

Regular physical examinations should be encouraged. See Appendix IV for a suggested schedule. Useful references to help you formulate a health history are Bates (14), Foster, Hunsberger, and Anderson (69), Hoole, Greenberg, and Pickard (94), and Sherman (182).

The examination is conducted much as for the adult. However, it is crucial that the examiner knows and understands the special emotional needs, developmental changes, age and maturation level of the person, and physiologic differences specific to adolescence.

Honest and genuine interest in the adolescent and not "speaking down" as though the young person is a child are essential. Confidentiality and trust are key issues. Be sure to express honestly to the teen what part of the interview and examination can be kept in strict confidence and what may need to be shared. Specific age of the person and the nature of the findings will determine these factors. Above all, do not say, "This is completely confidential," only to say later, "I believe we better share that."

Physical complaints and emotional symptoms may relate to underlying problems of drug abuse, alcoholism, sexual uncertainties and stress, pregnancy or fear of pregnancy, fear of or actual sexually transmitted disease, depression, family or peer adjustment problems, school problems, or concerns about future plans.

Because the adolescent may be extremely shy about his or her body, every effort must be made to protect privacy within the confines of the situation. With the advent of the female nurse practitioner and physician's assistant conducting examinations on male patients, the traditional "embarrassment roles" are switched. Much has been written on the conduct of the male examiner with the female patient but not on the reverse. The younger the adolescent male in terms of sexuality development, the more concern he has about a female examiner seeing and touching his body parts that are considered private (130). The female examiner ought to provide proper draping and emphasize the touching as little as possible. She may make the preliminary statement, "It is important that I palpate your scrotum to detect . . . . I know this is a tender area and I will proceed as quickly as possible while being thorough in my exam."

The blood pressure should be at adult levels. The athlete in training may have a slower pulse rate than his or her peers.

Pallor, especially in girls, should be a clue to check hemoglobin levels.

The teen needs frequent dental visits because most have caries. Many young adolescents whose parents have insurance for the service or have sufficient funds have orthodontic work in progress.

Because myopia seems to increase during these years, increased reading and study encourage eye strain. Many teens are now being fitted with contact lenses (182).

Although breast neoplasms are not common to this age group, females should be taught breast self-examination. Also, the girl should not be surprised if there is some asymmetric development. Some increase in breast tissue can also be expected in adolescent males. Excessive growth should be referred for evaluation. Both male and female breasts should be examined (182).

The heart should be found at the fifth left intercostal space as in the adult, and most functional murmurs should be outgrown. Serum cholesterol and triglyceride levels should be obtained if there is a family history of cardiovascular disease, and preventive dietary and exercise regimens should be discussed.

Striae may be found on the abdomen of females because of the rapid weight gain and loss experienced by fad diets followed by return to overeating (14, 182).

The examiner should be acutely aware not only of the pattern of sexual development of both males and females, but of the concerns and questions that may be voiced. The presence of the testes in the scrotum is of primary importance because undescended testicles at this age can mean sterility (182).

Papanicolaou (Pap) smears and pelvic examinations are done when the adolescent becomes sexually active. These procedures, done the first time with explanation and as much gentleness as possible, can set a positive tone for future examinations (182).

Some have suggested that urine cultures be taken periodically on females between the ages of 15 to 18 because of the number of asymptomatic urinary infections (182).

Scoliosis is common in teenagers, so a close look for asymmetry of the musculoskeletal system is essential, and any severe, persistent pain in the long bone area should also be referred (182).

Nutritional Needs

Teach parents and teenagers the following information about normal nutrition. Refer also to Box 11–2 (89, 224) and Appendix I. During this time of accelerated physical and emotional development the body's metabolic rate increases; accordingly, nutritional needs increase. The peak requirements occur in the year of maximum growth, which takes place between the tenth and twelfth years in girls and approximately 2 years later in boys. The calorie and protein requirements during this

---

■ BOX 11-2.
Recommended Nutritional Intake for Adolescents*

Food	Nonpregnant Adolescent (No. Servings)	Pregnant Adolescent (No. Servings)
Dairy products: one serving equals 1 cup milk, 1 ounce hard cheese, $1\frac{1}{4}$ cups cottage cheese, $\frac{1}{3}$ cup dry milk, or $1\frac{3}{4}$ cup ice cream (use low fat milk)	4 (ages 12–18) 2–3 (ages 19–22)	4
Meat and meat alternatives: one serving equals 2 eggs, 2 ounces lean meat, 1 cup beans or split peas, 4 tablespoons peanut butter, 2 ounces cheddar cheese, or $\frac{1}{2}$ cup cottage cheese	2–3	3
Fruits, vegetables, or juices: one serving equals $\frac{1}{2}$ cup or 1 medium fresh fruit or vegetable.	4–5	At least 5
Breads and cereals: one serving equals 1 slice of bread, $\frac{1}{2}$ cup cooked cereal, $\frac{3}{4}$ cup ready-to-eat cereal, or $\frac{1}{2}$ to $\frac{3}{4}$ cup cooked macaroni, spaghetti, rice, or grits, pasta	6–11 (6 servings for females)	6–11
Fats, oils, sweets	Use sparingly	Use sparingly

*Suggested amounts should support adequate weight gain

year are higher than at almost any other time of life. The adolescent female's requirements are equalled or surpassed only during pregnancy and lactation (see Box 11–2). Even after the obvious period of accelerated growth has ended, nutritional intake must be adequate for muscle development and bone mineralization, which continue (23, 135, 224). The adolescent's nutritional status encompasses the life span; it begins with the nutritional experience of childhood and determines the nutritional potential of adulthood.

Both males and females have an increased appetite; they are constantly hungry. A fast-growing boy may never feel full. His stomach capacity may be too small to accommodate the amount of food he requires to meet growth needs unless he eats at frequent intervals. Adolescent females between 11 and 14 years of age may need 2200 kcal per day; males of the same age need 2700 kcal. Females between 15 and 18 years of age need 2100 kcal and males need 2800 kcal (172, 224). However, stage of sexual maturation, rate of physical growth, and amount of physical and social activity should be considered before determining exact caloric needs. In addition, the nutritional needs differ for the pregnant and nonpregnant adolescent.

Protein helps to maintain a positive nitrogen balance within the body during the metabolic process (89, 224). Protein needs increase to between 45 to 56 g daily; approximately 15% of the total caloric intake should be derived from protein consumed in adequate quantities. Protein may be obtained from milk, cheese, eggs, meat, legumes, nuts, and whole grains. There is an additional need for iron during adolescence because of the increased muscle and soft tissue growth and the rapid growth demands of an expanding red cell mass. Girls may be especially susceptible to iron deficiency at menarche (224).

Calcium is needed for bone growth and continued teeth formation; intake should be increased to 1200 mg daily. If the adolescent drinks a quart of milk daily, this dietary requirement can be easily met (224).

Underweight and overweight are probably the two most common but overlooked symptoms of malnutrition. Assess the adolescent; teach the adolescent and parents as indicated to foster health.

Underweight

Being underweight can be caused by an inadequate intake of calories or poor use of the energy. It is often accompanied by fatigue, irritability, anorexia, and digestive disturbances such as constipation or diarrhea. Poor muscular development evidenced by posture and hypochromic anemia may also be observed. In children and adolescents growth and development may be delayed. Even with the recommended dietary intakes, malabsorption of protein, fat, or carbohydrate can result in undernutrition. Underweight may be a symptom of an undiagnosed disease (69). The most severe form of underweight is seen in individuals with anorexia nervosa

and bulimia. You may be the first person to assess these conditions in the adolescent.

Anorexia nervosa is a *syndrome*, occurring usually in females between the ages of 12 to 18, although onset may occur in the twenties and thirties, *in which the person voluntarily refuses to eat, presumably because of lack of hunger but related to distorted body image and conflictual relationships.*

Symptoms and signs of anorexia nervosa are presented in Box 11–3 (10, 57, 68, 108, 122, 127, 229).

Men may also suffer from this disease but may be even more reticent than women to reveal symptoms or seek treatment (57, 108, 127).

Bulimia may be associated with anorexia nervosa and is a *syndrome characterized by voluntary restriction of food intake followed by extreme overeating and self-induced vomiting and laxative abuse.*

Symptoms and signs for bulimia are presented in Box 11–4 (59, 68, 122, 131, 229).

Anorexia nervosa is more common than bulimia among adolescents, although the latter is increasing in incidence. Often both syndromes exist together (68). Impaired psychologic functioning, disturbed body image, confused or inaccurate perceptions about body functions, and a sense of incompetence and helplessness are present in all anorectic and bulimic clients (55, 68, 69, 147). There are several theories about causation and dynamics of anorexia nervosa (68, 69, 108, 127, 147, 224).

■ BOX 11-3
Signs and Symptoms of Anorexia Nervosa

- Refusal to eat or eating only small amounts yet feeling guilt about eating
- Denial of hunger (hunger becomes a battle of wills) yet preoccupied with food (plays with food when eating; collects recipes)
- Intense fear of becoming obese, even when underweight; refusal to maintain body weight; compulsive exercise and weighing
- Large (at least 20% to 25%) weight loss with no physical illness evident
- Abuse of laxatives and/or diuretics
- Distorted body image; perception of self as fat even when below normal weight
- Vital sign changes: bradycardia, hypotension, hypothermia
- Interruption of normal reproductive system processes in females—at least three consecutive menses missed when otherwise expected to occur
- Malnutrition adversely affecting (a) the skeleton, causing decalcification, decreased bone mass, and osteoporosis; (b) muscular development; and (c) cardiac and liver function, arrhythmia, and body metabolic functions, which may decrease as a result of liver involvement
- Skin dry, pale, yellow-tinged; lanugo present; hair loss
- Enlargement of brain ventricles, with shrinkage of brain tissue surrounding them; depression, irritability

---

BOX 11-4
Signs and Symptoms of Bulimia

- Binge eating—consuming excessively large amount of food—followed by self-induced vomiting or laxative and/or diuretic abuse (at least twice weekly); secretive eating
- Fear of inability to stop eating voluntarily
- A feeling of lack of control over the eating behavior during eating binges
- Preoccupation with food and guilt about eating
- Weight fluctuations and fluid and electrolyte imbalance due to binges, fasts, and vomiting/laxatives
- Use of crash diets to control weight
- Weakness, headaches, fatigue, depression
- Orthostatic hypotension due to fluid depletion
- Scars on dorsum of hand from induced vomiting
- Loss of tooth enamel and esophageal and gastric bleeding in vomiters
- Chest pain from esophageal reflux or spasm
- Parotid gland enlargement in vomiters
- Increased peristalsis, rectal bleeding, constipation if laxative abuser
- Menstrual irregularities

The person usually is treated on an outpatient basis; however, hospitalization, with nutritional support and intense psychotherapy, is recommended when loss of 25% or more of body weight leaves the person physically, emotionally, and socially compromised to the point of being in a life-threatening situation. The anorectic person should be hospitalized if there is a low serum electrolyte or fluid level; depression with suicidal thoughts or attempts; substantial disorganization of the family; or failure of outpatient treatment. These criteria also apply to the bulimic person; the additional criterion is spontaneous vomiting after binges. Hospitalization may also be helpful in diffusing parent-adolescent tensions and the resultant power struggle and in preventing suicide (10, 57, 68, 108, 127, 229).

The goals of treatment for the anorectic and bulimic client are to maintain normal weight, treat the hypokalemia and metabolic alkalosis, change attitudes toward food, and develop more effective coping skills to overcome the underlying conflicts. The nursing approach is holistic: you will work with the interdisciplinary team and the psychologic, physiologic, family, spiritual, and sociocultural dimensions of the person to promote adaptive behavior. Treatment involves any of the following methods: behavior modification, insight-oriented, supportive, group, or family therapy. For further information refer to articles at the end of the chapter (10, 57, 58, 68, 108, 122, 127, 147).

Both the family and the adolescent need therapy. Goals of family therapy include reducing pathogenic conflict and anxiety within the family relationships, becoming more aware of and better meeting each other's emotional needs, promoting more appropriate role be-havior for each gender and generation, and strengthening the capacity of the adolescent and family as a whole to cope with various problems (68, 69).

Overweight

Being overweight is rarely the result of an endocrine, metabolic, or neurologic disturbance. Teach adolescents and parents the following information. Genetic predisposition to obesity may exist as shown by studies that correlate parental weight more closely with the weight of their natural children than with those of adopted children (224). *Often weight status is a result of lifelong food and activity habits.* Children grow up associating food with much more than nourishment for their bodies. Food means celebration, consolation, reward, or punishment. People give and receive food as symbols of their love. Food and drink are chief forms of entertainment both at home and "on the town." We have learned to expect an offer of at least a beverage when we visit friends. This misuse of food, accompanied by a decrease in physical activity levels during the twentieth century, has led to a steady increase in the prevalence of obesity. Energy input is greater than energy output.

Various theories are proposed regarding the deposition of fat in the body. Apparently obese persons have either more fat cells (hyperplastic obesity), or the fat cells are bigger than those of normal-weight persons (hypertrophic obesity). Hyperplastic obesity is usually associated with early onset obesity, and hypertrophic obesity is usually associated with adult-onset obesity. Critical times for development of proliferation of fat cells may be the last prenatal trimester, the first 3 years of life, and adolescence. African-American infants usually are fatter than Caucasian infants, but this reverses later in childhood. Socioeconomic class may also affect weight. Males living in poverty are thin as children and grow to be thin adults. By contrast, females living in poverty are thin children who become fat women. Affluence results in overweight children who become slim adults (20, 69, 89, 122, 224). Childhood obesity does not always lead to adult obesity. Early onset obesity may be caused by a metabolic genetic defect that is compounded by excess caloric intake, with later-onset obesity caused by excess caloric intake. Onset of obesity in later life may have a situational basis; crises trigger fat cell hypertrophy or upset in appetite-control mechanisms (55, 160, 220, 224).

According to most research, **obesity** *exists if more than 20% of the male's body weight and 30% of the female's body weight is adipose tissue.* (Normal values of adipose tissue are 12% to 18% for men and 18% to 24% for women.) Another means of determining the degree of obesity is to measure skinfold thickness near the midpoint of the upper arm with a skinfold caliper. Skinfold thickness exceeding 15 mm in males and 25 mm in females indicates obesity (20, 224).

It has been estimated that 10% to 30% of adolescents are obese and approximately 80% of these teens will remain obese as adults (160, 220). As with most abnormal states of health, prevention of obesity is better than treatment. A pound of body fat contains approximately 3500 calories. An intake in excess of need of even 100 calories a day will add up to 3000 calories a month, or almost 1 pound of body weight. With the obese adolescent, food intake and activity habits should be assessed with weight loss and/or control in mind. Numerous approaches exist for the treatment of obesity; few of these methods are successful with the adolescent. There are various approaches for treating obesity, including diet, exercise, medication, behavior modification, surgery, and mechanical methods (20, 168, 224).

Both prescription and over-the-counter appetite depressants are available. Many of these contain caffeine, which can cause an elevated heart rate and high blood pressure. Many over-the-counter dietary aids contain bulk-producing agents and a sympathomimetic with anorectic action. The sympathomimetic in these aids (propanolamine) is capable of producing nervousness, restlessness, insomnia, and headaches; the bulk-producing agents have a laxative effect. Like other drugs, these appetite depressants can be addictive and have other side effects that might produce health problems. Thyroid hormone is beneficial only to persons who are in a hypometabolic state. Because thyroid hormone medication can inhibit thyroxin production in metabolically normal persons, it can be detrimental to their efforts at weight reduction. Thyroid hormones can also have adverse effects on the cardiovascular system. Similarly, the use of diuretics by a person who needs to lose fat is both misleading and dangerous. The person loses necessary fluid and electrolytes instead (220, 224).

Diet plans vary from balanced low-calorie diets to nutritionally poor fad diets. Some of the dietary plans encourage total fasting (therapeutic starvation); other plans change the type and amount of food, the frequency of eating episodes, and the speed at which food is eaten. Caloric restriction does not work well with adolescents. Teens want rapid, easy results. Eating also is an important part of the adolescent socialization pattern. Thus limiting caloric intake or restricting foods eaten may alter their social interaction.

Mechanical methods, often advertised in popular magazines, include sauna suits, special exercise outfits, mechanical spot reducers, and steam baths. Because overweight is a problem of energy input and output, these methods have no long-term benefit.

Surgery is a drastic approach to weight reduction. Intestinal bypass and similar surgical procedures prevent the absorption of glucose for energy and that of many vitamins, minerals, and electrolytes. Severe complications can result from this surgery even years after an apparent uneventful recovery. Gastric partitioning decreases the size of the stomach and slows the stomach's emptying ability; individuals feel full and curtail their food intake.

Insertion of a gastric balloon is also being used in conjunction with dietary control and behavior modification. A polyurethane balloon is inserted into the stomach and is inflated with air. The balloon occupies approximately 25% of the stomach capacity and thus produces satiety. None of the surgeries alters the cause of obesity—eating habits—but these procedures may be used in cases of life-threatening obesity when all other attempts have failed (73, 160, 190).

Because obese people tend to gauge their eating according to external environmental cues rather than hunger, programs using behavior modification on eating habits have been used with some success (122, 222, 224). By learning to change problem behaviors associated with eating or exercise, they can change habits and maintain their subsequent weight loss. Through daily school physical education classes, exercise programs should be designed.

An eating pattern assessment is described by White (222), as are areas for psychologic, physiologic, and sociocultural assessment. Based on assessment, the following suggestions, if followed, can help most obese adolescents lose weight:

1. Consciously ask self before eating, "Am I really hungry?"
2. Eat only at mealtimes and at the table; avoid snacks. To lose 1 pound weekly, dietary intake must be reduced by 500 calories daily.
3. Count the mouthfuls, cut food into small pieces, and eat slowly to eat less. Set down eating utensils between each bite of food.
4. Keep a food diary, with the goal of reinforcing the adherence to the traditional food groups and avoid empty calories (20, 69, 153).
5. Engage in planned, regular exercise such as bicycle riding, walking the pet dog, gardening, yard work, calistehenics, or swimming.
6. Maintain proper posture and an overall attractive appearance.

Families should be given the following suggestions to help the adolescent achieve weight loss:

1. Limit purchases and cooking and baking of carbohydrate foods or snacks.
2. Remove tempting snacks such as candy and cookies from the home.
3. Ban eating in front of the television or reading while eating.
4. Make dining at the table a pleasant time.
5. Avoid using food as reward or punishment.
6. Serve food in individual portions on the plate rather than in bowls on the table to avoid second helpings, and serve food on smaller plates.
7. Praise even a small weight loss; avoid nagging (20, 69).
8. Participate in physical activity with the adolescent when possible.

Further, you can reinforce the permanence of new food habits and achievement of weight loss through your continued guidance and realistic praise. The key to successful treatment may be in improving the adolescent's self-image. If emotional problems exist, you will need to counsel the adolescent or refer him or her to an appropriate source. Regardless of the methods of treatment used, parental understanding and cooperation are needed, and you are one member of the health team with whom both parents and the adolescent can discuss their concerns. Your listening, discussing, teaching, and referral when necessary can help the adolescent prevent or overcome the health hazard of obesity. You can also work with the school system to establish daily physical exercise programs that stimulate the teen to remain physically active. Use of dietary instructions, checking of weight, low-calorie refreshments, behavior modification techniques, exercise, and individual support can be helpful.

Obesity presents physical health hazards and problems with social and emotional adjustment. The obese adolescent is frequently rejected by the peer group and harassed by his or her parents. Many overweight teenagers withdraw from social interactions and develop feelings of inadequacy and inferiority. Physical health problems such as abnormal menstrual cycles, orthopedic difficulties, kidney stones, and gallbladder disease develop. If obesity persists into adulthood, the incidence of diabetes mellitus, cardiovascular diseases, and other illnesses increases.

Preventing adolescent obesity through education of the child and the parents and treating it when it occurs can eliminate future health problems. More information on types, effects, and treatment of obesity can be found in various references (4, 20, 42, 45, 89, 128, 220, 224).

Adolescent Pregnancy

Adolescent pregnancy, discussed later in the chapter, presents another health problem related to nutrition as well as to other physical, social, and emotional factors. Clearly, many teenagers lack the physiologic maturity needed to withstand the stresses of pregnancy. The adolescent's nutritional intake may be only barely sufficient to support her own development—not adequate to satisfy two nutritional requirements (69, 89, 201, 224).

Exercise, Play, and Rest

Exercise and rest must be balanced. Teach adolescents and parents the following information.

Exercise and Play Activities

Three types of play predominate in this age group: cooperative play, exemplified in games; team play, exemplified in sports; and construction play, exemplified in hobbies. All of these types of play can promote growth in the adolescent (135).

Teenage boys are concerned with activities that require physical abilities and demonstrate their manliness. This age group probably spends more time and energy practicing and participating in sport-related activities than any other age group. Many boys attempt to participate in sports like basketball, football, baseball, hockey, and soccer, or work on cars or machines. There is growing acceptance, however, of the boy who wants to cook, garden, or do other activities which traditionally were not so popular or acceptable.

Adolescent girls are less apt to participate in team sports after the onset of puberty. Although the female role is changing, some cultures still expect girls to develop the traditional interests in social functions and domestic skills such as cooking, cleaning, and serving. Although girls are involved in swimming, gymnastics, jogging, ice skating, dancing, and horseback or bicycle riding, some teenage girls in the United States are on football or rugby teams or practice weight lifting. Those who try out for and succeed on boys' teams are challenging long-accepted ideas about femininity, masculinity, strength and endurance of each gender, and competition. There is no physiologic reason why girls should not play aggressive sports; the uterus is well protected, and a blow to the breast does not result in long-term harm. In fact, the male reproductive organs are actually more vulnerable to injury than the female reproductive organs. The key is that we have not wanted to raise girls to be aggressive. Although aggressive behavior in females is specific to the competitive sports, female athletes describe themselves as acting in the socially expected way in nonathletic situations (134).

Help parents and teens realize that competitive activities prepare young people to develop a process of self-appraisal that will last them throughout their lives (Fig. 11–1). Learning to win and to lose can also be important in developing self-respect and concern for others. Physical activities provide a way for adolescents to enjoy the stimulation of conflict in a socially acceptable manner. Participation in sports training programs in junior and senior high schools can also help decrease the gap between biologic and psychosocial maturation while providing exercise. Some form of physical activity should be encouraged to promote physical development, prevent overweight, formulate a realistic body image, and promote peer acceptance. Being an observer on the sidelines will not fulfill these needs.

As women join the labor force in growing numbers, the importance of the sports experience increases since the working woman, like the working man, is involved in a structure in which rules are modeled on competitive sports teams. The worker must be able to play the game: follow rules, get along with all kinds of people, and not disparage colleagues or talk back to the boss (134). In nursing these attributes are increasingly important for the successful professional in the health care system. The emphasis in nursing education on the individual nurse and individual patient has often caused real frustration and conflict for the individual nurse in the work setting. A sense of the competition and teamwork that exists in the

Figure 11-1. Team sports provide adolescents with a socially accepted outlet for competitive feelings and conflict and promote physical and psychosocial development. (Top: Copyright © Mike Valeri, FPG International. Bottom: Copyright © Robert Bennett, FPG International.)

real world is as essential in nursing as in other occupations and professions. Perhaps in the future the professional female nurse who has participated in competitive team sports as a child and adolescent will adjust better to system demands while maintaining quality of practice.

Rest and Sleep

During adolescence bedtime becomes variable; the adolescent is busy with an active social life. The teen is ex-

pending large amounts of energy and functioning with an inadequate oxygen supply; both contribute to fatigue and need for additional rest. In addition, protein synthesis occurs more readily during sleep. Because of the growth spurt during adolescence, protein synthesis needs are increased (69, 135). Increased rest may also be needed to prevent illness.

Limit setting may be necessary to ensure adequate opportunities for rest. Rest is not necessarily sleep. A period of time spent with some quiet activity is also beneficial. Every afternoon should not be filled with extracurricular activities or home responsibilities, and when there is school the next morning, the adolescent should be in bed at a reasonable hour.

PSYCHOSOCIAL CONCEPTS

Cognitive Development

Formal Operations Stage

Tests of mental ability indicate that adolescence is the time when the mind has great ability to acquire and use knowledge. One of the adolescent's developmental tasks is to develop a workable philosophy of life, a task requiring time-consuming abstract and analytic thinking and inductive and deductive reasoning.

The adolescent uses available information to combine ideas into concepts and concepts into constructs, develop theories, and look for supporting facts; consider alternate solutions to problems; project his or her thinking into the future; and try to categorize thoughts into usable forms. He or she is capable of highly imaginative thinking, which, if not stifled, can evolve into significant contributions in many fields—science, art, music. The adolescent's theories at this point may be oversimplified and lack originality, but he or she is setting up the structure for adult thinking patterns, typical of the Period of Formal Operations. The adolescent can solve hypothetical, mental, and verbal problems; use scientific reasoning; deal with the past, present, and future; and understand causality. The Formal Operations Period differs from Concrete Operations in that a much larger range of symbolic processes and logic is used (83, 161, 213).

Keniston (106, 107) describes cognitive development of youth or late adolescence as proceeding through a complex transition of dualism such as a simple understanding of right and wrong and either-or of an issue to an awareness of multiplicity, a realization of relativism, and a more existential sense of truth. Keniston believes that an aspect of this stage of cognitive development is to think about thinking: the ability to achieve a new level of consciousness, an awareness of consciousness, and a decrease in self-consciousness that permits intellectual tricks, phenomenologic games, and a higher level of creativity. This stage involves being very aware of inner processes, focusing on states of consciousness as something to control and alter, and thinking about the ideal self and society (106, 107).

The abstract level of thinking described by Keniston can be considered a part of the period of Formal Operations (106, 107). Even though there are no overall differences between female and male adolescents' intelligence, females have shown greater verbal skills, whereas males have shown more facility with quantitative and spatial problems. These differences are apparently the result of interest, social expectations, and training rather than different innate mental abilities (83, 134).

In the United States the emphasis in education and the work world is on logical, analytic, critical, and convergent thinking. The goal of these linear thinking processes is precision, exactness, consistency, sequence, and correctness of response. The source of such thinking is the left hemisphere of the brain. Yet original concepts do not necessarily arise from logical thinking. Thinking that is creative or novel is marked by exploration, intentional ambiguity, problem solving, and originality. Creativity is a multivariaet mental process, divergent, intuitive, and holistic in nature; its source is the right hemisphere of the brain. It is an intellectual skill in which the person creates new ideas rather than imitating existing knowledge.

Creativity can be encouraged when the educational process requires the following (41):

1. Written assignments that necessitate original work, independent learning, self-initiation, and experimentation
2. Reading assignments that emphasize questions of inquiry, synthesis, and evaluation rather than factual recall
3. Group work to encourage brainstorming or exposure to creative ideas of others
4. Oral questions that are divergent or ask for viewpoints during lectures
5. Tests that include both divergent and convergent questions that engage the student in reflective, exploratory thought (questions should become increasing complex in nature; ideally the questions are worded so that there is not just one right answer but answers that can be innovative and express thoughtfulness)
6. A creative atmosphere, whereby the learner is autonomous, self-reliant, internally controlled, and self- evaluated (the curriculum emphasizes process, and the teacher provides a supportive atmosphere and recognizes creativity; in such an environment one would observe puzzlement and frustration but also eagerness, humor, laughter, and enjoyment related to the task at hand)

Parents sometimes underestimate the cognitive abilities of the adolescent. Help them work with the adolescent from an intellectual and creative perspective. Parents can learn from adolescents, just as adolescents learn from parents. Help the adolescent learn how to use cognitive skills in a way that will not antagonize parents.

The adolescent does not always develop intellectual potential by staying in school. School dropout occurs for a variety of reasons, not just because of socioeconomic disadvantage (124). School dropout has many negative consequences. Sherraden's article (183) describes school dropout in detail. Providing special classrooms for the teen during pregnancy and after delivery so that she can bring the baby for day care while she attends class is one way to prevent school dropout for that population (95, 114).

Peer-Group Influences

The **peer group,** *friends of the same age,* influences the adolescent to a greater extent than parents, mass media, teachers, popular heroes, religious leaders, or other adults. This finding contradicts a survey 20 years ago that showed parents and teachers to have greater influence than peers (134).

Because peer groups are so important, the adolescent has intense loyalty to them. Social relationships take precedence over family and counteract feelings of emptiness, isolation, and loneliness. Significance is attached to activities deemed important by peers. Peers serve as models or instructors for skills not yet acquired. Usually some peers are near the same cognitive level as the learner; their explanations may be more understandable. When student peers of varying cognitive levels discuss problems, less advanced students may gain insights and correct inaccuracies in thinking. The more advanced students also profit; they must think through their own reasoning to explain a concept (217).

Peer groups provide a sense of acceptance, prestige, belonging, approval, and opportunities for learning how to behave. Adolescents believe they have to have immediate, useful function; the real business of life is ahead of them. The peer group provides a sense of immediacy, concentrating on the here-and-now, what happened last night, who is doing what today, what homework is due tomorrow. Thus the adolescent is given reason for *being* today, a sense of *importance right now,* and not just dreams or fears about what he or she might become in some vague future time (55, 116, 135, 220). In addition, relationships with peers provide learning for later adult roles.

The peer group helps the adolescent define personal identity as he or she adapts to a changing body image, more mature relationships with others, and heightened sexual feelings. The peer group has well-defined types of behavior for masculinity and femininity, although adults may not recognize the distinctions. As the adolescent tries a variety of acceptable behaviors within the safety of the group, he or she incorporates new ideas into the body image and self-concept. The adolescent who is rejected by peers may be adversely affected since he or she does not learn the high degree of social skill and ability to form relationships that are necessary for the adult culture (135, 143, 144).

Peer group relations are beneficial, but they can also direct the adolescent into antisocial behavior because of pressure to conform and the need to gain approval. The adolescent may participate in drug and alcohol abuse, sexual intercourse, or various delinquent acts not because he or she wants to or enjoys them, but rather to prove self, to vent aggression, or to gain superiority over younger or fringe members of the group. He or she may even gain pleasure from sadistic activities toward others. Parents have reason to be concerned about their adolescent's peers and to guide their child into wholesome activities and groups that will reinforce the values they have taught. Help parents and teachers understand peer groups and work through crises related to peer relations (16).

Peer-Group Dialect

This dialect is a communication pattern seen in the adolescent period. Slang, or jargon, is one of the trademarks of adolescence and may be considered a **peer-group dialect.** *It is a highly informal language that consists of coined terminology and of new or extended interpretations attached to traditional terms.*

Slang is used for various reasons. It provides a sense of belonging to the peer group and a small, compact vocabulary for a teenager who does not want to waste energy on words. Slang also excludes authority figures and other outsiders and permits expression of hostility, anger, and rebellion. Unknowing adults do not understand the digs given with well-timed pieces of slang. Other adults sense the flippancy of underlying feelings but to their chagrin can do little other than try to understand. By the time they learn the meanings of the current terms, new meanings have evolved.

You can help parents understand the purposes of teenage dialect and the importance of not trying to imitate or retaliate verbally. In addition, encourage parents to enter into discussion with their teenager to understand more fully him or her and the teen-age dialect.

Use of Leisure Time

Leisure time with the peer group is important for normal social development and adjustment. The adolescent spends an increasing amount of time away from home, either in school, in other activities, or with peers, as he or she successfully achieves greater independence. School is a social center, even though abstract learning is a burden to some students. In school students seek recognition from others and determine their status within the group, depending on success in scholastic, athletic, or other organizations and activities.

Dating Pattern

Dating is one use of leisure time and is influenced greatly by the peer group but also varies according to the culture and social class and religious and family beliefs. Dating prepares the adolescent for intimate bonds with others, marriage, and family life. The adolescent learns social skills in dealing with the opposite sex, in what situations and with whom he or she feels least and most comfortable, and what is expected sexually.

In the United States dating may begin as early as age 10 or 11 years, especially with pressures from peers and family to attract the opposite sex. Generally, however, girls in junior high school are more mature than boys. Girls may seek male companionship, but boys frequently prefer activities with other males. Many fellows at this age are women haters. Near age 15, boys begin to catch up with girls in physical and emotional maturity, and their interests become better correlated. Social pursuits take on more meaning for boys.

Not all American adolescents assume this dating pattern. Some begin early to date one person and continue that pattern until marriage. Others do not date until young adulthood. A few will prefer homosexual relationships. Isolated homosexual encounters are not unusual, especially among males, and do not mean the person will remain a homosexual. The dynamics behind homosexuality are more complex. Because the person is usually a young adult when homosexuality is declared the chosen sexual pattern, the topic is discussed in greater detail in Chapter 12. However, the adolescent may have always felt more comfortable with or more cared for by the same-sexed person.

When dating begins, the emphasis is first on commonly shared activities. Later the emphasis includes a sharing, close relationship. Similarly, dating may start with groups of couples, move to double dates, and finally involve single couples. With each step, the adolescent learns more about and feels more comfortable with the opposite sex. He or she also learns personal acceptability to others. Going steady has become popular because it provides a readily available partner for social activities, but it can be detrimental if it stops the adolescent from searching for the qualities he or she wants in a future mate or involves sexual experimentation that he or she is unprepared to handle.

As you work with adolescents, you should assess the stage of peer-group development and dating patterns. A few years will make a considerable difference in attitudes toward the opposite sex. You must be able to build your teaching on current interests and attitudes. The same age groups in different localities may also be in different stages. Adolescents from another culture may sharply contrast in pattern with American adolescents. For example, in Egypt the male is not supposed to have any intimate physical contact with the female until marriage. In America certain physical contact is expected.

Leisure Activities

Sports, dancing, hobbies, reading, listening to the radio or stereo, talking on the telephone, daydreaming, experimenting with hairstyles, cosmetics, or new clothes, or just loafing have been teenagers' favorite activities for decades. Motorcycle riding, driving and working on cars, watching television, and playing video games are also popular. Political activism draws some youth; various causes rise and then fade in interest as the youth matures. "Everybody's doing it" is seemingly a strong influence on the adolescent's interests and activities.

Socioeconomic and educational levels determine to some extent how youth use free time. Upper-class youths may travel extensively, go boating, and attend cultural events or debutante parties. Middle-class emphasis is on participation in activities. During adolescence these youths are involved in church- or school-related functions such as sports, theater, and musical organizations. Lower-class youths may spend more time in unstructured ways such as standing on the corner, talking to peers, or finding ways to earn extra money. In many homes, however, the absence of money does not mean the absence of healthy leisure activity. Smoking and using alcohol and drugs cannot be attributed primarily to lower-class youths, for a great deal of money is required to supply some of these habits. Shoplifting, for example, is sometimes done for "kicks."

Many parents consider a party in the home for a group of teenagers a safe use of leisure time. This is undoubtedly true if parents and other adults are on the premises and can give guidance as needed and if the parents are not themselves supplying the teens with alcohol and drugs. However, the latter sometimes happens; parents rationalize by saying they prefer their youngster be at home (or at a friend's home) if they are using or abusing alcohol and drugs. They may even drive home teens who are unsafe to drive. Usually, however, drug and alcohol parties are hosted by teens when parents are out of town; teenagers chip in for beer for an "open" party (any number of people may attend) (180). When behavior becomes boisterous, police are often called by the neighbors, but they find the situation difficult to handle because there is no responsible authority figure on the premises. The police in one community give the following guidelines to help parents and teens *host and attend* parties. You may wish to share these suggestions with parents (79).

1. Parents should set the ground rules before the party to express feelings and concerns about the party, ask who will attend and whether adults will be present, and learn what is expected of their adolescent. The address and phone number of the host should be known by the parents of the teens who are attending.
2. Notify neighbors that you will be hosting a party, and encourage your teen to call or send a note to close neighbors notifying them of the party and asking them to let the family know if there is too much noise.
3. Notify the police when planning a large party. They can protect you, your guests, and your neighbors. Discuss with the police an agreeable plan for guest parking.

4. Plan to have plenty of food and nonalcoholic beverages on hand.

5. Plan activities with your teenager before the party so that the party can end before guests become bored (3 or 4 hours are suggested as sufficient party time).

6. Limit party attendance and times. Either send out invitations or have the teenager personally invite guests beforehand. Discourage crashers; ask them to leave. Open house parties are difficult for parents and teenagers to control. Set time limits for the party that enable guests to be home at a reasonable time, definitely before a legal curfew. Suggested closing hours are grades 7 and 8, 10:30 PM; grades 9 and 10, 11:30 PM; grades 11 and 12, 12:00 PM. Check curfew times for your locale. Transportation home for each teen who attends should be planned in advance by parents and the adolescent.

7. A parent should be at home during the entire time of the party. The parent's presence helps keep the party running smoothly; it also gives the parent an opportunity to meet the teenager's friends. Invite other adults to help supervise.

8. Decide what part of the house will be used for the party. Pick out where your guests will be most comfortable and you can maintain adequate supervision. Avoid having the bedroom area as part of the party area.

9. Do not offer alcohol to guests under the age of 21 or allow guests to use drugs in your home. This sounds prudish in this permissive era. However, you may be brought to court on criminal charges or have to pay monetary damages in a civil lawsuit if you furnish alcohol or drugs to minors. Be alert to the signs of alcohol or drug use.

10. Do not allow any guest who leaves the party to return to discourage teenagers from leaving the party to drink or to use drugs elsewhere and then return to the party.

11. Guests who try to bring alcohol or drugs or who otherwise refuse to cooperate with your expectations should be asked to leave. Notify the parents of any teenager who arrives at the party drunk or under the influence of any drug to ensure his or her safe transportation home. Do not let anyone drive under the influence of alcohol or drugs.

12. Teenagers frequently party at homes when parents are away. Typically, the greatest problems occur when parents are not at home. Tell your neighbors when you are going to be out of town.

13. Many parties occur spontaneously. Parents and teens should understand before the party that these guidelines are in effect at all parties. If, despite your precautions, things get out of hand, do not hesitate to call the local police department for help.

14. Emphasize to parents the importance of their being role models through minimum drinking of alcoholic beverages or use of drugs.

In some states there is legal parental responsibility in the home. A parent commits the crime of endangering the welfare of a child less than 17 years of age if he or she recklessly fails to exercise reasonable diligence in the care or control of a child to prevent him or her from behavior, environment, or associations that are injurious to the welfare of the child or to the welfare of others. In some states a person commits the crime of unlawful transactions with a child if he or she knowingly permits a minor child to enter or remain in a place where illegal activities in controlled substances are maintained or conducted. Parents have responsibility (possibly in all states) if a minor is killed or injured after leaving their home in which an illegal substance was consumed. Juvenile officers identify an adult doing an act "knowingly and recklessly" when a minor is involved as a criterion for possible prosecution. In the opinion of attorneys and judges, parents could be subject to suit for damages for careless or imprudent behavior (79).

The teenager may also feel more secure when the parent is actively interested in knowing where he or she will be and what he or she will be doing even though rebellion may ensue. Parents should be awake or have the teen awaken them when arriving home from a party. This is a good sharing time. Peers are important, but if peer activity and values are in opposition to what has been learned as acceptable, the adolescent feels conflict. Parental limits can reduce feelings of conflict and give an excuse to avoid an activity in which he or she does not want to engage. Parental limits appropriate to the situation and not unduly constraining develop ego strength within the adolescent.

Explore with parents the adolescent's need for constructive use of leisure time and the importance of participation in peer activities.

For some teenagers there is little leisure time. They may have considerable home responsibility such as occurs in rural communities or work to earn money to help support the family. Other youths are active in volunteer work. Ideally, the adolescent has some time free for personal pursuits, to stand around with friends, and to sit and daydream.

Emotional Development

Emotional Characteristics

Emotional characteristics of the personality cannot be separated from family, physical, intellectual, and social development. Emotionally, the adolescent is characterized by mood swings and extremes of behavior. Table 11–1 lists typical contradictions (63, 64, 74, 116, 125, 134). Box 11–5 lists major worries of teenagers; these concerns contribute to emotional lability and identity confusion (200). Emotional development requires an interweaving and organization of opposing tendencies into a sense of unity and continuity. This process occurs during adolescence in a complex and truly impressive

TABLE 11-1. CONTRASTING EMOTIONAL RESPONSES OF ADOLESCENTS

Independent Behaviors	Dependent Behaviors
Happy, easygoing, loving, gregarious, self-confident, sense of humor	Sad, irritable, angry, unloving, withdrawn, fearful, worried
Energetic, self-assertive, independent	Apathetic, passive, dependent
Questioning, critical or cynical of others	Strong allegiance to or idolization of others
Exhibitionistic or at ease with self	Excessively modest or self-conscious
Interested in logical or intellectual pursuits	Daydreaming, fantasizing
Cooperative, seeking responsibility, impatient to be involved or finish project	Rebellious, evading work, dawdling, ritualistic behavior, dropout from society
Suggestible to outside influences, including ideologies	Unaccepting of new ideas
Desirous for adult privileges	Apprehensive about adult responsibilities

way to move the person toward psychologic maturity (74).

Share this information with parents and the adolescent. Through using principles of communication and crisis intervention and through your use of self as a role model, you will be able to help the adolescent work through identity diffusion and achieve a sense of ego identity and an appropriate sense of independence.

We regularly hear of the rebellious, emotionally labile, egocentric adolescent but do not stereotype all adolescents into that mold. Some, perhaps more than we know of, can delay gratification, behave as adults, and have positive relationships with family and authority figures.

■ BOX 11-5
Major Concerns of Teenagers

- Their appearance
- Divorce of parents
- Having good marriage and family life
- School performance
- Choosing career; finding steady employment
- Being successful in life
- Having strong friendships; how others will treat them
- Paying for college
- Making lots of money
- Finding purpose and meaning in life
- Contracting AIDS
- Drug and alcohol use by self, friends
- Hunger and poverty in United States and the world
- Societal violence

Data from reference 200.

Developmental Crisis

The psychosexual crisis of adolescence is identity formation versus identity diffusion: "Who am I?" "How do I feel?" "Where am I going?" "What meaning is there in life?" **Identity** means that an *individual believes he or she is a specific unique person;* he or she has emerged as an adult. **Identity formation** *results through synthesis of biopsychosocial characteristics from a number of sources, for example, earlier gender identity, parents, friends, social class, ethnic, religious, and occupational groups* (62, 63).

A number of influences can interfere with identity formation (62, 63, 64, 116, 134):

1. Telescoping of generations, with many adult privileges granted early so that the differences between adult and child are obscured and there is no ideal to which to aspire
2. Contradictory American value system of individualism versus conformity in which both are highly valued and youth believe that adults advocate individualism but then conform
3. Nuclear family structure; the adolescent perceives most adults as parent figures and has primarily parents as targets for conflicts and aggressions
4. Middle-class cultural emphasis in child rearing, with inconsistencies between proclaimed and actual parental concern
5. Emphasis on sexual matters and encouragement to experiment without frank talking about sexuality with parents
6. Diminishing hold of Judeo-Christian traditions and ethics throughout society so that the adolescent sees that failure to live by the rules is not necessarily followed by unpleasant consequences
7. Increasing emphasis on education for socioeconomic gain, which prolongs dependency on parents when the youth is physically mature
8. Lack of specific sex-defined responsibilities (Blurring of the traditional male-female tasks has its positive and negative counterparts; although eventually allowing more individual freedom, it can be very confusing to the adolescent who must decide how to act as a male or female.)
9. Rapid changes in the adolescent subculture and all society, with emphasis on conforming to peers
10. Diverse definitions of adulthood: after 12 the adolescent pays adult airline fares; after 16 he or she can drive; after 18 he or she can vote

Identity formation implies an *internal stability, sameness, or continuity, which resists extreme change and preserves itself from oblivion in the face of stress or contradictions.* It implies emerging from this era with a sense of wholeness, knowing the self as a unique person, feeling responsibility, loyalty, and commitment to a value system. There are three types of identity, which are closely interwoven: (1) **personal,** or **real identity—**

what the person believes self to be; (2) **ideal identity—** *what he or she would like to be;* and (3) **claimed identity—** *what he or she wants others to think he or she is.*

Identity formation is enhanced by having support not only from parents but also from another adult who has a stable identity and who upholds sociocultural and moral standards of behavior (62, 63). If the adolescent has successfully coped with the previous developmental crisis and feels comfortable with personal identity, he or she will be able to appreciate the parents on a fairly realistic basis, seeing and accepting both their strengths and shortcomings. The values, beliefs, and guidelines they have given him or her are internalized. The adolescent needs parents less for direction and support; he or she must now decide what is acceptable and unacceptable behavior.

Students from different ethnic and racial backgrounds have unique needs and ways of adapting to stressors and unique aspects of the developmental crisis of identity formation. Some may feel isolated and alienated in relation to mainstream culture values. Parents, school teachers, and health care professionals can help these teens work through values and cognitive and emotional conflicts (226).

Identity diffusion *results if the adolescent fails to achieve a sense of identity* (62, 63). He or she feels self-conscious and has doubts and confusion about self as a human being and his or her roles in life. With identity diffusion, he or she feels impotent, insecure, disillusioned, and alienated. Some researchers believe girls enter puberty and adolescence feeling self-confidence and high self-esteem and because of classroom and socialization processes, are more likely than boys to enter the twenties feeling low self-esteem and insecure (38). Erikson (62, 63) believes such feelings exist in both males and females until identity formation occurs.

Identity diffusion is manifested in other ways as well. The adolescent feels that he or she is losing grip with reality. He or she is impatient but unable to initiate action. The teenager vacillates in decision making; he or she cannot delay gratification and appears brazen or arrogant. Behavior at work, with peers, and in sexual contacts is distorted. The adolescent is apprehensive about and avoids adult behavior, fearing loss of uniqueness by entering adulthood. The real danger of identity diffusion looms when a youth finds a negative solution to the quest for identity. He or she gives up, feels defeated, and pursues antisocial behavior since "it's better to be bad than nobody at all." Identity diffusion is more likely to occur if the teenager has close contact with an adult who is still confused about personal identity and who is in rebellion against society (62–64).

Assist parents to work with the adolescent who feels identity diffusion. Most adolescents reach physical maturity before they achieve ego identity or the emotional maturity expected as a sign of having completed the adolescent era. One study showed that individuals between 17 and 20 years of age report significantly more ego diffusion than those between 21 and 24. Females report less ego diffusion in all age groups than males (63).

References by Norris and Kunes-Carroll (146) and by Oldaker (148) describe nursing diagnoses pertinent to the adolescent who is having difficulty with identity formation.

Self-Concept and Body-Image Development

Development of self-concept and body image is closely akin to cognitive organization of experiences and identity formation. The adolescent cannot be viewed only in the context of the present; earlier experiences have an impact that continues to affect him or her. The earlier experiences that were helpful enabled the adolescent to feel good about the body and self. If the youngster enters adolescence feeling negative about self or the body, this will be a difficult period.

Other factors influence the adolescent's self-concept, including age of maturation, degree of attractiveness, name or nickname, size and physique appropriate to gender, degree of identification with the same-sexed parent, level of aspiration and ability to reach ideals, peer relationships, and culture (12, 16, 77, 116, 138).

The rapid growth of the adolescent period is an important factor in body-image revision. Girls and boys are sometimes described as "all legs." They are often clumsy and awkward. Because the growth changes cannot be denied, the adolescent is forced to alter the mental picture of self to function. More important than the growth changes themselves is the meaning given to them. The mother who says, "That's all right, Tom, we all have our clumsy moments," is providing the understanding that a comment such as "Can't you ever walk through the room without knocking something down?" denies. The adolescent needs this understanding because he or she fears rejection and is oversensitive to the opinions of others. Physical changes in height, weight, and body build cause a change in self-perception and in how the adolescent uses his or her body. To some male adolescents, the last chance to get taller is very significant.

The body is part of one's inner and outer world. Many of the experiences of the inner world are based on stimuli from the external world, especially from the body surface. Therefore the adolescent focuses attention on body surface. He or she spends a great deal of time in front of mirrors and for body hygiene, grooming, and clothing. These are normal ways for the early adolescent to integrate a changing body image. If the teen does not seem to care about appearance, he or she may have already decided, "I'm so ugly, so what's the use?"

Growth and physical changes draw the adolescent's attention to the body part that is changing, and he or she becomes more sensitive to it. This can cause a distorted self-view. He or she may overemphasize a defect and underevaluate self as a person. The body acts as a source of acceptance or rejection by others. If the adolescent does not get much acceptance for self and his or her body, he or she may try to compensate for real or imagined defects through sports, vocational or academic success, a religious commitment, or a date or group of friends that enhances prestige. The adolescent is idealistic and may not be able to achieve an ideal body. Thus he or she may discredit self by seeing the body and self as defective, inferior, or incapable.

If the adolescent does have a disability or defect, peers and adults may react with fear, pity, repulsion, or curiosity. The adolescent may retain and later reflect these impressions since a person tends to perceive self as others perceive him or her. If the adolescent develops a negative self-image, motivation, behavior, and eventual life-style may also be inharmonious and out of step with social expectations.

By late adolescence self-image is complete, self-esteem should be high, and self-concept should have stabilized. The person feels autonomous but no longer believes he or she is so unique that no one has ever experienced what he or she is currently experiencing. The late adolescent no longer believes everyone is watching or being critical of his or her physical or personality characteristics. Egocentricity has declined. Interactions with the opposite sex are more comfortable, although awareness of gender is keen.

Your understanding of the importance of the value the adolescent places on self can help you work with the adolescent, parents, teachers, and community leaders. Your goal is to avoid building a false self-image in the adolescent; rather, help him or her evaluate strengths and weaknesses, accept the weaknesses, and build on the strengths. You will have to listen carefully to the adolescent's statements about self. You will have to sense when you might effectively speak and work with him or her and when silence is best. Share an understanding of influencing factors on body-image and self-concept development with parents, teachers, and other adults so that they can positively influence adolescents.

You may wish to use a therapeutic group such as reality therapy or rational thinking group, using cognitive restructuring exercises to help adolescents think more positively about themselves and reduce anxiety. Small group sessions outside the regular classroom have been found effective in enhancing self-concepts of junior high students. Group sessions can focus on personal and social awareness and how to cope with age-related problems.

Sexuality Development

Sexuality *encompasses not only the individual's physical characteristics and the act of sexual intercourse but also the following:* (1) *search for identity as a whole person,* including a sexual person; (2) *role behavior of men and women;* (3) *attitudes, behaviors, and feelings toward self, each gender, and sexual behavior;* (4) *relationships, affection, and caring between people;* (5) *the need to touch and be touched;* and (6) *recognition and acceptance of self and others as sexual beings* (197). One of the greatest concerns to the adolescent is sexual feelings and activities. Because of hormonal and physiologic changes and environmental stimuli, the adolescent is almost constantly preoccupied with feelings of developing sexuality.

Sexual desire is under the domination of the cerebral cortex. Differences in sexual desire exist in young males and females, and desire is influenced by cultural and family expectations for sexual performance. The female experiences a more generalized pleasurable response to erotic stimulation but does not necessarily desire coitus. The male experiences a stronger desire for coitus because of a localized genital sensation in response to erotic stimulation, which is accompanied by production of spermatozoa and secretions from accessory glands that build up pressure and excite the ejaculatory response. The male is stimulated to seek relief by ejaculation (116, 134).

Menarche is experienced by the girl as an affectively charged event related to her emerging identity as an adult woman with reproductive ability. Menarche may be perceived as frightening and shameful by some girls; previous factual sex education does not necessarily offset such feelings. Often information in classes is not assimilated because of high anxiety in the girl during the class. The girl is likely to turn to her mother for instruction at the time of menarche, even if the two of them are not close emotionally.

Family and cultural traditions are needed to mark the menarche as a transition from childhood to adulthood. Menarche is anticipated as an important event, but in the United States no formal customs mark it, and no obvious change in the girl's social status occurs. The girl may get little help from her mother, other female adults, or peers in working through feelings related to menarche. Often menses is perceived as an excretory function, and advertisements treat it as a disease.

Nocturnal emissions are often a great concern for the boys.

Both sexes are concerned about development and appearance of secondary sex characteristics, their overall appearance, their awkwardness, and their sex appeal, or lack of it, to the opposite sex (16, 77, 116, 134).

The most common form of sexual outlet for both sexes, but especially males, is **masturbation,** *manipulation of the genitals for sexual stimulation*. Public education about the normality of masturbation is reducing guilt about the practice and fears of mental illness (116).

Intercourse is an increasing sexual activity among adolescents. Premarital sexual activity is often used as a means to get close, sometimes with strangers, and may result in feelings of guilt, remorse, anxiety, and self-recrimination. The feelings associated with the superficial act may be damaging to the adolescent's self-concept and possibly to later success in a marital relationship. Adolescent males and females often report that the initial coitus was not pleasurable. In spite of overt sophistication and widespread availability of information on birth control devices, pregnancy or fear of pregnancy is the deciding factor in close to half of all high school marriages. The number of pregnant teenage females who are not marrying is significantly increasing, which has implications for the future care and well-being of the baby and implications for future intimate relations of the teenage girl. If teenagers do marry, the marriage is considerably more likely to end in separation and divorce than is true for the general population, which also has a high divorce rate, because of the unstable sense of self (77, 116).

You can teach parents and adolescents of both sexes that they and other people are not like disposable plastic cartons and that an intimate and important experience is cheapened and coarsened when it is removed from love. Some youths argue that sex can be pleasurable if one hardly knows or even loathes one's partner, but most youths are likely to get emotionally involved in the sexual act, and their feelings will be bruised when the act leads nowhere. A wide variety of sexual experience before marriage may cause the person to feel bored with a single partner later (16, 116).

Americans have to relearn the satisfaction of self-denial and anticipation. The adolescent will not be harmed by knowing about the body and sexuality and yet not engaging in intercourse. A certain amount of tension can be endured; in fact, it can be useful to become

mature and creative. The values of self-discipline and self-denial with anticipation must be taught before adolescence begins, however (16, 116). Such teaching comes from how parents live more so than from sex education courses and is the most critical teaching. In fact, sex education should be directed toward the parents as much as toward their offspring, for what they teach—or do not teach—is the main factor in their child's eventual behavior (201).

Other countries are also having their problems with teenage sexuality. In Kenya, East Africa, adolescent sexual development has for years been controlled by tribal customs. Recently, however, Western permissiveness has crept in, especially among the teenagers in the larger cities. Pregnancy among girls from 14 to 18, with a rash of self-induced abortions, has caused leaders to insist on some sex education for their youth. Small pilot programs, sponsored jointly by government and church groups in connection with African educators, are making some impact at the secondary education level (230).

Adaptive Mechanisms

The **ego** is the *sum total of those mental processes that maintain psychic cohesion and reality contact; it is the mediator between the inner impulses and outer world*. It is that part of the personality that becomes integrated and strengthened in adolescence and has the following functions (116):

1. Associating concepts or situations that belong together but are historically remote or spatially separated
2. Developing a realization that one's way of master-

 Research Abstract

Mischel, W., Y. Shoda, and M. Rodriquez, Delay of Gratification in Children, Science, 244 (1989), 933-938.

The ability to learn present self-control for the sake of a future reward is essential for many areas of life.

The purpose of this study was to examine differences among children in the ability to delay gratification and the effects of these differences on early adolescents. A longitudinal study was done in which 4-year-olds were tested for the ability to take their mind off a tempting treat and develop strategies to delay eating the treat. These same individuals were tested 10 years later, and their parents were interviewed about personality and behavioral characteristics of the 14-year-olds. Results indicated that preschool children who had been able to wait longer for the treat were seen by their parents as higher in self-esteem, more competent, and better able to resist temptation and cope with frustration and stress. Their Scholastic Aptitude Test scores were higher. They had more friends, expressed ideas more clearly, were more attentive, used and responded to reason, and were better able to plan than the adolescents who as preschoolers could not wait as long for the treat.

Preschoolers who had resisted the treat the longest period of time had developed a variety of strategies to distract

themselves from thinking about the treat: (1) putting hands over eyes, (2) talking and singing to self, (3) flapping hands and feet, and (4) sleeping. The more the preschooler thought about the treat, the less able he or she was to resist it. When children did think about the treat those who thought of it in abstract terms (e.g., thinking of marshmallows as fluffy clouds) or who mentally framed the treat like a picture were able to resist the treat the longest. When the known treat was completely out of sight, the child had more difficulty with waiting than if it were in view but covered.

Additional studies with third and sixth grade children and with children who have behavioral problems confirmed the result that children who are most successful in delaying gratification develop distracting strategies in new situations. As children mature, they become more knowledgeable about the ability to delay gratification. Third grade children can delay better if a treat is covered and if they think about what they have to do to wait. Sixth grade children find that focusing on abstract qualities of the treat is the best strategy to help them resist the treat.

ing experience is a variant of the group's way and is acceptable
3. Subsuming contradictory values and attitudes
4. Maintaining a sense of unity and centrality of self
5. Testing perceptions and selecting memories
6. Reasoning, judging, and planning
7. Mediating among impulses, wishes, and actions and integrating feelings
8. Choosing meaningful stimuli and useful conditions
9. Maintaining reality

When a strong ego exists, the person can do all these tasks. He or she has entered adulthood psychologically. Adolescence provides the experiences necessary for such maturity.

Ego changes occur in the adolescent because of broadening social involvement, deepening intellectual pursuits, close peer activity, rapid physical growth, and social role changes, all of which cause frustrations at times. **Frustration** is the *feeling of helplessness and anxiety that results when one is prevented from getting what one wants.* Adaptive mechanisms leading to resolution of frustration and reconciling personal impulses with social expectations are beneficial because they permit the self to settle dissonant drives and to cope with strong feelings. All adaptive mechanisms permit one to develop a self, an identity, and to defend the self-image against attack. These mechanisms are harmful only when one pattern is used to the exclusion of others for handling many diverse situations or when several mechanisms are used persistently to cope with a single situation. Such behavior is defensive rather than adaptive, distorts reality, and indicates emotional disturbance.

The adaptive mechanisms used in adolescence are the same ones used (and defined) in previous developmental eras, although they now may be used in a different way.

Compensation, a form of compromise, *sublimation,* and *identification* are particularly useful because they often improve interaction with others. They are woven into the personality to make permanent character changes, and they help the person reach appropriate goals.

Teach parents that adaptive abilities of the adolescent are strongly influenced by inner resources built up through the years of parental love, esteem, and guidance. The parents' use of adaptive mechanisms and general mental health will influence the offspring. Are the parents living a double standard? Has the teenager seen the parents enjoy a job well done or is financial reward the key issue? Do the parents covertly wish the teenager to act out what they could never do?

Even with mature parents, the adolescent will at times find personal adaptive abilities taxed. But the chances for channeling action-oriented energy and idealism through acceptable adaptive behavior are much greater if parents set a positive example.

Other factors influence ability to adapt to stress and the adaptive mechanisms that will be used. Adolescents from upper and middle socioeconomic levels report that the life events that were most stressful to them agreed with what adults consider the most stressful life change (125). Upper-class adolescents included "quitting school" and "parent losing a job" as more stressful than individuals of other ages and socioeconomic levels; and the importance of education and occupation are related to socioeconomic level. Middle-class adolescents viewed drug and alcohol abuse and hassling with parents as more stressful, which is reflective of middle-class moral values. Middle-class adolescents revealed more reliance on physical appearance than upper-class teenagers; the advantages of family status and more money for clothing and entertaining may make the upper-class adolescent less dependent on appearance for social acceptance. Items written in as stressful life events for both classes were "wrecking the car," "not getting selected for an activity," "brother getting someone pregnant," and "sister getting pregnant." Age in this sample was not a significant variable in scaling the events, but the number of events experienced increased with age. Girls perceive more events as more stressful than boys (125).

Moral-Spiritual Development

Refer to Kohlberg's Theory of Moral Development presented in Table 5–4. According to Kohlberg (111), the adolescent probably is in the Conventional Level most of the time. However, the adolescent may at times show behavior appropriate to the second stage of the Preconventional Level or the first stage of the Post-Conventional Level. Munhall (137) found that the average normal reasoning for baccalaureate nursing students was at the Conventional Level.

The early adolescent typically is in the conformist stage; structure and order of society take on meaning for the person, and rules are followed because they exist (analogous to Kohlberg's Conventional Level). The late adolescent is in the conscientious stage, in which the person develops a set of principles for self that is used to guide personal ideals, actions, and achievements. Rational thought becomes important to personal growth (analogous to Kohlberg's Post-Conventional Level, stage one) (134, 161). The young adolescent must examine parental moral and religious verbal standards against practice and decide if they are worth incorporating into his or her own life. He or she may appear to discard standards of behavior previously accepted, although basic parental standards likely will be maintained. In addition, he or she must compare the religious versus the scientific views. Although moral-spiritual views of sensitivity, caring, and commitment may be prevalent in family teaching, the adolescent in the United States is also a part of the scientific, technological, industrial society that emphasizes achievement, fragmentation, and regimentation. Often youth will identify with one of the two philosophies (64). These two views can be satisfactorily combined but only with sufficient time and experience, which the adolescent has not had (16, 116, 134).

If the adolescent matures in religious belief, he or she must comprehend abstractions. Often when he or she is capable of the first religious insights, the negativism tied with rebellion to authority prevents this experience.

Probably by age 16 the youth will make a decision. He or she will accept or reject the family religion. If the parents represent two faiths, the teen may choose one or the other or neither. He or she may be influenced by a friend or someone who is admired. He or she may have a religious awakening experience in the form of a definite crisis called, by some, **conversion,** or **getting saved.** *This connotes an emotional and mental decision to conform to some religious pattern.* The form may be a definite but not dramatic decision at a confirmation or first communion. Another form is the gradual awakening, one which is not completely accomplished in adolescence.

Help parents and adolescents realize that the adolescent who does find strength in the supernatural, who can rely on a power greater than self, can find much consolation in this turbulent period of awkward physical and emotional growth. If he or she can pray for help, ask forgiveness, and believe he or she receives both, a more positive self-image develops. In this period of clique and group dominance, the church is a place to meet friends, to share recreation and fellowship, and to sense a belonging difficult to find in some large high schools.

Adolescents whose faith is mixed with some God fearing are probably less likely to experiment in behavior they have been taught will bring them harm. Adolescents who have been taught that they are part of a divine plan and who have been given a specific moral code may better answer the essential questions, "Who am I?" "Where am I going?" "What meaning is there in life?" However, adolescents who have been raised very strictly may instead develop a reaction formation pattern of adjustment—rebelling and pursuing the previously forbidden activities.

The following methods of moral development have been most widely used: setting an example, persuading, limiting choices, dramatizing, establishing rules and regulations, teaching religious or cultural dogma, and appealing to conscience. Advice, approval, commands, lessons, sermons, warnings, criticisms, and interrogation have produced few results in the field of ethical development. Recent experiments show that a Socratic approach, which promotes moral development and clarifies values, produces fruitful results that have not been achieved by simply handing down rules of conduct. You can be instrumental in working with parents and teachers to use the Socratic approach and other value clarification exercises (111).

Late Adolescence: Transition Period to Young Adulthood

In some cultures parents select schooling, occupations, and the marriage partner for their offspring. In the United States the youth is usually free to make some or all of these decisions.

By the time the youth is a junior or senior in high school, he or she should be thinking about the future: whether to pursue a mechanical or academic job; to attend some form of higher education; to live at home or elsewhere; to travel; to marry soon, later, or not at all; to have children soon, later, or not at all. Answers to these questions will influence the adolescent's transition into young adulthood.

Those who seem not to be making the transition into young adulthood—who continue to rebel against society, who wander from job to job or from college to college, who rely heavily on drugs and alcohol or sexual exploitation for emotional "highs," who cannot seem to make decisions about the future— may be the children of affluent parents and may not have had to become independent. The parents continue to dole out money and demands. The money is taken; the demands are ignored.

Establishing a Separate Residence

This step is one marker of reaching young adulthood. The late adolescent often spends less time at home and prepares for separation from parents. If there is intense intrafamily conflict, if the adolescent feels unwanted, or if the adolescent is still struggling with dependence on parents or identity diffusion, a different mode of separation may occur.

In an effort to find self and think about the future or to escape abuse, incest, or other home problems, the adolescent may become either a walkaway or a runaway. The **teen walkaway** *leaves home before finishing high school or before reaching legal age; however, parents generally know where the child is and are resigned to the child's new living arrangements.* The **teen runaway** *leaves home without overt notice and his or her whereabouts are unknown to parents, friends, or police.* Some walkaways may continue high school or get some type of job while living with relatives, friends, or a boyfriend or girlfriend. The problem with the walkaway is that the adolescent can achieve developmental tasks better in a stable family situation in which parents continue to give support and assist him or her as necessary while treating the offspring in an adult manner. If the newly found living situation is unstable or emotionally unsupportive or if the adolescent has no means of financial support, he or she may be forced into prostitution or juvenile offenses (21, 116).

You may have an opportunity to discuss residence

situations with the adolescent. If you can get to the person before he or she walks or runs away, help him or her consider the intolerability of parental demands and the family situation. Discuss alternative ways of handling the problem. You may contact a high school counselor or potential employer. Although either the walkaway or runaway situation should be avoided if possible, the teen should be encouraged to report incest or abuse so that the teen's parents and other siblings can receive proper therapy and an appropriate, healthy living situation can be found for the teen.

Health care is a problem for adolescent runaways. Refer to the article by Manov and Lowther (121), which describes general health problems and sex-related health concerns such as pregnancy, sexually transmitted diseases, prostitution, alcohol abuse, and child abuse and incest. The following intervention strategies are described: (1) clarification of the health care provider's attitudes and values; (2) establishment of trust; (3) use of effective interviewing skills; (4) ability to provide maximum medical treatment and information when the client presents self for care; and (5) establishment of foundations for future interactions and care (121).

Career Selection

This selection has often been haphazard. High school counselors often do more record keeping than realistic guiding toward career choices. Often youth are influenced by parental wishes or friend's choices. Because of changes in societal role expectations for men and women, jobs or college study programs that were once considered exclusively "male" or "female" are now open to both. A woman may now comfortably major in mathematics, architecture, or medicine. A man may study home economics or nursing. A woman may be a lineman for the telephone company, and a man may be an operator.

Although these changes are positive, understand that the selection is more vast and thus more confusing to adolescents. You can guide them to testing centers in which their skills and interests are measured and jobs are recommended. You may direct them to members of various professions who can tell them about their jobs. You also must be aware of the national adolescent mood. Group biases and fads should not dictate career choices that do not coincide with the person's skills.

Occupation represents much more than a set of skills and functions; it is a way of life. Occupation provides and determines much of the physical and social environment in which a person lives, his or her status within the community, and a pattern for living. Occupational choice is usually a function or a reflection of the entire personality, but the occupation, in turn, plays a part in shaping the personality by providing associates, roles, goals, ideals, mores, life-style, and perhaps even a spouse.

For many youth the college years are a time to consider various careers, to decide what type of people he or she wishes to associate with and imitate, and to measure self against others with similar aspirations.

Although college attendance and pursuit of a profession are still the ideal of many, growing emphasis and opportunity exist for vocational and technical training. Many will enter jobs right out of high school.

You can be a key person in helping adolescents clarify values and attitudes related to occupational selection and in talking with parents about their concerns.

Moral-Spiritual Development

This development may take on a special significance if the adolescent period is extended into the twenties because of college education or military duty. Instead of settling into the tasks coexistent with marriage, job, and family, the adolescent has a period in which a great deal of thinking can be accomplished. He or she has passed the physically awkward stage so that time and energy formerly spent in making the transition into physical adulthood can be turned toward philosophy.

The mid-twenties apparently is the least religious period in life. College youth and late adolescents often reject affiliation with their childhood church. Perhaps it is part of their break from dependence to independence. They also are secure in pursuing their ambitions; they are not yet aware that their goals may not be met. They do not yet have children whom they want to educate to a religion; and they have not developed a perspective about the importance of their own upbringing. Yet these late adolescents are often altruistic: they wish to help others, defend a cause, and do not hesitate to devote many hours of the day to their goals.

Veterans, especially combat returnees or prisoners of war, are in a difficult position. The protective childhood religion of fantasy, left in some, is forcibly removed as they experience violence, torture, hatred—the worst of human nature. If they salvage a religious experience, it is one of maturity.

Explore moral-spiritual development with adolescents and parents. Your own behavior may be the best teacher.

Developmental Tasks

The following developmental tasks should be met by the end of adolescence (54, 86):

1. Accepting the changing body size, shape, and function and understanding the meaning of physical maturity
2. Learning to handle the body in a variety of physical skills and to maintain good health
3. Achieving a satisfying and socially accepted feminine or masculine role, recognizing how these roles have similarities and distinctions
4. Finding the self as a member of one or more peer

groups and developing skills in relating to a variety of people, including those of the opposite sex

5. Achieving independence from parents and other adults while maintaining an affectionate relationship with them
6. Selecting an occupation in line with interests and abilities (although the choice of occupation may later change) and preparing for economic independence
7. Preparing to settle down, frequently for marriage and family life or for a close relationship with another, by developing a responsible attitude, acquiring needed knowledge, making appropriate decisions, and forming a relationship based on love rather than infatuation
8. Developing the intellectual and work skills and social sensitivities of a competent citizen
9. Desiring and achieving socially responsible behavior in the cultural setting
10. Developing a workable philosophy, a mature set of values, and worthy ideals and assuming standards of morality

Until these tasks are accomplished, the person remains immature, an adolescent regardless of chronologic age. How you interact with, or teach other adults to interact with, the adolescent will contribute to the adolescent's maturity.

Common Health Problems and Nursing Applications

Scope of the Nursing Role

Your role in caring for the adolescent may be many faceted. Astute assessment is needed; knowledge from this chapter and communication principles described in Chapter 17 may be useful in gaining information from a client or family who may be hesitant to disclose about self. *Nursing diagnoses* that may be applicable to the adolescent are listed in Box 11–6. Interventions that may involve direct care to the ill adolescent or involves various health promotion measures are described in the previous or following sections.

■ **BOX 11-6.**
Selected Nursing Diagnoses Related to the Adolescent[a]

Pattern 1: Exchanging

Altered Nutrition: More than body requirements
Altered Nutrition: Less than body requirements
Altered Nutrition: Potential for more than body requirements
Potential for Infection
Potential for Injury
Potential for Trauma
Potential Impaired Skin Integrity

Pattern 2: Communicating

Impaired Verbal Communication

Pattern 3: Relating

Impaired Social Interaction
Social Isolation
Altered Sexuality Patterns

Pattern 4: Valuing

Spiritual Distress

Pattern 5: Choosing

Ineffective Individual Coping
Impaired Adjustment
Defensive Coping
Ineffective Denial
Decisional Conflict
Health Seeking Behaviors

Pattern 6: Moving

Fatigue
Potential Activity Intolerance
Sleep Pattern Disturbance
Diversional Activity
Altered Health Maintenance
Altered Growth and Development

Pattern 7: Perceiving

Body Image Disturbance
Self-esteem Disturbance
Chronic Low Self-esteem
Situational Low Self-esteem
Personal Identity Disturbance
Sensory/Perceptual Alterations
Hopelessness
Powerlessness

Pattern 8: Knowing

Knowledge Deficit

Pattern 9: Feeling

Pain
Dysfunctional Grieving
Anticipatory Grieving
Posttrauma Response
Anxiety
Fear

[a]Other NANDA diagnoses are applicable to the ill adolescent.
From North American Nursing Diagnosis Association, *NANDA Nursing Diagnosis Taxonomy I* (Rev.). St. Louis: North American Nursing Diagnosis Association, 1990.

A mature or maturing body and an immature emotional state make the adolescent a source of misunderstanding, fear, and laughter. Mood swings, rebellious behavior, and adherence to colorful fads baffle many adults, who then cannot look beyond the superficial behavior to identify health needs. Yet health care needs of today's adolescents are great.

Millions of teenagers in the United States between the ages of 13 and 19 years are sexually active. Many adolescent girls from 13 to 19 years of age become pregnant each year. A number of adolescents will run away from home. A significant number of youths will die from motor vehicle and other accidents and from homicide and suicide (229). Other health problems abound, including sexually transmitted diseases, substance abuse, chronic illness, and obesity and nutritional deficiency (3) (the latter two previously discussed). Although the scope of this book does not allow discussion of needs assessment and intervention for adolescents with physical disabilities, you may wish to consult several references for information. Hedahl (88) describes how a college health program can assist the adolescent with physical disabilities.

Health Promotion and Health Protection

Immunizations

Immunizations are a part of health protection to the adolescent, although they may be overlooked by that time of life. You should take a careful health history. If the immunizations discussed in relation to other age groups have not been received, they should be given as indicated. If the adolescent has been routinely immunized, combined tetanus and diphtheria toxoids (adult-type Td) should be given near 14 to 16 years of age and every 10 years thereafter. This preparation contains less diphtheria antigen than the DTP preparations given to children (69, 207).

The oral form of polio virus (OPV) is recommended for all children younger than 18 years of age unless contraindicated. Influenza virus vaccine, pneumococcal polysaccharide vaccine, and hepatitis B vaccine should be given to adolescents in selected high-risk groups. For clean wounds, no tetanus booster is needed by a fully immunized person unless more than 10 years have elapsed since the last dose. For dirty or contaminated wounds, a booster dose can be given if more than 5 years have elapsed since the last dose. Pertussis vaccine should not be given to anyone over 6 years of age. Periodic testing for tuberculosis should be included in all adolescent immunization programs (6–8, 69, 220).

Your actions and teaching in relation to immunizations are important for the teenager's health now and in the adult years.

Safety Promotion and Accident Prevention

Accidents, homicide, and suicide are responsible for approximately 75% of all deaths between the ages of 15 and 24. Motor vehicle accidents account for nearly half of the deaths of adolescents between the ages of 16 and 19 and are more common among young drivers who use alcohol, marijuana, and other drugs while driving (29, 156, 208, 220). One of the biggest adolescent-parent hurdles comes with learning to drive. The adolescent needs to learn this skill; yet the arguments between parents and their children concerning how to drive, what vehicle to drive, and where to go or not to go often keep parents in a state of anxiety and children in a state of rebellion.

Head and spinal cord injuries, skeletal injuries, abrasions, and burns may all result from an accident involving a car, motorcycle, motor scooter, moped, all-terrain vehicle, snowmobile, or minibike. Sports-related accidents such as drowning, football, hockey, gymnastic and soccer injuries, and firearm mishaps are also common. Contusions, dislocations, sprains, strains, overuse syndromes, and stress fractures occur frequently (75). In the adolescent the epiphyses of the skeletal system have not yet closed, and the extremities are poorly protected by stabilizing musculature. These two physical factors, combined with poor coordination and imperfect sport skills, probably account for the numerous injuries (220, 225).

Homicide is the second leading cause of death in the 15- to 24-year-old group and is the leading cause of death among non-Caucasian youths in this age group. Handguns are the most frequently used weapons (5). The media report that every 36 minutes a youth is injured or killed by a gun.

Suicide, the third leading cause of death, is discussed on pp. 398 to 400.

Safety Education

Safety courses, including driver education, knowledge of safety programs in the community, instruction in water safety, routine safety practices, and emergency care measures, should be required for every adolescent. Many accidents and deaths could be avoided if the adolescent were better equipped to handle the new freedom. As an informed citizen in the community or in relation to your job, you can initiate and teach in such programs with the school, church, clinic, industry, Red Cross, or other civic organizations. If you do not teach, you can insist on qualified and objective instruction. Parents and youths should be informed about the dangers and the exercise and prestige value involved with certain sports and privileges. A teenage safety checklist can be obtained from the National Society for Crippled Children and Adults, 2023 W. Ogden Ave., Chicago, IL, 60612, to help the adolescent be aware of how to improve safety behavior.

Because of the sports activities in which adolescents are involved, they may sometimes experience musculoskeletal chest pain, minor strains or sprains to a joint, and minor ankle strain. You should know how to advise for these conditions.

Musculoskeletal chest pain *arises from the bony*

structures of the rib cage and upper-limb girdle, along with the related skeletal muscles. Age does not automatically rule out heart-related problems. Although musculoskeletal pain is usually aggravated by activity that involves movement or pressure on the chest cage rather than by general exertion (such as stair climbing), a thorough lung and cardiac examination is merited. Putting heat to the area (unless it is a fresh injury), resting the area, and taking an antipyretic can be recommended (94).

Minor strains and sprains to a joint involve a *mild trauma that results in minimal stretching of involved ligaments and contusion of the surrounding tissues.* The treatment is immobilization of the affected joint and use of an ice pack for 24 to 36 hours. Local heat can then be used if needed. Aspirin, if tolerated, can be used for its analgesic and anti-inflammatory effects (94).

A **minor ankle sprain** involving *stretching of the ligament without tearing* can be treated the same as minor strains and sprains with the addition of an Ace bandage and possibly keeping weight off the ankle longer than 24 to 36 hours through the use of crutches (94).

Common Health Problems: Prevention and Treatment

As you care for the adolescent, refer to Appendices III and IV for a schedule of health screening measures. Several references describe how to conduct physical assessments with the adolescent (14, 69, 94, 120, 182).

In addition to the hazards of accidents, health problems other than obesity and teenage pregnancy, already discussed, are also apparent among adolescents. These conditions are styes (hordeolum), nosebleed (epistaxis), acne vulgaris, dental caries and gingivitis, athlete's foot (tinea pedis), infectious mononucleosis, hepatitis, Rocky Mountain spotted fever, and Lyme disease. Table 11–2 summarizes definition, symptoms and signs, and prevention and treatment for these conditions (69, 94, 120, 182).

Neoplasms, both benign and malignant, are the fourth leading cause of death (220). Females exposed to diethylstilbestrol (DES) in utero should be watched closely for adenocarcinoma of the vagina. Males exposed to DES in utero have an increase in urinary tract abnormalities and a higher incidence of infertility (220). Dysplasia of the cervix, a precursor of cervical carcinoma, is a sexually transmitted disease that is occurring with increased frequency in adolescent females. Sexually active females should receive annual Pap smears (188). Testicular cancer, Hodgkin's disease, and certain bone cancers are not uncommon in this age group.

Cardiovascular disease is the fifth leading cause of death. Although essential hypertension is consistently higher in African-American adults than in Caucasian adults, the same does not hold true for adolescents. According to one study, blood pressure levels in Caucasian youths equaled or exceeded that of African-American youths (202).

Allergic dermatitis, cysts, and keloid formation of the earlobes are also seen with more frequency since ear piercing has become popular. Inner ear damage from exposure to rock music is increasing and can be assessed by pure tone audiometry. The adolescent is also subject to postural defects, fatigue, anemia, and respiratory problems. Discuss prevention of these problems with adolescents.

Suicide

Suicide now ranks as the third most frequent cause of death in adolescence (9, 19, 76, 78, 85, 87, 93, 208, 220, 229). The media report that teen suicides have doubled since 1970. Suicide in adolescents is frequently reported as an accidental death. Motor vehicle accidents, drug and alcohol overdose, firearm accidents, and even homicides can be disguised suicides (19, 85). Psychologic, social, and physiologic stressors are the apparent causes for the rising number of suicides. Television dramatizations on the nightly news or in movies of teenage suicides appear to contribute to an increased wave of teenage suicide attempts and successes (70, 194).

Adolescents who attempt suicide often come from families who have nonproductive communication patterns, inconsistent positive reinforcement behaviors, and a high level of conflict or child abuse. Suicides occur in rich and poor, urban and rural families. Adolescent suicides occur most frequently in 15- to 25-year-old Caucasian males; African- American male incidence is lower. Females are now using forms of suicide usually associated with males and account for 40% of all successful suicides (44, 194). The males, however, are more successful, more violent, and less likely to give warning before the suicidal act (44).

Frequently physical fatigue contributes to emotional stress that precipitates a suicide attempt (44, 194). Most adolescents have short bouts with suicidal preoccupations in the presence of these stresses. Sometimes even a small disappointment or frustration can lead to an impulsive suicidal attempt. Often the impulsive acts are committed to force parents to pay attention to the adolescent's pleas for help and get needs met. Because the adolescent often feels great ambivalence toward parents, he or she rejects parents and yet solicits love, sometimes by attempting suicide. In reality the parents may be giving all the love they can. In other situations the adolescent may be experiencing (1) an intense sense of loss, external or internal, real or imagined, that is believed permanent or (2) anger at parents, teachers, or another significant person, and hurting self is a way to get even and make the other sorry for not treating the person right. Death is not seen as irreversible. If there is a history of family suicide, the adolescent may attempt

TABLE 11-2. COMMON HEALTH PROBLEMS OF ADOLESCENTS

Problem	Definition	Symptoms/Signs	Prevention/Treatment
Hordeolum (stye)	Localized infection of sebaceous gland on eyelid margin	Painful, reddened swelling on eyelid; sometimes drainage.	Apply hot compresses. Administer antibiotic drops.
Epistaxis (nose bleed)	Spontaneous bleeding from nose caused by ruptured blood vessel	Bleeding from nose	Prevent dry and cracking nasal mucosa by keeping humidity level sufficient. If nose bleeds, sit with head slightly forward and pinch nostrils for at least 15 min. Use cold compresses.
Acne vulgaris	Comedones, pimples, and cysts formed from increased activity of sebaceous glands	"Blackheads," "whiteheads," and additional lesions, especially on face, chest, back	Use good hygiene techniques and cleansing agents. Apply topical preparations. Administer oral medications.
Dental caries and gingivitis	Decay of teeth and disease of gums	Broken, dark teeth; bleeding inflamed gums	Use good dental hygiene. Check periodically with a dental hygienist for education and treatment.
Tinea pedis (athlete's foot)	Fungal infection affecting feet, especially toe webs	Intense itching; cracking; peeling	Soak feet and dry well. Apply antifungal agent. Wear clean cotton socks.
Infectious mononucleosis (mono)	Condition caused by Epstein-Barr virus	Fever, sore throat, enlarged lymph nodes; general malaise; enlarged spleen; sometimes jaundice	Treat symptoms: use rest, increased fluid intake, antipyretic, good nutrition.
Hepatitis A	Inflammation of hepatocytes of liver caused by viruses, bacteria, drugs, chemicals; transmitted via fecal contamination of food or water with subsequent close person-to-person contact (25% of hepatitis cases)	Fatigue, anorexia, swollen glands; aversion to smoking (if smokes); short incubation period: 15–45 days	Prevention: stay in good physical condition. If condition develops, prevent transfer. Treat symptoms.
Hepatitis B	Transmitted via blood, primarily parentally, although person-to-person contact possible (50% of hepatitis cases)	Prodromal stage: 2 to 20 days; jaundice phase: 2 to 8 wk; recovery phase: 2–24 wk	Vaccine is available; take recommended precautions. Treat symptoms. Avoid complications.
Hepatitis C (non A, non B) and other types	Diagnosed by deduction (25% of hepatitis cases)	Hepatitis symptoms; history of transfusion; no serologic evidence	Treat symptoms.
Rocky Mountain spotted fever	Acute febrile disease caused by *Rickettsia rickettsii*; passed to human by bite of infected tick	Symptoms start in 2 days to 2 wk: headache, fever, rash on hands and feet, pain in back and leg muscles	Prevention: be aware of problem and appropriate removal of ticks. Treatment: administer tetracycline.
Lyme disease	Tick-borne disease introduced by the spirochete *Borrelia burgdorferi* from animal host to human (ticks are only 1–2 mm in size)	Early (3 or 4 days after bite): ring-like rash at bite site (approximately 4 inches in diameter) then secondary lesion, flulike symptoms, sometimes cardiac problems (10%); in 4 wk neurologic problems (in 15%); in 6 wk to 1 yr, arthralgias and synovitis (in 50%)	Administer antibiotic (doxycycline). Provide rest and healthy diet. Treat symptoms. Prevent through education.

reunion with the deceased, often on the anniversary of the suicide. Other reasons for suicide are discussed in references at the end of the chapter (29, 34, 44, 78, 85, 87, 115, 126, 159, 185, 192, 229).

Signs of suicide are often subtle to detect, but a composite of behaviors should be a clue that the teen is experiencing severe stress. Box 11–7 lists behaviors as-

sociated with or indicators of suicide attempts (85, 159, 194, 229). Do not be afraid to ask if the youth has thought of suicide. The stressed person welcomes this query and the fact that you are taking the statements and behavior seriously.

The suicidal adolescent may be a loner at school and feel unable to meet scholastic expectations of par-

---

■ BOX 11-7.
Some Signs That Indicate Risk
for Suicide Attempt

- Radical personality changes such as persistent sadness, loss of interest in usual activities, feelings of guilt, worthlessness, helplessness, failure
- Withdrawal from family, friends, school, and regular activities
- Experiencing major disappointment, loss, or humiliation
- Falling grades or a decline in the quality of schoolwork; inability to compete
- Noticeable changes in eating or sleeping habits or energy level; neglect of personal appearance
- Physical symptoms often related to emotional disturbances such as stomachache, headache, or fatigue
- Difficulty in concentrating
- Verbal hints of despair, death; statements such as, "I won't be a problem for you much longer," and "Nothing matters"
- Puts affairs in order—gives away favorite possessions, throws things out, cleans up his or her room
- Suddenly becomes cheerful after prolonged depression—the final decision has been made, which is in itself a form of relief
- Suicide attempts, even those that are meant to fail

---

ents. School performance often drops; there may be frequent absences. If peers state that a friend is suicidal, investigate their concerns. No threat should be ignored. Depression is found in two thirds of suicidal adolescents; depression may be masked by restlessness, aggression, acting out, excessive smoking, social withdrawal, impulsiveness, mood swings, poor concentration, somatic complaints, loss of energy, and change in daily habits. The adolescent feels bored, apathetic, loses interest in usually pleasurable activities, has a negative self-image, and feels unloved, guilty, hopeless, and frequently, physically fatigued (29, 55, 60, 81, 85, 87, 126, 229).

Rarely does the adolescent plan a suicide because he or she really wants to die. At times, however, when death is desired, the adolescent is engaging in self-destructive behavior as a punishment for guilt over actions or thoughts that he or she has committed or experienced. Ten percent of adolescent who attempt suicide make further attempts within a year (9, 78).

Screen for emotionally distressed adolescents and be available to listen to and ask about their problems. Take a careful history to identify the underlying stresses. Refer to several references for guidelines in assessing family and school indicators, personality traits, and danger signs (29, 56, 81, 85, 87, 126, 169, 229). If you believe you are unable to handle the situation, discuss it with the teen and refer him or her to a guidance counselor, school psychologist, or private or school physician. Frequently the adolescent will turn to an adult with

whom he or she has had a personal relationship or sees as an advocate for youth. This relationship may help the adolescent through the present crisis. As a nurse, you can accept, support, inform, and serve as an advocate for youth, working with parents and adolescents (173, 220, 229).

Follow-up care with the family and adolescent after suicidal gestures is important. Some adolescents who attempt suicide ultimately do commit suicide.

If the adolescent makes a suicide attempt, crisis intervention is essential after the necessary medical and physical care is given. The goals, once life is assured, are to help the person work through feelings that led to and resulted from the suicide attempt, feel hope, identify the problem, see alternative ways of handling it, and mobilize supportive others to continue caring contact with the client. The family also needs your support and help in working through their feelings of anxiety, shame, guilt, and anger. Several references describe effective intervention for the suicidal person and **postvention,** *care of the surviving family, friends, and peers of a successful suicide victim* (138).

Alcoholism and Alcohol Abuse

Alcohol intake among adolescents also has greatly increased in recent years. Statistics vary with the geographic area and researcher. Ten percent to 20% of adolescents are problem drinkers (65, 140, 199, 216). Frequent, heavy drinking patterns often begin in the eighth grade and peak between the ages of 18 and 22 years. Over a million Americans from the ages of 10 to 19 are addicted to liquor (69, 134, 140, 216). Most states restrict the purchase and consumption of alcohol to people over 18 or 21 years of age, but this does little to prevent the underage drinker from acquiring alcohol when desired.

Drinking habits between male and female adolescents differ considerably. Males who occasionally drink tend to drink beer and whiskey, and they drink away from home. Most of the females who occasionally drink prefer drinking wine at home under parental supervision.

Adolescents drink because drinking is a widespread social custom in this country and drinking makes them feel more mature. The adolescent's drinking behavior is closely related to the drinking behavior of the parents and to peer-group pressure (180).

Adolescents who drink regularly generally start drinking at an unusually early age, and they use alcohol specifically for its mind-altering effects to participate in some activity that they would otherwise consider difficult or as a defense against depression, anxiety, fear, and anger. They become tolerant to the drug, and use of sedatives with alcohol is common. By the time they reach late adolescence, they may well be alcoholics (105, 123, 140, 203, 216, 220). (The person is often also abusing illicit drugs.) There are several programs in the

United States for the rehabilitation of youthful alcoholics such as Alateen.

The use of alcohol by adolescents has compounded the problem of motor vehicle injuries in youth. Overindulgence in alcohol impairs the ability of these inexperienced drivers and encourages risk taking while the adolescent is behind the wheel of the vehicle. Alcohol may also be involved in suicide attempts and drug-related deaths.

Medical hazards of alcohol abuse are numerous. All body systems may eventually become involved because of the toxic effects of alcohol, including the following conditions (65, 69, 138, 140, 229):

1. Gastritis (nausea, vomiting, headache, gastric pain; may vomit blood or ropy, thick mucus)
2. Pancreatitis (severe abdominal pain, nausea, vomiting)
3. Hepatitis (fever, jaundice, abdominal edema, ankle and foot edema, tenderness in area of liver)
4. Gastric and duodenal ulcers (vomiting of blood, severe pain, indurated abdomen; obstruction and perforation of stomach or intestine may occur)
5. Impotency (inability to maintain or sustain erection)
6. Neuritis (tingling, burning, itching, numbness, weakness, and finally paralysis of limbs if untreated)
7. Fatty liver (enlarged liver on palpation; symptoms of hepatits may persist)
8. Cirrhosis (weight loss, chronic nausea, vomiting, weakness; impotency; abdominal pain; bloated, indurated abdomen; hemorrhage; seventh leading cause of death)
9. Esophageal varices (varicose veins of the esophagus; internal hemorrhage may cause death)
10. Degeneration of cerebellum (permanent loss of motor coordination, unsteady walk, tremors)
11. Esophageal cancer (difficulty swallowing, sense of blockage behind sternum)
12. Delirium tremens (withdrawal from alcohol causes tremors, sweating, nausea, insomnia, confusion, delusions, hallucinations and convulsions; may be fatal 10% of the time)
13. Birth defects (fetal alcohol syndrome; infant is underweight, has small brain and head size, may have cleft palate and congenital heart defect; slow growth in childhood; slower mental development)

Various other health problems, injuries, or death may result from alcohol abuse, including (1) automobile accidents; (2) suicide (over 60% of fatal accidents and suicides involve alcohol); (3) fire deaths (50%); (4) choking on foods (25% of these deaths); (5) freezing to death (20% of these deaths); (6) drowning (20% of these deaths); (7) accidental asphyxiations (20%); and (8) falls (20% of all falls) (5, 69).

Social problems, which may in turn cause physical and emotional health problems (and death) that arise from alcohol abuse include child and spouse abuse and homicide (70% of all violent crimes involve alcohol) (5).

Avoid lecturing to adolescents about the hazards of drinking and driving and the medical effects of drinking. Help the person to clarify values about healthful activities and see the detrimental effects of drinking—physically, emotionally, mentally, and socially. Point out people who have suffered the ill effects of excessive alcohol intake. Teach adolescents how to identify hazards and to act responsibly to avoid injury to themselves and others.

Care of the alcoholic person and family is complex; specific measures vary with the stage of alcoholism and manifestations of the disease. For additional information on the needs of and nursing care for alcoholism, refer to references at the end of the chapter (11, 17, 85, 105, 135, 140, 180, 199, 203, 216, 220, 229).

Conditions Associated With Sexual Activity

Sexual decision making and premarital coitus were controlled in the past by family, social, and religious rules and restrictions. Today sexual activity is almost completely regarded as an individual responsibility. Because of the emotional and social characteristics of adolescents, the individual may have neither the readiness or desire to engage in sexual activity nor the decision-making skills *and* ego strength to behave counter to the peer group and abstain. Educationwise, there is not much to help the adolescent develop the necessary decision-making or value-clarification skills or the emotional strengths to be autonomous from the group or to avoid what is perceived as expected behavior. Add to that the stimulating influence of mass media, and the adolescent may feel caught. Growing up in poor neighborhoods seems to increase teenage pregnancy rates, especially for African-Americans (124).

The areas related to the adolescent's sexual activity that influence health are those involving sexually transmitted diseases and the use of contraceptives, pregnancy, and abortion. A careful history is essential (139).

Sexually Transmitted Diseases. **Sexually transmitted diseases (STD),** are *infections grouped together because they spread by transfer of infectious organisms from person to person during sexual contact.* STD is currently replacing the term *venereal disease* (VD), defined as a *condition of the genital organs usually acquired through sexual intercourse.* The very words *venereal disease* produce responses of fear, shame, guilt, anger, and disgust in most individuals. These feelings may impede a person from seeking medical help or telling who his or her contacts were, even though the person may know rationally that treatment is needed for self and the contacts. The term *sexually transmitted disease* is broader in scope; it covers diseases not included in the traditional definition.

Sexually transmitted diseases are a public health epidemic and a major problem because of high communicability. Reports of new cases represent a percentage of those affected (33, 69, 109, 117, 197). Enormous human suffering, the cost of hundreds of millions of dollars, and the tremendous demands on health care facilities all result. The problem is rooted in ignorance, apathy, and neglect. Women and children bear an inordinate share of the problem—sterility, ectopic pregnancy, fetal and infant deaths, birth defects, and mental retardation. Cancer of the cervix may be linked to the sexually transmitted herpes II virus (26, 27, 109). Some of the specific reasons for the increase in recent years include changing sexual patterns, changing attitudes and cultural mores regarding sexual behavior, lack of understanding about STD, the feeling of "it can't happen to me," breakdown of the family unit, increased mobility within the population, and the widespread use of contraceptives (16, 116, 229). Adolescents have many reasons for wanting to be sexually active, including to (1) enhance self-esteem; (2) have someone care about them; (3) experiment; (4) be accepted by peers; (5) feel grownup; (6) be close and touched by another; (7) feel pleasure or have fun; (8) seek revenge; (9) determine normality; (10) love and be loved; and (11) gain control over another (69, 197, 229).

The four most common sexually transmitted diseases are herpes genitalis, syphilis, gonorrhea, and acquired immuno-deficiency syndrome (AIDS). The increasing incidence of syphilis is not as well known as the increasing incidence of AIDS (69). The disease AIDS is discussed primarily in Chapter 12, although reference is made to AIDS in Chapter 10 and later in this chapter. Table 11–3 compares the causes, common symptoms, prognosis, and treatment to assist you as you assess and care for clients (25–28, 33, 69, 94, 103, 110, 117, 197, 229). Other sexually transmitted diseases are discussed in the following pages to assist you in nursing care.

Other sexually transmitted diseases include vaginitis, chlamydia, genital warts, and pubic lice. Vaginitis can be grouped into four categories—candidal, trichomonal, nonspecific, and chlamydial— that may or may not be related to sexual activity (94).

Candidal vaginitis is an *inflammatory process caused by a common skin fungus, Candida albicans.* This condition may accompany diabetes mellitus or be related to the use of antibiotics, birth control pills, bath oils, lack of moisture-absorbing underpants, or sexual intercourse. The most common sign is a copious, cheesy vaginal discharge, accompanied by an intense vulval inflammation and itching or burning. In addition to the application of cool compresses, a vaginal cream is prescribed and used one or two times daily for 2 to 7 days (94).

Trichomonal vaginitis is an *inflammatory process caused by the common flagellate parasite Trichomonas vaginalis.* The most common sign is frothy, bubbly, greenish-yellow, foul-smelling vaginal discharge with minimal vulval inflammation but some itching. The nonpregnant female is treated with oral medication; if pregnant, she is treated with a vaginal cream (94).

Nonspecific vaginitis is an *inflammation caused by more than one bacteria but especially Haemophilus vaginalis.* The most common sign is a small amount of yellowish-white vaginal discharge that has a "fishy" smell. Itching is usually not intense. Treatment consists of an initial douche followed by vaginal cream applied two times a day for 7 days *or* oral medication. If the oral medication is used, the sexual partner should have identical treatment (94).

Chlamydia trachomatis is a *vaginal infection caused by an intracellular parasite, C. trachomatis, which often causes no symptoms in the woman but is transmitted to sexual partners or the infant at birth.* The woman may have vaginal discharge or pelvic inflammatory disease. Antibiotic treatment (tetracycline, erythromycin) is effective. The infected male may develop urethritis or epididymitis. He may complain of painful urination and frequency. A discharge may be milky and purulent but does not culture out as gonorrhea. This condition is treated with an oral antibiotic. Usually there are no complications. The infected infant may develop conjunctivitis or pneumonia. Chlamydia is the *most common* sexually transmitted disease in the world and the most commonly diagnosed cause of sterility. Babies born to women with the disease have a 60% chance of contracting the disease (103, 117).

Genital warts are *caused by the human papilloma virus and are seen on the foreskin and penis in males (especially in uncircumcised males) and on the perineum and vaginal mucosa in females.* They can appear from 1 to 3 months after contact. Unless a large number of warts are present, they can be treated by repeated topical application of a medication, followed in 3 to 5 hours by a sitz bath. This is repeated at weekly intervals until warts are gone (94).

Phthirus pubis, *pubic lice,* or *"crabs,"* should be treated with gamma benzene hexachloride cream or lotion. The application should be repeated in 7 to 10 days. Sexual contacts should be treated simultaneously, and any family and close contacts should be examined carefully but treated only if infested. Sometimes oral antihistamines are prescribed to relieve intense itching (94).

Contraceptive Practices. **Contraception,** or **birth control,** is the *use of various devices, chemicals, or abortion to prevent or terminate pregnancy.* The adolescent may choose contraception to avoid pregnancy while continuing sexual activity. Contraceptive practices are summarized in Table 11–4 and additional information may be obtained from various references at the end of this chapter (43, 46, 69, 82, 84, 94, 133, 162, 170, 219, 220). Although contraceptives may prevent pregnancy (and sexually transmitted diseases when the contraceptive device is the condom), they have unwanted side effects or disadvantages. *The only way to avoid both pregnancy and the unwanted side effects is sexual abstinence.* Your approach and the structure of the health care environment are critical to the teenage female ad-

TABLE 11-3. COMPARISON OF GONORRHEA, SYPHILIS, AND HERPES GENITALIS

	Gonorrhea	Syphilis	Herpes Genitalis (Herpes 2) (HSV-2 Infection)
Cause	*Neisseria gonorrhoea*	Treponema pallidum	Herpes simplex virus, type 2
Incubation period	3 to 9 days	10 to 90 days; average 3 wk	Several days to 3 wk
Symptoms	Male: asymptomatic at times, including when organism lodged rectally; urethritis—thin, watery, white urethral discharge, becoming purulent; dysuria Female: asymptomatic in 60% to 90% of cases, including when organism lodged rectally; dysuria and vaginal discharge common symptoms; trichomoniasis vaginalis present in 50% of cases Both sexes: gonococcemia, systemic gonorrhea, with skin lesions, malaise, fever, tachycardia	Male and female Stage one (primary): chancre—solitary, indurated, painless, ulceration on genitalia 10 to 28 days after sexual contact; lesion occasionally on mouth, nipples, anus; lesion healing within 4 to 6 wk; treponemes multiplying rapidly Stage two (secondary): rash covering skin, mouth, and genitalia (red-copper color on white skin, gray-blue on black skin; red rash on palms and soles); hair loss; eyes and ears inflamed; lymphadenitis, low-grade fever; sore throat; pain from bone involvement; albuminuria; liver and spleen enlarged, jaundice, nausea; blood test positive after 5 wk Stage three (latent): symptoms gone in 2 to 6 wk; symptoms possibly absent from a few months to a lifetime; blood test positive; person is noninfectious, but possible for syphilitic pregnant woman to give birth to congenitally syphilitic child Stage four (tertiary): complications after 3 to 30 yr in 30% of untreated cases; symptoms affecting heart, blood vessels, brain, spinal cord, eyes, skin, and bones; blood test positive NOTE: Symptoms from all stages may be present at once.	Male and female: Beginning infectious stage: after intercourse with infected partner, itchy, tingling, numb, when virus beneath skin Active infectious symptomatic stage: blister-like sores that ulcerate on skin, mucous membranes, vagina, cervix, penis, anal area; fever, headache, muscle aches, general malaise, vaginal discharge, enlarged lymph glands; dyspareunia (painful intercourse); lesions heal 5 to 7 days but are sites for secondary infection; symptoms last several weeks Infectious dormant stage: lesions heal; no symptoms; blisters within vagina or urethra may go undetected; may be transmitted sexually at this time. Recurring symptomatic stage: usually recurrence of repeated painful attacks because virus remains dormant near base of spine between attacks; duration of time between attacks varies; may be precipitated by emotional stress, ovulation, onset of menses, poor diet, excess sun or wind, lack of sleep, friction from clothes
Prognosis	Male: usually treated successfully Female: sterility Both sexes: arthritis, endocarditis No immunity to future infections Reinfection common	Can be treated successfully; no immunity; transmitted to fetus via placenta unless mother treated before 16 weeks' gestation If untreated: aortic aneurysm, heart failure; complete or partial paralysis or crippling; personality changes; blindness, gumma, lesions of granulation tissue, causing tissue breakdown and impaired circulation; pain from bone involvement; convulsions Death: congenital syphilis or death for fetus	Incurable: one half to 1 million new cases annually with several million recurrence. Complications: herpes keratitis, eye infection (results from rubbing eye after touching herpes sore); repeated attacks and blindness possible Females: five times more likely to develop cervical cancer Pregnant women: pregnancy often ends in abortion, stillbirth, prematurity, neonatal infection, or death; fetal infection may occur in utero Infant: virus transmitted through placenta or by direct contact at birth; 50% chance of being born with disease unless delivered by cesarean section; 75% infected neonates blind or have brain damage; death may occur.
Treatment	Aqueous penicillin Some drug-resistant strains of organisms developing	Penicillin G benzathine or procaine penicillin	Aseptic technic in care of patient; cleansing lesions with soap and water; use of drying medications Experimental drugs reported to reduce symptoms

(continued)

TABLE 11-3. COMPARISON OF GONORRHEA, SYPHILIS, AND HERPES GENITALIS (Continued)

	Gonorrhea	Syphilis	Herpes Genitalis (Herpes 2) (HSV-2 Infection)
Treatment (cont.)			Antibiotics for secondary infection. Incurable but zovirax suppresses signs and symptoms. Psychologic counseling. Prevention of further spread by avoiding any contact with genitals and sexual intercourse while lesions are present unless male wears condom

TABLE 11-4. CONTRACEPTIVE MEASURES: EFFECTIVENESS AND DISADVANTAGES

Name	Description	Effectiveness	Disadvantages
Oral contraceptives	Pills used to suppress chemically ovulation; new low dose pill available, with one tenth amount of hormones, thus fewer side effects	Highly effective, two pregnancies in 100	Fewer serious effects than previously seen; screen for nausea, edema, depression, anemia, blood clots, myocardial infarction, and liver cancer; smokers have increased triglycerides, total cholesterol, and lipoproteins and greater cardiovascular disease risk
Intrauterine device (IUD: (Progestasert)	Metal coil inserted in uterus, preventing implantation of fertilized ovum	Very effective, five pregnancies in 100	Cramping and bleeding between periods, heavy periods, anemia, perforation of uterus, and pelvic infection
Spermicidal chemicals	Chemical substances inserted in vagina before intercourse	Less effective, 5 to 24 pregnancies in 100; effective if used with diaphragm	Irritation of penis or vagina
Billings ovulation method	Changes in cervical discharge show presence of ovulation	Very effective when followed and abstinence maintained during fertile time	Accurate observation by the woman is necessary
Diaphragm	Small occlusive device inserted over cervix before intercourse	Very effective when properly placed and checked often	Irritation of cervix; aesthetic objections
Condom	Occlusive device placed over penis before ejaculation	Effective when properly used, 9 to 10 pregnancies in 100	Aesthetic objections; possibly impaired sensation in male
Rhythm	Abstinence of intercourse before and during ovulation; increased body temperature during fertile days	Less effective, 5 to 24 pregnancies in 100	Pregnancy unless menstrual periods regular, ovulation closely observed, and abstinence adhered to
Sponge	Two-inch circular sponge of soft polyurethane saturated with spermicide; sponge inserted vaginally, removed by string loop	If left in 6 hr after intercourse, 88% to 90% effective	Not well tested; concern about TDA in sponge being a possible carcinogen to liver and breasts; not for use during menses or may cause toxic shock syndrome
Prostaglandins	Chemicals that regulate intracellular metabolism administered parenterally or orally for contraception or to induce abortions	Effectiveness uncertain	Nausea, vomiting, diarrhea, and pelvic pain
Luteinizing hormone releasing hormone (LHRH)	Daily injection of hormone decreases sperm; substance inhibits pituitary gland's release of hormone that controls ovulation and spermatogenesis	In women 98% effective; useful in men and women	Experimental; data on men still limited
Injections	150-mg injection of a progestogen, medroxy progesterone acetate (Depo-Provera); 200-mg injection of a progestogen, Norigest	Injections 98% effective for 3 mo	Licensed for use in 84 countries; not approved by FDA in United States; experimental

TABLE 11-4. CONTRACEPTIVE MEASURES: EFFECTIVENESS AND DISADVANTAGES (Continued)

Name	Description	Effectiveness	Disadvantages
Implants	Levo-norgestrel (progestin) inserted via silicone rubber, matchstick-size tubes into woman's arm	Implants last 5 yr; continual release of synthetic hormone inhibits ovulation, thickens cervical mucus, and impedes sperm passage; removed if woman desires pregnancy	Experimental in Europe and Asia; FDA approved in United States
Hysterectomy	Surgical removal of uterus; usually done for pathologic condition of uterus rather than for sterilization only	Completely effective; ovum and hormonal production unchanged; menstruation ceases	Mortality rate higher than after tubal ligation; possible postoperative complications; irreversible procedure.
Tubal ligation	Surgical interference with tubal continuity and transport of an ovum	Effectiveness depending on type of procedure done, 0.5 to 3 pregnancies in 100; ovum maturation, menstruation, and hormonal production unchanged	Occasional recanalization (fallopian tube ends regrowing together) causing fertility; adhesions, infection, or swelling of tubes postoperatively
Vasectomy	Surgical severing of the vas deferens (sperm duct) from each testicle	Effectiveness depending on type of procedure done; failure rate low; less expensive and time consuming and easier to obtain than female sterilization; no risk to life; no effect on hormone production of testes or sexual functioning	Bleeding, infection, and pain postoperatively in 2% to 4%; occasional recanalization of severed ends of vas deferens causing fertility; uncertain reversibility

Note: A combination of contraceptive practices may be used by the couple.

hering to instructions about contraceptive practices or abstinence (141).

Approximately one half of the teens in the United States have sexual intercourse by age 18; education and contraceptive services have not kept abreast of the changing sexual mores. Some youth, however, do not use contraceptives because of misconceptions or ignorance about them, inability to secure appropriate contraceptives, inability to plan ahead for their actions, a belief that using contraceptives marks them as promiscuous, or rebelliousness. Males are less likely to recognize risk of pregnancy as a result of sexual activity, have less information about contraceptives, and are less supportive of contraceptive use than females. The attitude of the male may indeed influence the female toward sexual activity without contraceptive use, even though she realizes the hazards and wishes to avoid them (46, 69, 191).

Adolescent Pregnancy. Adolescent pregnancy is at epidemic proportions. The United States exceeds other nations in incidence: more than 1 million teenage girls between 15 and 19 become pregnant annually; 70% to 85% of the pregnancies are unplanned. African-American teen pregnancy rates are higher, although 8% of Caucasians in the 15-to-19 age group become pregnant. Many teenage mothers are unmarried.

The main factor in the difference between incidence of teen pregnancy in the United States and Sweden, France, the Netherlands, England, Wales, and Canada is American attitudes toward sex. Although the media constantly offer messages that suggest sex, almost nothing that teenagers see or hear about sex informs them about contraceptives or the importance of avoiding pregnancy. These other countries apparently are more tolerant of teenage sexual activity than the United States and are more open about sex in general. The lowest pregnancy rates exist in countries with the most liberal attitudes toward sex (209).

Unintended pregnancy causes much human misery—for the pregnant teen and her family and often for the offspring. (Refer to Chapter 6 also for effects of teen pregnancy.) Effects on the teen father are less well known (69, 149).

Various factors influence whether the adolescent becomes pregnant. Although some pregnancies may be accidental, four other themes may underlie the mask of "accident" (229):

1. Self-destruction or self-hate
2. Rebellion, anger, hate, reverse aggressiveness toward parents and authority
3. Lack of responsibility for self and personal behavior, related to identity diffusion or confusion
4. Plea for attention and help, either from parents, the boy involved, or others

Other factors and combinations of factors may also contribute to the teenage girl's becoming pregnant. Box 11–8 summarizes these factors (24, 69, 149, 165–167, 201, 229).

The early adolescent is not physically, socially, emotionally, educationally, or economically ready for pregnancy or parenthood. The late adolescent is physically mature but may not be ready for pregnancy emotionally, socially, or economically. These latter factors override the biologic advantages of early pregnancy and may account, in part, for the lack of health care that is sought during pregnancy (166). In turn, health providers

---

■ **BOX 11-8.**
**Factors Influencing Incidence
of Adolescent Pregnancy**

Developmental Factors

• Low self-esteem
• Need to be close to someone; to relieve loneliness
• Recent experience of significant loss or change
• Early physical sexual maturation
• Egocentrism
• School dropout or truancy; school underachiever
• Personal fable (feeling that "it won't happen to me")
• Responsiveness to peers' sexual behavior
• Independence from family
• Need to prove own womanhood
• Denial of personal sexuality or sexual behavior
• Self-punishment for earlier sexual activity or pregnancy for which feels shame, guilt

Societal Factors

• Variety of adult sexual behavior values
• Implied acceptance of intercourse outside of marriage
• Importance of involvement in heterosexual relationships stressed by the media
• Inadequate access to contraception
• Access to public financial support for teen parents and offspring

Family and Friends

• Difficult mother-daughter relationship
• Desire to break symbiotic tie between self and mother
• Lack of religious affiliation
• Mother, sister, or close relative pregnant as teen
• Sexually permissive behavior norms of the larger peer group
• Sexually permissive values and behavior of close friends; immediate peer group sexually active
• Inadequate communication in heterosexual relationships
• Fulfillment of mother's prophecy if she expects such behavior
• History of sexual abuse or incest
• Few, if any, girlfriends
• Older boyfriend
• Substance abuse or use in family or peer group

---

count for the majority of teenage births. Teenagers at highest risk of adverse pregnancy outcomes, specifically those less than 17 years old, are more likely to be African-American, live in rural areas (especially if Caucasian), and receive inadequate prenatal care (especially if Caucasian) than older first time mothers. Risks are highest for 11- to 14-year-old teens. However, sexual activity is still atypical in the United States at such early ages; very peculiar social circumstances (e.g., extreme isolation from the social and economic mainstream, rape, or incest) may account for these pregnancies and births and the negative outcomes. Early fertility implies early menarche, which is associated with short stature, a risk factor for poor neonatal outcome. The excessive rates of short gestation, low-birth weight, and neonatal mortality may result from a variety of physiologic consequences of environmental disadvantage, not primarily from inherent and intractable biologic developmental limits (69, 149, 166).

The late adolescent male is more likely to be involved in the pregnancy and be supportive to the girl than his younger counterpart. Urban teenage African-American fathers are more involved with their children and the children's mothers than stereotypes suggest (113, 195). The more mature the adolescent girl and boy when they become parents, the more likely they will manifest positive parenting characteristics described in Chapter 7. The younger the adolescent, the more likely it is that negative parenting behaviors will occur, with one possible exception. During middle adolescence, Caucasian mothers who are poor are more likely to exhibit picking, poking, and pinching behaviors toward the infant. Often the adolescent parent expects behavior beyond the developmental ability of the baby, which creates intense frustration and anger that result in child abuse or neglect. You may be able to assess these behaviors and intervene with support, teaching, and counseling. Agencies that have adolescent pregnancy programs should provide both teen fathers and mothers with parenting classes and child development information (186).

A major problem in adolescent parenting is that many teenage girls who become mothers have themselves come from single-parent homes or homes in which active participation by the father is lacking. Further, the teenage father often gives no real support—emotional or financial. The maternal grandmother is the one who is expected to raise the child; if she cannot, the adolescent single parent is likely to lack the emotional maturity or knowledge to demonstrate positive parenting characteristics (69). If the teenage couple marries, divorce often occurs within the first or second year so that the baby is in a single-parent home. Smith's article (186) discusses the nurse's meeting psychosocial needs of the teenage mother and father.

There are ways to help the teenage mother be a more effective and loving mother and also feel more

often do not understand the needs underlying the adolescents' behavior and thereby fail to provide the necessary services.

Neonatal risks associated with teen-age maternity are not uniform but are high. The risks vary by age of the adolescent mother, amount of prenatal care, and racial identification. In the United States socioeconomically advantaged teenagers, with healthy and unimpaired physical growth and development, rarely bear children. Disadvantaged Americans, on the other hand, often initiate child bearing by their late teens and currently acsecure and comfortable with parenting. Having a warm, caring woman visit the teen in her home during the infancy stage to assist with infant care, model nurturant child care, explain normal development, and encourage expression of the mother's feelings of frustration and anxiety improves the teen's parenting behavior. In addition, a drop-in center where the teen can take her baby for a few hours to be free of child care for a while and to gain emotional support and information is also a useful community support (149). The teen parent needs multiple support from family, school, peers, church, the media, the community, and legal system (201).

Abortion. **Abortion** is a *method of terminating a pregnancy through expulsion or extraction of the fetus,* usually for economic, emotional, or social reasons. Poor women who economically cannot take care of another child often resort to this drastic form of birth control when they believe they cannot possibly meet the demands of parenting. Abortion carries possible risks to the physical and psychologic health of the female, although the legal abortion is statistically safer than the illegal abortion. However, more widespread use of abstinence or contraception would reduce the need for abortion. You may be involved in helping the female who is pregnant, the parents, and even the father of the baby to determine their values and feelings about remaining pregnant versus having an abortion. The persons involved should decide; it is not appropriate for you to give advice. Rather give full information, be nonjudgmental of the people, and listen. The people involved will be capable of arriving at a decision.

Incest. A universal taboo in all cultures is **incest,** *sexual intercourse between persons in the family too closely related to marry legally.* Incest has been present at epidemic levels for some time but is now being admitted more freely by the victims as they speak of the resultant emotional and physical pain. (The woman may be in her thirties, forties, or fifties before she can talk about incest that occurred in early childhood.) In your assessment be aware that the adolescent, either male or female, but especially the female, is at risk for incest or for youth prostitution (21). The child and adolescent will tell you if you pick up the initial verbal cues or if you ask if he or she has been the victim of such activity. The risk to boys is not as well documented as that to girls but may be equally common, with either the mother or the father as the abuser. Incestuous relations usually begin when the child is 6 to 12 years of age and continue through adolescence (91). The behavior and consequent signs and symptoms that occur are like those of the sexually abused child described in Chapter 10. Incest may involve stepparents or step siblings, grandparents, or the uncles or cousins.

In adolescence the signs and symptoms may include runaway attempts, drug and alcohol abuse, hyster-ical seizures, indiscriminate sexual activity, and early pregnancy. Destructive effects of incest continue into adult life, long after contact has ceased. Adult women have persistent and often severe impairments in self-esteem, intimate relationships, and sexual functioning. Incest victims also have a higher-than-normal risk for repeated victimization (battering and rape). Marriage to an abusive spouse, with potential repetition of abuse in the next generation, is a frequent outcome (21, 91). Of all the entanglements, incest between siblings apparently is the least psychologically harmful (21).

In incestuous families the man is often the sole economic support. The woman often is isolated and cannot drive a car. The family does not have visitors. The woman and other children are frequently beaten and abused; the daughter(s) singled out for the sexual relationship is usually spared the beatings, but she clearly understands what happens if she incurs her father's displeasure. Incestuous fathers are described as family tyrants but when confronted with the behavior, will appear pathetic, meek, bewildered, and ingratiating. They are exquisitely sensitive to power and seldom try to intimidate anyone of equal or greater status. Instead, with the health care professional, the man will attempt to gain the professional person's sympathy and deny, minimize, or rationalize their behavior (21, 24, 91, 97, 164).

Inexperienced professionals may incorrectly blame the mother for the incest. However, typically the mother is ill or disabled and unable to care for herself or her children. The mother usually cannot be independent and tries to preserve the marriage at any cost, including conscious or unconscious sacrifice of a daughter. Incestuous fathers do not assume maternal caretaking roles when wives are disabled. Rather they expect the eldest daughter to assume the "little mother" role for housework and child care responsibilities. The daughter's sexual relationship with the father often evolves as an extension of her other duties. When the oldest daughter becomes resistant, the father turns his attention to the next daughter—or nieces, stepchildren, or granddaughters. The father continues sexual activity with the wife on demand during this time; it is his choice if he limits sexual activity only to the daughters (21, 91, 97).

Father-daughter incest should be suspected in any family that includes (1) a violent or domineering and suspicious father, (2) a battered, chronically ill or disabled mother, and (3) a daughter who appears to have assumed major adult responsibilities. If incest has been reported with one daughter, it should be suspected with all of the other daughters. Incest should also be suspected as a precipitant in the runaway, delinquent, drug abuse, or suicidal behavior of adolescent girls. The main obstacle to obtaining a history of incest in the clinician's reluctance to ask about it. False accusations of sexual abuse or incest are rare; however, the girl commonly retracts a true allegation because of family pressure (21, 91, 97).

Discovery of incest is a family crisis. *Immediate crisis intervention is essential.* Typically the behavior has been going on many years, and the family's defenses are organized around preservation of the incest secret. Disclosure interrupts patterns of functioning. The father faces loss of sexual activity, which has become an addiction, and the possible loss of a wife and family; social stigmatization; and possible criminal sanctions (these seldom are applied). The mother faces possible loss of a husband, social stigmatization, and the terrifying prospect of raising her family alone, which she is ill prepared to do. The man denies his behavior and maintains his innocence. The wife is torn between husband and daughter, and unless she is given rapid support, her initial belief of the daughter gives way to rallying to the husband's side in 1 or 2 weeks. The daughter then finds herself discredited, shamed, punished for bringing trouble on the family, and still unprotected from sexual abuse. Suicide and runaway behavior are likely at this time as the offspring is being segregated and driven out of the family (91, 97).

Professionals frequently accept the father's denial and rationalizations and support the family secret. They may believe that incest is harmless, consensual, with the daughter a willing or initiating participant, and the result of the man's being deprived of adult sexual expression. Traditional psychodynamic treatment will not be effective. An active, directive, even coercive approach is necessary. Treatment requires ongoing cooperation between the therapist and agencies of the state—both law enforcement and child protective services (91).

It may be necessary to remove the offspring from the home to ensure his or her safety. However, this intervention is destructive because it (1) makes the adolescent (child) feel he or she has done something wrong and is being punished by banishment from the family, (2) reinforces the couple's bonding against the offspring, and (3) makes it difficult to find appropriate placement for him or her. If the safety of the adolescent (child) is in question, it is preferable to have the father leave during this period. Unfortunately, child protective services do not have legal authority to remove a parent, but a court order may be obtained, and the court can establish supervised visitation, mandated treatment, and family support.

All family members need intensive support. All too frequently this recommended approach is ignored or not implemented (91).

Crisis support for the offspring involves the following (91):

1. Reassure the adolescent (or child) that there are protective adults outside of the family that believe his or her story and will not allow further exploitation to occur.
2. Praise the adolescent (child) for the courage to reveal the incest secret.

3. Assure the offspring he or she is not to blame for the incest and that he or she is helping, not hurting, the family by seeking outside help.
4. Tell the offspring explicitly that many children retract their initial complaint because of pressure or fear; encourage him or her not to do so, with the assurance he or she will not be abandoned by authorities if he or she does.

Crisis support for the mother involves encouragement and assistance to do the following (91):

1. Continue to believe the offspring, even if this is painful.
2. Resist the tendency to bond with the husband against the offspring.
3. Talk about his or her feelings of shame, guilt, anger, fear, inadequacy.
4. Explore ways he or she can handle the issues of survival and seek needed help.
5. Obtain treatment for health problems.

Crisis support for the father involves helping him face that the secret has been broken, that he must admit and give up his sexual relationship with his daughter before his problem can be resolved and the family restored (91).

Group treatment for the mother, father, and offspring is more effective than family or individual therapy alone, although individual therapy can be combined with group therapy. Family therapy may be used in the late stages of treatment. The best motivator for the offender to remain in therapy is the court mandate. Self-help activities can supplement other therapy. The family's intense need for support may be met by frequent peer contact such as through Parents United, Daughters and Sons United, or other such agencies (91, 97).

Restoration of the incestuous family centers on the mother-daughter relationship. Safety for the daughter comes not just from improving the marital relationship, but by helping the mother feel strong enough to protect herself and her children and by ensuring that the daughter feels sure she can turn to her mother for protection (91).

The father is ready to return to the family when he has admitted and taken full responsibility for the incest, apologized to the daughter(s) in the presence of all family members, and promised never to abuse the children or wife again. When he is ready to return to the family, they may or may not be ready to receive him. A decision for divorce may be as valid as family reunion. The best gauge for measuring successful treatment is the daughter's feeling of safety, the disappearance of her distress symptoms, and her resumption of normal development (91).

Rape and *other sexual abuse* may be part of the adolescent's experience as a victim. Burgess (21, 22) describes three types of sex rings: child sex initiation rings, youth prostitution rings, and syndicated pornography and prostitution rings.

As you work with sexual assault victims, be aware of various types of assault and entanglements that exist so that you can better detect verbal and nonverbal cues, give immediate assistance, and refer the person (and parents) to receive the necessary medical and legal assistance. References at the end of the chapter are helpful (21, 22, 24, 80, 91, 97, 138, 164).

Drug-Abuse Problems

Drug abuse (illicit and prescription) is an epidemic adolescent health problem that is not new. The history of drug abuse is long throughout the world. The problem continues to intensify in America, a drug-conscious nation, compared to other countries. It is an epidemic with serious consequences for future generations. A major problem is the increasing number of infants born with addiction to one or several drugs (1, 35, 96, 132, 150). Every age group takes a certain amount of medication at one time or another. Usually these drugs are taken for therapeutic reasons. However, reports show that schoolchildren, adolescents, and young adults are increasingly using drugs that cause dependence and toxicity (69, 96, 112, 176, 193).

Drug abuse is the *use of any drug in excess or for the feeling it arouses.* A **drug** is a *substance that has an effect on the body or mind.* Excessive use of certain drugs causes **drug dependence,** a *physical need or psychologic desire for continuous or repeated use of the drug.* **Addiction** is *present when physical withdrawal symptoms result if the person does not repeatedly receive a drug and can involve* **tolerance,** *having to take increasingly larger doses to get the same effect.*

Reasons for drug abuse are many: curiosity; peer pressure; need to overcome feelings of insecurity and aloneness and to be a part of the group; need for acceptance; easy availability; imitation of family; rebellion, escape, or exhilaration; need for a crutch; unhappy home life; sense of alienation or identity problem; or an attempt at maturity or sophistication. Gradually the drug subculture replaces interest in family, school, church, hobbies, or other organizational activity. The beliefs and attitudes of the drug subculture are learned from experienced drug users and are fortified by certain rock-and-roll songs and stars (1, 13, 32, 36, 39, 105, 140, 180, 189, 216, 229).

Drug abuse and addiction affect all ethnic and racial groups (13). Entire communities are affected. In large cities much of the drug trade also involves street gangs, which have become ghetto-based drug trafficking organizations. Even rural communities are affected. Total community effort is needed to stop or prevent the problem (176, 193).

Drug dependence is epidemic among the wealthy as well as among the middle class and poor. Children of wealthy parents may develop such traits as poor impulse control, poor frustration tolerance, depression, and poor coping ability. As a result, drugs may be used to cope. Predictably, these traits make children from wealthy homes a difficult population to treat. When drug abuse is the presenting problem, the financial ability to buy drugs of high quality, subcultural acceptance of their use, and at least a relative immunity from legal consequences do not motivate behavioral change (214).

Ingestion of alcohol and illicit drugs depresses the cerebral cortex, a still immature reasoning and intellectual center in the teens, and releases inhibitions in the limbic system, the center of love, pleasure, anger, pain, and other emotions. The limbic system seeks instant and constant gratification or stimulation and contributes to the adolescent's sense of boredom. Thus some adolescents go to extremes in seeking television, alcohol, hard drugs, hard rock, and aggressive video games. There is loosening of social controls and increase in aggressive and sexual behavior when the limbic system is stimulated. Box 11–9 describes the primary or general signs of drug abuse (1, 35, 65, 67, 69, 92, 99, 100, 105, 132, 140, 150, 177, 184, 187, 216, 229).

Therapy is usually entered into as a result of family pressure— often in the form of threatened financial loss such as the withdrawal of allowance or inheritance—or a crisis event such as attempted suicide or arrest. The behavior and illness of the young drug abuser control the entire family, causing family illness. Parents must regain control of their home, forcing the youth to face the illness by seeking treatment. Love and care in a family is essential, but that alone will not cure the drug abuse problem or the craziness that results in a family in which a member is a drug abuser, nor will parental strictness solve the problems. Professional treatment should be obtained in a center that treats the whole person and family, using an interdisciplinary team approach, and that provides after discharge care to the person and family. Intensive treatment over time to the entire family system creates the attitude change that is essential for remaining healthy and functional and for ongoing maturity. A combination of drug detoxification, methadone maintenance, and emotional, cognitive, didactic, and experiential therapies is helpful to reduce symptoms and work through underlying character and interactional pathology (214). Adolescent treatment centers typically prohibit use of stereo and rock music, television, video games, drugs, cigarettes, alcohol, and even rock-star T-shirts. Instead, the teens participate in a structured schedule that involves nutritious foods, jogging and other exercise, group discussions, individual therapy, reading, art and music therapy, school work, responsibility to follow rules, goal setting, and a milieu that builds a spiritual foundation similar to the 12 steps of Alcoholics Anonymous (229).

If after discharge the youth returns to his or her drug-using friends, there will be a return to drug abuse

■ **BOX 11-9.**
Primary and General Signs and Symptoms of Drug Abuse Among Adolescents

- Decrease in quality of schoolwork without a valid reason; Reasons given may be boredom, not caring about school, not liking the teachers
- Personality changes, lack of empathy, becoming more irritable, less attentive, less affectionate, secretive, unpredictable, uncooperative, apathetic, depressed, withdrawn, hostile, sullen, easily provoked, insensitive to punishment
- Less responsible behavior, not doing chores or school homework, school tardiness or absenteeism, forgetful of family occasions such as birthdays
- Change in activity, lack of participation in family activities, school or church functions, sports, prior hobbies, or organizational activities
- Change in friends, new friends who are unkempt in appearance or sarcastic in their attitude; secretive or protective about these friends, not giving any information
- Change in appearance or dress, in vocabulary, in music tastes to match those of new friends, imitating acid rock-and-roll stars
- More difficult to communicate with, refuses to discuss friends, activities, drug issues; insists it is all right to experiment with drugs; defends rights of youth, insists adults hassle youth; prefers to talk about bad habits of adults
- Rebellious, resistant to authority, antisocial behavior, persistent lying; seeks immediate gratification; feels no remorse
- Irrational behavior, frequent explosive episodes, driving recklessly, unexpectedly stupid behavior
- Loss of money, credit cards, checks, jewelry, household silver, coins in the home that cannot be accounted for
- Addition of drugs, clothes, money, albums, tapes, or stereo equipment suddenly found in the home
- Presence of whiskey bottles, marijuana seeds or plants, hemostats, rolling papers, drug buttons, and marijuana lead buttons; also may be unusual belt buckles, pins, bumper stickers, or T-shirts and magazines in the car, truck, or home
- Preoccupation with the occult, various pseudoreligious cults, satanism, or witchcraft; evidence of tattoo writing of 666, drawing of pentagrams on self or elsewhere, or misrepresentation of religious objects
- Signs of physical change or deterioration, including pale face; dilated pupils; red eyes; chewing heavily scented gum; using heavy perfumes; using eyewash or drops to remove the red; heightened sensitivity to touch, smell or taste; weight loss, even with increased appetite (marijuana smoking causes the "munchies"—extra snacking)
- Signs of mental change or deterioration, including disordered thinking or illogical patterns, decreased ability to remember or to think in rapid thought processes and responses; severe lack of motivation

and all the consequences. It is not easy for the youth to give up drugs or to overcome the drug abuse reputation at school, among peers, or elsewhere. It may be very difficult to work into a new group of friends unless during the treatment program the youth and family were helped to establish new interests, new hobbies, new social ties and friendships, and new organizational connections. Remaining drug free may mean giving up the prior boyfriend or girlfriend, certain favorite clothes or possessions, certain words in the vocabulary, and certain mannerisms or aspects of appearance. The change in attitudes, self-concept, and body image must be total enough so the person feels like a new person and is strong enough in that identity that the new self is maintained in the face of inevitable peer, school, family, and other stressors. The ability to give up aspects of the old self and maintain the new identity begins in the treatment center but can only be accomplished with love, support, and encouragement (not nagging) from family and other loved ones. *The person must feel that he or she is gaining more than what is being lost to maintain the changes begun in treatment and to move forward in maturity.* To remain drug-free involves more than just "saying no" or a one-time seminar (52). Support groups in the school, church, and community for the teens who do not want to use alcohol or drugs are essential to prevent the loneliness and ostracism some teens feel when they go against peers. Illicit drug trade can be stopped best by community action; which reduces supply to individuals (176).

Table 11–5 will assist you in assessing the **specific signs** (objective evidence) and **symptoms** (subjective evidence) **resulting from drugs commonly abused.** Often the youth is taking a mixture of these drugs since use of any of them is likely to increase use of other drugs. Assessment becomes more complex. At times neither the person nor friends know for sure what drugs have been used. Various references at the end of this chapter give information on drug abuse (1, 28, 51, 59, 92, 99, 105, 134, 140, 175, 177, 184, 189, 193, 212, 216, 229).

Because the use of cocaine (or crack) is a serious health and social problem, a discussion in addition to the information under "Stimulant Abuser" in Table 11–5 is presented in the following pages.

Cocaine is an *alkaloid extracted from the leaves of the coca bush, which grows mainly on the eastern slope of the Andes mountain in Peru and Bolivia.* It is sold on the streets as a hydrochloride salt; it is a fine, white crystalline powder known as "coke," "snow," "flake," "blow." Freebase cocaine resembles rock candy chunks. Street cocaine is diluted with cornstarch, talcum powder, sugar, amphetamines, and quinine. Its purity is usually 5% to 50%; it may be 80%. Cocaine is taken by (1) snorting (inhaled through a straw or a rolled-up dollar bill or a coke spoon), (2) freebasing (smoked in a small water pipe filled with rum instead of water), or (3) mainlining (taken intravenously) (1, 30, 35, 96, 176, 189, 193).

TABLE 11-5. SYMPTOMS OF COMMON FORMS OF DRUG ABUSE

Type	Signs and Symptoms
Inhalant Abuser Squeezes airplane glue into paper bag, holds nose, inhales fumes; may sniff gasoline, lighter fluid, refrigerants, aerosols, anesthetics, or cleaning agents	1. Odor of substance on person's clothes or breath, in plastic or paper bags 2. Secretions from nose or eyes 3. Euphoria; weightlessness; distorted sense of time and space 4. Distorted perception, diplopia, tinnitus 5. Muscular weakness; staggers as if drunk 6. Drowsy, sleepy after 35 to 45 min, or unconscious 7. Severe anemia if persistent use 8. Hallucinations; violent behavior 9. Dependence emotionally, not physically 10. Kidney, liver, and brain damage or death from excess inhalation
Depressant Abuser Uses barbiturates, sedative-hypnotics, and tranquilizers, which depress central nervous system	1. Varied onset and duration of effects according to preparation used and route of administration 2. Symptoms of alcohol intoxication with no odor of alcohol on breath 3. Sleepy, drowsy, irritable 4. Interest in usual activities diminished; poor hygiene; depression; slow speech 5. Sudden behavior changes; impaired judgment 6. Pulse rate and blood pressure lowered. 7. Respirations slow and shallow 8. Confusion and disorganized behavior 9. Drugs ingested, one after another, without user's awareness of action 10. Tolerance possible 11. Dependence and physical addiction, with consequent withdrawal symptoms 12. Liver, brain, and kidney damage from long-term use 13. Coma, death from overdosage
Stimulant Abuser Uses *caffeine* orally; *amphetamines* orally or intravenously; *ice* (recrystallized, smokable methamphetamine); *cocaine* by snorting or intravenously; or other drugs that stimulate the central nervous system	1. Needles and syringes present, usually concealed; scars on body 2. Euphoria, increased alertness, energetic, talkative, decreased sense of fatigue 3. Insomnia, anorexia 4. Pupils dilated 5. Pulse rate increased 6. Mouth and nose dry, halitosis 7. Speech slurred 8. Agitated, excessive activity, irritable, suspicious 9. Disoriented, confused, hallucinates, violent, psychotic 10. Dependence psychologically; tolerance 11. Addicting physically 12. Injuries occurring from activity while under drug effects or death from large doses 13. Caffeine may cause symptoms described in signs 2 through 8; may be chronic caffeinism 14. Cocaine causes nasal congestion and hole in nasal septum when snorted (snuffed); habitual abuse causes cerebral atrophy 15. Ice: absorbed through lungs; immediate effect; stays in body; all symptoms more severe than for cocaine
Narcotic Abuser Uses drugs from the opiate plant (heroin or morphine) that relieve pain and induce euphoria and sleep	1. Traces of white powder around nostrils from inhaling heroin ("Persian Brown," dark red-brown granular powder from Iran, is more potent; may be smoked or snorted) 2. Scars on the body from injecting narcotic into vein or under skin 3. Needles and syringes left in hidden places at home or school 4. Flushed skin, tingling sensations; may become pale, clammy, and increasingly cyanotic 5. Euphoria 6. Lethargic, drowsy, nodding, reduced physical activity; slow respirations 7. Pupils constricted and unresponsive to light; reduced visual acuity 8. Concentration impaired, apathy 9. Vomiting, constipation, urinary retention 10. Pulmonary complications from snorting powder 11. Physical deterioration from poor health practices 12. Tolerance

(continued)

TABLE 11-5. SYMPTOMS OF COMMON FORMS OF DRUG ABUSE (Continued)

Type	Signs and Symptoms
	13. Dependence physically and psychologically
	14. Death from overdosage; 10% of addicts die in 10 to 12 mo; death six times rate for general population, adjusted for age
Marijuana Abuser	1. Nervous system
Uses marijuana (cannabis), Indian hemp, which produces varying grades of hallucinogenic material: hashish, pure cannabis resin, the most powerful grade from leaves and flowering tops of female plants; ganja, less potent preparation of flowering tops and stems of female plant and resin attached to them; bhang, least potent preparation of fried mature leaves and flowering tops of male and female plants; THC in fat part of cell prevents nutrients from crossing cell membrane; RNA production and new cell growth reduced; *all* cell function interfered with	Stored in fat portion of cells; remains in brain 6 wk after cessation of smoking
	Speech comprehension, ability to express ideas, and ability to understand relationships impaired because of damage to the cerebral cortex
	Memory, decision making, handling complex tasks, ability to concentrate or focus impaired because of effects on cells in the hypocampus and cerebrum
	Emotional swings, depression, pessimism, irritability, low frustration tolerance, and temper outbursts because of cell damage in limbic system
	Does not learn adaptive skills or how to cope with stressors
	Lack of motivation, fatigue, moodiness, depression, inability to cope, loss of interest in vigorous activity or all previously enjoyed activities occur because of THC effects on various parts of the brain; fails to continue in emotional development.
	Insomnia because of damage to cells in the hypothalamus
	Vision blurred and irregular visual perception because of damage to cells in the occipital areas
	Body coordination, maintenance of posture and balance, ability to perform sports or drive a car impaired because of damage to cells in the cerebellum
	2. Respiratory system
	Upper respiratory infections common because of destruction to mucosal cells from the smoke (more destructive than tobacco smoke)
	Sinusitis, inflammation of the lining of one or more of the sinuses, from nasal infection
	Bronchitis, with low-grade fever, chest pain, chronic cough, and yellow-green sputum, common because of inflammation to the bronchial tree caused by smoke inhalation
	Lung cancer more likely because of the numerous chemicals in marijuana (smoking three to five joints a week is equivalent to smoking 16 cigarettes daily for 7 days a week)
	Emphysema and chronic obstructive pulmonary diseases from long-time smoking and deep inhalation; lung function permanently damaged
	3. Cardiovascular system
	Cardiac arrythmias and tachycardia related to the dose of THC absorbed (one joint immediately raises heart rate by as much as 50%)
	Hypertension, which may contribute to aneurysm formation or cardiovascular accident, common
	Myocardial infarction possible
	4. Congested conjunctiva associated with hypertension
	5. Reproductive system
	Infertility in males from moderate to heavy use because production of testosterone is reduced and low sperm production or production of abnormal sperm occurs.
	Impotence, inability to ejaculate sperm
	Gynecomastia, enlarged breast formation, in puberty when secondary sex characteristics are being developed (lower testosterone level causes fat deposits around the breast tissue)
	Hirsutism in females, with increased androgen production resulting in male secondary sex characteristics (increased hair growth on face and arms, deeper voice), irregular menstrual cycles, serious acne, and lack of development of female secondary sexual characteristics
	Infertility in the female because of damage to the ova; menstrual cycle irregularity

TABLE 11-5. SYMPTOMS OF COMMON FORMS OF DRUG ABUSE (Continued)

Type	Signs and Symptoms
	Pregnancy, if present when marijuana is smoked, endangers the embryo and fetus, increasing chance of congenital defects and fetal mortality because THC crosses the placental barrier Lactation, if breast-feeding while smoking marijuana, endangers baby's health because THC transfers through breast milk 6. Immune system suppressed; prone to infections 7. Endocrine system impaired for 11–16-year-olds. 8. Marijuana combined with PCP causes psychosis; if taken with other substances, effect of each drug multiplied
Psychedelic Drug Abuser Uses lysergic acid from ergot, which can be converted to LSD or lysergic acid diethylamide tartrate (LSD 25), a potent hallucinogen that is chemically synthesized and alters mood, perception, and thinking; phencyclidine (angel dust) or PCP; mescaline (peyote cactus); psilocybin (mushroom)	1. Euphoria, impaired judgment, anxiety, hyperactive 2. Suspicious, psychotic 3. Pupils dilated; high blood pressure; weight loss 4. Hallucinations, illusions, trancelike state; amnesia 5. Senses of sight, hearing, touch, body image, and time distorted; dissociation from reality 6. Depression, confusion, disorientation, delirium 7. Fear, excitement, terror 8. Exaggerated feeling of strength, power, invulnerability 9. Incoordination, muscular rigidity, dizzy, seizures 10. Flashback effects reexperienced without further use of drug 11. Chromosomal changes possible 12. Coma, death from cardiorespiratory failure or cerebral hemorrhage 13. PCP makes person insensitive to severe pain, so serious injury or death may occur

Cocaine creates tolerance and is addicting because of the sense of stimulation (rush) that comes from activation of nerve cells in the brain that release dopamine. The sense of pleasure or good feeling is so great that the person develops a stronger compulsion for cocaine each time he or she uses it so that addiction results. Chronic cocaine use blocks the ability of the brain cells to release dopamine without increasing amounts of cocaine. The person feels terrible without the drug. Finally, there is the **kindling effect,** *a small amount of cocaine can trigger unexpectedly severe dopamine reactions,* resulting in seizures or bursts of psychotic behavior (1, 30, 31, 35, 96, 132, 150, 176, 189, 193, 227).

Physical changes that occur from cocaine use are as follows (1, 30, 31, 35, 96, 132, 150, 176, 189, 193):

1. Cardiovascular: tachycardia, arrhythmias, hypertension
2. Respiratory: nasal stuffiness, tachypnea, shortness of breath, runny nose
3. Musculoskeletal: twitching, tremors, weight loss
4. Gastrointestinal: nausea, constipation, anorexia
5. Genitourinary: difficult urination, impotency
6. Dermatologic: pallor, cold sweats
7. Ophthalmologic: dilated pupils, blurred vision
8. Central nervous system: fever, insomnia, fatigue, headache, seizures
9. Reproductive: abnormal spermatozoa

Medical hazards that result from cocaine use include the following (1, 28, 30, 31, 35, 51, 59, 96, 132, 150, 176, 189, 193):

1. Nasal septum and mucous membrane destruction from inhalation
2. Bronchitis, with infection, hemorrhage, and blocking of the respiratory tract from inhalation of foreign particles
3. Respiratory failure from vasoconstriction of blood vessels in the lung, cyanosis, shortness of breath, dyspnea, pulmonary edema, respiratory collapse, and death
4. Cardiac arrhythmias, tachycardia, myocardial infarction, cardiac arrest, sudden death
5. Seizures from freebasing and mainlining, which cause strong, explosive stimulation; convulsions, which may result in death
6. Phlebitis from repeated injections in the veins; resulting thrombus can cause an embolus, causing myocardial infarction, pulmonary embolus, renal embolus, or cerebrovascular accident
7. Endocarditis from mainlining with bacterial-contaminated needles, causing infection of heart valves; fatality rate, 50%
8. Hepatitis from mainlining with blood-contaminated needles, causing tender, enlarged liver, jaundice; repeated attacks can be fatal
9. Brain abscess from mainlining with bacterial-contaminated needles, causing fever, convulsions, paralysis, and possible death
10. AIDS from mainlining with blood-contaminated needles; 75% of all intravenous addicts have been exposed to the virus, 5% to 10% or more will develop the fatal disease.

CASE SITUATION: Adolescent Drug Abuse

Jess, 17, was taken for treatment to an adolescent chemical abuse unit. "My parents, when they put me in (the hospital), they thought I was just drinking and using pot. When they got my toxscreen back, my mom almost fainted."

The drug-screening analysis showed that marijuana, Valium, Demerol, Dilaudid, and codeine all had been ingested within a week. "All I did was live to get high—and, I guess you could say, get high to live," he said.

"I used to work at the home of a doctor who had a medicine cabinet full of everything anybody could dream of. He had a bunch of narcotics and stuff, and I thought I was in heaven. But I could go out right now and get drugs in about 15 minutes if I wanted. People, they're waiting for you to buy it. Around 10, I started drinking a little bit—just tasting it, and getting that warm feeling. The first time I got high, I was 12, and I loved it. There wasn't no stopping me then. I got high all I could. I used to wake up and think, "How can I get high today?"

His friends put pressure on him to try other drugs. "I told myself I'd never do any pills, never drop any acid, but those promises went by the wayside." He first took Quaaludes in the ninth grade and dropped acid that year at a concert. Soon he was drinking a lot and taking speed and Valium and other depressants.

"If I drank any beer, I'd want another one. If I got drunk, I'd want to get high; if I got high, I'd want to get pills. When I started out, I thought it was just cool, and that feeling was great. Instead of dealing with normal, everyday problems, I'd run off and get high. It got so I was picking fights just so I could stomp out of the house and get high."

He became a connoisseur. "I didn't buy dope at school. There's no good dope at school."

He also became more difficult to handle at home and at school.

"That period of time, I started fighting a lot with my parents. My grades dropped. I got into fistfights at school. I was real rebellious. I usually was high during class."

"I think it was real obvious to my teachers, because of the way I dressed and the way I acted in class. All the guys I hung around with had real long hair, moccasin boots, heavy metal T-shirts, and leather pants."

"I was pretty much an A student, and they (grades) dropped to low Cs and Ds. I was really withdrawing into myself."

"I wasn't myself when I was stoned. For years, I didn't even know how to feel (emotions). I've left home a few times."

"One time I was on LSD and I took a razor blade and cut my leg up. I still have the scars from that. I blanked out a lot. I'd come home beaten-up looking, and didn't know why."

Jess spent 8 weeks in treatment and now says he's been straight for over a year.

"It's a dependency," he said. "There's no way to eliminate it. You just try to control it. If I smoked a joint today or took a drink, I'd be right back."

Jess agrees with other former addicts: part of the problem is the naiveté of the parents.

"My parents, when I started getting in trouble, weren't going to admit it." Advice for parents who uncover a drug problem is simple: "Get some help. Not just for your kids, but for the parents and siblings also, because the whole family gets crazy. It's a family disease."

"I'll have to be on the lookout for the rest of my life to avoid falling back into drug use. I've learned just to be myself, and people will like me—and I never would have believed that before."

Crack or **rock** is an *extremely potent, highly addictive, inhalant form of cocaine.* It is beige or slightly brown, white or yellowish white, and it is sold in pellet-sized chips called "rocks" or in small plastic vials, in an envelope, or in foil wrap. It can be smoked using a glass pipe or a tin can; the user inhales the vapor from the heated crack. It may be mixed with marijuana or tobacco, or it may be mixed with PCP (angel dust), which is called "space blasting," or with other drugs. Some users smoke in a "base house," "crack house," or "rock house" in which the person pays a fee to use the house, pipes, and torches. The well-to-do individual may use crack in his or her suburban or urban home (30, 36, 189).

The frightening aspect about crack is that the person may become addicted the first time of use or in a matter of weeks. The addiction is as powerful as heroin addiction. The intense high feeling is produced in 4 to 6 seconds and lasts 5 to 7 minutes. The high is followed by an intensely uncomfortable low feeling so that the person will do anything to get more crack. The person may become violent toward friends or family; the person may become paranoid or psychotic, or the person may commit suicide. Death may occur in the user because of heart or respiratory failure. The first dose may cost only a few dollars, but a binge that lasts 1 or 3 days and is repeated weekly may cost hundreds or thousands of dollars. Crack becomes the most, the only, important thing in life so that all other aspects of life suffer: family relations, friendship, jobs, emotional status, social status, ability to think or behave rationally, personal hygiene or self-care, activities of daily living. If the user is a pregnant woman, there is risk of miscarriage, stillbirth, an addicted baby, impaired physical and mental development in the child, or respiratory failure or strokes in the baby (30, 36, 140, 189).

Nursing Role in Health Promotion

The adolescent is between childhood and adulthood. Allow him or her to handle as much personal health care and business as possible, yet be aware of the psychosocial and physical problems with which he or she cannot cope without help. Watch for hidden fears that may be expressed in unconventional language. For example, the high school junior may state concern about her figure. Underlying this statement may be a fear that she will not adequately develop secondary sex characteristics. She may believe she is not physiologically normal or sexually attractive and will not be able to have children. With adequate assessment, you may discover that she is simply physically slow in developing. Explaining that not all adolescents develop at the same rate and that she is normal may rid her mind of great anxiety.

Today's adolescent, because of improved communications, knows more about life than did former generations. He or she is bombarded with information but does not have the maturity to handle it. Do not assume that because of apparent sophistication he or she understands the basis of health promotion. The adolescent may be able to discuss foreign policy but thinks that syphilis is caught from toilet seats.

Some teenagers, especially those with understanding and helpful families, go through adolescence with relative ease; it is a busy, happy period. But the increases in teenage suicide and in escape activities such as drugs and alcohol speak for those who do not have this experience. Adolescents are looking for adults who can be admired, trusted, and leveled with and who genuinely care. Parents are still important as figures to identify with, but the teenagers now look more outside the home—to teachers, community, and national leaders. They idealize such people, and if the leaders are found to be liars or thieves, their idealism turns to bitterness. As a nurse, you will be one of the community leaders with the opportunity, through living and teaching health promotion, to influence these impressionable minds.

Counseling the Adolescent for Health Promotion

Help the person clarify values, beliefs, and attitudes that are important and be more analytic in thinking as first steps in bringing behavior into congruence and to reduce a sense of conflict. Tauer (197) describes value clarification exercises.

Teach the adolescent effective decision-making skills so that the person learns how to develop a plan of action toward some goal. The decision-making model involves (1) defining the problem; (2) gathering and processing information; (3) identifying possible solutions and alternatives of action; (4) making a decision about action; (5) trying out the decision; (6) evaluating whether the decision, actions, and consequences were effective or desirable; (7) rethinking other alternate solutions with new information; and (8) acting on these new decisions. Having the adolescent write out answers when setting goals, thinking of possible solutions, and analyzing consequences can help make an abstract process more concrete and more useful to the person who needs signs of structure (197).

McCreary-Jahasz and Kavanaugh show a model for sexual decision making that you can use to help the person clarify values, make decisions, and understand consequences related to sexual behavior (83, 166).

Promote warm, accepting, supportive, nonjudgmental feelings, and honest feedback as the adolescent struggles with decisions. Help him or her make effective choices by fostering a sense of self- importance (he or she is a valuable and valued individual). Helping the person look ahead to the future in terms of values, goals, and consequences of behavior can strengthen a sense of what is significant in life and a resolve to live so the values and goals are fulfilled and positive consequences are achieved.

Both individual and group counseling are useful. In the group setting the adolescent may be asked to bring a close friend or parent to share the experience. Some concerns and conflicts, however, are best worked through with the individual. Group sessions are effective for the following reasons (138, 197):

1. The person realizes concerns, feelings, and sense of confusion are not unique to him or her.
2. Experiences and successful solutions to problems can be shared with others who are at different points of development.
3. Ideas and roles can be tried out in the group before being tried in real life.
4. Values can be clarified and decisions made with support and feedback from others.

Tauer (197) describes a number of group exercises that can be used. Additional information on counseling methods is also available (121, 138).

Care Related to Sexuality

Personal Attitudes. First examine personal attitudes toward yourself as a sexual being, the sexuality of others, family, love, and changing mores regarding sexual intercourse before you do any sex education through formal or informal teaching, counseling, or discussion. How objective are you? Can you talk calmly about biologic reproduction and use the proper anatomic terms? Can you relate biologic information to the scope of family life? Can you emotionally accept that masturbation, homosexuality, intimacy between unmarried persons, unwed pregnancy, sexually transmitted diseases, and unusual sexual practices exist? Can you listen to others talk about these subjects? If you cannot, let some other nurse do sex education.

The adolescent may be trying to understand another kind of sexual experience in his or her own family. For example, a number of adolescents have to deal with the formerly hidden primary sexual orientation of their parents. Either parent may, during this time, announce a same-sexed preference, so in addition to the adolescent's working out his or her own sexual identity, the identity of the parent must be reworked. If you cannot handle these issues, let some other appropriate professional provide sex education and counseling about being lesbian or gay (40).

Realize that no one can do all areas of nursing intervention. Your astute assessment, case finding, and ability to refer the adolescent elsewhere are still major contributions toward helping him or her stay healthy. The rapport necessary to work with the adolescent in any area is highly sensitive, and if he or she has no rapport with the family, your attitudes are crucial.

Promoting Education. You can promote education about sexuality, family, pregnancy, contraceptives, and sexually transmitted diseases through your own intervention and by working with parents and school officials so that objective, accurate information can be given in the schools. Most adults favor sex education in school and on television as a way to reduce the problem of teenage pregnancy.

Teenagers need the opportunity to identify what they consider important problems and a chance to discuss their feelings, attitudes, and ideas and to obtain factual information and guidance with effective solutions (Fig. 11–2). The sex act should be discussed as part of a relationship between individuals requiring a deep sense of love, trust, and intimacy and not just as a means of biologic gratification. Sexual behavior is not solely a physical phenomenon but one of great psychosocial significance. The consequences of sexual activity must be explored honestly. More progressive schools include this in the curriculum, and the teacher or school nurse must be comfortable, knowledgeable, and able to promote discussion. Studies show that 15- and 16-year-olds that have participated in sex education are less likely to engage in sexual behavior. Sex education courses given outside the home supplement the influence of parental guidance and teaching (198).

Such sex education and related discussions can also be offered through church youth groups, the Red Cross, local YMCA or YWCA, or other public organizations. Again, you can initiate and participate in such programs.

Perhaps most important, you can encourage the teenager and family to talk together and can teach the

Figure 11-2. Nurses should encourage adolescents to discuss health concerns and provide teaching for the issues that are important to this age group. (Courtesty of Mary Ann Scoloveno.)

parents how and what to teach, where to get information, and the significance of formal sex education beginning in the home. References at the end of the chapter can be helpful in sexuality counseling (69, 83, 113, 116, 134, 166, 197, 201).

Care and Counseling. You may work directly with a pregnant teenager or one with a sexually transmitted disease as a school or clinic nurse or in your primary-care practice. That person needs your acceptance, support, and confidentiality as you do careful interviewing to learn his or her history of sexual activity, symptoms, and contacts. Effective interviewing, communication, and crisis intervention discussed by Murray and Huelskoetter (138) are essential to reduce unwanted consequences of sexual activity. Because of the stigma and legal problems associated with unwed pregnancy, abortion, and sexually transmitted diseases, fear of reprisals, and the quixotic personality of the adolescent, your behavior at the first meeting is crucial. You may not get another chance for thorough assessment or beginning intervention.

Basically, the teen with a sexually transmitted disease wants your help and comfort; he or she is a troubled person. Information is needed about the type of disease, symptoms, the contagious nature, consequences of untreated disease, and where to get treatment. In all of these diseases, both male and female partners (along with any other person who has had sexual contact with these partners) should be treated by medication and use of hygiene measures and by counseling and teaching. You are in a key position to determine signs and symptoms and to help make a differential diagnosis. Refer to references at the end of the chapter that were cited earlier. You can also teach about the importance of continued body hygiene, avoiding unprescribed douching or other self-medication, the danger of continued reinfection from sexual intercourse, and the long-term damage to genital tissue from any sexually transmitted disease or repeated abortions. Remind your clients that the *symptoms* of the disease may go away, but the *disease* may not. Hence a complete round of treatment is essential. Further, there are two reliable ways to prevent infection or reinfection: abstinence or the male's use of a condom. One sexual contact is all that is necessary to acquire sexually transmitted diseases.

The girl wants to confirm whether pregnancy exists and talk about personal feelings, family reactions, and what to do next. Explain what services are available and answer her questions about the consequences of remaining pregnant, keeping or placing the baby for adoption, or terminating pregnancy.

Comprehensive maternity services for pregnant adolescents can reduce maternal and neonatal complications, including prematurity, low birthweight, congenital defects, and infant death so often found in this age group. Various references at the end of this chapter are helpful (63, 69, 88, 167, 201, 224, 229).

An adolescent girl may want to know about methods of abortion and services available. Reputable abortion clinics do counseling before the abortion so that the girl does not regret her decision, but you can begin counseling. The questions you raise and guidance you give can help her make necessary decisions (138).

Many states have the law that a minor can be treated for sexually transmitted diseases and other conditions without parental consent. Although this law prevents parents from being with their child in a serious situation, it does enable minors to receive treatment without fear of parental retribution and without having to wait until parents feel ready. Encourage the adolescent to confide in the parents if at all possible and to seek their support. In turn, encourage the parents to be supportive. Consent and confidentiality are key concerns in all areas of health care of the adolescent: emergency care and treatment for drug abuse, alcoholism, sexually transmitted disease, pregnancy, and other problems. Be familiar with local and state legislation and federal policies dealing with legal age and treatment of minors.

Reforming the Present Health Care System. Reforming the present health care system seems essential since present public health services are frequently incapable of kindly or completely handling the problems resulting from adolescents' sexual activity, either because of policy, philosophy, understaffing, or underfinancing. You can participate in change by working through your professional organization and as an informed citizen. You can promote a deeper awareness of the adolescent as an individual with unique needs and work to extend education and counseling services, including peer-group counseling and teenage advisory boards. Further, you can help establish community services to work with the adolescent or youth in a health care crisis. The disabled adolescent also requires special care and teaching needs.

Working with the Drug Abuser and Alcoholic

Personal Attitudes. You must work through your attitudes about drug use and abuse to assess the person accurately or intervene objectively. Why does a drug problem exist? Do you believe drugs are the answer to problems? How frequently do you use drugs? Do you use amphetamines or barbiturates? Have you ever tried marijuana, LSD, or heroin? What are the multiple influences causing persons to seek answers through using illegal drugs? What are the moral, spiritual, emotional, and physical implications of excessive drug use, whether the drugs are illegal or prescribed? What treatment do drug abusers deserve? How does the alcoholic differ from the drug abuser? Until you can face these questions, you will not be able to help the adolescent drug abuser or alcoholic.

An accepting attitude toward the drug abuser and alcoholic as a person is essential while at the same time you help him or her become motivated and able to cope with stresses without relying on drugs or alcohol. You will need to use effective communication and assessment, but since these problems are complex, you need to work with others. The treatment team should consist of other health care professionals, representatives from law enforcement and religious agencies, and self-help groups established in various cities by previous drug or alcohol abusers who have been rehabilitated and now seek to rehabilitate others.

Various references at the end of this chapter, which were cited previously, provide more detailed information to aid you in your care.

Members of society impose heavy responsibilities on the young adult. With your intervention, some adolescents who could not otherwise meet these forthcoming demands will exert a positive force in society.

Knowledge. Knowledge about drugs—current ones available on the street, their symptoms and long-term effects, legislation related to each—is necessary for assessment, realistic teaching, and counseling. Also learn about the effects of alcohol. Know local community agencies that do emergency or follow-up care and rehabilitation with drug abusers and alcoholics.

Help teenagers understand that problems of drug abuse and alcoholism can be avoided in several ways. They must get accurate information and make decisions based on knowledge rather than on emotion, have the courage to say "no," and know and respect the laws. They must also participate in worthwhile, satisfying activities, have a constructive relationship with parents, and recognize that the normal, healthy person does not need regular medication except when prescribed by a doctor. Help youths realize the unanticipated consequences of drug and alcohol abuse: loss of friends; alienation from family; loss of scholastic, social, or career opportunities; economic difficulties; criminal activities; legal penalties; poor health; and loss of identity rather than finding the self.

Every person with whom you work is a potential drug abuser or addict, and all drugs and chemical substances have a potential for harm from allergy, side effects, toxicity, or overdosage. Different drugs taken simultaneously may have an unpredictable or increased effect. In addition, taking unprescribed drugs may mask signs and symptoms of serious disease, thus postponing necessary diagnosis and treatment. Hence a major responsibility on your part is to teach others how to take drugs safely, the importance of taking only prescribed drugs as directed, and the hazards of drugs. Adolescents may not realize that drugs obtained illegally have an unknown purity and strength and are frequently produced under unsanitary conditions. They may not realize that when injections are given without sterile technique, infectious hepatitis, AIDS, tetanus, or vein damage may result. Help parents realize the impact their behavior and attitudes toward drug and alcohol use have on their children.

REFERENCES

1. Acee, A., and D. Smith, Crack, *American Journal of Nursing,* 87, no. 5 (1987), 614–617.
2. Acock, A., and J. Kiecolt, Is It Family Structure or Socio-economic Status? Family Structure During Adolescence and Adult Adjustment, *Social Forces,* 68, no. 2 (1989), 553–571.
3. Adams, B., Adolescent Health Care: Needs, Priorities, and Services, *Nursing Clinics of North American,* 18, no. 2 (1983), 237–248.
4. Adeyanju, M., et al., A Three-year Study of Obesity and Its Relationship to High Blood Pressure in Adolescents, *Journal of School Health,* 57, no. 3 (1987), 109–113.
5. Alcohol-Related Deaths May Be More Common Than Thought, *Nation's Health,* (September 1987), 3.
6. American Academy of Pediatrics, Committee on Infectious Diseases: Prevention of Hepatitis B Virus Infections, *Pediatrics,* 75, no. 2 (1985), 362–364.
7. ——, Committee on Infectious Diseases: Recommendations for Using Pneumococcal Vaccine in Children, *Pediatrics,* 75, no. 6 (1985), 1153–1158.
8. ——, *Report of the Committee on Infectious Diseases.* Elk Grove Village, Ill: American Academy of Pediatrics, 1988.
9. Andrus, J., et al., Surveillance of Attempted Suicide Among Adolescents in Oregon, 1988, *American Journal of Public Health,* 81, no. 8 (1991), 1067–1069.
10. Anorexia May Have Effect on Brain, Bones, Studies Show, *Health Scene,* (Fall 1987), 3.
11. Atkin, C., Effects of Televised Alcohol Messages on Teenage Drinking Problems, *Journal of Adolescent Health Care,* 11, no. 1 (1990), 10–24.
12. Austin, J., V. Champion, and O. Tzeng, Cross-Cultural Relationships Between Self-Concept and Body Image in High School Age Boys, *Archives of Psychiatric Nursing,* 3, no. 4 (1989), 234–240.
13. Bachman, J., et al., Racial/Ethnic Differences in Smoking, Drinking, and Illicit Drug Use Among American High School Seniors, 1976–89, *American Journal of Public Health,* 81, no. 3 (1991), 372–377.
14. Bates, B., *A Guide to Physical Examination and History Taking* (4th ed.). Philadelphia: J.B. Lippincott, 1987.
15. Berry, R., Home Care of the Child with AIDS, *Pediatric Nursing,* 4 (July-August, 1988), 341–344.
16. Bettelheim, B., and A. Freedgood, *A Good Enough Parent: A Book on Child-Rearing.* New York: Random, 1988.
17. Bettes, B., et al., Ethnicity and Psychosocial Factors in Alcohol and Tobacco Use in Adolescence, *Child Development,* 61, no. 2 (1990), 557–565.
18. Boggs, K., Pubertal Stress and Social Support-Seeking Behavior in Early Adolescents, *Journal of Pediatric Nursing,* 3, no. 4 (1988), 229–236.
19. Bolger, N., et al., The Onset of Suicidal Ideation in Childhood and Adolescence, *Journal of Youth and Adolescence,* 18, no. 2 (1989), 175–190.
20. Boyd, M., Living With Overweight, *Perspectives in Psychiatric Care,* 25, no. 3, 4 (1989), 48–52.
21. Burgess, A., and H.J. Birnbaum, Youth Prostitution, *American Journal of Nursing,* 82, no. 5(1982), 832–834.
22. ——, and L. Holmstrom, The Rape Victim in the Emergency Ward, *American Journal of Nursing,* 73, no. 10 (1973), 1741–1745.
23. Burgess, J., *Children, Adolescents and Nutrition.* New York: Grollier, 1988.
24. Butler, J., and L. Burton, Rethinking Teenage Childbearing: Is Sexual Abuse a Missing Link? *Family Relations* (January 1990), 73–79.
25. Canadian Guidelines for the Treatment of Sexually Transmitted Diseases in Neonates, Children, Adolescents, and Adults, *Canadian Disease Weekly Report* (April 1988), 1452.
26. Center for Disease Control: 1985 STD Treatment Guidelines, *MMWR* (October 18, 1985), 34, 35, 45.
27. Centers for Disease Control: *AIDS Weekly Surveillance Report - United States.* Atlanta: Centers for Disease Control, July 18, 1988.
28. Chirgwin, K., et al., HIV Infection, Genital Ulcer Disease, and Crack Cocaine Use Among Patients Attending a Clinic for Sexually Transmitted Diseases, *American Journal of Public Health,* 81, no. 12 (1991), 1576–1579.
29. Clemen-Stone, S., D.G. Eigsti, and S.L. McGuire, *Comprehensive Family and Community Health Nursing* (3rd ed.). St. Louis: Mosby–Year Book, 1991.
30. Cocaine, Glamorous Status Symbol of the "Jet Set," Is Fast Becoming Many Students' Drug of Choice, *Chronicle of Higher Education,* 31, no. 11 (November 12, 1985), 33–35.
31. Cocaine Toxicity, *National Institute of Drug Abuse Notes,* Washington, D.C.: U.S. Department of Health and Human Services, 1990, pp. 2, 3.

32. College Alcohol Problem Not a Class Act, *University News* (St. Louis U.), February 17, 1989, p. 3.

33. Congenital Syphilis Soars in N.Y.C.: Sex-for-Drugs Trade Pushes U.S. Syphilis Rates Up, *Nation's Health* (January 1990), 17.

34. Cookfair, J., *Nursing Process and Practice in the Community*. St. Louis: Mosby–Year Book, 1991.

35. The Crack Children, *Newsweek,* (February 12, 1990), 60–63.

36. *Crack: The New Cocaine.* Phoenix; DIN Publications, 1989.

37. Craft, M., Health Care Preferences of Rural Adolescents: Types of Service and Companion Choices, *Journal of Pediatric Nursing,* 2, no. 1 (1987), 3–12.

38. Daley, S., Little Girls Lose Their Self-Esteem on Way to Adolescence, Study Finds, *New York Times,* January 9, 1991, p.10.

39. Dangerous Alliance: Family Dysfunction, Adolescent Curiosity Leads Teens to Drugs, *West Citizen Journal* (St. Louis County), June 23, 1989, p. 1.

40. Deevy, S., When Mom or Dad Comes Out: Helping Adolescents Cope with Homophobia, *Journal of Psychosocial Nursing,* 27, no. 10 (1989), 35–36.

41. Demetrulias, D., and R. Shaw, Encouraging Divergent Thinking, *Nurse Educator,* 10, 6 (1985), 12–17.

42. Desmond, S.M., et al., Black and White Adolescents; Perceptions of Their Weight, *Journal of School Health,* 59, no. 8 (1989), 353–358.

43. Dickerson, J., Oral Contraceptives: Another Look, *American Journal of Nursing,* 83, no. 10 (1983), 1392–1398.

44. Diekstra, R.F., and K. Hawton, *Suicide in Adolescence.* Boston: Martinus Nighoff, 1987.

45. Dietz, W.H., You Are What You Eat—What You Eat is What You Are, *Journal of Adolescent Health Care,* 11, no. 1 (1990), 76–81.

46. Dirubbo, N., The Condom Barrier, *American Journal of Nursing,* 87, no. 10 (1987), 1306–1309.

47. Does Your College Bound Teenager Need a Measles Shot, *American Journal of Nursing,* 87, no. 6 (1987), 766–768.

48. Dorn, L.D., et al., Perceptions of Puberty: Adolescent, Parent, and Health Care Personnel, *Developmental Psychology,* 26, no. 2 (1990). 322–329.

49. Dornbusch, S., The Sociology of Adolescence, *Annual Review of Sociology,* 15, (1989), 233–259.

50. Drewnowski, A., S. Hopkins, and R. Kessler, The Prevalence of Bulimia Nervosa in the US College Student Population, *American Journal of Public Health,* 78 (1988), 1322–1325.

51. The Drug Advisory, St. Louis: National Council on Alcoholism and Drug Dependence, 1990.

52. The Drug War: The Wrong Efforts Aimed at Lesser Problems, *Nation's Health* (March 1990), 20.

53. Dukes, R., and B.D. Lorch, The Effects of School, Family, Self-Concept, and Behavior on Adolescent Suicide Ideation, *Journal of Adolescence,* 12, no. 3 (1989), 239– 251.

54. Duvall, E., and B. Miller, *Marriage and Family Development* (6th ed.). New York: Harper & Row, 1984.

55. Dworetzky, J., and N. Davis, *Human Development: A Lifespan Approach.* St. Paul: West Publishing, 1989.

56. Earls, F., Studying Adolescent Suicidal Ideation and Behavior in Primary Care Settings, *Suicide and Life Threatening Behavior,* 19, no. 1 (1989), 99–107.

57. Eating Disorders—Not for Women Only, *Health Scene* (Fall 1987), 10.

58. Edmonds, M., Overcoming Eating Disorders: A Group Experience, *Journal of Psychosocial Nursing,* 24, no. 8 (1986), 19–25.

59. Effects of Drug Use on Immune System, *National Institute of Drug Abuse Notes.* Washington, D.C.: U.S. Department of Health and Human Services, 1986, pp. 4–6.

60. Elkind, D., The Facts About Teen Suicide, *Parents,* 65, no. 1 (1990), 111.

61. Elliott, D., L. Goldberg, and D.B. Girard, Obesity: Pathophysiology and Practical Management, *Journal of General Internal Medicine,* 2, (1987), 188–196.

62. Erikson, E.H., *Childhood and Society* (2nd ed.). New York: W.W. Norton, 1963.

63. - —, *Identity: Youth and Crisis.* New York: W.W. Norton, 1968.

64. ——, Memorandum on Youth. In Sze W., ed., *Human Life Cycle.* New York: Jason Aronson, 1975, pp. 351–359.

65. *Fact Sheet: Alcohol and Drug Use by Teenagers.* Jefferson City, Mo: Missouri Department of Mental Health, 1991.

66. Fenzel, M., Role Strain in Early Adolescence: A Model for Investigating School Transition Stress, *Journal of Early Adolescence,* 9, no. 1–2 (1989), 13–33.

67. The Fire of Ice, *Newsweek* (November 29, 1989), 37.

68. Flood, M., Addictive Eating Disorders, *Nursing Clinics of North America,* 24, no. 1 (1989), 45–53.

69. Foster, R., M. Hunsberger, and J. Anderson, *Family-Centered Nursing Care of Children.* Philadelphia: W.B. Saunders, 1989.

70. Friedrick, N., et al., Sex Differences in Depression in Early Adolescents, *Psychological Reports,* 62 (1988), 475–481.

71. Garbarino, J., E. Guttman, and J. Seeley, *The Psychologically Battered Child: Strategies for Identification, Assessment, and Intervention.* San Francisco: Jossey-Bass, 1987.

72. Garrison, C., The Study of Suicidal Behavior in the Schools, *Suicide and Life Threatening Behavior,* 19, no. 1 (1989), 120–130.

73. Gastric Balloon for Treatment of Obesity, *Medical Letter,* 28 (1986), 77–78.

74. Gesell, A., F. Ilg, and L. Ames, *Youth: The Years from Ten to Sixteen.* New York: Harper Brothers, 1956.

75. Goldberg, B., Injury Patterns in Youth Sports, *Physician and Sports Medicine,* 17, no. 3 (1989), 174–176.

76. Gould, M., et al., Suicide Clusters: An Examination of Age-Specific Effects, *American Journal of Public Health,* 80, no. 2 (1990), 211–212.

77. Grieve, N., et al., Self-Esteem and Sex-Role Attitudes: A Comparison of Italian and Anglo-Australian Adolescent Girls, *Psychology of Women Quarterly,* 12, no. 6 (1988), 175–189.

78. Grossman, D., C. Milligan, and R. Deyo, Risk Factors for Suicide Attempts Among Navajo Adolescents, *American Journal of Public Health,* 80, no. 2 (1990), 870–874.

79. Guidelines for Teenage Parties, *Olivette Advisory* (Olivette, Mo.), 6, no. 4 (January 1983).

80. Guio, M.V., et al., Child Victimization, Pornography, and Prostitution, *Crime and Justice,* 3 (1980), 65–81.

81. Hall, J., and P. Stevens, AIDS: A Guide to Suicide Assessment, *Archives of Psychiatric Nursing,* 1, no. 2 (1988), 115–120.

82. Hall, P., and S. Holch, Injectable Contraceptive, *World Health* (May 1982), 2–4.

83. Hammes, M., and E. Duryee, Cognitive Development and The Dynamics of Decision-Making Among Adolescents, *Journal of School Health,* 56, no. 6 (1986), 224–226.

84. Hatcher, R., et al., *Contraceptive Technology—1990–1992* (15th ed.). New York: Irvington, 1992.

85. Hatton, C., and S. Valente, *Suicide: Assessment and Intervention.* Norwalk, Conn: Appleton-Century-Crofts, 1984.

86. Havighurst, R., *Developmental Tasks and Education* (3rd ed.). New York: David McKay, 1972.

87. Hawton, K., *Suicide and Attempted Suicide Among Children and Adolescents.* Beverly Hills, Calif: Sage Publishers, 1990.

88. Hedahl, K., Assisting the Adolescent With Physical Disabilities Through a College Health Program, *Nursing Clinics of North America,* 15, no. 2 (1983), 357–374.

89. Hegarty, V., *Decisions in Nutrition.* St. Louis: Times Mirror/Mosby College Publishers, 1988.

90. Heiney, S., Helping Children Through Painful Procedures, *American Journal of Nursing,* 91, no. 11 (1991), 20–24.

91. Herman, J., Recognition and Treatment of Incestuous Families, *International Journal of Family Therapy,* 5, no. 2 (1983), 81–91.

92. *Heroin: The Junk Equation.* Phoenix: D.I.N., 1985.

93. Hoffman, L., et al., *Developmental Psychology Today* (5th ed.). New York: Random, 1988.

94. Hoole, A.J., R.A. Greenberg, and A.G. Pickard, Jr., *Patient Care Guidelines for Nurse Practitioners* (3rd ed.). Boston: Little, Brown, 1988.

95. Horwitz, E., World, Here We Come (An Alternate Public School for Pregnant and Parenting Teens), *AAWW Outlook,* 85, no. 3 (1991), 14–19.

96. House, M., Cocaine, *American Journal of Nursing,* 90, no. 4 (1990), 41–45.

97. Hubbard, G., Perceived Life Changes for Children and Adolescents Following Disclosure of Father-Daughter Incest, *Journal of Child and Adolescent Psychiatric and Mental Health Nursing,* 2, no. 2 (1989), 78–82.

98. Hulka, B.D., et al., Protection Against Endometrial Carcinoma by Combination Product Oral Contraceptives, *Journal American Medical Association,* 247 (January 22–29, 1989), 475–477.

99. *Ice: Speed, Smoke, and Fire.* Phoenix: D.I.N., 1991.

100. *Inhalants: Just Say No.* Washington, D.C.: National Institute on Drug Abuse, 1986.

101. Jackson, P.L., and M.J. Ott, Precocious Puberty: The Role of the School Nurse, *School Nurse,* 6, no. 1 (1990), 16–18.

102. Joe, G., and D. Simpson, Mortality Rates Among Opioid Addicts in a Longitudinal Study, *American Journal of Public Health,* 77, no. 3 (1987), 347–348.

103. Johnson, J., Sexually Transmitted Diseases in Adolescents, *Primary Care,* (March 14, 1987), 100–120.

104. Jones, J., A Proposed Model of Relapse Prevention for Adolescents Who Abuse Alcohol, *Journal of Child and Adolescent Psychiatric and Mental Health Nursing,* 3, no. 4 (1990), 139–143.

105. Kafka, R., and P. London, Communication in Relationships and Adolescent Substance Use: The Influence of Parents and Friends, *Adolescence,* 26, no. 103 (Fall 1991), 587–597.

106. Keniston, K., Youth: A New Stage of Life, *American Scholar,* 39 (1970), 631–654.

107. ——, Youth as a Stage of Life. In Sze, W., ed., *Human Life Cycle.* New York: Jason Aronson, 1975, 332–349.

108. Kiecolt-Glaser, J., and K. Davis, Post-Adolescent Onset Male Anorexia, *Journal of Psychosocial Nursing,* 22, no. 1 (1982).

109. Kirkis, E., and M. Grier, *Nurse's Guide to Infection Control Practice.* Philadelphia: W.B. Saunders, 1988.

110. Kirshnit, C., M. Ham, and M. Richards, The Sporting Life: Athletic Activities During Early Adolescence, *Journal of Youth and Adolescence,* 18, no. 6 (1989), 601–615.

111. Kohlberg, L., Moral Stages and Moralization: The Cognitive Development Approach. In Lickera, T., ed., *Moral Development and Behavior.* New York: Holt, Rineholt, & Winston, 1976.

112. Kokkeui, A., and C. Stefanos, The Epidemiology of Licit and Illicit Substance Use Among High School Students in Greece, *American Journal of Public Health,* 81, no. 1 (1991), 48–52.

113. Lamb, M., *The Father's Role.* New York: John Wiley, 1986.

114. Lee, D., and L. Bermann, Teen-age Parents Talk About School: Meanings for the Cirriculum, *Educational Forum,* 31, no. 4 (1987), 355–375.

115. Levy, J., and E. Deykin, Suicidality, Depression, and Substance Abuse in Adolescence, *American Journal of Psychiatry,* 146, no. 11 (1989), 1462–1467.

116. Lidz, T., *The Person—His and Her Development Throughout the Life Cycle* (2nd ed.). New York: Basic Books, 1983.

117. Loucks, A., Chlamydia: An Unheralded Epidemic, *American Journal of Nursing,* 87, no. 7 (1987), 920–922.

118. Lynam, M.J., and L. Tenn, Communication: A Tool for the Negotiation of Independence in Families with Adolescents, *Journal of Advanced Nursing,* 14, no. 8 (1989), 653–660.

119. Manning, M., Disappearing Childhood: 6 Going on 16, *Kappa Delta Pi Record* (Fall 1985), 14–18.

120. Manning, M., Health Assessment of the Early Adolescent: Challenges and Clinical Issues, *Nursing Clinics of North America,* 25, no. 4 (1990), 823–831.

121. Manov, A., and L. Lowther, A Health Care Approach for Hard-to-Reach Adolescent Runaways, *Nursing Clinics of North America,* 18, no. 2 (1983), 333–341.

122. Marchi, M., and P. Cohen, Early Childhood Eating Behaviors and Adolescent Eating Disorders, *Journal American Academy of Child-Adolescent Psychiatry,* 29, no. 1 (1990), 112–117.

123. Martin, M., and M. Pritchard, Factors Associated with Alcohol Use in Later Adolescence, *Journal of Studies on Alcohol,* 52, no. 1 (1991), 5–9.

124. Mayer, S., and C. Jencks, Growing Up in Poor Neighborhoods: How Much Does It Matter? *Science,* 241 (March 17, 1989), 242–246.

125. McBride, A., *How To Enjoy a Good Life With Your Teenager.* Tucson, Ariz: Fischer Books, 1989.

126. Meares, P., Depression in Childhood and Adolescence, *Social Work,* 32, no. 6 (1987), 512–515.

127. Melton, J., A Boy With Anorexia Nervosa, *American Journal of Nursing,* 74, no. 9 (1974), 1649–1651.

128. Mickley, D., Evaluating Common Eating Disorders: 10 Questions to Ask Your Patient, *Physician Assistant,* 13, no. 9 (1989), 147–148, 153, 156.

129. Miller, K., Adolescents' Same Sex and Opposite Sex Peer Relations: Sex Differences in Popularity, Perceived Social Competence, and Social Cognitive Skills, *Journal of Adolescent Research,* 5, no. 2 (1990), 222–241.

130. Mitchell, J., Adolescents Concern About Physical Examination by a Female, *Nursing Research,* 29, no. 3 (1980), 165–169.

131. Mitchell, J., et al., Characteristics of 275 Patients With Bulimia, *American Journal of Psychiatry,* 142, no. 4 (1985), 482–485.

132. Mittleman, H., R. Mittleman, and B. Elser, Cocaine, *American Journal of Nursing,* 84, no. 9 (1984), 1092–1101.

133. Monier, B., Contraceptives: A Look at the Future, *American Journal of Nursing,* 89, no. 4 (1989), 197–199.

134. Moshman, D., J. Glover, and R. Bruning, *Development Psychology.* Boston: Little, Brown, 1987.

135. Mott, S., S. James, and A. Sperhac, *Nursing Care of Children and Families* (2nd ed.). Redwood City, Calif: Addison-Wesley, 1990.

136. Mullis, R., and K. McKinley, Gender Role Orientation of Adolescent Females: Effects on Self-Esteem and Locus of Control, *Journal of Adolescent Research,* 4, no. 4 (1989), 506–516.

137. Munhall, P., Moral Reasoning Levels of Nursing Students and Faculty in a Baccalaureate Nursing Program, *Image,* 12, no. 3 (1980), 57–61.

138. Murray, R., and M.M. Huelskoetter, *Psychiatric/Mental Health Nursing: Giving Emotional Care* (3rd ed.). Norwalk, Conn: Appleton & Lange, 1989.

139. Muscari, M., Obtaining the Adolescent Sexual History, *Pediatric Nursing,* 5 (October 13, 1987), 307–310.

140. Myers, D., and A. Anderson, Adolescent Addiction: Assessment and Identification, *Journal of Pediatric Health Care,* 5, no. 2 (1991), 86–93.

141. Nathanson, C., and M. Becker, The Influence of Client-Provider Relationships on Teenage Women's Subsequent Use of Contraception, *American Journal of Public Health,* 75, no. 1 (1985), 33–38.

142. National Center for Health Statistics, *Health,* No. PHS 84–1232. Washington D.C.: U.S. Government Printing Office, 1987.

143. Newman, B., The Changing Nature of the Parent-Adolescent Relationship From Early to Late Adolescence, *Adolescence,* 24, no. 96 (1989), 915–924.

144. ———, and Philip Newman, *Development Through Life: A Psychosocial Approach* (5th ed.). Pacific Grove, Calif: Brooks/Cole, 1991.

145. Nkowane, B., et al., Measles Outbreak in a Vaccinated School Population: Epidemiology, Chains of Transmission, and the Role of Vaccine Failures, *American Journal of Public Health,* 77, no. 4 (1987). 434–438.

146. Norris, J., and M. Kunes-Carroll, Self-Esteem Disturbance, *Nursing Clinics of North America,* 20, no. 4 (1985), 745–761.

147. Oehler, J., and M. Burnes, Anorexia, Bulimia, and Sexuality: Case Study of an Adolescent Inpatient Group, *Archives of Psychiatric Nursing,* 1, no. 3 (1987), 163–171.

148. Oldaker, S., Identity Confusion: Nursing Diagnoses for Adolescents, *Nursing Clinics of North America,* 20, no. 4 (1985), 763–773.

149. Osofsky, J., A. Culp, and L. Ware, Intervention Challenges With Adolescent Mothers and Their Infants, *Psychiatry,* 51, no. 8 (1988), 236–241.

150. Oswald, L., Cocaine Addiction: The Hidden Dimension, *Archives of Psychiatric Nursing,* 3, no. 3 (1989), 134–141.

151. Ott, M.J., and P.L. Jackson, Precocious Puberty: Identifying Early Sexual Development, *Nurse Practitioner: American Journal of Primary Health Care,* 14, no. 11 (1989), 21, 24–28, 30.

152. Otto, L., America's Youth: A Changing Profile, *Family Relations,* 37, no. 4 (1988), 385–391.

153. Overeaters Anonymous: A Self-Help Group, *American Journal of Nursing,* 81, no. 3 (1981), 560–563.

154. Pardeck, J., and J. Pardeck, Family Factors Related to Adolescent Autonomy, *Adolescence,* 25, no. 98 (1990), 311–319.

155. Parish, T., Evaluations of Family by Youth: Do They Vary as a Function of Family Structure, Gender, and Birth Order? *Adolescence,* 25, no. 98 (1990), 353–356.

156. Paxman, J.M., and R.J. Zuckerman, *Laws and Policies Affecting Adolescent Health.* Geneva: World Health Organization, 1987.

157. Pender, N.J., Expressing Health Through Lifestyle Patterns, *Nursing Science Quarterly,* 3, no. 3 (1990), 115–122.

158. Petersen, A., Those Gangly Years, *Psychology Today,* 21, no. 9 (1987), 28–35.

159. Pfeffer, C., *The Suicidal Child.* New York: Guilford Press, 1986.

160. Phipps, W., et al., eds., *Medical-Surgical Nursing: Concepts and Clinical Practice* (4th ed.). St. Louis: Mosby–Year Book, 1991.

161. Piaget, J., The Growth of Logical Thinking from Childhood to Adolescence. New York: Basic Books, 1961.

162. Pill Benefits Outweigh Risks in Young Women, Says Report, *Nation's Health,* 11, no. 2 (1981), 4.

163. Plant, M.A., J. Orford, and M. Grant, The Effects on Children and Adolescents of Parents' Excessive Drinking: An International Review, *Public Health Reports,* 104, no. 5 (1989), 433–442.

164. Polk-Walker, G., What Really Happened? Incidence and Factor Assessment of Abused Children and Adolescents, *Journal of Psychosocial Nursing,* 28, no. 11 (1990), 17–22.

165. Poole, C., Adolescent Pregnancy and Unfinished Developmental Tasks of Childhood, *Journal of School Health,* 57, no. 7 (1987), 271–273.

166. Proctor, S., A Developmental Approach to Pregnancy Prevention With Early Adolescent Females, *Journal of School Health,* 56, no. 1 (1986), 313–316.

167. Romig, C., and G. Thompson, Teen-age Pregnancy: A Family Systems Approach, *American Journal of Family Therapy,* 16, (1988), 133–143.

168. Rotheram-Borus, M.J., Ethnic Differences in Adolescents' Identity Status and Associated Behavior Problems. *Journal of Adolescence,* 12, no. 4 (1989), 361–374.

169. ——, Evaluation of Suicide Risk Among Youths in Community Settings, *Suicide and Life Threatening Behavior,* 19, no. 1 (1989), 108–119.

170. Rothman, K., Spermicide Use and Down's Syndrome, *American Journal of Public Health,* 72, no. 4 (1982), 399–401.

171. Runyon, N., and P. Jackson, Divorce: The Impact on Children, *Perspectives in Psychiatric Care,* 24, nos. 3–4, (1987/1988), 101–105.

172. Rush, K.L., The School Nurse and Sport Nutrition for the Adolescent Athlete, *Journal of School Health,* 60, no. 8 (1990), 425–427.

173. Ryerson, D., Suicide Awareness Education in Schools: The Development of a Core Program and Subsequent Modifications for Special Populations or Institutions. *Death Studies,* 14, no. 4 (1990), 371–390.

174. Sachs, B., Reproductive Decisions in Adolescence, *Nursing Clinics of North America,* 18, no. 2 (1986), 69–72.

175. Samkoff, J., and S. Baker, Recent Trends in Fatal Poisoning by Opiates in the United States, *American Journal of Public Health,* 72, no. 11 (1982), 1251–1256.

176. Saying No to Crack Gangs, *Newsweek* (March 28, 1988), 29.

177. Schaffner, A., and D. Dieterich, Streetwise Narcotic Safety: Precautions in Home Care, *American Journal of Nursing,* 86, no. 6 (1986), 707–708.

178. Scherer, P., How AIDS Attacks the Brain, *American Journal of Nursing,* 90, no. 1 (1990), 44–52.

179. Scherwets, P., An Alcohol Treatment Team, *American Journal of Nursing,* 82, no. 12 (1982), 1878–1879.

180. Schwart, R.H., et al., Drinking Patterns and Social Consequences: A Study of Middle-Class Adolescents in Two Private Pediatric Practices, *Pediatrics,* 77 (1986), 139–143.

181. Sebald, H., Adolescents' Peer Orientation: Changes in the Support System During the Past Three Decades, *Adolescence,* 24, no. 96 (1989), 937–946.

182. Sherman, J., and S. Fields, *Guide to Patient Evaluation* (5th ed.). Garden City, NY: Medical Examination, 1987.

183. Sherraden, M., School Dropouts in Perspective, *Education Forum,* 51, no. 1 (1986), 15–31.

184. Short-Term Marijuana Effects of National Concern, Says IOM, *Nation's Health,* 12, no. 4 (1982), 10.

185. Slap, G.B., et al., Risk Factors for Attempted Suicide During Adolescence, *Pediatrics,* 84, no. 5 (1989), 762–772.

186. Smith, D., Meeting the Psychosocial Needs of Teenage Mothers and Fathers, *Nursing Clinics of North America,* 19, no. 2 (1984), 369–379.

187. Spence, W., *Hallucinogens: Trip or Trap?* Waco, Tex: Health Ed., 1988.

188. Spitzer, M., and B. Krumholz, Pap Screening for Teenagers: A Lifesaving Precaution, *Contemporary Pediatrics,* 4, no. 5 (1987), 41–49.

189. Staus, H., From Crack to Ecstasy, *American Heath* (June 1987), 50–53.

190. Steinhard, A.J., G.H. Foster, and R.F. Grossman, Surgical Treatment of Obesity, *Advanced Psychosomatic Medicine,* 15, (1986), 140–166.

191. Stewart, D., Sexuality and the Adolescent: Issues for the Clinician, *Primary Care,* 1 (March 14, 1987), 83–99.

192. Stiffman, A., Suicide Attempts in Runaway Youths, *Suicide and Life Threatening Behavior,* 19, no. 2 (1989), 147–159.

193. The Streets Are Filled With Coke, *U.S. News and World Report* (March 5, 1990), 24–26.

194. Study Shows That TV Suicide Dramas May Contribute to Teen Suicide, *Journal of Child Adolescent Psychotherapy,* 4, no. 2 (1987), 139–140.

195. Study: Teenage Fathers Are Involved With Babies Too, *Nation's Health* (September 1986), 11.

196. Szyalo, V., Approaching Adolescents About a Pelvic Exam, *American Journal of Nursing,* 88, no. 11 (1988), 1502– 1506.

197. Tauer, K., Promoting Effective Decision-Making in Sexually Active Adolescents, *Nursing Clinics of North America,* 18, no. 2 (1983), 275–292.

198. Taylor, M.O., Teaching Parents About Their Impaired Adolescent's Sexuality, *American Journal of Maternal Child Nursing,* 14, no. 2 (1989), 109–112.

199. Teen Alcoholism Prevalent, Often Not Diagnosed, *Child and Adolescent Psychotherapy,* 4, no. 1 (1987), 53.

200. Teens Identify Worst Worries—Top 10, *Union Banner* (December 28, 1988), 10.

201. Thomas, B.H., H. Mitchell, and M.C. Devlin, *Pregnancy During Adolescence: Family Centered Nursing Care of Children.* Philadelphia: W.B. Sanders, 1989.

202. Thomas, S., and M. Groer, Relationships of Demographic, Life-Style, and Stress Variables to Blood Pressure in Adolescents, *Nursing Research,* 35, no. 3 (1986), 169–172.

203. Thompson, K., Effects of Early Alcohol Use on Adolescents' Relations With Peers and Self-Esteem: Patterns Over Time, *Adolescence,* 24, no. 96 (1989), 837–849.

204. Thorne, B., A Nurse Helps Prevent Sports Injuries, *American Journal of Maternal-Child Nursing,* 7, no. 4 (1982), 236–239.

205. Tierney, R., et al., Comprehensive School Suicide Prevention Programs, *Death Studies,* 14, no. 4 (1990), 347–370.

206. Turner, J., and D. Helms, *Lifespan Development* (3rd ed.). New York: Holt, Rinehart & Winston, 1987.

207. United States Department of Health and Human Services, *Public Health Service: Parents' Guide to Childhood Immunizations.* Atlanta: Centers for Disease Control, 1988.

208. ——, *Office of Maternal and Child Health: Child Health USA '89,* No. HRS–MCH 8915. Washington D.C.: Bureau of Maternal and Child Health Resources Development, 1989.

209. U.S. Far Exceeds Other Nations in Teen Pregnancy, *Health Link* (March 1987), 45–46.

210. Valente, S., Children, Adolescents, and Nuclear War Anxiety, *Journal of Child Psychiatric Nursing,* 1, no. 1 (1988), 36–41.

211. Values and Morality: Why Good Kids Do Bad Things, *Adolescent Counselor* (February-March 1988), 25–26.

212. Vourakis, C., and G. Bennett, Angel Dust: Not Heaven Sent, *American Journal of Nursing,* 79, no. 4 (1979), 649–653.

213. Wadsworth, B., *Piaget's Theory of Cognitive and Affective Development* (4th ed.). New York: Longman, 1989.

214. Walker, L., Coping With Drug Abuse by Children of the Wealthy; A New High-Risk Group, *Perspectives of Psychiatric Care,* 20, no. 2 (1982), 66–68.

215. Wallerstein, J., Children After Divorce: Wounds That Don't Heal, *Perspectives in Psychiatric Care,* 24, nos. 3–4 (1987/1988), 107–113.

216. Washburn, P., Identification, Assessment, and Referral of Adolescent Drug Abusers, *Pediatric Nursing,* 17, no. 2 (1991), 137–140.

217. Webb, P., Piaget: Implications for Teaching, *Theory Into Practice,* 19, no. 2 (1980), 93–97.

218. Webb, S., Some Developmental Issues of Adolescent: Children of Alcoholics, *Adolescent Counselor* (February-March 1989), 47.

219. Webber, L., et al., The Interaction of Cigarette Smoking, Oral Contraceptive Use,and Cardiovascular Risk Factor Variables in Children: The Bogalusa Heart Study, *American Journal of Public Health,* 72, no. 3 (1982), 266–274.

220. Whaley, L., and D. Wong, *Nursing Care of Infants and Children* (4th ed.). St. Louis: C.V. Mosby, 1990.

221. Whatley, J.H., Effects of Health Locus of Control and Social Network on Adolescent Risk Taking, *Pediatric Nursing,* 17, no. 2 (1991), 145–148.

222. White, J.H., Behavioral Intervention for the Obese Client, *Nursing Practice,* 11, (1986), 27–34.

223. Wilbur, R., Medicine for Addicts: Drugs That Fight Coke, *American Health* (June 1987), 44–49.

224. Williams, S.R., *Nutrition and Diet Therapy* (6th ed.). St. Louis: Times Mirror/Mosby, 1989.

225. Wintemute, G., et al., Drowning in Childhood and Adolescence: A Population-Based Study, *American Journal of Public Health,* 77, no. 7 (1987), 830–832.

226. Wright, D., ed., *Responding to the Needs of Today's Minority Students.* San Francisco: Jossey-Bass, 1987.

227. Yazigi, R., R. Odem, and K. Polakoski, Demonstration of Specific Binding of Cocaine to Human Spermatozoa, *Journal of American Medical Association,* 286, no. 14 (October 9, 1991), 1956–1959.

228. Yorker, B., The Prosecution of Child Sexual Abuse Cases, *Journal of Child Psychiatric Nursing,* 1, no. 2 (1988), 50–57.

229. Youngs, B., *A Parent's Survival Guide: Helping Your Teenager Deal With Stress.* Los Angeles: Jeremy P. Tarcher, 1986.

PERSONAL INTERVIEW

230. Leonard, J., Coordinator of Sex Education Program in Kenya, 1983.

Part IV

The Developing Person and Family: Young Adulthood Through Death

Chapter 12

Assessment and Health Promotion for the Young Adult

When I was a child I spoke as a child, I understood as a child, I thought as a child, but when I became a man (an adult), I put away childish things.
—I Corinthians 13:11

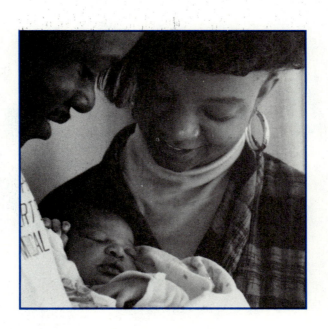

KEY TERMS

Average weight

Desirable weights

Sexuality

Gender identity

Gender role

Absolutist position

Hedonistic view

Relativistic position

Human sexual response cycle

    Vasocongestion

    Myotonia

Four phases of the cycle

    Excitement phase

    Plateau phase

    Orgasm

    Resolution phase

Mittelschmerz

Premenstrual syndrome

Homosexuals

    Homosexual man (gay)

    Homosexual woman (lesbian)

Transsexuals

Cohabitation

Biologic rhythms

    Exogenous rhythms

    Endogenous rhythms

    Circadian rhythm

Chronopharmacology

Sleep

Electroencephalogram

    Alpha rhythm

    Delta rhythm

    Sleep spindles

    K-complexes

NREM sleep

REM sleep

NREM stage I sleep

NREM stage II sleep

NREM stage III sleep

NREM stage IV sleep

Insomnia

    Primary insomnia

    Sleep onset

    Sleep maintenance

    Terminal insomnia

Physical fitness

Vascularization

Substance abuse

Burnout

Leisure

Life structure

Intimacy

Homogamy

Isolation or self-absorption

Body image

Singlehood

Announcement phase

Moratorium period

Focusing period

Amniocentesis

Infertility

Surrogate parent

Upper respiratory infection

Influenza

Essential hypertension

Mitral valve prolapse syndrome

Iron deficiency anemia

Atopic dermatitis

Folliculitis

Furuncles

Carbuncles

Urticaria

Scabies

Simple diarrhea

Cystitis

Acute pyelonephritis

Chronic fatigue syndrome

Acquired immunodeficiency syndrome

Hepatitis B

Dental caries

Periodontal disease

Lactose intolerance

Anxiety

Tension headaches

Migraine headaches

Aura

Functional bowel disease

Pediculosis

Biofeedback training

Stress reactions

Battered woman syndrome

Incest

Divorce

OBJECTIVES

Study of this chapter will enable you to:

1. Discuss young adulthood as a developmental crisis and how and why the present young adult generation differs from earlier generations.
2. Explore with middle-aged and older adults their feelings about and ways to be helpful to young adults.
3. List the developmental tasks of the young adult's family, and describe your role in helping families to meet these tasks.
4. Assess the physical characteristics of a young adult.
5. Explain facts from sex behavior research when asked for information about sexuality.
6. Teach nutritional requirements to the young adult male and female, including the pregnant and lactating female.
7. Identify various body rhythms, and give examples of body rhythms that maintain adaptation.
8. Describe factors that influence biologic rhythms, illness, and dyssynchrony that may result.
9. Discuss nursing measures to assist the person's maintenance of normal biologic rhythms during illness.
10. Compare the stages of the sleep cycle, effects of deprivation of the different stages of sleep, and sleep disturbances that occur.
11. Discuss with the young adult his or her need for rest, sleep, exercise, and leisure.
12. Assess emotional characteristics, self-concept and body image, and adaptive mechanisms of a young adult, and determine nursing implications.
13. Explore the meaning of intimacy versus isolation.
14. Contrast the life-style options of the young adult and their influence on health status and your plans for his or her care.
15. Discuss how cognitive characteristics, social concerns, and moral-spiritual-philosophic development influence the total behavior and well-being of the young adult.
16. State the developmental tasks of the young adult, and describe your role in helping him or her achieve them.
17. Assess a young adult who has one of the health problems described in this chapter, write a care plan, and work effectively with him or her to enhance health status.

When does young adulthood begin in the United States?

The person must be 18 to vote, 30 to be a senator, 35 to be the president. The woman may have her first child at 15 or at 35, or she may have none. Even with these variations the generally accepted age for young adulthood in America is about 25 to 45 years.

Childhood and adolescence are the periods for growing up; adulthood is the time for settling down. The changes in young adulthood relate more to sociocultural forces and expectations and to value and cognitive changes than to physical development. The young adult generally has more contact with people of different ages than previously. This experience tends to influence the young adult toward a more conservative, traditional viewpoint (84).

The young adult is expected to enter new roles of responsibility at work, at home, and in society and to develop values, attitudes, and interests in keeping with these roles. The young adult may have difficulty simultaneously handling work, school, marriage, home, and child rearing. He or she may work primarily at one of these tasks at a time, neglecting the others, which then adds to the difficulties (84).

During the twenties the tasks include finding an occupation, staying in one place, and establishing a new family, which involves focusing affections on one person with whom daily details of life are shared and assuming responsibility for offspring whose care is a continuous operation.

The definition, expectations, and stresses of young adulthood are influenced by socioeconomic status, urban or rural residence, ethnic and educational background, various life events, and the historical era. This generation of young adults is unique. They were born in the fifties, sixties, and seventies and have experienced economic growth and related abundance of material goods and technology, rapid social changes, and sophisticated medical care. They have never known a world without the threat of nuclear war, pollution, overpopulation, and threatened loss of natural resources. Instant media coverage of events has made the world a small and familiar place and has focused attention on outer space. Changes in the role of women, the decreasing birth rate, and increasing longevity are modifying the timing of developmental milestones in many people. Small wonder that the older generations feel a distance between themselves and young adults (238).

Further, the person who is 25 or 30 (the young-young adult) works at developmental tasks differently from the person who is 35, 40, or 45 (the old-young adult).

FAMILY DEVELOPMENT AND RELATIONSHIPS

The major family goal is the reorganization of the family into a continuing unity while releasing maturing young people into lives of their own. Most families actively prepare their children to leave home.

Family Relationships

In America the young adult is expected to be independent from the parents' home and care, although if the person has an extended education, he or she may choose to remain living with the parents to save expenses. Sometimes the young adult does not leave the parents' home as quickly as parents would like. With the increasing number of separations and divorces, the tight job market, and increasing apartment rental rates, the young adult child may move back home, sometimes with children. Emancipation from parents may not occur for years. Parents may resent the intrusion. As one mother said, "My son is 27, and I don't think he's ever going to leave home. I'm tired of being his cook, his cleaning maid, his laundress, his therapist, and his bank." If the young adult does live at home, he or she should expect, and be expected, to assume a share of the home responsibilities and to adjust life-style to that of the parents, to whom the home belongs. Sometimes the adult offspring can be a real help to the parents. Eventually the parents may have to ask the adult offspring to move out so that both parents and offspring can resume achieving their developmental tasks (84).

Some parents delay this emancipation process because of their own needs to hold onto their offspring. They may have a strong desire to be needed by or wish to continue living vicariously through their children. However, families have much less control over the life-style, vocational choice, and friends or eventual mate of their offspring than they did in earlier generations. For emancipation to occur, the parents must trust their offspring, and the offspring must feel the parents' concern, support, and confidence in his or her ability to work things through.

You can help parents understand that, although they are releasing their own children, new members are being drawn into the family circle through their offspring's marriage or close relationships. That the young adult is ready to leave home indicates the parents have done their job.

In a family with several children, the parents may anticipate having the older children leave. The parents then have less responsibility, and the remaining children get the benefit of a less crowded home and more parental attention. At the same time, the emancipated offspring can still use home as a place to return during times of stress.

Often family expenses are at a peak during this period as parents pay for education, weddings, or finance their offspring while they get established in their own home or profession. Young adults will earn what they can, but they may not be able to be financially independent even if they are no longer living at home. Both parents may work to meet financial obligations. As young adult offspring establish families, parents should take the complementary roles of letting go and standing by with encouragement, reassurance, and appreciation.

Often the main source of conflict between the parents and young adult offspring is the difference in philosophy and life-style between the two generations. The parents who sacrificed for their children to have a nice home, material things, education, leisure activities, and travel may now be criticized for how they look, act, and believe. In fact, the young adult may insist that he or she will *never* live like the parents.

Help the parents resolve within themselves that their grown children will not be carbon copies of them. However, the parents can secretly take solace in knowing that usually the basic values they instilled within their children will remain their basic guidelines, although outward behavior may seem different. This becomes even truer as the young adult becomes middle-aged. Help the parents to realize the importance of their acceptance and understanding of their offspring and of not deliberately provoking arguments over ideologies.

The parents need help in providing a secure home base, both as a model for the young adult and to reduce feelings of threat in the younger children. While the parents are withstanding the criticism of their grown children, they must remain cognizant that younger children in the home will be feeling conflict, too. The parents are still identification models to them, but young children and adolescents value highly the attitudes and judgments of young adult siblings, who, in turn, can have a definite influence on younger children. The parents can help the younger children realize that there are many ways to live and that they will encourage each to find his or her own way when the time comes.

Gradually the parents themselves must shift from a household with children to a husband-wife pair again as the last young adult establishes a home. Family structure, roles, and responsibilities change, and use of space and other resources change.

Use the above knowledge to teach and counsel families as they work through concerns about family relationships.

Family Developmental Tasks

In summary, the following tasks must be accomplished by the family of the young adult. Your listening, teaching, and counseling may assist the family to meet these tasks.

1. Rearrange the home physically and reallocate resources (space, material objects) to meet the needs of remaining members.
2. Meet the expenses of releasing the offspring and redistribute the budget.
3. Redistribute the responsibilities among grown and growing children and finally between the husband and wife or between the adult members living in the household on the basis of interests, ability, and availability.
4. Maintain communication within the family to contribute to harmony and happiness while remaining available to young adult and other offspring.
5. Enjoy companionship and sexual intimacy as a husband-wife team while incorporating changes.
6. Widen the family circle to include the close friends or spouses of the offspring and the entire family of in-laws.
7. Reconcile conflicting loyalties and philosophies of life (84).

PHYSIOLOGIC CONCEPTS

Although body and mind changes continue through life, most physical and mental structures have completed growth when the person reaches young adulthood. Changes that occur during adult life are different from those in childhood; they are slower and smaller in increment.

Physical Characteristics

Weight and Height

Norms denote a set standard of development or the average achievement of a group. However, an average adult person has never really been described. Each person is an individual, and normal values cover a wide range in healthy individuals. Height and weight depend on many factors: heredity, sex, socioeconomic level, geographic area, food habits and preferences, level of activity, and emotional and physical environments. Weight loss or gain is unpredictable in this age group, and norms for height and weight are difficult to determine. Most height and weight tables do not consider the individual and specific influencing factors. Tables usually record either average weight for a given height and age or ideal or desirable weight for a specific height. The **average weight** is a *mathematic norm, found by adding the weights of many people and dividing by the number in the sample*. **Desirable weights** are *usually 15 to 25 pounds (6.8 to 11.3 kg) below average weights for both sexes* and are associated with the lowest mortality rates for a given group (290, 352).

Height and weight tables are frequently prepared by insurance companies; their standards do not represent the total population but represent only people who buy insurance. In an example of tables based on insurance statistics, 25-year-old females in shoes with 1-inch heels ranged in height from 4 feet, 10 inches to 6 feet (147 to 183 cm); males of the same age ranged from 5 feet, 2 inches to 6 feet, 4 inches (137.5 to 193 cm). Consideration was not given to an increasing number of males over 6 feet, 4 inches in height. The weights associated with these heights did consider body frame: the clothed weight for females varied from 102 to 179 pounds (46.4 to 81.5 kg) and for males, from 128 to 207 pounds (58.3 to 94 kg). According to a table reflecting mean heights and weights, a female between the ages of 23 and 50 years should weigh 120 pounds (55 kg) and average 5 feet, 4 inches (163 cm) in height. A male of the same age should weigh 154 pounds (70 kg) and average 5 feet 10 inches (178 cm) in height (290, 352).

Musculoskeletal System

Skeletal growth for the young adult is completed by age 25 when the epiphyseal line calcifies and fuses with the mainshaft of the long bones. The vertebral column continues to grow until the individual reaches the age of 30; 3 to 5 mm may be added to an individual's height. Smaller leg bones, the sternum, pelvic bones, and vertebrae attain adult distribution of the red marrow by approximately 25 years of age. By the early forties, the bones will have lost some mass and density. The process begins earlier in women. With increasing age, the cartilage in all joints has a more limited ability to regenerate itself. Normally, posture is erect.

Body systems are functioning at their peak efficiency, and the individual has reached optimum physiologic and motor functions and stamina. Peak muscle strength is attained, and maximum physical potential occurs between the ages of 19 and 30. It is during young-young adulthood that most athletes accomplish their greatest achievements. After this peak period, a 10% loss of strength occurs between the ages of 30 and 60; this loss usually occurs in the back and leg muscles. However, a person can maintain peak performance through the thirties and much of the forties with regular exercise and dietary moderation (192, 238).

Skin

The skin of the young adult is smooth, and skin turgor is taut. Acne usually disappears because sex hormones have less influence on secretion of oils from sebaceous glands of the skin (85). The skin of the African-American may manifest some conditions that are not seen or are manifested differently in Caucasians such as hypopigmentation, keloids, pigmentary disorders, pseudofolliculitis (razor bumps), and alopecia. Refer to the article on African-American skin problems for a pictorial and descriptive summary (321). In late-young adulthood the skin begins to lose moisture, becoming more dry and wrinkled. Smile lines and lines at the corners of the eyes are usually noticeable (85).

Cardiovascular System

Heart and **circulatory** changes occur gradually with age, depending on exercise and diet patterns. During young adulthood, the total *blood volume* is 70 to 85 ml/kg of body weight. Maximum *cardiac output* is achieved and peaks between 20 and 30 years of age. The male's heart weighs an average of 10 ounces and the female's an average of 8 ounces. Heart rate averages 72 beats per minute; the *blood pressure* gradually increases, reaching 100 to 120 mm Hg systolic and 60 to 80 mm Hg diastolic. Heart and blood vessels are fully mature, and cholesterol levels increase. Arteries become less elastic. Hemorrhoids and other varicose veins may become health problems, especially in the childbearing woman (123, 132, 238).

Respiratory System

Since birth, the lungs have increased in weight 20 times. Breathing becomes slower and deeper, 12 to 20 breaths per minute. The maximum breathing capacity decreases between ages 20 and 40. Breathing rate and capacity will differ according to the size of the individual (259).

Gastrointestinal System

The digestive organs function smoothly during this period of life. The amount of ptyalin decreases after 20 years of age, and digestive juices decrease after 30 years of age. *Dental maturity* is achieved in the early twenties with emergence of the last four molars (wisdom teeth) (259). Some people must have their wisdom teeth removed because they become impacted and cause pain.

Neurologic System

The **brain** continues to grow into adolescence and young adulthood and reaches its maximum weight during adulthood. Mature patterns of brain wave activity occur after the age of 20; maturation continues to age 30 (85).

Visual and auditory sensory perceptions should be at peak. Gradually during young adulthood the lens of the eyes lose elasticity and begin to have difficulty changing shape and focusing on close objects. Women in this age group can detect high auditory tones better than men (259). Some young adults wear corrective glasses, contact lenses, or hearing aids. Assess for them when you are giving emergency care, especially if the person is unconscious, so that they are not lost or the person does not suffer eye or ear injury. Information on how to remove contact lenses from another person's eyes can be obtained from your local optometry association or optometrist.

Endocrine System

Adrenal secretion of cortisol (hydrocortisone) decreases approximately 30% over the entire adult life span. Because plasma cortisol levels remain constant, the person maintains good response to stress in young adulthood. A decrease in **basal metabolic rate** (body's consumption of oxygen) occurs gradually, which is related to decrease in the mass of muscle tissue (primarily large oxygen-consuming tissue). A gradual decrease in thyroid hormone is an adjustment to the progressively slower rate at which it is broken down and removed from the blood. The blood level of thyroxine (T_4) falls approximately 15% over the adult life span. The blood level of triiodothyronine (T_3), the active thyroid hormone, declines only when the person is ill and not eating (259).

Use the above knowledge in assessment or in health teaching with young adults.

Sexuality and Sexual Development

Sexual Maturity

Sexual maturity for men is usually reached in the late teens, but their sexual drive remains high through young adulthood. In healthy women menstruation is well established and regular by this time. Female organs are fully matured; the uterus reaches maximum weight by the age of 30. The woman is well equipped for childbearing. The optimum period for reproduction is between 20 and 30 years of age. Many of the dangers associated with adolescent pregnancy or pregnancy in the late thirties or early forties are not present. The Leydig cells, source of male hormones, decline in number after the age of 25 (85, 259).

Sexuality may be defined as a *deep, pervasive aspect of the total person, the sum total of one's feelings and behavior as a male or female, the expression of which goes beyond genital response.* Sexuality includes **gender identity,** the *sense of self as male, female, bisexual (feeling comfortable with both sexes), homosexual, or ambivalent (transsexual).* Gender identity also includes **gender role,** *what the person does overtly to indicate to self and others maleness, femaleness, bisexuality, or ambivalence* (330). Throughout the life cycle physiological, emotional, social, and cultural forces condition sexuality. Today's society offers many choices in sexual behavior patterns.

You will encounter three basic values taken by young adults toward sexuality: absolutist, hedonistic, and relativistic. The **absolutist position** *states that sexuality exists for the purpose of reproduction.* The **hedonistic view** *has pleasure and pursuit as its central value* and is interested in ultimate fulfillment of human sexual potentials. The **relativistic position** *is based on research and has become the basis for the new morality, which says that acts should be judged on the basis of their effects* (200). You will have your private set of values, but you must recognize that others' values may be as valid as yours.

During adulthood a number of sexual patterns may exist, ranging from heterosexuality, bisexuality, and homosexuality to masturbation and abstinence. Few people are totally homosexual or heterosexual; most people feel attracted or sexually responsive at some time to both sexes. Within each of these patterns the person may achieve a full and satisfactory life or be plagued with lack of interest, impotence, or guilt. Young adulthood is the time to reap the rewards or disasters of past sex education. Changes in sexual interest and behavior occur through the life cycle and can be a cause of conflict unless the partners involved can talk about their feelings, needs, and desires. Many misunderstandings arise because of basic differences between the male and female in sexual response. The more each can learn about the other partner, the greater will be the chance of working out a compatible relationship for successful courtship, marriage, and intimacy. The person cannot assume that the partner knows his or her wishes or vice versa. Each must declare his or her needs.

Sexuality Education

Often the popular literature available for reading promotes misinformation, and you should be prepared to give accurate information. Because people feel freer now to discuss sexual matters, you may be questioned frequently by the person recuperating from an illness, by the man or wife after delivery, or by the healthy young adult who feels dissatisfied with personal knowledge or sexual pattern. Various references provide in-depth information on this subject (23, 29, 101, 106, 124, 155, 161, 277, 298, 361). An organization that offers workshops and publications is American Association of Sex Educators, Counselors, and Therapists (AASECT).

The following are facts, based on current research, that you can teach young adults (23, 85, 155, 211, 218, 361):

1. Sexual mores and norms vary among ethnic groups, socioeconomic classes, and even from couple to couple. Sexual activity that is mutually satisfying to the couple and not harmful to themselves and others is acceptable.

2. Sexual activity varies considerably among people in relation to sex drive, frequency of orgasm, or need for rest after intercourse.

3. Various factors and feelings are as influential on men as on women in determining sexual expression. Sexual function, especially in men, is not an uninhibited, mechanical, automatic act requiring only appropriate stimulus and intact physical equipment.

4. Heterosexual intercourse is a reproductive act, but people do not only engage in sexual intercourse for reproduction. Many sexual acts are nongenital in nature but involve people sharing touch, affection, and pleasure.

5. The more sexually active person maintains the sex drive longer into later years.

6. The human sexual drive has no greater impact on the total person than any other biologic function. Sex is not the prevailing instinct in humans, and physical or mental disease does not result from unmet sexual needs.

7. Erotic dreams that culminate in orgasms occur in 85% of all men at any age and commonly in women, increasing in older women.

8. The woman is not inherently passive and the man aggressive. Maximum gratification requires that each partner is both passive and aggressive in participating mutually and cooperatively in sexual intercourse.

9. Women have as strong a sex desire as men, sometimes stronger.

10. Women have greater orgastic capacity than men with regard to duration and frequency of orgasm. The female can have several orgasms within a brief period of time.

11. Female orgasm is normally initiated by clitoral stimulation, but it is a total body response rather than clitoral or vaginal in nature.

12. The woman may need stimulation to the clitoris, other than that received during intercourse, to achieve orgasm. Some studies show that a large percentage of women regularly do not have orgasm in sexual intercourse. Overall sexual response is enhanced for the woman when there is warm, loving behavior from the partner before, during, and after intercourse, when foreplay between partners increases arousal, and when she has worked through strict parental admonitions against touching self, enjoying her body, masturbation, or sexual intercourse.

13. Simultaneous orgasm of both partners may be desired but is an unrealistic goal and occurs only under the most ideal circumstances. It does not determine sexual achievement or satisfaction.

14. No physiologic reason exists for abstinence during menses since menstrual flow is from the uterus, no tissue damage occurs to the vagina, and the woman's sex drive is not necessarily diminished.

15. No relationship exists between penile size and ability of the man to satisfy the woman, and little correlation exists between penile and body size and sexual potency. However, the woman's reaction to penile size or her feelings with penile penetration do affect the man's ability for orgasm and satisfaction.

16. No single most accepted position for sexual activity exists. Any position is correct, normal, healthy, and proper if it satisfies both partners.

17. Achievement of satisfactory sexual response is the result of interaction of many physical, emotional, developmental, and cultural influences and of the total relationship between the man and woman.

18. Chronically ill or disabled persons learn to live with physical changes and to adapt to express their sexual interests. Underlying fantasies, anxiety, guilt, attitudes toward self, and history of relationships with people affect sexual functioning.

19. Decreased sexual desire may be related to physical or emotional illness, prescribed medications, use of alcohol or other drugs, changed behavior in the partner, or fatigue from the stress and demands of employment or professional life—for either men or women.

20. Making love and having sex are not necessarily the same, although ideally they occur together.

Additionally, you may wish to share the following information. In the normal male spermatozoa are produced in optimum numbers and motility when ejaculation occurs two or three times weekly. A decreased or increased frequency of ejaculation is associated with decreased number of sperm (298).

Menstruation is a part of sexuality in women. Discomforts and disabilities associated with menstruation may be caused by social, cultural, and emotional factors and hard physical labor, not just by changing hormone levels. Many women learn to react to menstruation as "the curse" and treat it as an illness with medication and bed rest. Different sociocultural backgrounds teach women different responses. Women who strongly identify with traditional sexual roles are more likely to experience menstruation as a disabling illness. Periods of emotional stress, either happy or upsetting, can cause irregular menses (200).

Human Sexual Response

The human sexual response cycle involves physiologic reactions, psychologic components, and psychosocial influences or behavior. You may be asked to discuss the following information.

The two main physiologic reactions of the cycle are **vasocongestion,** *engorged blood vessels,* and **myotonia,** *increased muscular tension.*

The **four phases of the cycle** are *excitement, plateau, orgasm, and resolution,* and the phases vary with each person and from time to time. The **excitement phase** develops from any source of body or psychic stimuli, and if adequate stimulation occurs, the intensity of excitement increases rapidly. This phase may be interrupted, prolonged, or ended by distracting stimuli. The **plateau phase** is a consolidation period that follows excitement, during which sexual tension intensifies. **Orgasm** is the climax of sexual tension increase that lasts for a few seconds during which vasocongestion and myotonia are released through forceful muscle contractions. The **resolution phase** returns the body to the preexcitement physiology. The woman may begin another cycle immediately if stimulated, but the man is unable to be restimulated for approximately 30 minutes (211).

Physiologic requisites for the human sexual response include (1) an intact circulatory system to provide for vasocongestive responses and (2) an intact central and peripheral nervous system to provide for sensory appreciation and muscular innervation and to support vasocongestive changes (361). For a detailed account of changes that occur in both the genital system organs and other body systems during the four phases of the human sexual response, see references at the end of this chapter (66, 155, 211, 298, 361).

You may be asked subtly or directly about *sexual activity during pregnancy*. Be prepared to share the following information.

Intercourse can continue during pregnancy, although either partner may prefer other intimate behaviors: the woman because of comfort and fear that her appearance may be displeasing to the man and the man because of concern about discomfort to the woman or fetal distress or because he finds her body less attractive as pregnancy progresses. Although infection from intercourse is a possibility during pregnancy, this problem also applies to the nonpregnant state (66). Genital cleanliness is always an important measure in preventing infection. Concern for the partner's well-being is also an important concern. Signs of infection should always be reported early to a physician so that treatment can be given.

Sexual response during and after pregnancy varies slightly from the usual pattern. During orgasm, spasm of the third-trimester uterus may occur for as long as a minute. Fetal heart tones are slowed during this period, but normally no evidence of prolonged fetal distress occurs. Vasocongestion is also increased during sexual activity in genital organs and the breasts. During the resolution phase the vasocongested pelvis often is not completely relieved; as a result, the woman has a continual feeling of sexual stimulation. Residual pelvic vasocongestion and pressure in the pelvis from the second- and third-trimester uterus cause a high level of sexual tension (211).

Teach couples that coital activity is prohibited if there is any threat to fetal viability throughout the pregnancy and during the postpartum period if there is concern about episiotomy breakdown or endometriosis. If there is potential aggravation by the physical nature of coitus with penile penetration, only that form of sexual activity should be avoided. If the problem is one of potential uterine contractility, abstinence from all orgasmic sexual activity, including masturbation by the female, should be recommended. If prostaglandins in semen contribute to the problem, the male should wear a condom during intercourse. If the problem is a combination of the above, all sexual activity with the female is contraindicated; however, sexual activity directed at the male may continue (66).

Couples should always receive specific instruction about continuing sexual intercourse during the last month of pregnancy, depending on the condition of the woman.

Teach couples that such orogenital sexual activity as blowing air into the vagina should be avoided during pregnancy and for at least 6 weeks postpartum. Inflation of air into the vagina may cause air embolism; death has occurred in minutes after air is blown into the vagina. (Air embolism is also the reason that douching is avoided during pregnancy and postdelivery) (66). By the fourth or fifth week postpartum, sexual tensions are similar to nonpregnant levels, but physiologically the woman has not returned to the nonpregnant state. By the third postpartum month, physiological status has returned to prepregnancy levels (211).

Premenstrual Phenomena

Two periodic cyclic occurrences may occur in the menstrual history: mittelschmerz and premenstrual syndrome.

Mittleschmerz (the German word for *middle*

pain) is a *sharp, brief pain associated with ovulation.* Because a slight fever may accompany this pain, it may be confused with appendicitis until a white blood count is done. Using *mittelschmerz* as a guide for the practice of rhythm is unreliable; pain might be related to flatulence (298).

The **premenstrual syndrome (PMS)** is a *group of signs and symptoms occurring approximately a week premenses and associated with fluid retention:* mild cerebral edema and edema of fingers, feet, thighs, legs, hips, breasts, abdomen, and around the eyes. Box 12–1 shows physiologic symptoms and signs and emotional reactions that are reported by some women. Symptoms are more likely to appear or increase as women enter the thirties or reach age 40 (298).

Not all these signs and symptoms appear together; they are variable in degree, and they decrease after menses begins (37, 44, 144, 174, 175, 214, 298, 336, 361). Be empathic to the woman who describes these symptoms or feelings. Help the spouse and other family members recognize their significance, the importance of

 BOX 12-1.
Common Signs and Symptoms of Premenstrual Syndrome

Physiologic Symptoms and Signs

- Abdominal distention
- Acne or hives
- Appetite change, craving for salty or sweet foods
- Breast tenderness
- Clumsiness
- Constipation
- Diarrhea
- Dizziness
- Edema
- Fatigue, increased need for sleep
- Headache or backache
- Lower alcohol tolerance
- Menstrual cramps
- Nausea
- Prone to infection
- Sex drive changes
- Thirst
- Weight gain

Psychologic Reactions

- Apprehension or anxiety
- Confusion
- Forgetfulness
- Frequent crying
- Indecisiveness
- Irritability
- Restlessness
- Sadness or depression
- Suspiciousness
- Tenseness
- Withdrawal

medical treatment, and that their caring and reduced stress may contribute to a decrease in symptomatology.

Estimates are that fewer than 10% of women have severe symptoms or disability resulting from mittelschmerz, PMS, or menstruation. (Recent media publicity would suggest that women are incompetent or commit crimes or suicide during this time of the menstrual cycle.) The cause of either condition is uncertain; there may be several causes. Theories that have been proposed include too little estrogen or too little progesterone. More recent studies show that PMS symptoms may appear because of how neurochemicals and hormones interact with estrogen and progesterone, and these interactions are affected by nutrition and stress. Other factors may be emotional conflicts related to femininity or other emotional stress (44, 61, 174, 175, 215, 300, 336). Woods (360) found that negative attitudes toward menstruation and a stressful social milieu increase PMS symptoms. Regardless of cause, symptoms are not evidence of biologic or emotional inferiority. For the majority of women, the menstrual cycle is an ongoing but insignificant part of their lives—one that causes little discomfort (215).

A study by May (215) showed that, although some women felt depression as part of PMS, others were at their happiest mood. Sometimes women did not remember feelings, mood, or symptoms during the postmenstrual cycle. May's impression was that there are two common areas of anxiety about menstruation that could be associated with a motivated ignoring of that process and its emotional correlates. The first involves experiencing menstruation as a sign of helplessness, of being controlled by body processes in a way that insults one's cherished sense of strength and free will. The second area of anxious response stems from the tendency, rooted in centuries of tradition, to think of menstruation as both dirty and dangerous. This study suggested that these underlying emotional or symbolic relationships, the complex interaction of physiologic or psychologic events, were involved in menstrual mood.

No consistent relationship between premenstrual mood and cognitive function has been found. The magnitude of the premenstrual mood change is not great enough to affect intellectual functioning (164, 174, 175, 300).

Treatment for PMS may be symptomatic, using progesterone, diuretics, antidepressants, or other drugs. Some of the time these drugs are not necessary. Dietary measures may also be suggested.

Teach women that the following measures can offset symptoms (44, 144, 174, 175, 275, 276, 298, 300, 336).

1. Consume less caffeine in beverages, colas, and over-the-counter drugs, less sugar, alcohol, and salt, especially during the premenstrual period.
2. Eat four to six small meals a day rather than two or three meals to minimize the risk of hypoglycemia that accompanies PMS.
3. Snack on complex carbohydrates such as fresh fruits, vegetable sticks, and whole wheat crackers, which provide energy without excessive sugar.
4. Drink six to eight glasses of water to help prevent fluid retention by flushing excess salt from the body.
5. Limit fat intake (especially in red meats), which builds hormones that cause breast tenderness and fluid retention. Choose dairy products low in fat.
6. Eat more whole grains, nuts, and raw greens, which are high in vitamin B, magnesium, and potassium, and add Vitamin B_6 and calcium to reduce symptoms.
7. Develop a variety of interests, including maintaining exercise routines, so that focus is not on self and body symptoms during this period.
8. Walk and perform other physical exercise four times weekly to reduce symptoms of mood swings, increased appetite, crying, breast tenderness, craving for sweets, fluid retention, and depression (exercise raises beta-endorphin levels, which in turn increase feelings of well-being and improve the glucose tolerance curve).
9. Get extra rest and use relaxation techniques, meditation, and massage. Treat yourself to a relaxing and creative activity.
10. Discuss your feelings with family and friends so that they can be more understanding of your behavior.
11. Join a self-help group to gain other ideas on how to more effectively cope with symptoms.

Ovulation

Share the following information about ovulation, especially to couples who desire natural family planning (298, 361). Ovulation normally occurs in every menstrual cycle but not necessarily midcycle. The ovum is capable of being fertilized for 24 hours postovulation.

The mucous cycle by which to predict ovulation is as follows. It begins with menstruation. The period is usually followed by a few "dry days," variable in number, when no mucus is seen or felt. As the ovum begins to ripen, some mucus is felt at the vaginal opening and can be seen if the woman wipes the vaginal area with toilet tissue. This mucus is generally yellow or white, but definitely opaque and sticky. When the blood estrogen level (derived from the ripening ovum) reaches a critical point, the glands of the cervix respond with a different mucus. This fertile mucus starts out cloudy and is not sticky and becomes very clear, like raw egg white. After ovulation, progesterone causes the abrupt cessation of the clear, slippery, fertile mucus and produces its own mucus, which is sticky, much less preponderant, and sometimes not present at the vagina. Progesterone prepares the uterine lining for the reception of the egg if the egg has been fertilized. Usually the egg is ovulated within 24 hours of the peak of wetness, but this interval may be as long as 48 hours. Although the sticky mucus does not allow a sperm to live very long, the sperm could possibly survive long enough to reach a freshly ovulated egg through a lingering fertile mucous channel. If this method will be used to avoid pregnancy, there should be abstinence from intercourse from the beginning of the slippery fertile mucus until the height of wetness ("peak day" when there may be so much wetness that mucus is not seen but moisture is noted on the underclothing) *plus a full 72 hours* to assure that the ovum will not be impregnated.

Because the lifetime of the sperm depends on the presence of the fertile mucus, all genital contact between the partners must be avoided. The first drop of semen (the one that escapes before ejaculation) has the highest concentration of sperm. A woman can conceive even if only one drop of semen touches her external genital organ; sperm are powerful, and the mucus is equally potent.

Teach that spotting or bleeding may occur between menses and may be associated with ovulation, a cervical polyp, postintercourse in the presence of cervicitis, or carcinoma. Any abnormal pattern of bleeding should be investigated by a gynecologist.

Sexual Dysfunctions

Sexual dysfunctions affect both the male and female for various reasons. Several references provide additional information on sexual dysfunctions (12, 23, 211, 212, 240, 361). Your education and referral can assist couples in obtaining effective diagnosis and treatment.

Female Circumcision

Female circumcision may be appalling to you, but it is a widespread culturally and religiously based practice in some parts of the world such as some countries in the Middle East, Africa, Indonesia, and Malay. The circumcision may occur the eighth day after birth, the tenth day after birth, at age 3 or 4 years, or at 8 or 10 years as part of prepuberty rites to womanhood. You may care for circumcised women, especially in maternity and gynecologic services, who have migrated to this country. There are several types of circumcisions, classified on the basis of severity. All types of this practice usually are followed by a variety of complications. Initially there is shock, hemorrhage, sepsis, and lacerations to surrounding tissue. Shortly thereafter retention of urine and tetanus may occur. Dysmenorrhea, urinary tract infections, pelvic inflammatory disease, and infertility are common. After marriage, painful intercourse, forceful cutting of the circumcision scar, perineal lacerations, infections, hemorrhage, frigidity, and severe anxiety occur. During childbirth the scar tissue must be cut during the second stage of labor, or mother and baby may die because of obstruction to delivery, sepsis, or hemorrhage (294).

In most countries where female circumcision occurs, it is a way to control women sexually, economically, and religiously and to control the heritage line and inheritance. The tradition is practiced among Christians, Muslims, and Jews in some parts of Africa.

Some nurses in Kenya report their efforts to stop this practice. They report that Western approaches will not work in eliminating this problem because the practice is so traditional. It is accepted by women because in countries where it is practiced, the uncircumcised woman would not be considered for marriage. These nurses report that as the population becomes generally better educated, traditional practices, including circumcision, decline. Thus the nurses are heavily committed to promoting general and health education so that a better educated population will pass legislation prohibiting the practice.

When you care for women from the non-Western part of the world, assess for circumcision and its effects; be nonjudgmental to the woman. Focus on care that will prevent further complications. Help her gain understanding why this practice may be harmful to her daughter(s). Since the male is the decision maker in these cultures, you will have to establish a working relationship with him if any changes are to be made for the female children. Be aware that female circumcision may be being practiced in this country outside of the traditional health care system. You may encounter the woman after her circumcision in the emergency room, the maternity service, the clinic, or the home. Work through your own feelings with a supervisor or counselor. This woman needs a sensitive caretaker. Refer to the article by Shaw (294) for greater detail in the maternity care needed by circumcised women.

Variations in Sexual Behavior

The identity crisis that occurs during adolescence may not be completely resolved by the time the person enters young adulthood chronologically. Identity confusion may lead to confusion over sexual identity and may precipitate homosexual and heterosexual experimentation and arouse homosexual fears and curiosity.

Homosexuality. **Homosexuals** are *people who are regularly aroused by and who engage in sexual activity with members of their own sex*. Being a **homosexual man** (*gay*) or a **homosexual woman** (*lesbian*) is becoming more socially acceptable in the United States, although persons with this sexual orientation may still suffer rejection and discrimination (113). Members of some religious groups believe homosexuality is a sin. However, homosexuality was accepted by some ancient cultures.

Many theories attempt to explain the causes of homosexual behavior. Freud believed that bisexuality is inherent in all people and that homosexuality was not an illness. Today an increasing number of researchers believe a tiny bundle of neurons deep in the hypothalamus is linked to this orientation since this section in the brain is less than half normal size in homosexual males. However, the studies identifying hypothalamic bundles were done on cadavers; it is unknown whether tissue atrophy is a cause or a result of homosexual orientation, or atrophy may be the disease that caused death. Genetics and biochemistry are also implicated in causation. Others believe several factors, including developmental and emotional ones, are involved in the development of this orientation and that a biologic explanation is inadequate. Other researchers believe faulty parenting and the home environment contribute to homosexual orientation; case studies indicate such a correlation (163, 209, 212).

Whether homosexuality is biologic in origin and set at birth, learned from a parent who is gay or lesbian, the result of the first sexual experience being homosexual, or the result of child-rearing practices is not known. However, *homosexual experiences are a part of normal growth and development in childhood and early adolescence* (106, 320). Most people can report having had a close emotional attachment, with or without sexual contact, to a peer or adult that involved sexual feelings (23, 209). Sullivan (320) theorized that the normal homosexual period in life is the chum stage in preadolescence (see Chapter 10) when the person first cares for someone as much as he or she cares for self. Although the chum stage involves a very close emotional experience, it may include some fondling or exploration between the two chums. Sullivan (320) believed that if the person did not have a chum in preadolescence or adolescence, he or she would enter young adulthood still seeking a chum in the same sex. However, at this point the societal expectation is heterosexuality, and the person's behavior is interpreted in a sexual rather than emotional way. The person is labeled homosexual. If the person is rejected by, or is uncomfortable with, persons of the opposite gender, he or she may receive the greatest acceptance (friendship) from others of the same gender. That reinforces the homosexual preference. The person feels more comfortable being close to or intimate with someone of the same gender.

Research by Masters and Johnson (212) showed that the sexual response in homosexuals is the same as that of heterosexuals. Family interactions of homosexual partners and heterosexual partners without children are similar (23). Gays and lesbians can be nurturing parents to their children if at some point they decide to leave a heterosexual marital relationship (or mixed-orientation relationship) for a stable gay or lesbian relationship (38).

Bell, Weinberg, and Hammersmith (23) found in their studies that homosexual men and women can be categorized as follows:

1. Close coupled—involved in a quasi-marriage, affectionate with a same-sexed partner
2. Open coupled—involved in marital relationships, with interest in sexual contacts other than with the partner and feelings of regret about the homosexuality

3. Functional—single individuals with a high number of partners and level of sexual activity and low regret about homosexuality
4. Dysfunctional—single individuals with a high number of partners, many sexual problems, and much regret about their homosexuality
5. Asexual—single, uncoupled individuals, with low interest in sexual activity, few partners, and significant regret about their homosexuality

It is important to realize that people who identify themselves as homosexual evidence a complexity and diversity of life-styles, interests, problems, and relationships comparable to those of heterosexuals and to enable people to become increasingly reconciled to themselves and to others. There is also a wide spectrum of emotional experience on the homosexual-heterosexual continuum. Contrary to the stereotype, sexual intercourse is not the predominant concern; meaningful relationships are the key (23, 38, 163, 209).

Both male and female homosexuals vary widely in their emotional and social adjustment, just as heterosexuals do. Some people will demonstrate a homosexual orientation only under extreme conditions such as imprisonment. Some have their total life adjustment dominated by homosexuality and live in a homosexual subculture. For some sexual behavior is only an aspect of their total life experience; they may remain discrete and secretive about their homosexuality. Others will seek out heterosexual activity, marry, and have families (38, 152, 163).

The lesbian has not been studied as much as the gay man. It is still more socially acceptable for two women to live together in one dwelling than for two men. There may also be less societal fear of gay women than of gay men. As a result, less is known about their feelings, reactions, life-styles, or health problems (314).

The occurrence of sexually transmitted diseases such as pediculosis, gonorrhea, syphilis, urethritis, anorectal warts and infection, herpes genitalis, acquired immunodeficiency disease (AIDS), intestinal infections, shigellosis, and hepatitis has been publicized. The rapidly increasing incidence of AIDS has caused some homosexuals to change their sexual practices, to limit number of sexual partners, or to increase use of condoms. Heterosexual partners also get these diseases through sexual intercourse, and all homosexuals do not get them (55, 77, 305, 351). Refer to Chapter 11; sexually transmitted diseases do not occur only in adolescence but are likely to occur first in those years. Refer also to the section on health problems in this chapter.

It is essential that you convey a nonjudgmental attitude toward the person who is gay or lesbian. This person needs your respect and acceptance as a human being who is more than a bundle of sexual activity. This person may be a business executive, minister, inventor, delivery person, artist, homemaker, or parent. The person may be contributing as much to society's betterment as any heterosexual person. If this person indicates a desire to change to a heterosexual identity or to relate more comfortably to people of both sexes, refer the person to a counselor who can help the person grow in ability to relate or acquire a new identity without labeling, moralizing, rejecting, or becoming impatient as the person works through emotional and spiritual pain. Further, assist lesbians and gays to obtain needed health care (314).

Parents of homosexual offspring are often not considered, but they may also need help in coping with the homosexuality. Parents of gay or lesbian offspring may feel too embarrassed to talk about their feelings; some believe that they have lost a child; some grieve at the prospect of not having a grandchild; some fear meeting a same-sexed lover. Acceptance of the fact that their child is a homosexual may be a long time in coming, but most parents eventually reach that point. Listen to their feelings and concerns; help them focus on a wholesome relationship; caution against punitive behavior toward the offspring, and refer them to a counselor to work through spiritual and emotional conflicts related to the situation. You can refer parents to the Parents of Gays organization. A list of local chapters is available by writing 201 W. 13th Street, New York, NY 10011, or Box 24528, Los Angeles, CA 90024. You may also refer parents to the Federation of Parents and Friends of Lesbians and Gays, Inc. (Parent's FLAG), P.O. Box 20308, Denver, CO 80220. This organization has a booklet entitled *About Our Children,* published in several languages simultaneously. The organization also sponsors a newsletter, national projects, and regional meetings.

Transsexuality. **Transsexuals** are *people who lack harmony between their anatomic sex and their psychologic sex.* A disorder of gender identity occurs. Hormone therapy and surgery are used for people with this problem. Both therapies are directed at making the anatomic sex compatible with the psychologic sex (240).

To care for persons with sexual-identity confusion, you must first determine your own feelings toward yourself as a sexual person and then your feelings toward them. These people need someone to listen to their fears and insecurities and a consistent, accepting approach. You may not be able to work with these people, but you can make appropriate referrals. If problems of gender identity are assessed in a child, you should encourage early treatment. Without intervention, the majority of people will become more deeply frustrated by their lack of gender identity.

Sexual Experimentation Outside Marriage. Sexual activity outside marriage may include homosexuality, group sexual experiences, premarital intercourse, cohabitation, or infidelity.

The moral, emotional, and psychologic aspects of premarital sexual behavior have been widely discussed.

Sexual intimacy without a sense of commitment and love, responsibility, and care for the other means using another to meet one's needs, taking the other as an object rather than as a person. Such activity and attitudes can be poor preparation for marriage and establishing a lasting relationship and personal maturity. Compatibility between two people is in the head, not the pelvis. The rationalization of finding a compatible partner through premarital sexual intimacy is unfounded.

Yet **cohabitation,** *two persons of the opposite sex living together without being married,* is not unusual. Sometimes the arrangement of the young adult man and woman living together is asexual. They are friends and for economic, companionship, or convenience reasons wish to share an apartment. Sometimes the person may have had no siblings or no siblings of the opposite gender, and the person wants the experience of living with someone of the opposite gender who would be like a sibling. In such a situation both work to keep the relationship asexual.

Young adults sometimes live together in an effort to avoid some of the problems they saw in their parents' marriage or to test the degree of the partner's commitment before actually becoming married. Those goals may be achieved for some, but the danger is that one partner may take the commitment very seriously and the other may use the situation only as a convenient living arrangement. The uncaring person may suddenly decide to leave, an easy process since no legal ties are involved, and the other person is left with much the same hurt as a married person going through a divorce.

American society probably expects too much of marriage. The partners in the ideal marriage are supposed to stay passionately and exclusively in love with each other for the rest of their lives. Yet infidelity is a growing problem in an increasingly liberal society.

Various factors contribute to infidelity: the need to prove masculinity or femininity; difficulty in maintaining a steady and continuing relationship; feelings of insecurity, rejection, or jealousy; and a sense of loss when heightened passions of the initial stages of love do not remain constant. Believing that one can love two people simultaneously, getting great satisfaction from doing something forbidden and secretly, or wishing to recapture one's youth may also be involved.

Staying married to one person and living with the frustrations, conflicts, and boredom that any close and lengthy relationship imposes requires constant work by both parties. Couples are unrealistic when they think that marriage will suddenly shield them from further attraction to members of the opposite sex. The mature couple will expect to feel physically attracted to others at times and will have to resolve the feelings within themselves through discussion with and understanding from their partner or with the help of a counselor.

American society offers no alternative to the family unit. Although society as a whole is in a state of flux, the family unit seems fundamental. The strains that infidelity places on it are damaging for most people (36).

Personal Attitudes

To incorporate human sexuality into nursing practice, you must accept your own sexuality and understand sexuality as a significant aspect of development. Then you can acknowledge the concerns of the clients, recognize your strengths and limits in working with people who have sexual concerns, help these people cope with threats to sexuality, and counsel, inform, or refer them as indicated.

Supporting, caring, and nurturing are nursing behaviors. But at times you will have other feelings and may feel guilty about being sexually attracted to (or repulsed by) a client. These are honest feelings to acknowledge. After all, every thought and behavior will not result in intimacy or rejection. Feeling positively toward someone can help you give effective care. If you have negative feelings about someone, you can deal with these feelings if you can recognize the possible reasons for your feelings. If necessary, someone else can be assigned to care for the person. Actually, when you begin to understand another person, most likely you will find that person interesting, even if that person might not be an individual you would choose for a friend. When someone is perceived as unique and interesting, it becomes easier to give effective care and form a relationship.

The patient may express sexual behavior by brushing against you, trying to feel breasts or hips, or referring to sexual topics in conversation. Recognize the behavior as an energy outlet or as a way to validate himself or herself as a person. If the patient is observed masturbating, do not make a joke of this discovery. Realize that this is an acceptable sexual release and provide privacy. However, if a patient becomes obnoxious either in words or actions, you must tell him or her what behavior is appropriate in the particular situation.

Sexual History

If you feel comfortable and if there is sufficient rapport between you and the client, take a sexual history, especially with clients who have conditions that interfere with sexual activity. Follow these guidelines when you are taking a sexual history:

1. Ensure privacy and establish confidentiality of statements.
2. Progress from topics that are easy to discuss to those that are more difficult to discuss.
3. Ask the person how he or she acquired sexual information before asking about sexual experience.
4. Precede questions by informational statements about the generality of the experience, when appropriate, to reassure the person and reduce anxiety, shame, and evasiveness.

5. Observe nonverbal behavior while you listen to the person's statements.
6. Do not ask questions just to satisfy your curiosity.

The following are topics to include in the sexual history:

1. How sex education was obtained
2. Accuracy of sex education
3. Menstrual history if female or nocturnal emission history if male
4. Past and present ideas on self as a sexual being, including ideas on body image, masturbation, coitus, childbirth, parenting
5. Attitudes of marital versus nonmarital sexual experiences
6. Sexual dreams and fantasies
7. Ability to communicate sexual needs and desires
8. Partner's (if one exists) sexual values and behavior

If necessary, use several interviews to obtain information and be sure to include any specific questions or concerns that the person voices. Respect the person's desire not to talk about sexual matters and moral, spiritual, or aesthetic convictions. Know the terminology and have a nonjudgmental attitude when the person talks about sexuality concerns. Your matter-of-fact attitude helps the adult feel less embarrassed. Be aware of how illness and drugs can affect sexual function. Do not assume that chronic or disabling disease or mutilating surgery ends the person's sexual life.

Give accurate information and counseling when the person or family asks questions or indicates concerns. You may wish to prepare instructional units for a specific teaching plan to share with patients with various conditions, especially chronic diseases, and with their families to help them better understand how to meet sexual needs. Give gentle encouragement related to pursuit of sexual activity rather than personal advice or judgment. Know community resources for consultation or referral when necessary.

References at the end of the chapter will also be helpful on how to work with rape victims (6, 29, 154, 240).

Nutritional Needs

As the nutrition of childhood set the stage for the health of the young adult, so now the stage is being set for health in middle and old age. Growth is essentially finished by young adulthood. Activity level may stabilize or diminish. Caloric intake should be based on occupation, amount of physical activity or mental effort, emotional state, age, body size, climate, individual metabolism, and presence of disease. (A *calorie* or *kilocalorie* [kcal] is a unit of measure of the amount of energy required to raise 1 kg of water 1° C.) Women have a 5% to 10% lower metabolism than men of comparable height and weight; thus in the healthy, nonpregnant state women need lower caloric intake. The greater the body surface, the higher is the basal metabolic rate. However, the obese person requires fewer calories for size because adipose tissue consumes less oxygen than muscles; thus less energy is expended comparatively. Table 12–1 shows caloric expenditure for activity. However, the actual caloric consumption depends not only on type of activity but also on duration of activity and weight of the person (142, 352).

Normal Nutrition

Table 12–2 lists the recommended daily number of servings for each food group for young adults and for pregnant and lactating women (142, 244, 330, 352). Appendix I shows the requirements for vitamins and minerals, comparing adults to children (142, 330, 352). Appendix II lists the functions and sources of the various nutrients (148, 173, 330, 352). The December 1990, supplement (Vol. 80) to the *American Journal of Public Health,* "Hispanic Health and Nutrition Survey, 1982–1984" also presents information pertinent to Latinos.

Theoretically, a man between the ages of 25 and 45, living in the United States under the usual environmental stresses, weighing 154 pounds (40 kg) and standing 69 inches (172 cm) tall, will consume approximately 2700 calories daily to maintain nutritional status and weight; 56 g of his food should be *protein.*

A woman between the ages of 25 and 45, living in the United States under the usual environmental stresses, weighing 128 pounds (58.2 kg), and standing 65 inches (162 cm) tall, will consume approximately 2000 *calories* daily to maintain nutritional status and weight; 45 to 65 g of her food should be *protein.* That same woman when *pregnant* should increase her calories by at least 300 daily and her protein by 30 g. Weight gain during pregnancy should be 22 to 27 pounds. Rigid calorie restriction may be dangerous. When *lactating,*

her calorie intake should increase by 500, her protein intake by 30 g and calcium intake should be 1200 mg for optimum health (352). Refer to Chapter 6 for additional information.

Nutrition Assessment

Incorporate nutritional status into nursing assessment and the health history. Ask questions related to the following list to guide your assessment with the person or family (142, 352):

1. Knowledge of nutrients, food groups, balanced diet, and their relationship to health
2. Knowledge of nutrient requirements at present level of growth and development and whether nutrient needs are being met
3. Associations with food and how they influence food and eating patterns
4. What increases or decreases appetite
5. Cultural background, including religious beliefs, ethnic patterns, and geographic area, and how these beliefs influence food intake and likes and dislikes
6. Relationship of life-style and activity to food intake
7. Income level and food buying power; influence of income on dietary habits
8. Knowledge of alternatives to high-cost foods
9. Usual daily pattern of intake: times of day, types, amounts
10. Which is main meal of day
11. Eating environment
12. Special diet requirements
13. Food allergies
14. Relationship of eating patterns of family or significant others to individual's habits and patterns
15. Medications and methods used to aid digestion and nutrition intake; influence of other medications on nutritional intake
16. Condition of teeth and chewing ability
17. Use, condition, and fit of dentures
18. Types of food individual has difficulty chewing or swallowing
19. Condition of oral cavity and structures
20. Disabilities that interfere with nutritional intake
21. Assistance or special devices needed for feeding

Schweiger, Lang, and Schweiger (289) and Meissner (228) give descriptive and pictorial assessment guides for the oral cavity, which can be included in a nutritional assessment and at other times of nursing care.

Nutrition-Disease Relationships

Although overt clinical symptoms of *vitamin or mineral deficiencies* are seldom observed in most Americans, you will see individuals and families in whom you suspect inadequate nutrition. Pallor; listlessness; brittle, dull nails and hair; dental caries; complaints of constipation and poor resistance to common infections; and over- or

TABLE 12-1. ENERGY EXPENDITURE FOR ACTIVITY

Type of Activity	Kcal/Hr	
	Men	*Women*
Sedentary Sitting, working on leisurely activity with little arm movement	100	80
Light House or office work, sitting and standing, some arm movement	160	110
Moderate Housecleaning, gardening, laundry, carpentry, walking moderately fast, vigorous arm movement with sitting activity	240	170
Vigorous Heavy housecleaning, walking fast, golfing, bowling	350	250
Strenuous Swimming, athletic games, running, dancing, skiing	>350	>350

TABLE 12-2. RECOMMENDED NUTRITIONAL INTAKE FOR YOUNG ADULTS

Foods	Young Adult	Pregnant Woman	Lactating Woman
Traditional Basic Four			
Milk and milk products	2 or more cups	3 or 4 cups	4 or more cups
Meat, fish, or protein equivalent	2 (2 or 3 ounce) servings	3 (2 or 3 ounce) servings	3 or 4 (2 or 3 ounce) servings
Fruits and vegetables (including a high vitamin C source)	4 ($\frac{1}{2}$ cup) servings	4 or 5 ($\frac{1}{2}$ cup) servings	4 or 5 ($\frac{1}{2}$ cup) servings
Grain, bread, and cereals	4 servings	4 or more servings	4 or more servings
Suggested Change			
Milk and milk products	2 or 3 cups	3 or 4 cups	4 or more cups
Meat, fish, poultry, dry beans, eggs, nuts	2 or 3 (2 or 3 ounce) servings	3 (2 or 3 ounce) servings	3 or 4 (2 or 3 ounce) servings
Fruits	2–4 ($\frac{1}{2}$ cup) servings	2–4 ($\frac{1}{2}$ cup) servings	2–4 ($\frac{1}{2}$ cup) servings
Vegetables	3–5 ($\frac{1}{2}$ cup) servings	3–5 ($\frac{1}{2}$ cup) servings	3–5 ($\frac{1}{2}$ cup) servings
Breads, cereal, rice, pastas	6–11 servings	6–11 servings	6–11 servings
Fats, Oils, Sweets			
Use sparingly for all age groups.			

under-weight suggest a need for a complete diet history (352).

Laboratory evaluations of blood and urine supply meaningful information for a nutritional assessment. Hemoglobin, hematocrit, serum proteins and lipids (including cholesterol), glucose, sodium, and potassium levels are all important diagnostic tools.

One glaring deficiency you may find, however, is the lack of iron in women. A sizable percentage of women do not ingest sufficient dietary iron daily. The male can suffice with 10 mg of iron daily, but the female needs 18 mg (142, 352, 353).

Your assistance will be sought when dietary problems occur during early pregnancy, usually the transitory nausea and vomiting, commonly called *morning sickness*. Physiologic and psychologic factors contribute to this condition. Small frequent meals of fairly dry, easily digested energy foods such as carbohydrates are usually tolerated. Separating intake of liquids and solids and drinking flavored or carbonated beverages instead of plain water may also help. Constipation resulting from pressure of the expanding uterus on the lower portion of the intestine occurs in later pregnancy. Increased fluid intake and use of dried fruits, fresh fruits and juices, and whole-grain cereals should induce regularity of elimination. Laxatives should be avoided unless prescribed by a physician.

Americans have a vast array of food from which to pick, yet malnutrition may result from being overfed but undernourished. Additionally, *six of the 10 leading causes of death in the United States are connected to eating habits:* heart disease, cancer, stroke and hypertension, diabetes, arteriosclerosis, and cirrhosis of the liver. Formerly thought of as middle-aged diseases, some of these diseases are taking the lives of young adults.

Many Americans are more aware of the need for a nutritional diet, yet many other Americans eat too few fruits, vegetables, and grains and too much salt, fat, and sugar. The result is a big drop in vitamin and mineral intake. Television advertises heavily in the sugar, fat, and salt areas. Young adult working wives and single individuals are not spending time in the kitchen. Instead, they are paying the higher prices for the instant, often less nutritious foods. In fact, some young adults have grown up on the junk food they have seen advertised on television and on the ever growing "instant" dinners prepared by their parents or bought at the fast-food restaurants.

Because of the claim that saturated fat and cholesterol are related to cardiovascular disease, some manufacturers have responded with low-cholesterol and poly-unsaturated products. Fish, poultry, shellfish, and the leanest red meat have the lowest cholesterol–saturated fat index. Some African tribes consume enormous amounts of animal fats but rarely show signs of coronary disease, but the African tribal life-style differs drastically from that of the American life-style. Eating the recommended food groups, exercising, and losing weight are ways to increase the level of high-density lipoproteins that remove cholesterol from the arterial walls and to decrease low-density lipoproteins that contribute to disease (142, 298, 352). In American society you can be helpful in recommending that young adults steer away from too much sugar, excess salt, an abundance of animal products and red meats, and a steady diet of foods in which there are additives and preservatives (especially nitrates and nitrites).

Other diseases thought related to diet are diverticular disease of the colon and colon cancer, appendicitis, hiatus hernia, hemorrhoids, and varicose veins, again diseases affecting young adults. One theory relates these diseases to lack of fiber in the diet. Fiber (found mainly in plant foods) increases stool weight and transit time. Pressure is thus relieved all along the gastrointestinal tract so that these problems are not so likely to arise. Possibly potential carcinogens formed in the gastrointestinal tract do not have a chance to develop to the harmful level (142, 352). You can suggest an increase in fiber through eating bran or other foods (whole wheat bread, whole grain cereals, raw fruits or vegetables) so that young adults can cut down on disease proneness and improve their elimination pattern.

Obesity

Obesity is a persistent problem and is usually related to restricted activity (more than 3 hours of sitting daily was associated with obesity in one study) (328, 329), psychologic and body-image problems, worry, diabetes, hypertension, cardiovascular disease, pain, and premature mortality (142, 352). However, overweight people in Laffrey's study (189) perceived themselves as healthy as their normal weight peers. Often the active adolescent becomes the sedentary young adult but does not lower caloric intake. Thus more calories are eaten than are needed for energy. Those who have less education, and lower family income and are married are also more likely to be obese, especially African-American women (170). In an attempt to lose weight, the young adult may try a variety of approaches.

You can help dieters by insisting that any special diet must be analyzed for its nutritional value and overall effect on the body. Additionally, you might suggest a group approach and behavior modification techniques. Many people can lose weight, but they gain it back as soon as they abandon their diets. Often an increase in exercise is recommended rather than a continual decrease in calories for the following reasons:

1. Appetite is decreased after exercise because of lowered blood supply to the gastrointestinal tract.
2. Exercise may decrease tension and stress, resulting in less frequent eating for nonnutritive purposes.
3. Adequate energy or caloric intake is necessary for efficient use of protein for growth and tissue maintenance.
4. Basal metabolic rate decreases after a period of caloric restriction.
5. Caloric restriction combined with mild exercise can result in greater fat loss and reduced loss of lean body mass than caloric restriction alone.
6. Nutritional adequacy of diets low in energy value (less than 1800 to 2000 kcal) is questioned since many of the essential nutrients, especially minerals, are found in relatively low concentrations in foods.

Generally, a low-potency vitamin-mineral supplement is recommended for persons on calorie-restricted diets (148). Treatments for the obese person are discussed by several authors (40, 262).

Vegetarianism

In contrast to the obese person, the vegetarian is seldom obese. Vegetarianism has grown popular with young adults, but it is not new. Certain religious groups (e.g., the Seventh-Day Adventists) have been effectively practicing a form of vegetarianism for years. In addition to religious reasons, people are vegetarians for moral reasons (opposed to killing animals for food), for economic reasons (cannot afford animal protein), and for health reasons (may believe that a significant amount of animal food is detrimental or that a large amount of plant food is beneficial). Young adults probably fall mainly into the last category.

People who consider themselves vegetarians range from those who eat limited amounts of meat, milk products, or fish and animal products to vegetarians who eat only vegetables, fruits, legumes, nuts, and grains. Ovo-vegetarians consume eggs, and lacto-vegetarians consume milk products in addition to plant foods.

Depending on the extent of the vegetarian's dietary restrictions, certain precautions must be taken to maintain an adequate intake of required nutrients. If animal proteins, eggs, or milk is inadequate in the diet, the person may need supplementary calcium, iron, zinc, and vitamins B_2 and B_{12}. Soy milk fortified with vitamin D can supply that vitamin. Iron supplements may be needed, even if enriched grain products are used. If caloric and protein intake is minimal, serum albumin and total serum protein may be low (142, 352).

Eight amino acids are essential nutrients that must be obtained daily in the diet: isoleucine, tryptophan, threonine, leucine, lysine, methionine, valine, and phenylalanine. Cystine and tyrosine are quasiessential. In addition, infants must have arginine and histidine. The bioavailability of protein depends on proper balance of essential amino acids. Dietary deficiency of any substance may enhance our vulnerability to herpes, anxiety, overeating, high blood pressure, insomnia, and other disorders. There is increasing evidence that specific amino acids play important roles in central nervous system function and therefore behavior. Some medical disorders such as a few of the many types of schizophrenia may be helped through dietary manipulations of amino acids (258, 330, 352).

A wide variety of legumes, grain, nuts, seeds, vegetables, milk, and eggs can supply adequate amounts of required nutrients. Although the proteins in these foods are considered incomplete (in contrast to the complete proteins—meat, fish, poultry, and dairy products—which contain all essential amino acids) certain proteins such as those found in cereals (lysine) and those in legumes (methionine) complement each other when eaten together (142, 258, 352). For example, peanut butter or chili beans (high in lysine but low in methionine) can be served with whole wheat bread or corn bread (low in lysine but high in methionine). Other complementary combinations are beans and wheat in baked beans and brown bread or refried beans and rice or corn tortillas; lentil and rice in soup; beans and rice in casserole or bean curd and rice or lentils and rice; peas and rye in split pea soup and rye bread; and peas and rice in black-eyed peas and rice. Further, amino acids in milk products and eggs complement plant proteins. Such combinations are cereals and milk in breakfast cereal with milk; pasta and cheese in macaroni and cheese or pizza; bread and cheese in a cheese sandwich; rice and milk in rice cooked in milk instead of water; bread and egg in poached egg on toast; peanuts and milk in a peanut butter sandwich and yogurt (142, 258). Pure vegetarians who consume no milk and no eggs will need vitamin B_{12} supplements. A helpful guide in complementing proteins can be found in several references (25, 142, 258, 352).

Nutrition Education

You may be able to advise young adults about nutrition in a variety of settings. Even though this is a "I'll-do-it-my-way culture," you will find that young adults will question you about various diets, the value of vitamin supplements, and the value of certain foods. Keep in mind the basic foods as you suggest a diet pattern, and adjust your information to the vegetarians or those who have allergies or specific ethnic or cultural preferences. These suggestions, if followed, will contribute to nutritional health (142, 258, 352):

1. Increase consumption of fruits, vegetables, and whole grains.
2. Decrease consumption of foods or beverages high in refined sugars; instead drink more water and fruit juices.
3. Do not add salt to foods during cooking or at the table and avoid snack foods with visible salt or foods prepared in brine; instead use herbs, spices, and lemon for seasoning.
4. Decrease consumption of foods high in total fat and animal fat and partially replace saturated fats (beef, pork, butter, fatty meats) whether obtained from animal or vegetable sources with polyunsaturated fats (fish, poultry, veal, lean meats, margarine, vegetable sources).
5. Substitute low-fat and nonfat milk for whole milk and low-fat dairy products for high-fat products (except for young children).
6. Reduce use of luncheon or variety meats (e.g., sausage, salami).
7. Use skim or low-fat milk and cheeses instead of whole milk and cream.
8. Avoid deep fat frying; use baking, boiling, broiling, roasting, or stewing, which help remove fat.
9. Avoid excessive intake of any nutrient or food since excess consumption of, and in turn deficiency of, any substance can contribute to disease.
10. Avoid more than a minimum intake of alcohol.

Suggest that young adults take vitamins and mineral supplements only with a practitioner's sanction and after a complete blood and urine analysis has been done. Suggest that exercise is as important as food intake when considering the number of calories needed. Suggest exercise not only to burn off calories but to maintain muscle tone, elimination, and circulation, to regulate sleep, and to release tension.

Keep in mind the young adult who may need suggestions on economical but nutritious foods. Using powdered skim milk, less expensive cuts of meat, and home cooked cereals does not sacrifice nutrition but does save money.

Teach about the need for fiber in the diet, which can prevent constipation and help reduce the incidence of cancer of the colon, diverticulosis, appendicitis, gallstones, and heart disease. However, having only one source of fiber such as bran while excluding the fiber from vegetables and fruits can produce problems. Some fibers contribute to constipation if they are not diluted with substantial amounts of water (142, 262, 352).

Teach about the adverse effects of caffeine. Effects of caffeine can be detrimental to health. Hallal gives pertinent information in an article entitled "Caffeine" in the April 1986 issue of the *American Journal of Nursing* (pp. 423–425). Warn also that herbal teas may contain strong drugs that can cause severe problems. Those containing catnip, juniper, hydrangea, jimson weed, lobelia, nutmeg, and wormwood can be toxic to the central nervous system and can cause severe reactions, including hallucinations. People with allergies should stay away from teas containing camomile, goldenrod, marigold, and yarrow. Also be aware that some herbal teas have as much as twice the caffeine as a regular cup of coffee.

Hospitalized young adults may be suffering from nutritional deficiencies resulting from a specific diet. Be aware that hospital-induced malnutrition exists. Patients whose meals are withheld because they are undergoing various diagnostic tests or treatments, especially over a long period of time, are candidates for this problem.

Biologic Rhythms

Rhythms occur throughout the life cycle of each individual. From the time of birth different body structures and functions develop rhythmicity at different rates. By the time the individual reaches young adulthood, biologic rhythms are established by body chemistry and by the suprachiasmatic nucleus, a tiny cluster of cells buried deep in the brain. **Biologic rhythms** are *self-sustaining, repetitive, rhythmic patterns found in plants, animals, and man.* The rhythms are found throughout our external and internal environment and can be exogenous or endogenous.

Exogenous rhythms *depend on the rhythm of external environmental events* such as seasonal variations, lunar revolution, or night-and-day cycle that function as time givers. These events help to synchronize internal rhythms with external environmental stimuli and establish an internal time pattern or biologic clock.

Endogenous rhythms such as sleep-wake and sleep-dream cycles arise *within the organism*. Endogenous and exogenous rhythms are usually synchronized.

Many internal rhythms do not readily alter their repetitive patterns, however, even when the external stimuli are removed. For instance, when a person shifts to sleeping by day and waking at night, as frequently happens with nurses, a transient or temporary desynchronization occurs. Body temperature and adrenal hormone levels are usually low during the sleep cycle. With the shift in sleep and waking, the person is awake and making demands on the body during the usual sleep period. Three weeks may be needed before internal rhythms adapt to the shift. A similar period of desynchronization occurs when a person makes a flight crossing time zones (10, 22, 167).

Within any 24-hour period, physiologic and psychologic functions reach maximum and minimum limits. When a physiologic function approaches a high or low limit, the body's feedback mechanisms attempt to counterregulate the action. *This form of endogenous rhythm that reoccurs in a cyclic pattern within a 20- to 28-hour period is a* **circadian rhythm.** Body temperature, blood pressure, pulse, respirations, urine production, and hormone, blood sugar, hemoglobin, and amino acid levels demonstrate this rhythmic pattern. Similar variations or rhythms in the levels of alertness, fatigue, tenseness, and irritability can also be demonstrated.

In humans mental efficiency and performance apparently are related to the rhythms of body temperature and catecholamine excretion in the adult. The body temperature rises and drops by approximately 2 degrees over each 24-hour period. The body temperature begins to decline near 10 P.M., is lowest on awaking, gradually rises during the morning, levels off in the afternoon, and then drops again in the evening (Fig. 12–1). The level of adrenocortical hormone secretion appears correlated with body temperature rhythms and the individual's state of alertness and wakefulness. The level of adrenocortical hormones rises early in the morning, peaks around the time we typically awaken, and then drops to a low point by late evening (87, 98, 137, 167, 311). Usually the best mental and physical performances coincide with peak temperature, and the least desirable perform-

ances coincide with intervals of lowest body temperature. In addition, studies have shown that the lowest excretory rates of epinephrine in day-active people correlate with the time of maximum fatigue and poorest performance. Physical strength crests at different times of the day (64, 167, 322).

Researchers have theorized that many disasters have resulted from failure to consider human biology. For example, at the nuclear accident at Three Mile Island, the three young men in the control area worked on a shift system called slow rotation—days for a week, evenings for a week, and late nights for a week. At the time of the disasters at Bopal and Chernobyl, people were working unusual shifts. Work schedules with changing shift rotation causes a desynchronization of circadian rhythms, altering performance levels (117, 167).

Circadian Rhythms in Illness

An interrelationship exists between circadian rhythms and mental or physical illness. The pattern of living taught by the culture also affects body rhythms. A few examples of how circadian rhythms influence the health of young adults are presented next. (For more extensive discussion, refer to references (10, 75, 87, 98, 105, 137, 273, 280, 304).

Diagnostic cues are influenced by biologic rhythms. Observing the integration of the body's rhythms (or lack of such integration) can be used to determine the person's health status. Diagnosis and treatment of some illnesses can be determined from the study of circadian rhythms or biologic time. In some instances the illness alters the pattern of circadian rhythm. Other illnesses show exaggerated or decreased symptoms at a particular biologic time. Blood pressure and temperature values, laboratory findings, and biopsy specimens for cell study differ according to the biologic time of day. For instance, growth hormone levels in the blood are highest during the night hours; therefore routine blood values taken at 8 A.M. will not give a total picture. The percentage of red blood cells drops approximately $4\frac{1}{2}$% late

Figure 12-1. Diurnal cycle of temperature variations. (From Berger, K.J., and M.B. Williams, *Fundamentals of Nursing: Collaborating for Optimal Health.* Norwalk, Conn: Appleton & Lange, 1992, 446.)

at night; a decrease in red blood cells of 5% prompts blood transfusions in some hospitals. Concentrations of white blood cells peak in the morning and early afternoon (76, 140, 188). Ambiguous laboratory findings, the need for repeated medical tests, and the potential for unnecessary medical therapies can be avoided if the person's normal biologic rhythms are considered first.

Rhythmic time cycles appear to influence many aspects of human life. Births and deaths occur more frequently at night and during the early morning. Persons with ulcers and allergies suffer more in the nighttime and in spring; allergic responses, including asthmatic attacks, occur more frequently at night and in the early morning hours. There are certain yearly peaks in the number of suicides, psychotic episodes, and accidents. Eventually knowledge about circadian rhythms and biologic time may serve as a major tool in preventive health programs.

Depression has a number of causes but may be directly related to biologic rhythms of depressed people. Altered biochemical rhythms, diurnal (daytime) mood swings, and altered sleep cycles have been noted. Researchers have hypothesized that abnormalities of sleep patterns in some types of depression are due to abnormal internal phase relationships of circadian rhythms. The circadian rhythm of rapid eye movement (REM) sleep may occur abnormally early (86, 167, 242, 265, 304). Depressed persons usually experience insomnia or periods of predawn wakefulness. Their sleep cycles are shortened and fragmented, and they are easily disturbed by environmental changes. Successful treatment frequently comes in the form of antidepressant drugs that slow biologic clocks (i.e., lithium carbonate) or speed biologic clocks (i.e., imipramine) (240).

Various mental functions and the emotion, behaviors, and autonomic responses associated with them depend on certain chemicals secreted at the synapses of the neurons in specific pathways of the brain. Several brain neurotransmitters (norepinephrine, dopamine, serotonin, and acetylcholine) undergo cyclic changes in amount of chemical present. These fluctuations are thought related to factors concerned with periodicity and emotion (119, 322).

Cells in almost every tissue of the body divide or reproduce in a circadian rhythm. Normal cells show intervals of accelerated reproductive activity. In human beings, for example, skin and liver cells are more active at night. Cancer cells do not reproduce at the same rate as normal cells; abnormal mitosis (cell-reproduction) rhythms and, in many instances, a complete lack of circadian rhythms have been reported. Further, timing has been found crucial for surgical treatment or chemotherapy of cancer patients; recovery is linked to time of day of the treatment (119).

Research suggests that people who are desynchronized or constantly consuming foods and drugs that change the phase of their circadian rhythms may be a high-risk group for cancer (119). Health teaching should include the need to decrease the intake of coffee, tea, and certain barbiturates that may be carcinogens.

Adrenal hormone production in man is cyclic. The blood and urine concentrations of adrenocorticosteroid hormones in persons on schedules of diurnal activity and nocturnal sleep drop at night and rise to highest levels in early morning. The course of the adrenal cycle may also be followed by measuring the eosinophil (white blood cell) level; eosinophils decrease as the blood level of adrenal hormones increases.

Light is probably the synchronizer of the adrenocorticosteroid rhythm. This factor has implications for people who are night workers or who have varying degrees of blindness. Because adrenal hormones control other circadian rhythms within the body, knowledge of their cycle is important in the study and treatment of numerous conditions.

Low blood levels of adrenal hormones affect the nervous system and cause increased sensitivity to sounds, tastes, and smell. Sensory acuity reaches its maximum at the time of lowest steroid levels. A sudden drop in acuity occurs in the early morning as steroid levels begin to rise. A person is therefore better able to detect taste, smell, or sound at the end of the day. Daily fatigue from lack of sleep and neurologically related symptoms associated with adrenal insufficiency (Addison's disease) may be related to low levels of adrenal hormones.

Adrenal rhythm is also important in handling certain allergies. Sensitivity to histamine follows a circadian rhythm: it peaks near the time of evening or night when adrenocorticosteroids are reaching their lowest levels. Nasal congestion from hayfever, skin reactions from drug sensitivity, and breathing crises in asthma patients occur more frequently during the evening or night. Suggest to individuals with hayfever and asthma that they do their gardening and weeding in the morning when their adrenocorticosteroid levels are at their highest.

Nursing Assessment and Intervention

Nursing care should be planned with biologic rhythms in mind. Because our cyclic functioning is synchronized with environmental stimuli, physiologic disequilibrium occurs whenever we are confronted with environmental or schedule changes. Transient desynchronization may occur whenever a person is exposed to the hospital or nursing home stimuli. New noise levels; lighting patterns; schedules for eating, sleeping, and personal hygiene; and unfamiliar persons intruding on the person's privacy may all contribute to this desynchronization. Disturbed mental and physical well-being and increased subjective fatigue reflect the conflict between the internal time pattern and external events. Several days usually are required before the person adapts to the environment and thereby regains synchronization—normal biologic rhythms.

You can control some external factors such as meals, baths, and various tests, make them more nearly similar to the patient's normal (outside) routine, and lessen the stress to which the patient is subjected. Obtaining and using a nursing history comprise one method of lessening this stress.

Your *nursing history* should be directed at getting information about the patient's preillness or prehospitalization patterns for sleep, rest, food and fluid intake, elimination, and personal hygiene. Questions such as Do you consider yourself a "day" person or a "night" person? Do you feel cheerful when you first wake up? What time of day do you feel most alert? What hours do you prefer to work? Why do you prefer these hours? How do you feel when something causes you to change your routine? will provide you information about the patient's daily patterns (31, 261, 264, 306). Once this information has been obtained, nursing actions can be initiated that support these established patterns and possibly prevent total disruption of body rhythms during hospitalization.

After the patient has been hospitalized for a few days, certain objective data are available that will assist you in determining a rough estimate of the person's circadian patterns. The routine graphic record supplies information about the patient's vital signs. Using this source, you might be able to identify peaks and lows in blood pressure, pulse, or temperature curves. Also, an intake and output record that shows both the time and the amount voided will aid in determining the patient's daily urinary-excretory pattern. In addition to the postadmission nursing history, a daily log of sleep and waking hours, meal times, hunger periods, voiding and defecation patterns, diurnal moods, and other circadian rhythms recorded for 28 days before hospitalization can help determine the person's cyclic patterns. Diagnostic tests and certain forms of medical and nursing therapy can then be appropriately prescribed by using the person's own baseline rhythms' measurements. Determination of each patient's rhythms before, during, and after hospitalization or illness eventually will be possible when more simplified, economic, and accurate measurement devices are available.

The client's *medication schedule* can also reflect your understanding of biologic rhythms. Drug effectiveness can be altered by the time of day that the particular drug is administered. Aspirin administered at 7 A.M. will remain in the body 22 hours; aspirin ingested at 7 P.M. will last 17 hours. Some antihistamines last only 6 to 8 hours if taken at night but are effective 15 to 17 hours when taken at 7 A.M. Digitalis (a cardiac glycoside) is several times more effective when administered in the early morning than when administered at other times. The dosage of analgesics needed to relieve pain during the evening or dark hours is more than that needed during the daytime. Sensitivity to pain increases in the evening (341, 355).

One area of **chronopharmacology** (*study of cel-lular rhythms in relationship to drug therapy*) that has been researched extensively is the relationship of adrenocortical function and corticosteroid drug administration. The secretion of corticosteroids by the adrenal cortex has a 24-hour rhythm, with the highest corticosteroid values expected after the usual time of awakening. When corticosteroids are administered either daily or on alternate days, adrenal suppression and possibly growth disturbance can be minimized by timing to the circadian crest in adrenocortical function. Morning doses of prednisolone (a glucocorticoid) are less likely to cause alterations in the rhythmic pattern of urinary excretion than twice-daily divided doses or a single dose in the late evening (16, 97).

Circadian rhythms are also important factors in determining drug toxicity. A distinct 24-hour rhythm of vulnerability or resistance to drugs has been identified. Before setting a drug's toxic level, both the person's biologic clock and the drug dosage must be considered. At present, problems exist in determining toxicity levels. Federal research guidelines do not consider the circadian rhythms of the animals being tested. Noctural animals are tested in the daytime; animals are tested before they have had time to adjust to a new laboratory environment; animals are tested in light and dark cycles that are not regulated; and animals whose feeding schedules are not fixed and recorded are tested. All these factors can cause altered rhythms in animals and altered vulnerability or resistance to the drug being tested (98).

Without the aid of suitable measurement devices, it is impossible to determine a person's biologic clock. Drug administration is therefore usually based on other factors. Most medications are given before or after meals, at bedtime, or at the convenience of the nursing personnel and patients. In the future, as knowledge of the internal clock increases, you, the nurse, will find yourself altering drug administration times to suit the person's biologic time. Perhaps you will be in charge of a master computer that, after analyzing information about each person's biologic clock, will send the appropriate medication dose at the appropriate time.

Vital signs routine should be based on circadian rhythm patterns rather than on tradition or convenience of the agency staff. Both a person's internal and skin temperature shows a systematic rise and fall over a 24-hour period, a cycle difficult to alter in normal adults. Body temperature usually peaks between 4 P.M. and 6 P.M. and reaches its lowest point around 4 A.M. in people who are active by day and sleep by night. When the internal temperature is normally peaking, other body functions such as pulse rate, blood pressure, and cardiac output (volume of blood pumped by the heart) are also changing. Pulse rate is high when the temperature is highest and drops during the night. The human heart rate will vary as much as 20 or 30 beats per minute in 24 hours. Blood pressure shows a marked fall during the first hour of sleep, followed by a gradual rise throughout the daily cycle, with a peak between 5 and 7 P.M. Cardiac output reaches minimum levels between 2 and 4 A.M., the period of lowest temperature findings (75, 102, 273, 280).

Work Schedules

Work schedules should be developed with biologic rhythms in mind. You can also establish your own circadian patterns to help you gain insight into physical feelings and behaviors and can use this information to plan your days to advantage. You might choose to cope with the most difficult patient assignment during the time of peak mental and physical performance, for example.

Nurses and many industrial and law enforcement personnel are frequently required to change shifts every week or month. Night and rotating shift workers are at an excessive risk for accidents and injuries on the job because of disrupted circadian rhythms. Sleep cycles are interrupted. There is difficulty in falling asleep, a shorter duration of sleep, poorer quality of sleep, and persistent fatigue. Alertness and other physiologic processes suffer. Eating habits are disrupted; diets are poorer; and digestion is interfered with. Constipation, gastric and peptic ulcers, and gastritis are more common. Social activities and interactions, essential to physical and mental health, are interrupted. Family life and relationships are interfered with; shift workers have difficulty fulfilling family and parental roles. Rotating shift assignments are thus relevant to worker's health and quality of work performance (10, 105, 167, 179, 199, 304, 358). Altering the sleep-wake sequence requires time for the person to make adjustments and regain synchrony.

If shift rotation cannot be eliminated, individuals should be required to rotate no more frequently than once a month. Consistently working at night allows a person to acquire a new sleep-wake rhythm. Therefore night work should be made more attractive to persons who can adapt to the shift and are willing to remain on it permanently. Those who cannot adapt should be exempt from rotation.

Health teaching of any rotating-shift worker concerning the possible consequences of such a routine should not be overlooked. Night workers taking medications should be aware that the effects of medications may vary somewhat from those they usually experience when working days. The susceptibility to various degrees of drug metabolism occurs throughout the day but even more when a person is experiencing jet lag or the early phase of shift rotation. Individuals with a chronic illness such as diabetes, epilepsy, or hypertension and cardiac problems must consider these factors when they plan their medication regimen.

Rest and Sleep

Sleep is a *complex biologic rhythm, intricately related to rest and other biologic rhythms.* Help clients realize that factors such as emotional and physical status, occupation, and amount of physical activity determine the need for rest and sleep. For example, workers who alternate between day and night shifts frequently feel more exhausted and may need more sleep than people who keep regular hours. Surgery, illness, pregnancy, and the postpartum state all require that the individual receive more sleep. Mothers of infants, toddlers, and preschoolers may need daytime naps.

Some young people find themselves caught in a whirlwind of activities. Jobs, social activities, family responsibilities, and educational pursuits occupy their every minute. The young adult can adjust to this pace and maintain it for a length of time without damaging physical or mental health. The person may think he or she is immune to the laws of nature and can go long periods without sleep. If the person finds that he or she is not functioning well on a certain amount of sleep, the schedule should be adjusted to allow for more hours of rest. He or she also must be cognizant of the biologic rhythms for rest and activity. Setting aside certain periods for quiet activities such as reading, sewing, watching television, or various hobbies is restful but not as beneficial as sleep.

Each person has his or her own sleep needs and cycle, and research is helping us better understand the different stages of sleep and the importance of sleep to well-being. The tradition that young adults should have 7 to 8 hours of sleep seems valid, although some get along fine with less. When left to the body's natural pace, the person is likely to sleep every 25 hours (262).

Normal Sleep Pattern

Sleep is a complex phenomenon (30, 31, 57, 99, 185, 229, 259, 262). The functional component of the brainstem that exerts influence on consciousness and the wake-sleep cycle is called the *reticular activating system* (*RAS*). The RAS activates the state of consciousness and functions as a deactivation mechanism to decrease alertness and to produce sleep. **Electroencephalograms (EEGs),** *recordings of brainwave activity,* vary with the awake and asleep states and at different intrasleep cycles (Fig. 12–2). When a person is wide awake and alert, the EEG recordings show rapid, irregular waves. High-frequency beta and alpha waves predominate. As he or she begins to rest, the wave pattern changes to an **alpha rhythm,** *a regular pattern of low voltage, with frequencies of 8 to 12 cycles per second.* During sleep a **delta rhythm** occurs, *a slow pattern of high voltage and 1 to 2 cycles per second.* At certain stages of sleep, **sleep spindles,** *sudden short bursts of sharply pointed alpha waves of 14 to 16 cycles per second,* and **K-complexes,** *jagged tightly peaked waves,* occur.

Sleep is divided into **NREM** *nonrapid eye movement* and **REM** stages. NREM sleep is divided into four stages—light to deep. REM sleep follows the deepest NREM sleep as the person ascends to stage II sleep and occurs before repeated descent through stages II, III,

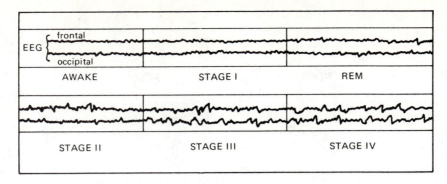

Figure 12-2. Changes in electroencephalogram during sleep.

and IV. In **NREM stage I sleep,** the *person makes a transition from wakefulness to sleep* in approximately 5 minutes. The alpha rhythm is present, but the waves are more uneven and smaller than in later stages. The person is drowsy and relaxed, has fleeting thoughts, is somewhat aware of the environment, can be easily awakened, and may think he or she has been awake. The pulse rate is decreased. **NREM stage II sleep** is the *beginning of deeper sleep* and fills 40% to 50% of total sleep time. The person is more relaxed than in the prior stage but can be easily awakened. Sleep spindles and K-complexes appear in the brain waves at intervals. **NREM stage III sleep** is a *period of progressively deeper sleep* and begins 30 to 45 minutes after sleep onset. EEG waves become more regular; delta waves appear; sleep spindles are present; muscles are more relaxed; vital signs and metabolic activity are lowered to basal rates; and the person is difficult to awaken. **NREM stage IV sleep** is *very deep sleep, occurs approximately 40 minutes after stage I, and rests and restores the body physically.* This stage is of as great importance as REM sleep. Delta waves are the dominant EEG pattern. The person is very relaxed and seldom moves, is difficult to arouse, and responds slowly if awakened. Physiologic measures are below normal. Sleep walking and enuresis may occur during this stage. After strenuous physical exercise, this stage is greatly needed.

REM sleep is called *active or paradoxic sleep* and is the *stage of rapid eye movements and dreaming that occurs before descending to the deeper sleep of stages II, III, and IV.* This stage is of great importance. In REM sleep the EEG readings are active and similar to stage I sleep, but various physiologic differences from other sleep stages are present. These differences, in addition to rapid, side-to-side eye movements are:

1. Muscular relaxation and absent tendon reflexes, with occasional twitching, so that the body is in immobility-like paralysis.
2. Respiratory rate increased 7% to 20% alternating between rapid and slow with brief apneic periods.
3. Pulse rate irregular and increased 5%.
4. Blood pressure fluctuations up to 30mm Hg.
5. High oxygen consumption by the brain.
6. Increased production of 17 hydroxycorticoid steroids, posterior pituitary hormones, and catecholamines.
7. Increased gastric secretions.
8. Penile erections in men of all ages.

REM sleep occurs in 70- to 90-minute cycles that increase as the night progresses. It rests and restores mentally and is important for learning and psychologic functioning. It allows for review of the day's events, categorizing and integrating of information into the brain's storage systems, and problem solving. During psychologic stress this stage is vital. Dreams that occur during REM sleep allow for wish fulfillment and release of potentially harmful thoughts, feelings, and impulses so that they do not affect the waking personality.

In a 7- or 8-hour period the person will have 60- to 90-minute cycles of sleep descending from stage I to IV and back to REM sleep. After 10 to 15 minutes of REM sleep, the person again descends to stage IV. The person may ascend to REM sleep three or five times a night, but each time he or she spends a longer period of time in it. In the first third of the night he or she spends more time in stage IV sleep; in the last third of the night more time is spent in REM sleep. Dreams in the early REM stages are shorter, are less interesting, and contain aspects of the preceding day's activities. As the night progresses, the dreams become longer, more vivid and exciting, and less concerned with daily life. Stages III and IV together comprise approximately 20% of sleep time until old age when deep sleep almost disappears.

Variations in Sleep Patterns

The percentage of time a person spends in sleep differs with age and with body temperature at the time of falling asleep. If the person's body temperature is at its high point in the biologic rhythm, he or she will sleep two times longer than if the temperature is at a low point in the biologic rhythm. REM sleep remains constant throughout adult life, comprising 20% to 25% of sleep, in contrast to 40% to 50% of sleep for babies. But the percentage of time spent in stage IV sleep decreases 15% to

30% with age so that the aged person sleeps less time and awakens more frequently. Elderly women's sleep patterns change approximately 10 years later than men's patterns. The aged person's adjustment to sleep seems dependent on arteriosclerotic changes so that the alert aged person sleeps about the same as the young adult. The aged person with cerebral arteriosclerotic changes sleeps 20% less than the young adult (60, 262, 274).

REM sleep is related to the onset of certain diseases. Convulsions are more likely to occur in the epileptic individual just before awakening, which is during REM sleep. Because the pulse is irregular during REM sleep, myocardial infarctions and arrhythmias are more likely to occur. Gastric secretion is increased during the REM state. The person with a peptic ulcer has more pain at these times (223, 262, 274).

Sedatives, antidepressants, and amphetamines significantly decrease REM sleep. If the person continually takes a sedative, there is a gradual return to the usual amount of REM sleep. But when the drug is withdrawn, REM sleep is markedly withdrawn, causing insomnia and nightmares, irritability, fatigue, and sensitivity to pain, all of which persist up to 5 weeks. Thus sedatives should be given sparingly, including to the young adult, although different sedatives cause different effects, and effects differ from person to person. You should learn from the person if he or she is regularly on sedatives. If the person is, he or she must continue them to avoid withdrawal symptoms while receiving health care (194, 311).

If REM deprivation and the rebound of more REM sleep later occur because of administration of sedatives, the patient with any health problem, but especially cardiovascular disease, should have sedative administration stopped before discharge. At home the person will not have the close observation needed during the prolonged periods of REM sleep when myocardial infarction is more likely to occur. Further, in contrast to popular belief, alcoholic beverages should not be used to promote sleep. Alcohol speeds the onset of sleep but interferes with REM sleep, which may contribute to hangover feelings.

Sleep Deprivation

Sleep deprivation should be avoided by the young adult. The person may feel rested if he or she awakens after 4 or 5 hours of sleep, but there has been insufficient time for REM sleep. If the person is awakened frequently, the sleep cycle must be started all over again. Physical and psychologic changes associated with sleep deprivation are shown in Box 12–2 (185, 256, 259, 262).

When the person decides to recover lost sleep by sleeping longer hours, he or she will spend more time in REM sleep. Twelve to 14 hours of sleep help to overcome brief periods of sleep deprivation. Studies indicate a minimum of 5 hours sleep daily is needed and for

---

■ **BOX 12-2.**
Physical and Psychologic Changes With Sleep Deprivation

Physical Changes

- Lack of alertness
- Feeling pressure on head
- Nystagmus; ptosis of eyelids
- Uncoordination; tremors
- Slowed reflexes
- Fatigue
- Bradypnea
- Cardiac arrhythmias
- Poorer performance
- Increased errors
- Physical discomfort; hypochondriasis

Psychologic Changes

- Anxiety; insecurity
- Introspective; unable to respond to support from others; irritable
- Apathy; withdrawal
- Depression
- Increased aggressiveness
- Suspicious
- Decreased mental agility
- Illusions
- Decreased concentration
- Loss of creativity
- Poor judgment
- Memory failure
- Confusion; disorientation
- Hallucinations
- Bizarre behavior; psychosis

---

most people 7 to 8 hours are needed to avoid sleep deprivation (185). After 48 hours of sleep loss, the body produces a stress chemical related structurally to LSD-25, which may account for behavioral changes. After 4 days of sleep deprivation, the body does not produce adenosine triphosphate (ATP), the catalyst for energy release, which may be a factor in fatigue. With total sleep deprivation, confusion, hallucinations, and psychosis ocur (85, 116, 345).

Thus the client, who needs all stages of sleep for physical and psychologic restoration, *should not be awakened during the night if at all possible*. Observe the person before awakening by studying eye movements under the lids. If he or she is in REM sleep, wait a few minutes for it to end before awakening the person since this is a short and important stage. Sleep has priority over taking vital signs, especially since the vital sign measurement is affected by the stage of sleep and therefore cannot be compared accurately to daytime measurements. Since steroids are released during REM sleep, disturbance of REM sleep causes steroid release to be out of synchrony with other biologic rhythms, affecting all areas of function in the person.

Being frequently awakened during the night such as happens to young parents with young children produces the same effects as sleeping fewer hours, even if the total length of time asleep is the usual amount. Blocks of uninterrupted sleep are a definite physical and psychologic need.

Help parents work out a system that responds to baby's need but also allows each parent to get as much uninterrupted sleep as possible. Use the above information on sleep stages and effects of sleep interruption and deprivation to teach the young adults.

Sleep Disturbances

Millions of people in the United States do not get normal sleep daily. They either sleep too much or not enough, suffer night terrors, or stop breathing for a minute or two during sleep. The cost of sleep disorders is enormous; some people pay a great deal for pills and potions to maintain normal sleep (259).

Insomnia, a *disorder of initiating and maintaining sleep,* is sometimes a problem for young adults. **Primary insomnia** is a *sleep problem that exists in the absence of any major medical or psychiatric condition.* Other types of insomnia are **sleep onset** *(difficulty falling asleep),* **sleep maintenance** *(awakening in the middle of the night),* and **terminal insomnia** *(early morning awakening).* Factors that may lead to insomnia include (1) disturbed circadian rhythms, (2) physical symptoms such as pain, dyspnea, and fever, (3) environmental disturbances, (4) emotional stress, and (5) stimulant drugs (259, 262).

Knowing the quantity and quality of sleep is useful in determining the existence of insomnia. Individual sleep requirements vary, and an individual's satisfaction with the length and quality of sleep is the basis for assessing the presence of insomnia.

You can help the insomniac by being an interested, calm listener and by suggesting that the following measures be tried (99, 138, 262).

1. Maintain a regular schedule of prebedtime relaxation, sleep, and wakefulness to keep biorhythms in synchrony.
2. Avoid strenuous activity in the evening before retiring; instead rely on soothing but enjoyable stimuli such as a backrub for muscular and emotional relaxation, quiet music, warm bath, progressive relaxation to loosen tight muscles, or a nonstimulating book or hobby.
3. Try a glass of warm milk, which contains l-tryptophan, a chemical that increases brain serotonin and induces sleep.
4. Improve the sleeping environment: make the bedroom dark, quiet, and as comfortable as possible so it is associated only with pleasurable feelings.
5. Purposefully relax after going to bed. Stretch out, get comfortable, let the body become heavy and warm.
6. Use pleasant imagery; let the mind "float."
7. Suggest that the person sleep on the back on a firm mattress. If the person sleeps on the side, a small pillow should be tucked between the waist and the mattress to provide proper support. Sleeping on the abdomen is not recommended because the head is turned sharply to one side all night, affecting neck joints and the lower back. In addition, pressure on one side of the face can irritate the jaw. Sleeping with one arm under the pillow stresses the jaw and may interfere with circulation or pinch a nerve in the wrist.
8. If not asleep in 20 minutes, get out of bed and go to another room. Stay calm. Do something boring or relaxing until you are sleepy.

Tranquilizers and sedatives are a last resort. For the ill person, first try a monotonous, rhythmic stimulus such as the backrub, quiet music, a dim light, eyeshades and earplugs, a wrinklefree bed, or reading a dull book that is conducive to sleep if it does not irritate the person since the cerebral cortex has nothing for which to stay alert. In effect, with monotony or boredom, the cerebral cortex does not respond to the reticular formation.

Assess the ill person's sleep pattern and help him or her adhere to the normal pattern. The hospital routine of "pass the pills at 9:00 and be asleep by 9:30" fits very few individuals.

If the person does complain of sleep problems, the problems should be explored with the goal of eventual correction. Refer the person to a sleep research center so that, through electronic monitoring of the sleep cycle and close surveillance, the problem can be identified and treated.

Physical Fitness—Exercise

Physical fitness is a *combination of strength, endurance, flexibility, balance, speed, agility, and power* and reflects ability to work for a sustained period with vigor and pleasure, without undue fatigue, and with energy left for enjoying hobbies and recreational activities and for meeting emergencies. Fitness relates to how the person looks and feels, both physically and mentally. Basic to fitness are regular physical exercise, proper nutrition, adequate rest and relaxation, conscientious health practices, and good medical and dental care.

Pregnant women can continue exercise routines unless they are contraindicated medically. The guidelines are as follows:

1. Avoid competitive exercise; do not push excessively.
2. Avoid workouts in hot, humid weather.

3. Strenuous exercise should not last longer than 15 minutes.
4. Pulse rate should not exceed 140 beats per minute.
5. Body temperature should not rise above 100.4° F (38° C) during exercise.
6. After the fourth month of pregnancy, no exercises should be performed while lying on the back (239).

Jogging makes joints in good condition stronger. Jogging as a regular form of exercise can aggravate old injuries of the back, hips, knees, and ankles since jogging puts as much as five times normal body weight on lower joints and extremities. Jogging can cause abnormal wear on joints and muscles. The person who jogs must also engage in exercise for the upper extremities and other muscles. Weight lifting can strengthen. Aerobic exercise, brisk walking, jumping rope, and bicycling may actually be better exercise than jogging. These activities stress bone to promote bone building, thickness, and strength and increase circulation throughout the body (5, 258, 323).

Swimming is probably the best overall activity because it increases strength and endurance and stimulates heart and blood vessels, lungs, and many muscle groups without putting excess stress on the person because of less gravity pull in the water. Further, swimming keeps joints supple, aids weight loss or weight control, and reduces hypertension. Perhaps more important, it is an enjoyable activity, either alone or with others.

Regular physical activity has been viewed as a natural tranquilizer, for it reduces anxiety and muscular tension. Some studies show that regular physical exercise improves a number of personality characteristics, correlating with composure, extraversion, self-confidence, assertiveness, persistence, adventuresomeness, and superego strength (85, 258).

Exercise periods are frequently not planned by young adults. Some will get abundant exercises in their jobs, but many will not. Those who do not can check with the local Y.M.C.A. or Y.W.C.A. organizations, community recreation departments, continuing education departments of 2-year colleges, or commercial gymnasiums and health salons for exercise programs appropriate to their life-styles and physical conditions.

After the person has had a thorough physical examination and has been cleared by a physician, three sessions weekly of 30 minutes are recommended for developing muscle tone and strength and increasing cardiovascular efficiency. Teach that very fast walking that increases heartbeat to 70% to 85% of maximum heart rate (MHR) is considered the best exercise of all; people who cannot jog or run can usually walk 20 to 30 minutes on alternate days. Exercise intensity is monitored by assessing MHR during exercise. MHR is calculated by subtracting the person's age from 220. During exercise the pulse should be 60% to 80% of that level. (For example, the 40-year-old should have a pulse rate

of 108 to 144 during exercise. Activities that are good physical exercise include fast walking, calisthenics, jogging, swimming, jumping rope, and games like tennis if they are played regularly (259). A health self-appraisal questionnaire and program can help the person determine the present state of health and fitness and implications for the years ahead (256, 261).

One of the 1990 health objectives established by the U.S. Department of Health and Human Services (DHHS) was for 60% of adults 18 to 65 years of age to be participating regularly in vigorous physical exercise. No valid or practical measurement system is available that will allow assessment of leisure time physical activity participation of large populations. Consequently, it has been difficult to assess progress toward the 1990 goal; an accurate baseline from which to measure potential progress does not exist. A diary technique for measuring aggregate population physical activity participation was used in a study of adults through the Institute for Social Research to arrive at a possible baseline. An activity index was developed based on intensity of the activity and time of participation so that an index energy expenditure could be calculated. The activities are listed under the intensity of light, moderate, or heavy, as shown below. American adults are quite sedentary. Over a period of 1 week, 31% undertake no leisure time physical activity; 14% expend more than 1600 kcal/week in leisure time physical activity; and only 10% meet the DHHS physical activity requirements (85, 238, 262).

Light Intensity Activities
- Bowling
- Fishing
- Boating or sailing
- Horseback riding
- Gardening indoors
- Pet care
- Swinging

Moderate Intensity Activities
- Golfing
- Frisbee or catch
- Exercises or yoga
- Hunting
- Walking
- Hiking
- Bicycling
- Swimming
- Carpentry
- Gardening outdoors
- Grounds improvement
- Social dancing

Heavy Intensity Activities
- Team sports
- Racquet ball
- Skating or skiing
- Jogging
- Lessons in body movements
- Aerobic dance

Gender Differences

Women and men sometimes share the same physical exercise activities; sometimes interests and energy levels are different, and partners may engage in exercise activities separately. Women may have as much endurance as men, especially with training, but there are some physiologic differences that account for differences in performance in physical exercise activities or athletic events.

Men have greater upper-body strength due primarily to their longer arms, broader shoulders, and higher muscle fiber counts. Muscle can be conditioned by exercise, but muscle fiber count cannot be increased. Whether men exercise or not, their muscle fibers gain bulk from the hormone testosterone. In men the heart and lungs, which average 10% larger than those in females, provide more powerful and efficient circulation. The delivery of oxygen to men's muscles, a factor crucial to speed, is further enhanced by the higher concentration of hemoglobin in the blood. Finally, the longer limbs provide them with greater leverage and extension.

The aspects of female physiology that result in women's athletic advantages are not as self-evident as in males. Women's bodies contain an average of 9% more adipose tissue than in the male body. This tissue is deposited not only on the thighs, buttocks, and breasts, but in a subcutaneous layer that covers the entire body. It is this adipose tissue that makes the woman more buoyant and better insulated against cold, both of which are advantages in long-distance swimming. (The record for swimming the English Channel—7 hours and 40 minutes—is held by a woman, Penny Dean.) Body adipose tissue may also be one of the reasons few female runners report the pain and weakness that most male runners encounter. The body is conditioned to call on stored fats once its supply of glycogen, which fuels the muscles, has been exhausted. Since women have greater reserves of body fat, they are able to compete in athletics longer. Females perspire in smaller amounts and less quickly than males. Perspiring is the body's way of avoiding overheating. Yet women may tolerate heat better than men. Not only can body temperature rise in a woman several degrees higher before she begins to sweat, but women sweat more efficiently because of the even distribution of their sweat glands. In women **vascularization,** *capacity for bringing blood to the surface for cooling,* is also more efficient. The female has certain structural advantages for all types of running and swimming events. In swimming, narrower shoulders offer less resistance through water. Even at identical heights (and ideal weights), female bodies are lighter than male bodies, leaving them with less weight to carry while running (360).

Foot Care
Foot care is not considered often enough in an exercise program. The feet, during walking, will meet the surface at $1\frac{1}{2}$ to 2 times the body weight and up to 3 times its weight when running. Proper shoe fit, which includes heel height, stability, and cushion, wedge support, and forefoot cushion, must be considered. Also, proper fitting and absorbent socks are important, along with proper washing and careful drying of feet after exercise (80).

PSYCHOSOCIAL CONCEPTS

Cognitive Development
Different learning abilities are required in different life stages. Youth is the time for acquisition; young adulthood is the time for achievement; middle age is the time for responsibility; and old age is the time for reintegration (91, 200).

Theories About Cognitive Development
Cognitive theories are described here; refer also to Chapter 5. Erikson (90) theorized that the basis for adult cognitive performance is laid during the school years when the child accomplishes the task of industry, learns how to learn and win recognition by producing and achieving, and learns to enjoy learning. The child learns an attitude that lasts into adulthood: how much effort a task takes and how long and hard he or she should work for what is desired or expected. The sense of industry is useful in adult life, both in coping with new experiences and in functioning as a worker, family member, citizen, and lifelong learner.

Current researchers and theorists propose that learning continues throughout the adult years. Longitudinal studies indicate that the brain continues to change in structure and complexity until age 40 or 50 years. The brain shows increasing myelinization until middle age, which permits more integrated modes of social response and stable or increasing intellectual functions (85, 238, 333, 334).

Becoming mature in young adulthood involves intellectual growth, becoming more adaptive and knowledgeable about self, forming values, and developing increasing depth in analytic and synthetic thinking, logical reasoning, and imagination. There are multiple and different intelligences besides academic aptitude, including leadership ability, creative and performing arts abilities, and ability to manage self, others, and a career. Further, developing social and interpersonal skills and personal friendships may have a powerfully maturing effect on intellectual skills (91, 200).

Influences on Learning
Influences differ somewhat from childhood to adulthood and include (1) level of knowledge in society generally, (2) personal values and perceptions and previously learned associations, (3) level of education, (4) available life opportunities, (5) interests, (6) participation by the person in the learning activity, (7) the learning environment, and (8) life experiences (200, 238). As a result of these influences, the person develops a preferred way of learning or cognitive style—a characteristic way of perceiving, organizing, and evaluating information (241).

Formal Operations Stage
The young adult remains in the Formal Operations stage, according to Piaget. The adult is creative in thought. He or she begins at the abstract level and com-

pares the idea mentally or verbally with previous memories, knowledge, or experience. The person combines or integrates a number of steps of a task mentally instead of thinking about or doing each step as a separate unit. He or she considers the multiplicity and relativism of issues and alternatives to a situation, synthesizing and integrating ideas or information into the memory, beliefs, or solutions so that the end result is a unique product. Adult thought is different from adolescent thought in that the adult can differentiate among many perspectives and the adult is objective, realistic, and less egocentric. Thinking and learning are problem centered, not just subject centered. Reality is considered only a part of all that is possible. The person can imagine and reason about events that are not occurring in reality but that are possible or in which he or she does not even believe. Hypotheses are generated; conjectures are deduced from hypotheses, and observations are conducted to disconfirm the expectations. The thought system works independent of its context and can be applied to diverse data. The person can evaluate the validity of a train of reasoning independent of its factual content. A concrete proposition can be replaced by an arbitrary sign of symbolic logic such as p or q. Probability, proportionality, and combining of thought systems occur (35, 341, 344).

Arlin (15) cites Gruber as proposing that some people continue to develop cognitively beyond the Formal Operations proposed by Piaget into a *fifth stage* of cognitive development that progresses through adulthood. The stage of Formal Operations describes strategies used in problem solving. The *problem-finding stage* goes beyond the problem-solving stage and is characterized by creative thought in the form of discovered problems, the formation of generic problems, the raising of general questions from ill-defined problems, use of intuition and hunches, and the development of significant scientific thought.

The person may use different thinking for scientific operations, business transactions, artistic activities, and intimate interpersonal interactions. Thus mature thinkers can accept and live with contradictions and conflicts and engage in a number of activities. However, at times the adult will of necessity do thinking typical of Concrete Operations. At times the adult may regress to the Preoperational Stage (some never get beyond this period), as shown by superstitious, egocentric, or illogical thinking. The adult may not have the ability to perform Formal Operations.

A further distinction in types of adult thinking separates the *managers,* those who have a better developed right brain and who synthesize data to see the overall picture, from the *planners,* those who have a better developed left brain and who analyze sequentially and look closely to the minute details. Women tend to have a better integrated brain and usually combine both manager and planner thinking (85, 238).

The young adult continues to learn both formally and informally to enhance cognitive and job skills and self-knowledge. Learning may be pursued in "on-the-job training," job-sponsored orientation courses, trade schools, college studies, or continuing education courses. Environmental stimulation is important in continued learning. Increasingly young adults are changing their minds about their life work and change directions after several years of study or work in the original field. Formal operations or abstract thinking appears linked to the content areas in which the person has extensive training. Berzonsky, cited in Webb (344), proposed that after concrete operations, a person may acquire abstract thinking in behavioral, symbolic, semantic, or figural content areas, depending on experience.

Gender Differences

Gender differences may be the result of gender bias in research. Cognitive ability in men and women has been considered unequal and has been described on the basis of different functions in each cerebral hemisphere, although brain structure is the same in men and women. The left hemisphere is dominant in 97% of people for language, logical reasoning, and mathematical calculation. The right hemisphere is nonverbal and mute: it knows but cannot tell what it knows without processing the knowledge through the left hemisphere. The right hemisphere processes spatial and visual abstractions, recognition of faces, body image, music, art forms, and intuitive, preconscious, and fantasy processes. At birth asymmetry in the left hemisphere is more marked in the male. Female infants have a somewhat larger area of visual cortex in the right hemisphere than male infants, which implies an anatomic advantage for nonverbal ideation. The female's brain matures earlier; thus the two hemispheres are more integrated in the female as indicated by less impairment of intellectual function in women who have suffered either right or left hemisphere damage. Males are more vulnerable to brain damage. On tests women use verbal strategies to solve spatial problems because of the greater interplay between the two hemispheres. In adulthood women are better able to coordinate activities of both hemispheres; thus they can think intuitively and globally. Men are better at activities in which the two hemispheres do not compete such as problem solving or determining spatial relationships (20, 21, 49, 238, 250).

Nonconformity to sex-role stereotypes is positively related to IQ. The more assertive and active woman has greater intellectual ability and more interests. The less aggressive man focuses less on developing physique and develops intellectual ability and interests to a greater extent (20).

Cognitive abilities have often been related to personality traits and interpersonal orientation. Sex-role socialization has been related to cognitive style. Some researchers believe the level of information processing a person attains exerts a profound influence on personality and on ability to integrate and differentiate in problem solving (21, 49, 238).

Claims about sex differences in other cognitive abilities such as creativity, analytic ability, and reasoning also apparently are the result of differences in verbal, quantitative, or visual-spatial abilities or in opportunity to develop such abilities—in either gender (21, 49, 220).

Both female and male young adults who are in formal education are causing shifts in the educational system. They are more vocal, persuasive, and determined about what they consider pertinent. They are stimulating diversity and quality in the higher-education patterns. The young adult wants to learn more about something or learn to do something better and wants a voice in planning education. The nontraditional education offered by some colleges is more an attitude than a system; the students' needs are first and the institution's convenience second. Competent performance and concern for the learner of any age rather than just obtaining degrees are being emphasized in adult education, including noncollegiate programs. Full educational opportunity through life is the goal of many young adults, enabling each to meet potential personally and as a citizen. The young adult is concerned about the most important principles or concepts to learn to provide the balance between the timely and timeless in this modern world.

The confident young adult takes pride in being mentally astute, creative, progressive, and alert to events. He or she normally has the mental capacity to make social and occupational contributions, is self-directive and curious, and likes to match wits with others in productive dialogue.

Both men and women have similar basic needs, their own unique cognitive abilities and talents, and often unspoken ideas and feelings longing for self-expression. From young childhood on, both females and males should be considered cognitively capable to their maximum potential and should have the opportunity, including in the adult years, to meet that maximum potential.

Teaching the Adult

Information on cognitive development and the principles of learning described in Chapter 17 should be considered whenever you are teaching adults. Avoid "canned" audiovisual presentations. Emphasize a sharing of ideas and experiences, role play, and practical application of information. In some cases you will be helping the person to unlearn old habits, attitudes, or information to acquire new habits and attitudes.

If you teach illiterate young adults, you must compensate for their inability to read and write. Slow, precise speech and gestures and the use of pictures and audiovisual aids are more crucial than with literate adults. Demonstration and *return demonstration* assure learning. Do not underestimate the importance of your behavior and personality as a motivating force, especially if some members of the person's family do not consider learning important.

Work and Leisure Activities

Although the following discussion focuses on work outside of the home, implying paid employment, we do not demean or overlook the young adult woman or man who chooses to stay at home and rear a family. *Homemaking and child rearing are essential and important work;* each is fatiguing and stressful in its own way. In fact, staying at home can be hazardous to health. The many noise and air pollutants or chemical toxins that come from appliances, building materials, cleaning products, and combinations of materials or supplies used in a home should be discussed (108).

Work Options and Attitudes

There are many work options and attitudes: for example, the young adult "workaholic" executive who puts in 70 to 80 hours weekly at the job, thinks about the job most of the remaining hours, feels guilty when not working, and channels much anger and aggression through work; the factory worker who, while feeding a certain part into the assembly line, is planning what he or she will do the minute he or she leaves the factory— to this person work is only a means of livelihood; the blue-collar worker who has more stress than the executive; and the young adult who, after several years, has lost interest in the job and is trying to decide whether to "stick it out" 35 more years to retirement or risk going into another field that appears challenging. There are also completely opposite attitudes about the same kind of work. For example, one young adult will choose to be a police officer or fire department employee because he or she cares more about adventure and challenge than money. Another will say, "Why should I put my life on the line when the public does not think enough of me to pay decent wages?" Then there are those people who work long hours and who are highly involved in their work but who are not workaholics. They feel exhilarated about the flow of work, the challenge, their goals, and the use of skills involved, and they feel creative, active, and motivated. These feelings are more likely to come from work than leisure. These people contribute a great deal to the advancement of their vocation or profession generally and to the individuals they serve (73).

In addition to agricultural, skilled and semi-skilled workers, blue-collar and white-collar workers, managerial or executive personnel, and professionals, a new classification exists—the knowledge worker. Because of expanding technology, rapid change, the burgeoning size of industries and megaindustries, and the knowledge explosion, some people are hired to do job planning and to create, innovate, and make decisions within the organization. The ultimate goal of the knowledge worker is cost containment for the company, improved efficiency of the worker, a more marketable product, and a more willing buyer. If you are a knowledge worker, your task is less well defined. For example, you might be helping the health care agency develop long-range plans and goals; you might be a consultant; or you might be observing other nurses at work to determine a more effective way to deliver nursing care and avoid nonnursing tasks. You must cope with unanticipated changes, predict changes, and collaborate with others.

You may find the worker—all the way from the executive level to the delivery person—a victim of **substance abuse,** *ingesting excessive alcohol or drugs or engaged in pushing illicit drugs* on the job. Substance abuse is a response to stress, often job related. The implications of substance abuse are grave, including job errors, accidents to self or others, poor job performance, a product that does not meet standard results, and increased insurance and worker's compensation benefits to employees, all of which increases the cost of the product to the consumer. In addition, the lives of family, friends, and coworkers are affected. Work with the personnel director, safety director, employee assistance programs, administrative personnel, and the affected individual (and family, if possible) to help the person get the necessary medical treatment. A recovered employee saves the company money. The employee keeps a job, and it is more expensive to hire and train a new worker in many situations.

Nurses may also suffer from substance abuse, but they are no more likely to have such problems than are other employees (319). Several references are pertinent to understanding and assisting the colleague who is chemically dependent (53, 100, 128, 312, 319). Refer also to the discussion of alcoholism and drug abuse later in this chapter.

More and more young adult women are entering the work force. Sometimes the move is a necessity (e.g., if she is single, divorced, and with children or if her husband has only seasonal work or a low-paying job). Many women are working to maintain occupational skills, self-esteem, and independence. If a woman is trying to work in addition to carrying on the traditional wife-mother-housekeeper roles, she will likely feel conflict. Finding day-care facilities for young children can be a problem. If the family can learn to work together on various home roles, the working wife–mother can be a real asset to the family because she will bring home her attitude of self-confidence and satisfaction. Also, the children will probably be more adaptive as they mature if they learn various household responsibilities and see their mother and father in a variety of roles instead of those stereotyped by traditional society (i.e., Mom sews, cooks, cleans; Dad mows the lawn, paints the house, repairs the car). Further, the children will learn that it is essential to become well prepared for adult work roles. The woman and the rest of the family, need some time free from responsibility (20).

Balancing work and family life responsibilities is often stressful for the woman who is a single parent or who is a member of a two-career family. There is never enough time and often too much to do (82, 98, 236, 293). Employers are beginning to confront these dilemmas. Some employers, to attract and keep competent workers, are offering flexible work schedules, job sharing, on-the-site day care, and both paternity leaves and extended maternity leaves. These suggestions can be shared with the parent who has the greatest responsibility for balancing home and work (217):

1. Identify priorities. Discuss with the spouse, or the children if they are old enough, what tasks must be done, what can be delegated (either on the job or to a service company in the home), and who can take on which responsibilities to even the load.
2. Allocate tasks. Design a system for assigning tasks, based on skill, age, availability, and fairness. Rotate tasks, if possible, or assign tasks that are especially requested.
3. Use a support network. Family, friends, neighbors, and child care providers can be asked for assistance on a regular basis or for help in emergencies.
4. Assess progress. Plan frequent review sessions to discuss effectiveness of the plan and problem areas to avoid resentments or rebellions or someone's taking advantage.

Differences between male and female personalities and behavior in young adulthood are related to occupation and whether the woman is solely a homemaker and mother. The young adult who is employed develops characteristics appropriate to achievement in the outside world—confidence, assurance, dependability—and is controlled, goal-oriented, self-satisfied. These gains may be accompanied by certain costs: detachment, compulsiveness, being less relaxed, being less responsive to humor, being less sensitive aesthetically, and being less interesting as a person. The woman who is a homemaker-mother shows a deeper understanding of relationships, feels more secure, shows more warmth, nurturance, tenderness, and giving and yet is inclined to guilt feelings and worry (20). Often the profession or career demands a combination of seemingly opposite characteristics—competitiveness and nurturance.

Fellow employees must be aware that women often look differently at the same work situation and respond to different rewards in the workplace than men and that they bring a perspective and judgment level that is not based solely on competition and aggressiveness. Further, equipment or protective clothing that fits men may well be hazardous to women because of size, weight, muscle stretching involved, or poor fit. The employer can benefit from the qualities and expertise women bring to the work force. In turn, women need to use the skills learned in the homemaking role and skills based on mathematics, technology, and information-computer systems (20, 238). Technologic change will increasingly compete with a rising demand for human services, especially in health, law, and recreation. Technology can help free people for service work. However, in a technologic age, skills related to caring for or serving others are often neglected. Colleges are already preparing for computer-addicted students with few human relation skills since human relation skills will be as essential in the future as technologic ones.

Regardless of the various attitudes about work, it remains a central part of the adult self-concept in most Americans, and a close relationship exists between occupational and family satisfaction (Fig. 12–3). If the person is dissatisfied in one, either work or family life, he or she will try to compensate in the other (91).

Because you are a nurse and view the person holistically, you may be asked for assistance by the manager, executive level employees, or the employers. They may find it difficult to understand the young adult worker who acts differently than the middle-aged or older worker; the behavior of the young adult who has newly achieved an executive position may be poorly understood by employees who are middle-aged and near retirement. Help them understand that each generation of worker has a different value system and responds to different values and different motivational stimuli (91, 238).

Because you are a nurse, others will seek you out as someone who can assist with safety and health problems, listen to and counsel about job problems, help another make decisions pertinent to occupation, and assist

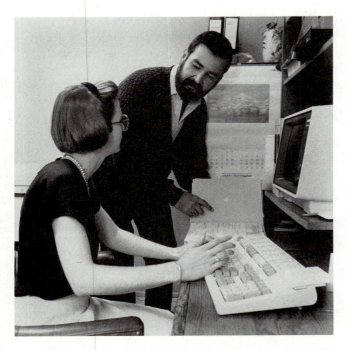

Figure 12-3. Career development is a central component of the life structure for many individuals. (From Berger, K.J., and M.B. Williams, *Fundamentals of Nursing: Collaborating for Optimal Health.* Norwalk Conn: Appleton & Lange, 1992, 266.)

in resolving conflicts related to the work setting or homemaker—career woman—mother roles. Through your counseling and education role, you can assist both the individual employee and administrative or management personnel to realize the importance of feelings of self-respect in relation to employment. Management consultants have learned that low self-esteem in the worker lowers productivity, morale, and profits. You can be instrumental in helping the work system promote workers' feelings of self-esteem and about the importance of their work.

You may also become an advocate for the woman who is undergoing sexual harassment on the job. Increasingly women workers are gaining the courage to talk publicly about and to seek legal aid for sexual harassment in factories, mines, offices, migrant farm fields, and health care facilities. Harassment can range from a passing caress to threats of or actual rape. Yet women or men who are harassed on the job may not complain, whether it is about the hug that the supervisor gives everyone daily—wanted or not—or about actual body contact because of fear of lack of confidentiality, fear of greater or more subtle harassment or retaliation, and fear of poor evaluations, loss of pay raises, or actual job loss (83).

Each work place should have policies and procedures established to handle complaints of harassment on the job. Ideally the work atmosphere should be such that, first, harassment would not occur, and second, everyone would be concerned about the problem and know how to handle it. The article by H. Heinrick (143) suggests how to cope with sexual harassment from clients.

The problems of sexism and sexual harassment in the workplace and in society in general is not limited to the United States. Black (33) describes how Japanese feminists are challenging the apathetic attitudes to sexism and consequent harassment in their society.

You must resolve your own job-related conflicts before you can help others. By using the above information and insights you gain from being a professional who works with and learns from many other people, you are indeed in a key position to assist the worker—whether you work in an occupational health setting, a clinic, or the emergency room or in a psychiatric–mental health, obstetric, medical, or surgical unit.

Burnout

Burnout, the *feeling of worthlessness, of not being appreciated, a sense of hopelessness, or loss of creativity,* is discussed primarily in relation to a job. The person who continually stays at home, with or without child care, can also suffer burnout. Some people propose that the homemaker's or mother's work should be assigned monetary worth since our society equates one's worth with earning power. Certainly the wife, husband, homemaker, mother, and father roles are each work and worthy, and the worth of each has not yet been calculated. However, a look at history and all cultures tells us we cannot survive without these roles, regardless of how they are acted out.

The choice of vocation, occupation, or profession depends to a great extent on the person's self-concept, personality, and opportunities and not only on abilities and interests. The young adult provides a livelihood for self and dependents through a chosen job or profession. This work can create feelings of happiness, pleasure, and fulfillment or feelings of being frustrated, blocked, and dehumanized. Job satisfaction increases with the level of job skill, variety of work, and opportunity for decision making. Job dissatisfaction increases with automation, lack of attention to the individual worker, and controlled decisions. Income and comfort factors, although important, do not play as big a role as challenge factors in job satisfaction. McCloskey (219) found that women nurses believed that autonomy, social integration, and connectedness related to their employment were major factors for job contentment.

Stress response (burnout) to the unrewarding, demanding work situation may become so great that the person undergoes physiologic and psychologic changes in response to work. There is inadequate emotional and physical energy for tasks, responsibilities, and roles. The physical and emotional exhaustion is accompanied by a sense of frustration and loss of control, a sense of tedium and apathy about first the job and then other aspects of life, anger about what is perceived as excessive work demands, guilt about not doing a good job or neglecting the family, depression, a number of somatic complaints, reduced productivity, disillusionment about the job, increased absenteeism, job turnover, low self-esteem, and poor morale. Although at first these feelings are related to the job, later they are also directed toward the family, home, friends, and other interests (110, 217, 241).

Professional health care professionals, including nurses, may suffer from burnout, especially if the nurse works in a high-stress area such as critical care, emergency, high-risk nursery, or a regularly understaffed unit or does frequent shift rotation that causes dyssynchrony of circadian rhythms and the consequences described on p. 446. Because of the physiologic and emotional toll of the workplace, especially if there are rotating shifts, there may be a number of consequent health problems and excess use of alcohol, tranquilizers, sleeping pills, and other drugs (217, 354). Personal motivation toward work and the physical effort of work should be considered in determining the impact of the job on the health of the pregnant woman and on the possibility of a preterm, low-birthweight delivery (156).

It is important to assess yourself in relation to work satisfaction and response to the stresses at work. Several references assist in job self-assessment, including Chapter 26 of *Psychiatric/Mental Nursing: Giving Emotional*

Care (240) and the references by Buechler (45), Kramer (181), and Pines and Aronson (260). Ways to overcome burnout are described by Freudenberger (110), Kramer (181, 182), Murray and Huelskoetter (240), Rich and Rich (266), and Schmalenberg and Kramer (287).

Kramer and her colleagues (181, 182, 287) investigated the process of new graduate nurses' socialization into the first work experience and termed the reaction *reality shock*. The new graduate often suffers from the discovery that values learned in nursing school conflict with those in the work setting. They proposed strategies to help the nurse become bicultural: (1) adjust at work while maintaining some of the ideals learned in school; (2) maintain the personal and professional identity in the work subculture while reacting appropriately on the job; and (3) initiate new ideas and values into the work subculture. These strategies and the renewed sense of hope and growth help prevent burnout (181, 182, 287).

Each of us must realize that every job has stresses and that stress can be viewed as a challenge. We all must realize, too, that every job, no matter how exciting it appears, has boredom and repetitive, routine, and noncreative aspects; it is unlikely that those aspects can be eliminated entirely. Thus each of us must be continually mindful of the satisfaction obtained from all pursuits of life; healthy ways to expand interests, hobbies, or social contacts; and ways to make the job more satisfying or interesting, if possible. Further, developing a sense of humor and a philosophic, spiritual outlook can give a balance to life that results in positive feelings about self, work, and others.

Leisure

Many young American adults are in pursuit of leisure—and rightly so. As job hours per week are being cut (especially in automated jobs), the time for leisure increases. Additionally, the work ethic is decreasing. Socialization of the current young adults has fostered a leisure ethic.

Leisure is *freedom from obligations and formal duties of paid work and opportunity to pursue, at one's own pace, mental nourishment, enlivenment, pleasure, and relief from fatigue of work.* Leisure may be as active as backpacking up a mountain or as quiet as fishing alone in a huge lake. Some people never know leisure, and others manage a certain leisure even as they work. Various factors influence the use of leisure time: gender; amount of family, home, work, or community responsibilities; mental status; income and socioeconomic class; and past interests.

Some people have never learned to pursue a hobby or an activity just for the "fun of it." Others have learned hobbies or have pursued recreational interests but use the same competitive spirit in the hobby or recreation as in work. Others pursue hobbies as the "current thing to do" but feel no real sense of pleasure.

Leisure gadgetry has invaded the marketplace. Electronic games have replaced household appliances as America's favorite gadgets. Technology affects leisure through changes in both products and values. As technology dictates specialized work, the games increasingly create specialized players and skills. The electronic games that reward aggressive and competitive behavior teach values and behavior that will be carried over to other leisure activities and the work force. The result may be contradictory to the meaning of leisure and even to meaning in life.

The real answer to the work-leisure dilemma is that the worker and the player are one. The unhappy worker will not automatically become the happy player. Challenging work makes leisure a time of refreshment. Successful leisure prepares the worker for more challenge.

Maintaining friendships is a healthy use of leisure time. It takes time, self-disclosure, and sharing of interests to form friendships. Gradually, a sense of reliability and confidentiality grows as a core to the friendship. Some conflict may surface and is natural as intimacy deepens. Getting closer to friends, rather than making more friends, is the way to reduce loneliness. Avoid developing all the friendships at the workplace. In today's competitive world people at work may not be able to be close. It is wiser to start out being more formal and distant until the trusting relationship evolves. In a world in which women juggle career, love, and family, time may limit the size of the friendship circle. Several close friends should be made. Successful friendship combines the freedom to depend on one another with the freedom to be independent. If free time is too limited, fewer friendships can be formed, because you will have little to give to anybody emotionally.

Doing volunteer work with a favorite charity or community group is a way to use nonwork time that can promote a sense of leisure and enjoyment while simultaneously using skills and talents to improve life for others. The rewards are dual—to the self and to society.

Help the client realize the importance of leisure as a part of balanced living. The young adult needs to develop a variety of interests as preparation for the years ahead to maintain physical and mental health.

Emotional Development

Emotional development in young adulthood is an ongoing, dynamic process, an extension of childhood and adolescent developmental influences and processes. Development is still influenced by the environment, but the environment is different. The fundamental developmental issues continue as central aspects of adult life but in an altered form. Thus trust, autonomy, initiative, industry, and identity all are reworked and elaborated, based on current experiences (90, 91, 200).

Young adulthood is a time when there is increased clarity and consistency of personality, a stabilization of self and identity, established preferences of interests and

activities, increased coping ability, less defensiveness, decrease in youthful illusions, fantasy, and impulsiveness, more responsiveness to and responsibility for self and others, more giving than taking, and more appreciation of surroundings, and it is a time to develop expanded resources for happiness. There are restrictions and continuities not previously experienced, some sacrifice of freedom and spontaneity, and less opportunity for variety, novelty, and impulsive adventure. However, there is more challenge to develop empathy (i.e., a depth of feeling and understanding), to learn in detail how systems work, and to reevaluate self and the world. If behavior is not too heavily bound by defenses against anxiety, it becomes more varied as experience accumulates (90, 91, 200).

Certainly adult experiences, life-style, and geographic changes can contribute to personality development and change. Yet the psychosocial development of the adolescent maintains a pattern or direction into young adulthood, as shown in a study of youth activists in the 1960s and others (85). In a longitudinal study of psychosocial development, it was found that most behavior and personality characteristics of the school-age child 6 to 10 years old were good predictors of early adult behavior and personality. However, various life experiences modify behavior and personality in adulthood. A major modifying variable is gender. Degrees of childhood passivity and dependency remained continuous for women but not for men (238). The longitudinal study by Maas and Kuyper (206) also shows the influence of childhood experiences on adult personality and the continuity of adult personality characteristics over the years. Expression of one emotion such as anger has also been consistently manifested across the lifespan of the person (324).

Theories of Emotional Development

Various stage theorists (Second Force) referred to in Chapter 5 also have research findings on which to base their beliefs about adult personality development. The findings of Jung, Vaillant, Gould, Sheehy, Levinson, Sullivan and Erikson are discussed in the following pages.

Jung (169) believes that the personality develops along different lines during the first and second halves of the life cycle. The first period, until approximately age 40 or 45 years, is a time of outward expansion. Maturational forces direct the growth of the ego and the unfolding of capacities for dealing with the external world. Young people learn to get along with others and try to win as many of society's rewards as possible. They establish careers and families, and they do what they can to advance up the social ladder of success. To do so, it is usually necessary for women to develop their feminine traits and skills and men their masculine ones, although in present society women who are successful must combine the traditional feminine and masculine traits into a unique, nonthreatening whole. During this phase a certain amount of one-sidedness is necessary and even valuable, for the young person needs to dedicate self to the task of mastering the outer world. It is not especially advantageous for young people to be too preoccupied with their self-doubts, fantasies, and inner nature. The task is to meet the demands of the external environment confidently and assertively. As one can imagine, extroverts, rather than introverts, may have an easier time in adjusting during this period.

From his longitudinal study of adult men, Vaillant (333, 334) proposes that development continues through adulthood in a number of ways: emotionally, mentally, socially in relationships, and in career. Simultaneously, the developing and successful adult also demonstrates what Freud calls the psychopathology of everyday life. All have special adaptational problems and mechanisms. Vaillant believes that emotional health and development are evolutionary, not static. Isolated traumatic events rarely mold individual lives; rather development comes from continued interaction between choice of adaptive mechanisms and sustained relationships with others. Poor adaptation, which lowers the threshold for perceiving or handling stress, leads to anxiety, depression, and physical illness. Vaillant's study identifies mature defenses—altruism, humor, suppression or minimization of discomforts, anticipation, sublimation—that promote adaptation. Successful adapters have had good relationships with parents, are energetic and alert, feel good about themselves, love their work, have very close relationships with wives and friends, and sublimate aggression into enthusiastic pursuits of projects, work, or competitive sports. His findings seem applicable to adult women as well.

Gould (125) describes life stages and key issues or tasks in late adolescence and young adulthood. Gould believes there is an increasing need throughout adulthood to win permission from the self to continue development. The direction of change through adulthood is becoming more tolerant of self and more appreciative of the surrounding world. Although Gould does not list specific assumptions about adult development, he sees adulthood as a time of thoughtful confrontation with the self—letting go of an idealized image, the desire to be perfect, and acknowledging the realistic image of self and personal feelings. Conflicts between past and present beliefs are resolved. Through constant examination and reformulation of beliefs embedded in feelings, the person can substitute a conception of adulthood for childhood legacy and fantasies. Whereas children mark the passing years by their changing bodies, adults change their minds, deepen their insights about self, and mature emotionally.

Sheehy (295, 296) believes that development occurs throughout adulthood and is influenced by external events or crises, the historical period, membership in the culture, and social roles and by the internal realism of the person—the values, goals, and aspirations. Sheehy ties developmental stages in late adolescence and young adulthood to Erikson's development stages.

Levinson (197, 198), like Vaillant, studied only men in formulating a concept of adult developmental stages. However, he believes the stages are age linked and universal; thus they should be applicable to women. In each period biologic, psychodynamic, cultural, social, and other timetables operate in only partial synchronization, which makes for developmental difficulties. The organizing concept of **life structure** *refers to a pattern of the person's life at a specific time* and is used to focus on the boundary between the individual and society. In its external aspects life structure refers to roles, memberships, interests, conditions or style, of living, and long-term goals. In the internal aspects life structure includes the personal meanings of external patterns, inner identities, core values, fantasies, and psychodynamic qualities that shape the person.

Sullivan (320) believes young adulthood is normally the time when the sexuality of human development is powerful, and there is a need to find adequate and satisfying expression. Now is the time of expanding experiences with people. If for some reason the person is thwarted in expression or sublimation of sexual feelings, perhaps because of illness or injury that causes a felt or imagined change in body, sexual concerns may become paramount.

Developmental Crisis

According to Erikson (90), the psychosexual crisis is intimacy versus self-isolation. **Intimacy** is *reaching out and using the self to form a commitment to and an intense, lasting relationship with another person or even a cause, an institution, or creative effort (90)*. In an intimate experience there is mutual trust, sharing of feelings, and responsibility to and cooperation with each other. The physical satisfaction and psychologic security of another are more important than one's own. The person is involved with people, work, hobbies, and community issues. He or she has poise and ease in the lifestyle because identity is firm. There is a steady conviction of who he or she is, a unity of personality that will improve through life. Intimacy is a situation involving two people that permits acceptance of all aspects of the other and a collaboration in which the person adjusts behavior to the other's behavior and needs in pursuit of mutual satisfaction (320).

A person's mental health is dependent on the ability to enter into a relationship and experience self-disclosure; in so doing, the support and maintenance of the relationship alleviates feelings of loneliness. Women, more so than men, are concerned with relationships and are interested in the process rather than the product of something. They also recognize their vulnerability and can acknowledge the need to change more readily than men. Women self-disclose more easily than men (49, 220). Such people are less lonely. Interpersonal dependency, an element of the normal adult personality, encompasses attachment and dependency. Anxious or insecure attachment develops when a natural desire for a close relationship with another is accompanied by apprehension that the relationship will end. If anxiety is transferred to the other person, the response may be a withdrawal from the relationship, contributing to feelings of loneliness. If a healthy balance between dependence and independence exists, social relationships and intimacy are maintained more easily, and the risk of experiencing loneliness and isolation decreases (90, 91, 200).

Although intimacy includes orgasm, it means far more than the physical or genital contact so often described in how-to sex manuals. With the intimate person the young adult is able to regulate cycles of work, recreation, and procreation (if chosen) and to work toward satisfactory stages of development for all offspring and the ongoing development and self and the partner. Intimacy is a paradox. Although the person shares his or her identity with another for mutual satisfaction or support (via self-abandon in orgasm or in another shared emotional experience), he or she does not fear loss of personal identity. Each does not absorb the other's personality.

Many in late adolescence or early young adulthood do fear a loss of personal identity in an intimate relationship. So do identical twins (166). You can explore intimacy issues with the young adults. In an increasingly complex society the search for self-definition is a difficult one. Identity is not always solidly possessed by the time one is 20 or even 25 years old. Achieving a true sense of intimacy seems very illusive to many of this generation. The media encourages self-seeking sexual gratification. Movies, novels, plays, and pornographic books glorify sex for kicks, and peer groups may pressure each other into sexual activity before they are ready for it. Many are puzzled, hurt, or dismayed when they find such sexual encounters are very disappointing. It is easy to *say* that understanding or insight into one's own sexuality is possible only when the self is fully defined. It is much more difficult to *act* on this principle. To come to the realization that sex is not a synonym for sexual intercourse may be a long and painful road.

Love

Love is the feeling accompanying intimacy (90, 320) (Fig. 12–4). The young adult often has difficulty determining what love is. A classic description of love as stated by the Apostle Paul in I Corinthians 13:4–7 has been the basis for many statements on love by poets, novelists, humanists, philosophers, psychiatrists, theologians, and common people:

> Love is patient and kind; love is not jealous or boastful; it is not arrogant or rude. Love does not insist on its own way; it is not irritable or resentful; it does not rejoice at wrong, but rejoices in the right. Love bears all things, believes all things, hopes all things, endures all things.

Figure 12-4. The principal developmental task of young adults is the formation of close relationships with significant others. (Courtesy of Carol Weingarten.)

One of the most important things the person can learn within the family as a child and adolescent is to love. By the time the person reaches the midtwenties, the person should be experienced in the emotion of love. If there was deprivation or distortion of love in the home when he or she was young, the adult will find it difficult to achieve mature love in an intimate relationship. By this time, the person should realize that one does not *fall* in love; one *learns* to love; one *grows* into love.

As a nurse, you will have many opportunities for discussions, individual and group counseling, and education on marriage, establishing a home, the relationship between spouses, and the relationship between parents and children. When you help people sort through feelings about life and love, you are indirectly making a contribution to the health and stability of them and their offspring.

Marriage

The socially accepted way for two people in love to be intimate is in marriage, a social contract or institution implying binding rules and responsibilities that cannot be ignored without some penalty. Marriage is endorsed in some form by all cultures in all periods of history because it formalizes and symbolizes the importance of family. Social stability depends on family stability. Marriage is more than getting a piece of paper.

There are norms in every society to prevent people from entering lightly into the wedded state (e.g., age limits, financial and property settlements, ceremony, witnesses, and public registration and announcement). One of the major functions of marriage is to control and limit sexuality and provide the framework for a long-term relationship between a man and a woman. Marriage gives rights in four areas: sexuality, birth and rearing of children, domestic and economic services, and property.

Most young people recognize that marriage is a decisive commitment. It marks the start of a new way of living and the achievement of a different status in life. A bride and groom have reason to experience anxiety. Marriage is both a special commitment and a voluntary choice made by them, and the consequences must be accepted in advance. But the potential sources of disturbance and danger are overshadowed by the recognition of marriage as a new source of strength and support in which the well-being of each is bound with the fate of the other.

The pattern and sequence of a person's life history influence whom, when, and why he or she marries. Apparently many people do not really know the person they are marrying and do not realize how greatly the partner's personality will influence their own. The problems of marital adjustment and family living have their roots and basis in the choice of the partner (200).

Mates often choose each other on the basis of unconscious needs, which they strive to meet through a mate whose personality complements rather than replicates one's own, or out of fear and loneliness or on the basis of physical attraction. The person chooses someone for an intimate relationship whose life-style and personality pattern strengthen and encourage personal development.

Although the person tends to marry an individual who lives and works nearby and has similar social, religious, and racial backgrounds, in America an increasing number of mixed marriages are occurring, an outgrowth of more liberal social attitudes. A number of factors influence the success of the marriage that crosses religious, ethnic, socioeconomic, or racial boundaries:

1. Motive for marriage
2. Desire, commitment, and effort to bridge the gulf between the couple and their families
3. Ability and maturity of the two people to live with and resolve their differences and problems
4. Reaction of the parental families, who may secretly or openly support **homogamy** (*marriage between a couple with similar or identical backgrounds*)

In America every married couple belongs to three families: to each other, to his family, and to her family. If the young adults are to establish a strong family unit of their own and avoid in-law interference, their loyalties must be to their *own* family before his or hers. The following guidelines may be helpful:

1. In-laws should not take priority over the spouse and home of the couple. If friends of either husband or wife are offensive to the partner, be prepared to minimize this friendship. Husband and wife together build new friendships.
2. Be faithful to the spouse. If one person engages in an extramarital affair, it is possible to repair the brokenness, but a feeling of mistrust may remain and is difficult to overcome.
3. Be mindful of sensitive areas, those which are sources of irritation in each other's life. Each needs to *work* at coping with the other's idiosyncrasies or habits and try to meet the other's preferences to keep love in the relationship.
4. Manage money and material possessions or they will manage the couple. Money and things are important, but the focus in a relationship should be on the person.
5. Maintain a spirit of courtship, spontaneity, and freshness to keep love in a marriage.

Marriage is becoming recognized as a close and loving partnership between two people rather than only a social institution in which the husband is the undisputed head of the house and the wife a child bearer. The current concept of companionship suggests intimacy and affection in a free and equal relationship. This concept imposes high standards. The success of the marriage depends ultimately on each feeling self-worth, each respecting the other, and on the two discovering and being able to fulfill mutual physical and psychologic needs.

Whether the young couple is going through the regular channels of engagement and marriage or through less traditional ways of living together, the following tasks must be accomplished if the couple will remain a viable, intimate unit:

1. Establishing themselves as a collaborative pair in their own eyes and in the eyes of mutual friends and both families; spending time together
2. Working through intimate systems of communication that allow for exchange of confidences and feelings and an increased degree of empathy and ability to predict each other's responses
3. Planning ahead for a stable relationship and arriving at a consensus about how their life should be lived; being committed to each other
4. Giving each other positive reinforcement, expressing appreciation and affection, to release love rather than focus on problems
5. Dealing with crises in a positive way

You may ask certain questions to ascertain readiness for marriage in the young adult or self. Can you take responsibility for your own behavior? Are you emotionally weaned from your parents? Have both of you thought about what lies ahead: both the disagreements

—— CASE SITUATION: Young Adult Development—Marriage and Commitment ——

James Chaney, 26 years old, received his bachelor's degree in nursing this year after combining fulltime employment as an attendant at a local hospital and part-time school attendance for 5 years. He has recently accepted a position at the hospital as a nurse in the surgical intensive care unit. James and his wife, Mary, have been married for 2 years. Mary, 25 years old, is finishing her bachelor's degree in accounting while she continues employment with an insurance firm. James and Mary plan to wait a few years before starting a family since both realize the importance of graduate education in their fields. They would also like to move from their apartment to a home with more space and a yard.

To save money to achieve their future plans, both James and Mary work extra hours when asked. This has frequently interfered with their studies. They also find they have little time for leisure activities and less time together. Communication is sometimes in the form of memos pasted on the refrigerator. Increasingly, the stresses of balancing school, work, and home demands have resulted in arguments, often over minor issues.

When a long-anticipated vacation must be canceled because of unexpected expenses, James and Mary are disappointed and angry. However, they decide to plan a week of inexpensive activities in the local area that will allow them to spend time together uninterrupted. They decide to tell no one that they have remained at home. The resulting vacation is truly restful and meaningful, as they share favorite activities and explore their dreams and goals for the future.

---

and the agreements, days of sickness and health, periods of depression and happiness, financial difficulties? Have you considered whether or not to have children? Have you had any education about child rearing to know what it entails? Do you understand female and male sexuality—the differences and the similarities? What do you each want out of marriage? What can you each give to marriage? Do you have mutual agreement on boundaries? Does it include group sex, nonmarital play, or complete monogamy? You can explore these and other questions in premarital counseling or courses in family living.

Isolation, or **self-absorption,** is the *inability to be intimate, spontaneous, or close with another, thus becoming withdrawn, lonely, and conceited and behaving in a stereotyped manner* (90). The isolated person often experiences a long succession of unsuccessful relationships, overextending self without any real interest or feeling, and then being unable to sustain close friendships. No real exchange of fellowship occurs, which is why encounter groups appeal to the isolated person. The forced fellowship and explorative closeness temporarily remove the sting of alienation.

The isolated person lives a facade, making pretentious claims. He or she may be naively childlike, easily disillusioned and embittered and may avoid the issues of life when possible. The person is distrustful, pessimistic, ruthless, and vacillating in behavior. Because he or she cannot see beyond personal needs and desires, he or she is progressively more alone. The person may establish a pattern of pseudointimate relationships in which he or she is initially friendly, but then sabotages the relationship as it grows closer to avoid true intimacy. For example, the person may have a history of numer-

ous dating partners or broken engagements but can never get to the intense stage of preparation for or settling into marriage. The person may not marry to remain liberated and to pursue a career and personal pleasures. There is avoidance of a need for a bond with another. If he or she does marry, the partner is likely to find personal emotional needs unmet while giving considerably of the self to the isolated, self-absorbed person (90, 200).

You may counsel the self-absorbed person and help him or her achieve the tasks of intimacy. You may also be a role model of commitment to serving others. Use principles of communication and relationship described by Murray and Huelskoetter (240).

Moral-Spiritual Development

The young adult may be either in the Conventional or Postconventional Level of moral development (see Chapter 5). In the Postconventional Level he or she follows the principles defined as appropriate for life. There are two stages in this level. In both stages the person has passed beyond living a certain way just because the majority of people do. Yet in stage I of this level the person adheres to the legal viewpoint of society. The person believes, however, that laws can be changed as people's needs change, and he or she is able to transcend the thinking of a specific social order and develop universal principles about justice, equality, and human rights. In stage 2 the person still operates as in stage 1 but is able to incorporate injustice, pain, and death as an integral part of existence (177).

Kohlberg (177) espouses that the reason for the behavior indicates the level of moral development and that for a person to be at any level, the reasons for behavior should be consistent to the stage 50% of the time. Therefore it would appear difficult for the average young adult, concerned about family, achieving in a career, paying the bills, and so on, to be in the Postconventional Level. Although the person may follow principles some of the time, conflicting situations and demands arise. To be consistently in the Postconventional Level takes considerable ego strength, a firm emotional and spiritual identity, and a willingness to stand up to societal forces. It may take years of maturing before the adult can be that courageous and consistent in Western society. For example, how does the young adult handle the dishonesty seen on the job? How does the mother handle the child viewing violence on television or demanding that clothes be the same designer outfits the other children are wearing? How does the couple react when a friend brags that he is having extramarital sexual experiences?

Probably only a few adults ever get to the second stage: 5% to 10% may reach stage 1 of the postconventional level; 20% to 25% stay in the conventional level, and the rest stay locked into the preconventional level described in Chapters 5 and 11 (177). However, studies indicate that moral judgment can change during adulthood (208).

Today's young adults have grown up with the influence of science and technology. As early as World War II some prophesied that the children born then would be postreligious, disinterested in other worlds, and concerned only in the secular existence of the present. Although some young adults fit this description and others are rejecting the institutional church, many have retained a desire and ability to apply spiritual and moral principles in this world. Increasingly parents with young children are joining a church or synagogue, seeking religion and a way to instill values in the child(ren).

In young adulthood there is a humanizing of values and a trend toward relativism as conflicts are encountered. The person increasingly discovers the meaning of values and their relation to achievement of social purposes, and he or she brings both personal experiences and motives to affirm and promote a value system. The person's values, whatever they are, become increasingly his or her own and a part of a unified philosophy of life. At the same time, there is expanding empathy for others and their value systems (200).

The spiritual awakening often experienced during adolescence, which might have receded with seeking of success, may now take on a more mature aspect as the young adult becomes firmly established in another life stage. If the person has children, he or she must rear them with some underlying philosophy. Their moral-spiritual questions must be answered. The young adult's religious teaching, perhaps previously rejected, may now be accepted as "not so bad after all." Or the young adult may build a new version of it.

Several qualities contribute to a spiritually mature disposition. The disposition is:

1. *Individualized and integrated*. The person translates the abstract knowledge into practical action. It helps him or her reach goals and attain harmony in various aspects of living.
2. *Consistent*. It produces basic standards of morality and conduct.
3. *Comprehensive, dynamic, and flexible*. It never stops searching for new attitudes and ideas. The person can hold ideas tentatively until confirmed or until evidence produces a more valid belief.

Because new and different ideas are always available, the mature disposition can continue for a lifetime. The person realizes that there is always more to learn (91, 218).

One of the dilemmas for the interfaith or interculture couple is what values and religion, if any, to follow in the home and to teach the children; how to celebrate holidays; what rituals and traditions to follow (e.g., Hanukkah or Christmas). Even when the couple makes a choice, there may be conflicts with relatives. Grandparents often have difficulty accepting that their child married someone of another faith or culture. Such marriages can work, and the children can have a firm moral and spiritual development. It is important for both spouses and families to discuss their feelings openly from the beginning. The couple should learn as much as possible about each other's religion or culture and talk to their families and friends about their experiences. It is critical that each family group remain open and accepting of the other. In turn, the children can learn deeper dimensions of spirituality, moral values, and their cultural background.

Although spiritual development and moral development follow sequential steps and are often thought of simultaneously, there is no significant link between specific religious affiliation or education and moral development. Moral development is linked positively with empathy, the capacity to understand another's viewpoint, and the ability to act reciprocally with another while maintaining personal values and principles. Being with people who are at a higher moral level stimulates the person to ask questions, consider his or her actions, and move to a higher moral level (177).

Adaptive Mechanisms

The young adult seeks stability while he or she is adapting to new or changing events. When the young adult is physically and emotionally healthy, total functioning is smooth (91, 200, 252). Adaptation to the environment, satisfaction of needs, and social interaction proceed relatively effortlessly and with minimum discomfort. The young adult behaves as though he or she is in control of impulses and drives and in harmony with superego ideals and demands. He or she can tolerate frustration of needs and is capable of making choices that seem best for total equilibrium (252). The person is emotionally mature for this life stage.

Emotional maturity is not exclusively related to physical health. Under stress, the healthiest people might momentarily have irrational impulses; in contrast, the extremely ill have periods of lucidity. Emotional health and maturity have an infinite gradation of behavior on a continuum rather than a rigid division between healthy and ill. Concepts of maturity are generated by culture. What is normal in one society may be abnormal in another.

In coping with stress in the environment, the young adult uses any of the previously discussed adaptive mechanisms. Use of these mechanisms such as *denial* or *regression* becomes abnormal or maladaptive only when the person uses the same mechanism of behavior too frequently, in too many situations, or for too long a duration.

Self-Concept and Body-Image Development

Self-concept and body image, defined in Chapters 5 and 7 and discussed in each developmental era, are now redefined and expanded to fit the young adult perspective.

The person's perception of self physically, emotionally, and socially, based on reactions of others that have been internalized, self-expectations, perceived abilities, attitudes, habits, knowledge, and other characteristics affect how that person will handle situations and relate to others. How the person behaves depends on whether he or she feels positively or negatively about self, whether the person believes others view him or her positively or negatively, and how he or she believes others expect the person to behave in this situation. The reactions of the family members, including spouse, and the employment situation are strong influences on the young adult's self-concept. Additionally, the person discloses different aspects of self to various people and in various situations, depending on needs, what is considered socially acceptable, reactions of others, and past experience with self-disclosure (195, 200, 227, 239, 263).

Body image, *a part of self-concept, is a mental picture of the body's appearance integrated into the parietotemporal area of the cortex. Body image includes the surface, internal, and postural picture of the body and values, attitudes, emotions, and personality reactions of the person in relation to the body as an object in space, separate from others.* This image is flexible, subject to constant revision, and may not be reflective of actual body structure. Body image shifts back and forth at different times of the day and at different times in the life cycle (195, 200, 239).

Under normal conditions the body is the focus of an individual's identity, and its limits more or less clearly define a boundary that separates the person from the environment. One's body has spatial and time sense and yields experiences that cannot be shared directly with others. A person's body is the primary channel of contact with the world, and it is a nucleus around which values are synthesized. Any disturbance to the body influences total self-concept (239).

Contributing Influences

Many factors contribute to the body image (195, 200, 239, 263):

1. Parental and social reaction to the person's body
2. The person's interpretation of others' reactions to him or her
3. The anatomic appearance and physiologic function of the body, including sex, age, kinesthetic and other sensorimotor stimuli, and illness or deformity
4. Attitudes and emotions toward and familiarity with the body
5. Internal drives, dependency needs, motivational state, and ideals to which the person aspires
6. Identification with the bodies of others who were considered ideal (a little bit of each person significant to the person is incorporated into the self-concept and personality)
7. Perception of space and objects immediately surrounding the body such as a chair or car; the sense of body boundaries
8. Objects attached to the body such as clothing, a wig, false eyelashes, a prosthesis, jewelry, makeup, or perfume
9. Activities the body performs in various roles, occupations, or recreations

The kinesthetic receptors in the muscles, tendons, and joints and the labyrinth receptors in the inner ear inform the person about his or her position in space. By means of perceptual alterations in position, the postural image of the body constantly changes. Every new posture and movement is incorporated by the cortex into a **schema** *(image)* in relation to or association with previously made schemata. Thus the image of the body changes with changing movements—walking, sitting, gestures, changes in appearance, and changes in the pace of walking (195, 200).

Self-produced movement aids visual accuracy. When a person's body parts are moved passively instead of actively (e.g. sitting in a wheelchair instead of walking), perceptual accuracy about space and the self as an object in space is hindered. Athletes, ballet dancers, and other agile people are more accurate than most in estimating the dimensions of the body parts that are involved in movement (195, 200). Adults fitted with distortion glasses adapt to the perceived distortion if they are permitted to walk around in the environment wearing the glasses. If they are moved passively in a wheelchair, little or no adaptation takes place. Thus activity appears to enhance sensory information in a way that passive movements do not. If a person undergoes body changes, he or she must actively explore and move the involved part to reintegrate it (195, 200, 263).

Self-Knowledge. How do you visualize your body as you walk, run, stand, sit, or gesture? How do you feel about yourself as you go through various motions? What emotions are expressed by your movements? How do you think others visualize you at that time? Movement of the body parts, gestures, and appearance communicate a message to the observer (e.g., the client, or family member) that may or may not be intended. The message you convey about yourself to another may aid or hinder the establishment of a therapeutic relationship. You must be realistically aware of the posture and movement of your body and what they may be conveying to another.

Self-knowledge is not necessarily the same as knowledge gained about the self from others. Each person sees self differently from how others see him or her, although the most mature person is able to view self as others do. New attributes or ideas are integrated into the old ones, but all ideas received are not necessarily integrated. Before any perception about the self can affect or be integrated into one's self-concept, the perceptions must be considered good or necessary to the self. If the person believes that he or she is competent, a statement about incompetence will not be integrated into the self-image unless he or she is repeatedly told about being incompetent. However, if the person has a negative self-image, it will also take many statements of his or her worth before they can be accepted and integrated into the self-concept.

A person has definite ideas and feelings about his or her own body, what is satisfying and what is frustrating. The person discovers that he or she has certain abilities and disabilities, likes and dislikes. He or she thinks of self as shy or outgoing and irritable or calm and learns something of how he or she affects others. What the person thinks of self has remarkable power in influencing behavior and the interpretation of other's behavior, the choice of associates, and goals pursued.

Feelings about certain self-attributes vary according to the importance placed on them and how central or close they are to the essence of self. Events such as illness or injury involving the face and torso are usually more threatening than those involving the limbs since the face and the torso are first integrated into the young child's self-perception. The extremities are seen as part of the self later and are therefore usually less highly valued in comparison (195, 200, 239, 263).

One's feelings about one's characteristics also depend on whether a characteristic or body part is viewed as a functional tool for living or as a central personal attribute. For example, teeth can be viewed as a tool for eating or as central to the face, smile, youth, and person-

ality. Dentures can be accepted and integrated as part of the body image more easily if they are viewed as a tool rather than if they are thought of as a sign of decline and old age. The person's work may also be viewed as a tool, function, or way to earn a living and help others or as central to the self. For example, is your image that of a woman or man who works as a nurse and does other things as well, or is your whole image primarily that of being a nurse? Age and sex are also characteristics that differ in degree of centrality or importance to the person (195, 200).

Also involved in self-concept and body image are the body parts supposedly considered strategically important in the character of the ethnic group or race (e.g., the German backbone, the Jewish nose, or the dark skin of the Black person). The body part with special significance, which would also include the afflicted limb in a disabled person, is believed heavier, larger, or more conspicuous and seems to the bearer of it to be the focus of others' attention, although it may not be.

The location and history of family residence, religion, socioeconomic background, and even attempts at climbing to another social class level are integrated into the adult self-concept but not the body image (200).

Body image in the adult is a social creation. Normality is judged by appearance, and ways of using the body are prescribed by society. Approval and acceptance are given for normal appearance and proper behavior. Self-concept continually influences and enlarges the person's world, mastery of and interaction with it, and ability to respond to the many experiences it offers. This integration, largely unconscious, is constantly evolving and can be identified in the person's values, attitudes, and feelings about self. The experiences with the body are interpreted in terms of feelings, earlier views of the self, and group or cultural norms (103, 195, 200, 239, 263).

In the adult there is a close interdependence between body image and personality, self-concept, and identity. A mature body image and mature behavior are built on having coped with the changing demands of each previous developmental crisis, particularly as these crises relate to dominant body parts—the mouth, limbs, and genitalia. If each of these body zones and their functioning are not integrated in turn into the total body image, the adult person's body image will remain immature in some respects. The immature body image may interfere with securing adult satisfactions and may be evidenced by personality disturbance. The young adult who can accept the body without undue preoccupation with its function or control of these functions is free for other experiences (195, 200, 239, 263).

You need to remember and use information about self-concepts and body image, for as a nurse your feedback to others is important. If you are to help another elevate self-esteem or feel positively about his or her body, you must give repeated positive reinforcement and help the person overcome unrealistic guilt and shame (36). Saying something positive or recognizing abilities once or twice will not be enough. The self-concept, whether wholesome or not, is difficult to change since the person perceives others' comments and behavior in relation to an already established image to avoid conflict and anxiety within self. The person with a sense of trust, self-confidence, or positive self-concept is less threatened by others' ideas, remarks, or behavior. He or she is more flexible, able to change, and admit new attributes to self.

Stereotyped Ideas About Correlation Between Personality and Body Type. Certain characteristics are attributed to a person on the basis of how he or she looks. You should be aware of how a client might perceive you on the basis of your shape. The stereotypes are numerous: the skinny are perceived as pinched and mean; the fat are perceived as gluttonous, unattractive, insensitive, or very jolly; the broad, overweight person is perceived as calm and passive; the thin, narrow person is perceived as active, excitable, tense, or reacting quickly. Reactions to body build are important to the individual, both in terms of how the person is treated by others and in terms of what others expect of him or her.

Certainly these perceptions have implications for you. Individualized care can hardly be given if you see only the physique of the person and label him or her accordingly. On the other hand, the client and family may be reacting to you on the basis of how they expect someone with your specific physique to behave.

In America there is much emphasis on the ideal adult figure. In one study on degree of satisfaction reported by people about aspects of the body, large women wanted to be smaller but not as small as small women. Small women wanted to be larger but not as large as large women. Small size was desirable for all body parts except the breasts. The small range of variation for the ideal size of the different body parts as stated by the women in the study indicates that cultural stereotype of the ideal female figure sets limits for acceptable size that are narrower than those produced by nature and eating habits. Few women have the physical dimensions that were identified as ideal, and none rated positively all their body parts (103, 195, 200).

Women's status and security are in some cases highly conditioned by their perceived and demonstrated attractiveness to males, irrespective of skills, interests, and values. Because most women do not attain the ideal proportions, they may not feel beautiful. The internalized ideal is indirectly responsible for much insecurity among women (103).

Men rate large size and height as desirable. Large muscular men rated their bodies as best liked by the self and as more active than small men. Tall height symbolizes dominion, self-confidence, leadership, and power (200).

Women have a more clearly defined and stable body concept than men. Girls seem to have an earlier realistic appreciation than boys of the smallness of their own bodies in relation to adults and of a sexual definition of self and a more realistic concept of the body thereafter. The difference between male and female body images seems related partly to different anatomic structure and body functions but also to the contrasts between males and females in their upbringing, style of life, and role in culture (103, 200).

Presumably persons having a well-integrated body image react to people and situations differently from those with a poorly integrated body image. The person with a firm ego boundary or body image more likely will be an independent person, with definite goals and forceful, striving ways of approaching tasks. He or she will be an influential member of the group. Under stress, these persons are more likely to develop diseases of the periphery of the body—skin and muscles. Persons with a poorly integrated body image or poorly defined body boundaries are more likely to be passive, less achievement minded, less goal striving. These persons are less influential in a group and more susceptible to the influence of others and external pressure. Under stress, the maximum physiologic response occurs internally, taking the form, for example, of heart disease or gastrointestinal disease (200).

Stereotyped Ideas Affecting Self-Concept in Women and Men. In America the woman is stereotyped to be an underachiever in education and occupation. Dependent, passive, and subordinate are terms frequently associated with women. Yet most people recognize the quiet strength in many women. The woman is believed cooperative and creative (as long as she is doing handicrafts). If she is academically or occupationally successful, she is considered aggressive or unfeminine.

The man is stereotyped as aggressive and competitive, even in a service role. Weakness is not accepted. If the man is gentle and passive, he is labeled a "sissy" or effeminate (20, 21).

The classic studies by Margaret Mead (225) show that the personality traits we have traditionally called masculine and feminine in the United States are an artifact of culture, not biology. In her study of three different groups of people, she found that in the first group men and women were equally cooperative, unaggressive, and responsive to the needs and demands of others. Sex drive was not a driving force for men or women. In the second group both men and women were equally ruthless, aggressive, violent, sexually active, and with maternal cherishing aspects of personality at a minimum. In the third group the ideal is the reversal of American culture, with the woman the dominant, impersonal, and managing partner and the man the less responsible and emotionally dependent person (225). Knowledge of these studies should help men and women feel freer to explore and incorporate a wide range of behaviors into the self-concept. The women's liberation movement and new occupational trends apparently are giving some impetus to this area.

Consciousness-raising groups for women also can help work through anger related to social reactions and differential treatment of men and women. Such groups can reaffirm a positive self-concept in the woman and teach ways to cope with sexism (240). You can initiate and lead such groups.

Body-Image Changes in Illness

A wide variety of messages about the body are constantly fed into the self-image for rejection, acceptance with integration, or revision. You will see disturbances in the person's body image after loss of a body function, structure, or quality—teeth, hair, vision, hearing, breast, internal organs, or youth—that necessitate adjustment of the person's body image. Because the body image provides a base for identity, almost any change in body structure or function is experienced as a threat, especially in America where wholeness, beauty, and health are highly valued.

A threat to body image is related to the person's pattern of adaptation. Some behavior patterns may depend heavily on certain organs of the body. If these organs become diseased or must be removed, the threat is greater than if an organ unimportant to the person is affected. The degree to which this loss of body control creates loss of customary control of self, physical environment, time, and contacts with others is very closely related to the degree of threat felt. To understand the nature of the threat, you must assess the pattern of adaptation, the value of this pattern for the person, and the usual coping mechanisms. The person with limited adaptive abilities, who easily feels helpless and powerless, will experience greater threat with a change in body structure or function.

Any adaptation to alterations in body size, function, or structure depends on the nature and meaning of the threat to the person, previous coping pattern, response from others, and the help you provide in helping him or her undergo change. The phases of crisis discussed in *Psychiatric/Mental Health Nursing,* Chapter 8, are a normal sequence of behavior in response to body image changes (240).

The Adult Undergoing Body Changes

Assessment. Assessment during illness, injury, or disability that necessitates eventual changes to self-image is often difficult because of the abstractness of self-image. But if you listen closely to the person, validate statements for less obvious meanings, and explore feelings with him or her you can gain considerable information for worthwhile intervention. Direct or probing questions about the following items do *not* obtain any information, but through open-ended questions you should gradually be able to obtain information about the fol-

lowing aspects that relate to body image. Assessment could include determining the person's response to the following (103, 239, 240):

1. Feelings about the self before and since the condition occurred
2. Values about personal hygiene
3. Values on beauty, self-control, wholeness, activity
4. Value of others' reactions
5. Meaning of the body part affected
6. Meaning of hospitalization, treatment, and care
7. Awareness of extent of condition
8. Effect of condition on person, roles, daily activities, family, and use of leisure time
9. Perception of others' reaction to person with this condition
10. Problems in adjusting to condition
11. Mechanisms used in adapting to condition and its implication

Observation of the client must be combined with purposeful conversation. Observe movements, posture, gestures, and expressions as he or she answers your questions or talks about self to validate the consistency between what is said and what is meant.

Nursing Intervention. Measures to help someone with a threat to or change of body image involves assisting the person reintegrate the self-view and self-esteem in relation to his or her condition. You can help the person in the following ways (234, 239, 240):

1. Encourage talking about feelings in relation to the changed body function or structure. Talking about feelings is the first step to reintegration of body image.
2. Assist client, without pressure, to become reacquainted with self by looking at the dressing or wound, feeling the cast, bandage, or injured part, or looking at self in mirror. The client who wants to "show the scar" should be allowed to do so. Reaction from you and the family can make a difference in how the person accepts the changed body.
3. Provide opportunity for gaining information about the body, both the intact and changed parts, and its strengths and limits.
4. Provide opportunity to learn mastery of the body, resume activities of daily care and living routines as indicated, move about, become involved with others, resume roles, and handle equipment.
5. Give recognition for what the person can do. Avoid criticism, derogation, or a nonverbal reaction of disgust or shame.
6. Help him or her see self as a whole person in spite of losses or changes.
7. Encourage talking about unresolved experiences, distortions, or fears in relation to body image.

You will be encountering many young adults with body-image distortions or changes as a result of accidental or war injuries, disease, weight gain or loss, pregnancy, or identity problems. You can make a significant contribution to the health of this person for the remainder of life by giving assistance through physical care, listening, counseling, teaching, and working with the people important to his or her life.

Be aware that health care professionals and certain treatment practices contribute to a negative self-concept and sexual stereotypes, and often the health care system treats the client (well or ill) as an unthinking, incompetent object. Although there may be some attitudinal changes occurring, many men and women still hold traditional stereotyped beliefs about sex-related behavior.

You will encounter health professionals in every field who are influenced by a sexist orientation when working with you and clients. By your behavior, use of problem solving, verbal facility, and nonverbal messages you can work to change sexist attitudes. Your efforts are important for your own positive self-concept and for unbiased care of each person—thus promoting a positive self-concept.

Life-Style Options

The increased pace of life in America has brought people an unparalleled degree of social alienation at all levels of society. Choosing a life-style very different from one's child-rearing experiences is an attempt to ward off alienation and organize one's life around meaning. The young adult has many options. He or she may decide to base the style of living around age (the youth cult); work (the company man or woman executive); leisure (the surf bum); drugs; or marriage and family.

Singlehood, *remaining unmarried and following a specific life-style,* is not new. Maiden aunts, bachelors, and single school teachers are traditional, as are those whose religion calls for singlehood. But remaining unmarried is increasingly an option, either as an end in itself or as a newly prolonged phase of postadolescence.

The single person may be in emotional isolation unable to establish a close relationship, and alienated from self and others or may feel depressed about the life situation. However, not all singles fit this description. The single person can accomplish the task of intimacy through emotional investment of self in others. Many are extroverts, have several very close friends with whom they share activities, have a meaningful career, and have a harmonious rather than conflictual relationship with parents. If they marry, they want to feel that they have chosen the right partner and have spent time living just for themselves so that they do not resent the responsibilities of marriage.

Many prefer to remain single as they pursue prolonged education and strive to become established in their occupational field. Others find that being free of relationships and to sample a variety of life-styles and travel as they please before settling down to raise a family is an important part of establishing a comfortable identity. They avoid living out their lives in the same manner and location as their parents and may live in apartment complexes for singles only, following a life-style that is supposed to convey freedom. For whatever reasons, the number of single people in this country is on the rise, especially in the 20 to 34 age group.

Trends suggest that young people are marrying later than they did in the 1960s. There still exists a great deal of cultural and family pressure for this age group to marry by the midtwenties. Americans so value family life that unmarried adults sometimes have been treated as immature and incomplete or even as failures and willful renegades who cannot or will not take up a respectable and responsible family role. Single adults have had to take reduced credit ratings and higher insurance rates just because they are single. Pressure from "embarrassed" families and friends leads many of these individuals to marry prematurely lest they be considered lifetime misfits.

The single person may need help in understanding that life-style choice is not irresponsible, that he or she can make significant contributions as a citizen, and that marriage and parenthood are only one way to demonstrate emotional maturity. If the person is single because of isolation and self-absorption, psychiatric counseling may be needed, not for singlehood, but because of feelings about self and others. Several books listed in the references give suggestions for managing alone (29, 82, 240, 258, 272). Haber (131) describes family therapy with single young adults. For additional information on singlehood, refer to Chapter 4.

Family Planning: The Expectancy Phase and Parenthood

Parenthood is an option for either the couple or a single person. It was not until the early 1960s that people felt in control of family planning. Birth control methods were often not successful either aesthetically or mechanically. But today oral contraceptives for the female and more skilled vasectomy procedures for the male make it possible for couples to say "We don't want children now." "We don't want children ever." "We want to try to have two children spaced 3 years apart."

Information presented in Chapter 11, Table 11–5, that summarizes contraceptives and various references at the end of this chapter will help you teach about all aspects of family planning (120, 237, 252, 298). Chapter 4 presents information useful for understanding the family with whom you are working.

You may be in a position to use decision theory with a couple who has many questions about having a family. In this method the couple writes their separate values in a hierarchy of importance and then examines the costs and benefits associated with their decision to have or not to have children. This approach is a variation of the old decision-making method of listing all the reasons *for* on one side and all the reasons *against* on the other side to get an accurate view of the components involved in the decision.

Reasons for Childbearing

The couple may have a child for a variety of reasons: (1) extension of self; (2) to offset loneliness; (3) sense of pride or joy; (4) psychologic fulfillment of having a child; (5) having someone to love self; (6) attempt to hold a marriage together; (7) feeling of power, generated by ability to create life; (8) representation of wealth; (9) to secure replacements for the work force; (10) to have an heir for family name and wealth; and (11) religious convictions (298). Whether the couple chooses to have only one child or more children is related to more than fertility and religious background. Life-styles, finances, career, available support systems, and emotional maturity are factors. The woman who has had the opportunity to pursue career and social activities may be more ready emotionally to settle down, commit self to the responsibilities of child care and parenting, in contrast to the female in the teens, twenties, or even early thirties (298, 349). End-of-chapter references give several perspectives on this decision (6, 154, 156, 298, 303, 308, 310).

Developmental Tasks for the Couple During the Expectancy Stage

You are in a position to assist the couple in understanding the changes that childbearing will create and the following developmental tasks for this stage of family life (42, 84, 325):

1. Rearrange the home to provide space, facilities, and supplies for the expected baby.
2. Rework the budget and determine how to obtain and spend income to accommodate changing needs and maintain the family unit financially.
3. Evaluate the changing roles, division of labor, how responsibilities of child care will be divided, who has the final authority, and whether the woman should continue working outside the home if she has a career or profession.
4. Adapt patterns of sexual relationships to the pregnancy.
5. Rework the communication system between the couple; explore feelings about the pregnancy and ideas about childrearing, and work to resolve the differences.
6. Acquire knowledge about pregnancy, childbirth, and parenthood.
7. Rework the communication system and relationships with family, friends, and community activities, based on the reality of the pregnancy and their reactions.
8. Use family and community resources as needed.
9. Examine and expand the philosophy of life to include responsibilities of childbearing and childrearing.

Developmental tasks that must be mastered during pregnancy and the intrapartum period to ensure readiness for the maternal role are as follows (277):

1. *Pregnancy validation,* accepting the reality of the pregnancy, working through feelings of ambivalence
2. *Fetal embodiment,* incorporating the fetus and enlarging body into the body image
3. *Fetal distinction,* seeing the fetus as a separate entity, fantasizing what the baby will be like
4. *Role transition,* after birth, an increasing readiness to take on the task of parenthood.

A number of authors have researched transition to parenthood, feelings, symptoms, body-image changes, and needs for social support during pregnancy. Events during pregnancy affect family functioning and child care after birth. Refer to references at the end of the chapter for more information (1, 42, 43, 48, 71, 72, 78, 94, 95, 207, 231, 232, 247, 298, 325, 338, 339, 342).

Father's Response. Some research indicates that attachment of the father to baby begins during pregnancy, rather than after birth, and that a strong marital relationship and vicariously experienced physical symptoms resembling pregnancy strengthen attachment (couvade syndrome) (63, 94, 95, 205).

Studies indicate a characteristic pattern of development of subjective emotional involvement in pregnancy among first-time expectant fathers. Three phases occur: an announcement phase, a moratorium, and a focusing period (214).

The **announcement phase** is *when pregnancy is suspected and confirmed*. If the man desired the pregnancy, he shows desire and excitement. If he did not want the pregnancy, he shows pain and shock (214).

During the **moratorium period,** the *man suppresses thoughts about the pregnancy*. This period can last from a few days to months and usually ends when the pregnancy is obvious. This period is characterized by emotional distance, a feeling the pregnancy is not real, concentration on himself and other life concerns, and sometimes leaving home. The man's emotional distance allows him to work through ambivalence and jealousy of the woman's ability to bear a child, but his distance causes her to feel unloved, rejected, angry, and uncared for. Marital tension exists. Pregnancy often emphasizes the disparity in the couple's life pace and focus. Gradually the man faces the financial and life-style implications of the pregnancy. If the man feels financially insecure, unstable with his partner, or wishes to extend the childless period, he resents pregnancy and spends a longer time in the moratorium stage. Most men eventually become enthusiastic about the pregnancy and baby when they feel the baby move or hear the heartbeat. If the man does not become enthusiastic and supportive, the couple may then be at risk for marital and parenting problems (214).

The **focusing period** occurs *when the man perceives the pregnancy as real and important in his life.* This begins approximately 25 to 30 weeks' gestation and extends until labor onset. The man redefines himself as father; he begins to feel more in tune with and is more helpful to his wife. He begins to read or talk about parenting and child development, notices other children, and is willing to participate in childbirth classes and purchasing baby supplies. He constructs a mental image of baby, sometimes different from the woman's mental image of the baby. The circle of friends may change to those who have children. He may feel fear about the coming labor and birth and feel responsible for a successful birth (214). The man who participates in pregnancy and birth experiences greater closeness with the infant and spouse and heightened self-esteem and esteem for the spouse. The man's readiness for pregnancy may significantly influence emergence of father involvement. The man's unconscious feelings and his earliest memories of childhood play an important role in his emotional reaction and adjustment to pregnancy and childbirth (135, 168, 205, 325).

Mother's Response. Certainly one would expect that an even stronger attachment would occur in the woman as she physically experiences the fetus and physical symptoms related to pregnancy and that her feelings for the child are stronger if she has a loving, supportive partner. Be aware also that some men have difficulty accepting the responsibility implied by a pregnant partner and do not want to be involved in childcare (135, 168).

Nursing Roles

An important decision for the expectant parents is whether to attend childbirth education classes. Encourage the pregnant woman and her partner to attend childbirth education classes during pregnancy that are taught by the American Society for Prophylaxis in Obstetrics (ASPO) certified childbirth educators. Insist that they be allowed to use the techniques and practical suggestions they learned during the labor and delivery process. The woman who is well supported during pregnancy experiences fewer complications during labor and delivery. The woman who has had childbirth education during pregnancy and can practice Lamaze techniques during labor uses less medication and is more likely to choose rooming-in with the baby.

Your support, acceptance, flexibility, helping the couple to use what they learned and practiced in prenatal classes, letting them assume responsibility for decisions when possible, assistance to mother, and teaching during the postpartum period are crucial to family-centered care. To clarify your patterns of caring for clients, refer to Cronenwett and Brickman (71) for a discussion of four models that professionals use in maintaining par-

ent and infant health. Cultural considerations are important as well (160).

Refer to a maternity nursing book for specific information on prenatal care, the labor and delivery process, and postpartum care—for both the normal and high-risk pregnancy and delivery. Refer also to the "Symposium on Maternal and Newborn Nursing," *Nursing Clinics of North America,* March 1982. Helpful references are also found at the end of Chapter 7 and at the end of this chapter (42, 101, 231, 232, 269, 316, 325).

Be aware that in contrast to the societal romanticized view of pregnancy and care of the pregnant woman, the pregnant woman may be a victim of battering. Articles by Helton and colleagues (145–147) are informative references on assessment, how to assist the woman in the decision to leave the partner, and resources for help. Sonkin, Martin, and Walker (309) described assessment of and intervention with the male batterer. Refer also to pp. 483 to 487 in this chapter for general information on spouse abuse and the male batterer.

Other Approaches to Parenthood

Some couples delay childbearing until they are in their thirties or early forties. The woman may wish to pursue her education, a career, or a profession; the couple may choose to travel, start a business, become financially established, or have a variety of experiences before they settle down with one or two children. With genetic counseling, the surgical ability to undo vasectomy and tubal ligation, improved prenatal and neonatal care, and reduced risk of maternal or neonatal complications, pregnancy is safe for the mother in her thirties and even early forties (141, 293, 298, 339). Because of concern about congenital abnormalities, **amniocentesis,** a *procedure in which a small amount of amniotic fluid is removed for analysis,* can be done in the early prenatal period. This allows the couple to begin the adjustment if the child has an abnormality—or to terminate the pregnancy if the abnormality is severe. Many of the risks of late parenthood are related to preexisting disease, if any, rather than to late conception. Of equal concern are the emotional and social implications, especially after birth when the couple's life revolves around baby rather than work or earlier interests (298).

Maternal age does not affect maternal role behaviors, and the sense of challenge, role strain, and self-image in the mother role is similar during the first year for the childbearing women of all ages. Mercer's study (231) of the process of maternal role attainment in three age groups (15 to 19 years, 20 to 29 years, and 30 to 42 years) over the first year of motherhood found that love for the baby, gratification in the maternal role, observed maternal behavior, and self-reported ways of handling irritating child behaviors remained the same over the year.

The single person may desire to be a parent. The single woman may, through pregnancy or adoption, choose to have a child(ren). More is being written about the single woman who decides to become a mother and remain single. Some are well-educated, professional women in the late thirties or forties who believe they have no chance of becoming married, for various societal reasons, but who wish to have the experience of motherhood. Some single men who will not be biological fathers are also choosing to have the experience of fatherhood through adoption (301). The number of both African-American and Caucasian single women who are choosing to be mothers and heads of the family is increasing. A few single men have also decided to adopt a child to be a parent. The decision to parent without a father or mother figure for the child should be carefully considered, for the child needs both female and male caregivers and the characteristics, responses, and relationships that each can give. The woman may choose to remain single but maintain a relationship with the biologic father or with a man who can act as father to the child. The man may have a close relationship with a woman who can assist in mothering, or he may decide to nurture alone.

You are in a key position to help the person as he or she thinks through why there is a wish to have a child and remain single. Who the support system will be, who can act in the father or mother role to the child, the consequences of a single mother or father to the child during school years or adolescence, and the social, familial, and economic consequences of single parenthood should be discussed. Poverty is more common among single mothers, and fewer single mothers finish high school. Implications related to the cultural and religious background of the person must also be considered.

Family planning is sometimes made difficult by **infertility,** *inability to achieve pregnancy after 1 year of regular, unprotected intercourse or the inability to carry a pregnancy to a term, live birth,* which is a health problem for 15% of women of childbearing age. Both partners should be given diagnostic tests together since 50% of infertility factors are in women and 50% are in men. Infertility can create great psychologic problems for the woman and man, between the couple, and between families of each partner. The problem becomes compounded by the increasing difficulty in adopting a local healthy baby in most communities since 90% of single mothers retain their babies. Artificial insemination and a surrogate mother are alternatives that may not always be acceptable to the couple. Menning (230) describes the emotional reactions in detail.

Sandelowski and colleagues (281, 282) found that infertile couples felt ambiguity or uncertainty about identity, life pursuits and control, and the infertility cause, diagnostic procedures, and cure. Even when pregnancy was achieved, ambiguity and a sense of unrealness about the pregnancy and its outcome were still the most prevalent feelings.

References listed at the end of the chapter describe fertility and diagnostic and treatment procedures for the woman and man (230, 281, 282, 298, 361). You may refer your client to local infertility clinics or the American Fertility Society, 1688 13th Avenue South, Birmingham, AL 35256. Another organization, Resolve, formed by people with infertility problems, gives counsel and support to people in 26 metropolitan areas. You may obtain more information by writing Resolve, Department P, Box 474, Belmont, MA 02178.

The couple who cannot biologically have a child may consider a **surrogate parent,** *a woman who, for a fee, will conceive through insemination, carry, and deliver a child for the woman who cannot conceive.* Many ethical concerns arise with this practice: the meaning of family, psychologic effects on the surrogate and contracting parents, relationship between fetus and pregnant woman, the possibility that the child who is born may not meet the desires of the contracting parents, care of the deformed child, and effect on the child when he or she learns about the surrogate parent. Does the couple have a right to children by any means? What are the cultural, moral, and religious implications? Further, legal aspects are also tenuous. As of now, there are no answers, just many questions. You can help a couple considering the surrogate parent method work through the above issues and questions according to their spiritual, cultural, and family values and beliefs, and their personal philosophies, values, and beliefs.

Developmental Tasks

The specific developmental tasks of the youth as he or she is making the transition from adolescence into young adulthood are discussed in Chapter 11 and can be summarized as choosing a vocation, getting appropriate education, establishing a residence, and formulating ideas about selection of a mate or someone with whom to have a close relationship.

For the young adult in general, the following tasks must be achieved, regardless of the station in life (84, 91):

1. Accepting self and stabilizing self-concept and body image
2. Acknowledging and resolving conflicts between the emerging self and conformity to the social order
3. Establishing independence from parental home and financial aid
4. Becoming established in a vocation or profession that provides personal satisfaction, economic independence, and a feeling of making a worthwhile contribution to society
5. Learning to appraise and express love responsibly through more than sexual contacts
6. Establishing an intimate bond with another, either through marriage or with a close friend
7. Establishing and maintaining a home and managing a time schedule and life stresses
8. Finding a congenial social and friendship group

Research Abstract

Tucker, B., and C. Huerta, A Study of Developmental Tasks as Perceived by Young Adult Mexican-American Females, Lifelong Learning: An Omnibus of Practice and Research*, 10, no. 4 (1987), 4–7*

A major limitation of much current research on human development is that often middle-class Caucasians are the subjects. Thus the results may not be generalizable to other populations. Little research has been done on developmental tasks as experienced by other ethnic groups.

Developmental tasks described by R. Havighurst and by D. Levinson for early adulthood and the tasks of intimacy in young adulthood as described by E. Erikson provided the framework for this study. The purpose of the study was to obtain information about these previously defined developmental tasks as experienced by Mexican-American women.

A pilot study sample was composed of 15 Mexican-American women aged 18 to 34 years. Seven were married with one to three children; eight were single or divorced. Educational levels were as follows: 16% had a high school diploma; 32% had completed 1 to 2 years of college; 42% had completed 3 to 4 years of college; and 7% had postbaccalaureate education. Naturalistic inquiry by interview (20 minutes average) was the method used to collect data. Six tasks were typical of this sample: (1) establishing a stable relationship; (2) obtaining education for a career—a most definite goal for the unmarried women; (3) establishing independence and economic and personal freedom; (4) rearing a family; (5) maintaining friendships; and (6) participating in civic or community activities.

A sample of 100 Mexican-American women between the ages of 18 and 34 years was then studied. From the pilot study results, a survey questionnaire was developed, using a four-point, Likert-type scale for rating the six tasks according to perceived importance. The questionnaire was administered to women in college classes or at places of employment.

Analysis of variance (ANOVA) was used to explore group differences in the data. Each of the developmental tasks was analyzed by age, marital status, educational level, and parenthood. In the age groups 63% were 18 to 24 years, 29% were 25 to 29 years, and 7% were 30 to 34 years. Most were single (65%); 30% were married, and 5% were divorced. No one had more than five children; 6% had three to five children; 24% had one or two, and 70% had none. Most had at least some college education; 32% had 1 or 2 years; 42% had 3 or 4 years; and 7% had postbaccalaureate education.

Results may have been skewed by the characteristics of this sample, but these subjects revealed developmental tasks that agree with those identified by Havighurst, Levinson, and Erikson, although there were also significant differences for the different groups. The task of obtaining an education had the highest overall ranking, in contrast to earlier studies, although married women gave less priority to this task. The task of establishing a relationship, which is important cross-culturally, was of high importance to all the women. The task of establishing independence was important to all women, in contrast to the stereotype that Mexican-American women are subservient, interested only in marriage and parenthood. The task of maintaining friendship was perceived as less important by more highly educated, professional women. In breaking out of the usual homemaker role, there may also be a decreased need for social support. The task of having children was considered more important by women who were parents, but the women who were surveyed did not feel bound to the traditional roles of wife and mother. Civic and community participation had the lowest perceived level of importance; and women with children were least concerned with this task.

Implications of the results for adult educators are discussed. Further, the results may not be generalizable because of the higher-than-average educational level of the participants.

9. Deciding whether or not to have a family and carry out tasks of parenting
10. Resolving changed relationship with the parental families
11. Formulating a meaningful philosophy of life and reassessing priorities and values
12. Becoming involved as a citizen in the community
13. Achieving a more realistic outlook about other cultures, mores, and political systems

McCoy (221), using the stages of development proposed by the life-stage theorists discussed earlier, formulated similar developmental tasks for each stage. They are depicted in Table 12–3.

You can assist young adults in meeting these developmental tasks through use of therapeutic communication principles, counseling, teaching, and crisis intervention. An in-depth source of information to help you understand and work with the married and young adult family and with families across generations is the text by Kramer (180).

Common Health Problems and Nursing Applications

Health Promotion and Health Protection

Your role in caring for the young adult may be many faceted. Assessment based on knowledge presented throughout this chapter is the basis for formulating *nursing diagnoses*. Nursing diagnoses that may be applicable to the young adult are listed in Box 12–3. Health promotion interventions to assist the young adult and the family to meet physical, cognitive, emotional, social, and spiritual needs are described in the following, and in the previous, sections.

Immunizations

The young adult may need immunizations, depending on his or her history. Five to 20% of young adults remain susceptible to measles, rubella, or both. The American College Health Association recommends that colleges

TABLE 12-3. DEVELOPMENTAL TASKS AND OUTCOMES FOR THE STAGES OF YOUNG ADULTHOOD

Developmental Stages	Developmental Tasks	Outcomes Sought
Becoming adults, 23–28 yr old	1. Select mate. 2. Settle in work, begin career ladder. 3. Parent. 4. Become involved in community. 5. Consume wisely. 6. Own home. 7. Socially interact. 8. Achieve autonomy. 9. Problem solve. 10. Manage stress accompanying change.	1. Successful marriage. 2. Career satisfaction and advancement. 3. Effective parents; healthy offspring. 4. Informed, participating citizen. 5. Sound consumer behavior. 6. Satisfying home environment. 7. Social skills. 8. Fulfilled single state, autonomy. 9. Successful problem solving. 10. Successful stress management; personal growth.
Catch-30, 29–34 yr old	1. Search for personal values. 2. Reappraise relationships. 3. Progress in career. 4. Accept growing children. 5. Put down roots; achieve "permanent" home. 6. Problem solve. 7. Manage stress accompanying change.	1. Examined and owned values. 2. Authentic personal relationships. 3. Career satisfaction, economic reward, a sense of competence and achievement. 4. Growth-producing parent-child relationship. 5. Sound consumer behavior. 6. Successful problem solving. 7. Successful stress management; personal growth.
Midlife reexamination, 35–43 yr old	1. Search for meaning. 2. Reassess marriage. 3. Reexamine work. 4. Relate to teenage children. 5. Relate to aging parents. 6. Reassess personal priorities and values. 7. Adjust to single life. 8. Problem solve. 9. Manage stress accompanying change.	1. Coping with existential anxiety. 2. Satisfying marriages. 3. Appropriate career decisions. 4. Improved parent-child relations. 5. Improved child-parent relations. 6. Autonomous behavior. 7. Fulfilled single state. 8. Successful problem solving. 9. Successful stress management; personal growth.

Modified from McCoy V., Adult Life Cycle Tasks Adult Continuing Education Program Response, *Lifelong Learning in the Adult Years* (October 1977), 16.

and universities require student documentation of immunity (including tuberculin testing) to preventable diseases as a prerequisite to registration. Adults should be vaccinated against influenza, hepatitis B, rubella (German measles), and regular measles and should receive a tetanus booster every 10 years. Mumps vaccine is especially recommended for adult males (70, 354).

Common Health Problems: Prevention and Treatment

Physical Problems

Health problems and risks, preventive behavior and response to illness are influenced by gender and life-style. Refer to references at the end of the chapter for specific information on gender-related health issues (9, 69, 104, 172, 196, 253, 298, 304, 347, 362). Table 12–4 summarizes common health problems encountered by the young adult (13, 54, 115, 138, 159, 172, 262, 298, 351, 354).

Acquired Immunodeficiency Syndrome. **AIDS** was defined by the Centers for Disease Control (CDC) in 1987 *as a disabling or life-threatening illness caused by human immunodeficiency virus (HIV) and characterized by HIV encephalopathy; HIV wasting syndrome, or*

certain diseases resulting from immunodeficiency in a person with laboratory evidence for HIV infection or without certain other causes of immunodeficiency (305).

AIDS was first reported in the United States in 1981 but more likely occurred in 1977. Currently the World Health Organization (WHO) predicts up to 30 million World AIDS cases by the year 2000. WHO estimates there have been 1.3 million AIDS cases up to early 1991 and that there are at least 8 to 10 million adults infected with the virus. With 10 million of these predicted infections expected in children by the year 2000, AIDS will be a major global cause of death, if not the biggest killer in some countries (350).

The HIV epidemic has hit urban America the hardest, but everyone is at risk for the disease, regardless of life-style or employment and whether gay or lesbian, bisexual, or heterosexual (354). In 1989 11% of the increase in AIDS cases occurred in gay or bisexual men; 20% in intravenous drug users; 36% in heterosexuals; and 38% in newborns, showing that although most AIDS patients were still gay men and IV drug users, the lesser rate increase among homosexuals and IV drug users was proof that the virus was not bound to certain groups. This trend is seen worldwide. The media have reported about babies in Romania who are AIDS-infected; and in

---

■ BOX 12-3.
Selected Nursing Diagnoses Related to the Young Adult[a]

Pattern 1: Exchanging

Altered Nutrition: More than body requirements
Altered Nutrition: Less than body requirements
Altered Nutrition: Potential for more than body requirements
Potential for Infection
Potential for Injury
Potential for Impaired Skin Integrity

Pattern 2: Communicating

Impaired Verbal Communication

Pattern 3: Relating

Impaired Social Interaction
Social Isolation
Altered Role Performance
Altered Parenting
Potential Altered Parenting
Altered Family Processes
Parental Role Conflict
Altered Sexuality Patterns

Pattern 4: Valuing

Spiritual Distress

Pattern 5: Choosing

Ineffective Individual Coping
Impaired Adjustment
Defensive Coping
Ineffective Denial
Ineffective Family Coping: Disabling
Ineffective Family Coping: Compromised
Family Coping: Potential for Growth
Decisional Conflict
Health Seeking Behaviors

Pattern 6: Moving

Fatigue
Potential Activity Intolerance
Sleep Pattern Disturbance
Diversional Activity Deficit
Impaired Home Maintenance Management
Altered Health Maintenance

Pattern 7: Perceiving

Body Image Disturbance
Self-esteem Disturbance
Chronic Low Self-esteem
Situational Low Self-esteem
Personal Identity Disturbance
Sensory/Perceptual Alterations
Hopelessness
Powerlessness

Pattern 8: Knowing

Knowledge Deficit

Pattern 9: Feeling

Pain
Chronic Pain
Dysfunctional Grieving
Anticipatory Grieving
Potential for Violence: Self-directed or directed at others
Post-trauma Response
Rape-trauma Syndrome
Anxiety
Fear

[a]Other NANDA diagnoses are applicable to the ill young adult.
From North American Nursing Diagnosis Association, *NANDA Nursing Diagnosis Taxonomy I* (Rev.). St. Louis: North American Nursing Association, 1990.

Eastern and Central Africa 10% to 20% of urban heterosexuals have AIDS (362). Health care professionals are not immune; in fact, it is imperative that they take protective measures constantly.

In spite of action taken by the Public Health Service to isolate the causative virus, screen the nation's blood supply, and educate the public, the available data appear ominous. The AIDS virus infects and destroys white blood cells known as T-helper cells. These particular cells regulate the body's immune system, and if they are destroyed, the capacity to fight disease is gone. In addition, the HIV virus can affect the cells in the central nervous system (285, 286).

Infection with the AIDS virus does not always lead to AIDS, but if the person test positive for HIV he or she can transmit the virus to another human being.

Transmission of the blood-borne virus occurs through the following ways:

1. Sexual intercourse with an infected person, male or female
2. Contact with contaminated blood equipment such as sharing equipment for IV drug abuse
3. From a mother to her unborn fetus during pregnancy or during birth or while breast-feeding

The virus has been isolated in semen, vaginal secretions,

TABLE 12-4. COMMON HEALTH PROBLEMS FOR YOUNG ADULTS

Problem	Definition	Symptoms/Signs	Prevention/Treatment
Upper respiratory infection (URI or common cold)	Acute infection of the upper respiratory tract lasting several days	General malaise; nasal stuffiness and discharge, mild sore throat, watery eyes; sometimes ear discomfort	If bacterial: antibiotic; otherwise, symptomatic treatment—antipyretic, antihistimine, decongestants
Influenza	Acute contagious viral illness often occurring in epidemics	Fever, malaise, myalgia and respiratory symptoms; sometimes cough, rhinitis, and scattered rales	Prevention: immunization. Treatment: antipyretic, increase fluid intake, rest; for influenza: amantadine hydrochloride
Hypertension (uncomplicated), **essential**	Pertinent elevation of arterial blood pressure >150/100 but <200/110 present on three weekly determinations, without secondary cause found	Sometimes none; sometimes headache, dizziness, light headedness	Appropriate lab workup along with other testing; diet; weight reduction; exercise; possibly medication
Mitral valve prolapse	Insufficiency of valve to open and close appropriately	Usually in young adult female; chest pain, arrhythmias, palpitations, tachycardia, sense of fullness in neck and head, feeling faint, anxious	Medication, adequate rest; reduction of stress in life to extent possible
Iron deficiency anemia	Blood hemoglobin level of 10 g/dl or less, compared to normal value of 12–16 g/dl (for women)	Usually caused by menses; sometimes no signs; fatigue, irritability, depression, weakness, dizziness, headache, pallor of skin and conjunctivae, brittle nails	Prevention: blood screen, iron rich foods; treatment: iron preparation (ferrous sulfate)
Atopic dermatitis of adulthood	Dry, thickened skin, accentuating normal folds (different appearance than in infancy)	Hyperpigmentation, especially on flexor areas of extremities, eyelids, dorsi of hands and feet, and back of neck	Keeping skin dry in humid conditions; mild, nondrying soap; hydrocortisone cream
Folliculitis	Localized infection of hair follicle	Irritated area around hair follicle	Washing well; hot compresses
Furuncle (boil)	Infected area that has draining point	Raised red area with exudate	Hot compresses; antibiotics; sometimes incision and drainage
Carbuncle	Large group of furuncles with several draining points	Raised red areas with multiple exudate areas	Hot compresses; antibiotics; incision and drainage
Urticaria (hives)	Allergic reaction, usually to drugs, food, inhalants, or insect bites	Itching, red raised welts, usually on trunk or extremities	Cool compresses; sometimes antihistamine or epinephrine; trying to find offending agent
Scabies	Dermatitis caused by mite burrowing into skin and consequent allergic reaction	Severe itching; punctate excoriation	Lindane (Kwell) treatment (all sexual and household contacts too)
Simple diarrhea of adulthood	Gastrointestinal upset due to viral infection, psychologic disturbance, dietary changes, laxatives	Frequent loose, watery stools that are not greasy, bloody, or purulent	Clear liquid diet; antidiarrhea preparation (e.g., loperamide hydrochloride [Imodium])
Cystitis	Inflammation of bladder (often seen in young, adult women)	Dysuria, frequency, bladder spasms	Appropriate antibiotics after clean-catch urinalysis and culture; increased water intake (at least eight 8-ounce glasses daily); sometimes antispasmotic medication
Acute pyelonephritis	Cystitis plus inflammation of kidneys and collection system	Dysuria, frequency, flank pain, chills, nausea, vomiting	Appropriate antibiotic treatment plus antipyretic and antinausea medicine if necessary
Chronic fatigue syndrome (CFS)	Debilitating fatigue that lasts at least 6 mo	Eight of the following must persist or recur over 6 months: chills or low-grade fever; sore throat; tender lymph nodes; muscle pain and weakness; extreme fatigue; headaches; joint pain without swelling; neurologic problems (confusion, memory loss); sleep disorders	No known prevention; common sense treatment—adequate rest, nutritious diet, small amounts of exercise; rationing of energy; dealing emotionally with disease; possibly tricyclic antidepressants

blood, saliva, and tears. Even though the virus has been found in saliva and tears, there are no known documented cases of transmission other than by the ways just listed (285, 286).

In an individual more than 4 months of age, the AIDS antibody test can determine whether or not a person has been exposed to the AIDS virus. This does not mean that the person will necessarily develop AIDS. Unfortunately, the antibodies are not protective to the person like the antibodies to other disease organisms. It is not yet understood why this is so, but research is seeking an answer. It is also suggested that large amounts of virus are required to cause the infection and possibly cofactors are necessary for invasion to occur. The cofactors that have been suggested are an already decreased immune system, alcohol use, recreational drugs, poor nutrition, inadequate rest or exercise, severe stress, and other infections (285, 286).

HIV disease appears to have four relatively distinct stages in the young adult: early or acute period with flulike and respiratory symptoms lasting for a few weeks; middle or asymptomatic period of minor or no clinical problems lasting for months or sometimes years; transitional, symptomatic period lasting an intermediate length of time; and late or crisis period lasting months or occasionally years. Mean time from infection to disease is 8 years and from disease to death is 18 months (18, 285, 286). One of the drugs that seems to prolong life is zidovudine, or AZT. It attacks the virus after it has invaded the cell but before it has integrated itself into the cell's chromosones. Another drug, Ditiocarb sodium, shows promise in boosting the natural immune system (18). Currently there are experimental attempts to slow down the progress of the disease and to develop a vaccine (126).

Public education is the only way of dealing with this public health menace. It is estimated that 1 to $1\frac{1}{2}$ million Americans have been infected with the AIDS virus. Of this group, approximately 10,000 people are known to have the disease, leaving the remainder capable of transmitting the virus for several years. The incubation period of the virus varies from months to as many as 10 years; thus preventive education is the key factor. New ways of educating must be tried, including teaching groups at schools, occupational sites, and churches and at gay bars and gay or lesbian organizations and developing organizations for Latinos and African-Americans since they may not attend general meetings. Television could be used to promote responsible sexual behavior, including abstinence and use of condoms to prevent sexually transmitted diseases. Further, some cities distribute free needles and syringes to drug users, using a monitoring system that is designed to prevent the spread of AIDS. This action appears to reduce sharing of needles between infected and noninfected drug users and provides a time for education (18, 55, 92, 130, 305, 351, 354). However, educational programs that em-

phasize hope and not just fear and include social and community issues and disease facts are most effective (92).

The prevention of AIDS is dependent on behavior that reduces or eliminates the possibility of contracting or transmitting the disease. The Public Health Service recommends these behaviors (55, 77, 92, 217):

1. Do not have sexual intercourse with multiple persons or with persons who had multiple partners (including prostitutes). The more partners you have, the greater your risk.
2. Avoid sexual intercourse with persons with AIDS, with people at risk for AIDS, or persons who have had a positive result on the AIDS antibody test. However, if you do have sexual intercourse with a person you think may be infected, protect yourself by taking precautions to prevent contact with that person's body fluids. (*Body fluids* include blood, semen, urine, feces, saliva, and vaginal secretions.) *Use of a condom* will reduce the chances of spreading the virus. The intact correctly applied rubber condom is effective against transmission of sexually transmitted disease. Dirubbo (77) specifies types and their use; directions are given for teaching clients so that the condom will be used correctly. Avoid practices such as anal intercourse that may injure body tissues and make it easier for the virus to enter the bloodstream. Oral-genital contact should also be avoided, as should open-mouthed, intimate kissing.
3. Do not use IV drugs. If you do, do not share needles or syringes.
4. Consult your doctor for counseling if you believe that you may be at increased risk for infection by the AIDS virus. Consider taking the AIDS antibody test, which will enable you to know your status and take appropriate action.

Persons in the following groups are at increased risk for infection from the AIDS virus (305, 350, 351, 362):

1. Homosexual and bisexual men (or men who have had sexual intercourse with another man since 1977)
2. People who inject illegal IV drugs or who have done so in the past
3. Persons with symptoms of AIDS or AIDS-related illnesses
4. Persons from Haiti and Central African countries, where heterosexual transmission is believed more common than in the United States
5. Male or female prostitutes and their sex partners
6. Sexual partners of persons infected with the AIDS virus
7. Persons with hemophilia who have received clotting factor products
8. Infants of high-risk or infected mothers

If hospital infection control practices are followed when health care providers care for patients with AIDS or work with their biologic specimens, there is low risk of occupationally acquiring the opportunistic infections associated with AIDS: (1) HIV through serum conversion, (2) cytomegalovirus (CMV), or (3) hepatitis B virus (HBV) or herpes simplex virus type 2 (HSV-2). Seroconversion to HIV is most likely to follow a contaminated needle-stick injury. Health care professionals who use rubber gloves are effectively protected against transmission of HIV when the gloves are correctly fitted and worn and are intact (77, 92). In addition, thorough handwashing is mandatory. A face mask should be worn when required. Sharp objects, if contaminated, should be carefully handled. Contaminated instruments should be sterilized or disposed of properly.

The 10 warning symptoms of HIV infection in adults are as follows:

1. Swollen glands, especially in neck, armpits, or groin
2. Blotches or rashes, usually pink to purple, that grow in size, are harder than surrounding areas, and may appear under skin, in the mouth, nose, rectum, and among other body sites
3. Unexpected weight loss of more than 10 pounds within 2 months
4. Fever persisting for more than 1 week and night sweats
5. Cough that is persistent and dry
6. Diarrhea
7. Malaise and persistent fatigue
8. Thrush or white coating on tongue
9. Easy bruising
10. Blurred vision or persistent headaches

These symptoms may indicate early stages of various diseases that may lead to death such as Kaposi's sarcoma and *Pneumocystis carinii* pneumonia (285, 286).

As a nurse, you may care for the person with AIDS in the hospital, in his or her home, or in a special home designated for AIDS clients and families. You will be a resource to relatives, partners, and friends of AIDS clients. Care will be determined by body parts affected, mind set, and neurologic and other physical and emotional symptoms and signs. Remember the extreme isolation and loneliness that most clients will experience as they deal with a disease with such stigma. Seek various educational tools for use (92, 178, 202, 251, 305, 327). A toll-free hotline has been set up by the Public Health Service. Publications are issued by public health organizations and agencies such as the American Red Cross. Information written in the appropriate language and at appropriate learning levels is essential to affect any person's attitude and behavior.

The following references provide additional information on all aspects of HIV and AIDS: 18, 39, 55, 92, 96, 126, 130, 178, 202, 251, 292, 327, 351, and 362.

Refer also the Chapter 11 for information on other

sexually transmitted diseases that can be contracted by the adult. Smeltzer and Whipple (305) also give information. Another useful reference for information about AIDS and other sexually transmitted diseases (bacterial vaginosis, *Chlamydia trachomatis* infection, gonorrhea, pelvic inflammatory disease, genital herpes simplex, genital warts), including information about exposure to them during pregnancy and about chronic ones, is *Nursing Clinics of North America,* December 1988, Vol. 23, no. 4.

Hepatitis. **Hepatitis B,** a *type of inflammation of the liver,* is believed on the rise. The disease, which causes 80% of the world's primary liver cancer and a high incidence of cirrhosis, is often undetected. The disease itself can cause death. Some people never develop the main symptom, jaundice. Approximately 10% become carriers of the disease who in turn infect others. The CDC urges that anyone at risk for the disease get vaccinated. People at high risk include health care providers, male homosexuals, persons with multiple sex partners, IV drug users, institutionalized mentally ill persons, prisoners, and kidney dialysis clients (351, 354).

Accidents. Accidents are a leading cause of death for young adult men and the second leading cause of death for young adult women, with motor vehicle accidents producing the most deaths in both sexes. Among the young male population, industrial accidents and drownings also rank high as major causes of accidental death. Other injuries typical in young adulthood are fractures, dislocations, lacerations, abrasions, and contusions (149, 159, 337). These injuries require restriction of activity, which also presents the young adult with social and economic problems.

Because accidents and their resultant injuries are serious health hazards for the young adult, safety education should be a prime concern for you in all occupational settings. You should initiate and actively participate in safety programs in various settings: employment, school, or recreation. Young adults should be reminded of the safety rules for swimming and other sports and be encouraged to drive defensively. The groundwork in safety education should be established when the individual is young. Old habits and patterns are difficult to change.

Dental Problems. Not so commonly considered health problems for the young adult are **dental caries** *(decay)* and **periodontal disease,** *characterized by spongy, bleeding, hypertrophied gums, later receding of gums and bone, and eventual loss of teeth.* Twice yearly visits to the dentist for regular care increase the likelihood of avoiding dentures or health problems of the mouth in later life. Proper diet and tooth and mouth care should be taught to the young adult (142, 289, 352).

Malignancies. **Cancer of the mouth** begins to appear in the young adult age group. Oral cancer has a poorer survival rate than cancer of the breast, colon, rectum, or prostate; therefore early detection is essential. The nurse should examine the mucous membranes of the mouth as part of the physical assessment and report and record any abnormalities (11, 259, 288, 332).

Cancer is the leading cause of death in women between 25 and 44 years of age. The risk of cancer of the reproductive organs of women increases with age. African-American women are more likely than Caucasian women to suffer **cervical cancer.** It also occurs more frequently in smokers and women passively exposed to cigarette smoke (34, 59, 93, 136, 191). Periodic pelvic examinations and cytologic smears are essential in all women who are sexually active or over the age of 20. Pelvic examinations are also indicated for women with physical symptoms such as excessive menstrual flow, watery discharge, or bleeding between periods. The history of the person is especially significant if her mother took diethystilbestrol (DES). It is estimated that between 1941 and 1971 2 to 4 million women received the drug during pregnancy, particularly in the North and Midwest. The majority of their daughters will develop an abnormal glandular cell growth called *vaginal adenosis,* a possible precursor to cancer. They may also have difficulty becoming pregnant and retaining the pregnancy (133, 193, 259).

Breast cancer is rare under the age of 25, but the risk increases steadily after the age of 30. All young women should be taught and encouraged to do self-breast examinations since most breast cancers are first found by the individual woman. In addition, examination by a physician or nurse practitioner should be done annually. Many women are hesitant to do self-breast examinations: fear, lack of knowledge, modesty, health orientation, education level, and age contribute to this reluctance. Women are likely to practice self-examination of the breasts if they have a positive self-concept, if they are aware of the benefits, and if barriers are minimized, and if they perform other preventive health measures. Media coverage of someone who has successfully recovered from a mastectomy increases the incidence of self-examination (17, 56, 68, 291, 297).

You should teach the following information about self-breast examination. Examination should include systematic inspection and palpation. The woman should sit in front of a well-lit mirror and, with arms hanging, inspect each breast for asymmetry or irregularities. The woman should then raise her hands above her head and observe for retraction or distortion of the nipple, which is common in breast carcinoma. Then with hands on her hips, the woman should forcefully contract the pectoral muscles; through this maneuver a lesion adherent to the pectoral muscles can be seen to move. Finally, the woman should bend forward with her hands up to determine if there is fixation of the breast to the chest wall. While lying in a supine position, keeping under her head the hand closest to the breast being examined, the woman should palpate each breast. Using the palm of her free hand in a circular motion, she should feel all tissue systematically to determine the presence of either a fixed or movable nodule. After both breasts are examined, she should repeat the palpation process while standing. The examination should be done monthly, at a specific time of the month, so that the woman is familiar enough with her breasts to detect any abnormalities (158, 160).

During young adulthood the man should be taught to examine his scrotum and penis regularly since **cancer of the testes** may occur and may be detected by palpating unusual nodules. Teach the following information about the examination. The examination should be done immediately after a shower or warm bath when both the scrotum and the examiner's hands are warm. The scrotum should be held in the palms of the hand and palpated with the thumb and fingers of both hands. Each testicle should be examined individually. Locate the epididymis (found on top of and extending down behind the testicle); it should be soft and slightly tender. The spermatic cord should be examined next; it ascends from the epididymis and has a firm, smooth, tubular texture (111, 245, 356). It is important to become familiar with the consistency of normal testicular structures so that changes can be detected. In later young adulthood an annual rectal examination is helpful to detect prostatic enlargement and possible cancer of the prostate gland, although prostatic cancer is more common in later adulthood. In addition, proctosigmoidoscopy (examination of the rectum and lower colon with a lighted instrument) should be done on both men and women as part of the annual or biennial physical examination in an attempt to detect early rectal cancer. This examination is done less frequently on people with a low cancer risk level (159). See Appendix III for recommended physical examination procedures to do for this age group.

Teach clients the *warning signs* of cancer (Box 12–4). Often it seems that the public is oblivious to health hazards in spite of information presented in the media. For example, **skin cancer** is increasing in incidence, primarily because of overexposure to sunlight. In the early stages skin cancer can usually be cured. Teach

---

■ BOX 12-4.
Seven Warning Signs of Cancer

Change in bowel or bladder habits
A sore that does not heal
Unusual bleeding or discharge
Thickening or lump in breast or elsewhere
Indigestion or difficulty in swallowing
Obvious change in wart or mole
Nagging cough or hoarseness

Used by permission, American Cancer Society, Inc., *Cancer Facts and Figures—1991.*

protection through use of a sunscreen or covering skin when exposed to ultraviolet rays, including on an overcast day, especially from 11 A.M. to 2 P.M. Teach also signs that should be considered *suspicious* and reported to a physician:

1. Changes in a dark-colored mole or spot
2. Pink or flesh-colored nodule that slowly grows larger
3. Open or crusted sore that does not heal
4. Red, rough patch or bump that persists
5. Mole that grows, changes, hurts, bleeds, or itches
6. Mole that is larger in size than a pencil eraser and has irregular borders or variegated colors with shadings of red-white or blue-black
7. Elevation or bulge in a mole that was flat
8. Mole on the bottom of the feet or in an area of repeated trauma

Daily habits may contribute to risk for cancer in other ways. For example, risks for lung and hematopoietic cancers apparently are increased in adulthood after childhood exposure to parental smoking (270). Tell women that incidence of breast cancer or fibrocystic disease is higher in those who consume increased amounts of caffeine (270). Consuming two or more cups of caffeinated coffee a day may be associated with increased risk of colon or bladder cancer (270). Realize that some cultural groups are more prone to cancer. For example, Sievers and Fisher (302) found that environmental and cultural factors (e.g., diet, life-style stress, exposure to pollutants) contribute significantly to increased incidence of cancer. American Indians, in comparison to Caucasians, have lower rates for cancer of the lung, breast, and colon and higher rates for gallbladder, kidney, and cervical cancer, possibly related to genetics, diet, or life-style. American Indians have a higher rate of alcoholism than Caucasians. Although Oriental populations have a low rate of breast and colon cancer, those who have migrated to Western countries experience higher frequency of carcinoma of each anatomic site than prevails in their original country.

Gastrointestinal Conditions. **Lactose intolerance** or **milk malabsorption syndrome** may first become apparent in young adulthood. In a *large percentage of ethnic people of dark skins, the lactose (milk in sugar) is not hydrolyzed because they lack sufficient amounts of the enzyme lactose.* Ingesting milk or milk products can cause severe discomfort. The syndrome is more fully described in Chapter 1. Englert and Guillon (89) also describe the syndrome in detail.

The person may obtain relief by using LactAid (Sugar Lo Company, Pleasantville, N.J.), which is a concentrated form of this enzyme. Ten drops added to a quart of milk and refrigeration for 1 day afterward will reduce lactose by 90%. Lactobacillus milk also marketed for this condition is less likely to cause symptoms. A lactosefree diet is the best treatment. The person should

avoid all milk and milk products and check labels for whey or other lactose ingredients in foods that would not normally be considered as milk foods or products. For example, other foods to avoid include (89, 157, 257):

1. Cream of rice; instant cream of wheat
2. Breads, rolls, biscuits, crackers, muffins, and pancakes
3. Packaged bread crumbs, breading, or croutons
4. Fruits dried, frozen, or canned with lactose
5. Fruits or vegetables prepared with cheese, milk, milk products, butter, or margarine
6. Creamed or breaded meats, fish, or poultry
7. Lunchmeats that contain milk products, frankfurters, sweetbreads, canned soup

Life-style and Physical Illness. Life is rooted in and organized around a person's changing culture and society, whether the changes are dramatic or subtle. Coping with extreme change taxes the person physically and psychologically and may be responsible for physical disease. Research shows relationships between physical adaptation and illness and sociocultural experiences. Death rates from cancer, diabetes, tuberculosis, heart disease, and multiple sclerosis for urban populations are inversely proportional to income, implying that stresses of poverty may be a cause of disease (74, 159, 240).

The adult is most likely to fall ill when he or she is experiencing the "giving up–given up complex": feelings of lowered self-esteem, discouragement, despair, humiliation, depression, powerlessness to change or cope with a situation, imagined helplessness, loss of gratifying roles, sense of uncertain future, and memories of earlier periods of giving up. Apparently such feelings modify the capacity of the organism to cope with concurrent pathogenic factors. Biologically, the central nervous system fails in its task of processing the emergency defense system so that the person has a higher statistical tendency toward illness or death. Conversely, contentment, happiness, faith, confidence, and success are associated with health (24, 74, 162, 210, 258).

Anxiety is a combination of *fearfulness, nervousness, apprehension, and restlessness* that is often associated with a family or personal crisis and sometimes with a physical or mental illness. The symptoms may include loss of appetite (or increased appetite), lack of sleeping ability, increased perspiration, a "thumping of the heart," headaches, weakness, or fatigue. Occasionally trembling hands and tightly drawn facial muscles are noticeable. Table 12–5 summarizes the levels of anxiety (240).

More information on how to assess anxiety is available in other texts. Supportive therapy and crisis intervention provide the best treatment. The young adult may need short-term treatment with an antianxiety medication, but this should only be an adjunct to understanding, counseling, and eliminating the cause of anxiety (240, 271).

Tension headaches are often associated with pe-

TABLE 12-5. LEVELS OF ANXIETY AND THEIR MANIFESTATIONS

Level of Anxiety	Physiologic	Cognitive	Emotional
Mild	Tension of needs motivates behavior. Individual adapts to variety of internal and external stimuli.	Attentive, alert, perceptive to variety of stimuli; effective problem solving.	No intense feelings; self-concept not threatened. Use of ego adaptive mechanisms minimal, flexible. Behavior appropriate to situation.
Moderate[a]	Some symptoms may be present.	Perceptual field narrows; responds to directions. Tangible problems solved fairly effectively, at least with direction and support. Selective inattention—focus on stimuli that do not add to anxiety.	Impatient, irritable, forgetful, demanding, crying, angry. Uses various adaptive mechanisms to protect from feelings and meaning of behavior.
Severe[b]	Alarm Stage changes intensify, and Stage of Resistance may progress to Stage of Exhaustion.	Perceptual field narrows; stimuli distorted; focuses in on scattered details. Selective inattention prevails. Learning and problem solving ineffective. Clarification or restatement needed repeatedly. Misinterprets statements. Unable to follow directions or remember main points. Unable to plan or make decisions; needs assistance with details. Consciousness and lucidity reduced.	Self-concept threatened; sense of helplessness; mood changes. Erratic or inappropriate behavior; may be aware of inappropriate behavior but unable to improve. Many ego defense mechanisms used; dissociation and amnesia may be used. Disorientation, confusion, hallucinations, and delusions may be present.
Panic[c]	Severe symptoms of Exhaustion Stage may be ignored.	Sensory ability and attention reduced so that only object of anxiety noticed. May fail to notice specific object of concern or disastrous event but will be preoccupied with trivial detail.	Self-concept overwhelmed. Ego defense mechanisms ineffective; behavior often inappropriate and uncontrollable. Behavior focused on finding relief; may scream, cry, pray, thrash limbs, run, hit others, hurt self. Often easily distracted; cannot attend or concentrate. No learning, problem solving, decision making, or realistic judgments. May become immobilized, assume fetal position, become mute, or be unresponsive to directions. Needs protection.

Data from reference 240.

[a]Physiologic cognitive, and emotional changes of Alarm and Resistance States of the General Adaptation Syndrome (see Figs. 17–2 and 17–6). Individual functions in normal pattern but may not feel as healthy physically or emotionally as usual. Illness may result if feeling persists.

[b]Psychoses or physical illness or injury may result.

[c]Psychoses may occur.

riods of stress and are usually described as a *bandlike pressure across the forehead and around the back of the skull.* The pain is usually described as dull and aching, with an accompanying feeling of tightness. It may last for long periods. The examiner may find the muscles in the posterior neck and the scalp are sore because these headaches are essentially a *musculoskeletal phenomenon.* Relief usually comes with reassurance, mild analgesics, massage, or manipulation, and elimination of some of the tension (3, 159, 162).

Migraine headaches are believed *vascular in origin. Arterial spasm followed by dilation is thought to cause the pain, which is usually of a throbbing, unilat-*

eral *nature.* Often the headaches are preceded by an **aura,** an *inherent warning,* usually visual, during which surroundings may look different than usual, followed by some neurologic signs such as tingling and weakness of the extremities. The headache may last 1 hour to several days and is sometimes associated with nausea and vomiting. Often a family history of similar episodes is found (159, 162, 259).

Several prescription medications are used to try to avert an impending migraine. Caffeine is also thought to help prevent the onset. Once the headache is established, however, relief usually comes only with rest in a dark room and a strong analgesic such as meperidine

(Demerol) or codeine. Various alternate methods used with some success are nutrition, chiropractic, and biofeedback. Sometimes readjustment of the temporomandibular joint will cause migraines to disappear (159).

Functional bowel disease or **irritable colon syndrome** is characterized by *four to six small, loose, watery bowel movements daily along with lower abdominal discomfort and a sensation of the need for further defecation.* It is often associated with tense and anxious young adults. Prevention of recurrence is in the form of stress reduction and reassurance of the nature of the problem. Antidiarrheal agents are not indicated. A mild tranquilizer may be used temporarily (159, 259, 262).

Life-style influences illness in yet another way. Multiple living arrangements, sexual experimentation, and mobility from group to group are responsible for a number of conditions. They include the present epidemics of sexually transmitted diseases and insect infestation such as *body and pubic lice* (**pediculosis**), bedbugs, or ticks; airborne diseases such as respiratory infections; and skin infections such as staphylococcal or fungal infections. Other conditions are hepatitis from fecal contamination of food and water or use of unsterile equipment in drug abuse; gastrointestinal disorders from unhygienic food preparation; and malnutrition from lack of proper food intake (159).

One life-style that involves geographic mobility, transient and inadequate housing, hard work, poor nutrition, and inadequate immunizations or other health promotion measures is that of the **migrant farm worker.** The migrant worker has unique and numerous health care needs because of the following: (1) the opportunity for prevention of certain illnesses is nonexistent; (2) prenatal and maternal care is lacking; (3) chronic health problems are numerous; (4) economic resources are scant; and (5) contacts with the health care system are sporadic and temporary. Specific ways to work with Mexican-American seasonal workers and their families are described by O'Brien (250). (Migrant workers from other cultural backgrounds would have some of the same needs as those described by O'Brien). Refer also to Chapter 1.

Be attuned to cultural differences, including language difficulties, definitions of health and illness, food preferences, lines of authority, health practices, job-related diseases, and general life-style of your clients.

Health problems in women and the related issues of sex-stereotyped treatment are experienced, especially by women from minority groups, be they African-American, Hispanic, Asian-Pacific, or American Indian. Painter (254) describes the socioeconomic and health disadvantages of African-American women in America related to the historical roots of slavery and complex problems of racism and sexism. The adaptations that African-American women (and men) have made to adverse socioeconomic conditions have produced relationships within the family that, in many cases, do not conform to the gender roles and values prevalent in the dominant Caucasian society. African-American women deserve praise for their resourcefulness and ability in maintaining the family unit against overwhelming odds. Although the infant mortality rate for African-American babies is $1\frac{1}{2}$ times that of Caucasian babies in the United States, African-American families have tried to give the best possible care to their children within often unresponsive social and health care systems.

The American Indian has an infant mortality rate as high as that for African-American children, and the deficiency of medical care facilities for both nonreservation rural Indians and reservation Indians is great. Yet these mothers, especially when they incorporate cultural practices in child rearing, give the best possible care to their children, often under poverty conditions.

In contrast, in the United States women who are in higher socioeconomic levels, who are high achievers, and who have professional or executive positions have a 29% better life expectancy than other women. The same trend is true for men who are in the higher socioeconomic levels, who are achievers, and who have professional or executive positions. Thus it appears that many health and related social and economic issues are not just women's issues, but they are equally relevant to men (49, 184).

You can use this information for health promotion. Illness can be prevented through counseling susceptible persons not to make too many life changes in too short a time since the more rapid the pace, the more disorganized the individual becomes. Listen to what the person says, note whether he or she is well or ill, and note the degree of change occurring in his or her life. If unavoidably rapid change and a high degree of stress are occurring, a detailed, frequent follow-up program that uses the principles of crisis intervention may prevent the onset of illness or complications of an already present condition.

Explore ways, being nonjudgmental, to improve hygienic conditions for young adults. Sincere interest, factual information, and willingness to give care without preaching are essential to health promotion for young adults.

Biofeedback. The young adult is likely to be interested in and benefit from **biofeedback training,** *learning to control body functions once considered involuntary* such as heartbeat, blood pressure, breathing, and muscle contractions (see Chapter 17 for further discussion). Learning biofeedback is much like learning other skills of muscular coordination and physical activity. Involved is controlled production of alpha waves, the brain waves typical of relaxation and reverie, the fringe of consciousness. Biofeedback has been used to treat a variety of conditions (3, 240, 258, 283).

Meditation has also become a popular method to

relax and to produce physiologic changes that are healthful such as lower metabolism, pulse, respirations, and blood pressure. You may teach meditation techniques to clients. Acupressure and yoga are other self-care measures.

Emotional Health Problems

Stress reactions, *physiologic and psychologic changes resulting in unusually or disturbed adaptive behavior patterns,* result when the young adult is unable to cope with the newly acquired tasks and responsibilities. Mate selection, marriage, childrearing, college, job demands, social expectations, and independent decision making are all stressors that carry threats of insecurity and possibly some degree of failure. Some of these stress reactions take the form of physical illnesses just described. Others take the form of self-destructive behavior such as suicide, alcoholism, drug abuse and addiction, eating disorders, and smoking. Other stress reactions include abuse of spouse.

Self-destructive behavior, in the form of death by suicide, is increasing in spite of the many religious, cultural, and moral taboos. Thousands of people take their own lives or attempt suicide yearly.

Suicide. Suicide is the fourth leading overall cause of death among young adults in the United States (331). Although medicine has decreased the threat of many physical illnesses, the present-day life-style has increased the physical, mental, and emotional stress on individuals. Suicide statistics might actually prove higher if all accidental deaths were investigated more closely for clues of suicidal intent. Many people deliberately conceal their suicide under the guise of an accident: driving their car off the road, combining alcohol and barbiturates, or discharging a gun while cleaning it (6, 109, 139, 154).

Women make the majority of unsuccessful suicide attempts, whereas men complete suicide more frequently. Both physiologic and psychologic factors influence the choice of method for suicide. Women tend to use less lethal methods such as aspirin or barbiturate overdose, poisoning, or cutting the wrists. Men usually use the more lethal methods: gunshot wounds of the head or hanging. Women may see attempted suicide as a means of expressing aggression or manipulating relationships or events in the environment; therefore they select the less lethal methods. Degree of physical strength and the subconscious fear of disfigurement may also influence women's choice of methods (6, 109, 139, 154). Most of the time the person does not really desire death but rather a way out of an apparently hopeless or intolerable situation.

Statistics indicate that suicide occurs less frequently among married persons. Suicide is higher among single (especially males) and widowed individuals and highest among the divorced. Apparently the married person does not suffer from the social isolation and total lack of someone with whom to communicate as do the single, divorced, or widowed individuals. But the suicide rate in married persons less than 24 years of age is higher than for single persons. Perhaps these people sought marriage as an attempt to escape from their unmanageable situations. When marriage does not immediately solve their problems or creates new stresses, they end their lives (6, 109, 154, 307).

Occupation is also an important factor in suicide rates. Professional groups such as dentists, psychiatrists, and physicians are considered high-risk groups, although the underlying causes for this are undetermined. The required strenuous educational courses or the stressful demands and responsibilities of their positions may be factors.

Consider three factors when planning primary prevention of suicide among young adults. Educate the public about emotional needs of the person and early signs of suicide so that high-risk persons can be more easily identified by family and friends. To compensate for the effects of separating from home and encountering a variety of stressors, a close and significant relationship between high-risk persons and a caring person should be established. The person needs opportunity to talk through frustration, anger, and despair and to formulate life plans. Finally, encourage young adults to participate in group and extracurricular activities that prevent social isolation.

Nursing responsibility for the suicidal person extends to the industrial setting, clinic, general or psychiatric hospital, and the general community. You are in contact with and in the position to identify persons who may be potential candidates for suicide: unwed mothers, divorcees, widows and widowers, alcoholics, the terminally ill, and depressed people. Watch for signs of depression. If the person speaks of overwhelming sadness, worthlessness, hopelessness, or emptiness and complains of sleep and gastrointestinal disturbances, lack of energy, or chronic illness, he or she is in a depressed state. Decreased muscle tone with slumped shoulders, slowed gait, drooped faces, and decreased interest in work, personal appearance, religion, family and friends, or special events are also signs of depression. The person prefers being alone and is self-preoccupied. He or she is unable to carry out ordinary tasks or make simple decisions. Once identified, these signs of depression must be communicated to others: friends, relatives, a physician, or other persons concerned with the potentially suicidal person.

The person is more prone to attempt suicide *when the depression is lifting* and energy is greater. Listen closely to the person who speaks of being alienated, in an impossible situation, or of the future looking bleak and unchangeable, even after saying the situation is improving. He or she is a high-risk suicidal candidate, as is the person who talks of suicide, who has made an attempt, who is in crisis, or who is an alcoholic or a drug abuser (6, 154, 240).

Your responsibility in individual suicide prevention varies according to the setting, the source, and extent of distress. You will need to protect the person against self-destructive behavior by reducing environmental hazards; but emotional support is of greater importance while the person works through problems. The principles of crisis intervention, therapeutic communication, and nurse-client relationship are discussed in psychiatric nursing texts (240). Show the person verbally and nonverbally that someone—you—understands, respects, and cares about him or her.

You must know your own feelings about suicide and other self-destructive behavior. If you have more than transient depression, you cannot help another. You must see yourself and each person as an individual who possesses dignity and worth. Acceptance, understanding, and respect must be shown each person. Above all, you must be available and willing to listen. You can always listen long enough to assess and refer, even if you cannot work with the situation.

Alcoholism. Alcoholism, a complex disease, is also a form of self-destructive behavior. One suicide in every five is that of an alcoholic (6, 154). In addition, many alcoholics literally drink themselves to death or die as a result of physical debilitation or injuries sustained while under the influence of alcohol.

In the United States there is much ambivalence about drinking. Some states prohibit the purchase and consumption of alcohol until the age of 21; other states have lowered the age to 18. Drinking frequently starts during preadolescence or early adolescence, is introduced by the parents, and follows the pattern of the person's parents. Thus with drinking behavior and expectancies poorly defined during the young years, lack of cultural norms of alcohol consumption, and individual biochemical predispositions, the state is set for alcoholism in later life.

Alcoholism may occur during any life period. Male alcoholics outnumber female alcoholics; however, identification of female alcoholics is increasing yearly. The alcoholic's life span is shortened approximately 12 years, and most alcoholics show physical and cognitive complications because of their prolonged drinking. In addition, millions of dollars are lost yearly in business as a result of absenteeism, lowered work efficiency, and accidents.

Alcoholism is a disease with physiologic, psychologic, and sociologic aspects. Excessive drinking causes physiologic addiction and psychologic dependence. Not drinking causes mild to severe withdrawal symptoms. Alcohol is used to relieve worry and guilt, and it falsely leads to an increased sense of adequacy and sociability. In turn, the person becomes more anxious and guilty when learning of his or her behavior while drinking. He

or she drinks again to forget and deny. The vicious cycle becomes worse; behavior, performance, and health deteriorate until he or she is forced to seek help or dies. References at the end of this chapter give more information on the causes, psychodynamics, symptoms, and treatment of alcoholism (8, 88, 107, 171, 240, 284). Alcoholism in nurse colleagues is a concern. Several references give more information (53, 128, 243, 312, 326).

The same stress-producing situations that lead to suicide may also promote alcoholism in the young adult. Early case finding and early treatment are important in alcoholism, both for the ill individual and for the family members. A growing concern is the effect of the alcoholic parent on the development of the child(ren) (150). You can be active in both case finding and treatment.

Acceptance of the alcoholic as a sick person and providing support for those close to him or her are as important as the technical care you give during or after detoxification. You might write for the self-administered test for alcoholism that is available through National Council for Alcoholism or Alcoholics Anonymous. A certain score indicates alcoholic tendencies.

Drug Abuse and Addiction. These are other forms of self-destructive behavior. Drug use and the nurse's responsibility are discussed in Chapter 11. The same information is applicable to the young adult. Drug abuse is increasing in the young adult, including all levels of workers.

As with alcoholism, male addicts are more numerous than female ones. Symptoms of drug addiction differ with the type of drug, amount used, and personality of the user (see Table 11–5). Symptoms may also differ for the young adult at work. Box 12–5 summarizes signs and symptoms seen in the worker who is abusing drugs–sometimes in the workplace.

Treatment for drug abuse and addiction involves helping the person work through emotional problems, seeing that he or she has proper medical and nutritional regimens, helping him or her return to a community where the dangers of becoming addicted again are not too great, and helping him or her get involved in worthwhile work or activities.

Eating Disorders. **Eating disorders** (anorexia and bulimia) currently are identified more frequently in young adults. Refer to Chapter 11 for information also pertinent to the young adult who has this condition. Several references provide helpful information (204, 235, 268).

Smoking. Smoking is considered suicidal behavior because nicotine causes many harmful physiologic effects and is habit forming. Many people, even some with serious respiratory and vascular disorders, continue to smoke heavily despite the warnings from their physicians and reports from the Surgeon General's office about the harmful effects of smoking. Various reasons are given for smoking: smoking is relaxing; it prevents

<table>
<tr><td>

■ **BOX 12-5.**
Signs and Symptoms of Drug Abuse
in the Young Adult

- Late to work frequently; late in producing assignments
- Increased absenteeism (Abusers miss twice as much work as nonabusing employees.)
- Increased productivity in work for a short period (Cocaine will cause some people to perform better than normal or more creatively for a short time; overachievement can be used to compensate for or cover up initial stages of abuse.)
- Falling productivity, poorer quality work, disorganized thinking and work outcome, missed deadlines
- Forgetfulness, failure to follow instructions properly, to carry out usual steps of a procedure
- Personality change, increasing irritability, depression, suspicion
- Chronic runny nose from cocaine inhalation or sniffing glue or other chemicals that cause irritation of the nasal mucous membrane; regular complaints of a cold
- Nodding or sleeping on the job
- Accident proneness, clumsy at work, poor gross or fine motor coordination on the job, reports of accidents in the auto or at home
- Clandestine meetings and discussions with other employees (users become dealers for fellow employees and withdraw from supervisory staff.)

</td></tr>
</table>

rette smoking. To achieve this goal, you will have to do more than give information about morbidity and mortality rates. Explore his or her ideas of health and personal vulnerability to adverse effects from smoking. The social dynamics of smoking must also be considered. Smoking may mean being an adult or a way to get peer approval or to identify with the in-group, and exchanging cigarettes is a gesture of solidarity. It is important not to ridicule the smoker or interpret his or her behavior and smoking norms. Rather, deglamourize gestures of smoking, and hold up as models of adulthood those individuals who do not smoke. Further, realize that to give up smoking represents a loss. Help the person who is trying to stop smoking to acknowledge feelings of loss and grief related to giving up a part of self and social lifestyles. Instead of emphasizing that the person is "giving up" smoking, help the person verbalize feelings and identify what is being gained by a smoking cessation program. Encourage the person to find a substitute other than eating to overcome the sense of emptiness. Help the person find ways of rewarding self for not smoking. Further, you can give the person positive feedback for not smoking. Give the person time to change habits. If the person has smoked for many years, it is not easy to stop (62, 122, 222, 258, 267).

Battered or Abused Women. Battering is a social and emotional health problem of all socioeconomic levels that has gained increasing public attention. Wife beating has always been a problem: woman was the man's property and beating was accepted behavior in some cultures. Traditionally the woman was too ashamed or too helpless to admit the problem or seek help. Further, no help existed. Perhaps acknowledgment of and efforts to overcome child abuse and the women's liberation movement together helped to initiate change. Efforts are being made in some cities to make the police and legal system more aware of the **battered woman syndrome,** *a symptom complex of violence in which a woman has received deliberate and severe injury more than three times from the husband or a man with whom she has a close relationship.* Further, attempts have been made to make the police and legal system more protective to the woman who has been treated violently and more punitive to the violent man. Emergency shelters for battered women and their children are increasingly being established in urban areas so that the woman who seeks help does not have to return home or be at home when the man who was released shortly after arrest returns home even more violent than before. Crisis telephone lines have been established and publicized by the media, and hundreds of women have memorized these numbers. In some communities rap sessions and referrals are available for battered women. Assistance to women seeking divorce is inadequate in most cities because of the cost and bureaucratic red tape (6, 153).

nervousness and overeating; and it gives the person something to do with his or her hands in social gatherings. All these reasons may stem from internal tensions and may well be the young person's way of dealing with stress. If the pattern of smoking is not altered during the stage of young adulthood, it may be impossible for changes to be made later in life.

More women than men now smoke cigarettes. Smoking in younger women has significantly increased the number of cardiac deaths and the incidence of lung cancer in women. Other health problems are also attributed to smoking. Smoking more than 10 cigarettes a day during pregnancy can cause low-birthweight babies, premature births, spontaneous abortions, bleeding, fetal and neonatal deaths, and abnormal sperm and chromosomal damage in the newborn. Additional problems are periodontal disease, carcinoma in situ of the cervix, chronic respiratory disease, and shortened life expectancy. Offspring of the person who smokes are subject to more respiratory infections and allergies (14, 58, 118, 161, 165, 233, 279, 318, 326).

Less well known, but equally dangerous, is that chemicals found in cigarette smoke are also commonplace in many work environments. Thus the person who smokes may suffer double jeopardy. Further, the person who smokes has more occupational accidents and injuries and uses more sick time and health benefits (278).

Work with the young adult to reduce or stop ciga-

You can work with other health and legal professionals to identify and overcome the problem of abused women. *Assessment of a family and woman* suffering adult abuse often reveals the following typical characteristics (46, 129, 145–147, 153, 186, 249, 270, 309):

1. The family and the woman are isolated socially or physically from neighbors, relatives, and friends.
2. The woman feels increasing helplessness, guilt, isolation, and low self-esteem. She feels trapped and has been forced to be dependent on the man.
3. The woman may range in age from 17 to 76 and may suffer violent injury for months or years.
4. The woman's educational and occupational status is often higher than that of the man.
5. Most beatings begin early in marriage and increase in frequency and intensity over the decades.
6. Most violence occurs in the evening, on weekends, and in the kitchen.
7. Generally there are no witnesses.
8. The woman is frequently unable to leave the home because of lack of money, transportation, a place to go, support people, or support agencies in the community. Further, she has learned helplessness behaviors and feels unable to try to escape.
9. The injuries from abuse may not be visible, but if abuse is present, the woman usually talks about the problem freely when asked directly if abuse is occurring.
10. With increasing incidence of abuse and the physical and emotional consequences of abuse, the woman becomes more passive, less flexible, less able to think logically, more apathetic, depressed, and possibly suicidal.
11. Eventually the frustration, stress, and anger may be externalized into physical behavior that is more than protective of the self or the child(ren); she may in turn become violent to the point of killing the battering partner.

Women remain in a threatening situation for many complex and interrelated reasons (Box 12–6) (153, 176). An astute assessment will uncover at least some of these characteristics and factors if present. Box 12–7 describes some "red flags" that can help you identify a battered adult in an emergency room or intensive care, occupational, or other medical setting (46, 129, 145–147, 249).

Increasingly the literature is discussing *marital* (not just date) *rape* as a problem in young adulthood. Marital rape meets the criteria for criminal sexual conduct. The difference is that the rapist and his victim are married; thus the man may be immune from prosecution. Often the women have been child victims of sexual abuse or incest, and there are physical, psychosomatic, and emotional effects. Some of the content related to the abused or battered woman applies in this situation. Often children in these marriages are also raped or molested (6, 51, 154, 348).

Incest, *sexual intercourse between biologically re-*

BOX 12-6.
Reasons Why Women Are Unable to Leave a Violent Situation

- Lacking economic independence and being without money
- Being forbidden to leave the house or visit or call others
- Fearing being alone, being unable to support self and children, or the man's finding and harming her after she left him (Personal safety is a continual issue.)
- Lacking emotional or social support (Often parents encouraged her to return to the abusive partner.)
- Believing that she is unworthy of anything better
- Having nowhere to go or being turned away from a public shelter
- Believing traditional norms related to women's role, marriage, religion, and violence; believing the woman is less than human
- Believing there are positive aspects of the relationship that the woman believes are worth preserving; emotional dependency in the relationship
- Desiring a father for her children; wanting to protect the children from greater harm
- Feeling disbelief, sense of horror, and shock about the man's violent behavior to her and denial or rationalizations that it would happen again
- Believing the man's promise that he will not hit again; thinking she can change him
- Finding the police unresponsive to calls for help (Many women have kept extensive records of the number of times legal action was taken with unsatisfactory results.)
- Taking responsibility for the violence, feeling guilty and that his behavior is her fault (Often the man would say, "Look what you made me do.")
- Feeling helpless; being unable to counter the power, authority, and threats of the man (Often the women were forced out or locked out of the home in the middle of the night in winter without clothing or money.)
- Increasing force or violence, which was condoned by police or society, from failing to comply with the husband's wishes or demands
- Relying on the sexual relation to punish him, to prevent battering, and to prove self-worth (Sexual enjoyment lessened as battering increased.)
- Wanting to protect the man's reputation in the community or in the job
- Having several small children and the related child care responsibility, often coupled with need to protect the children against the man's violence
- Fearing the unknown aspect that would come with leaving the home and man (welfare, homelessness, unemployment, single parenting) (Often there is a predictability about his behavior versus the unpredictability of the future.)
- Introjecting the societal attitude that the victim is to blame
- Believing that all marriages are like this (violent), especially if the woman grew up in a violent home

BOX 12-7.
Identification of Wife Abuse in the Health Care Setting

Multiple Injuries

Multiple abrasions and contusions to different anatomic sites should alert health care providers. There are relatively few ways of sustaining such injuries.

Body Map

Many incidents of abuse involve injury to the face, neck, chest, breasts, or abdomen, whereas most accidents involve the extremities.

Rape

Most women are raped by a male intimate, and many times rape is yet another incident of ongoing physical abuse.

Severity of Injury

Severity varies among abused victims. Presentation of medically insignificant trauma to the emergency service may alert medical personnel that ongoing assault and impending danger comprise the real emergency for which she is seeking aid.

Pregnancy

Abused women are more likely to be beaten when pregnant. There is a higher rate of miscarriage among battered women.

Trauma History

A history of trauma can be the key indicator! Both asking about previous injuries and looking at her medical records are important. Records may indicate repeated visits and injuries to the same site.

Suicide Attempts

Studies indicate that battering is a frequent precipitant of female suicide attempts; conversely, women who attempt suicide are likely to have a history of domestic violence.

Inconsistent Description of Injuries

Injuries do not fit with the woman's description of the genesis of injury.

Vague and Non-specific Complaints

Complaints include, for example, anxiety, depression, and sleeplessness and may indicate intrafamilial crisis.

Heavy Use of Alcohol and Drugs

Victims are more likely than nonvictims to use alcohol and drugs, and partners are much more likely to use alcohol and drugs excessively.

lated persons, is another form of battering that may affect either the man or the woman, but more commonly the woman. Woman victims of incest outnumber men 10 to 1. Incest is considered one form of sexual abuse, although adult family members may convey that incestual behavior is normal.

Symptoms and problems in adulthood resulting from childhood *sexual abuse and incest* are:

1. Chronic depression, hopelessness related to shame and guilt.
2. Drug and alcohol abuse.
3. Various physical complaints, including symptoms of panic attacks, headaches, hysterical seizures.
4. Problems with trusting or intimate relationships with the opposite gender.
5. Character disorders such as borderline or narcissistic states.
6. Multiple personality disorders.
7. Sexual dysfunction and gynecologic problems.

This problem is expected to affect more young adults in the future, based on the statistics currently of childhood sexual abuse and incest (6, 129, 154, 183, 186).

Why do women leave the violent situation? Often the leaving occurs when the woman feels suicidal but does not want to kill herself because of concern about the children's welfare; or the woman may fear for the life of the unborn child, if pregnant, or for that of her other children. Fear of being killed may be a motivator; acknowledging that the situation will never improve is important. The shock of a particular beating or the horror of being beaten while pregnant may be the turning point (an estimated 25% to 45% of pregnant women are battered). She realizes she has no power to make him change. At some point the woman may have received enough subtle or overt encouragement to leave or a new vision of what marriage and family life should be, coupled with a renewed sense of self-worth and the feeling she "doesn't have to take it anymore." The ideal of mutuality believed to be part of love and marriage cannot be reconciled with the experience of the authority and power of the male. The woman realizes that at this point the man no longer asks for forgiveness, shows no remorse (as he might have after the first beating), and usually denies he behaved violently. There comes a decision point, and then a plan may be made. Some women, however, leave abruptly to prevent being murdered (153).

Women may or may not be in acute distress when they leave. Despite the desperate situations and the difficulty in finding aid, these women are not typically helpless. Generally, they continually scheme how to stop the battering, either by examining personal behavior or planning ways to escape and how to get and keep some money. They take steps to please their partners and to satisfy their demands while protecting and caring for the children. Often they are the primary wage earner in the home. They may describe how they actively defended themselves; if they did not, it was not because they felt helpless but because other negative consequences or a worse beating would ensue (153).

The *typical adult and parental behavior of the male batterer,* in order of incidence, according to the research by Sonkin, Martin, and Walker (309), is as follows:

1. Has battered a previous partner
2. Is employed, frequently under stress at work
3. Has children who have viewed the domestic violence and his battering behavior
4. Was under the influence of alcohol or drugs at the last battering incident
5. Uses physical punishment on his children
6. Has been violent with others not in their family, outside the home
7. Has been violent both when and when not under the influence of drugs and alcohol
8. Has a family history of suicide (attempted and completed)
9. Has been violent only when under the influence of alcohol and drugs
10. Has been violent only when not under the influence of alcohol or drugs
11. Lack of close friends or someone with whom to talk

Psychologic violence by the man against the woman can be categorized as follows (309):

1. Explicit threats
2. Extreme controlling type of behavior, taking her everywhere; saying when she must come home; knowing her whereabouts, companions, and life activities
3. Pathologic jealousy; continually questioning her about her behavior; making accusations without cause; highly suspicious
4. Mental degradation; calling her names or telling her she is incompetent, stupid, and no good
5. Isolating behavior (Because of his jealousy, suspicion, and dependence, he controls the woman's behaviors so that she in turn becomes extremely isolated and dependent on him.)

The man who batters the female partner has the following typical childhood history, in order of incidence, according to research by Sonkin, Martin, and Walker (309):

1. Received physical punishment as a child
2. Saw his mother abused or treated violently by his father
3. Attacked one of the parents
4. Was physically abused as a child
5. Was sexually abused as a child

The male batterer comes from all walks of life and cultures. Personality characteristics of the male batterer that are typical include:

1. Denying of or minimizing the violent behavior and its effects (The batterer may actually lose memory of the event because of his rage.)
2. Blaming the behavior of the woman or others as the cause of the violent scenes
3. Periodic uncontrollable anger and rage, which is externalized into physical and verbal behavior
4. Dependency on the partner as sole source of love, support, intimacy, and problem solving, resulting from the controlling and isolating behavior that entwined him and the partner and children
5. Sense of alienation from others and society (he considers himself a loner and therefore his "own boss"—means he can do whatever he wants in his home.)
6. Jealousy of and suspiciousness of his partner, children, and finally everyone else
7. Low self-esteem; lack of confidence in his ability to keep his partner, lack of skill or ability to ask for what is wanted in a nonthreatening way

Some stresses predispose to family violence and male battering of the woman and children. These stresses are listed in Box 12–8.

Because you are a nurse, you are in a position to (1) make a thorough and holistic assessment, using the prior content; (2) provide necessary crisis and emergency care; (3) encourage the battered woman to share her secret with you, another nurse, a social worker, confidante, or religious leader; (4) educate the public and abused women about the myths of abuse (Box 12–9) (176); help her secure help from social service agencies, legal aid societies, counselors, health centers, and the welfare office; and (5) encourage separation from her husband if her life is in danger. Work with the individual woman to the extent possible for her to talk through her feelings of shame, guilt, embarrassment, anger, and fear. Help her gain courage to make decisions, including de-

---

■ **BOX 12-8.**
Stresses That Predispose to Family Violence

- Financial pressures, low pay, high cost of living
- Family separation
- Geographic mobility, loss of friends, social supports, and familiarity
- Isolation and communication barriers
- Cultural differences; living in a strange environment or with unfamiliar customs, creating higher mutual dependence
- Lack of family support
- Living abroad such as in military families
- Inability to separate administrative or work roles from home life (Behavior that is functional at work may not be at home.)
- Lack of privacy at work or at home
- Job pressures or competitiveness; lack of support from supervisor

cisions on how to protect herself and her children, how to leave her husband, and where to go.

Group therapy and individual therapy are effective for the woman victim (50–52, 129, 147, 153, 154, 176, 201, 270, 349). Group therapy may be more effective than individual therapy for the man (27, 246, 309). Intervention must take into account incest, marital rape, and battering. Work also with the children, if possible. Research shows that children (ages 2 to 12 years) of battered women have deep feelings of fear about safety and abandonment, anger, confusion, social isolation, and aggression. Themes in the children's play reveal conflicts about overpowering adults, identification with the same-sex parent, and that children are learning abnormal behavior and roles that could be carried into their adult relationships and life-style (153). You can also work with others to establish emergency centers or crisis phone lines for the woman and to exert pressure to reform the current legal and judicial system so it will be more equitable to women.

Social support and the meaning a person attaches to stressful events can influence whether the person becomes ill or remains healthy—physically and emotionally—in a situation. The battered woman who extricates herself from her violent situation has strengthened her ability to survive, to resolve crisis, and to move forward (153).

The problem of spouse abuse, like that of child abuse discussed in Chapters 6 and 9, violent television programming discussed in Chapter 10, and elder abuse discussed in Chapter 14, is part of overall societal violence. Each nurse, as a citizen and health care provider, must work in whatever way possible to decrease violence, its causes and effects. Refer to several references for additional information (46, 51, 129, 147, 153, 154, 176, 183, 186, 201, 270, 307). Check also with the legal services of your area for information.

Many communities have shelters or homes for abused women sponsored by the Salvation Army, Women's Self-Help Centers, or family service agencies. These homes provide peer discussion and support, help the woman work through her feelings in a positive way and build self-esteem, and give education about how to cope with the situation and to find an alternative lifestyle. Some communities have organizations that also work with the abusing man in an effort to help him recognize angry and frustrated feelings in self, realize it is not acceptable to vent feelings through violent behavior to the spouse, and learn alternate coping and behavior patterns.

Hoff (153) describes the shelter experience for battered women and their children, the difficulties of poor and homeless women and children, the struggles of moving to a life without violence, the complexities of starting new relationships, and the effects on the children. Hoff calls the battered woman who removes herself from a violent situation not just a victim, but also a survivor. A 5-year follow-up study of the women showed their continued resilience despite hardships. Most still felt shock that someone who supposedly loved them beat them, but they also sensed victory, self-mastery, and recognition of their survival ability.

Social Health Problems

Divorce. **Divorce** is the *termination of marriage, preceded by a period of emotional distress in the marriage, separation, and legal procedures.* Divorce is a crisis for those involved and can affect society in general as well as the physical and emotional health of the persons involved (6, 131, 240).

Some young people enter marriage to escape the problems of young adulthood. Marriage provides them with a ready-made role, and it supposedly solves the problem of isolation. However, if marriage takes place before the individual has developed a strong sense of identity and independence, intimacy cannot be achieved.

Most divorces (one in three marriages) occur in the first 3 to 5 years of married life and involve persons less than 29 years of age. These couples are frequently from lower economic groups and have married at an early age. They tend to have less education and money and fewer personal resources than couples from higher economic groups. Approximately one in four children live with a single parent as a result (187).

Marriage often breaks down because of the partner's inability to satisfy deep mutual needs in a close demanding relationship. One of the partners may be overly dependent and seek in the other a mother or father. Dependent behavior may at first meet the needs of the more independent partner. But as the dependent person matures, the relationship is changed. If the stronger partner neither understands nor allows this change, divorce may follow.

Emotional deprivation in childhood is also a poor foundation for marriage. The deprived person grows up without sufficient experience of feeling acknowledged, wanted, appreciated, or loved. He or she has low self-esteem and is too sensitively tuned to rejection and not adequately responsive to acceptance and approval. He or she can easily misinterpret the partner's behavior, feel exploited, and have difficulty accepting any form of appreciation and love. The person from a home in which the parents' marital relationship was one of detachment, disharmony, or conflict or in which abuse or divorce occurred is poorly prepared for marriage. He or she has no healthy or loving marital model to follow. The person may try to model the marriage after another's happy marriage; however, the person learns most thoroughly that which is lived during childhood.

The divorce rate reflects the ease in which a divorce can be obtained. The lack of commitment to people and relationships when the going gets tough, seen also in other areas of life, and the dichotomy between the ro-

■ **BOX 12-9.**
Myths and Realities About Battered Women

Myth 1: Battered Women Are a Small Percentage of the Overall Population.

Fact: Domestic violence is the most underreported crime in the United States. The Federal Bureau of Investigation estimates that 60% of all married women experience physical violence by their husbands at some time during their marriage. There are an estimated 2 to 6 million female victims of family violence each year.

Myth 2: Battered Women Are Masochistic.

Fact: Battered women are *not* masochistic. The prevailing belief has always been that only women who "liked it and deserved it" were battered; that women experienced some pleasure, often akin to sexual pleasure, through being beaten by the men they love. Because this is such a prevailing stereotype, many battered women begin to wonder if indeed they are masochistic.

Myth 3: Battered Women Are Crazy.

Fact: Battered women are not crazy, although battering may contribute to mental illness. This myth places the blame for battering on the woman's negative personality characteristics and takes the focus off the batterer. Further, being abused and beaten may result in what apparently is abnormal behavior—the woman's attempt to adapt.

Myth 4: Middle-Class Women Are Not Battered As Frequently or as Violently as Poorer Women.

Fact: Women from lower socioeconomic classes are more likely to come in contact with community agencies, so their problems are more visible. Middle- and upper-class women often fear that disclosure will result in social embarrassment and harm to their own or their husband's career or that people will not believe them. This is often true when the husband is held in high esteem in the community.

Myth 5: Women From Ethnic or Racial Minority Groups Are Battered More Frequently Than Caucasian Women.

Fact: Studies show that battering crosses all ethnic lines, with no one group suffering more than another.

Myth 6: Battered Women Are Uneducated and Have Few Job Skills.

Fact: Educational levels of battered women range from grade school through completion of professional and doctoral degrees. Many successful career women would be willing to give up their careers if to do so would eliminate battering. Changing jobs or staying home to ease the situation usually has no effect on their partner's behavior, and sometimes battering worsens.

Myth 7: Batterers Are Unsuccessful and Lack Resources to Cope With the World.

Fact: It has been suggested that men who feel less capable than women resort to violence. Contrary findings were reported in England, where the highest incidence of wife-beating was among physicians, service professionals, and police. Affluent batterers include attorneys, professors, and salesmen. Many of these men donate a great deal of their time to community activities and could not maintain their involvement in these projects without the support of their wives.

Myth 8: Batterers Are People With Personality Disorders.

Fact: If batterers could simply be considered antisocial personalities, individual therapy could be used to differentiate batterers from other men. Unfortunately, it is not that simple. One trait they share is the ability to use charm as a manipulative technique. Manipulation, acting out of anger, exhilaration felt when they dominate and beat the woman, and denial of the behavior are characteristic of people with personality disorders.

Myth 9: Police Can Protect Battered Women.

Fact: At most, only 10% of battered women call the police. Of those who did, many believe the police officers were ineffective. When the police left, the men continued the assault with vigor. In St. Louis a pro-arrest policy is improving police response to domestic violence. Several thousand women are murdered annually by male partners, often as a part of the battering act. At least one half of the injuries presented by women at an emergency room are the result of battering. Battering may also be the basis for a suicide attempt.

Myth 10: Batterers Are Violent in All Their Relationships.

Fact: Most men who batter their wives are generally not violent in other aspects of their lives. Although being violent in public has definite, negative consequences, there are few consequences in domestic cases.

Myth 11: The Batterer Is Not a Loving Partner.

Fact: Batterers are often described by women during the honeymoon phase of the cycle of violence as fun-loving, playful, attentive, sensitive, exciting, and affectionate. The woman may describe some very positive characteristics in the man that cause her truly to love him.

Myth 12: Long-Standing Battering Relationships can Change for the Better.

Fact: Relationships that have rested on the man's having power over the woman are stubbornly resistant to an equal power-sharing arrangement. Even with the best of

■ Box 12-9.
Continued

help, such relationships usually do not become battering-free.

Myth 13: Once a Batterer, Always a Batterer.

Fact: Batterers can be taught to change their aggressive responses. However, very few batterers are willing to get help. If the batterer does not get treatment and if he is divorced and then remarries, he is likely to batter the next women he marries also.

Myth 14: Battered Women Can Always Leave Home.

Fact: Many battered women have no place to go and no means of survival outside the framework of their marriage. They also may have small children to care for, whom they would not want to leave home alone with the father. Because battering weakens a woman's self-esteem, she may believe she is incapable of managing on her own.

Myth 15: Battered Women Are Weak and Come From a Bad Background.

Fact: Typically the battered woman in Hoff's study (154) had a warm, loving relationship as a child with the mother and a negative, destructive relationship with the father. Not all battered women were abused as children. Women who experienced violence before they were battered by their mates showed resilience and strength. But long-standing abuse breeds self-degradation and despair so that a women feels unworthy of the continued love of even her mother and unable to reach out for help. The battered woman should be considered a survivor type of person.

Myth 16: Battering May Occur Only Once or Infrequently and Could Be Predicted, and Thus Prevented by the Woman.

Fact: For most of the battered women in several studies, the violence was frequent, extended over time, and often unexpected and included many similar incidents. Often violence occurred concomitantly with the man's rages, drunkenness, and/or financial insecurity and during the woman's pregnancy. Often each beating was worse than the previous one. Women consistently report doing everything possible to avoid violence; they try to second-guess the husband. "It's like walking on eggshells." Women have been socialized into the nurturing role, so they doggedly try to succeed in it as wife and mother, regardless of the circumstances. Further, society and medical and psychiatric services and professionals reinforce the belief that the woman's troubles are the result of her own inadequacies and failures (men are taught that the source of stress is other than self). Although the battered woman may think of hurting or killing the man as a punishment, the woman is often inhibited from such action by concern for the children, if present, and fear of consequences for self. Yet there have been times that the women retaliated; most women found that if they fought back, the man became even more violent.

manticized ideal of marriage and the fact that much of married life has a routine and sameness about it contributes to separation and divorce. Further, our youth are not educated for family life in any formal sense, and what they learn in the home may be poor preparation for marriage and good preparation for the divorce court.

When marriage fails and bonds are broken, aloneness, anger, mistrust, hostility, guilt, shame, a sense of betrayal, fear, disappointment, loss of identity, anxiety, and depression, alone or in combination, can appear both in the divorcee and the one initiating the divorce. Eventually there may be a feeling of relief. There must be an interval of adjustment to the physical and emotional loss. Often the second marriage is a rebound affair: a partner is selected as soon as possible to help assuage the feelings from the divorce and relieve the loneliness. Second and subsequent remarriages can be successful, but they carry a higher risk of instability and are more likely to end in divorce because of (1) the person's lack of ability to form a mutually satisfactory new relationship; (2) the past experiences, vulnerability, guilt, and insecurity that cannot be easily removed; (3) the hassles of her kids, his kids, and our kids; (4) child

and wife support; and (5) interference from the ex-spouse. Psychologic effects of divorce vary because of the following factors: (1) family psychodynamics before divorce; (2) nature of the marital breakup; (3) relationship between the ex-spouses after the divorce; (4) developmental age and coping skills of the children, if any, during the time of marital disharmony and divorce; and (5) coping skills of each ex-spouse. If the offspring are adolescents, expression and control of aggressive and sexual impulses, dependency-independency issues, deidealization of the parents, peer acceptance and social approval, and premature responsibilities of adulthood may intensify.

Children, even 15 or more years later, suffer from the consequences—emotional and social—of divorce. The problems of low self-esteem, depression, anxiety about intimacy and relationships, mistrust of others and close relationships, depression, guilt, and fantasies about the parents' reunion remain strong for many years (226, 343). Thus some researchers believe it is critical for parents to work at resolving marital conflicts, to recommit to each other, and ultimately to improve the relationship and gain greater maturity. Health care professionals and society must provide support systems so that parents can work out their stresses in other than divorce courts (36, 226, 343).

If the divorce cannot be prevented, the parents and children should be given emotional support. (Mothers and children may also have to struggle to meet physical needs and may need help in getting financial support.) The losses must be resolved, a new identity must be formed, and the children involved should have the option of continued close relationships with both parents (19, 65, 82, 131, 343).

If the person embarks on a second marriage with an understanding of how he or she has matured and of the reasons the first marriage failed, the second marriage may be satisfactory. If the mistakes of the first marriage are repeated in finding a partner, the second marriage is also likely to fail. The person may meander from one relationship to another, hoping for satisfaction, but always finding frustration and disappointment because he or she carries within self the seeds of failure. Ideally, the second marriage should be entered into with time (at least 1 year) and thought. The success of the second marriage depends on finding another person with whom common needs can be met and whose personality development matches that of the divorcee (19, 82, 131, 240).

Recently more emphasis has been given to helping people through the emotions involved in divorce. Divorce has been likened to death except that contact is often maintained, especially if small children are involved (19, 65, 82, 131, 240, 343).

A support group for the divorced woman is Displaced Homemakers Network, which has chapters around the country. The national office can be contacted at 1010 Vermont Avenue NW, Washington, D.C. 20005. Helping divorced women identify and pursue personal goals is important. Primary needs of divorced women are economic independence, education, managing parenting, maintaining friendships, establishing a partner relationship, and obtaining adequate housing, school, and environment for self and children. Mental health goals are a low priority, although the theme of accepting the divorce and establishing a happy life-style as a single-parent family would encompass mental health. Support groups for the divorced woman can assist her in meeting needs and securing goals. Refer to Duffy (81) to understand better the needs of the woman who heads the household and ways to assist her.

Hewlett (151) discusses how laws intended to make life better for women and divorce fairer ended up hurting women. The standard of living after divorce falls for the woman; it increases for the man. Many divorced women have had difficulty with custody rights and with obtaining child support.

Groups for children of divorcing and divorced parents can help the child work through the feelings of loss, anger, guilt, and ambivalence about relationships with parents—and often eventually stepparents and stepsiblings. The key is for the parents to continue showing love to their child(ren) and to maintain open communication between them about the offspring.

The ideal situation is for the departing parent to be pictured in the best possible light by the one with whom the child remains and for unimpeded contact to be maintained. The child should be given honest information at whatever level he or she can understand. The child must know that he or she did not cause the divorce. Delinquency, lack of gender identification, and eventually inability to form a lasting relationship may result in the child unless he or she is handled with care.

The divorce rate has increased in the United States, but that is not necessarily a symptom of decay of the institutions of marriage and family. Most couples who marry plan to stay married, and those who seek divorce usually also seek remarriage. The rate does reflect a departure from the prison-like life of some past marriages in which the partners remained locked together in misery by conventions of respectability or religion.

Abortion. Changing legislation and changing social attitudes toward women's rights, sexual mores, and human life are present in the United States. Many young adult women, married and unmarried and of all socioeconomic classes, are having abortions to terminate unwanted pregnancies; many other unmarried women are choosing to keep their babies. Although abortion can be the treatment of choice at times, it is no panacea and should not be considered lightly. Abortion occasionally induces physical complications such as hemorrhage or later cervical incompetency. Emotional anguish, guilt, unhappiness, or self-directed anger sometimes follows the decision to have an abortion. The mature young adult must consider the consequences of sexual activity.

As a nurse, you may experience considerable emotional turmoil unless you think through the abortion issue. Women or men seeking your counsel on this issue need to hear a professional presentation. If you feel incapable of this counsel, refer the person to someone who can counsel.

As a nurse, realize that the health state of the young adult and the type of health care sought are influenced by the person's background, knowledge, experience, philosophy, and life-style. Young adults with health problems might more readily seek care and information if they could find programs compatible with their expectations and life-styles. You can initiate programs that are specifically aimed at young adults since they seem to accept the treatment plan more readily when they understand the rationale and expected effects. Keep the previously discussed health problems and unmet physiologic needs in mind as you talk with young adults and plan and give care. Young adulthood ends in the forties when the person should have a stable position in society and the knowledge of what he or she can make out of life. Your efforts at teaching and counseling can enhance the young adult's awareness of health promotion and establish a program to make that position more stable.

Continuing Adjustments.   One couple invited others to a celebration of their twenty-fifth wedding anniversary with the following words (363):

> We continue to adjust to each other, an adjustment that started 25 years ago, and will never stop because we each continue to grow and change. We will always be different.
>
> Don't mistake it for a solid marriage. There is no such thing. Marriage is more like an airplane than a rock. You have to commit the thing to flight, and then it creaks and groans, and keeping it airborne depends entirely on attitude. Working at it, though, we can fly forever. Only the two of us know how hard it has been or how worthwhile.
>
> Celebrate with us. . . .

REFERENCES

1. Aaronson, L., Perceived and Received Support: Effects on Health Behavior During Pregnancy, *Nursing Research,* 38, no. 1 (1989), 4–9.
2. Abraham, I., and H.V. Krowchuk, Unemployment and Health: Health Promotion for the Jobless Male, *Nursing Clinics of North America,* 21, no. 1 (1986), 39–50.
3. Abramowitz, S., and N. Bell, Biofeedback, Self-Control, and Tension Headache, *Journal of Psychosomatic Research,* 29, no. 1 (1985), 95–99.
4. Abrams, D.I., Routine Care and Psychosocial Support of the Patient With Acquired Immunodeficiency Syndrome, *Medical Clinics of North America,* 70, no. 3 (1986), 707–720.
5. Aerobics for Type A's, *Health* (April 1990), 16.
6. Aguilera, D., and J. Messick, *Crisis Intervention: Theory and Methodology* (6th ed.). St. Louis: C.V. Mosby, 1989.
7. Aldrich, M.S., and J.B. Chauncey, Are Morning Headaches Part of Obstructive Sleep Apnea Syndrome? *Archives of Internal Medicine,* 150, no. 6 (1990), 1265–1267.
8. Allan, C., and D.J. Cooke, Stressful Life Events and Alcohol Misuse in Women: A Critical Review, *Journal of Studies in Alcohol,* 46, no. 2 (1985), 147–152.
9. Allen, D., and M. Wheatley, Nursing and Men's Health: Some Critical Considerations, *Nursing Clinics of North America,* 21, no. 1 (1986), 3–13.
10. Alward, R. R., and T. H. Monk, A Comparison of Rotating Shift and Permanent Night Nurses, *International Journal of Nursing Studies,* 27, no. 3 (1990), 297–302.
11. American Cancer Society. *Cancer Facts and Figures—1988.* New York: American Cancer Society, 1988.
12. American Psychiatric Association, *Diagnostic and Statistical Manual of Mental Disorders* (3rd ed.). Washington, D.C.: American Psychiatric Association, 1987.
13. Anderson, U.K., Mitral Valve Prolapse: A Diagnosis for Primary Nursing Intervention, *Journal of Cardiovascular Nursing,* I, no. 3 (1987), 41–51.
14. Anthony, H.M., Reactive Changes in the Blood of Smokers and the Development of Arterial Diseases and COPD: A Review, *Review of Environmental Health,* 8, no. 1–4 (1989), 25–86.
15. Arlin, P., Cognitive Development in Adulthood: A Fifth Stage? *Developmental Psychology,* 11, no. 5 (1975), 602–606.
16. Aronson, J.K., Chronopharmacology: Reflections on Time and a New Text, *Lancet,* 335, no. 8704 (1990), 1515–1516.
17. Bargagliotti, T., D. Lauver, and M. Angerame, Overadherence With Breast Self-Examination, *Image: Journal of Nursing Scholarship,* 23, no. 1 (1991), 63.
18. Barrick, B., Light at the End of a Decade, *American Journal of Nursing,* 90, no. 11 (1990), 37–40.
19. Barron, C., Causal Explanations and Emotional Health of Women During Divorce, *Archives of Psychiatric Nursing,* 3, no. 5 (1989), 266–271.
20. Basow, S., *Sex Role Stereotypes: Traditions and Alternatives.* Monterey, Calif: Brooks/Cole, 1980.
21. Batz, J., Casting the Sex Roles, *Universitas* (Spring 1990), 5–9.
22. Beh, H.C., and P.J. McLaughlin, Mental Performance of Air Crew Following Layovers on Transzonal Flights, *Ergonomics,* 34, no. 2 (1991), 123–136.
23. Bell, A., M. Weinberg, and S. Hammersmith, *Sexual Preference: Its Development in Men and Women.* Bloomington, Ind: Indiana University Press, 1981.
24. Bell, J.B., Stressful Life Events and Coping Methods in Mental Health and Wellness Behaviors, *Nursing Research,* 26 (1981), 236–241.
25. Bender, A.E., *Health or Hoax: The Truth About Health Foods and Diets.* Goring-on-Thames, England: Elvenden Press, 1986.
26. Benjamin, H., and C. Ihlenfeld, Transsexualism, *American Journal of Nursing,* 73, no. 3 (1973), 457–461.
27. Bennett, G., Group Therapy for Men Who Batter Women: Some Promising Developments, *Holistic Nursing Practice,* 1, no. 2 (1987), 33–42.
28. Benson, H., *Beyond the Relaxation Response.* New York: William Morrow, 1988.
29. Bernhard, L., and A. Dan, Redefining Sexuality From Women's Own Experiences, *Nursing Clinics of North America,* 21, no. 1 (1986), 125–136.
30. Bes, F., et al., The Distribution of Slow-Wave Sleep Across the Night: A Comparison for Infants, Children, and Adults, *Sleep,* 14, no. 1 (1991), 5–12.
31. Biddle, C., and T.R. Oaster, The Nature of Sleep, *AANA Journal,* 58, no. 1 (1990), 36–44.
32. Binkley, S., et al., Human Daily Rhythms Measured for One Year, *Physiological Behavior,* 48, no. 2 (1990), 293–298.
33. Black, A., Game of Life, *Elle* (January 1992), 62–63.
34. Black-White Differences in Cervical Cancer Mortality—United States, 1980–1987, *Journal of the American Medical Association,* 263, no. 22 (1990), 3001–3002.
35. Blackburn, J., The Influences of Personality, Curriculum, and Memory Correlates in Formal Reasoning in Young Adults and Elderly Persons, *Journal of Gerontology,* 39, no. 2 (1984), 207–208.
36. Borysenka, J., Ridden With Guilt, *Health* (March 1990), 78–81.

37. Boyle, C., G. Berkowitz, and J. Kelsey, Epidemiology of Premenstrual Symptoms, *American Journal of Public Health,* 77, no. 3 (1987), 349.

38. Bozett, F., *Gay and Lesbian Parents.* New York: Praeger, 1987.

39. Bradley-Springer, L., Nutritional Support in HIV Infection: A Multilevel Analysis, *Image,* 23, no. 3 (1991), 155–159.

40. Brentin, L., and A. Sieh, Caring for the Morbidly Obese, *American Journal of Nursing,* 91, no. 8 (1991), 41–43.

41. Brewer, M.J., To Sleep or Not to Sleep: The Consequences of Sleep Deprivation, *Critical Care Nurse,* 5, no. 6 (1985), 35–41.

42. Broom, B., Consensus About the Marital Relationship During Transition to Parenthood, *Nursing Research,* 33, no. 4 (1984), 223–228.

43. Brown, M., Social Support During Pregnancy: A Undimensional or Multidimensional Construct? *Nursing Research,* 35, no. 1 (1986), 4–9.

44. ——, and P. Zimmer, Personal and Family Impact of Premenstrual Symptoms, *Journal of Obstetric, Gynecologic, and Neonatal Nursing,* 15, no. 1 (1986), 31.

45. Buechler, A., Help for the Burned Out Nurse?, *Nursing Outlook,* 33, no. 4 (1985), 181–182.

46. Bullock, L., and J. McFarlane, The Birth-Weight/Battering Connection, *American Journal of Nursing,* 89, no. 9 (1989), 1153–1155.

47. ——, et al., The Prevalence and Characteristics of Battered Women in a Primary Care Setting, *Nurse Practitioner,* 14, no. 6 (1989), 47–56.

48. Cabral, H., et al., Foreign-Born and US-Born Black Women: Differences in Health Behaviors and Birth Outcomes, *American Journal of Public Health,* 80, no. 1 (1990), 70–72.

49. Campbell, A., ed., *The Opposite Sex: The Complete Illustrated Guide to Differences Between the Sexes.* New York: Salem House, 1989.

50. Campbell, J., A Survivor Group for Battered Women, *Advances in Nursing Science,* 8, no. 2 (1986), 13–20.

51. ——, and P. Alford, The Dark Consequences of Marital Rape, *American Journal of Nursing,* 89, no. 7 (1989), 846–849.

52. ——, and D.J. Sheridan, Emergency Nursing Interventions With Battered Women, *Journal of Emergency Nursing,* 15, no. 1 (1989), 12–17.

53. Cannon, B., and J. Brown, Nurses' Attitudes Toward Impaired Colleagues, *Image,* 20, no. 2 (1988), 96–101.

54. Carney, R.M., et al., Major Depression, Panic Disorder, and Mitral Valve Prolapse in Patients Who Complain of Chest Pain, *American Journal of Medicine,* 89, no. 6 (1990), 757–760.

55. Cates, W., and S. Bowen, Education for AIDS Prevention: Not Our Only Voluntary Weapon, *American Journal of Public Health,* 79, no. 7 (1989), 871–874.

56. Champion, V.L., Breast Self-Examination in Women 35 and Older: A Prospective Study, *Journal of Behavioral Medicine,* 13, no. 6 (1990), 523–538.

57. Chase, M., H. Morales, and R. Francisco, The Atonia and Myoclonia of Active (REM) Sleep, *Annual Review of Psychology,* 41 (1990), 557–584.

58. Chassin, L., et al., The Natural History of Cigarette Smoking: Predicting Young-Adult Smoking Outcomes From Adolescent Smoking Patterns, *Health Psychology,* 9, no. 6 (1990), 701–716.

59. Chronic Disease Reports: Deaths from Cervical Cancer—United States, 1984–1986, *The Journal of the American Medical Association,* 262, no. 15, (1989), 2067–2071.

60. Clapin-French, E., Sleep Patterns of Aged Persons in Long-Term Care Facilities, *Journal of Advanced Nursing,* 11, no. 57 (1986).

61. Clare, A.W., Pre-Menstrual Syndrome: Single or Multiple Causes? *Canadian Journal of Psychiatry,* 30 (1985), 474–480.

62. Clark, J.M., S. Haverty, and S. Kendall, Helping People to Stop Smoking: A Study of the Nurse's Role, *Journal of Advanced Nursing,* 15, no. 3 (1990), 357–363.

63. Clinton, J., Expectant Fathers at Risk for Couvade, *Nursing Research,* 35, no. 5 (1986), 290–294.

64. Clodore, M., et al., Psychophysiological Effects of Early Morning Bright Light Exposure in Young Adults, *Psychoneuroendocrinology,* 15, no. 3 (1990), 193–205.

65. Cohen, M., *Long Distance Parenting: A Guide for Divorced Parents.* New York: Nal-Dutten, 1989.

66. Cohn, S., Sexuality in Pregnancy: A Review of the Literature, *Nursing Clinics of North America,* 17, no. 1 (1982), 91–98.

67. Colarusso, C., and R. Nemeroff, *Adult Development.* New York: Plenum Press, 1981.

68. Coleman, E.A., and H. Pennypacker, Evaluating Breast Self-Examination Performance, *Journal of Nursing Quality Assurance,* 5, no. 3 (1991), 65–69.

69. Collier, P., Health Behaviors of Women, *Nursing Clinics of North America,* 17, no. 1 (1982), 121–126.

70. Cornell, C., Tuberculosis in Hospital Employees, *American Journal of Nursing,* 88, no. 4 (1988), 484–486.

71. Cronenwett, L., Parental Network Structure and Perceived Support After Birth of First Child, *Nursing Research,* 34, no. 6 (1985), 347–352.

72. ——, and P. Brickman, Models of Helping and Coping in Childbirth, *Nursing Research,* 32, no. 2 (1983), 84–88.

73. Csikszentmihalyi, M., *Flow: The Psychology of Optimal Experience.* New York: Harper & Row, 1990.

74. Custer, M., Stress, Life Events, and the Epidemiology of Wellness, *Journal of Community Health Nursing,* 2, no. 4 (1985), 215–222.

75. Davis, C., and M.J. Lentz, Circadian Rhythms: Charting Oral Temperatures to Spot Abnormalities, *Journal of Gerontological Nursing,* 15, no. 4 (1989), 34–41.

76. Decousus, H., et al., Circadian Dynamics of Coagulation and Chronopathology of Cardiovascular and Cerebrovascular Events. Future Therapeutic Implications for the Treatment of these Disorders? *Annual of New York Academic Science,* 618 (1991), 159–165.

77. Dirubbo, N., The Condom Barrier, *American Journal of Nursing,* 87, no. 10 (1987), 1306–1309.

78. Drake, M., et al., Spouses' Body Image Change During and After Pregnancy: A Replication in Canada, *Image,* 20, no. 2 (1988), 88–92.

79. Drew, B.J., Cardiac Rhythm Responses: Review of 22 Years of Nursing Research, Part 2, *Heart and Lung Journal of Critical Care,* 18, no. 2 (1989), 184–191.

80. Drimmer, A., If the Shoe Fits, Wear It, *St. Louis Manager* (March 1986), 24–26.

81. Duffy, M., When a Woman Heads a Household, *Nursing Outlook,* 30, no. 5 (1982), 468–473.

82. ——, C. Mowbray, and M. Hudes, Personal Goals of Recently Divorced Women, *Image,* 22, no. 1 (1990), 14–17.

83. Duldt, B., Sexual Harassment in Nursing, *Nursing Outlook,* 30, no. 6 (1982), 336–343.

84. Duvall, E., and B. Miller, *Marriage and Family Development* (6th ed.). New York: Harper & Row, 1984.

85. Dworetzky, J., and N. Davis, *Human Development: A Lifespan Approach.* St. Paul: West Publishing, 1989.

86. Eastman, C.I., Natural Summer and Winter Sunlight Exposure Patterns in Seasonal Affective Disorder, *Physiological Behavior,* 48, no. 5 (1990), 611–616.

87. ——, and K.J. Miescke, Entrainment of Circadian Rhythms with 26-h Bright Light and Sleep-wake Schedules, *American Journal of Physiology,* 259, no. 6 (1990), 1189–1197.

88. Eells, M.A., Interventions With Alcoholics and Their Families, *Nursing Clinics of North America,* 21, no. 3 (1986), 493–504.

89. Englert, D., and J. Guillon, For Want of Lactose, *American Journal of Nursing,* 86, no. 8 (1986), 902–906.

90. Erikson, E., *Childhood and Society* (2nd ed.). New York: W.W. Norton, 1963.

91. ——, ed., *Adulthood.* New York: W.W. Norton, 1978.

92. Evans, C., Reducing AIDS Anxiety on the Unit With Preventive Infection Control, *Journal of Psychosocial Nursing,* 28, no. 1 (1990), 36–39.

93. Fackelmann, K., More Cervical Cancer in Passive Smokers, *Science News,* 135, no. 11 (1989), 166.

94. Fawcett, J., and R. York, Spouses' Physical and Psychological Symptoms During Pregnancy and the Post-Partum, *Nursing Research,* 35, no. 3 (1986), 144–148.

95. ——, et al., Spouses' Body Image Changes During and After Pregnancy: A Replication and Extension, *Nursing Research,* 35, no. 4 (1986), 220–223.

96. Fedor, M.A., AIDS: Advocacy and Activism, *Nursing and Health Care,* 12, no. 4 (1991), 177.

97. Fehm, H.L., and J. Born, Evidence for Entrainment of Nocturnal Cortisol Secretion to Sleep Processes in Human Beings, *Neuroendocrinology,* 53, no. 2 (1991), 171–176.

98. Felton, G., Human Biologic Rhythms, *Annual Review of Nursing Research,* 5 (1987), 45–77.

99. Finlay, G., Sleep and Intensive Care, *Intensive Care Nursing,* 7, no. 1 (1991), 61–68.

100. Finley, B., The Role of The Psychiatric Nurse in a Community Substance Abuse Prevention Program, *Nursing Clinics of North America,* 24, no. 1 (1989), 121–136.

101. Fischman, S., et al., Changes in Sexual Relationships in Post-partum Couples, *Journal of Obstetric, Gynecologic, and Neonatal Nursing,* 15, no. 1 (1986), 58.

102. Folkard, S., D.S. Minors, and J.M. Waterhouse, "Demasking" the Temperature Rhythm After Simulated Time Zone Transitions, *Journal of Biological Rhythms,* 6, no. 1 (1991), 81–92.

103. Fontaine, K., The Conspiracy of Culture: Women's Issues in Body Size, *Nursing Clinics of North America,* 26, no. 3 (1991), 669–676.

104. Forrester, D., Myths of Masculinity: Impact Upon Men's Health, *Nursing Clinics of North America,* 21, no. 1 (1986), 15–24.

105. Fossey, E., Shiftwork Can Seriously Damage Your Health! *Professional Nurse,* 5, no. 9 (1990), 476–480.

106. Frank, D., E. Downard, and A. Lang, Androgyny, Sexual Satisfaction, and Women, *Journal of Psychosocial Nursing,* 24, no. 7 (1986), 11–15.

107. Frank, S., M. Tuer, and S. Jacobson, Psychological Predictors of Young Adults' Drinking Behaviors, *Journal of Personality and Social Psychology,* 59, no. 4 (1990), 770–780.

108. Freedman, T., Warning: Staying at Home Can Be Dangerous to Your Health, *Common Cause* (June 1982), 13–17.

109. Fremouw, W., M. dePerczel, and T. Ellis, *Suicide Risk: Assessment and Response Guidelines.* Elmsford, NY: Pergamon Press, 1990.

110. Freudenberger, H., *Burn-out: High Cost of High Achievement.* New York: Doubleday, 1980.

111. Friman, P.C., and J.W. Finney, Health Education for Testicular Cancer, *Health Education Quarterly,* 17, no. 4 (1990), 443–453.

112. Fuerst M., Free Yourself From Chronic Fatigue, *Prevention* (January 1990), 58–64.

113. Gantz, J., *Whose Child Cries: Children of Gay Parents Talk About Their Lives.* Rolling Hills Estates, Calif: View Press, 1983.

114. Garrison, J., Part 7: Gay in America, A Special Report: Creating New Families, *San Francisco Examiner,* June 12, 1989, Sec. A, p. 17.

115. Garrity, T., et al., The Association Between Type A Behavior and Change in Coronary Risk Factors Among Young Adults, *American Journal of Public Health,* 80, no. 11 (1990), 1354–1357.

116. Gillin, J., and W. Byerley, Medical Intelligence—Drug Therapy: The Diagnosis and Management of Insomnia, *New England Journal of Medicine,* 322, no. 4 (1990), 239–248.

117. Gillooly, P.B., et al., Circadian Variation in Human Performance Evaluated by the Walter Reed Performance Assessment Battery, *Chronobiology International,* 7, no. 2 (1990), 143–153.

118. Glantz, S.A., and W.W. Parmley, Passive Smoking and Heart Disease: Epidemiology, Physiology, and Biochemistry, *Circulation,* 83, no. 1 (1991), 1–12.

119. Glass, L., *From Clocks to Chaos: The Rhythms of Life.* Princeton, NJ: Princeton University Press, 1988.

120. Glasser, M., Males' Use of Public Health Department Family Planning Services, *American Journal of Public Health,* 80, no. 5 (1990), 611–612.

121. Glenn, B.L., and L.A. Moore, Relationship of Self-Concept, Health Locus of Control, and Perceived Cancer Treatment Options to the Practice of Breast Self-Examination, *Cancer Nursing,* 13, no. 6 (1990), 361–365.

122. Glynn, T., et al., Essential Elements of Self-Help/Minimal Intervention Strategies for Smoking Cessation, *Health Education Quarterly,* 17, no. 3 (1990), 329–345.

123. Goldstein, I.B., and D. Shapiro, The Beat-to-Beat Blood Pressure Response to Postural Change in Young and Elderly Healthy Adult Males, *Journal of Behavioral Medicine,* 13, no. 5 (1990), 437–448.

124. Goleman, D., Death of a Sex Drive, *Health* (June 1991), 53–57.

125. Gould, R., Adult Life Stages: Growth Toward Self-Tolerance, *Psychology Today*, 8, no. 7 (February 1975), 74–78.

126. GPA Prepares Ground for Vaccine Trials, *Global AIDS News*, Preliminary Issue (1991), 1–2.

127. Gray, M.E., Factors Related to Practice of Breast Self-Examination in Rural Women, *Cancer Nursing*, 13, no. 2 (1990), 100–107.

128. Green, P., The Chemically Dependent Nurse, *Nursing Clinics of North America*, 24, no. 1 (1989), 81–94.

129. Greenfield, M., Disclosing Incest: The Relationships That Make It Possible, *Journal of Psychosocial Nursing*, 28, no. 7 (1990), 20–23.

130. Gruen, S.M. et al., Setting Up a School-Based Sexual Education Program to Help Prevent AIDS and Other Sexually Transmitted Diseases, *Nurse Practitioner*, 16, no. 8 (1991), 47–51.

131. Haber, J., A Family Systems Model for Divorce and the Loss of Self, *Archives of Psychiatric Nursing*, 4, no. 4 (1991), 228–234.

132. Hahn, W.K., J.A. Brooks, and R. Hite, Blood Pressure Norms for *Healthy Young Adults:* Relation to Sex, Age, and Reported Parental Hypertension, *Research in Nursing and Health*, 12, no. 1 (1989), 53–56.

133. Hale, E., The Controversial Pap Test, *FDA Consumer*, 23, no. 7 (1989), 20–23.

134. Hansen, S., Single Custodial Fathers and the Parent-Child Relationship, *Nursing Research* 30, no. 4 (1981), 202–204.

135. Hanson, S., and F. Bozett, eds., *Dimensions of Fatherhood*. Beverly Hills, Calif: Sage Publications, 1985.

136. Harlan, L., A. Berstein, and L. Kessler, Cervical Cancer Screening: Who Is Not Screened and Why? *American Journal of Public Health*, 81, no. 7 (1991), 885–890.

137. Harma, M., et al., The Relation of Age to the Adjustment of the Circadian Rhythms of Oral Temperature and Sleepiness to Shift Work, *Chronobiology International*, 7, no. 3 (1990), 227–233.

138. Hart, L., M. Freel, and F. Milde, Fatigue, *Nursing Clinics of North America*, 25, no. 4 (1990), 967–976.

139. Hatton, C., and S. Valente, *Suicide: Assessment and Intervention*. Norwalk, Conn: Appleton-Century-Crofts, 1984.

140. Haus, E., et al., Circadian Variations in Blood Coagulation Parameters, Alpha-antitrypsin Antigen and Platelet Aggregation and Retention in Clinically Healthy Subjects, *Chronobiology International*, 7, no. 3 (1990), 203–216.

141. Having It All, *Elle* (January 1992), 42–47.

142. Hegarty, V., *Decisions in Nutrition*. St. Louis: Times Mirror/Mosby College Publishing, 1988.

143. Heinrick, K., Effective Responses to Sexual Harassment, *Nursing Outlook*, 35, no. 2 (1987), 70–72.

144. Heitkemper, M., et al., GI Symptoms, Function, and Psychophysiological Arousal in Dysmenorrheic Women, *Nursing Research* 40, no. 1 (1991), 20–28.

145. Helton, A., Battering During Pregnancy, *American Journal of Nursing*, 86, no. 8 (1986), 910–913.

146. Helton, A., et al., Battered and Pregnant: A Prevalence Study, *American Journal of Public Health*, 77, no. 10 (1987), 1337–1339.

147. Helton, A.M., and F.G. Snodgrass, Battering During Pregnancy: Intervention Strategies, *Birth*, 14, no. 3 (1987), 142–147.

148. Henley, E.C., and S. Bohl, Nutrition Across the Woman's Life Cycle, *Nursing Clinics of North America* 12, no. 1 (1982), 99–110.

149. Herman, J.M., and V.K. Sonntag, Diving Accidents: Mechanism of Injury and Treatment of the Patient, *Critical Care Nursing Clinics of North America*, 3, no. 2 (1991), 331–337.

150. Hetherington, S., Children of Alcoholics: An Emerging Issue, *Archives of Psychiatric Nursing*, 1, no. 4 (1988), 251–255.

151. Hewlett, S., *A Lesser Life: The Myth of Women's Liberation*. New York: Warner Books, 1987.

152. Hill, I., ed., *The Bisexual Spouse*. McLean, VA: Barlina Books, 1988.

153. Hoff, L., *Battered Women As Survivors*. New York: Routledge, 1990.

154. ———, *People in Crisis: Understanding and Helping* (3rd ed.). Redwood City, Calif: Addison-Wesley, 1989.

155. Hogan, R., *Human Sexuality: A Nursing Perspective* (2nd ed.). Norwalk, Conn: Appleton-Century-Crofts, 1985.

156. Homer, C., S. James, and E. Siegel, Work Related Psychosocial Stress and Risk of Preterm, Low Birthweight Delivery, *American Journal of Public Health*, 80, no.2 (1990), 173–177.

157. Hongladorom, G., and M. Russell, An Ethnic Difference— Lactose Intolerance, *Nursing Outlook*, 24, no. 12 (1976), 764-765.

158. Hooks, S.R., The Role of Health Education in Prevention of Breast Cancer, *Health Education*, 21, no. 5 (1990), 33–40.

159. Hoole, A., R. Greenberg, and C. G. Pickard, *Patient Care Guidelines for Nurse Practitioners* (3rd ed.). Boston: Little, Brown, 1988.

160. Horn, B., Cultural Concepts and Postpartal Care, *Journal of Transcultural Nursing*, 2, no. 1 (1990), 48–51.

161. Humble, C., et al., Passive Smoking and 20-Year Cardiovascular Disease Mortality Among Nonsmoking Wives, Evans County Georgia, *American Journal of Public Health*, 80, no. 5 (1990), 599–601.

162. Hyman, R.B., and P. Woag, Stressful Life Events and Illness Onset: A Review of Crucial Variables, *Research in Nursing and Health*, 5 (1982), 155–163.

163. Isay, R., *Being Homosexual: Gay Men and Their Development*. New York: Farrar, Strauss, Giroux, 1990.

164. Jensen, B.K., Menstrual Cycle Effects on Task Performance Examined in the Context of Stress Research, *Acta Psychologica*, 50, (1981), 159–178.

165. John, E.M., D.A. Savitz, and D.P. Sandler, Prenatal Exposure to Parents' Smoking and Childhood Cancer, *American Journal of Epidemiology*, 133, no. 2 (1991), 123–132.

166. Johnson, E., and G. Johnson, Premature Developmental Jumps: The Effects of Early Intimacy on the Adult Lives of Identical Twins, *Perspectives in Psychiatric Care*, 20, no. 2 (1982), 87–90.

167. Jones, G., Biological Clocks: Testing Our Internal Timing, *Science: The Teacher*, 58, no. 3 (1991), 16–20.

168. Jordan, P., Laboring for Relevance: Expectant and New Fatherhood, *Nursing Research*, 39, no. 1 (1990), 11–16.

169. Jung, C., Psychological Types. In Adler, G., et al., eds., *Collected Works of Carl G. Jung, Vol 6. Princeton, NJ: Princeton University Press, 1971.*

170. Kahn, H., D. Williamson, and J. Stevens, Race and Weight Change in US Women: The Roles of Socioeconomic and Marital Status, *American Journal of Public Health,* 81, no. 3 (1991), 319–323.

171. Kaplan, H., Substance Abuse Patterns and Their Relationships to Family Attitudes and Values, *Health Values,* 11, no. 2 (1987), 40–46.

172. Keller, K.B., and L. Lemberg, Myocardial Infarction in the Young Adult, *Heart and Lung: Journal of Critical Care,* 20, no. 1 (1991), 95–97.

173. Kennedy-Caldwell, C., and M. Hansen, Metabolism of Vitamins and Trace Minerals, *Nursing Clinics of North America,* 18, no. 1 (1983), 29–45.

174. Keye, W., Premenstrual Syndrome, *Postgraduate Medicine,* 83, (1988), 167–173.

175. Kinch, R.A., and E.G. Robinson, Symposium: Premenstrual Syndrome—Current Knowledge and New Directions, *Canadian Journal of Psychiatry,* 30, no. 7 (1985), 467–468.

176. King, M.C. and J. Ryan, Abused Women: Dispelling Myths and Encouraging Interventions, *Nurse Practitioner,* 14, no. 5 (1989), 47–58.

177. Kohlberg, L., *Recent Research in Moral Development.* New York: Holt, Rinehart & Winston, 1971.

178. Korniewicz, D.M., M. O'Brien, E. Larson, Coping with AIDS and HIV: Psychosocial Adaptation, *Journal of Psychosocial Nursing,* 28, no. 3 (1990), 14–21.

179. Kostreva, M., and P. Genevier, Nurse Preferences Vs. Circadian Rhythms in Scheduling, *Nursing Management,* 20, no. 7 (1989), 50–51, 54, 56, 58, 60, 62.

180. Kramer, J., *Family Interfaces: Transgenerational Patterns.* New York: Brunner/Mazel, 1985.

181. Kramer, M., *Reality Shock: Why Nurses Leave Nursing.* St. Louis: C.V. Mosby, 1974.

182. ——, and C. Schmalenberg, Bicultural Training and New Graduate Role Transformation: Part I. *Nursing Digest,* 5 (Winter 1978), 1–47.

183. Kreidler, M., and R. Carbon, Breaking the Incest Cycle: The Group as a Surrogate Family, *Journal of Psychosocial Nursing,* 29, no. 4 (1991), 28–32.

184. Kreps, J., Stop Calling Them Women's Issues, *Graduate Women,* 75, no. 6 (1981), 36.

185. Kryger, M.H., R. Roth, and W.B. Dement, *Principles and Practice of Sleep Medicine.* Philadelphia: W.B. Saunders, 1989.

186. Kuhn, L., The Aftermath of Childhood Incest and Sexual Abuse, *Res Medica,* 3, no. 2 (1986), 15–18.

187. Kutner, L., *Parent and Child: Getting Through to Each Other.* New York: William Morrow, 1991.

188. LaDou, J., Rhythmic Variations in Medical Monitoring Tests, *Occupational Medicine,* 5, no. 3 (1990), 479–489.

189. Laffrey, S., Normal and Underweight Adults: Perceived Weight and Health Behavior Characteristics, *Nursing Research,* 35, no. 3 (1988), 173–177.

190. Lancaster, J., Coping Mechanisms for the Working Mother, *American Journal of Nursing,* 75, no. 8 (August 1975), 1322–1323.

191. Layde, P., Smoking and Cervican Cancer: Cause or Coincidence? *Journal of the American Medical Association,* 261, no. 11 (1989), 1631–1632.

192. Lefevre, J., et al., Motor Performance During Adolescence and Age Thirty as Related to Age at Peak Height Velocity, *Annual of Human Biology,* 17, no. 5 (1990), 423–435.

193. Lehmann, A., DES: A Living Legacy—What Can Nurse Do About It? *Canadian Nursing,* 79 (December 1983), 34.

194. Lehne, R., et al., *Pharmacology for Nursing Care.* Philadelphia: W.B. Saunders, 1990.

195. Lerner, R., and J. Jovanovic, The Role of Body Image in Psychosocial Development Across the Life Span. In Cash, T., and T. Pruzinsky, eds., *Body Images: Development, Deviance, and Change.* New York: Guilford Press, 1990.

196. Leslie, L., Changing Factors and Changing Needs in Women's Health Care, *Nursing Clinics of North America,* 21, no. 1 (1986), 111–123.

197. Levinson, D., *The Seasons of a Man's Life.* New York: Ballantine Books, 1978.

198. ——, et al., Periods in the Adult Development of Men: Ages 18 to 45, *Counseling Psychologist,* 6, no. 1 (1976), 21–25.

199. Licopantio, E., Shift Work in Nursing and Circadian Rhythms, *Imprint,* 36, no. 2 (1989), 161, 163, 165.

200. Lidz, T., *The Person: His and Her Development Throughout the Life Cycle* (2nd ed.). New York: Basic Books, 1983.

201. Limandri, B., The Therapeutic Relationship with Abused Women: Nurses' Responses That Facilitate or Inhibit Change, *Journal of Psychosocial Nursing,* 25, no. 2 (1987), 9–16.

202. Lone, P., A Place to Call Home, *American Journal of Nursing,* 89, no. 4 (1989), 490–491.

203. Loucks, A., Chlamydia: An Unheralded Epidemic, *American Journal of Nursing,* 87, no. 7 (1987), 920–922.

204. Love, C., and H. Seaton, Eating Disorders, *Nursing Clinics of North America,* 26, no. 3 (1991), 677–697.

205. Lynn, D., *The Father: His Role in Child Development.* Monterey, Calif: Brooks Cole, 1974.

206. Maas, H., and J. Kuyper, *From Thirty to Seventy.* San Francisco: Jossey-Bass, 1974.

207. Majewski, J., Conflicts, Satisfactions, and Attitudes During Transition to the Maternal Role, *Nursing Research* 35, no. 1 (1986), 10–14.

208. Marchand-Jodoin, L., and J. Samson, Kohlberg's Theory Applied to the Moral and Sexual Development of Adults, *Journal of Moral Education,* 11, no. 4 (October 1982), 247–258.

209. Marmor, J., ed., *Homosexual Behavior: A Modern Reappraisal.* New York: Basic Books, 1980.

210. Mason, J., and M. McGinnis, "Health People 2000": An Overview of the National Health Promotion and Disease Prevention Objectives, *Public Health Reports,* 105, no. 5 (1990), 441–446.

211. Masters, W., and V. Johnson, *The Human Sexual Response.* New York: Bantam, 1981.

212. ——, *Homosexuality in Perspective.* Boston: Little, Brown, 1979.

213. Maugh, T., Fighting the Plague: 27 New Drugs to Stop a Killer, *American Health* (June 1987), 73 ff.

214. May, K., Three Phases of Father Involvement in Pregnancy, *Nursing Research,* 31, no. 8 (1982), 337–342.

215. May, R.R., Mood Shifts and the Menstrual Cycle, *Journal of Psychosomatic Research,* 20 (1985), 125–130.

216. McArthur, M., Reality Therapy With Rape Victims, *Archives of Psychiatric Nursing,* 4, no. 6 (1990), 360–365.

217. McBride, A., Mental Health Effects of Women's Multiple Roles, *Image,* 20, no. 1 (1988), 41–47.

218. McBride, L., Mistaking Religion for Spirituality, *Pastoral Forum,* 9, no. 1 (1990), 10–11.

219. McCloskey, J., Two Requirements for Job Contentment, *Image,* 22, no. 3 (1990), 140–143.

220. McCollum, E., Talking Man to Man, *New Choices* (June 1991), 87.

221. McCoy, V., Adult Life Cycle Tasks/Adult Continuing Education Program Response, *Lifelong Learning in the Adult Years* (October 1977), 16.

222. McKool, K., Facilitating Smoking Cessation, *Journal of Cardiovascular Nursing,* 1, no. 4 (1987), 28–40.

223. McNeil, B.J., et al., Sleep Questionnaire, *American Journal of Nursing,* 86, no. 1 (1986), 261.

224. Mead, G.H., *Mind, Self, and Society.* Chicago: University of Chicago Press, 1962.

225. Mead, M., *Sex and Temperament in Three Primitive Societies.* New York: William Morrow, 1935.

226. Medved, D., *The Case Against Divorce.* Atlanta: Ivy Books, 1990.

227. Meisenhelder, J., Self-Esteem in Women: The Influence of Employment and Perceptions of Husband's Appraisals, *Image,* 18, no. 1 (1986), 8–13.

228. Meissner, J., A Simple Guide for Assessing Oral Health, *Nursing '80,* 10, no. 4 (1980), 84–85.

229. Mendolson, W.B., *Human Sleep: Research and Clinical Care.* New York: Plenum Medical, 1987.

230. Menning, B., The Psychosocial Impact of Infertility, *Nursing Clinics of North America,* 17, no. 1 (1982), 155–163.

231. Mercer, R., The Process of Maternal Role Attachment Over the First Year, *Nursing Research* 34, no. 4 (1985), 198–203.

232. ———, and S. Ferketich, Predictors of Family Functioning Eight Months Following Birth, *Nursing Research,* 39, no. 2 (1990), 76–81.

233. Miller, G.H., The Impact of Passive Smoking: Cancer Deaths among Nonsmoking Women, *Cancer Detection Previews,* 14, no. 5 (1990), 497–503.

234. Miller, K., Body Image Therapy, *Nursing Clinics of North America,* 26, no. 3 (1991), 727–736.

235. Miller, K., Compulsive Overeating, *Nursing Clinics of North America,* 26, no. 3 (1991), 699–705.

236. Mommy Vs. Mommy, *Newsweek* (June 4, 1990), 84–87.

237. Monier, M., and M. Laird, Contraceptives: A Look at the Future, *American Journal of Nursing,* 89, no. 4 (1989), 497–498.

238. Moshman, D., J. Glover, and R. Bruning, *Developmental Psychology.* Boston: Little, Brown, 1987.

239. Murray, R., Self-Concept. In Potter, P., and A. Perry, eds., *Fundamentals of Nursing: Concepts, Process, and Practice* (2nd ed.). St. Louis: C.V. Mosby, 1989, 722–747.

240. ———, and M.M. Huelskoetter, *Psychiatric/Mental Health Nursing: Giving Emotional Care* (3rd ed.). Norwalk, Conn: Appleton & Lange, 1991.

241. Myers, I., and M. McCaulley, *Manual: A Guide to the Development and Use of the Myers-Briggs Type Indicator.* Palo Alto, Calif: Consulting Psychologists Press, 1985.

242. Nadis, S., Rhythm and Blues, *Technology Review,* 94, no. 1 (1991), 22–25.

243. Naegele, M., Drug and Alcohol Abuse in Nursing: An Occupational Hazard, *Nursing Life* (January-February 1988), 42–54.

244. National Academy of Sciences, *Recommended Daily Allowances* (10th ed.). Washington, DC: The Academy, 1989.

245. Neef, N., et al., Testicular Self-Examination by Young Men: An Analysis of Characteristics Associated With Practice, *Journal of American College Health,* 39, no. 4 (1991), 187–190.

246. Nikstaitis, G., Therapy for Men Who Batter, *Journal of Psychosocial Nursing,* 23, no. 7 (1985), 33–36.

247. Norbeck, J., and N. Anderson, Psychosocial Predictors of Pregnancy Outcomes in Low Income Black, Hispanic, and White Women, *Nursing Research,* 38, no. 4 (1989), 204–209.

248. Norris, A., Cognitive Analysis of Contraceptive Behavior, *Image,* 20, no. 3 (1988), 135–139.

249. Nuttall, S.E., L.J. Greaves, and B. Lent, Wife Battering: An Emerging Problem in Public Health, *Canadian Journal of Public Health,* 76, no. 10 (1985), 297–299.

250. O'Brien, M.E., Reaching the Migrant Worker, *American Journal of Nursing,* 83, no. 6 (1983), 895–897.

251. O'Donnell, T.G., and S.L. Bernicer, Parents as Caregivers: AIDS, *Journal of Psychosocial Nursing,* 28, no. 6 (1990), 14–17.

252. Oelbaum, C., Hallmarks of Adult Wellness, *American Journal of Nursing,* 74, no. 9 (September 1974), 1623–1625.

253. Ossler, C., Men's Work Environments and Health Risks, *Nursing Clinics of North America,* 21, no. 1 (1986), 25–36.

254. Painter, D., The Black Woman in American History, In Lussier, V., and J. Walstedt, eds., *Women's Lives: Perspectives in Progress and Change,* Boston: Little, Brown, 1979.

255. Panel Recommends Hepatitis B Vaccine for Health Workers, Some Heterosexuals, *Nation's Health* (July 1985), 12.

256. Parish, J.M., and J.W. Shepard, Cardiovascular Effects of Sleep Disorders, *Chest: The Cardiopulmonary Journal,* 97, no. 5 (1990), 1220–1226.

257. Payne, D., et al., Effectiveness of Milk Products in Dietary Management of Lactose Malabsorption, *American Journal of Clinical Nutrition,* 34 (1981), 2711–2715.

258. Pender, N., *Health Promotion in Nursing Practice* (2nd ed.). Norwalk, Conn: Appleton & Lange, 1987.

259. Phipps, W., et al., eds., *Medical-Surgical Nursing: Concepts and Clinical Practice* (4th ed.). St. Louis: Mosby–Year Book, 1991.

260. Pines, A., and E. Aronson, *Burn-out: From Tedium to Personal Growth.* New York: Macmillan, 1981.

261. Pinnell, N., and M. deMeneses, *Nursing Process: Theory, Application, and Related Processes.* Norwalk, Conn: Appleton-Century-Crofts, 1986.

262. Potter, P., and A. Perry, *Fundamentals of Nursing: Concepts, Process, and Practice* (2nd ed.). St. Louis: C.V. Mosby, 1989.

263. Pruzinsky, T., and T. Cash, Integrative Themes in Body Image Development, Deviance, and Change. In Cash, T., and T. Pruzinksy, eds., *Body Images: Development, Deviance, and Change*. New York: Guilford Press, 1990.

264. Reilly, T., Human Circadian Rhythms and Exercise, *Critical Review of Biomedical Engineering*, 18, no. 3 (1990), 165–180.

265. Reynolds, C.F., et al., Sleep, Gender, and Depression: An Analysis of Gender Effects on the Electroencephalographic Sleep of 302 Depressed Outpatients, *Biologic Psychiatry*, 28, no. 8 (1990), 673–684.

266. Rich, V., and A. Rich, Personality, Hardiness and Burnout in Female Staff Nurses, *Image*, 19, no. 2 (1987), 63–66.

267. Richard, E., and A. Shepard, Giving Up Smoking: A Lesson in Loss Therapy, *American Journal of Nursing*, 81, no. 4 (1981), 755–757.

268. Riley, E., Eating Disorders as Addictive Behavior, *Nursing Clinics of North America*, 26, no. 3 (1991), 715–726.

269. Rising, S., The Fourth Stage of Labor: Family Reintegration, *American Journal of Nursing*, 74, no. 5 (1974), 870.

270. Roberts, A., *Battered Women and Their Families: Intervention Strategies and Treatment Programs*. New York: Springer, 1984.

271. Robinson, L., Stress and Anxiety, *Nursing Clinics of North America*, 25, no. 4 (1990), 935–944.

272. Rosenthal, K., and H. Keshet. *Fathers Without Partners*, Totowa, NJ: Rowman & Littlefield, 1981.

273. Rosenthal, N.E., et al., Phase-Shifting Effects of Bright Morning Light as Treatment for Delayed Sleep Phase Syndrome, *Sleep*, 13, no. 4 (1990), 354–361.

274. Ross, M.S., et al., When Sleep Won't Come: Helping Our Elderly Clients, *Canadian Nurse*, 82, no. 14 (1986).

275. Rossignol, A., Caffeine-Containing Beverages and Premenstrual Syndrome in Young Women, *American Journal of Public Health*, 75, no. 11 (1985), 1335–1337.

276. Rossignol, A., et al., Tea and Premenstrual Syndrome in the People's Republic of China, *American Journal of Public Health*, 79, no. 1 (1989), 67–69.

277. Rubin, R., Maternal Tasks in Pregnancy, *Maternal-Child Nursing Journal*, 4, no. 3 (Fall 1975), 143–153.

278. Ryan, J., C. Zwerling, and E. Orav, Occupational Risks Associated With Cigarette Smoking: A Prospective Study, *American Journal of Public Health*, 82, no. 1 (1992), 29–32.

279. Samet, J.M., New Effects of Active and Passive Smoking on Reproduction? *American Journal of Epidemiology*, 133, no. 4 (1991), 348–350.

280. Samples, J.F., et al., Using Nursing Research. Circadian Rhythms: Basis for Screening for Fever. New York: UNLN Publication, No. 15–2232 (1989), 92–96.

281. Sandelowski, M., The Color Gray: Ambiguity and Infertility, *Image*, 19, no. 2 (1987), 70–74.

282. ——, and D. Holditch-Davis, Mazing: Infertile Couples and the Quest for a Child, *Image*, 21, no. 4 (1989), 220–226.

283. Scandrett, S.L., et al., A Comparative Study of Biofeedback and Progressive Relaxation in Anxious Patients, *Issues in Mental Health Nursing*, 8, no. 3 (1986), 255–271.

284. Scavnicky-Mylant, M., The Process of Coping Among Young Adult Children of Alcoholics, *Issues in Mental Health Nursing*, 11, no. 2 (1990), 125–139.

285. Scherer, P., How AIDS Attacks the Brain, *American Journal of Nursing*, 90, no. 1 (1990), 41–52.

286. Scherer, P., How HIV Attacks the Peripheral Nervous System, *American Journal of Nursing*, 9, no. 5 (1990), 66–70.

287. Schmalenburg, C., and M. Kramer, *Coping With Reality Shock: Voices of Experience*. Wakefield, Mass: Nursing Resources, 1979.

288. Schulmeister, L., Join the Fight Against Oral Cancer, *Nursing '87*, 17, no. 5 (1987), 66–67.

289. Schweiger, J., J. Lang, and J. Schweiger, Oral Assessment: How To Do It, *American Journal of Nursing*, 80, no. 4 (1980), 654–657.

290. Sciacca, J., et al., Body Mass Index and Perceived Weight Status in Young Adults, *Journal of Community Health*, 16, no. 3 (1991), 159–168.

291. Screening for Breast Cancer . . . U.S. Preventive Services Task Force Guidelines, *Journal of the American Academy of Physician Assistants*, 3, no. 8 (1990), 624–628.

292. Seidell, J., et al., The Relation Between Overweight and Subjective Health According to Age, Social Class, Slimming Behavior, and Smoking Habits in Dutch Adults, *American Journal of Public Health*, 76, no. 12. (1986), 1410–1415.

293. Sekaran, U., *Dual Career Families: Contemporary Organizational and Counseling Issues*. San Francisco, Calif: Jossey-Bass, 1986.

294. Shaw, E., Female Circumcision, *American Journal of Nursing*, 83, no. 6 (1983), 684–687.

295. Sheehy, G, *Passages: Predictable Crises of Adult Life*. New York: Bantam Books, 1976.

296. ——, Introducing the Postponing Generation: The Truth About Today's Young Men, *Esquire Magazine* (October 1979), 264–272.

297. Shepperd, S.L., et al., Determinants of Breast Self- Examination Among Women of Lower Income and Lower Education, *Journal of Behavioral Medicine*, 13, no. 4 (1990), 359–371.

298. Sherwen, L., M. Scoloreno, and C. Weingartern, *Nursing Care of the Childbearing Family*. Norwalk, Conn: Appleton-Lange, 1991.

299. Shopland, D., S. Niemcryk, and K. Marconi, Geographic and Gender Variations in Tobacco Use, *American Journal of Public Health*, 82, no. 1 (1992), 103–106.

300. Seigel, J., Premenstrual Syndrome: Psychiatric, Psychological, and Psychosocial Perspectives, *Health and Social Work*, 3, (1987), 284–288.

301. Siegelman, M., Parental Backgrounds of Homosexual and Heterosexual Men: A Cross-National Replication, *Archives of Sexual Behavior*, 10 (1981), 505–573.

302. Sievers, M., and J. Fisher, Cancer in North American Indians, *American Journal of Public Health*, 73, no. 5 (1983), 485–486.

303. Single Mothers' Perceptions of the Newborns, *American Journal of Nursing*, 85, no. 12 (1985), 1397.

304. Skipper, J.K., F.D. Jung, and L.C. Coffey, Nurses and Shiftwork: Effects on Physical Health and Mental Depression, *Journal of Advanced Nursing*, 15, no. 7 (1990), 835-842.

305. Smeltzer, S., and B. Whipple, Women and HIV Infection, *Image*, 23, no. 4 (1991), 249–256.

306. Smith, C., C. Reilly, and K. Midkiff, Evaluation of Three

Circadian Rhythms Questionnaires With Suggestions for an Improved Measure of Morningness, *Journal of Applied Psychology,* 74, no. 5 (1989), 728–738.

307. Smith, J., J. Mercy, and J. Conn, Marital Status and the Risk of Suicide, *American Journal of Public Health,* 78, no. 1 (1988), 78–80.

308. Smith, S., Big Families Can Be Happy, Too, *Newsweek* (January 14, 1985), 12–13.

309. Sonkin, D., D. Martin, and L. Walker, *The Male Batterer: A Treatment Approach.* New York: Springer, 1985.

310. A Special Needs Child Affects Marriage, *Home Life,* 46, no. 2 (1991), 44–45.

311. Spencer, M.B., et al., Circadian Rhythmicity and Sleep of Aircrew During Polar Schedules, *Aviation and Space Environment Medicine,* 62, no. 1 (1991), 3–13.

312. Stefanik-Campisi, C., and T. Marion, Case Management and Follow-up of a Chemically Impaired Nurse, *Perspectives in Psychiatric Care,* 23, nos. 3–4, (1987/1988), 114–119.

313. Stein, T., Homosexuality and New Family Forms: Issues in Psychotherapy, *Psychiatric Annals,* 19, no. 1 (1988), 12–20.

314. Stevens, P., and J. Hall, Stigma, Health Beliefs, and Experiences With Health Care in Lesbian Women, *Image,* 20, no. 2 (1988), 69–73.

315. Stinnett, N., and J. DeFrain, *Secrets of Strong Families.* New York: Berkley Books, 1985.

316. Strickland, O., The Occurrence of Symptoms in Expectant Fathers, *Nursing Research,* 36, no. 3 (1987), 184–189.

317. Strickland, S., Critical Health Issues in the Workplace . . . Alcohol and Substance Abuse, *American Association of Occupational Health Nursing,* 34, no. 9 (1986), 443–444.

318. Subar, A.F., L.C. Harlan, and M.E. Mattson, Food and Nutrient Intake Differences Between Smokers and Non-Smokers in the US, *American Journal of Public Health,* 80, no. 11 (1990), 1323–1329.

319. Sullivan, E., A Descriptive Study of Nurses Recovering From Chemical Addiction, *Archives of Psychiatric Nursing,* 1, no. 3 (1987), 194–200.

320. Sullivan, H.S., *The Interpersonal Theory of Psychiatry,* New York: W.W. Norton, 1953.

321. Sykes, J.A., P. Kelly, and J.A. Kennedy, Jr., Black Skin Problems, *American Journal of Nursing,* 79, no. 6 (1979), 1092–1094.

322. Testu, F., Diurnal Variations of Performance and Information Processing, *Chronobiologia,* 13, no. 4 (1986), 319–326.

323. Tips for Joggers, *Health Scenes* (Fall 1987), 12.

324. Thomas, S., and R. Williams, Perceived Stress, Trait Anger, Modes of Anger Expression, and Health Status of College Men and Women, *Nursing Research* 40, no. 5 (1991), 303–307.

325. Tomlinson, P., Spousal Differences in Marital Satisfaction During Transition to Parenthood, *Nursing Research,* 36, no. 4 (1987), 239–242.

326. Trinkoff, A., W. Eaton, and J. Anthony, The Prevalence of Substance Abuse Among Registered Nurses, *Nursing Research,* 40, no. 3 (1991), 172–175.

327. Trudeau, M., Dark Nights and Bright Mornings: Caring for a Person with AIDS, *Journal of Psychosocial Nursing,* 29, no. 1 (1991), 32–33.

328. Tucker, L., and M. Bagwell, Television Viewing and Obesity in Adult Females, *American Journal of Public Health,* 81, no. 7 (1991), 908–911.

329. Tucker, L., and G. Friedman, Television Viewing and Obesity in Adult Males, *American Journal of Public Health,* 79, no. 4 (1989), 516–518.

330. Urdung, L., ed., *Mosby's Medical and Nursing Dictionary.* St. Louis: C.V. Mosby, 1983.

331. U.S. Bureau of the Census, *Statistical Abstract of the United States: 1989.* Washington, DC: U.S. Government Printing Office, 1989.

332. U.S. Department of Health and Human Services, *Smoking and Health: A National Status Report.* Bethesda, Md: National Cancer Institute, 1987.

333. Vaillant, G., How the Best and the Brightest Came of Age, *Psychology Today,* 11, no. 9 (1977), 34ff.

334. ———, The Normal Boy in Later Life: How Adaptation Fosters Growth, *Harvard Magazine,* 55, no. 6 (1977), 234–239.

335. Van Cauter, E., and F. Turek, Strategies for Resetting the Human Circadian Clock, *New England Journal of Medicine,* 322, no. 18 (1990), 1306–1308.

336. Van Den Akker, O., and A. Steptoe, Psychophysiological Responses in Women Reporting Severe Premenstrual Symptoms, *Psychosomatic Medicine,* 51 (1989), 319–328.

337. Vegega, M.E., and T.M. Klein, Alcohol Related Traffic Fatalities Among Adolescents and Young Adults— United States, 1982–1989, *Journal American Medical Association,* 265, no. 15 (1991), 1930.

338. Ventura, J., Parent Coping, A Replication, *Nursing Research,* 35, no. 2 (1986), 77–80.

339. Ventura, S., First Births to Older Mothers, 1970–86, *American Journal of Public Health,* 79, no. 12 (1989), 1675–1677.

340. Von-Roemeling, R., The Therapeutic Index of Cytotoxic Chemotherapy Depends Upon Circadian Drug Timing, *Annual of New York Academic Science,* 618 (1991), 292–311.

341. Wadsworth, B., *Piaget's Theory of Cognitive and Affective Development* (4th ed.). New York: Longman, 1989.

342. Walker, L., H. Cran, and E. Thompson, Maternal Role Attainment and Identity in the Postpartum Period: Stability and Change, *Nursing Research* 35, no. 2 (1986), 68–71.

343. Wallerstein, J., and S. Blakeslee, *Second Chances: Men, Women and Children a Decade After Divorce—Who Wins, Who Loses, and Why.* New York: Picknor & Fields, 1990.

344. Webb, P., Piaget: Implications for Teaching, *Theory Into Practice,* 19, no. 2 (1980), 93–97.

345. Webb, W., A Further Analysis of Age and Sleep Deprivation Effects, *Psychophysiology,* 22, no. 2 (1985), 156–161.

346. Webster, D., Changing Definitions, Changing Times, *Nursing Clinics of North America,* 21, no. 1 (1986), 87–97.

347. ———, and G. Ipema, Women and Mental Health: A Model for Practice, *Nursing Clinics of North America,* 21, no. 1 (1986), 127–150.

348. Weingourt, R., Wife Rape in a Sample of Psychiatric Patients, *Image,* 22, no. 3 (1990), 144–147.

349. When Childbearing Is Postponed, *Medical Aspects of Human Sexuality,* 19, no. 8 (1986), 108–110.

350. WHO Predicts Up to 30 Million World AIDS Cases by Year 2000, *Nation's Health* (January 1991), 1.

351. Williams, A., Women at Risk: An AIDS Educational Needs Assessment, *Image,* 23, no. 4 (1991), 208–213.

352. Williams, S., *Nutrition and Diet Therapy* (6th ed.). St. Louis: Times Mirror/Mosby, 1989.

353. ——, Nutritional Guidance in Prenatal Care. In Worthington-Roberts, B., S. Williams, and J. Vermeersch, eds., *Nutrition in Pregnancy and Lactation* (4th ed.). St. Louis: C.V. Mosby, 1989.

354. Williamson, K., et al., Occupational Health Hazards for Nurses—Part II, *Image,* 20, no. 3 (1988), 162–168.

355. Willis, J., Keeping Time to Circadian Rhythms, *FDA Consumer,* 24, no. 6 (1990), 18–21.

356. Willson, P.C., and A.F. Judkins, Testicular and Breast Self-Examinations: Nurses' Impact on Early Cancer Detection, *Dimensions in Oncology Nursing,* 4, no. 3 (1990), 27–32.

357. Windom, R., Adult Immunization Should Be Routine, Too, *Public Health Reports,* 102, no. 3 (1987), 245–246.

358. Wojtczak-Jaroszowa, J., and D. Jarvsz, Time-Related Distribution of Occupational Accidents, *Journal of Safety Research,* 18, no. 1 (1987), 33–41.

359. Women and Athletic Endurance, *Graduate Woman,* 79, no. 4 (1985), 5.

360. Woods, N., Relationship of Socialization and Stress to Premenstrual Symptoms, Disability and Menstrual Attitudes, *Nursing Research,* 34, no. 3 (1985), 145–149.

361. Woods, N., *Human Sexuality in Health and Illness* (3rd ed.). St. Louis: C.V. Mosby, 1984.

362. Yelin, E., et al., The Impact of HIV-Related Illness on Employment, *American Journal of Public Health,* 81, no. 1 (1991), 79–84.

INTERVIEW

363. Heuermann, P., and J. Personal Correspondence—Twenty-Fifth Wedding Anniversary Invitation, August 1988, Des Moines, Ia.

Chapter 13

Assessment and Health Promotion for the Middle-Aged Person

Middle age really is "middle." We're in the middle of our career and in the middle of the generations—still caring for the children and also doing more for the parents.
—Ruth Beckmann Murray

KEY TERMS

Middle age	Presbyopia	Gout or hyperuricemia	Generativity
Generation gap	Sleep apnea	Diabetes type II	Mentor
Social mobility	Sinusitis	Acute bacterial prostatitis	Stagnation or self-absorption
Widow(er) hood	Hiatal hernia	Chronic prostatitis	Maturity
Filial responsibility	Duodenal peptic ulcer	Lumbosacral strain	Adult socialization
Menopause	Angina pectoris	Foot balance	Midlife crisis
Perimenopausal years	Secondary hypertension	Callus	Midlife transition
Climacteric	Hyperthyroidism	Sexual dysfunction	

OBJECTIVES

Study of this chapter will enable you to:

1. Explore with a middle-aged person ideas about his or her generation, life-style, and the conflict between the generations.
2. Discuss the family relationships and sexuality development of the middle-aged adult, conflicts that must be resolved, and your role in helping the family work through concerns and conflicts.
3. List the developmental tasks for the middle-aged family, and give examples of how these can be accomplished.
4. Discuss the emotional, social, economic, and life-style changes usually encountered by the widow(er).
5. Describe the hormonal changes of middle age and the resultant changes in appearance and body image, physiologically and emotionally.
6. Discuss the nutritional, rest, leisure, work, and exercise needs of the middle-aged adult, factors that interfere with meeting those needs, and your role in helping him or her meet these needs.
7. Describe how the middle-aged adult's cognitive skills and emotional and moral development influence your nursing care plan.
8. State the developmental crisis of this era and its significance to social welfare.
9. Contrast the behavior of generativity, or maturity, and self-absorption, or stagnation, and related adaptive mechanisms.
10. Describe the developmental tasks for this person and your role in helping him or her accomplish these tasks.
11. Explore with a middle-aged adult ways to avoid injury and health problems.
12. Assess the body image, physical, mental, and emotional characteristics, and family relationships of a middle-aged person.
13. Plan and give effective care to a middle-aged person by using scientific principles and considering

special needs and reaction to illness and hospitalization.

The next generation complains about what we are and do. They say they'll do better. They should! They're standing on our shoulders.

Middle age does not exist in every culture; in the United States and other countries it is attributed to improved nutrition, control of communicable disease, discovery and control of familial disease, and other medical advances. Life has been stretched in the middle; what used to be old age is now middle age.

Further, as the work structure and roles and technologic development become more complex, as family life and child-rearing patterns change toward smaller families and a longer postparental period, the periods of childhood and youth are lengthened. Life is divided into more stages with more precise time periods and special developmental tasks for each age group. Thus in the past several decades, middle age has become a distinct life period. New concepts of adulthood involve a change in definitions of sex and age roles. Midlife development implies growth of the personality to encompass some characteristics that had stereotypically in the past been assigned to the opposite sex. Thus biology diminishes its influence on much of what had been held to be immutably biologic characteristics. Individuals may also work out more flexible adaptations (33). Middle adulthood is a time of widening social interest in which the family becomes increasingly oriented to its responsibility to the greater society. Parental attention is directed toward assisting integration of offspring's wishes with social requirements.

Defining middle age is a nebulous task. Chronologically, **middle age** *covers the years of approximately 45 to 65 and even 70, but each person will also consider the physiologic age condition of the body and psychologic age—how old he or she acts and feels.* Point of view alters definition: a child may think age 45 is old; the 45-year-old may consider himself or herself young. In the mid-1960s people placed early middle age between 40 and 55 and late middle age between 56 and 64

(37, 72). Many people today consider themselves young until nearly age 50 and middle-aged until around 70 years. Age assignment varies according to social class; the poorer person perceives the prime or midpoint of life to vary from the midtwenties to midthirties.

Because of changing demographics, an increasing number of Americans are considered middle-aged. They earn most of the money, pay a major portion of the bills and most of the taxes, and make many of the decisions. Thus the power in government, politics, education, religion, science, business, industry, and communication is often wielded not by the young or the old, but by the middle-aged.

Middle age is a time of relatively good physical and mental health, new personal freedom, and maximum command of self and influence over the social environment. At work the person has increasing ability to make decisions, hold high-status jobs, and earn a maximum income. The person has expanding family networks and social roles, and married life for postparental couples can be as harmonious and satisfying as the early married years.

In his book *Time Flies,* Bill Cosby has popularized becoming middle-aged. Some of the toils and deficits may be exaggerated, but the book conveys a middle-aged adult's attitude—the ability to see his or her strengths and limits and to accept, with a sense of humor, those normal changes that are part of development (27).

FAMILY DEVELOPMENT AND RELATIONSHIPS

Relationship With Children

The **generation gap,** the *conflict between parents and adolescents,* may have always existed to some degree (72, 81). The experience of elders, and therefore their values and expectations, differs from that of their offspring. Actually the generation lines are blurring. Some present middle-aged adults, perhaps out of fear of their own mortality, are looking and acting more like their children. These adults would rather think of themselves as carefree, innocent, and young. The changing attitudes, values, behavior, and dress of middle-aged persons reflect our cultural emphasis on youth and beauty versus wisdom and our more informal society (25).

However, Carlson (20) and Kaplan (64) say the term *generation gap,* which was coined in the 1960s, is inaccurate. The generations are not really in conflict with each other; rather each generation is concerned about the other, although for different reasons. In fact, the younger and older generations can successfully combine efforts to work for legislation, policy changes, or social justice.

The middle-aged adult was born sometime between the late 1920s and early 1940s, experiencing as a child or adolescent the Great Depression and World War II. He or she learned that interdependence of nations, economic security, and material possessions may be lost for reasons beyond personal control. Values and behavior have been influenced by growing up with inadequate material resources after the Great Depression and during World War II and by rapid social and technologic changes that occurred after World War II and during the 1950s.

The nuclear family is no longer prominent in the United States, and we discount learning from elders. The offspring cannot be fully prepared for the future by the parent generation. Youth must develop new patterns of behavior based on their own experience and that of peers. The present affluence, emphasis on age differences, independence, blurring of gender differences, and insistence on a unique life-style of today's youth add to the conflict—both value conflicts and parents' envy of their offspring. Youth's seeking of control over self and cultural institutions and living various life-style options may be better understood by younger middle-aged persons. Negative reactions of offspring reawaken in parents personal conflicts engendered by the remembrances of early personal commitments to ideals that became compromised over the years to fit narrower concerns. The addition of innate parental feelings of affection, admiration, and compassion for youth to the negative feelings produces an ambivalence (33, 72, 79).

Social mobility, *in which the child moves away from the social position, educational level, class, occupation, or ethnicity of parents,* causes offspring overtly to forsake parental teaching and seek new models of behavior. The mass media and societal trends help to set standards and expectations about behavior that may be counter to parental teaching or wishes. Rapid social changes and awareness that much about the future is unknown threaten established faiths and stimulate attraction to new ideologies and exceptional behavior.

As a nurse you may discuss with middle-aged persons what they as adults have to offer their children. They are the only generation to ever know, experience, and incorporate such rapid changes into daily life and the job. They can give their offspring imaginative, innovative, and dedicated adult care, a safe and flexible environment in which children can be given support, feel secure, grow, and discover themselves and the world. Reaffirm that it is up to the parents to teach *not what* to learn but *how to learn, not what to be* committed to but the *value of commitment.* Tell parents that research shows the continuity of values from generation to generation within a family. Typically the values of young adults are more similar to their parents' values than to those of other adults or peers (33). Help youth ask questions adults do not think of but yet to trust their parents enough to work on the answers together. The middle-aged parent can be encouraged to listen and exchange information and ideas honestly and with a sense of humor. The parent can accept youth's rejection of the faulty areas of society while supporting the values, principles, and institutions he or she knows are sound and necessary. As parent and offspring learn together to cope with the future, the parent will be able to assist youth to reach responsible, independent adulthood without a false maturity or alienation. The adult cannot abdicate the role of parent. If the parent works to maintain open communication, the generation gap may be minimum. Your work with families can promote greater harmony.

The *divorce of offspring* is an increasing area of concern for middle-aged parents. The parents may feel shock (or relief if they did not like the child's spouse). They may believe that their effort and help in getting the child "out of the nest" through marriage or helping the couple set up a home were to no avail. This feeling may be especially strong if the divorced family member decides to live at home again. The parents may blame their child or the in-laws and may criticize the couple for not working on the marital problems like the middle-aged parents have done (44).

If younger children are still at home, their needs and desires may be temporarily neglected because the emphasis is on the divorce crisis. Furthermore, the younger children may have to give back a room to the divorced brother or sister. The parents, in an attempt to make the divorced family member feel comfortable, may negate their own new patterns of freedom. Additionally, they may question their child-rearing ability and be too embarrassed, guilt ridden, or depressed to talk about the situation with others. If the divorced son or daughter is in a financial crisis, the parents' money may also go to help him or her instead of as originally planned. If the divorcing couple has children, an additional strain will be added to the middle-aged grandparents who wonder what their future relationship with their grandchildren will be. Relations may be strained between the in-laws as each family wonders how to interact with the other. Recent cordiality and affection may turn to anger and criticism.

The divorce may not have a completely negative effect on the middle-aged parents. If the parents have a healthy self-esteem and an ability to proceed cautiously, they may help their offspring to gain the essential maturity that he or she was previously lacking. However, the crisis and stages of grief that accompany divorce and loss of a family member are still keenly felt.

Young adults may return home to live with parents for reasons other than separation or divorce. Some new college graduates cannot find a job of their choice or are finding that their first jobs are not paying enough for them to cover high rents along with other costs of living, so they are living with parents until they can accumulate some money or can move to higher income jobs. Some young adult children return home more than once until they finally become independent (96).

This may cause stress since most middle-aged par-

ents look forward to having children leave the home—the so-called "empty nest" (90). The middle-aged adult wants space, time, and financial resources to pursue personal, organizational, and civic goals rather than to continue child-care responsibilities. Prolonged dependence of young adult offspring may also create conflict with grandparents and other children who are still at home.

The **grandparent role** has a different dimension in middle age than in later maturity. For example, if the adult offspring is divorced and brings young grandchildren into the middle-aged adult's home or if the offspring is unmarried and has children, the sense of responsibility and loss of independence are heightened. The middle-aged woman, especially, may resent the demands and constraints placed on her by having young children, including grandchildren, in the home fulltime. The middle-aged person is not necessarily happy about being a grandparent since that may indicate old age. If there are grandchildren, the relationship to the grandchild is informal and playful; the child is a source of fun, leisure activity, and self-indulgence. Emphasis is on mutual satisfaction, authority lines are irrelevant, and the child is seen as a unit of consumption (90). Such a relationship is less likely if the grandchild lives in the home with the middle-aged person. Further, having extra children and grandchildren in the home interferes with the relationship with the spouse. Normal developmental tasks cannot be met. The return of children into the home and the resultant demands may also serve to prevent the middle-aged woman from attempting to pursue new career goals, either because of a defensive withdrawal from an anxiety-producing new situation or because her conflict about roles prevents her from finding reasonable creative solutions to meet her own needs (72).

A growing number of grandparents are raising their grandchildren because their children are dead, divorced, or incapacitated from drugs or another devastating habit. Two groups addressing this issue are Grandparents Raising Grandchildren, P.O. Box 104, Coffeyville, TX 76034, and Sylvie de Toledo, Grandparents as Parents, Psychiatric Clinic for Youth, 2801 Atlantic Inc., Long Beach, CA 90801.

Increasingly you will be caring for middle-aged parents who are being threatened emotionally or are having social or financial problems because of their children's separation or divorce. Use the principles of communication and crisis intervention described in Chapters 5 and 8 of *Psychiatric/Mental Health Nursing; Giving Emotional Care* (86). Parents should be cautioned to proceed carefully with financial assistance. Few young adults pay back family loans. Further, there seldom are tax benefits to giving such assistance. The middle-aged grandparents may also need encouragement in securing visitation rights when divorce or death has severed the relationship (44). Help the middle-aged couple regain a sense of self-esteem, a sense of confidence in setting limits so that they can pursue their own life goals, and a method of working through decisions and problems with the young adult offspring.

Relationship with Spouse

Equally important as rearing the children and establishing wholesome affectional ties with them, and later with the grandchildren, is the middle-aged adult's relationship with the spouse.

A *happy marriage* has security and stability, although there are also struggles. The couple knows each other well; they no longer have to pretend to each other. Children can be a source of pleasure rather than concern since conflicts that arose between partners about rearing or disciplining children vanish when the children leave home. Each knows that his or her way of life and well-being depend on the other. Each has become accustomed to the way of the other. There is increased shared activity, and the sexual relationship can be better than before. Because the middle-aged adult is likely to have roots firmly implanted in the community of choice, he or she is able to cultivate warm friendships with members of the generation and with parents, the family of the spouse, and families of married children. Marriage can be secure economically, for the median income usually is above the national average. Middle-aged adults generally have more money in savings accounts and proportionately less debt than other age groups. Economic influence begins to wane as retirement nears, but the middle-aged working wife helps to offset this. Nationally, many working women are over 45 (28).

Although there is much discussion in the literature about the crisis of menopause and the "empty nest," menopause and middle age may bring both men and women an enriched sense of self and enhanced capacity to cope with life. It is a crisis in that behavioral changes are necessary but not a crisis in the negative sense of incapacitation.

In a study of 54 middle- and lower-middle-class men and women whose youngest child was about to leave home, Lowenthal and Chiriboga (75) found that the parents anticipated the departure with relief. The years before retirement were anticipated as promising, for responsibility for the children was over; adultlike peer relationships were sought with the children; job security was stable; and both partners felt more relaxed. In this study the men were more likely than the women to be dissatisfied with their work, perhaps as a kind of preparation for retirement or because they had longer experience in out-of-the-home work than women. The men spoke positively of their wives, describing them as warm, understanding, and competent homemakers. Women were twice as likely to speak of their husbands in negative terms, criticizing particularly the man's poor responsiveness to them. In a comparison of the views of both sexes, women had a somewhat more negative outlook than men and were more critical of themselves, their spouses, and their lives. These differences may be the result of the men's giving traditional responses and the women's feeling freer to state complex, negative, or ambivalent feelings (75). Empirical evidence still validates these results.

Negative, critical feelings can gradually erode what was apparently a happy relationship. At some point the husband and wife may feel they are each living with a stranger, although the potential still exists for a harmonious marriage. With everything seeming to go well for them, the middle-aged couple may now feel that the zest has gone out of their love life. The wife and husband may have drifted apart instead of growing closer together with the years. The wife feels neglected; the husband feels nagged; and both feel bored with each other. Why has their relationship changed so suddenly? It has not! It only seems that way. Their relationship is changing because they are changing. Marital crisis may result from feelings of disappointment with self, feeling depleted emotionally because of lack of communication with the spouse, seeking rebirth or changing directions, or seeking escape from reality and superego pressures (37, 72). In contrast, two factors found in one study were predictive of successful long-term marriages: (1) Congruence of perceptions between spouses of the marriage and each other and (2) sexual satisfaction (61).

Often the woman and man overlook that they still do really love each other. They simply have to get reacquainted. It may be difficult for the middle-aged man and woman to "tune in" to each other because both are encountering problems peculiar to their own gender. The woman may equate ability to bear children with capacity to enjoy sexual relationships, although they have nothing to do with each other. Whereas the woman needs the man's support to reinforce her femininity, he too is undergoing a crisis; he believes that he is losing his vigor, virility, and self-esteem, which are products primarily of psychologic reactions rather than physiologic inabilities. In the fifties there may be a reduction of male potency triggered by fears of incompetence and feelings of inability to satisfy his wife, who may be sexually more active after menopause. He may equate success on the job with success as a husband, believe that he is losing both, and covet his son's potency and youth.

Society and health care professionals have until recently ignored the sexual needs or problems of the married middle-aged adult. But the middle-aged person is an active sexual being. Physical changes in appearance and energy and the multiple stress of daily living may result in an increased desire for physical intimacy and the need for reassurance of continuing sexual attractiveness and competency. Intercourse is not valued for procreation but for body contact, to express love and trust, and to reaffirm an integral part of the self-concept. The person may fear loss of potency and rejection by the partner, but talking with the spouse about feelings and preferences related to sexual activity can promote increased closeness.

Men and women differ in their sexual behavior. Males reach their peak in their late teens and early twenties. Females peak in desire in the late thirties or forties and maintain that level of desire and activity past the menopause into middle age. The enjoyment of sexual relations in younger years, rather than the frequency, is a key factor for maintenance of desire and activity in the female, whereas frequency of relations and enjoyment are important factors for males (33, 77).

Disenchantment in any or all areas of life, with lack of enthusiasm for self and each other and for their physical relationship, may threaten the marriage in the middle years. Husband and wife are no longer distracted by daily activities of raising a family, and children are no longer present to act as buffers. There is increasing awareness of aging parents, aging friends, and signs of their own aging. Each becomes preoccupied with the self and anxious about losing youthfulness, vitality, sex appeal, and the partner's love. Each needs the other but may hesitate to reach out and demonstrate affection or intimacy. The end result may be for one or the other to reach outside the marriage to prove youthfulness, masculinity, or femininity.

The man who feels frustration in his marriage or that his wife is nagging or unattractive may pursue a younger woman to feel youthful, masculine, and admired. The woman may overcompensate for her felt loss of femininity by getting her face lifted, dressing more youthfully, acting like a teenager, and being flirtatious with her daughter's suitors.

Relationships with work colleagues may set the stage for an extramarital affair. This tendency is increased when the younger woman finds the company of an older man more interesting than that of the men in her own age group. Although divorce occurs during these years, the extramarital affair does not necessarily lead to the divorce courts. Divorce is major surgery, and the man may be reluctant to cut that much out of his life. Besides, he may find, having aroused the ardor of the younger woman, that he is no match for her physical demands. With increased consciousness of his age, he may return to his wife, particularly if she has in the meantime assessed her own situation and tried to change her behavior (33, 57, 72). Midlife crisis is discussed further in another section.

Be aware that there is an increasing number of over-40 divorces. The middle-aged man often remarries; fewer women are entering later maturity with the first marriage intact. (These women are also more likely to have a divorced daughter. Both generations have a lower standard of living as a result [120].) In the community mental health setting you will increasingly work with troubled families who are contemplating divorce or who have experienced separation and divorce.

Helping the couple regain closeness and happiness is worth the effort, for the mature years can be regarded as the payoff on an investment of many years together, many problems shared, and countless expressions of love exchanged. Each knows that his or her way of life and well-being depend on the other, so there is a willingness to change outlook, habits, and lovemaking, if necessary, to enhance their marriage. You can promote such changes.

You may teach or counsel the middle-aged adult who is having difficulty in relating to his or her spouse. Share the information in this chapter. Help the person determine, and then live out, the values of continuing to love and being patient and forgiving when the spouse has been unfaithful. Facilitate a desire to change behavior so that two people can grow together rather than apart. Work with the couple or refer them to counseling.

The following guidelines to couples may help them reduce stress in the marriage:

1. Talk daily to each other about feelings so that small problems are solved continually, rather than allowing emotional tensions to accumulate, creating a breaking-point scene.
2. Explore with each other feelings and ideas about possible, even if unlikely, life events that may occur—"what if" conversations. Such anticipatory worry helps the couple expand the repertoire of ideas and behavior so that if unexpected events occur, each will have more adaptive resources.
3. Vary schedules and chores, family goals or expectations, and roles and rules or make other periodic changes just to stay comfortable with change and to be prepared to adapt if a crisis requiring flexibility occurs.
4. Use each other as a resource. Talk to each other about individual problems, validate solutions, or ask each other about options for dealing with problems. Each must be willing to disclose about self to the other and be willing to support and help the other.
5. Maintain contact with others, including the extended family, who can help during a crisis. Sometimes the family does not exist or cannot be supportive; seek other resources such as a church or other support group.
6. In times of high stress or crisis, each should express the feelings of anger, grief, or helplessness to the other and to others who are caring. Expressing feelings about the circumstance, not about the spouse, allows conflict to surface and be handled.
7. Keep active with each other and with others, which prevents feelings of either stagnation during routine times or helplessness during stressful times.

Refer also to the section on midlife crisis later in the chapter for ideas on how to assist the couple.

Widow(er)hood, the *status change that results*

from death of husband (or wife), is a crisis in any life era, but it is more likely to occur first in middle age. The woman who is about to become a widow usually appreciates being able to participate in her husband's care but must feel that her husband will not suffer lack of care or support if she takes a few hours for her own rest. She needs someone to listen as she expresses feelings of anger, sadness, and guilt; the nurses may be better able to listen, support, and encourage than family or friends. The nurse can gently test her reactions to determine if she is ready for the shock of death by offering to call a clergyman or by asking if family members need to be prepared for deterioration of the husband's condition. If the woman appears brave and strong, allow her to keep her veneer of courage if that is holding her together. Realize the wife may feel much ambivalence—not wanting the husband to suffer pain and yet wanting him to be alert so that she can talk with him or praying that death will relieve his suffering and yet hoping for his survival. After death she may linger on the nursing unit—a place of support—rather than leaving for home, a very empty place.

The person's reaction to death of a spouse depends on personality and emotional makeup, the relationship between the couple (how long they have been married; how long the mate has been ill), and religious, cultural, and ethnic background.

The loss of a spouse may mean many things: loss of a sexual partner and lover, friend, companion, caretaker, an audience for unguarded spontaneous conversation, accountant, plumber, or gardener, depending on the roles performed by the mate. Managing finances is often a major problem, especially for the widow. Secondary losses involve reduced income, which frequently means moving to a new residence and strange environment, change in life-style and social involvements, return to the work force, and giving up any number of things previously taken for granted. Widowhood is a threat to self-concept and sense of wholeness; now the person is seen as "only one." Often the woman's identity if so tied to that of her husband that she feels completely lost, alone, and indecisive and as a nonperson after his death. If she has no one else close with whom to talk or from whom to receive help, she may believe she will lose her mind or become suicidal. The widow(er) misses having someone with whom he or she can share both happy occasions and sad news and problems. He or she can dial a crisis line to talk about a problem; it may be more difficult to tell about a source of happiness. The pet or houseplant is a poor substitute for a person. The emotional burden is increased if the woman still has children in the home to raise by herself. She has a hard time helping them work through their grief when she is in mourning. Friendship patterns and relations with in-laws also often change. The widow is a threat to women with husbands; they perceive her as competition, and she is a reminder of what they might experience. With friends the widow is the odd person in number, so social engagements become stressful and are a constant reminder of the lost partner. The widow also becomes aware that she is regarded as a sexual object to men who may offer her their sexual services at a time when she has decreased sexual desires but a great need for companionship and closeness. Yet in contrast to assumptions, one study showed that many widows are quite competent in managing their lives (94).

Although the widower is more accepted socially, he too will have painful gaps in his life. If the wife concentrated on keeping an orderly house, cooking regular and nutritious meals, and keeping his wardrobe in order, he may suddenly realize that what he had taken for granted is gone. Even more significant is the loss if his wife were a "sounding board" or confidante in business matters and if she were actively involved in raising children still in the home.

The bereavement of widowhood affects physical health; somatic complaints related to anxiety are not unusual. The widow(er) may experience symptoms similar to those of the deceased spouse.

One study showed that mortality rates, based on person-years at risk, were approximately the same for widowed as for married women but significantly higher for widowed than married men. Mortality rates among widowed males who remarried were very much lower than among those who did not remarry, but no significant difference was observable among widowed women who did or did not remarry (52). Another study showed that death, including from suicide, is more likely to occur during the first year of widowhood (65).

Your contact with the widow(er) can help to resolve the crisis. Encourage the bereaved to talk about feelings as you provide a supportive relationship (or help the widow[er] to find one). Death of a husband in middle age is more common than that of a wife; you will encounter more widows. Building up the widow's confidence and self-esteem, especially if she had lived a protected life, is essential. Help her identify people other than her children who can assist her with various tasks to avoid feelings of burden in any helper. Encourage her to try new experiences, expand interests, join community groups, do volunteer work, seek new friends, and become a person in her own right. Now is a good time to pursue activities formerly not done because the mate did not enjoy them. Encourage getting a medical checkup and following healthful practices in response to physical complaints, and help her recognize the somatic aspects of grief and mourning (55, 73, 86, 101). You may want to offer group crisis intervention through the local Red Cross, a church, or school. Several books and articles can be useful to the widow(ers) (15, 19, 41, 42, 60, 72, 83, 97).

Some national organizations that help widow(ers), include Naim, Parents Without Partners, THEOS, and the Older Women's League. Naim was founded by a couple in cooperation with a priest in Chicago. The chapters have well-planned monthly meetings about educational, spiritual, legal, and social needs of the widowed. Information can be obtained from Father Corcoran, Naim, St. Patrick's Roman Catholic Church, in Chicago (15).

Parents Without Partners, Inc., 8807 Colesville Rd, Silver Springs, MD 20010, is an international nonprofit, nonsectarian, educational, and social organization devoted to the welfare and interest of one-parent families and their children. Monthly meetings help the widow(er) get practical assistance and information and work through mourning (15).

They Help Each Other Spiritually (THEOS), 717 Liberty Avenue, Pittsburgh, PA 15222, is a national, nonsectarian organization designed primarily to help recently bereaved persons and the young and middle-aged adults who need to resolve the grief related to the death of a loved one. Monthly meetings deal with various problem areas: reorganizing life, working through grief and loneliness, coping with the feeling of being a "fifth wheel," raising children alone, finances, dating and remarriage, expressions of bitterness, anger, and fear, and integrating loss and grief into belief in God and spiritual life (15).

Another organization that is an informational resource to help the woman adapt and plan for the future is Older Women's League, 730 11th Street N.W., Suite 300, Washington, DC 20001. The middle-aged woman can get information about life insurance and Medicare and responses to other questions. Such information can help plan for later maturity.

Many of the problems that confront the widow(er) also confront the divorced person. Your intervention principles will be similar, although the words will be different.

Relationship With Aging Parents and Relatives

Because people are living longer, parents in later maturity and their adult offspring may expect more than 50 years of overlap; there is an increase in the number and duration of intergenerational linkages. The middle-aged person is in the middle in many ways—including in the middle of two demanding generations. Although childcare responsibilities may be decreasing, considerable care of or involvement with offspring may remain at the same time there is increasing care of, involvement with, and responsibility for aging parents, aunts, uncles, or grandparents. The adult daughter and elderly mother may have remained in a close relationship through the years; if so, that daughter is likely to become more involved in that parent's life as the years pass. The friendship and interdependency of the younger years develop into a relationship with an increasingly dependent mother (60). The middle-aged woman may be in additional close relationships with elderly relatives moreso than the middle-aged man or son.

The literature about middle-aged caregiving focuses on the caregiving to parents. However, sometimes the middle-aged adult is the caregiver for the child (e.g., when the adult offspring has a chronic illness, an injury causing permanent loss of some function, or, increasingly, acquired immunodeficiency syndrome (AIDS) (95).

Responsibility for Elderly Relatives

Three cultural trends affect the dilemma of caring for older dependent relatives:

1. Long-term societal emphasis on personal independence and social mobility of middle-aged and young adults, which creates physical separateness of generational households and new kinship patterns of intimacy at a distance
2. Focusing on the dynamics of the marriage bond and socialization of young children, with the emphasis on affection, compatibility, and personal growth of each person in the nuclear family as the most important aspects of family life
3. Longer life spans of older people and the problem of caring for the older generation when they become dependent (59)

Filial responsibility is an *attitude of personal responsibility toward the parents that emphasizes duty, protection, care, and financial support,* which are indicators of the family's traditional protective function. Middle-class Caucasian culture in the United States believes that good relationships between the aged and their adult children are dependent on the autonomy of the parents. They believe that a satisfactory role reversal between generations is not possible since the mores of society do not sanction it and both children and parents resent it. However, older persons expect children to assume responsibilities when they can no longer maintain their independence. Families do in fact continue to provide nurturance and companionship through visits and telephone calls; information, assistance in decision making, transportation, assistance with shopping, laundry, and household chores, immediate response to crisis, a buffer against bureaucracies, help in searching out services, and facilitation for continuity of individual-bureaucracy relations. In many ethnic or racial cultures structure and style for the younger generation(s) have evolved through an extended family system to provide support, assistance, protection, and mobility (50). Often inadequate family economic reserves and inadequate health insurance necessitate the middle-aged adult's having to be caregiver (49, 70, 117).

For the African-American, an extended family serves as a mechanism for meeting physical, emotional, and economic needs. However, most aged African-Americans do not live in extended families. Influences such as Black power, economic and social mobility, and self-fulfillment may have weakened the perceived filial obligations of younger African-Americans more than those of their Caucasian counterparts. These influences may be eroding parental care in other subcultures or ethnic and racial groups as well. Adult offspring may be anxious about their competence in taking care of elderly persons. The average American family does not have the structure, organization, or economic resources necessary to care for older persons over long periods of time. Members of other racial groups, in general, have fewer resources and opportunities than Caucasians. Some of the differences in adult children's support of filial responsibility may stem from the greater worries and fears they have with regard to being able to provide support for their parents (50). Yet many families have four or five generations; the young middle-aged person may have parents, grandparents, and great-grandparents. Further, elderly siblings, aunts, uncles, or cousins may also be living and need and expect help from the middle-aged adult. The person who is in the forties, fifties, or early sixties may be seen as possessing energy, free time, and money. Older relatives become more demanding just when the middle-aged adult believes he or she deserves time for self, a vacation, and an opportunity to pursue additional education or a social cause. The additional stress occurs when the older relatives want their needs met *right now;* they can create considerable guilt in the middle-aged adults.

Certainly the older and middle-aged generations can give a great deal to each other. The older generation(s) can share insights and wisdom about life. Sometimes they can give assistance financially or with various tasks. The older generation(s) can be a source of joy, pride, and inspiration. However, if they live long enough, the middle-aged adult will have someone who is increasingly dependent and in need of help. Sometimes the middle-aged adult realizes the dependence and need for help before the elderly person is ready to admit the need, and that can become a source of frustration and stress.

Caregiver Role

Care of a parent is a normative but stressful experience, although most people willingly help the parent and derive satisfaction from doing so. Various factors that influence the caregiving role include the following (4, 8, 22, 78, 111, 115, 116, 131, 134):

1. Seriousness of the elder's health status
2. The caregiver–care recipient relationship and living arrangement
3. Duration of the caregiving experience
4. Other roles and responsibilities of the caregiver
5. Overall coping effectiveness of the caregiver
6. Caregiver gender and age
7. Number of generations needing care
8. Help and support from others—family or social agencies
9. Information needed to carry out tasks related to physical care of the parent

Meeting parent's dependency needs may have many diverse effects (4, 8, 12, 13, 21, 43, 104, 105, 111, 134, 136):

1. Financial hardship
2. Physical symptoms such as sleeplessness and decline in physical health, especially in the primary caregiver
3. Emotional changes and symptoms in the caregiver and other family members, including frustration, inadequacy, anxiety, helplessness, depression, guilt, resentment, lowered morale, and emotional distance
4. Emotional exhaustion related to restrictions on time and freedom and increasing responsibility
5. A sense of isolation from social activities
6. Conflict because of competing demands, with diversion from care of other family members
7. Difficulty in setting priorities
8. Reduced family privacy
9. Inability to project future plans
10. Sense of losing control over life events
11. Interference with job responsibilities through late arrival, absenteeism, or early departure needed to take care of emergencies—or even routine tasks
12. Interference with life-style and social and recreational activities.

Thus the whole family and its relationships are affected.

The dilemma of care for the elderly inevitably has an emotional impact on their grown children. The *caregiver role* is a major one, especially for the woman. In fact, the word *caregiver* is an euphemism for *unpaid female relative.* The middle-aged woman who is the older daughter is most likely to do the caregiving. Caregiving apparently is a woman's career; care of the dependent parent is only one phase of the woman's caregiving career. The woman often is caring for children in the home simultaneously with caring for aged parents, grandparents, other aged family members, parents-in-law, and finally the husband in old age. Interestingly, women who work provide as much caregiving as women who do not work outside the home. Nonemployed daughters provide more tangible help, but employed daughters contribute in other ways, according to one study (78). Some may reduce the working hours; others quit their jobs, especially if the aged parent lives with them. Parent care makes the woman feel tied down and competes for time with the husband. Relations between husband and wife are affected because of financial or other help one person may give to the elderly parent(s), especially when done without consulting the other spouse. The needs of elderly parents may cause discord among their sons and daughters by recalling childhood rivalries and jealousies. A common phenomenon is when the middle-aged person resents those siblings who will not help care for the elderly parent(s) or other relatives. Further, if the middle-aged adult believes he or she was not well cared for by the parents as a child, continued resentment, anger, or hate may inhibit a nurturing attitude or even minimum assistance.

The meaning of caring for the dependent parent is different than for caring for the dependent child. The child's future holds promise for reducing dependency needs; the older parent will have increasing dependency needs. Parent care also stimulates anticipation of the final separation from the parent and of one's potential dependence on one's child. The way filial care is negotiated depends on the past and has implications for the future when the adult child is old.

Sometimes the adult child continues to care for the parent beyond physical and psychologic means to do so rather than to use formal support systems. Various dynamics are at work: (1) symbiotic ties, (2) gratification of being the burden bearer, (3) a fruitless search for parental approval that has never been received, and (4) expiation of guilt for having been a favorite child. The middle-aged adult may perceive caregiving as an acceptable, permanent, fulltime role that is altruistic and enhances self-esteem. Because this role gives meaning, a job or other roles may be discontinued, or this role may be a substitute for a failed marriage or for being widowed. Thus successful resolution of this crisis may be acceptance of what cannot be done as well as of what can and should be done. Box 13–1 lists signals indicating that the caregiver needs assistance. For the elderly, successful adaptation to dependence includes accepting what adult children cannot do (12).

The popular trend of expecting the middle-aged family to care for the dependent aged in their home assumes an emotional closeness and family cohesion that may not exist. The caregiving may instead contribute to a deterioration of relationships, even though a commitment to caring for family members is a value. Closeness may not be a basis for caregiving. Now can we assume that satisfactory family relationships in early and middle adulthood will persist without change into late adulthood. Apparently there is a periodic rebalancing in family ties throughout life. Bonds may either loosen or grow closer with the conflicts and demands inherent in the caregiving role (59).

A kind of psychologic distancing between parents and caregiving children may occur. The adult children may feel little affection for the parent, feeling rather a kind of grief, and may hesitate to cancel the caregiving burden out of a sense of respect and loyalty to the parent. The adult child, often a married daughter, does not feel enough gratification from the caregiving to offset the sense of burden, yet the cultural expectation of closeness and love for family members leads her to feel guilt or despair. The person may question whether she can care for the parent if she does not feel love and may be concerned about the cost of caregiving to personal emotional stability (59).

Adult offspring with disrupted marriages (divorce,

BOX 13-1.
Danger Signals Indicating Caregiver Needs Assistance

- Your relative's condition is worsening despite your best efforts.
- No matter what you do, it is not enough.
- You believe you are the only person in the world enduring this.
- You no longer have any time or place to be alone for even a brief respite.
- Things you used to do occasionally to help are now part of your daily routine.
- Family relationships are breaking down because of the caregiving pressures.
- Your caregiving duties are interfering with your work and social life to an unacceptable degree.
- You are going on in a "no-win situation" just to avoid admitting failure.
- You realize you are alone—and doing all the work because you have shut out everyone who offered to help.
- You refuse to think of yourself because "that would be selfish" (even though you are unselfish 99% of the time).
- Your coping methods have become destructive; you are overeating or undereating, abusing drugs or alcohol, or being harsh or abrasive with your relative.
- There are no more happy times; loving and caring have given way to exhaustion and resentment; and you no longer feel good about yourself or take pride in what you are doing.

---

widow(er)hood, or remarried) give significantly less help, perceive fewer parental needs, feel less filial obligations, and feel more limited in helping because of job responsibilities (22).

Future parallel situations may be drawn between the older parent or relative and the middle-aged person. Some of the impatience, aggravation, and desire to see less of the older person comes from the middle-aged adult's dawning realization that the older person is a picture of what the middle-aged person may become. The person who is in the prime of life may fear greatly the physical disabilities, illness, personality eccentricities, intellectual impairments, or social changes that old age brings.

Research findings document the strength of intergenerational ties, the continuity of responsible filial behavior, the frequency of contact between generations, the predominance of families rather than professionals in providing health and social services, the strenuous family efforts to avoid institutional placement of the old, and the central role played by families in caring for noninstitutionalized impaired elderly (8, 12, 59, 78, 112, 115, 128).

One of the most difficult decisions when parents become aged and dependent concerns the housing arrangement. The older daughter usually is the one to take the dependent parent into her home—a phenomenon called the "refilling of the empty nest" (12), or the unmarried adult child may move into the parent's home. When the parent(s) cannot manage living alone, the middle-aged person may not have the room to take the parent(s) into his or her home. Even if there is adequate space, if all members of the household are working, finding someone to stay during the day may be difficult, although such an arrangement or the use of adult day care is less cost prohibitive than placing the parent who is in poor health in an institution. Most communities do not have adequate, or any, day-care facilities for elderly adults. Placing the parent(s) in an institution may be the only answer, but it is typically considered the last resort. Refer to Chapter 14 for more information on what to consider in that event.

Considerable research has been done on the middle-aged adult's caregiving role to parents, the tasks faced by and the effect on the caregiver and the middle-aged adult's family relations, physical and emotional health, and life-style. For additional information see references 4, 8, 12, 13, 21, 43, 49, 59, 70, 78, 104, 105, 111, 112, 114–117, 128, 131, 134, 136 at the end of the chapter.

Nursing Role

You are in a key position to help the middle-aged adult work through the conflicts, feelings of frustration, guilt, and anger about the increased responsibility and past conflicts or old hurts from parents or siblings. The middle-aged adult who verbally expresses great irritation typically also loves the older relative very much. Assist the middle-aged adult to gain a sense of satisfaction from the help he or she gives and a greater understanding of the person being helped. The generation gap and negative feelings that exist between the middle-aged adult and elderly person can be overcome with love, realistic expectations, a sense of forgiveness, and the realization that sometimes it is all right to say "No" to the demands of the elderly. Refer also to Chapter 14 for specific information you can share about physiologic, emotional, cognitive, and social needs, changes, and characteristics of the elderly person. One study indicated that teaching the caregiver stress management and time management techniques may reduce the sense of burden moreso than participation in a support group (29). Encouraging the caregiver to maintain other roles outside of caregiving and family roles, although adding extra commitments to the sense of burden, may also increase the sense of caregiver well-being and health (116). Refer

---

■ Research Abstract

Farran, C., et al., Finding Meaning: An Alternative Paradigm for Alzheimer's Disease Family Caregivers, Gerontologist, 31, no. 4 (1991), 483–489.

Caregiving can be stressful; research shows that caregivers experience a sense of burden, depression, and decline in physical health. There are also caregivers who, although not intentionally seeking such a situation, may choose to make the best of the situation and to find positive outcomes.

Existentialism, or the Third Force Theory, was the framework for this study. The purpose of this study was to understand how caregivers grow emotionally and spiritually and find meaning in the caregiving situation and in the suffering that is part of being a caregiver.

The sample was comprised of 94 caregivers—wives (34%), husbands (32%), daughters (24%), sons (3%), and other family members (6%)—who ranged in age from 30 to 78 years. All care receivers were diagnosed with an irreversible, progressive form of dementia and ranged in age from 49 to 92 years. The sample was middle class and primarily Caucasian (81%).

A 2-hour structured interview about caregiving was carried out in the home. Qualitative techniques were used to analyze the data. The data were grouped into four major themes: (1) loss and powerlessness; (2) values, choices, and provisional and ultimate meaning; (3) caregiving resources; and (4) responsibilities of caregiving.

Results indicated that these caregivers express existential themes. Finding meaning is an individual process, and spouses may differ from others in developing a caregiving attitude. Suffering is experienced at physical, psychologic, social, and spiritual levels by caregivers. Suffering involves a sense of powerlessness— the inability to change one's circumstances.

Caregivers mourn their own losses as they experience changes in the relationship with the family member and realize their future plans have changed. Values form a basis for meaning. Experiential values focus on relationships and the feelings people have toward each other and are expressed as the caregiver focuses on who the person was in the past and enjoys the person for who he or she still is. Attitudinal values include philosophic or spiritual beliefs, and caregivers persevere in their efforts to provide care based on spiritual philosophy. Caregiving involves accepting the responsibility for making decisions about whether to be a caregiver and how to carry out these responsibilities. Caregivers may find provisional or short-term meaning from daily tasks, and ultimate meaning comes from exploring the deeper meanings in life.

Creative values are expressed in jobs, hobbies, or other creative activities. Caregivers are creative as they develop innovative approaches to daily problems. Each person must work through these values and meaning for self; this is an individual process not linked to race, gender, or relatedness to the care receiver. Caregivers can respond to the caregiving experience by making personal choices about life and caregiving, by valuing positive aspects of the caregiving experience, and by searching for meaning. Health care professionals can assist caregivers in these tasks. The caregiver spouse of a person with dementia must face the guilt of not caring for the impaired spouse and the guilt of not going forward with her or his own life. The caregiving role must be freely chosen, according to the Existential Framework.

to a counselor or spiritual leader if necessary. Counseling can promote a resolution of feelings that in turn fosters a more harmonious relationship between the middle-aged adult and parents.

One way to help the adult child to continue the caregiving role, set aside guilt, and gain more positive feedback is to offer a *relabeled perspective*. The cultural mandate of affection for aging parents is of recent origin. Historically, aged parents have been cared for on the basis of obligation. Being a good child means not feeling great affection but showing concern for the well-being of the parent and giving care to the limits of one's ability. Helping the adult child internalize this perspective helps him or her begin to cope with the stresses without being overwhelmed. Thus the parent cared for in the adult child's home has the advantage of a home environment. Further, outside resources can be used to support the adult child in the caregiving role. Often a little help will enable the person to make changes and use inner resources in a distressing situation. Having the caregiver keep a daily list of helping behaviors and of negative behaviors (not feelings) is a way of assisting the caregiver to see the role and behavior in a positive light and to gain reinforcement from the caregiving since almost always the helping behaviors far outnumber the negative behaviors. Such a log can provide a base for talking with the adult child about the interaction with the parent and ways to resolve feelings and improve the interaction (59).

Although some adult children are helped through this relabeling process, some ethnic or racial groups do not respond to this technique. For example, African-Americans have maintained a kind of behavioral closeness between generations that produces a different pattern of attitudes and less social and emotional distance between middle generation adults and their parents.

Death of Parents in Adulthood

A critical time for the adult is when both parents have died, regardless of whether the relationship between parent(s) and offspring was harmonious or conflictual. The first death of a parent signals finiteness and mortality of the self and of the other parent and other loved ones. Memories of childhood experiences are recalled. The person may wish deeply, even though simultaneously realizing it is impossible, to be able to relive some of those childhood days with the parent, to undo naughty behavior, to be a good child just once more, to sit on the parent's lap and be cuddled one more time, to return to the relatively carefree days and to relive holidays. Further, more recent memories are recalled—the joys that were shared and the disharmonious times that are normal in any relationship but that are likely to engender guilt. There may be deep yearning to hold the parent one more time. Mourning may be done not only for the parent but for previously lost loved ones, and some mourning is in anticipation of future losses of the other parent, other beloved relatives and friends, and self. When the other parent dies, the adult is an orphan. Now he or she is no longer anyone's "little boy" or "little girl." The person may feel forlorn and alone, especially if there are few other relatives or friends. Sometimes there are no other living relatives and no sons so that the adult offspring represents the last of the family line. The person may question who and what will be remembered and by whom. This is a time of spiritual and philosophical searching whether or not the adult child is alone, has siblings, or has other relatives.

If there was conflict between the adult offspring and parents to the point of one-sided or mutual hate and unforgiveness, grief feelings may be denied or repressed or may be especially guilt laden. Consequently, the mourning process is delayed and not resolved as effectively. There is a yearning that life experiences with the parent(s) could have been better or different, a wish that harsh feelings could have been smoothed, and a sadness over what was never present more so than a sadness over what has been lost. The adult survivor may fear that he or she in turn may have similarly parented children, if any, and anxiety may arise about how the third or current child generation will feel when this parent dies. Will the scene and feelings be replayed? Can that be prevented? Certainly this can be a time for the adult to take stock, undo past wrongs with his or her children (and others), resolve old conflicts, and become motivated to move ahead into more harmonious relations with family members and others.

Throughout the period of parental loss, you may be a key person in helping the adult survivor or adult orphan relive, express, and sort out feelings; accept that any close relationship will not always go smoothly; and finally achieve a balance between happy, sad, and angry memories and feelings in regard to the parent(s). Finally, through such counseling the person can mature to accept and like self and other significant persons better and to change behavior patterns so that future relationships are less thorny.

Little is written specifically about bereavement experienced when the adult's parents die. One useful book is *The Orphaned Adult: Confronting the Death of a Parent,* by Marc Angel (1).

Developmental Tasks

In summary, the following developmental tasks must be accomplished for the middle-aged family to survive and achieve happiness, harmony, and maturity (32):

1. Maintain a pleasant and comfortable home.
2. Assure security for later years, financially and emotionally.
3. Share household and other responsibilities, based on changing roles, interests, and abilities.
4. Maintain emotional and sexual intimacy as a couple

or regain emotional stability if death or divorce occurs.

5. Maintain contact with grown children and their families.
6. Decrease attention on child-care tasks and adapt to departure of the child(ren).
7. Meet the needs of elderly parent(s) in such a way as to make life satisfactory for both the parent(s) and middle-aged generations.
8. Participate in community life beyond the family, recommitting energy once taken by child care.
9. Use competencies built in earlier stages to expand or deepen interests and social or community involvement (32).

McCoy (79) has formulated developmental tasks and their outcomes for the stages of middle age, as shown in Table 13–1.

As a nurse you will have the opportunity and responsibility to help the middle-aged couple meet their developmental tasks.

PHYSIOLOGIC CONCEPTS

Physical Characteristics

The growth cycle continues with physical changes in the middle years, and different body parts age at a different rate. One day the person may suddenly become aware of being "old" or middle-aged. Not all people decline

alike. How quickly they decline depends on the stresses and strains they have undergone and on the health promotion measures that were maintained. If the person has always been active, he or she will continue with little slowdown. People from lower socioeconomic groups often show signs of aging earlier than people from more affluent socioeconomic groups because of their years of hard physical labor, poorer nutritional status, and lack of money for beauty aids to cover the signs of aging (33).

Now the person looks in the mirror and sees changes that others may have noticed some time ago. Gray, thinning hair, wrinkles, coarsening features, decreased muscular tone, weight gain, varicosities, and capillary breakage may be the first signs of impending age.

Because a number of your clients will be middle-aged, you are in a key position to help them understand the physiologic changes that occur in middle age, work through feelings about these changes, reintegrate the body image, and find specific ways to remain as healthy as possible. Use the following information to assist you in listening, teaching, reaffirming a positive self-concept, and counseling.

Hormonal Changes
Female Climacteric. This is the era of life known as the *menopause* for the woman or the *climacteric* for either sex. The terms are often used interchangeably. The **menopause** is the *permanent cessation of menstruation preceded by a gradually decreasing menstrual flow.*

TABLE 13-1. DEVELOPMENTAL TASKS OF MIDDLE AGE AND THEIR OUTCOMES

Developmental Stages	Developmental Tasks	Outcomes Sought
Restabilization, 44–55 years old	Adjust to realities of work.	Job adjustment
	Launch children.	Letting go of parental authority
	Adjust to empty nest.	Exploring new sources of satisfaction
	Become more deeply involved in social life.	Effective social relations
	Participate actively in community concerns.	Effective citizenship
	Handle increased demands of older parents.	Better personal and social adjustment of elderly
	Manage leisure time.	Creative use of leisure
	Manage budget to support college-age children and ailing parents.	Sound consumer behavior
	Adjust to single state.	Fulfilled single state
	Solve problems.	Successful problem solving
	Manage stress accompanying change.	Successful stress management, personal growth
Preparation for retirement, 56–64 years old	Adjust to health problems.	Healthier individuals
	Deepen personal relations.	Effective social skills
	Prepare for retirement.	Wise retirement planning
	Expand avocational interests.	Satisfaction of aesthetic urge; broadening of knowledge; enjoyment of travel
	Finance new leisure.	Sound consumer behavior
	Adjust to eventual loss of mate.	Adjustment to loss, fulfilled single state
	Use problem solving.	Successful problem solving
	Manage stress accompanying change.	Successful stress management, personal growth

Modified from McCoy, V., Adult Life Cycle Tasks/Adult Continuing Education Program Response, *Lifelong Learning in the Adult Years* (October 1977), 16.

The term **perimenopausal years** denotes a *time of gradual diminution of ovarian function and a gradual change in endocrine status* (90). The **climacteric** is the *period in life when important physiologic changes occur, with the cessation of the woman's reproductive ability, and the period of lessening sexual activity in the male* (99). Basic to the changing physiology of the middle years is the declining hormonal production (108).

Contrary to myth, depression or other symptomatology are neither inevitable nor clearly related to the perimenopausal or climacteric years (108). Most women feel relieved or neutral about menopause; only 3% view if negatively. Attitudes toward menopause improve as women move from pre- to postmenopause, and perception of health becomes more positive as menopause proceeds (34, 35, 108). The worst part about the menopause or climacteric may be not knowing what to expect since there is still a dearth of research and scientific knowledge about this normal period of life. Myths abound (24, 108).

Traditional homemakers in the United States experience greater difficulty with menopause. In societies in which women rise in status after menopause or generally enjoy high status regardless of reproductive stage, a menopausal syndrome is nonexistent. A woman's perception of her menopause experience is largely her perception of the physical, social, and psychologic changes she undergoes (35, 76, 108).

In a study of the impact of menopausal stage, current life change, and attitude toward traditional women's roles on perceived health status in women 40 to 55 years of age, well women perceived few current life changes. Apparently negative life changes have a greater impact on one's health perception than positive life changes, in contrast to general opinion that all life changes tax individuals' coping ability. However, the perception of the stressfulness of a life event could be biased by assessment of its positive or negative value. Attitude toward women's roles may be associated with perceived health status among midlife women (35).

Male Climacteric. This comes in the fifties or early sixties, although the symptoms may not be as pronounced as in the female climacteric. A man's "change of life" is passed almost imperceptibly, but he usually notices it when he makes comparisons with past feelings and performance. A few men may even complain of hot flashes, sweating, chills, dizziness, headaches, and heart palpitations. Unlike women, however, men do not lose their reproductive abilities, although the likelihood diminishes as age advances. The output of sex hormones of the gonads does not stop; it is merely reduced. The testes become less firm and smaller; cells in the tubules degenerate; and sperm production decreases. Because of decreased testosterone production, the man may need a longer time to achieve erection and may experience premature or less forceful ejaculation. Testosterone

level usually is lower in the middle-aged man who has high stress, lowered self-esteem, and depression. Testosterone therapy should be used cautiously because administration may increase prostatic hypertrophy and cancer development (48, 57, 77).

In approximately 20% of men hypertrophy of the prostate begins naturally late in middle age so that gradually the enlarging prostate around the urethra causes the embarrassment of frequent urination, dribbling, and nocturia. In addition, urinary stasis may predispose the man to urinary infections (102).

Menopause. The average age for onset of menopause is 51; the usual range is between 45 and 55 years, although it may occur as early as age 35 for approximately 1% of women. In the woman the process of aging causes changed secretion of the follicle-stimulating hormone (FSH), which brings about progressive and irreversible changes in the ovaries, leading to the menopause and loss of childbearing ability. The primordial follicles, which contain the ovum and grow into vesicular follicles with each menstrual cycle, become depleted, and their ability to mature declines. Finally, ovulation ceases since all ova are either degenerated or have ovulated. Thus the cyclic production of progesterone and estrogen fails to occur and levels rapidly fall below the amount necessary to induce endometrial bleeding. The menstrual cycle becomes irregular; periods of heavy bleeding may alternate with amenorrhea for 1 or 2 years, eventually ceasing altogether (48). Consistent or regular excessive bleeding may be a sign of pathology, not of the approaching menopause.

The pituitary continues to produce FSH and luteinizing hormone (LH), but the aging ovary is incapable of responding to its stimulation. With the pituitary no longer under the normal cyclic or feedback influence of ovarian hormones, it becomes more active, producing excessive gonadotropins, especially FSH. A disturbed endocrine balance influences some of the symptoms of menopause. While the ovaries are producing less estrogen and progesterone, the adrenals may continue to produce some hormones, thus helping to maintain younger feminine characteristics for some time (48).

During the perimenopausal period (approximately 5 years) some discomforts may occur in a small percentage of women. Vasomotor changes cause hot flashes associated with chilly sensations, dizziness, headaches, perspiration, palpitations, water retention, nausea, muscle cramps, fatigability, insomnia, and paresthesia of fingers and toes. Many symptoms, including irritability, depression, emotional lability, and palpitations, are frequently attributed to menopause. But in a study of 1630 men and women, only sweating and hot flushing were consistently related to menopause. Difficulties experienced during menopause may be associated with concurrent life change or recent loss, or marital, psychologic, or social stress (35). The cause of the symptoms apparently is more complex than simple estrogen deficit. Psychologic factors such as anger, anxiety, and excitement are considered as important in precipitating hot flashes in susceptible women as conditions giving rise to excess heat production or retention such as a warm environment, muscular work, or hot food. However, the symptoms may arise without any clear psychologic or heat-stimulating mechanism.

Related Changes. Decline of estrogen affects many body functions and increases the risks of heart disease and osteoporosis in women. The hormonal decline brings additional changes. The skin, subcutaneous tissue, and mucous membranes become dry and begin to atrophy. The loss of skin turgor and muscle tone results in wrinkles, pouches under the eyes, sagging jowls, and loss of muscle tone, including of the pelvic floor. The loss of tone of the bladder mucosa and sphincter and urethral tissue and supporting structures results in frequent, urgent urination, stress incontinence, and embarrassment, which may limit social activities. The uterus, ovaries, external genitalia, and breast tissue begin to atrophy. Atrophy, loss of elasticity of the vaginal mucosa, and less vaginal lubrication during sexual arousal may interfere with the pleasure of the sexual experience and cause dysuria after intercourse. Regular sexual intercourse helps to maintain an adequate vaginal outlet and to prevent shrinkage of the vaginal mucosa (48, 77). If the couple experiences difficulty with sexual response and if the sexual problems result from changes in lubrication, use of estrogen vaginal cream can be effective in maintaining lubrication and distensibility and preventing vaginitis, dyspareuria, and burning on urination. Because estrogen is absorbed via the vaginal mucosa, the same concerns that apply to treatment with oral estrogens may be relevant to this treatment.

Hormone Replacement Therapy. Administration of estrogen and progestin reverses the vasomotor symptoms, and use of a gradually decreasing dose avoids severe symptoms. Hormone treatment also reduces the risk of heart disease and osteoporosis. Such treatment may prolong occurrence of the symptoms and may be of little assistance in treating emotional symptoms except as a placebo (76, 107, 108).

Some middle-aged women whose vaginal smears show changes in vaginal cells—decreased number, small and round instead of large and quadrilateral, blue instead of pink, thinning, drying, inflamed, and scant in acid secretion—are described as *estrogen-dependent,* or *estrogen-sensitive.* Such a woman's mental and physical well-being has previously depended on a high level of estrogen, as manifested by the following signs: she had optimum feeling of well-being during pregnancy when estrogen level was high, depression several weeks after delivery when the estrogen level fell to normal, and great improvement of vasomotor and psychic symptoms associated with estrogen administration when approach-

ing menopause. If a trial dose of estrogen shows improvement physically and emotionally, this woman is a candidate for long-term low-dose estrogen treatment to improve the metabolic state, postpone and reduce osteoporosis, and promote a feeling of well-being (14, 76, 107). Studies also indicate that women have reduced heart disease because of this natural supply of estrogen. Prolonged estrogen therapy (more than 10 years) predisposes to cancer of the breast and endometrium, hypertension, myocardial infarction, and cerebrovascular accident. Thus women should take estrogen in the lowest possible doses and be carefully monitored. Breast carcinoma is the principal cause of death from cancer in women, with the highest mortality rate occurring between ages 55 and 74 (48, 121). Long-term studies have shown that the rise in incidence of endometrial cancer from the mid-1960s through mid-1970s was related to increased use of replacement estrogen treatment. With more careful estrogen prescription, there has been an associated decline in incidence rates of endometrial cancer in the United States (3, 53, 99).

Reinforce in the middle-aged woman that hormonal changes are normal, that they can be adapted to and lived with. Support groups may be helpful. Emphasize that estrogen products, whether facial and skin products or vaginal creams, should be purchased with medical guidance; likewise, replacement therapy is done only when deemed by the physician as essential.

All women receiving estrogen replacement therapy because ovaries were surgically removed or to relieve menopausal symptoms should be seen every 6 to 12 months for a Papanicolaou test, breast examination, and blood pressure reading. All menopausal women should be taught that any abnormal bleeding (if receiving estrogen-progestin therapy) or spotting 12 months after cessation of menses indicates an increased risk of carcinoma and should be reported immediately to a physician.

Metabolic Changes

Metabolic changes include decalcification and resorption of the bones, producing decreased bone density and a gradual osteoporosis. Osteoporosis occurs particularly in women who are underweight and small boned but also because women generally have bones with less density and they lose bone at an accelerated rate for 3 to 7 years after menopause. Cultural differences also exist. Caucasians and Orientals are more likely than Latinos and African-Americans to suffer bone porosity because their bones are generally smaller and lose mass more quickly. The bones of African-Americans have 10% greater density than those of Caucasians. The following men and women are at risk regardless of cultural background: people with low dietary calcium intakes, those who lead sedentary life-styles, and those who smoke and have high alcohol and caffeine intake (caffeine increases loss of calcium).

With the bone porosity and gradually shrinking intervertebral disks, the woman will eventually be 1 or 2 inches shorter, and the "dowager's hump" will form in the cervical upper thoracic area. By age 55 a woman runs 10 times the risk of bone fractures as the 55-year-old man. Most vulnerable to fractures are forearms, hips, and spinal vertebrae (7, 17, 48, 54, 133).

Some of the changes in the woman result because the level of androgen in the body remains constant while the estrogen is decreasing. Thus the woman is dismayed to find a small amount of hair growth, especially on the chin. She also experiences a loss of weight in the face and limbs at a time when diminishing muscle tone and additional adipose deposits make her look and feel larger in the middle. The coarseness of skin and sharpness of contours are the result of loss of some subcutaneous tissue (48).

Teaching should encompass safety and nutritional and exercise measures to prevent fractures. A confirmed diagnosis of postmenopausal osteoporosis and a demonstration of calcium malabsorption or intestinal lactose deficiency require the following diet supplementation: 1 to 2 g daily of elementary calcium alone or with 50,000 U of vitamin D or with no more than 60 mg daily of sodium fluoride may decrease the annual rate of cortical bone loss (132). Ideally nutrition and exercise are used before the midlife years to prevent or reduce osteoporotic effects.

Other Changes

Cell atrophy and changes in cell regulation and repair cause the number of cells to reduce gradually after approximately 30 years. The body starts to shrink minutely. Muscle mass decreases by 10% to 12% between the ages of 30 and 65 years. A gradual loss in efficiency of nerve conduction and muscle function contributes to gradual muscle atrophy and impaired sensation to heat and cold.

Changes also occur in the *special senses* (e.g., dimming of vision). **Presbyopia,** a *decreasing elasticity of the lens and decreasing power of accommodation,* occurs in middle age so that the person reads the morning paper at arm's length. The pupil takes in half as much light at 50 as at 20 years. Pupils react more slowly in late middle age. Glasses are often needed, but self-consciousness can delay getting the needed visual aid. Some degree of hearing is also gradually lost, especially for high-pitched sounds. Auditory reaction time slows; sound discrimination decreases. Other sensory acuity remains intact (28, 76, 108).

The *decreasing elasticity of blood vessels,* particularly in the coronary arteries, increases the middle-aged person's susceptibility to hypertension and cardiovascular disease. The woman becomes as prone to coronary disease as the man after the menopause; thus estrogen is an apparent protective agent. Serum cholesterol levels rise after the menopause, but administration of estrogen alters the serum cholesterol, alpha-lipoproteins, and cholesterol-phospholipid ratio to retard the process of atherosclerosis. Cardiac output and glomerular filtration rate gradually decrease (76, 108).

Tooth decay is not caused by aging but chiefly by circulatory changes, poor dietary habits, poor mouth hygiene, or poor dental care over the years. Hence the middle-aged person may have dentures or a partial plate or need dental care either for dental caries or periodontal disease.

You are in a key position to help the middle-aged adult work through feelings about the meaning of midlife changes and ways to prevent or minimize their effects.

Emotional Changes Related to Physical Changes

Depression, irritability, and a change in sexual desire may occur in response to physical changes and their meaning, but they do not automatically occur. Some women fear loss of sexual identity. Severe symptoms occur in fewer than 10% of women, so these symptoms may be minor and little noticed. Earlier personality patterns and attitudes are more responsible for the symptomatology than the cessation of glandular activity. Women who had previous low self-esteem and life satisfaction are more likely to have difficulties with menopause. Reactions to menopause are consistent with reactions to other life changes, including other reproductive turning points such as puberty. Women with high motherliness scores and heavy investment in childbearing react more severely to the menopause (54, 72, 100, 108).

Reactions to menopause vary across social classes and according to the availability of alternate roles. Middle- and upper-class women appear to find the cessation of childbearing more liberating than lower-class women, perhaps because more alternatives are open to them. In the relatively advantaged social classes younger women anticipating menopause express the most concern. Postmenopausal women generally take a more positive view than premenopausal women, agreeing that the menopause creates no major discontinuity in life and, except for the underlying biologic changes, women have a relative degree of control over their symptoms and need not inevitably have difficulties. In general, menopausal status is not associated consistently with measurable anxiety in any group (34, 54, 108).

Studies of normal women in middle age from working- and middle-class backgrounds who were in good physical health, married, and had at least one child showed that these women saw the menopause as a normal life event rather than as a threat to feminine identity. They minimized the significance of the menopause and regarded it as unlikely to cause much anxiety or stress. Some believed health improved after menopause, and 65% believed there was no effect on sex life. Any changes in sexual activity during the climacterium was seen as a function of the woman's (or couple's) attitudes. Half reported sexual relations as more enjoyable because menstruation and fear of pregnancy were removed. Few reported having symptoms sufficient to seek medical treatment, although 75% reported minor discomforts. A majority believed change in health or emotional status during the menopause reflected individual differences in coping with stress or idiosyncrative factors. Only 4 of the 100 regarded the menopause as a major source of worry. Women who had difficulties with the menarche, menses, or pregnancy were more likely to have menopausal problems. More than half indicated that the death of the husband was the greatest concern; other concerns were fear of cancer and the implications of getting older. In general, 80% attributed little or no change in their lives to menopause. Most believed the woman had control over the symptoms and need not have symptomatic difficulties (34, 88, 90, 108).

Cross-cultural studies of the male climacteric have not been done. A construction worker who gauges his age by physical strength may feel middle-aged or old before he reaches 40 or 45. The factory worker may not have as many frustrations of unattainable goals as a white-collar worker and thus may be less likely to undergo a midlife crisis. Another manual laborer who feels oppressed by his foreman and stifled by his job may fear the day when physical powers decline and he may lose his only source of security—his job. The African-American man apparently experiences a midlife crisis much like that of the Caucasian man. Bachelors and widowers who may be lonely and lack the warmth of family ties frequently suffer at least temporary loss of libido in the middle years and symptoms of midlife crisis related to fears of mortality and the meaninglessness of their life. Some men may experience again a long-dormant homosexual interest (57).

Refer to Chapter 12, pp. 466 to 467, for ways to help the person work through self-concept and body image changes and for ways to enhance self-concept.

Nutritional Needs

Basal metabolic rate gradually decreases by 2% every decade after age 20. For each decade after 25 years, there should be a reduction in caloric intake proportionate to activity level (132). The reduced basal energy requirements caused by losses in functioning protoplasm and the frequently reduced physical activity combine to create less demand for calories.

Teach that intake of carbohydrate and foods with high fat, saturated fat, and cholesterol content should be reduced, including the foods with "empty" calories: rich desserts, candies, fatty foods, gravies, sauces, and alcoholic and cola beverages. Intake of salty food should be limited; herbs, spices, and lemon juice can be used for flavoring. Overweight is not just a genetic factor (92) and should be avoided since it is a factor in diabetes, and cardiovascular, and hypertensive disease and in problems with mobility such as arthritis.

Dietary intake will be imbalanced nutritionally if meals are not wisely planned. For the healthy person daily diet should contain all of the food groups found in a variety of foods, with emphasis on protein, minerals, vitamins, low-cholesterol and low-calorie foods, and fiber. Refer to Box 12–2 for recommended daily servings (51, 102, 132). Plenty of fluids, especially water and juices, along with an adequate diet, will maintain weight control and vigor and help prevent "heartburn," constipation, and other minor discomforts caused by physiologic changes. Equally important, the person should chew food well, eat smaller portions, eat in a pleasant and unhurried atmosphere, and avoid eating when overtired.

There is no evidence that use of commercial vitamin-mineral preparations is necessary unless they are prescribed by a physician because of clinical signs of deficiency and insufficient diet. Adequate calcium intake is essential for both men (1000 mg/day) and women (1200 to 1500 mg/day; 2000 mg/day for the postmenopausal woman who is not treated with estrogen). Note that one glass of milk contains 300 mg of calcium, although there are many other sources of calcium (51, 98, 132) (see Appendix I).

Considerable information is available to the public about healthful nutrition; yet the American diet remains overloaded with sugar-filled and fatty foods. Only as values change will diet change. Health teaching must begin with understanding cultural concepts and values before a significant trend toward wise eating habits can begin. Joining self-help groups such as Weight Watchers or Take Off Pounds Sensibly (TOPS) is effective for many people. It is possible to change habits of overeating and to lose weight in middle age.

Teach the middle-aged person to avoid using extreme diets to decrease weight quickly and to avoid repeatedly losing weight that is then regained. Each gain-lose cycle reduces the total muscle mass with weight loss and increases body fat since regained weight is in the form of adipose tissue. Adipose tissue burns fewer calories than muscle, so each round of dieting makes it more difficult to lose weight and maintain weight loss. Extreme low-calorie diets should also be avoided because with them, the basic metabolic rate becomes lower so that, even with restricted calories, little weight is lost. Thus to lose weight it is essential to exercise—at least moderately for 40 minutes a day—and eat a healthy high-fiber, low-fat diet (see Box 13–2) (51, 54, 132).

Rest and Exercise

Middle age need not be a time when a person's body fails, but it is a period that requires better maintenance than was necessary in the earlier years.

Exercise

Exercise and erect posture may not increase longevity but they will enhance quality of life by keeping people healthy and independent (Fig. 13–1). A combination of the following activities appears optimum: brisk walking,

■ BOX 13-2.
Healthy-Eating Plan for the Middle-Aged Adult

Go Nutrient Dense and High Fiber

- Buy cereals that give you a larger portion for the calories.
- Serve meals loaded with complex carbohydrates such as pasta, rice (brown for more fiber), barley, and potatoes.
- Be creative with your potato toppings—plain yogurt mixed with herbs, picante sauce, or melted low-fat cheese.
- Use meats such as lean beef and skinless turkey and chicken not as the biggest part of the meal but more as condiments. Serve them in 2- to 3-ounce portions.
- Use romaine lettuce in salads instead of the pale, anemic-looking variety. Romaine lettuce has approximately eight times more vitamin A and double the iron of iceberg lettuce.
- Serve an iron-rich plant food such as a legume or dried fruit with a vitamin-C–rich food such as citrus fruit. Vitamin C helps your body use the iron more efficiently.
- Chop fruits and vegetables as little as possible, cook them just a short time, and minimize standing time. A number of vitamins are destroyed by air, light, and heat.
- Choose dark-green and bright orange vegetables and fruits. They tend to have more nutrients than the paler plant foods. One half cup of cooked, chopped broccoli, for instance, has more than double the vitamin A and eight times more vitamin C than the same amount of lighter green beans.
- Choose plain, low-fat yogurt and add your own fruit.
- Steam foods rather than cook them in large amounts of water, which can leach away important nutrients.
- Select whole-grain products more often than refined ones.
- Try to avoid empty calories (those giving you few nutrients) such as those found in alcohol or in desserts such as cake or pie.
- Work more fiber into your meals with peas and beans—mix them with rice or pasta, use them in meatless chili, or sprinkle them on salads.

Cut the Fat

- Reduce fat in the diet by eating ordinary foods and cutting back on just four things: fat used in prepared foods and in cooking, oils, red meats, and whole milk dairy products. These measures will reduce fat intake to approximately 20% of caloric intake.
- Avoid fried foods. Simulate the crunch of fried foods by oven- frying. For instance, dip fish or chicken in egg whites and then in bread or cracker crumbs and bake on a nonstick cookie sheet at 300°–350° F until done; or slice potatoes into spears and bake in the oven at 350° F for 30 min.
- Invest in a large nonstick frying pan that uses little or no oil when sautéing or pan frying. Lightly coat regular pans and casseroles with nonstick vegetable spray.
- Experiment with low-fat, low-calorie flavor enhancers such as Dijon mustard, horseradish, chopped green or red peppers, onions, and seasonings such as tarragon, dry mustard, dill, and curry powder.
- Chill sauces, gravies, and stews ahead of time so the hardened fat can be skimmed from the surface.
- Make sauces without fat by slowly mixing cold liquid directly into the flour or cornstarch. Stir until smooth and bring to a boil, stirring frequently.
- Use evaporated skimmed milk instead of cream in coffee and recipes.
- In place of sour cream, use low-fat or nonfat yogurt or low- fat cottage cheese that has been mixed in a blender with a little milk and lemon juice.

Ease More Fish Into Meals

- Try fish in your favorite meat and chicken recipes.
- Do not overcook fish. Cook fish for approximately 10 mins per inch of thickness—be it on the grill, under the broiler, or in an oven preheated to 450° F.
- Be creative—serve fish and shellfish in soups, salads, stews, pasta, and stirfry dishes.

Boost Milk Intake (Without Drinking a Drop)

If your system is not lactose intolerant, but you prefer not to drink milk as a beverage:

- Sneak nonfat dry milk powder into anything you can: soups, sauces, casseroles, meat loaf, and stews. Add a few teaspoons of it to coffee; this blend will taste like café au lait.
- Treat yourself to low-calorie puddings made with skim or low- fat milk.
- Make milk-based soups with skim milk.
- Use a blender to make a low-fat milk shake with a few ice cubes, skim or low-fat milk, fresh fruit, and low-calorie sweetner.
- Experiment with fun flavorings in low-fat milk—vanilla, rum extract, or even cocoa with a little artificial sweetner.
- Have cold breakfast cereals with milk and fresh fruit.
- In coffee or tea try low-fat milk instead of cream. If that is not palatable, try evaporated skim milk.

---

stretching, weight bearing, bicycling, rowing, swimming, aerobics, and resistance activities. Such exercise maintains muscle mass and strength; improves coordination and agility; stimulates bone formation and increased bone size and density; improves cardiovascular function and circulation; maintains body flexibility and collagen tissue elasticity; promotes deeper respirations; and promotes weight loss. In fact, the more a person exercises, the less will be his or her percentage of body fat, regardless of age (17, 48, 54, 133).

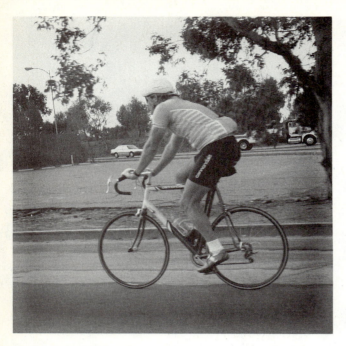

Figure 13-1.   Middle-aged adults should be encouraged to partici-
pate in healthy behaviors such as exercising. (From Berger, K.J., and
M.B. Williams. *Fundamentals of Nursing: Collaborating for Optimal
Health.* Norwalk, Conn: Appleton & Lange, 1992, 314.)

velopmental impetus and opportunities for personal
growth.

The middle-aged adult invests considerable energy
in occupational, home, and organizational activity and
in leisure-time pursuits. He or she often has fine physical
health. Although chronic disease is more prevalent than
in the young, there is ordinarily good resistance to communicable diseases, superior emotional stamina, and a
willingness to work despite minor illnesses. The person
brings economy of effort, singleness of purpose, and
perseverance to various roles.

Teach that, although physical changes do occur,
adopting sedentary habits will not maintain health. Balanced with rest and sleep must be physical activity to
keep the body posture and functioning at its optimum.
Capacity for intense and sustained effort diminishes, especially if engaged in irregularly, but judicious exercise
may modify and retard the aging process. In addition to
the physical benefits, regular and vigorous exertion is an
excellent outlet for emotional tensions. Even a half-hour
of brisk walking three times a week promotes better
health (102).

Teach about the value of exercise. The type of exercise does not matter as long as the person *likes* it, engages in it *regularly,* and it is *suitable* for personal
strength and physical condition. The middle-aged person should take certain precautions: (1) gradually increase the exercise until it is moderate in strenuousness,
(2) exercise consistently, and (3) avoid overexertion.
Ten minutes after strenuous exercise, the heart should
be beating normally again, respirations should be normal, and there should be no sense of fatigue. If the person is overweight, has a personal or family history of
cardiovascular disease, or has led a sedentary life, new
exercise routines should not be started until after a thorough physical checkup (54). Using exercise as an over-
compensation to prove youthfulness, health status, or
prevent old age is pointless. The person may benefit
from enrolling in an exercise program that is directed by
a health professional.

Sleep

Most middle-aged adults sleep without difficulty; the 7
to 8 hours of sleep comprise a normal pattern. Refer to
Chapter 12 for more information on normal sleep patterns. However, one kind of sleep disturbance—sleep
apnea—in middle age is being studied to a greater extent.

Sleep apnea, *more than five episodes of cessation
of air flow for at least 10 seconds each hour of sleep,* is
a problem that is being increasingly recognized. This
syndrome is found primarily in men over 50 and
postmenopausal women. Thirty-five to 40% of the elderly suffer sleep apnea. Often it is first detected because the person snores loudly or does daytime dozing.
Sleep apnea can be life threatening. There are three
types:

One of the most stable characteristics is *activity
level.* Although there is a general and gradual decline in
quickness and level of activity during the latter part of
life, people who were most active among their age
group during adolescence and young adulthood usually
are the most active among their age group during middle and old age. It is almost as though each person has
a physical and mental "clock" that runs at a fast or slow
rate throughout life. The rate at which an individual's
clock runs is reflected as well in various cognitive and
personality characteristics.

The physical strength of the man peaks around 21
and gradually diminishes to the late sixties when degenerative diseases begin to increase. (However, regular exercise maintains strength to a greater extent.) The ardu-
ous training program of the astronauts, a number of
whom have been over age 40, has shown that a man can
double his normal physical competence at ages much
beyond 21.

There is frequently a postmenopausal rise in energy
and activity possibly for several reasons (108). Less time
and energy go into child rearing. The children's leaving
home allows time for self and pursuits in creative, social,
or community projects. The person may feel more self-
confident and satisfied with life achievements and less
competitive. Less physical and psychic energy may be
used in various internal conflicts or in worrying unnecessarily about the details in life. New self-awareness and
flexibility can increase psychic and physical energy and
a feeling of well-being. This new energy permits a de-

1. Obstructive—respiratory effort continues despite pharyngeal obstruction to air flow
2. Central—no respiratory effort with air flow
3. Mixed—episodes of no respiratory effort initially are followed by respiratory effort and then air flow

The person may have the following symptoms: (1) excessive daytime sleepiness, (2) frequent nocturnal awakening, (3) insomnia, (4) loud snoring, (5) morning headaches, (6) intellectual deterioration, (7) irritability and personality changes, (8) impotence, (9) hypertension, and (10) arrhythmias. Weaver and Millman (127) give a detailed description of the signs and symptoms, associated physical conditions in pathology, diagnostic measures, and treatment. Refer also to Chapter 12 for more information.

Health Promotion and Health Protection

Injury and Accidents

The gradually changing physical characteristics and preoccupation with responsibilities may contribute to the middle-aged person's having accidents.

Fractures and dislocations are the leading cause of injuries for both sexes, with more men affected than women, probably because of occupational differences. Because of the middle-aged adult's changing physical abilities, motor vehicle accidents are the most common cause of accidental deaths in the later years, especially for men. Occupation-related accidents rank second, and falls in the home rank third as causes of death. However, women suffer less than one third as frequently as men from fatal falls during the middle years (76).

The middle-aged adult is a person at work in an industry, office, school, home, or out-of-doors. Accidents that disable for 1 week or more sharply increase for the worker after age 45 (32). Because of their interest in accident-protection legislation, industries and other occupational settings are increasingly health and safety conscious. Efforts must continue in this direction.

As a nurse you can teach about safety as it relates to remodeling a home, maintaining a yard, or establishing a work center. Handrails for stairways; a handgrip at the bathtub; conveniently located electric outlets; indirect, nonglare, and thorough lighting; and tools, equipment, and home or yard machines kept in proper working condition all provide ways to avoid an accident, especially in later middle age. Sensible middle-aged people plan for the gradual failing of their physical abilities by making the home as safe, convenient, and comfortable as possible as they rethink homemaking functions for the coming decades. Further, you can be instrumental in initiating or strengthening a safety program in an occupational or school setting.

Illness Prevention

Middle age is not automatically a period of physical or psychologic hazard or disease. No single disease or mental condition necessarily is related to the passage of time, according to an American Medical Association Subcommittee on Aging, although the middle-aged person should be carefully assessed for signs of illness (102). Major health problems of this era are cardiovascular disease, cancer, pulmonary disease, diabetes, obesity, alcoholism, anxiety, depression, and glaucoma.

You can help the person maintain energy and improve health by teaching the information presented in this chapter. The person can learn to moderate eating, drinking, or smoking habits and to use only medically prescribed drugs. Many measures promote health: regular physical examinations (see Appendix IV), pursuit of leisure activity, use of relaxation techniques, working through the emotional and family concerns related to middle age, affirming the worth of self as a middle-aged person, preparing for the later years, and confronting developmental tasks. The person also needs to prepare for possible accidents or illness.

Teach that the mounting statistical, experimental, and autopsy findings point to cigarette smoking as a causative factor in breast and lung cancer, cardiovascular disease, chronic obstructive pulmonary disease, and peptic ulcer. For the person who feels trapped, depressed, frustrated, or isolated, easily accessible escapes are alcoholism, drugs, or excess food intake. Assist the person in finding other ways to cope with stressors (86).

The medicine cabinet may look like a pharmaceutical display if the self-absorbed person retreats into hypochondriasis. Old injuries may become bothersome, and new injuries do not heal as quickly. Illness or accident proneness can also be a means of resolving serious difficulties or of escaping responsibilities. If understanding and help from others are negligible or nonexistent and the possibility of recouping losses or rearranging one's life seems unlikely, the brief care and attention given during illness or after injury may not offer sufficient gratification. Suicidal thoughts and attempted or actual suicide are a call for help or an escape from problems (86). The prop of ill health should not be removed without study and caution, for removing one syndrome may only result in discharge of emotional tension through another physical or emotional syndrome. Thus nursing intervention and medical treatment must be directed toward both physical and emotional factors.

Because nursing care is holistic, you can meet emotional and spiritual needs of the person while giving physical care and doing health teaching related to common health problems discussed in the following pages.

Common Health Problems: Prevention and Treatment

A variety of health problems may occur, although many middle-aged adults remain healthy. Refer to Table 13–2 for a summary of diseases that are frequently experienced and to a medical-surgical nursing text for more information on the following diseases.

TABLE 13-2. COMMON HEALTH PROBLEMS IN MIDDLE AGE

Problem	Definition	Symptoms/Signs	Prevention/Treatment
Sinusitis, nonbacterial and bacterial	Inflammation of mucous membrane lining paranasal sinuses; may be caused by bacteria, viruses, irritants, or allergies	Normal sinus drainage prohibited. Usually clear drainage in nonbacterial type. Purulent drainage in bacterial type, with fever (headache and tenderness of frontal and maxillary sinus to palpation frequent with bacterial involvement)	Oral antihistimine and decongestant for nonbacterial type. Addition of antibiotic for bacterial type
Hiatal hernia with esophagitis	Herniation of stomach through diaphragm with reflux of acid into esophagus	Substernal pain, usually worse when bending over or lying down. Sometimes nausea and vomiting	Maintenance of ideal weight. Avoidance of tight clothing. Eat frequently in small amounts. Elevation of head of bed
Duodenal peptic ulcer disease	Ulceration of duodenal mucosa	Pain in the epigastrum or right upper quadrant usually 1–2 hr after meals	Antacids or prescription drugs (e.g., cimetidine [Tagamet]). Small frequent meals. Avoidance of caffeine, alcohol, and spices
Angina pectoris	Imbalance between oxygen needed by myocardium and oxygen supplied	Pain in substernal region but sometimes in neck, back, and arms	Workup to determine accurate diagnosis. Nitroglycerin
Secondary hypertension	High blood pressure based on specific cause	Blood pressure >150/100	Following treatment plan based on cause of high blood pressure. Reduction of sodium and cholesterol in diet. Reduction of weight as needed. Relaxation techniques
Hyperthyroidism (Graves' disease)	Too much secretion of thyroid hormone	Can mimic heart problems with accelerated or irregular heart beat. Feeling of agitation	Antithyroid medications or radioactive iodine therapy
Hyperuricemia or Gout	High uric acid level, causing acute inflammatory arthritis (can also be chronic)	Usually red, hot tender joint; often in great toe but can be in other joints	Specific drugs. Rest. Elevation of joint(s). Cold compresses
Diabetes type II	Glucose intolerance corrected by means other than insulin	High blood sugar. Thirsty. Weight loss. Frequent urination	Diet. Exercise. Oral medication
Prostatitis, acute	Acute infection of prostate gland; often caused by organism *Escherichia coli*	Low back and perineal pain referred sometimes to inguinal region and testes. Extremely tender prostate	Sitz baths. Appropriate antibiotics
Prostatitis, chronic	Prolonged inflammation of prostate	Only slightly tender and enlarged prostate	Prostatic massage. Sitz baths. Increased sexual activity
Lumbosacral strain, mild	Strain and inflammation of ligaments and musculature in lumbosacral region	Muscle spasm over region but no radiation. No flank pain. Negative result from straight leg raising	Cold packs. Muscle relaxant medication. Analgesic. Bed rest. Chiropractic treatment. Education in bending and lifting techniques. Use of firm mattress

Respiratory conditions are a frequent cause for days absent from work. Generally middle-aged women have more disability days from work because of respiratory and other acute disorders; men have more disability days from injuries (56, 102).

Foot balance, the *ability to alter one's position so that body weight is carried through the foot with minimum effort,* is essential to prevent strain, foot aches and pain. Foot imbalance may result from contracted toes, improper position, size or shape of one or more bones of the foot, weak or rotating ankles, muscle strain, weak ligaments, poor body posture, overweight, arthritis, injuries, and improperly fitted or shaped shoes. Treatment by a podiatrist consists of careful assessment of the posture and provision of balance inlays for insertion into the shoes (135).

A **callus,** *thickening of the outer layers of the skin on the sole of the foot,* is formed in areas of excess pressure and friction. Calluses become painful when congestion and swelling from them press on nerve endings and underlying bursa become inflamed.

Foot problems may occur in middle age. Teach the person to observe for the following common signs of need for diagnostic evaluation and possible treatment (135):

1. Swelling of the feet and ankles
2. Cramps in the feet and the calf while walking or at night
3. Inability to keep the feet warm
4. Loss of the fat tissue on the padded surfaces of the feet
5. Chronic ulcers on the feet that fail to respond to treatment
6. Absence of or bounding pulse in the arteries of the feet
7. Showing of arteries in the foot on routine x-ray film
8. Burning in the soles of the feet.

Foot care should include the following:

1. Clean the feet with soap and water at least once daily; dust with foot powder or cornstarch.
2. Exercise the feet, extend the toes, and then flex rapidly for 1 or 2 minutes. Rotate the feet in circles at the ankles. Try picking up a pencil or marble with toes.
3. Walk barefoot on uneven surfaces, thick grass, or sandy beach.
4. Walk daily and properly. Keep toes pointed ahead and lift rather than push the foot, letting it come down flat on the ground, placing little weight on the heel.
5. Massage the feet to rest them after a tiring day.
6. Lie down with feet higher than head for approximately $\frac{1}{2}$ hour daily.
7. Avoid wearing poorly fitted shoes or shoes with high heels and pointed toes.

Teach that the callus or other foot problems should be treated by a podiatrist. If the person scrapes or cuts a callus, there is risk of infection (135).

Abnormal Pap smear findings in an asymptomatic female are reported as follows: suggesting inflammatory reaction, somewhat suggestive of malignancy, highly suggestive of malignancy, "diagnostic" of malignancy (56). The inflammatory changes should be treated after appropriate diagnostic workup. A Pap smear should be repeated 6 to 8 weeks after treatment; 90% of women with mild dysplasia revert to normal. Women who have

other findings are treated with medication, surgery, or radiation, as indicated, after thorough diagnostic study.

Sexual dysfunction, *severely diminished or absent orgasmic response,* may result from alcoholism, obesity, preoccupation with career or finances, mental or physical fatigue, boredom, fear of failing sexually, or chronic illness related to impaired circulation or neuropathy. For example, in one study of diabetic men, more than half of them were impotent, probably because of autonomic neuropathy involving the sacral parasympathetic fibers that supply the penis and bladder. Vascular disease affects potency because a high volume of blood flow is necessary to distend the vascular spaces of erectile tissue. Occlusion of the pudendal arteries or their tributaries may result in impotence. Hypertension with a blood pressure of 180/110 constitutes a contraindication to coitus because of increased risk of strokes. Antihypertensive drugs, other than diuretics, may cause impotence or inhibition of ejaculation. A past myocardial infarction may limit physical activity of any kind, but after a period of recovery most coronary patients resume sexual relations. Although hysterectomy does not affect sex drive, oophorectomy may because of the hormonal changes. However, hormone replacement may return sex drive. Adrenalectomy has a negative effect on libido because hormone production is diminished. Most men retain potency after prostatectomy unless the surgical approach has been through the sex-related nerve centers. If the prostate is malignant and surgery more radical, however, the man's possibilities of retaining potency are not as favorable (77). Increased expectations in this age of sexual liberation may also increase sexual problems along with other marital problems.

The middle-aged person may subtly, hesitantly, or openly discuss problems of sexual function with you. Listen carefully. Let the person know that such problems are not unusual. You may not know the answers, but your listening can help the person make a decision to seek medical care or counseling, realize the need to change behavior, or assist in attitude and value clarification about sexuality and sexual behavior. Refer the person or couple to a counselor who can help with physical and emotional problems. Your discussion with the physician of the person's problems with changed libido or impotence can also be helpful. Sometimes a change in medication dosage or modification in treatment regimen can reduce sexual dysfunction.

PSYCHOSOCIAL CONCEPTS

Factors That Influence Research Findings on Cognitive Ability

Because most studies on adult cognition have been cross-sectional, caution is necessary in interpreting the results since many factors are influential. For the middle-aged person especially, amount of education, experiential differences, fixed attitudes, the number of years since formal schooling was completed, and the general health status may negatively influence test scores. Because most intelligence tests are developed for children and adolescents, the kind of subtest given can influence the scores. The middle-aged adult scores higher on tests that require general information or vocabulary abilities. At age 60 intelligence quotient (IQ) test results are equal to or better than those of young adults. Only arithmetic reasoning shows a plateau through the adult years. Speed requirements of the test may mitigate against the IQ test scores; adults show a peak in speed of performance in the twenties and a gradual decrease in overall speed of performance through the years. Adults usually value accuracy and thoroughness more than speed (24, 28, 130).

In various studies physically fit and active men were found to have a higher intelligence score than men who engaged in little physical activity (24, 28, 103).

In the early 1970s Kangas and Bradway (63) did a 38-year follow-up study of people tested for intelligence as preschoolers, junior high school students, young adults, and early middle-aged adults. They found an increase in IQ across the four testing periods, indicating continued mental growth during middle age and possibly even beyond. Interesting sex differences emerged from these findings. Women whose IQs had been high as children gained less than those with medium or low preadult IQs and less than men with any level of preadult IQ. On the other hand, the higher the level of a man's preadult IQ, the greater was his adult gain. These findings have interesting implications in light of the theory that bright women fear success. Women who tested so high as girls inhibited their intellectual potential later in life. The recent study by the American Association of University Women reveals the same results (80). The phenomenon of different educational processes and expectations has meant that society in general and specific women both lost the benefit of talent and ability.

In the past decade more middle-aged women have returned to college for baccalaureate, graduate, doctoral, and post-doctoral degrees. They have shown themselves as capable as men scholastically and in applying intellectual ability in the workplace.

Cognitive Development

Cognitive processes in adulthood include reaction time, perception, memory, learning and problem solving, and creativity.

Reaction time or *speed of performance* is individual and generally stays the same or diminishes during late middle age. The speed of response is important primarily in test situations since much of the problem solving necessary in adulthood requires deliberation and accuracy rather than speed. Reaction time is related to complexity of the task, the habitual pattern of response to stimuli, and familiarity with the task. Time for new learning increases with age, but adults in their forties and fifties have the same ability to learn as they did in their twenties and thirties (24).

Memory is maintained through young and middle adulthood; no major age differences are evident. Some quantitative changes may occur. For example, a person in early adulthood who could recite a 10-digit span of numbers as a series of discrete units may recite eight digits grouped or categorized in late middle age. The ability to categorize or group information, to sharpen observational skills and give more attention to the phenomenon, to relate meaning to that to be remembered, and to use interactive imagery—imagining events in a story form with self in the interaction—are all ways to strengthen memory and aid learning (130). The middle-aged adult memorizes less readily material that is not well organized and seems to retain less from oral presentation of information than younger students (28). Travis (119) maintains that memory is not reliable in the adult years—or at any age. Most people forget or ignore episodes that do not fit the self-image or that are considered unimportant. People who think they remember an event from childhood or a number of years previously may be making up plausible scenarios, fantasies, or confabulations based on earlier reports or stories. The middle-aged adult who continues to use memory will retain a keen memory (130).

Learning occurs in adults of all ages. The highly intelligent person becomes even more learned. The capacity for intellectual growth is unimpaired and is enhanced by interest, motivation, flexibility, a sense of humor, confidence, and maturity attained through experience. Learning means more; it is not just learning for learning's sake. Knowledge is applied; motivation to learn is high for personal reasons. Reluctance to learn occurs if the new material does not appear relevant or does not serve the person as well as current information (24, 28, 130).

Problem-solving abilities remain throughout adulthood. There are no significant differences between 20-, 40-, and 60-year-olds in learning a task. Generally, better educated people perform better than less educated people in any age group. When there is no time limitation, there are no task differences in complex task solutions because young and middle-aged adults use different strategies. Young adults, knowing they can function quickly, may be more likely to use less efficient reasoning strategies such as trial and error. In late middle age, because people know they are becoming slower, they tend to think a problem through first so they can solve it in fewer tries (24, 28, 130).

The middle-aged adult is able to do all the cognitive strategies of Piaget's Stage of Formal Operations described in Chapters 11 and 12. Sometimes the practicality of a situation will call forth use of Concrete Operations; because not all problems in life can be solved by abstract reasoning, the middle-aged adult does both Operations realistically in problem solving. He or she also uses the fifth stage of cognitive development, problem finding, described in Chapter 11. Societal, occupational, and general life experiences are crucial to cognitive operations of the middle-aged person. Thus perceptions about the same situation, problem, or task can vary considerably in a group of middle-aged adults (125).

Cognitive characteristics that are developed in the young adult are used throughout middle age as well. Various patterns mark the development of *intellectual skills*. The mature adult can symbolize experience and behaves in a way that shows organization, integration, stability, and unity in the cognitive process. Representing experience symbolically as hunches, words, thoughts, or other symbols is part of becoming mature. The person can reflect on past and current experience and can imagine, anticipate, plan, and hope. The person develops an inner private world that gives him or her resources for happiness and potential for anxiety. The person can recall past defeats and triumphs and monitor ongoing thoughts for consistency and logic. When the person solves a problem, he or she can explain how it was solved. Because the mature adult is more imaginatively productive, he or she is capable of producing more images, thoughts, and combinations of ideas, is able to use reflection to gain perspectives about life, and is aware of personal beliefs, values, motives, and powers. The mature person is increasingly interested in other persons and warm, enduring relationships and is adaptable, independent, self-driving, conscientious, enthusiastic, and purposeful. The person can reflect about personal relationships and their sources of strain and satisfaction and concomitantly understand why other persons feel and act as they do (24, 28, 33, 37, 72).

Buhler (16) implies cognitive development as she describes the maintenance and change tendencies in life. Maintenance, through the restitution of deficiencies (need satisfaction) and upholding of the system's internal order, is necessary for cognitive function to occur. Change, involving self-limited adaptation and creative expansion, is part of the cognitive development of the adult. Maintenance and change occur with different emphases in various life stages. The child develops self-limiting adaptation as he or she learns; the adolescent and adult move into creative expansion; after middle age the person assesses the past and self and wants to restore inner order; and in old age the person either continues to follow previous adaptive and creative drives or regresses to need-satisfying tendencies.

The intellectually curious have an increased need and ability to spin new syntheses and theories, to make meaningful that which seems meaningless, to coordinate hypotheses formation and testing, to be systematic at problem solving, to seek environmental diversity, and to become more subtle, differentiated, integrated, and

complex. The mature person has a progressive integration; that is, he or she is continually open, flexible, curious, and actively engaged. If cognitive efficiency becomes disrupted, a mature person is able to recover from such disorganization more quickly than an immature person, even though the two do not differ in intelligence. The mature person becomes discriminating in decisions based on the facts at hand and can postpone, suppress, or ignore. The person can analyze and judge information, even that which is personally relevant, in terms of demands of the information itself without being influenced by either personal desires or persuasive opinions of others. Thought becomes objective and judgment independent (24, 28, 33, 37, 72).

Neugarten (90) believes that the person changes both cognitively and emotionally over time as the result of accumulated experience. The person abstracts from experiences and creates more encompassing and more refined categories for interpreting events. The middle-aged person differs cognitively from the young adult in that he or she was born in a different historical era and thereby has different formative experiences. The middle-aged adult thus has a greater apperceptive mass or store of past experience by which to evaluate events or make decisions. Through the adult years perspectives and insights broaden and deepen, and attitudes and behaviors change.

Although Gould (46) focuses more on personality than cognitive development, he sees adulthood as a time of thoughtful confrontation with the self—letting go of the idealized image, the desire to be perfect, and acknowledging the realistic image of self and personal feelings. The adult continues to gain new beliefs about self and the world. Conflicts between past and present beliefs are resolved.

Assist the middle-aged adult (and others) in understanding the cognitive changes and strengths of cognitive ability. Reinforce a positive self-image related to cognitive abilities.

Creativity

Dennis (30) found an age pattern for creative output. He found that scientists show a peak activity in early and middle adulthood. Unique, original, and inventive productions are more often created in the twenties, thirties, and forties than later in life. The more a creative act depends on accumulated experience, the more likely it is to occur in middle age or later life. People are less productive in total creative output in the twenties than in the thirties and forties. Poets, novelists, and scholars gain in productivity in middle and old age, and, although quantity may decrease, quality increases as a greater proportion of crystallized intelligence is used. Some creative works cannot be produced without the benefit of years of experience and living, absorbing the wisdom of the culture, and the resultant development of new insights.

Creativity is seen not only in famous people or young people. The average middle-aged adult may have many responsibilities and stresses; however, typically he or she approaches a situation, task, or learning experience in a creative way.

You can encourage the middle-aged adult to pursue creative ideas and activities and to approach roles, responsibilities, and tasks in a creative way. Help the middle-aged adult overcome any self-consciousness about the unique cognitive response to a situation.

With increasing emphasis on continued learning, the middle-aged person is frequently enrolled in refresher courses, continuing education courses, or workshops related to occupation or profession. He or she takes college credit and noncredit courses to deal with specific problems; learn specific content; learn for fun; find an academic program necessary for changing a profession or occupation; gain more personal satisfaction; relieve boredom, loneliness, or an unhappy situation; or broaden the mind and learn for the sake of learning. Rapid technologic changes in business or the professions cause obsolescence of knowledge and skills, which also forces middle-aged persons to continue to learn.

When you are teaching, use methods that capitalize on the learning strengths of mature adults, including active discussion and role play. Deemphasize memorizing and acquisition of large amounts of new information. Assist the learner to develop cognitive strategies that will help him or her synthesize, analyze, integrate, interpret, and apply knowledge. Your major role may be in convincing the middle-aged adult and others that he or she can learn since myths to the contrary are prevalent. Further, you can enhance learning by providing a conducive environment—one that considers sensory changes. Your verbal and visual presentations must also consider the sensory changes discussed previously.

Work and Leisure Activities

Work

Consider that this person grew up under the hardships of the Depression and with the Protestant ethic. Both stressed the economic and moral importance of work. Thus work became respected and sought. Being without a job or idle was a harbinger of problems and meant being lazy and worthless. How has the middle-aged adult adjusted to mechanization, waning of the work ethic, the demise of a full day's work for a full day's pay?

If the person is fortunate enough to be in a business or profession in which he or she works successfully for self or is allowed freedom within a specialized area of work, he or she will feel goal achievement for self, family, and community. He or she will experience the dignity of being productive and will enjoy an increasing self-esteem.

Unfortunately, most middle-aged adults are not in this position. Most are employed in a system in which the only value is in the production, not the person. Furthermore, only so much production is acceptable; unions have set rules whereby no more than a specified amount can be done within a specified time.

Many middle-aged women work outside of the home; thus they are especially in the middle in terms of the demands of various roles on their time and energy. The middle-aged woman is wife, mother, homemaker, grandmother, worker, and organization member. In one study (59), 21% of the women nationally who were caregivers also had child-care responsibility; 9% had quit their jobs; and 21% had work conflict. The middle-aged woman is often in the middle in terms of two competing values: (1) that traditional care of the elderly is a family responsibility and (2) that women should be free to work outside the home if they wish. Each family member feels the repercussions as the balance of roles and responsibilities changes. More middle-aged women are working today for a variety of reasons (59):

1. Inflation and the rising cost of living
2. Changes in attitudes about gender-appropriate roles as a result of the women's movements
3. The rising divorce rate that forces the woman to become economically independent
4. Fewer children in the home
5. Use of labor-saving devices for the home that results in free time
6. Increasing educational levels that stimulate career interests
7. Expectancy of a higher standard of living

Knowing the degree of work stability, extent to which work is satisfying, and the emotional factors that have operated in the person's concept of work and in the self-concept are all important in assessing how well the middle-aged person can function as a mentally and physically healthy person. As a professional person, you will have to resolve conflicts related to the work role. Hence you are in a position to assist the middle-aged person in talking about and resolving feelings and values related to work and other activity.

Because the demands on middle-aged adults are often overwhelming— work, home, family, church, social and civic organizations—teach the following steps for effective *time management:*

1. *Do it now.* Do not procrastinate with small tasks; schedule large projects.
2. *Clear the decks—and desks.* Eliminate clutter; organize the work place for efficiency.
3. *Stick to the job.* Avoid distractions.
4. *Do one thing at a time.* Finish one task before beginning another.
5. *Plan ahead.* Assemble what is needed for a task before initiating it.
6. *Consider limitations*—your own, equipment not

available for a project, and other responsibilities that will interfere.

7. *Learn to say "No"* and *suggest someone else* who would be able to handle the situation.
8. *Anticipate delays* that are inevitable in every task.
9. *Plan an alternative* way to do the job; have backup activity if a selected task cannot be done as scheduled.
10. *Use odd times.* Shop when stores are not crowded; carry a notebook to jot ideas while you wait.

Explore with the person various options to prepare for retirement—at 55, 62, 65, 70, or 75 years (Box 13–3). Assist the person to examine risks or the worst possible scenario if an option is chosen. Examine what it will take in effort and ability to make the option happen, strategies to fall back on if the option is not successful, the support system (financial, emotional, and social) to ensure success, and personal willingness both to take the risks and to enjoy the benefits (11). A part of planning for retirement is to study the financial plans that will ensure, to the extent possible, financial security in old age.

The decade of the fifties is a point of transition in development of consciousness about retirement. Mid-dle-aged persons least likely to anticipate retirement include those who:

1. Have unfinished agendas at work.
2. Have high job satisfaction.
3. Perceive retirement as financially unfeasible.
4. Retain their health (66).

Leadership Role

The middle-aged adult's cognitive stage is in favor of his or her being a designated or an informal leader if other factors are favorable. (Usually middle-aged leaders have developed necessary qualities form childhood on, but occasionally a person does not believe that he or she has this ability until there is a measure of success in the life work.)

The *leader* usually has the following characteristics: (1) adequate socioeconomic resources; (2) higher level of education or success than majority of group to be led; (3) realistic self- concept; (4) realistic goals and ability to encourage others toward those goals; (5) high frustration tolerance; (6) ability to express negative thoughts tactfully; (7) ability to accept success or failure gracefully; (8) ability to delegate authority; (9) understanding of group needs; and (10) flexibility in meeting group needs (28, 33, 72).

The middle-aged person may demonstrate this leadership ability on the job or in community or church organizations. Women who are most successful in leadership careers are those who have little conflict in the multiple roles of career woman, mother, and wife. Their husbands' support and encouragement are major assets (108).

You can encourage or reaffirm the middle-aged person in the leadership role. As a nurse, you may also assist him or her in working through feelings or conflicts related to the work setting or the job itself.

Leisure

The middle-aged person, taught little about how to enjoy free time, is now faced with increasing amounts of leisure because of advances in technology, earlier retirement, and increased longevity. The average middle-aged adult who has moved up the pay scale and whose children may be grown will have more money and more time to take trips or try new hobbies. Yet various factors hinder use of these new opportunities: value of work learned in younger years; cultural emphasis on intellectual pursuits so that play is considered childish and a poor use of time and talents; conditioning to at least appear busy; fears of regression and not wanting to return to work; lack of previous opportunity to learn creative pursuits or hobbies; and hesitation to try something new because of fear of failure (72).

As a nurse you can help the person avoid feelings of alienation that result from inability to use leisure time. Use the following suggestions with your middle-aged clients:

■ BOX 13-3.
Career Track Options in Late Middle Age

Coast Into Retirement

Do the job but no more; collect the paycheck; enjoy the final years.

Go for Last Promotion

Campaign to obtain final reward for all that was contributed to receive public acknowledgement of the importance of work done.

Try for Great Achievement

Work to outdo the present record, and others' records so that others will see you saved the best for last.

Survive Difficult Period

Recognize the company's difficult period; learn to survive and even prosper in the challenging time.

Retire Early

Take the attractive package being offered by the company so that the years of later maturity can be enjoyed.

Start Your Own Business

If tired of working for others, go into business for self (e.g., consulting in work arena, turning hobby into business).

1. Emphasize that play and recreation are essential to a healthy life.
2. Stress the indispensability of leisure as a part of many activities, whether work or creative endeavors. Leisure is both a state of mind and use of time away from work. Have the person analyze leisure activities, whether they bring pleasure, work off frustration, make up deficits in life, or create a sense of pressure or competition.
3. Help the person recognize the interplay of physical and intellectual endeavors and the contribution of them to mental health.
4. Differentiate compulsive, competitive, and aggressive work and play from healthy, natural work and play. Intrinsic in play are spontaneity, flexibility, creativity, zest, and joy.
5. Recognize the person's creative efforts to encourage further involvement in leisure activities.
6. Educate the person about the importance of preparing for retirement.
7. Inform the person of places, courses, or workshops at which he or she can learn new creative skills and use of talents.
8. Encourage the person to enjoy change, to participate in organizations, and to initiate stimulating contacts with others.
9. Encourage the person to stop the activity when it no longer meets personal needs (32, 72).

Emotional Development

The middle years, the climacteric, is a period of self-assessment, and greater introspection—a transitional period. In middle age (and beyond) the person perceives life as time left to live rather than time since birth. Time is seen as finite; death is a possibility. Middle-aged adults clock themselves by their positions in different life contexts—changes in body, family, career—rather than by chronologic age. Time is seen in two ways: (1) time to finish what the person wants to do and (2) how much meaning and pleasure can be obtained in the time that is left (90). The person makes the often agonizing reappraisal of how achievements measure up against goals and of the entire system of values. He or she realizes that the choices of the past have limited present choices. He or she can no longer dream of infinite possibilities. The person is forced to acknowledge that he or she has worked up to or short of personal capabilities. Goals may or may not have been reached; aspirations may have to be modified. The possibility for advancement becomes more remote. The person will have to go on with ever-brighter, ever-younger men and women crowding into the competitive economic, political, and social arena. In the United States success is highly valued and is measured by prestige, wealth, or power. To be without these by middle age causes stress, and the likelihood of achieving them diminishes with age. Con-

trary to an earlier trend, however, the middle-aged adult is again being perceived as a valuable worker because of the experience and knowledge he or she can contribute. Thus he or she is less likely to be replaced on the job by a younger employee just on the basis of age. Federal legislation prohibiting age discrimination contributes to this later trend.

Developmental Crisis

The psychosexual crisis of middle age, according to Erikson (36), is generativity versus self-absorption and stagnation. **Generativity** is a *concern about providing for others that is equal to the concern of providing for the self*. If other developmental stages were managed successfully, the person has a sense of parenthood and creativity; of being vital in establishing and guiding the next generation, the arts, or a profession; of feeling needed and being important to the welfare of humankind. The person can assume the responsibility of parenthood. As a husband or wife, each can see the strengths and weaknesses of the other and combine their energies toward common goals.

A biologic parent does not necessarily get to the psychosocial stage of generativity, and the unmarried person or the person without children can be very generative.

The middle-aged person who is generative takes on the major work of providing for others, directly or indirectly. There is a sense of enterprise, productivity, mastery, charity, altruism, and perseverance. The greatest bulk of social problems and needs falls on this person who can handle the responsibilities because of personal strengths, vigor, and experience. There is a strong feeling of care and concern for that which has been produced by love, necessity, or accident. He or she can collaborate with others to do the necessary work. Ideas about personal needs and goals converge with an understanding of the social community, and the ideas guide actions taken on behalf of future generations.

The generative middle-aged adult may be a mentor to a young adult. A **mentor** is an *experienced adult with patience and understanding who befriends, guides, and counsels a less-experienced and younger adult in the work world or in a social or an educational situation*. The mentor is usually approximately 10 years older, is confident, warm, and flexible, enjoys sharing knowledge and skills, is trustworthy, and promotes psychosocial development and success of the younger person. The mentor is found in business, management, nursing, or other careers or professions, sponsoring the younger person as an associate, creating a social heir, teaching him or her as much as possible for promotion into a position, or recommending the one being mentored for advancement. Several references present more information on mentoring (5, 18, 82, 106, 124).

The person's adaptive mechanisms and superego are strong but not rigid. There is an expansion of interests and investment in that for which the person is responsible. Youth and young adults usually are self-centered. With approaching middle age and the image of one's finite existence faintly in view, the person consciously reappraises and uses self. With introspection, the self seems less important, and the words *service, love of others,* and *compassion* gain new meaning. These concepts motivate action. In church work, social work, community· fund drives, cultural or artistic efforts, the profession, or political work, the person is active and often the leader. The person's goal is to leave the world a better place in which to live. A critical problem, however, is coming to terms with accomplishments and accepting responsibility that comes with achievement. In addition, he or she must come to terms with violations of the moral codes of society (e.g., tax loopholes used by some adults) and, with superego and ego in balance, develop a constructive philosophy and honest method of operation.

Some middle-aged adults believe the most important work of the person begins after parenthood ceases and is cognitive and emotional in nature: preserving culture, maintaining the annals of history, keeping alive human judgment, maintaining human skills, preserving and skillfully contriving the instruments of civilization, and teaching all this to oncoming generations. Although the young and middle-aged adult is involved in such functions, these qualities of the human mind are best manifested in the late middle years or thereafter.

The generative person feels a sense of comfort or ease in life-style. There is realistic gratification from a job well done and from what has been given to others. He or she accepts self and the body, realizing that although acceptance of self is originally based on acceptance from others, unless he or she accepts self, he or she cannot really expect acceptance from others.

The mature middle-aged person has tested ways of doing things. He or she can draw on much experience; thus he or she may have deep sincerity, mature judgment, and a sense of empathy. He or she has a sense of values or a philosophy underlying the life, giving a sense of stability and causing him or her to be reflective and cautious. The person recognizes that one of the most generative things he or she can give to society is the life led and the way he or she lives it. Consider the following statement by a 50-year-old man:

> Those were full years—raising the kids with all its joy and frustration. I'm glad they're on their own now. This is a new stage of life. I can go fishing; Mary can go out to lunch. We have more time together for fun, and now we have more time for working at the election polls and in volunteer activities.

The middle years can be wise and felicitous, or they can be foolish and frantic, fraught with doubts and despair.

If the developmental task of generativity is not achieved, a sense of **stagnation,** or **self-absorption,** enshrouds the person (36). Thus *he or she regresses to adolescent, or younger, behavior characterized by physical and psychologic invalidism.* This person hates the aging body and feels neither secure not adept at handling self physically or interpersonally. He or she has little to offer even if so inclined. He or she operates on a slim margin and soon burns out. The person is withdrawn, resigned, isolated, introspective, and rebellious, and because of personal preoccupations, he or she is unable to give of self to others. The person becomes like a child, indulging self. Relations with others are impoverished. The fear of old age may cause regression to inappropriate youthfulness in behavior or dress, infidelity, or absence of dignity. Although the person cannot admit the normal physical changes that are occurring, they are apparent to others. He or she fools no one but self.

Certainly the opposite can occur; the middle-aged person can become resigned to inappropriate old age too soon, seeing each physical change to an exaggerated degree. The chronic defeatism and depression that result from feeling too old also isolate the person in self-pity and egocentrism. Consider the following statement by a 50-year-old woman:

> I spent all those years raising the kids and doing housework while Bob moved up the professional ladder. We talked less and less about each other, only about the kids or his job. Now the kids are gone. I should be happy, but I'm lost. I can't carry on a decent conversation with Bob. I don't have any training for a job. And I look terrible! I sit around and eat too much. I wear high collars to hide my wrinkled neck, and no cosmetics will hide the dark circles under my eyes.

When one is self-absorbed, physically, psychologically, and socially, either overpliancy or rigidity in behavior and an intolerant, ruthless, or cynical attitude may develop. This person may lack stamina, self-confidence, and a value system. Immature adults have impaired and less socially organized intellectual skills; their intellectual skills are fused by personal emotions and are coordinated in strange and unrealistic ways. The immature person seeks private self-absorption and vicarious immersion in subjective problems of others (36, 37, 72).

Yet the characteristics of the self-absorbed person are health-endeavoring attempts and reparative efforts to cope or adapt. They may or may not work well, depending on the intensity of personality characteristics and the social and physical environment.

Maturity

Because **maturity,** *being fully developed as a person,* is not a quality of life reached at any one age or for all time, the characteristics described as generativity are general guidelines. If the person is doing what is appropriate for age, situation, and culture, he or she is acting maturely for the age. Attaining feelings of maturity and independence comes later for the professional than for technical workers or laborers because of prolonged education. Also, as the person grows older, the ideal level of maturity and autonomy may recede further into the future and never be fully achieved (33, 37, 58). Maturity is the achievement of efficiently organized psychic growth predicated on integration of experiences of solving environmentally stimulated conflicts. The external environment is a potent force on the person; conflicts are primarily socially incurred. The psychosocial organization in maturity shows a cultural direction. As one ages, the psychic interests broaden and are less selfish. Part of maturity is staying power, the power to see it through, which is different from starting power. Seeing it through is to use faith and persistence, to continue even against great odds. Characteristics of staying power include (1) integrity of consciousness and personhood; (2) remaining loyal to values, faith, philosophy, beliefs; (3) holding to a cause greater than self; and (4) giving up something worthwhile rather than worrying about present risks.

In adulthood there is no one set of appropriate personality characteristics or any one characteristic such as inflexibility or intolerance that is bad. The great person is inflexible or stands firm in the face of opposition at a crucial moment in history. The great person is intolerant of the evils he or she is trying to combat. Each of us leads a particular life at a particular time, place, and circumstance and with a particular personal history. Success in leading that life depends on a *pattern* of qualities appropriate to that life. No person can lead everyone's life. The mature person is reflective, restructures or processes information in the light of experience, and uses knowledge and expertise in a directed way to achieve desired ends. No one will reach the ideal of self-actualization described by Maslow (Chapter 5, pp. 168 to 169), yet each can reach his or her own ideal and peak of well-being and functioning relatively free of anxieties, cognitive distortions, and rigid habits and with a sense of the individuality and uniqueness of the self and others (58, 90).

The following characteristics of positive mental health and maturity were described by Jahoda (58):

1. Accepting personal strengths and limits, having a firm sense of identity, and living with the past without guilt
2. Striving for self-actualization and living up to the highest potential
3. Developing a philosophy of life and code of ethics, an ability to resist stress and tolerate anxiety, and an equilibrium of intrapsychic forces
4. Having a sense of autonomy, independence, and ability for self-direction
5. Having an adequate perception of reality and of fac-

tors affecting reality, having a social sensitivity, and treating others as worthy of concern
6. Mastering the environment: working, playing, solving problems, and adapting to the requirements of life
7. Valuing human relationships and feeling responsible to others.

Other authors have also identified criteria for emotional maturity (36, 37, 72, 90, 100). See Box 13–4.

Personality Development

Emotional or personality development has also been described by the stage theorists Jung (62), Sheehy (106), Gould (45–47), Levinson (71), and Vaillant (122, 123).

Jung divided personality development to correspond to the first and second halves of the life cycle. In the first half—until the age of 35 or 40—the person is in a period of expansion. Maturational forces direct the growth of the ego (the conscious or awareness of self and the external world); capacities unfold for dealing with the external world. The person learns to get along with others and tries to win as many of society's rewards as possible. A career and family are established. To achieve, it is usually necessary for men to overdevelop their masculinity and for women to overemphasize their feminine traits and skills. The young person dedicates self to mastery of the outer world. Being preoccupied with self-doubt, fantasy, and the inner nature is not advantageous to the young adult, for the task is to meet the demands of society confidently and assertively (62).

Jung believed that during the forties the personality begins to undergo a transformation. Earlier goals and ambitions have lost their meaning. The person may feel stagnant, incomplete, depressed, as if something crucial is missing, even if the person has been quite successful, since success has often been achieved at the cost of personality development. The person begins to turn inward, to examine the meaning of life. Separating self

---

■ BOX 13–4.
Criteria of Emotional Maturity

- Ability to deal constructively with reality
- Capacity to adapt to change
- Relative freedom from symptoms that are produced by tensions and anxieties
- Capacity to find more satisfaction in giving than receiving
- Capacity to relate to other people in a consistent manner with mutual satisfaction and helpfulness
- Capacity to sublimate, to direct one's instinctive hostile energy into creative and constructive outlets
- Capacity to love
- Ability to use intuition, the natural mental ability, associated with experience to comprehend life events and formulate answers

from ordinary conformity to the goals and values of mass society and achieving a measure of psychic balance are accomplished through individuation—finding one's individual way (62).

Jung recognized that, although middle-aged persons begin to turn inward, they still have much energy and resources for the generativity described by Erikson and for making personal changes. The person may begin new or long-forgotten projects and interests or even change careers. Men and women begin giving expression to their opposite sexual drives. Men become less aggressively ambitious and more concerned with interpersonal relationships. They begin to realize that achievement counts for less and friendship for more. Women tend to become more aggressive and independent. Such changes can create midlife marital problems. Although ongoing development may create tension and difficulties, Jung believed that the greatest failures come when adults cling to the goals and values of the first half of life, holding on to the glories and beauty of youth (62).

Neugarten's research (87–91) has found personality characteristics in middle-age are similar to those described by Jung (62).

Sheehy (106), Gould (45–47), Levinson (71), and Vaillant (124, 125) also describe midlife stages of development. These stage theorists confirm many of the characteristics already described and emphasize that this is a time of new stability and authenticity.

As you work with the middle-aged person use the concept of generativity versus self-absorption in assessment of the client's developmental level, and promote achievement of this developmental task through your listening, support, encouragement of activities, teaching, and counseling. The self-absorbed person should be referred to a long-term counselor. The generative person or mentor needs to hear that what he or she is doing is indeed a worthwhile contribution. Your own generativity can be a positive model for others. Your reinforcement of another's strengths facilitates further emotional development and maturity.

Body Image Development

The gradually occurring physical changes described earlier confront the person and are mirrored in others. The climacteric causes realignment of attitudes about the self that cuts into the personality and its definition. Other life stresses cause the person to view self and the body differently. The person not only realizes he or she is looking older but subjectively feels older as well. Work can bring a sense of stress if he or she feels less stamina and vigor to cope with the task at hand. Illness or death of loved ones creates a concern about personal health, sometimes to excess, and thoughts about one's own death are more frequent. The person begins to believe that he or she is coming out second-best to youth, for the previous self-image of the youthful, strong, and

healthy body with boundless energy becomes inadequate. Depression, irritability, and anxiety about femininity and masculinity result. In the United States, more so than in European or Asian cultures, youth and vigor are highly valued, a carryover from frontier days. The person's previous personality largely influences the intensity of these feelings and the symptoms associated with body-image changes. Difficulties are also caused by fear of the effects of the climacteric, folklore about sexuality, attitudes toward womanhood, social and advertising pressures in our culture, and emphasis on obsolescence (85).

Whether a man or a woman, the person who lacks self-confidence and who cannot accept the changing body has a compulsion to try cosmetics, clothes, hair styles, and the other trappings of youth in the hope that the physical attributes of youth will be attained. The person tries to regain a youthful figure and face, perhaps through surgery; tints the hair to cover signs of gray; and turns to hormone creams to restore the skin. These people are clients at times. There is nothing wrong with dressing attractively or changing the color of one's hair. But too few men or women realize that the color and texture of their skin have changed as the color of their hair faded and that their aging hands contrast considerably with the commercial coloring on the head. Women in the eighteenth century may have had a more realistic self-picture. They used white wigs or powdered their hair instead of dyeing it, perhaps because they recognized that white or gray hair softens the contours and flatters the face as the years go by.

Most people gradually adjust to their slowly changing body and accept the changes as part of maturity. The mature person realizes it is impossible to return to youth. To imitate youth denies the mature person's own past and experience. The excitement of the middle years lies in using adeptly the experience, insights, values, and realism acquired earlier. The person does not need to downgrade or agree continually with everything youth say and do. The middle-aged person feels good about self. Healthy signs are that he or she prefers this age and has no desire to relive the youthful years.

You can promote integration of a positive body image through your communication skills and teaching. Reaffirm the strengths of being middle-aged to the client, using information presented in this chapter and emphasizing the specific strengths of the person.

Adaptive Mechanisms

The adult may use any of the adaptive mechanisms described in previous chapters. **Adult socialization** is defined as the *processes through which an adult learns to perform the roles and behaviors expected of self and by others and to remain adaptive in a variety of situations.* The middle-aged adult is expected and normally considers self to be adaptive. The emphasis is on active, recip-

CASE SITUATION: Midlife Crisis

Louise, a 48-year-old architect, had an uneasy feeling about her relationship with her husband Charles, age 49, a teacher. The feeling had been there for some time, and she had tried a time or two to talk about it but had been rebuffed by Charles.

Louise believed that she and Charles were slowly drifting apart, each into his or her own profession. Yet the pronouncement by Charles seemed so sudden. As she joined him in the family room after dinner, he quietly looked at her and said, "I have something to tell you. I'm leaving. There's nothing here for me anymore. I'm almost 50. I've got to get on with things."

Louise was overcome with shock, grief, guilt, disbelief, helplessness, and worry. They had been married for 22½ years. She had often thought about all they could do together when they retired. Since they were childless, they would be free to travel. She panicked as she thought of life and aging without him. For days she slept and ate little but managed to go to work.

In the following months Louise and Charles met to talk several times. She wanted them to see a marriage counselor and work out their differences. As Charles continued to move his clothes, belongings, and favorite items from the home, he revealed that he would be living with another woman, a colleague from his school, and they would marry as soon as both divorces were finalized.

The divorce proceedings took over a year. During that time Louise sought counseling for herself. Gradually she revealed her situation to her family, other relatives, and friends. She often blamed herself for Charles' leave-taking and talked frequently of what a wonderful person he was. She maintained a hectic pace, caring for the home and yard and handling the responsibilities of her job. However, in the months after the initial separation, Louise also reestablished a daily exercise routine, which she had interrupted after Charles left home. She contacted a number of friends she had seen only occasionally in the past few years and began to attend the church of her childhood faith. She was pulling herself together—physically, emotionally, mentally, socially, and spiritually.

After the divorce was finalized, Louise continued to blame herself for several years. She worked hard, achieving recognition at the architectural firm where she was employed. She also maintained her home and neighborhood ties and became active in her church.

After 10 years Charles, who is remarried, still visits Louise occasionally and calls every few weeks. Louise has resolved the events of Charles' midlife crisis but has avoided opportunities to date or remarry. She believes the struggles and crises of the past decade, including various illnesses and the death of her parents, have prepared her for adaptation to her eventual retirement, aging, and dying. She still believes that she and Charles could reestablish a marriage and that it would be more love filled and happy. However, she remains fully committed to caring for a number of older friends; the responsibilities of her profession, home, and organizational and church membership; and to continuing to deepen her spiritual and emotional maturity.

---

rocal participation of the person; little preparation is directed to anticipating, accepting, or coping with failure. The ability to shift emotional investments from one activity to another, to remain open-minded, and to use past experience as a guide rather than as the rule is closely related to adaptive ability (37, 72).

The adult, having been rewarded for certain behaviors over the years, has established a wide variety of role-related behaviors, problem-solving techniques, adaptations to stress, and methods for making role transitions; they may not be adaptive to current demands or crises or to increasing role diffusion. There is a continuous need for socialization in adulthood, for a future orientation, for anticipating events, and for learning to respond to new demands (37, 72). Ongoing learning of adult roles occurs through observation, imitation, or identification with another, trial and error behavior, the media, books, or formal education.

Coping or adaptive mechanisms or ego defenses used in response to the emotional stress of the middle years depend on the person's capacity to adapt and satisfy personal needs, sense of identity, nature of interaction with others, sense of usefulness, and interest in the outside world.

The middle-aged adult must be able to channel emotional drives without losing initiative and vigor. During middle age the person is especially vulnerable to a number of disrupting events: physiologic changes and illness in self and loved ones, family stresses, changes in job or role demands or responsibilities, conflict between family generations, and societal changes. The person should be able to cope with ordinary personal upheavals and the frustrations and disappointments in life with only temporary disequilibrium. He or she should be able to participate enthusiastically in adult work and play and to experience adequate sexual satisfaction in a stable relationship. The person should be able to express a reasonable amount of aggression, anger, joy, and affection without undue effort, unnecessary guilt, or lack of adequate control (72). Further, the middle-aged adult is a role model of maturity for the young adult.

The person can retain a sense of balance by recognizing that each age has its unique joys and charms, and the entire life span is valued as equally precious. He or she can appreciate what is past, anticipate the future, and maintain a sense of permanence or stability. The person can adapt successfully to the stresses of middle age by achieving the developmental crisis.

As a nurse you can help the middle-aged adult prevent or overcome maladaptive mechanisms. As you extend empathy and reinforce a sense of emotional maturity and health, the person may feel more able to cope with life stressors and perceived failures. You may use principles and techniques of stress management and do and teach crisis intervention as described in *Psychiatric/Mental Health Nursing: Giving Emotional Care* (86). If you feel unable to listen to or work with the problems of someone who may be twice your age, refer the person to a counselor.

Midlife Crisis

The midlife crisis was first described by Jung (62). He believed that at approximately age 40 or 45, the psyche begins to undergo a transformation. The individual believes that the goals and ambitions that once seemed so eternal have lost their meaning. Quite often, the person feels depressed, stagnant, and incomplete, as if something crucial is missing. Jung observed that this happens even among people who have achieved a good measure of social success, for rewards have been won at the cost of a diminution of personality. Middle age can be seen as a transition or a crisis.

Midlife crisis is a *major and revolutionary turning point in one's life, involving changes in commitments to career and/or spouse and children and accompanied by significant and ongoing emotional turmoil for both the individual and others.* The term **midlife transition** has a different meaning; it includes *aspects of crisis, process, change, and alternating periods of stability and transition* (62).

For some midlife is one of the better periods of life: it is a *transition* from youth to later maturity; life expectancy is longer; psychologically and physically, midlife is healthier than ever in history; and parental responsibilities are decreasing. Most people are in their late forties or early fifties when the last child leaves home, leaving a couple of decades for the spouses to be together without the obligations of childrearing. The couple realizes that the myth of decreasing sexual powers is not true. Women in midlife may begin or continue their education or a career. Men see midlife as a time of continuing achievement. Experience, assurance, substance, skill,

success, and good judgment more than compensate for the disappearance of youthful looks and physical abilities.

Levinson (71) found in his study of men that the period of midlife transition is around ages 40 to 45. For a few the sense of change even in relation to body changes was slight, not particularly painful, and a manageable transition. However, for approximately 80% of the men the early forties evoked tumultuous struggles within the self and with the external world. This period involved for many a profound reappraisal. It involves false starts, emotional turmoil, and despair. At least one third of the male population in the United States between the ages of 40 and 60 years will experience some aspect of midlife crisis.

If the person has not resolved the identity crisis of adolescence and achieved mature intimacy in young adulthood, if the person fears the passage of time, physical changes, aging, and mortality, if the person cannot handle the meaning of life's routines and changes, midlife is seen as a *crisis.*

The person may declare he or she is bored. The nagging feeling that all is not right within the self and with the world can become a way to avoid facing the challenges presented by a deepening self-awareness and to avoid responsibility for personal immaturities or failures. Although many areas of life can be a source of boredom, the two most blamed as tedious and unsatisfying are marriage and work. Leaving either one may be a practical solution to a nagging expediency that was only partially satisfying. Often, however, the joblessness or job change or the affair or the divorce is a headlong flight from aging—an attempt to slow the passage of time by recapturing a lost sense of wholeness, by trying to gain total freedom to explore, and by changing goals and becoming a different sort of person. The new freedom may be found as equally stressful and full of rejection, competition, loneliness, meaninglessness, and personal dissatisfaction as the old routines. Often the structure and tedium of work or marriage look comfortable, pleasant, and meaningful only after either situation has been left behind. The identity crisis, when it is over, is seen to have been a denial of reality, not a new level of maturity. The "rational" goal seeking and need to change turn out to be compulsive and meaningless activity.

The psyche itself provides the way out of this crisis. It urges the person to turn inward and examine the meaning of his or her life. This turning inward is prompted by the unconscious, the region in which all the repressed and unlived aspects of the self have grown and now clamor to be heard. The unconscious calls out for recognition to bring about psychic balance and harmony. This often becomes apparent first in dreams. The unconscious speaks to us primarily through dreams. As middle-aged adults examine their lives and listen to unconscious messages, they sooner or later encounter images of the self, the symbols of wholeness and centeredness. The person must confront the negative aspects of self to become whole and find his or her true center (62).

The introspectiveness of middle age can cause a change in perceptions, felt needs, feelings toward others, and a heightened sense of disappointment without the balance of an increased awareness of achievements and positive aspects of life. The person may feel bitter, depressed, and desperate even though he or she has success, wealth, material possessions, and power.

Family experiences are undoubtedly integral to the direction of the midlife crisis. The midlife transition for men, often the husbands of menopausal women, brings new stresses. This period is often accompanied by sexual problems, sometimes leading to affairs, marital disruption, and the abandonment of the wife. Adolescent children may be sexually and aggressively provocative, challenging, or disappointing. Children leaving home for school or marriage change the family balance. Having no children can be a keen disappointment when the man realizes he has no heirs. Some women view their children's leaving home and marrying as an extension or expansion of parenting to include the wider interests and loci of their children. Far-flung needs of family members and expanded interests and activities lead to a different kind of parenting. Some women are restored to themselves and to their own development. Restored to themselves does not mean alone: women depend much more on their relationships for their development—not only for their emotional comfort and security but also to express the acting-on-the-world component of their aggression. The potential for autonomy, changes in relationships, and the development of their occupational skills, contacts, and self-image may start after childbearing is over (33, 37, 72). The woman's new-found autonomy, role changes, and increased interaction with or demands on the husband may be very threatening to the man.

In essence, the midlife crisis involves internal upheaval that may or may not be precipitated by such external events as job crisis, children's maturation, or marital difficulty. Often these events are the symptoms, rather than the causes, of the upheaval. Midlife crisis is not always experienced consciously. The feelings of rebellion, meaningless, and depression and the need for change may lead instead to altered behavior or attitudes in several life areas, involvement with a variety of causes, or escape into psychosomatic illness, alcoholism, and psychiatric illness (41).

It is healthier in the long range for the person to acknowledge the disruptive feelings and the diffusion of identity and to work through them rather than to deny them, and to seek a healthy and constructive outlet for these feelings. Colarusso and Nemeroff (24) describe in detail various issues in midlife for both men and women related to physical changes, changes in relationships

with spouse, family, and children, the relationship of the parent with the same and opposite-sexed child, work relationships and dissatisfactions, and time perspectives.

You can be instrumental in assisting the person in working through this crisis. You will use principles of communication and crisis intervention. Refer the person to a counselor who can work with the individual and family. The following guidelines may help the person who feels he or she is in midlife crisis. Share and use them as you work with others, or use them in your own life.

1. Do not be scared by the midlife crisis. Physical and psychologic changes are normal throughout life; see them as opportunities for maturing.

2. Face your feelings and your goals realistically. If you feel confused, see a counselor who can help you sort through your feelings and goals.

3. See your age as a positive asset. Acknowledge your strengths, the benefits of middle age. Take steps to adjust to your liabilities—or to correct them if you can. If a change in hair style or clothes makes you feel better, make that change.

4. Reconcile yourself to the fact that some or many of your hopes and dreams may never be realized and may not be attainable. Remain open to the opportunities that are available; they may exceed your dreams.

5. If the job is not satisfying, consider another job or another field after appraising yourself realistically; or be willing to relinquish some responsibility at work.

6. If you dread retirement, plan for it financially, along with leisure and other activities.

7. If job pressures are great, seek outlets through recreational activities or other diversions, become involved in community service, and renew spiritual study and religious affiliations.

8. Renew old friendships; initiate new ones. Invest in others and in the process enhance personal self-esteem and emotional well-being.

9. Try to be flexible and open-minded rather than dogmatic or inflexible in meeting and solving the problems you face.

10. If you are concerned about sexual potency, realize that the problem is typically transient. The more you worry, the worse it gets. Talk about your sexual feelings and concerns with your spouse. The love and concern you have for each other can frequently overcome any impotency. It is important for the woman to perceive sexuality apart from childbearing and menstruation and for the man to perceive sexuality apart from having children and love affairs. If you are so inclined, together read how-to sex manuals. Seek a marriage counselor if together you cannot work out problems of sexual dysfunction.

11. Share your feelings, concerns, frustrations, and problems with your spouse or confidante so that she or he can understand the changes you are experiencing. Keeping feelings to yourself can increase alienation and the difficulty of repairing the relationship.

12. Examine your attitudes as a parent; strike a balance between care and protection of offspring. Realize their normal need for independence.

13. Realize that frequently the middle-aged woman is becoming more assertive just when the middle-aged man is becoming more passive. Recognizing this as normal and talking about these changes can help the spouses better understand each other's needs and aspirations.

14. Get a physical examination to ensure that physical symptoms are not indicators of physical illness. Do not think that vitamins or health foods alone will cause you to feel differently.

15. Seek counseling for psychologic symptoms. The counselor may be a nurse, religious leader, mental health therapist, social worker, marriage counselor, psychologist, or psychiatrist.

You can give some specific suggestions to the spouse of the man in midlife crisis:

1. Recognize and acknowledge changes in him, but do not make value judgments. Do not say, "You look awful dressed in that. Who do you think you are, a young swinger?" Say instead, "I notice you're no longer wearing your regular suits and ties. Why is that?"

2. Make it easier for him to talk about his feelings and fears by listening to verbal and nonverbal messages. Avoid telling him how he should feel, dress, or behave.

3. Try not to make him feel guilty by hurling your fears or anger at him. His guilt about your fears will only cause him to withdraw and refuse to discuss his problems with you.

4. Emphasize to him that he does not have to leave to find what he is looking for. Try to find new joint interests, friends, or hobbies. Be willing to see a marriage counselor with him.

5. Focus on changing yourself. Become more alive by taking care of your appearance, keeping informed, and broadening your interests.

6. Avoid threatening his self-concept by appearing too competent in managing all areas of life while he neglects his usual family and home roles. Encourage him to maintain roles. Be prepared to pick up loose ends, however.

7. Try to reestablish the intimacy and closeness that you once shared. Be willing to compromise and change your own attitudes and behavior.

8. Try to maintain a certain spontaneity in your sexual life. Allow a sense of adventure to rekindle the relationship. If you can reestablish an active and satisfying sexual life at this point, you can both be certain that it will continue for many more years.

9. If he is coping with a midlife crisis symptom, focus on his strengths. But do not hand out empty praise. Instead find a real reason to praise him.

10. Do not adopt a motherly role toward him. Whereas sympathy and compassion are constructive, constant mothering and giving advice tend to diminish his sexual interest and ability to relate as husband.

11. Emphasize that the wife should not feel guilty when her husband develops any of the midlife crisis symptoms. It is not her fault. If handled with honesty and intelligence, the midlife crisis in men can be a positive turning point in a marriage, eventually creating a more constructive, satisfying, loving relationship.

Individuals considering midlife career or work changes must be able to assess their current job skills and applicability of them to new careers, explore alternatives within their current job position and external counseling services, and examine personal values. Career transition then becomes the response to seeking compatibility between self-image and the world of work (72). How the career change is negotiated depends in part on whether it is forced by external forces such as job layoff or technologic advances or voluntarily pursued because of value conflicts or as a means to personal, creative, economic, or social advancement. The person considering career change in life structure needs time, opportunity to talk, and help in working through the various facets of the situation.

Benefits from the midlife crisis include personality growth and deepening maturity because of personal introspection and desire to change behavior to feel better and improve one's life. Further, if the person in crisis can accept assistance, affection, and acceptance from loved ones, he or she can grow closer to them, and relationships deepen as a result. Sometimes the changes made in relation to a second career can enhance social status, financial well-being, or a sense of independence. The concern about mortality can motivate the person to take better care of health and to take time to pursue new interests or reinitiate old relationships. The person can experience an invigorating rebirth, generating new energies and new commitments.

Moral-Spiritual Development

The middle-aged person continues to integrate new concepts from widened sources into a religious philosophy if he or she has gained the spiritual maturity described in Chapter 12. He or she becomes less dogmatic in his or her beliefs. Faith and trust in God or another source of spiritual strength are increased. Religion offers comfort and happiness. The person is able to deal effectively with the religious aspects of upcoming surgery and its possible effects, illness, death of parents, or unexpected tragedy.

The middle-aged person may have become alienated from organized religion in early adulthood or may have drifted away from religious practices and spiritual study because of familial, occupational, and social role responsibilities. As the person becomes more introspective, studies self and life from new perspectives, ponders the meaning of life, and faces crises, he or she is likely to return to study of religious literature, practices of former years, and organized religious groups for strength, comfort, forgiveness, and joy. Spiritual beliefs and religion take on added importance. The middle-aged adult who becomes "born again" is likely to remain devout and active in his or her faith throughout life. If the person does not deepen spiritual insights, a sense of meaninglessness and despair is likely in old age.

Moral development is advanced whenever the person has an experience of sustained responsibility for the welfare of others. Middle age, if it is lived generatively, provides such an experience. Although the cognitive awareness of higher principles of living develops in adolescence, consistent commitment to their ethical applications develops in adulthood after the person has had time and opportunity to meet personal needs and to establish self in the family and community. Further, the level of cognitive development sets the upper limits for moral potential. If the adult remains in the state of Concrete Operations, he or she is unlikely to move beyond the Conventional Level of moral development (law and order reasoning) since the Postconventional Level requires a deep and broad understanding of events and a critical reasoning ability (68).

Although Kohlberg's work (68) on moral development was done on men, women generally come out at Stage 3 of the Conventional Level (Table 5–4), which emphasizes an interpersonal definition of morality rather than a societal definition of morality or an orientation to law and order. Perhaps the stage of moral development often seen in women, with concern for the well-being of others and a willingness to sacrifice self for others' well-being, is an aspect of Stage 5 of the Post Conventional Level.

Loevinger (74) sees middle age as the Autonomous Stage of Ego Development when the person evolves principles for self apart from the social world. The person deals with the differences between personal needs, principles by which to live, and duties demanded by society.

Gilligan (40), whose research centered on moral development in women, found that women define morality in terms of selfishness versus responsibility. Women subjects with high morality scores emphasized the importance of being responsible in behavior and of exercising care with and avoiding hurt to others. Men think more in terms of general justice and fairness; women think in terms of the needs of specific individuals. Gilligan's view of moral development is outlined in Table 13–3 according to three levels and the transition points from Level I to Level II and from Level II to Level III (40).

Developmental Tasks

Each period of life differs from the others, offering new experiences and opportunities and new tasks to surmount. The developmental tasks of middle age have a biologic basis in the gradual aging of the physical body, a cultural basis in social pressures and expectations, and an emotional origin in the individual life-style and self-concept that the mature adult has developed.

The following developmental tasks should be accomplished by middle-aged people (32, 37, 79, 87, 91). Through your care, counsel, and teaching, you can assist your clients to be aware of and to achieve these tasks.

TABLE 13-3. MORAL DEVELOPMENT IN WOMEN

Level	Characteristics
I. Orientation of individual survival	Concentrates on what is practical and best for self
Transition 1: from selfishness to responsibility	Realizes connection to others; thinks of responsible choice in terms of another as well as self
II. Goodness as self-sacrifice	Sacrifices personal wishes and needs to fulfill others' wants and to have others think well of her; feels responsible for others' actions; holds others responsible for her choices; dependent position; indirect efforts to control others often turns into manipulation through use of guilt
Transition 2: from goodness to truth	Makes decisions on personal intentions and consequences of actions rather than on how she thinks others will react; takes into account needs of self and others; wants to be good to others but also honest by being responsible to self
III. Morality of nonviolence	Establishes moral equality between self and others; assumes responsibility for choice in moral dilemmas; follows injunction to hurt no one, including self, in all situations

1. Maintain or establish healthful life patterns.
2. Discover and develop new satisfactions as a mate, give support to mate, enjoy joint activities, and develop a sense of unity and abiding intimacy.
3. Help growing and grown children to become happy and responsible adults and relinquish the central position in their affections, free the self from emotional dependence on children, take pride in their accomplishments, stand by to assist as needed, and accept their friends and mates.
4. Create a pleasant, comfortable home, appropriate to values, interests, time, energy, and resources; give, receive, and exchange hospitality; and take pride in accomplishments of self and spouse.
5. Find pleasure in generativity and recognition in work if employed; gain knowledge, proficiency, and wisdom; be able to lead or follow; balance work with other roles; and prepare for eventual retirement.
6. Reverse roles with aging parents and parents-in-law, assist them as needed without domineering, and act as a buffer between demands of aging parents and needs of young adults; prepare emotionally for the eventual death of parents unless they are already deceased.
7. Maintain a standard of living related to values, needs, and financial resources.
8. Achieve mature social and civic responsibility; be informed as a citizen; give time, energy, and resources to causes beyond self and home. Work cooperatively with others in the common responsibilities of citizenship; encourage others in their citizenship; stand for democratic practices and the welfare of the group as a whole in issues when vested interests may be at stake.
9. Develop or maintain an active organizational membership, deriving from it pleasure and a sense of belonging; refuse conflicting or too burdensome invitations with poise; work through intraorganizational tensions, power systems, and personality problems by becoming a mature statesperson in a diplomatic role, leading when necessary.
10. Accept and adjust to the physical changes of middle age, maintain healthful ways of living, attend to personal grooming, and relish maturity.
11. Make an art of friendship; cherish old friends and choose new; enjoy an active social life with friends, including friends of both sexes and of various ages; accept at least a few friends into close sharing of feelings to help avoid self-absorption.
12. Use leisure creatively and with satisfaction without yielding too much to social pressures and styles; learn to do some things well enough to become known for them among family, friends, and associates; enjoy use of talents; share some leisure-time activities with a mate or others and balance leisure activities with active and passive, collective and solitary, service-motivated and self-indulgent pursuits.
13. Acknowledge and confront the psychologic sense that the time left for cognitive, creative, emotional, social, and spiritual fulfillment is shorter and that fulfillment may never come.
14. Continue to formulate a philosophy of life and religious or philosophic affiliation, discovering new depths and meanings in God or a creator that include but also go beyond the fellowship of a particular religious denomination; gain satisfaction from altruistic activities or the concerns of a particular denomination; invest self in significant causes and movements; and recognize the finiteness of life.
15. Prepare for retirement with financial arrangements and development of hobbies and leisure activities, and rework philosophy and values.

The single or widowed middle-aged person will have basically the same developmental tasks but must find a sense of intimate sharing with friends or relatives.

Peck (100) sees the issues or conflicts that the person must work through in middle age as encompassing the following:

1. *Valuing wisdom gained from living and experience versus valuing physical powers and youth.* The person needs to accept his or her age, that youth cannot be regained, and that although physical strength and power may diminish, wisdom may accomplish more than physical strength anyway.
2. *Socializing versus sexualizing in human relationships.* The middle-aged adult, although still active sexually, now sees and relates to people as humans rather than just on the basis of men or women. The person relates to others without the gender self-consciousness of adolescence or young-young adulthood and sees the intrinsic dignity and worth of all people as social and spiritual beings.
3. *Emotional flexibility versus emotional impoverishment.* The middle-aged adult, although often accused of being rigid and unable to change, remains accepting of and empathic to others, open to people of different backgrounds, and open to changing personal behavior. The person becomes emotionally impoverished only if he or she withdraws from others, avoids learning from experience, refuses to change, or demonstrates the self-absorption described by Erikson (36).
4. *Mental flexibility versus mental rigidity.* The middle-aged adult, although accused of being closed to new ideas and excessively cautious, remains open to learning and flexible in problem-solving strategies. The person becomes mentally rigid if he or she avoids new experiences or learning opportunities or denies social, educational, or technologic changes.

Nursing Applications

Your role in caring for the middle-aged person and family has been described throughout the chapter. Assessment, using knowledge presented in this chapter, is the basis for formulating *nursing diagnoses*. Nursing diagnoses that may be applicable to the middle-aged adult are listed in Box 13-5. Interventions may involve the health promotion or direct care measures described throughout the chapter to assist the person and family in meeting physical, emotional, cognitive, spiritual, and social needs.

TRANSITION TO LATER MATURITY

The middle-aged adult has developed a sense of the life cycle; through introspection, he or she has gained a heightened sensitivity to the personal position within a complex social environment. Life is no longer seen as an infinite stretch of time into the future. The person anticipates and accepts the inevitable sequence of events that occur as the human matures, ages, and dies. The middle-aged adult realizes that the course of his or her life will be similar to the lives of others. Gender differences between men and women diminish in reality and per-

---

 BOX 13-5.
Selected Nursing Diagnoses Related to Middle Age[a]

Pattern 1: Exchanging

Altered Nutrition: More than body requirements
Altered Nutrition: Less than body requirements
Altered Nutrition: Potential for more than body requirements
Potential for Infection
Potential for Injury
Potential for Trauma
Potential Impaired Skin Integrity

Pattern 2: Communicating

Impaired Verbal Communication

Pattern 3: Relating

Impaired Social Interaction
Social Isolation
Altered Role Performance
Potential Altered Parenting
Altered Family Processes
Parental Role Conflict
Altered Sexuality Patterns

Pattern 4: Valuing

Spiritual Distress

Pattern 5: Choosing

Ineffective Individual Coping
Impaired Adjustment
Defensive Coping
Ineffective Denial
Ineffective Family Coping: Disabling
Ineffective Family Coping: Compromised
Family Coping: Potential for Growth
Decisional Conflict
Health Seeking Behaviors

Pattern 6: Moving

Impaired Physical Mobility
Activity Intolerance
Fatigue
Potential Activity Intolerance
Sleep Pattern Disturbance
Diversional Activity Deficit
Impaired Home Maintenance Management
Altered Health Maintenance

Pattern 7: Perceiving

Body Image Disturbance
Self-esteem Disturbance
Chronic Low Self-esteem
Situational Low Self-esteem
Sensory/Perceptual Alterations
Hopelessness
Powerlessness

Pattern 8: Knowing

Knowledge Deficit

Pattern 9: Feeling

Pain
Chronic Pain
Dysfunctional Grieving
Anticipatory Grieving
Potential for Violence: Self-directed or directed at others
Post-trauma Response
Anxiety
Fear

[a]Other NANDA nursing diagnoses are applicable to the ill middle-aged adults.
From North American Nursing Diagnosis Association, *NANDA Nursing Diagnosis Toxonomy I* (Rev.). St. Louis: North American Nursing Diagnosis Association, 1990.

ception. Turning points affect all and are inescapable. Personal mortality, achievements, and failures and personal strengths and limits must be faced if the person is to be prepared emotionally and developmentally for later maturity and the personal aging process. The person realizes that the direction in life has been set by prior decisions related to occupation, marriage, family life, and having or not having children. Although occupation and life-style can be changed, at least to some extent, the results of other earlier decisions cannot be changed. The consequences must be faced and resolved. The middle-aged person realizes he or she may not achieve all dreams, but remaining open to opportunities along the way may enable the person to achieve accomplishments never fantasized that are equally meaningful.

For example, if the young adult woman focused on career and did not marry and have children, at age 50 she may still marry, but having children—or adoption—is less likely. Having no children means not being a grandparent in old age. The need to be a parent, grandparent, or to nurture must be met in another way. In turn, the single or childless middle-aged woman may realize that she has been nurturing a larger number of people than some middle-aged women who focused their attention solely on the children.

The person in late midlife realizes that life's developmental markers and crises call forth changes in self-concept and sense of identity, necessitate incorporation of new social roles and behaviors, and precipitate new adaptations. But they do not destroy the sense of continuity within the person from youth to old age. This adaptability and a sense of continuity are essential for the achievement of ego integrity in the last years of life.

REFERENCES

1. Angel, M., *The Orphaned Adult: Confronting the Death of a Parent.* New York: Human Sciences Press, 1987.
2. Arlin, P.K., Cognitive Development in Adulthood: A Fifth Stage? *Developmental Psychology,* 11 (1975), 602–606.
3. Atunes, C.M., et al., Endometrial Cancer and Estrogen Use, *New England Journal of Medicine,* 300 (January 4, 1979), 9–13.
4. Baille, V., J. Norbeck, and L. Barnes, Stress, Social Support, and Psychological Distress of Family Caregivers of the Elderly, *Nursing Research,* 37, no. 4 (1988), 217–22.
5. Bajinck, I., et al., Nurses as Colleagues and Mentors, *Canadian Nurse,* 84, no. 2 (1988), 16–17.
6. Bates, B., *A Guide to Physical Examination and History Taking* (4th ed.). Philadelphia: J.B. Lippincott, 1987.
7. Bauer, R., et al., Risk of Postmenopausal Hip Fracture in Mexican-American Women, *American Journal of Public Health,* 76, no. 8 (1986), 1020–1021.
8. Baum, M., and M. Page, Caregiving and Multigenerational Families, *Gerontologist,* 31, no. 6 (1991), 762–769.
9. Berg, B., I've Got a Hunch, *New Choices* (May 1991), 74–77.
10. Berglas, C., *Mid-Life Crisis.* Lancaster, Pa: Technomic Publishing, 1987.
11. Bolles, R., The Decade of Decisions, *Modern Maturity* (March 1990), 36–45.
12. Brody, E., Parent Care as a Normative Family Stress, *Gerontologist,* 25, no. 1 (1985), 19–29.
13. Brody, E., et al., Work Status and Parent Care: A Comprehensive Study of Four Groups of Women, *Gerontologist,* 27, no. 3 (1987), 201–208.
14. Brody, J., M. Farmer, and L. White, Absence of Menopausal Effect on Hip Fracture Occurrence in White Females, *American Journal of Public Health,* 74, no. 12 (1984), 1397–1398.
15. Buchaman, R., The Widow and the Widower. In Grollman, E., ed., *Concerning Death: A Practical Guide for the Living.* Boston: Beacon Press, 1974, pp. 287–311.
16. Buhler, C., The Developmental Structure of Goal Setting in Group and Individual Studies. In Buhler, C., and F. Massarik, eds., *The Course of Human Life.* New York: Springer Publishing, 1968.
17. Building Better Bone, *Prevention* (May 1991), 54–59.
18. Burnard, P., Mentors: A Supporting Act, *Nursing Times,* 84, no. 46 (1988), 27–28.
19. Caine, L., *Being a Widow.* New York: Arbor House, 1988.
20. Carlson, E., The Phony War, *Modern Maturity* (February-March 1987), 34–44.
21. Cattanach, L., and J. Tebes, The Nature of Elder Impairment and Its Impact on Family Caregivers' Health and Psychosocial Functioning, *Gerontologist,* 31, no. 2 (1991), 246–255.
22. Cicerelli, V., A Comparison of Helping Behavior to Elderly Parents of Adult Children With Intact and Disrupted Marriages, *Gerontologist,* 23, no. 6 (1983), 619–625.
23. Clark, N., and W. Rakowski, Family Caregivers of Older Adults: Improving Helping Skills, *Gerontologist,* 23, no. 6 (1983), 637–641.
24. Colarusso, C., and R. Nemeroff, *Adult Development.* New York: Plenum Press, 1981.
25. Colen, B., The Generation Blur, *Health* (October 1989), 30–31.
26. Collison, C., and S. Miller, Using Images of the Future in Grief Work, *Image,* 19, no. 1 (1987), 9–11.
27. Cosby, B., *Time Flies.* Garden City, NY: Doubleday, 1987.
28. Cross, K., *Adults As Learners.* San Francisco: Jossey-Bass, 1981.
29. Dellasega, C., Coping With Caregiving: Stress Management for Caregivers of the Elderly, *Journal of Psychosocial Nursing,* 28, no. 1 (1990), 15–22.
30. Dennis, W., Creative Production Between the Ages of 20 and 80, *Journal of Gerontology,* 21, no. 1 (1966), 8.
31. Dresen, S., The Middle Years: The Sexually Active Middle Adult, *American Journal of Nursing,* 75, no. 6 (June 1975), 1001–1005.
32. Duvall, E., and B. Miller, *Marriage and Family Development* (6th ed.). New York: Harper & Row, 1984.
33. Dworetzky, J., and N. Davis, *Human Development: A Lifespan Approach.* St. Paul: West Publishing, 1989.

34. Eastman, P., Life After Menopause Liberating, Women Say, *AARP News Bulletin* (July-August 1988), 4–5.

35. Engel, N., Menopausal Stage, Current Life Change, Attitude Toward Women's Roles and Perceived Health Status, *Nursing Research,* 36, no. 6 (1987), 353–356.

36. Erikson, Erik, *Childhood and Society* (2nd ed.). New York: W.W. Norton, 1963.

37. Erikson, E., ed., *Adulthood*. New York: W.W. Norton, 1978.

38. Ferguson, T., Decision Making Without a Partner, *Archives of the Foundation of Thanatology,* 2, no. 1 (April 1970), 21–22.

39. Friday, N., *My Mother, Myself*. New York: Dell, 1977.

40. Gilligan, C., In a Different Voice: Women's Conceptions of Self and of Mortality, *Harvard Educational Review,* 47, no. 4 (1977), 481–517.

41. Golan, N., *Passing Through Transitions*. New York: The Free Press, 1983.

42. Goldberg, E., G. Comstock, and S. Harlow, Emotional Problems and Widowhood, *Journal of Gerontology: Social Sciences,* 43, no. 6 (1988), S 206–S 208.

43. Goldstein, V., G. Regnery, and E. Wellin, Caretaker Role Fatigue, *Nursing Outlook,* 29, no. 1 (1981), 24–34.

44. Gottlieb, D., I. Gottlieb, and M. Seavin, *What To Do When Your Son or Daughter Divorces*. New York: Bantam Books, 1988.

45. Gould, R., The Phases of Adult Life: A Study in Developmental Psychology, *American Journal of Psychiatry,* 129, no. 5 (1972), 521–531.

46. ———, Adult Life Stages: Growth Toward Self-Tolerance, *Psychology Today,* 8, no. 7 (February 1975), 74–78.

47. ———, Transformation in Mid-Life, *New York University Education Quarterly,* 10, no. 2 (1979), 2–9.

48. Guyton, A., *Textbook of Medical Physiology* (8th ed.). Philadelphia: W.B. Saunders, 1990.

49. Hamon, R., and R. Blieszner, Filial Responsibility Expectations Among Adult Child–Older Parent Pairs, *Journal of Gerontology: Psychological Sciences,* 45, no. 3 (1990), P 110–P 112.

50. Hanson, S., W. Sauer, and W. Seelbach, Racial and Cohort Variations in Filial Responsibility Norms, *Gerontologist,* 23, no. 6 (1983), 626–631.

51. Hegarty, V., *Decisions in Nutrition*. St. Louis: Times Mirror Mosby College Publishing, 1988.

52. Helsing, K., M. Szklo, and G. Comstock, Factors Associated with Mortality After Widowhood, *American Journal of Public Health,* 71, no. 8 (1981), 802–809.

53. Hershel, J., A. Walker, and K. Rothman, The Epidemic of Endometrial Cancer: A Commentary, *American Journal of Public Health,* 70, no. 2 (1980), 264–267.

54. High Health in the Middle Years, *Prevention* (July 1988), 35–47, 100–110.

55. Hoff, L., *People in Crisis: Understanding and Helping* (3rd ed.). Redwood City, Calif: Addison-Wesley, 1989.

56. Hoole, A.J., R.A. Greenberg, and C.G. Pickard, *Patient Care Guidelines for Nurse Practitioners* (3rd ed.). Boston: Little, Brown, 1988.

57. Irwin, T., *Male Menopause: Crisis in the Middle Years*. New York: Public Affairs Pamphlets, 1982.

58. Jahoda, M., *Current Concepts of Positive Mental Health*. New York: Basic Books, 1958.

59. Jarrett, W., Caregiving Within Kinship Systems: Is Affection Really Necessary? *Gerontologist,* 25, no. 1 (1985), 5–10.

60. Johnson, K., and T. Ferguson, *Trusting Ourselves: The Sourcebook on Psychology for Women*. New York: Atlantic Monthly Press, 1991.

61. Jones, S., and P. Jones, Predictors of Divorce in Long-Term Marriages, *Archives of Psychiatric Nursing,* 2, no. 5 (1988), 267–273.

62. Jung, C., *Modern Man in Search of a Soul*. New York: Harcourt, Brace & World, 1955.

63. Kangas, J., and K. Bradway, Intelligence at Middle Age: A 38-Year Follow-Up, *Developmental Psychology,* 5, no. 2 (1971), 333–337.

64. Kaplan, S., The New Generation Gap, *Common Cause Magazine* (March-April 1987), 13–15.

65. Kaprio, J., M. Koskenvuo, and H. Rita, Mortality After Bereavement: A Prospective Study of 95,647 Widowed Persons, *American Journal of Public Health,* 77, no. 3 (1987), 283–287.

66. Karp, D., The Social Construction of Retirement Among Professionals 50-60 Years Old, *Gerontologist,* 29, no. 6 (1989), 750–760.

67. Knowles, M., *The Adult Learner: A Neglected Species* (4th ed.). Houston: Gulf Publishing, 1990.

68. Kohlberg, L., *Recent Research in Moral Development*. New York: Holt, Rinehart & Winston, 1977.

69. Lauver, D., Irregular Bleeding in Women: Causes and Nursing Interventions, *American Journal of Nursing,* 3, no. 3 (1983), 396–401.

70. Lerner, M., et al., Adult Children as Caregivers: Egocentric Biases in Judgments of Sibling Contributions, *Gerontologist,* 31, no. 6 (1991), 746–755.

71. Levinson, D., *The Seasons of a Man's Life*. New York: Alfred A. Knopf, 1986.

72. Lidz, T., *The Person: His and Her Development Throughout the Life Cycle* (2nd ed.). New York: Basic Books, 1983.

73. Lindeman, E., Symptomology and Management of Acute Grief, *American Journal of Psychiatry,* 101 (1944), 141–148.

74. Loevinger, J., *Ego Development*. San Francisco: Jossey-Bass, 1976.

75. Lowenthal, M., and D. Chiriboga, Transition to the Empty Nest: Crisis, Challenge, or Relief? *Archives of General Psychiatry,* 26, no. 1 (1972), 8–14.

76. Mastering Menopause, *Prevention* (April 1990), 46–55.

77. Masters, W., and V. Johnson, *Human Sexual Response*. Boston: Little, Brown, 1981.

78. Matthews, S., J. Werkner, and P. Delaney, Relative Contributions of Help by Employed and Nonemployed Sisters to Their Elderly Parents, *Journal of Gerontology: Social Sciences,* 44, no. 1 (1989), S36–S44.

79. McCoy, V., Adult Life Cycle Tasks/Adult Continuing Education Program Response, *Lifelong Learning in the Adult Years* (October 1977), 16.

80. McKee, A., The AAUW Report: How Schools Shortchange Girls, *AAUW Report,* 86, no. 1 (1992), 1–9.

81. Mead, M., *Culture and Commitment: A Study of the Generation Gap. The New Relationships Between the Generations in the 1970's*. Garden City, NY: Natural History Press/Doubleday & Company, 1978.

82. Million, S., Training Mentors and Proteges: The Key to

Successful Mentoring, *Kappa Delta Pi Record* (Fall 1990), 21–26.

83. Morgan, D., Adjusting to Widowhood: Do Social Networks Really Make It Easier? *Gerontologist,* 29, no. 1 (1989), 101–107.

84. Muhlenkamp, A., M. Waller, and A. Bourne, Attitudes Toward Women in Menopause: A Vignette Approach, *Nursing Research,* 32, no. 1 (1983), 20–23.

85. Murray, R., Body Image Development in Adulthood, *Nursing Clinics of North America,* 7, no. 4 (1972), 622–624.

86. ——, and M. Huelskoetter, *Psychiatric/Mental Health Nursing: Giving Emotional Care* (3rd ed.). Norwalk, Conn: Appleton & Lange, 1991.

87. Neugarten, B., The Awareness of Middle Age. In Owen, R., ed., *Middle Age.* London: British Broadcasting Corporation, 1967.

88. ——, Women's Attitudes Toward Menopause. In Neugarten, B., ed., *Middle Age and Aging.* Chicago: University of Chicago Press, 1968.

89. ——, Dynamics of the Transition of Mid-Age to Old Age, *Journal of Geriatric Psychiatry,* 4 (1970), 71–87.

90. ——, Adaptation and the Life Cycle, *The Counseling Psychologist,* 6, no. 1 (1976), 16–20.

91. ——, and J. Moore, The Changing Age-Status System. In Neugarten, B., ed., *Middle Age and Aging.* Chicago: University of Chicago Press, 1968.

92. Newman, B., et al., Nongenetic Influences of Obesity on Other Cardiovascular Disease Risk Factors: An Analysis of Identical Twins, *American Journal of Public Health,* 80, no. 6 (1990), 675–678.

93. Nolan, J.E., Developmental Concern and the Health of Midlife Women, *Nursing Clinics of North America,* 21, no. 1 (1986), 151–159.

94. O'Bryant, S., and L. Morgan, Recent Widows' Kin Support and Orientations to Self-Sufficiency, *Gerontologist,* 30, no. 3 (1990), 391–397.

95. O'Donnell, T., and S. Bernier, Parents as Caregivers: When a Son Has AIDS, *Journal of Psychosocial Nursing,* 28, no. 6 (1990), 14–17.

96. Okimoto, J., and P. Stegall, *Boomerang Kids.* Boston: Little, Brown, P 1987.

97. Olson, T., and J. Hanover, Preparing Women to be Widows, *Health Values: Achieving High Level Wellness,* 9, no. 1 (1985), 8–11.

98. Osteoporosis: Estrogen Connection Clearer, *American Journal of Nursing,* 88, no. 1 (1988), 13.

99. Pearson, L., Climacteric, *American Journal of Nursing,* 82, no. 7 (1982), 1098–1102.

100. Peck, R.C., Psychological Developments in the Second Half of Life. In Neugarten, B., eds., *Middle Age and Aging.* Chicago: University of Chicago Press, 1968.

101. Peretz, D., Reaction to Loss. In Schoenberg, B., et al., eds., *Loss and Grief: Psychological Management in Medical Practice.* New York: Columbia University Press, 1970, pp. 20–35.

102. Phipps, W., et al., eds., *Medical-Surgical Nursing: Concepts and Clinical Practice* (4th ed.). St. Louis: Mosby–Year Book, 1991.

103. Powell, R., and R. Pohndorf, Comparison of Adult Exercisers and Nonexercisers on Fluid Intelligence and Selected Physiological Variables, *Research Quarterly,* 42, no. 1 (1971), 70–77.

104. Scharlach, A., and S. Boyd, Caregiving and Employment: Results of an Employee Survey, *Gerontologist,* 29, no. 3 (1989), 382–387.

105. Schulz, R., P. Visintainer, and G. Williamson, Psychiatric and Physical Morbidity Effects of Caregiving. *Journal of Gerontology: Psychological Sciences,* 45, no. 5 (1990), P181–P191.

106. Sheehy, G., *Passages.* New York: Bantam Books, 1984.

107. Should You Take Estrogen? *Prevention* (November 1989), 42–51.

108. Siegal, D., and P. Doress, *Ourselves, Growing Older: Women Aging With Knowledge and Power.* New York: Simon & Schuster, 1987.

109. Silverstone, B., and H. Hyman, *You and Your Aging Parent: A Family Guide to Emotional, Physical, and Financial Problems* (3rd ed.). New York: Pantheon Books, 1989.

110. Sinott, J., Everyday Thinking and Piagetian Operativity in Adults, *Human Development,* 18 (1975), 430–433.

111. Smith, G., M. Smith, and R. Toseland, Problems Identified by Family Caregivers in Counseling, *Gerontologist,* 31, no. 1 (1991), 15–22.

112. Soldo, B., and J. Myllyluoma, Caregivers Who Live With Dependent Elderly, *Gerontologist,* 23, no. 6 (1983), 1605–1610.

113. Speroff, L., PMS—Looking for New Answers to an Old Problem, *Contemporary OB-Gyn* (August 1983), 102–127.

114. St. George, J., and B. Dicicco-Bloom, Using Dramatizations to Train Caregivers for the Elderly, *Nursing Outlook,* 33, no. 5 (1985), 302–304.

115. Stoller, E., Males as Helpers: The Roles of Sons, Relatives, and Friends, *Gerontologist,* 30, no. 2 (1990), 228–235.

116. Stollar, E., and K. Pugliesi, Other Roles of Caregivers: Competing Responsibilities or Supportive Resources, *Journal of Gerontology: Social Sciences,* 44, no. 6 (1989), S231–S238.

117. Strawbridge, W., and M. Wallhagen, Impact of Family Conflict on Adult Child Caregivers, *Gerontologist,* 31, no. 6 (1991), 770–777.

118. Take Charge and Be Happy, *Prevention* (June 1990), 50–55, 136–140.

119. Travis C., The Freedom to Change, *Prime Time* (October 1980), 27–33.

120. Uhlenberg, P., T. Cooney, and R. Boyd, Divorce for Women After Midlife, *Journal of Gerontology: Social Services,* 45, no. 1 (1990), S3–S11.

121. U.S. Bureau of Census, *Statistical Abstract of the United States: 1990* (110th ed.). Washington, DC: Government Printing Office, 1990.

122. Vaillant, G., How the Best and the Brightest Came of Age, *Psychology Today,* 11, no. 9 (1977), 34ff.

123. ——, The Normal Boy in Later Life: How Adaptative Fosters Growth, *Harvard Magazine,* 55, no. 6 (1977), 234–239.

124. Vance, C., Is There a Mentor in Your Career Future? *Imprint,* 36, no. 5 (1989-1990), 41–42.

125. Wadsworth, B., *Piaget's Theory of Cognitive and Affective Development* (4th ed.). New York: Longman, 1989.

126. Warner, S., A Comparative Study of Widows' and Widowers' Perceived Social Support During the Past

Year of Bereavement, *Archives of Psychiatric Nursing,* 1, no. 4 (1987), 241–250.

127. Weaver, T., and R. Millman, Sleep Apnea, *American Journal of Nursing,* 86, no. 2 (1986), 146–150.

128. Weeks, J., and J. Cuellar, The Role of Family Members in the Helping Networks of Older People, *Gerontologist,* 21, no. 4 (1981), 388–394.

129. Weinhaus, E., and K. Friedman, *Stop Struggling With Your Teen.* New York: Penguin Books, 1989.

130. West, R., *Memory Fitness Over Forty.* Gainesville, Fla: Triad, 1985.

131. Whitbeck, L., R. Simmons, and R. Conger, The Effects of Early Family Relationships on Contemporary Relationship and Assistance Patterns Between Adult Children and Their Parents, *Journal of Gerontology: Social Sciences,* 46, no. 6 (1991), S330–S337.

132. Williams, S., *Nutrition and Diet Therapy* (6th ed.). St. Louis: Times-Mirror Mosby, 1989.

133. Win the Weight War, *Prevention* (June 1990), 42–49, 133–135.

134. Young, R., and E. Kahana, Specifying Caregiver Outcomes: Gender and Relationship Aspects of Caregiving Strain, *Gerontologist,* 29, no. 5 (1989), 660–666.

135. *Your Feet After Fifty.* Miami Beach, Fla: Foot Facts Publications, n.d.

136. Zarit, S., P. Todd, and J. Zarit, Subjective Burden of Husbands and Wives as Caregivers: A Longitudinal Study, *Gerontologist,* 26, no. 3 (1986), 260–266.

Chapter 14

Assessment and Health Promotion for the Person in Later Maturity

Old age, to the unlearned, is winter: to the learned, it is harvest time.
—*Yiddish Proverb*

KEY TERMS

Aging	Selective perception	Secondary anemia	Isolation
Biologic age	Situational reinforcement	Chronic lymphocytic leukemia	Compartmentalization
Social age	Erikson's Epigenetic Theory	Hodgkin's disease	Denial
Psychologic age	Peck's Theory	Benign prostatic hypertrophy	Rationalization
Cognitive age	Disengagement Theory	Osteoporosis	Somatization
Senescence	Activity Theory	Osteoarthritis	Counterphobia
Later maturity	Symbolic Interaction Theory	Congestive heart failure	Rigidity
Young-old	Lentigo senilis	Chronic occlusive arterial disease	Sublimation
Mid-old	Presbyopia	Stasis ulcer	Displacement
Old-old	Cataracts	Pitting edema	Projection
Gerontology	Glaucoma	Brawny edema	Insight
Geriatrics	Arcus senilis	Crystallized intelligence	Equanimity
Ageism	Presbycusis	Fluid intelligence	Perseverance
Wear and Tear Theory	Functional reach	Episodic memory	Self-reliance
Deprivation Theories	Dyspareunia	Ego integrity	Meaningfulness
Accumulation Theories	Herpes zoster (shingles)	Despair or self-disgust	Existential aloneness
Free Radical Theory	Parkinson's disease	Ego differentiation	Leisure time
Cross-Linkage Theory	Alzheimer's disease	Body transcendence	Prosumers
Biologic Clock Theories	Chronic obstructive pulmonary disease	Ego transcendence	Translocation syndrome
Immune Theory	Pernicious anemia	Regression	Remotivation
Glycation Theory			
Continuity Theory			

OBJECTIVES

Study of this chapter will enable you to:

1. Define terms and theories of aging related to understanding of the person in later maturity.
2. Explore personal and societal attitudes about growing old and your role in promoting positive attitudes.
3. Contrast relationships in the late years with those of other developmental eras, including with spouse, offspring, grandchildren, other family members, friends, pets, and other networks.
4. Contrast the status of either singlehood or widow(er) in later maturity to that status in early and midadulthood.
5. Describe signs and contributing factors to elder abuse and contrast with child and spouse abuse.
6. Describe physiologic adaptive mechanisms of aging and influences on sexuality, related health problems, and assessment and intervention to promote and maintain health, comfort, and safety.
7. Discuss the cognitive, emotional, body-image, and spiritual development and characteristics of the aged person, the interrelationship of them, and

your role in promoting health and a positive self-concept.

8. Contrast the adaptive mechanisms used by the person in this period with those used in other periods of life.
9. Describe the developmental crisis of later maturity, the relationship to previous developmental crises, and your role in helping the person meet this crisis.
10. List the developmental tasks for this era, and describe your contribution to their accomplishment.
11. Identify changing home, family, social, and work or leisure situations of this person and your responsibility in helping the person face retirement, loss of loved ones, and changes in roles and living arrangements. Discuss selection of an adequate nursing home or residence for seniors.
12. Describe major federal, state, and local programs to assist the elderly financially, socially, and in health care, and describe your professional and personal responsibility in this regard.
13. Demonstrate remotivation technique and discuss the value, purpose, and use of this and other group processes with the elderly.
14. Summarize the needs of the elderly, standards of

nursing care to assist in meeting those needs, and future trends in care of the person in later maturity.

15. Assess and work effectively with a person in later maturity, using the information presented in this chapter and showing empathy and genuine interest.

> I really don't like being labeled a golden-ager. I acknowledge my age and my limits, but I certainly didn't turn incompetent at 65.

When does later maturity begin? Historically, it was the designation of an eligible age for receipt of Social Security benefits that established 65 years old as the beginning age for this period in the life cycle. In reality, the age span for this period is continually changing. Images once associated with later maturity are no longer clear. The chronologic age of 65 no longer determines or predicts behaviors, life events, health status, work status, family status, interests, preoccupations, or needs. Individuals undergo aging at different rates, and their view of the aging process is influenced by many factors—culture, generation, and occupation. Not everyone 65 or 70 years old and older considers himself or herself old, but in the United States the person of that age is expected to assume roles appropriate to later maturity. Some individuals, especially members of ethnic minorities and lower socioeconomic levels, view the onset of old age as taking place earlier than age 65 (243, 255). Younger generations may misperceive how the old view themselves.

In 1860 2.7% of the population in the United States was more than 65 years of age. This figure changed dramatically during the next 125 years. By 1985 there were 28.5 million people in this age group, 12 % of the population. By 1988 the median age of people over 65 was approximately 73 years. Life expectancy for a person reaching 65 years in 1988 was more than 80 years. Life expectancy for a woman born in 1988 is 78.3 years and for a man, 71.4 years (210, 266). At present in the United States more than 5000 persons reach their sixty-fifth

birthday every day, and 55 reach 100 years daily. Those individuals reaching 65 live longer than in the past. In fact, the fastest growing segment of population in the United States is the group over 85 years old. In 1986 the 65-to-74 age group was 8 times larger than it was in 1900; the 75-to-84 age group was 12 times larger; and the group over 85 was 23 times larger (210). It is projected that by the year 2000 there will be more than 36 million Americans over 65, comprising as much as 13% of the population, with 4.9 million over 85 and approximately 100,000 people over age 100 (there were 20,000 in 1980) (9). By 2030 65 to 70 million people, or approximately 25% of the U.S. population, will be 65 years of age or over ($2\frac{1}{2}$ times their number in 1980). This rapid increase between the years 2000 and 2030 reflects the aging of the baby boom generation born in the 1960s (72, 93, 210, 244). Four-generation families will be the norm (Fig. 14–1); five-generation families will be increasing in number. This continued aging trend in the population requires changes in all aspects of our social structure—employment, housing, education, leisure activities, transportation, industrial development, and health care.

DEFINITIONS

Because the terms describing this age group are not clearly defined by the general public or health care professionals, it is important to clarify some of the terms used in this chapter (1, 72, 75, 244, 260, 285).

Aging, which *begins at conception and ends at death, is a process of growing older, regardless of chronologic age.*

Biologic age is the *person's present position with respect to the potential life span, which may be younger or older than chronologic age,* and encompasses measures of functional capacities of vital organ systems.

Social age, which *results from the person's life course through various social institutions,* refers to *roles*

Figure 14-1. Four-generation families, once unusual, will become the norm as the population ages.

and habits of the person with respect to other members of society. Social age may be age appropriate or older or younger than that of most people in the social group. Social age includes such aspects as the person's type of dress, language usage, and social deference to people in leadership positions.

Psychologic age refers to *behavioral capacity of the person to adapt to changing environmental demands and includes capacities of memory, learning, intelligence, skills, feelings, and motivation for exercising behavioral control or self-regulation.*

Cognitive age includes the *age the person feels and looks to self, plus the fit of behavior and interests to his or her chronologic age*. The person says, "I do most things as if I were _____ years old."

Senescence is the *mental and physical decline associated with the aging process*. The term describes a group of effects that lead to a decrease in efficient function.

Later maturity is the *last major segment of the life span; the stage begins at the age of 65 or 70 years*. The World Health Organization (WHO) divides this segment of life into the elderly (65 to 75), the old (76 to 90), and the very old (over 90). Some authors divide this group into **young-old,** *age 65 to 74* (235) or *65 or 70 to 80* (75); **mid-old,** *75 to 84* (235); and **old-old,** *85 and older* (235) or *80 and older* (75). The term **frail-old** is sometimes used instead of **old-old** or **very old.**

Senility is a *wastebasket term still used to denote physical and mental deterioration often associated with old age. It is used when other options have not been carefully considered.* The more common euphemism currently is Alzheimer's disease. Yet what looks like senility or Alzheimer's disease may be the result of drug reactions; malnutrition; dehydration; delirium; hypothyroidism; microstrokes and hypertension; toxicity in the system; disorders resulting from lack of communication and experiencing sensory deprivation for physical reasons or because of institutionalization; or the expectations of caregiver (287).

Gerontology is the *scientific study of the individual in later maturity and the aging process from a physiologic, pathologic, psychologic, sociologic, and economic point of view.*

Geriatrics is a *medical specialty concerned with the physiologic and pathologic changes of the individual in later maturity and includes study and treatment of the health problems of this age group.*

Later maturity is divided into three sequential segments. The first segment may be regarded as a *social-political* or *cultural-organizational perspective*. Offspring are in a creative period, and the mature adult is in the ruling, protective stance as he or she assumes parental hierarchical leadership over the family of families. The older person becomes concerned with the creation, ordering, and maintenance of a larger society. The second segment is characterized by a *reaffirmation of social,*

moral, and ethical standards necessary for establishment of pacific relationships among the oncoming generations as they are involved in rendering decisions, planning, erecting social guideposts, and selecting subordinate leaders. The judgmental functions of the mind are most highly developed at this time, created out of actual and vicarious experience with conflict situations and from cultural learning and values. The last segment of psychic maturity involves *retrospective examination,* the need to correlate the present with the past to determine the true nature of accomplishments, errors, and rediscoveries. Cultural vision is at its broadest possible development, embracing one nearly complete life cycle and its interrelatedness with a multitude of other life cycles. The person compares and contrasts his or her values with cultural values and through reasoning and intuition evaluates meaning and purpose and has an increased interest in the history of human development. Values of the adolescent are movement, agility, quantitative productivity, exhibitionistic sexual attractiveness, and artfulness. In contrast, values of the older adult are deliberation, caution, equality, modesty, and loyalty. Whereas the adolescent views self as the ambitious master of a dimly concerned manhood, the older adult views self with real humility as at least a participant in and at most a contributor to the improvement of society (78, 153).

SOCIETAL PERSPECTIVES ON AGING

> I may be old and wrinkled on the outside but I'm young and vulnerable on the inside.

Ageism refers to *any attitude, action, or institutional structure that discriminates against individuals on the basis of their age*. Ageist attitudes toward older adults are not new in the United States. Even during colonial days, the elderly were categorized as unnecessary and burdensome. Of growing concern is the ageism of the aged; the attitudes of some older people are discriminatory toward others who are in their own age group. Children appear most positive in their perception of elderly persons (72, 75).

In the United States old age frequently is characterized as a time of dependence and disease. Negative presentation of older adults, especially women, in movies, books, and magazines, in jokes, and on television contributes to negative beliefs and attitudes (12, 27, 146, 159, 196). Society's fear of the changes associated with aging such as gray hair, hearing loss, wrinkles, loss of muscle tone, slowness, and approaching death also contributes to negative attitudes.

Numerous unproven *myths* and age-related *stereotypes* pervade American culture. These myths and stereotypes obscure the truth and may prevent us from achieving our own potential as we grow older. Society stereotypes the older adult as being asexual, unemployable, unintelligent, and socially incompetent. Statements such as "You can't teach old dogs new tricks" and "dirty old men and women" typify the feelings of many. Instead of seeking the truth, most individuals accept myths that have been perpetuated through the years. Some of these myths and the contrasting realities are listed in Box 14–1.

Many of the myths and stereotypes associated with aging are culturally determined. The older adult in America lives in a culture oriented to youth, productivity, and rapid pace. Because of this orientation, older Americans may feel that they are not respected, valued, or needed.

There is no one criterion for successful aging. A study by Roos & Havens (222) of more than 3500 people in Manitoba, Canada, from 1971 to 1983 found few consistent predictors of successful aging. A book that provides suggestions for growing older and aging well is *Your Renaissance Years* by Robert Veninga, Little, Brown and Company, Publishers, 1991.

Culture, ethnicity, and socioeconomic level influence the role of the older adult in family relationships and determine health practices. For example, with the African-American, aging and death are viewed as natural processes; the older family members are held in esteem. In Asian cultures the older adults have an important role, and the young are expected to respect and care for them. Westernized children may have difficulty accepting this role. Many older adults continue to follow health practices that are linked to their cultural heritage. Respect for these cultural aspects of aging and cultural influences on health practices and healing methods must be shown (2, 8, 34, 44, 59, 64, 75, 97, 127, 130, 158, 163, 172, 216, 218, 223, 253).

THEORIES OF AGING

Although biologic and psychosocial theories of aging have been proposed, the specific cause of aging is unknown. Evolutionists relate senescence to the lack of se-

---

 ### Research Abstract

Seccombe, K., and M. Ishii-Kuntz, Perceptions of Problems Associated With Aging: Comparisons Among Four Older Age Cohorts, Gerontologist, 31, no. 4 (1991), 527–533.

The elderly are judged to be weak; in poor health; dependent; of lower competence, intelligence, and attractiveness than the young; asexual; and socially isolated. These negative sentiments are reported by children, college students, adults, and health care professionals who work with the elderly. These negative stereotypes have no biologic, sociologic, or psychologic basis.

The purpose of this study was to seek information about how perceptions of aging and concern over special problems faced by the aged vary among four adult age groups: the middle-aged (55 to 64 years), the young-old (65 to 74 years), the old (75 to 84 years), and the oldest-old (85 plus years).

The sample included 2329 noninstitutional adults living in different regions and types of communities. The survey involved interviews, and respondents were asked about their attitudes toward aging and sociodemographic questions.

The sample was not fully representative because the possibility of institutionalization increases with age (25% of people over age 85 reside in institutions). Although there were approximately equal numbers of middle-aged men and women, the gender ratio for the older groups included more women. Younger respondents more likely were college educated than older respondents. Most of the three older groups were retired; only 25% of the middle-aged adults were retired. Whereas 72% of the oldest-old were widowed, only 17% of the middle-aged adults, 25% of the young-old, and 55% of the old were widowed. Most of the oldest-old lived alone (74%), compared with 20% of the middle-aged, 40% of the young-old, and 53% of the old respondents. Further, the older the person, the more likely he or she was to report ill health.

A series of one-way analysis of variance (ANOVA) tests were performed to compare the perceptions of aging among the four age groups. Results indicated that definitions of old age varied among the age groups. The hypothesis was confirmed that the older the person, the more likely the person defined old age as older; the aging boundary was extended as the person approached it. Further, women are reported to age at an earlier age than men, related to women's being valued for physical attractiveness and sexuality and men being's valued for power, occupational achievement, and earning power.

The hypothesis that the media portray old people negatively was not confirmed..

There were significant differences among age groups about the problems for old people: money, loneliness, housing, fear of crime, and jobs. Consistent with the hypothesis, middle-aged adults reported these problems as more serious for the elderly than did the other age groups, and the oldest-old reported them as least problematic for the elderly. No differences between age groups were noted about the problems of poor health, lack of education, and insufficient medical care for the aged. The middle-aged group perceived personal problems experienced and general problems faced by the elderly as more serious than did the older age groups. The oldest-old respondents, especially Caucasians, were more optimistic about aging than younger groups, as were the married and widowed versus single elders. Further analysis with four regression equations for each age group indicated that elders with personal problems were more likely to view aging as problematic.

Implications of this study are that our youth-oriented society has exaggerated the obstacles faced by older persons. Further, because middle-aged adults have a less-than-positive attitude about aging, they experience anxiety about their own aging process. It is important to recognize that the elderly may be more accepting of and optimistic about their aging than is generally perceived. It is critical that health care providers, especially nurses, share this optimism and positive perception.

lection pressure in postreproductive years; they believe there is no universal cause for aging (29, 93, 102, 141, 233, 244, 260).

Biologic Theories

Biologic theories can be categorized as genetic, nongenetic cellular, and physiologic.

Genetic Theories

Genetic theories such as *DNA damage theories, random error theory, gene regulation theory, and somatic mutation by radiation* propose that aging results from change or damage to the genetic information involved in cellular protein formation. Accumulation of mutations or errors in cell reproduction cause death of the cell and eventually the organism.

Nongenetic Cellular Theories

These theories suggest that changes occur in the cellular proteins after their formation. Nongenetic theories include the wear-and-tear theory, deprivation theories, accumulation theories, free radical theory, and cross-linkage theory. The **Wear-and-Tear Theory,** or effects of temperature theory, is associated with the work of Hans Selye. According to this theory, *body systems wear out because of the stress of life and effects of metabolism.* This theory does not take into consideration the self-repair mechanisms of a living organism or the differences in life span within a species. **Deprivation Theories** assume that *aging is caused by deprivation of essential nutrients and oxygen to cells of the body.* It is likely that deprivation is the result of aging. **Accumulation Theories** suggest that *substances such as waste materials and lipofuscin accumulate in the cells of living organisms.* These substances interfere with cellular metabolism and ultimately cause cell death. These substances may also be a result rather than cause of senescence. **Free Radical Theory** hypothesizes that *free radicals (charged molecules) or chemicals that contain oxygen in a highly activated state and react with other molecules during normal metabolism cause aging.* There are many limitations to date on this research; the theory is not generally accepted. **Cross-Linkage Theory** hypothesizes that *bonds or cross-linkages develop between molecules and these bonds change the cellular properties physically and chemically.* Thus intracellular or extracellular material is chemically altered. In turn, cellular function is adversely affected. Protein elastin and collagen bonds have been studied, and this apparently is a viable theory.

Physiologic Theories

These theories explain aging on the basis of a breakdown of an organ system or impairment in neuroendocrine or physiologic control mechanisms. The **Biologic Clock Theory** suggests that *each organism contains genes that control the speed at which metabolic processes are performed. These genes act as a genetic clock,* dictating the occurrence of aging and dying. The **Immune Theory** proposes that *ability of the immune system to deal with foreign organisms or molecules diminishes with age,* with the greatest decline in thymus-derived immunity (T-cell or cellular immunity). Further, the production of antibodies by the immune system diminishes after adolescence, and protection from microorganisms and atypical mutant cells decreases. Normal cells sometimes are engulfed and digested; thus the person is more vulnerable to disease. This hypothesis appears reasonable.

Neuroendocrine Theory refers to the importance of the neurologic and endocrine systems. *Loss of neurons and endocrine cells reflects losses in ground substance, fluids, and hormones, causing cellular changes. The rate of adjustment or performance diminishes.* A slower response and eventually cell death are caused by impaired integrative functions at the neural and endocrine levels. In fact, cell death may be programmed, related to neuroendocrine factors. **Glycation Theory** suggests that the *process of nonenzymatic reactions that occur between reducing sugars and tissue proteins and nucleic acids results in dehydrated and rearranged irreversible structures as end products.* These glycated proteins exhibit loss of enzyme activity, inappropriate cross-linking, and decreased degradation of abnormal proteins. Glycation of collagen reduces elasticity and changes connective tissue. Thus glycation has profound cumulative effects through the life span. It is unknown if this is a cause or a result of aging.

Psychosocial Theories

Just as one biologic theory does not adequately address biologic aging, one single psychosocial theory of aging is not adequate to explain psychologic or social aging. The **Continuity Theory** proposes that *an individual's patterns of behavior are the result of a lifetime of experiences, and aging is the continuation of these lifelong adjustments or personality patterns.* Continuity Theory, as first proposed by Brim and Kagan, assumes neither a necessary reduction in activity levels (Disengagement Theory) nor the necessity of maintaining high activity levels (Activity Theory). They associated successful aging with the ability of the person to maintain patterns of behavior that existed before old age. Continuity in behavioral patterns and life-style exists over time, regardless of the actual level of activity present. Each of us has a powerful drive to maintain the sense of identity or continuity that allays fears of changing too fast or being changed against one's will by external forces. There is a simultaneous drive to develop and mature further, which fosters continuing change in at least small ways. Adult development is not in the genes but in the intricacies of life experiences. Two psychologic mechanisms, selective perception and situational reinforcement, are used to maintain a sense of continu-

■ BOX 14-1.
Myths and Misconceptions and Their Realities for the Elderly Person

Myth 1: Age 65 Is a Good Marker for Old Age.

Fact: Factors other than chronologic age cause the person to be old. Many people are more youthful than their parents were at age 65. With increased longevity, perhaps 70 or 75 should be the chronologic marker (72).

Myth 2: Most Old People Are in Bed or in Institutions and Are Ill Physically and Mentally.

Fact: Approximately 5% are institutionalized; 95% are living in the community. Although 67% of older persons outside institutions have one or more chronic conditions, 14% do not. Chronic conditions range from mild and correctable to more severe. Approximately 81% of the aged living in the community have no mobility limitations; 8% have trouble getting around; 6% need the help of another person; and 5% are homebound. The average number of restricted activity days is only twice that for young adults (72). Some report no physical illness, and some with physical disease processes do not consider themselves ill.

Myth 3: All Old People Are Alike.

Fact: Each older adult is unique and *quite diverse.* This segment of the life span covers more years than any other segment—sometimes more than 35 years. The older people are, the more varied are their physical capabilities, personal style, economic status, and life-style preferences. From birth, physical and mental elaboration continues through life to make people more and more unlike one another (102).

Myth 4: The Next Generation of Older Adults Will Be the Same as This Generation.

Fact: The next generation will be better educated, healthier, more mobile, more youthful in appearance, more accustomed to life-style change and technology, and more outspoken. The world is changing so quickly that each successive generation is vastly *different* from the ones that came before (72).

Myth 5: Old Age Brings Mental Deterioration.

Fact: Approximately 5% of older adults show serious mental impairment, and only 10% demonstrate even mild to moderate memory loss. Many professionals work past 65 to 70 years (72).

Myth 6: Old People Cannot Learn and Are Less Intelligent.

Fact: Older adults *can* and *do* learn. However, they may need a longer time period in which to respond to questions and stimuli. When learning problems occur, they are usually associated with a disease process. Intelligent people remain so (34, 75).

Myth 7: Most Older Adults Are Incompetent.

Fact: Older people may have a slower reaction time and take longer to do psychomotor tasks. However, they have more consistent output, less job turnover, greater job satisfaction, fewer accidents, and less absenteeism (72).

Myth 8: Most Older Adults Are Unhappy and Dissatisfied With Life.

Fact: How happy or sad the person feels reflects basic temperament throughout life, the adaptation to past and current life events, and social support. Positive social ties and realistic expectations buffer psychologic distress. Older people tend to be as satisfied with their lives as middle-aged people, even when lower incomes and poorer health are present (14, 196, 218).

Myth 9: The Elderly Are Self-Pitying, Apathetic, Irritable, and Hard to Live With.

Fact: Research shows that mood is related to the present situation and past personality. The older person is as likely as a younger one to have an interesting and pleasant personality (148).

Myth 10: The Elderly Are Inactive and Unproductive.

Fact: Many young children have working grandparents. Thirty-six percent of men over 65 years are employed in some type of job. Older women often do their housework into their eighties or nineties. Older workers have a job attendance record that is 20% better than young workers, and they also sustain fewer job-related injuries (148).

Myth 11: The Elderly Do Not Desire and Do Not Participate in Sexual Activity.

Fact: Recent research refutes this assertion (74, 148). Sexual activity may decline because of lack of a partner or misinformation about sexuality in late life. The person who has been sexually active all along is able to continue sexual activity, and sexual activity involves more than intercourse between the partners (148).

Myth 12: The Elderly Are Isolated, Abandoned, and Lonely, and They Are Unlikely to Participate in Activities.

Fact: Many elderly prefer to live in a separate household. Many elderly live with someone and do not feel lonely. Approximately 10% of people over 65 years never married and have adjusted to living alone. Elderly people who do not have children often have siblings or friends with whom they live. Other elderly live in institutions or residences for the aged where they make friends. The percentage of purposefully abandoned elderly is small; often the person who is a loner in old age has always been alone (71, 72, 148).

■ **Box 14-1.**
Continued

Myth 13: Retirement Is Disliked by All Old People and Causes Illness and Less Life-Satisfaction.

Fact: Although this may be true for some people, many older people look forward to retirement and are retiring before 65 so that they can continue other pursuits. Most are not sick from idleness and a sense of worthlessness. More than three fourths of them have satisfying lives (148).

Myth 14: Special Health Services for the Aged Are Useless Because the Aged Cannot Benefit Anyway.

Fact: At age 65 the average person can look forward to 15 more years of life. The elderly have fewer acute illnesses and accidental injuries, and these conditions are correctable, although older people take longer to recover than younger people do. Common chronic conditions are cardiovascular disease, cancer, arthritis, diabetes, sensory impairments, and depression, which can be treated so that the person can achieve maximum potential and comfort (72, 148).

ity. **Selective perception** means that *experiences are reacted to on the basis of their relative congruence with currently held values, beliefs, and attitudes.* Noncongruent ideas are screened out of awareness, ignored, or not attended to. **Situational reinforcement** means that the *behaviors used are those that are rewarded. Previously established behavior patterns tend to have a long history of reinforcement* (153).

Developmental Theories

Several developmental theories have addressed psychosocial aging. **Erikson's Epigenetic Theory** (79) suggests that *successful personality development in later life depends on the ability to resolve the psychosocial crisis known as integrity versus despair.* Erikson's theory is psychodynamic and is part of a life cycle approach that emphasizes that the developmental tasks of each stage must be met before the person can work through the next tasks. The theory is discussed in detail on pp. 575 to 576.

Peck's Theory (199) hypothesizes that *there are three psychologic developmental tasks of old age: ego differentiation versus work-role preoccupation, body transcendence versus body preoccupation, and ego transcendence versus ego preoccupation.* These issues are an extension and further development of Erikson's stage, with emphasis on change and growth in later life. Robert Havighurst (106) presents several major developmental tasks that must be mastered or achieved to meet the developmental needs of later maturity (see pp. 581 to 582). He uses an eclectic approach that combines previously developed concepts into one theory (106). According to all developmental theories, the older adult's behavior and response depend on how earlier developmental crises were handled.

Sociologic Theories

The Disengagement Theory, Activity Theory, and Interactionist Theory are sociologic theories. **Disengagement Theory,** proposed by Cumming and Henry (58), *suggests that all old people and society mutually withdraw, that the withdrawal is biologically and psychologically intrinsic and inevitable, and that it is necessary for aging and beneficial to society.* This voluntary withdrawal or separation from society is related to a decreased life space in the older adult, relinquishment of roles, decreased integration into society, fewer social interests, and increased preference for individual interactions and rewards. Cumming and Henry's Disengagement Theory suggests that society finds ways to minimize the social disruption that results from death of its members. In addition, individuals in a society undergo a self-disengagement process during the middle and later years of life. This process is characterized by a reduction in general energy levels, reduction in societal involvement, and an increased preoccupation with one's own needs and desires. Studies do not support the Disengagement Theory. The older person may be alone but enjoy the solitude, be mentally alert, and be responsive socially (160).

Cross-cultural studies show disengagement is not inevitable, and it is generally not applicable to family relationships. Thus Disengagement Theory as proposed by Cummings and Henry is considered factually incorrect, methodologically unsound, and dangerous as a basis for social policy (153, 238). Sill's research (238) reveals that awareness of **finitude,** *estimate of time remaining before death,* and physical incapacity were more important than age in predicting level of activity. The person who perceives self as near death begins to constrict life space; psychologic preparation for death may lead to disengagement.

Activity Theory, formulated by Havighurst, Maddox, and Palmore to refute Disengagement Theory, is the more popular of the two theories. *Basic concepts of the theory are that most elderly people maintain a level of activity and engagement commensurate with their earlier patterns of activity and past life-styles and that the maintenance of physical, mental, and social activity is usually necessary for successful aging* (34, 160, 197).

Activity Theory implies that the older adult has essentially the same psychologic and social needs as do middle-aged people. According to this theory, the older adult must compensate for the loss of roles experienced in later maturity. The older adult does not disengage but needs to maintain a moderately active life-style. In reality, the response to aging by most older adults is a combination of the two theories (153).

Mead first articulated the **Symbolic Interaction Theory** in 1934, from which many of our present theories have grown. This theory holds that *the person develops socially according to the continuous bombardment of self-reflections perceived from others.* The aged in our culture are generally seen as having little social validity, and if this attitude is perceived consistently, it can become a self-fulfilling prophecy. People may expect to become inept and forgetful. Social and cultural expectations may strongly color self-view and consequent behavior. Symbolic Interaction Theory attempts to consider the interrelationships of several dimensions of the aging process, including:

1. Sociocultural dimensions that set the limits on available alternatives for the person.
2. Contextual dimensions within which the individual's life course develops (e.g., includes biologic change, past experiences).
3. Personal evaluation of life experience, health status, and the future foci of energy and roles.

Biologic changes, psychologic changes, societal circumstances, and past and present experiences all are considered as relevant for explaining the aging process (173).

FAMILY DEVELOPMENT AND RELATIONSHIPS

The changing demographic profile of developed countries has been associated with an increased number of four- and five-generation families. In such families it is common to have two generations at or near old age, with the oldest person frequently over 75 years. The "generation in the middle" may extend into retirement years in many families. Thus the "young-old," facing the potential of diminished personal resources, may be the group increasingly called on to give additional support to aged kin—the old-old and very or frail-old.

Several authors have written about aging in different cultures, family relations between generations in different cultures and countries, and how worldwide social changes are affecting the elderly as family members. (1, 8, 34, 37, 44, 59, 64, 75, 82, 97, 127, 139, 158, 163, 172, 184, 218, 223, 250, 283).

Relationship With Spouse

In later life responsibilities of parenthood and employment diminish with few formal responsibilities to take their place. There is usually a corresponding decline in social contacts and activities. The factors that affect the social life of the elderly are found in personal social skills and in resources available in the private life. Marital status remains a major organizing force for personal life. With children gone and without daily contact with co-workers provided by employment, the elderly lose the basis for social integration. Declining health, limited income, and fewer daily responsibilities may create greater needs for social support. Thus having a spouse provides the possibility for increased companionship. Having a spouse also increases longevity, especially for older males, unless the male never married.

Interestingly, spouses may not increase in their support to each other into late life, perhaps because of increased **interiority** (*introspection*) with aging. Time may erode bases of respect, affection, and compatibility. Sometimes marriages have not been filled with mutual emotional or social support in earlier years, so there is no foundation for increasing mutual emotional support. Women are often the sole support for men; older women tend to feel the husband is not supportive emotionally or in health care. However, women tend to rely on a more extensive network of family and friends for support (62).

For the woman continually to have a spouse in the house or with her, wanting to share in her activities, can be distressing, even though it has been anticipated. The loss of privacy and solitude, doing tasks her own way and at her own pace, loss of independence, and loss of contact with friends may all be issues. However, the increased accommodation to meeting husband's needs is offset by increased opportunities for nurturing and being nurtured and for sharing mutual interests.

Your listening and teaching may assist the elderly person in making the necessary adjustments to the spouse.

Relationships With Offspring and Other Family Members

Historical trends toward smaller families, longer life spans, increasing employment of women, and increasingly high mobility of both young and old have important implications for children's being a primary resource in old age (264).

The number of children is related to the recency with which older parents have seen their child, the amount of assistance older parents receive, and factors influencing older parents' interaction with children. Parents with one child report fewer visits and less help received, especially if the only child is an employed daughter. Older parents expect children, especially the daughter(s), to assume an appreciable level of responsibility in meeting important health, economic, and emotional needs, regardless of how many offspring there are to share in the assistance. Assistance from children-in-law, grandchildren, siblings and siblings-in-law, and nieces and nephews increases as the number of offspring decreases. Geographic proximity is a stable predictor of older parent–child interaction, more than offspring gender or health status of the parent. Daughters who are primarily blue-collar workers provide more assistance to older parents and have more association with parents than corresponding sons. Parents receive more help from offspring as income for the offspring increases (34, 75).

Thomas (258) found that older parents receive and perceive their children's help in several ways. Younger parents receive more help with automobile maintenance and help in the form of gifts. Older parents receive help with shopping and transportation. Parents who most strongly valued family are most desirous of and satisfied with family support. Parents may tend to expect less help from children when they live at a distance or when they work outside the home. Further, they appreciate most the help that keeps them self-reliant or autonomous, maintains social integration, maximizes choice and expressive interactions, and forestalls reliance on more extensive services. Parents with greater degree of ill health express less satisfaction with children's help, possibly because it symbolizes dependency and loss of social integration.

Some elderly people have a limited number of family members; some couples have no children. The childless couple will probably have adapted to childlessness psychologically. However, they are especially vulnerable at crisis points such as episodes of poor health or death of spouse or housing companion. If those persons or couples cannot drive or have no transportation, they will have greater need for help, although they many hesitate to ask for help.

Your teaching and referrals may enable the elderly person with few relatives or resources to manage more effectively.

Grandparenthood

Grandparenthood has multiple meanings for the person, depending in part on age at the initial time of grandparenthood, and the number and accomplishments of the grandchildren are probably a source of status (143). The stage of grandparenthood may come to the middle-aged persons, depending on age of their own childbearing and age of their childrens' childbearing. The relatively young grandparent may either like and accept or resist the role and may not like the connection of age and being a grandparent. Relative youth of grandparents contributes to the complex patterns of help and relationships between the generations. The increasing divorce rate also adds to the complexity of grandparent relationships (126). The child may have eight sets of grandparents. The grandparents may be the main caretakers for the child(ren), or there may be a part-time commitment, sharing child care with their adult children (23, 81).

Grandparents are often happy with their role in that they can enjoy the young person and enter into a play-

ful, informal, companion, and confidant relationship (Fig. 14–2). The grandchild is seen as a source of leisure activity, someone for whom to purchase items that are also enjoyable to the grandparent. The grandparent typically does not want to take on an authoritarian or disciplinarian role but will, and has the experience to do so, if necessary. The number of **great-grandparents** and **great-great-grandparents** is increasing as more people live longer. The roles are emotionally fulfilling; these young family members provide a sense of personal and family renewal and transcendence; add diversion—to conversations if not activities; and mark longevity. Great-grandparents may be as active in the grandparenting role as they were as grandparents, but advanced age, geographic distance, and cohabitation, divorce, and remarriage of family members tend to limit their participation. Also, this generation feels removed from the very young, whereas the grandparent generation feels a special tie with the very young (65).

Social Relationships

Social networks of family, friends, and neighbors provide instrumental and expressive support. They contribute to well-being of the senior by promoting socialization and companionship, elevating morale and life satisfaction, buffering the effects of stressful events, providing a confidant, and facilitating coping skills and mastery. For example, social supports buffer the effects of stressful life events and represent more than the quantity or proximity of social ties but also the extent to which social ties fulfill needs of the senior. Also, the components of informal support networks—spouses, children, close relatives, distant kin (cousins, aunts, uncles, nieces, nephews), coworkers, close friends, neighbors, and acquaintances—have a variety of functions and vary in importance to the senior. Instrumental help is given in the form of advice, information, financial aid,

Figure 14-2. Grandparents often look forward to their role. (From Sherwen, L.N., M.A. Scoloveno, and C.T. Weingarten, *Nursing Care of the Childbearing Family.* Norwalk, Conn: Appleton & Lange, 1991, p. 764.)

and assistance with tasks. Socioemotional aid is given in the form of affection, sympathy, understanding, acceptance, esteem, and referral to services (50, 144). Planning for contact between the generations (e.g., with preschoolers or adolescents) also contributes to meaningful social interactions for both generations (40, 140, 151).

Frequency of use of social networks is not related to physical health. As income decreases, visiting with neighbors declines, but visits to close friends or relatives increase, as does the tendency to talk to family members about feelings and to talk to friends about events. The elderly rate helpfulness of children and other family members as important. Lower income increases the senior's reliance on friends and relatives and the value placed on their help. Higher income may provide resources that facilitate social visiting and a broader network of relationships. A higher frequency of social contacts and greater intensity of kin and friend relationships have been found for women in comparison to men. Apparently intimacy or close friendship ties and having a confidant are less important to the male (50, 137, 144).

Supportive ties become smaller and more unstable in old age, and social support may provide burdens for those who provide it to the senior. The closer the bond, the greater are the physical, emotional, and financial strains. Burdens and costs may result in being less willing or able to help, physical or psychologic distancing, increasing the social isolation of the dependent senior, or becoming enmeshed in the caregiver role to the exclusion of other relationships or roles. Informal networks ideally are integrated with formal support services (144).

An unregulated or informal social welfare system naturally exists in the average community or senior residence, which provides more services, security, and hope for the future than is provided by formal agencies. This system of informal assistance through family, friends, and neighbors is the major source of help for the elderly. Among and for seniors, there are three types of neighborhood exchange types: (1) high helpers, who exhibit a more formal quasi-professional style of helping without reciprocation; (2) mutual helpers, who show an interdependent style of give and take; and (3) neighborhood isolates, whose social ties and help sources are primarily outside the neighborhood. High helpers with neighbors are those who also do volunteer work or are active in self-help groups. Often these people have been in the helping professions in their work years; they also had a spiritual or religious orientation with serving others. Mutual helpers have more neighborhood contact and are generally quite outgoing. Isolates have little contact with others and view themselves as quiet people. They may be in poor health and in need of help themselves (98).

Many of the events of later life are exit events, involving continuous threat, stress, and loss such as widow(er)hood, chronic or poor health, retirement, change in residence, and lower income. Thus coping often becomes problem specific and also involves socialization, learning how to perform new roles, adjusting to changing roles, and relinquishing old roles. Socialization contributes to well-being by lending continuity and structure to the transitions encountered by people (273).

Often you will be able to assist the elderly in asking for and accepting help from others, or in becoming familiar with community resources.

Caregiver Role

The role of the middle-aged offspring in caring for the elderly parent has been described in Chapter 13. Refer to Chapter 13 and references at the end of that chapter and at the end of this chapter for more information on the caregiver role. Even as elders are being cared for, they are also a source of support—emotionally, socially, financially, by providing living arrangement—for the adult child (99, 180).

The caregiver in an elderly couple is most frequently the wife since women live longer than men and are usually younger than the spouse. If the woman is impaired, the husband is often the caregiver. The spouse is the primary source of help for married elderly with impaired capacity, and adult daughters are the major helpers when a spouse is not present or not able to sufficiently help. The probability of relying on friends is highest among impaired elderly who are unmarried and have few family members within an hour's travel. The more frail the person, the more likely a family member will be the primary caregiver rather than formal systems or nonrelated people (28, 46, 155, 211, 254). The majority of noninstitutionalized elderly are self-sufficient (147).

When the spouse cannot manage care for the elderly parent, children try to assist. Sons tend to become caregivers only in the absence of an available female sibling and are more likely to rely on their own spouses for support and help. Sons tend to provide less direct care assistance and to be less involved; hence they do not feel as stressed by the caregiving experience.

The elderly person who cares for a disabled spouse is a hidden victim, at risk for physical and emotional stresses of caregiving superimposed on stresses of the aging process. He or she is likely to experience a barrage of feelings and role overload, including being head of the household. The woman, as the spouse who is the caregiver, may also be chronically ill or disabled. Thus the family caregiver of the noninstitutionalized elderly is in need of help from supportive services. These services for the spouse could include a wives' support group sponsored by a senior center; home health care; adult day care; foster home placement; extended respite care; homemaker, transporter, and repairman services; and visitor or "relief" services. Several authors discuss the role of the spouse as the main caregiver with the disabled elderly. Pratt, Schmall, and Wright (208) discuss ethical concerns of family members in the caregiver role.

Be aware of feelings of the middle-aged or elderly caregiver and the family; needs and feelings of the elderly person; issues and conflicts for the family; and ways to help families manage the caregiving experience. Education and support group programs appear to hold great promise as a means for assisting family caregivers of older relatives. You will have an important role in implementing both of those interventions. A number of strategies can be helpful to the caregiver both in preventing decline in the caregiver and in administering care to the elder (34, 75).

Widow(er)hood

Because widow(er)hood may occur before late life, the feelings, problems, and issues pertinent to the widow(er) have been discussed in Chapter 13. Refer to Chapter 13 and the references at the end of this chapter for additional insights. Bereavement does not permanently affect health status for most seniors, although the grief reaction may induce physiologic symptoms initially. Stress appears to increase as the death approaches, and then health status may deteriorate. Regardless of the predeath mourning done by the survivor, the elderly widow(er) has great increase in psychologic distress (10, 69, 90, 150, 154, 181, 285).

Widow(er)hood disrupts couple-based relationships and obligations to a spouse and introduces emotional and material burdens on those relationships that outlive the marriage. Widow(er)hood, especially after a period of caregiving, may also introduce both a measure of freedom to make new contacts and a stimulus to do so. If the person moves to a smaller dwelling, increased housing density produces a greater increase in social contacts among the widowed than is seen in the married. Without the support that the spouse usually provides, the widowed may turn to friends and relatives as a source of replacement. The widowed may have greater intimacy with their friends than the married, for married people interact more with their spouses (121, 144, 179).

The elderly widowed are not more isolated than elderly married, and elderly women have some advantage over elderly men in their ability to develop or maintain social relationships. Patterns of social relationships established among the married apparently provide the parameters within which social relationships continue among the widowed. Both married and widowed women are more likely to talk to close friends and relatives and to talk to family about worries and to children about crises than are married or widowed men. Loss of spouse allows for expansion or addition of new roles; frequency of contact increases with widow(er)hood. Widow(er)hood results in greater involvement with informal social relationships than marriage (144, 261).

The widow who lives alone in her own home may be in need of a great deal of help. Neighbors often provide this help, especially if children reside out of town. Bryant (31) found that the childless widow, however, may not receive any more help from neighbors than widows with children in spite of greater needs. Perhaps adult children are able to elicit neighbor assistance; such re-

quests for extra help are not forthcoming if there are no children.

Your teaching, emotional support, referral to services, and encouragement to continue as active a life as possible are important to the widow(er) as she or he adjusts to losses and new roles. A helpful book for the widow is *Suddenly Alone: A Woman's Guide to Widowhood,* by P. Gates, Harper Perennial Publishers, 1991.

Divorce and the Elderly

Those who are separated from their spouses and those who are legally divorced total slightly over 5% of the population. Both the number of people who were ever divorced, who have been divorced before age 65 years, and who are over age 65 when divorce occurs are increasing. Also, the proportion of older persons who have ever experienced a divorce is considerably larger than the proportion who are currently divorced since many divorced people remarry. In the future fewer marriages will be terminated by death before old age. Also, an increased number of seniors will fall in the ever-divorced and currently divorced categories since those entering old age in the future will be more accepting of divorce as a solution to an unpleasant marriage (52). Further, in the future more elderly women will have economic independence because of their years in the work force, and this may encourage higher divorce rates (43, 265).

Being divorced in old age, or in any age, may negatively affect a person's economic position and may increase demands for social welfare support. Typically divorce is associated with a deterioration in the standard of living for women, although it has little effect for men. Further, family and kinship relationships are affected by divorce. The children or other relatives who would provide physical help and psychosocial support may not be available to one of the parents in his or her old age. Remarriage also establishes a new set of nuclear family relationships. The experience of being divorced can help the senior cope with bereavement. The person knows survival is possible after a marital relationship ends (43, 265).

Be prepared to give emotional support or crisis intervention to the older person who is encountering divorce or who is reworking the conflicts, dilemmas, and losses of having experienced divorce.

Singlehood

A small percentage (approximately 5% of elderly) of people remain single and never marry. They have no spouse or children. They may or may not have living family members. They may or may not live alone. The never-married elderly do not constitute a single "social type"; their situations are more complex. Like other elderly, they are affected by social opportunities and restraints and the cultural values and changes that impinge on their life situations. Some older people are homosexual. Some live in locations in which women outnumber men causing an imbalance in mate selection. Others may have chosen the single life-style as a means to some end such as a career. Some have had family responsibilities that precluded marriage or were otherwise unable to break out of their families of orientation. Others have been lifelong isolates and have had poor health or a stigmatized social identity. Possibly the factors for singlehood have been multiple. As practitioners, we should be sensitive to these differences and to their effects on the lives and identities of never married elderly (226).

There are five types of key personal relationships for never-married older women that help reduce social isolation and loneliness and increase life satisfaction and social support (225). They are:

1. *Blood ties*—nieces, nephews, siblings, aging parents. Often the woman gives assistance, which involves sacrifice.
2. *Constricted ties*—affiliation with a nonkin family; establishment of a quasi-parental tie with a younger person who is like a son or daughter; or a long-term relationship with a same-generation companion. These relationships are voluntary and positive, but there is no assurance of care from these individuals.
3. *Quasi-parental relations*—acting like a parent to younger nonrelatives. There is no biogenetic tie, but the relationship is modeled on parent-child tie.
4. *Companionate ties*—a marriagelike interdependency in which there is much involvement over time and a sense of obligation to care for each other.
5. *Friendship ties*—a close relationship that endures and provides security. Depending on the duration and closeness, the friend may provide help in time of need.

Issues of attachment may be different for the widowed and the never married, but this does not mean that there are no loss issues, although it is clear that there are some never-married elderly who do not develop such attachments. There is a range of attachments and bereavement experiences for the never married in late life, not just an absence of personal loss issues (226). Having lived independently all during adult life, the person may have developed effective adaptive mechanisms and a supportive social network (136). The assumption is that being married provides social, emotional, and sustenance needs. In fact, the single person who has planned carefully for retirement may be as satisfied with self and life and as secure in all aspects as the married person. The single person may be no more lonely than the married person. He or she does not experience the desolation of widow(er) hood or divorce (225, 226).

Few studies have been done on health status of the single senior. They generally conclude that the well-being of single people is equivalent to that of married persons, whereas widowed, divorced, and separated persons have lower well-being (273). A decline in functional capacity greatly increases the likelihood that the unmar-

ried older person will move in with others or become institutionalized (225, 284).

Single women tend to have greater education, occupational status, and intellectual ability than married women, suggesting that career orientation makes marriage less attractive for women. Single women are likely to be first-born, which leads to a less romantic view of marriage because of early roles as surrogate parents. Single men do not display the higher educational and occupational attainment found with single women, but they are more likely to be only children, suggesting socialization for greater achievement. Psychologic integrity and social independence are features of the single personality (226).

The single person views fluidity and variety in social relationships, rather than the exclusivity of marriage, as an advantage in promoting opportunities for personal growth while still protecting autonomy. Life-style is geared to preserving personal independence and the development of self, with privacy, self-expression through work, freedom of movement, and preoccupation with expanding experiences, philosophic insights, and imaginative conceptions of life as goals for the person. Single women are happier and better adjusted than single men; marital roles may be less beneficial and more stressful for women than for men. Although single women are happier than single men, they are nevertheless less happy than married women. The characteristic that best explains their relative unhappiness is greater dissatisfaction with family life. The lower well-being of the never married is attributable either to changes accompanying aging, which lessen the viability of single life-styles, or to less support of single living among other older people (225, 226, 273).

Be alert to special emotional and social needs of the single elderly, to their reticence at times to ask for help, and to the need for information about community resources. You may become a significant confidant.

Elderly and Pets

Pets are great companions for older people. In 1983 President Ronald Reagan signed a law guaranteeing the right to keep pets in government-assisted rental housing for the elderly and handicapped. A number of states have adopted laws to allow animals as permanent residents of hospitals and nursing homes. Pets are therapeutic in the home and in the center or institution for the elderly. They offer companionship and unconditional love, and a specially trained dog can offer assistance and security (e.g., as a brace for the neurologically impaired). Dogs can pull wheelchairs and even help load them into cars. Pets have a beneficial effect on physical health: they lower stress response and lower blood pressure. The touch from the pet and stroking the pet offer physiologic release and lower anxiety. Pets can promote verbal communication skills; birds can even talk back. Although animals and birds do carry disease, healthy pets can be obtained from well-run shelters and shops or the Humane Society. The person or family may need help in keeping the pet immunized, cleaned, and given the care that prevents unnecessary decline in the pet's health. You can be instrumental in promoting pet therapy (38, 112, 146, 281).

The death of a pet can precipitate a deep grief, and mourning will result because of the loss. Crisis counseling, giving the person a helping hand and a shoulder to cry on, may help the person work through the pet's death or work through feelings related to having to put the pet to sleep. Be aware that the senior who is wanting euthanasia for an apparently healthy pet may be contemplating suicide or suicide may follow the death of a pet. Death of a pet can be the last straw in a series of stresses and losses.

Elder Abuse

The Older Americans Act (Public Law 89–73), passed by Congress in 1965, was amended in 1987 (Public Law 100–175) to add services for prevention of elder abuse as a priority for government funding. In addition, state offices of aging were to identify nonprofit entities that were involved in prevention, identification, and treatment of abuse, neglect, and exploitation of older persons.

It is estimated that more than 1,000,000 older Americans are abused annually. The victim usually is a Caucasian female over 70 years old with moderate to severe physical or mental impairments. Usually the abuser is a relative (spouse or offspring) residing with her.

The four main types of abuse are:

1. Physical—the senior is beaten, shoved, slapped, restrained for long periods, or sexually molested.
2. Psychologic—the senior is treated like an infant, yelled at, cursed, not included in family activities, or isolated for long periods.
3. Financial—the senior's resources or money are taken or totally managed by the caregivers without consent, or the senior is forced to sign over legal title to property.
4. Neglect—the senior is not given the materials for meeting basic needs such as food, or necessary medication, eyeglasses, hearing aids, or medical treatment is withheld (34, 36, 75, 116, 205).

Hypotheses about the cause of elder abuse include (1) psychopathology in the caregiver, (2) stresses of caring for the impaired elder, and (3) dependency of the elder as a trigger for victimizing the person (34, 36, 75, 116, 205).

Signs and symptoms of the abused elder include:

1. Bruises, fractures, malnourished status.
2. Undue confusion not attributable to physiologic consequences of aging.
3. Conflicting explanation about the senior's condition.

4. Unusual fear exhibited by the senior in a presumed safe environment, in the home, or in the presence of the caregiver.
5. A report of the daily routine that has considerable gaps in the sequence.
6. Apparent impaired functioning or abnormal behavior in the caregiver.
7. Indifference or hostility displayed by caregiver in response to questions.

During assessment of potential abuse, avoid a censuring tone of voice or judgmental expression or stance. Show a willingness to listen to the caregiver's perspective. Solicit the caregiver's early memories of relationships with the senior to learn of long-term conflicts. Most abused seniors are reluctant and ashamed to report abuse because of (1) fear of retaliation, (2) exposure of offspring to community censure or legal punishment, and (3) fear of potential removal from their home.

In planning care and during intervention, be familiar with the reporting laws of your state and whether the law covers only known abuse or suspected abuse. In most states professionals who fail to report abuse may be fined, and they are accorded protection from civil and criminal liability if they report abuse.

Because the abused senior is an adult with full legal rights, intervention is not possible without the consent of the senior if the person is legally competent. If the client is in a life-threatening situation, is competent, and chooses to remain at home, the nurse must honor that decision after counseling the elder of the danger. If the person is legally incompetent and appears in immediate danger, the nurse should begin appropriate guardianship procedures.

Be aware that advocacy for the abused elder may be difficult; you may receive threats of harm from caregivers who resent the disruption of a previously convenient financial exploitation of an elderly relative. A common situation is when the elder refuses help and desires to remain in an environment that, by your standard, is unacceptable or unsafe. This can be very frustrating. Testifying in court to the nature of specific abusive situations can be anxiety provoking.

PHYSIOLOGIC CONCEPTS

Physical Characteristics

When we are born, regardless of our genetic background or external influences, we all have one thing in common—the element of aging. From the day of birth, we begin the aging process.

The rapidity and manifestations of aging in each individual depend on heredity, past illnesses, life-style, patterns of eating and exercise, presence of chronic illnesses, and level of lifetime stress. However, some generalized physiologic changes do occur; they include a decrease in rate of cell mitosis, a deterioration of specialized nondividing cells, an increased rigidity and loss of elasticity in connective tissue, and a loss of reserve functional capacity (29, 102, 244).

Certain other characteristics have been observed about aging (29, 75, 102, 111, 244):

1. The time of onset, type, and degree of aging differs between men and women and is more distinctive between the sexes in middle life than in the later years.
2. Senescent alterations in one organ or in the whole organism can be either premature or delayed in relation to the body's total chronology.
3. The progression of aging in cellular tissues is asymmetric: in one system the characteristics of old age may be displayed prominently (brain, bone, cardiovascular apparatus, lungs) and be less obvious elsewhere (liver, pancreas, gastrointestinal tract, muscles).
4. Certain pathology is a manifestation of aging.
5. A direct relationship exists between the sum of common aging traits and the length of survival.

General Appearance

The general appearance of the older adult is determined in part by the changes that occur in the skin, face, hair, and posture.

Skin. The overall appearance of the skin changes dramatically (Table 14–1). It develops creases and furrows and begins to sag. *Irregular areas of dark pigmentation* **(lentigo senilis)** that look like large freckles appear. These are especially common on the dorsum of hands, arms, and face. Some capillaries and small arteries on exposed portions of the skin surface become dilated. The coloring of fair-skinned older adults loses the pinkish flesh tone (7, 29, 75, 102, 244). Berliner's two articles

(17, 18) are excellent references and also contain pictures of various conditions seen in the older adult.

Because of changes in the skin cells and cellular elements, there is a loss of skin firmness and resiliency, with a decrease in the skin turgor. The elastin fibers in the skin become more brittle, and the outer epidermal layer becomes thinner as cells are depleted. Normal skin cells in an average 70-year-old live only 46 days as compared to 100 days for a 30-year-old. In addition, skin cells are replaced more slowly in the older adult. Because the *sebaceous glands,* which normally lubricate the skin with oil, decrease activity, the skin becomes dryer and rougher. The inability of the aging skin to retain fluids also contributes to dry, less flexible skin. The skin gradually loses its ability to regulate body temperature. There is a significant reduction in the number of sweat glands. This interferes with the body's ability to sweat freely, which can lead to heat exhaustion. Furthermore, the loss of subcutaneous fat, which functions as insulation for the body, can make the older adult susceptible to the cold. The loss of the subcutaneous fat also accounts for the characteristically emaciated look of old age (7, 29, 75, 102).

Avoid brisk rubbing, hot water, and use of excessive soap during baths. Pat skin dry; use lotions for dryness and itching. Avoid abrasions and long pressure on a local area.

Head. Even the appearance of the *face* changes as the nose and ears tend to become longer and broader and the chin line alters. Wrinkles on the face are pronounced because of the repeated stress produced by the activity of facial muscles. The predominant mood expressed by the facial muscles of the individual becomes permanently etched on the face in the form of wrinkles (smile or frown lines) above the eyebrows, around lips, over cheeks, and around the outer edges of the eye orbit.

TABLE 14-1. SKIN ALTERATIONS RELATED TO AGING

	Alteration	Manifestations
Epidermis	Increased fragility	Thinning
	Decreased cellular division	Wrinkling
	Decreased number of pigment cells	
	Larger pigment cells grouped together	Uneven pigmentation
	Increased permeability of surface cells	
Dermis	Decreased fat, water, and matrix content	Translucent tissue
	Decreased flexibility of collagen	Decreased elasticity
	Decreased number of fibroblasts and fiber	Thinning tissue
	Larger and coarser collagenous fibers	
Subcutaneous tissue (hypodermis)	Loss of fat, especially in face and limbs	Sagging tissue
	Decreased blood supply to skin	Wrinkling
		Decreased insulation
		Decreased padding
Adnexal structures	Decreased sebaceous gland activity	Dry, scaly skin
	Decreased sweat gland activity	Decreased ability to regulate body temperature
	Slowly growing nails	Yellowish color to nails
		Developing ridges on nails
	Increased deposit of calcium in nails	Thickening of nails

Shortening of the platysma muscle produces *neck* wrinkles (29, 75, 102).

Gray hair is the universal phenomenon associated with aging, but it is not a reliable indicator of age since some individuals begin graying as early as their teen years. In the older adults melanin production in the hair follicle diminishes. The hair gradually grays; the exact shade of gray depends on the original hair color. Eventually all the pigmented hair is replaced by nonpigmented hair; gradually the overall hair color turns pure white. Hair loss and thinning due to destruction or regression of the germ center that produces hair follicles occur. Both males and females are affected. The loss of hair occurs on the scalp, in the pubic and axillary areas, and on the extremities. In most older adults there is also increased growth of facial hair due to the change in androgen-estrogen ratio (29, 75, 102, 244).

Posture. The posture of the older adult is one of general flexion. The head is tilted forward; hips and knees are slightly flexed. Muscles in the torso are held rigidly. The older adult stands with the feet apart to provide a wide base of support. He/she takes shorter steps which may produce a shuffling gait. A shift in the center of gravity occurs as well, which affects movement and balance (29, 75, 244).

Neurologic System

Nervous System Changes. With aging there are major changes in the nervous system that occur normally and alter the individual's sensory response (29, 56, 102, 244):

1. Loss of nerve cells
2. Decrease in neurotransmitters
3. Slower nerve impulse transmission
4. Decrease in nerve conduction velocity
5. Decline in electric activity
6. Increase in sensory threshold
7. Decline in integration of sensory and motor function

All of these neurologic changes create problems for the older adult. For example, by the age of 70, upper body stiffness, slower voluntary movement, slower decision making, visual changes, and slowed startle response are seen. Because of these particular neurologic changes, older adults do not respond as quickly to changes in their external environment. This slower response affects many facets of their life (e.g., there is greater risk to overall safety, and drivers over 65 years of age are involved in a higher percentage of automobile accidents per mile driven than are drivers ages 25 to 54 years). The older adult's increase in sensory threshold affects pain and tactile perception and response to stimuli, resulting in increased susceptibility to burns or other injuries (29, 102, 244).

Brain. By age 90 the brain's weight has decreased 10% from its maximum. This weight loss is accompanied by a reduction in the cortical area and a decrease in the number of functioning neurons in the gray matter. The white matter is not significantly different than in young people. The void left by these anatomic changes is filled by expanding ventricular volumes in the form of cerebrospinal fluid. The anatomic and physiologic changes in the brain of the older adult are not always directly related to performance abilities. Declining human performance in advanced age may be due to deficits in systems peripheral to the central nervous system and/or to other behavioral factors (29, 56, 102, 244).

Vestibular and Kinesthetic Response. The response to vestibular and kinesthetic stimuli decreases with age. The vestibular division of the vestibulocochlear nerve is associated with balance and equilibrium. With aging there is a decrease in the number of nerve fibers, thus affecting balance and equilibrium. Reduction in the number of sensory cells in the utricle, saccule, and semicircular ducts further affects balance. These reductions may begin as early as 50 years of age but are especially noticeable after the age of 70. Vestibular sense receptors are located in muscles and tendons; these receptors relay information about joint motion and body position in space to the central nervous system. Loss of neurons in the cerebellum that receive the sensory information also contributes to diminished balance (29, 102).

Vision. Visual changes occur. Lacrimal glands produce fewer tears, causing the cornea to become dry and irritated. The lens thicken and yellow; objects take on a yellowish hue; and the cells within the lens lose water and shrink. The size of the pupil decreases; it is less responsive to light. Increased lens opacity causes light to scatter, causing sensitivity to glare and difficulty in adjusting from lighted to darker room. Visual contrast sensitivity for size and light decreases. These changes interfere with the ability to transmit and refract light. **Presbyopia,** *inability to change lens shape for near vision,* is present in most adults after the age of 45 or 50. Even with corrective lenses the individual may need longer to focus on near objects. Cataract development and glaucoma frequently occur in this age group. With **cataracts** the *lens becomes opaque,* accompanied by diminished vision and increased sensitivity to glare. **Glaucoma** is *caused by damage to the optic nerve from increased intraocular pressure.* These conditions and the other visual changes such as **arcus senilis,** the *accumulation of lipids on the cornea,* can be assessed during periodic eye examinations. The elderly with lens-opacifying disease have increased risk for macular degeneration, regardless of age, gender, or systolic blood pressure (29, 102, 117).

Color vision is also altered. The reception of short wavelengths (blue) is affected first, followed by middle wavelength hues (green, greenish yellow) and, last, by the long wavelengths (red). Thus for the older adult, colors such as green, blue, and violet are more difficult to see than are red, orange, and yellow. Pastels fade so that they are indistinguishable from each other; monotones, whites, and dark colors are also difficult to see. Brighter colors compensate for decline in color discrimination and yellowing and opacity of the lens (29, 75). These changes have implications for safety, for personal grooming and dress, for enjoyment (or lack of enjoyment) of the outdoors, and for interior decorating and design of the living environment.

Hearing. With age the pinna (external ear) becomes longer, wider, and less flexible; this change does not appear to affect hearing. However, as cerumen production diminishes and the wax becomes drier, blockage of the ear canal can occur. The presence of dried, packed wax can interfere with sound transmission. Any auditory changes that occurred in middle age continue through later life. The tympanic membrane becomes thinner and less resilient and may show some sclerotic changes. In some older adults calcification of the ossicles occurs. There are also changes in the organ of Corti, loss of nerve cells in the eighth cranial nerve, and an increased rate of time for passage of impulses in the auditory nerve.

Of all individuals over 65, 13% suffer severe **presbycusis,** *progressive loss of hearing and sound discrimination.* The consonants, especially *s, sh,* and *f,* are examples of high-frequency sounds that produce problems for the individual with presbycusis. In addition, the consonant sounds of *z, ch,* and *dg* are affected. The ability to locate the direction from which sound is coming diminishes, and older people have difficulty hearing individuals who speak rapidly or in high tones (29, 34, 75, 86, 102, 244).

Tactile acuity. Two-point threshold is one of the oldest measures of spacial acuity of the skin. Age-related deterioration of tactile acuity, like visual and hearing changes, begins in late middle age. Acuity of touch, however, varies with different body regions; the fingertip has more acuity than the forearm for texture and temperature in old age. Acuity is also related to space between stimuli; for example, the fingertip may be

sensitive to a single nodule but not as sensitive to the dots of Braille, to the glucose testing monitor used by the diabetic, or to other tactile aids used by the sensory handicapped (247).

Taste and Smell. With aging, there is a general decrease in taste perception. The exact cause is unknown. Studies report little, if any, decline in the actual number of taste buds; it is suggested that the diminished taste perception is linked to the changes in the processing of taste sensations in the central nervous system. Taste perception may also be affected by the diminished salivation that occurs in older persons. Usually older adults experience an increased preference for more sugar, salt, spices, and highly seasoned foods. The sense of smell begins to decline in most people by middle age and continues a gradual decline into old age. It is believed that the sense of smell decreases because the olfactory nerves have fewer cells. This diminished sense of smell combined with the decline in taste sensation may account for the loss of appetite experienced by many older adults. The inability to smell also presents hazards for the individual since he or she cannot quickly detect leaking gas, spoiled food, smoke, or burning food (29, 34, 75, 102, 108, 244).

Cardiovascular System

Although the cardiovascular system undergoes considerable changes with aging (Table 14–2), in the absence of heart disease it is usually able to maintain the daily cardiac and circulatory functions of the older adult. However, the cardiovascular system may not be able to meet the needs of the body when a disease process is present or when excess demands caused by stress or excessive exercise occurs. Obesity, physical inactivity, and abdominal fat distribution also reduce physiologic function (102).

Heart. Structural changes occur within the heart. The number and size of cardiac muscle cells are reduced, and the amount of collagen and fat deposits increase; the valves become more rigid, and the left ventricular wall increases in thickness. Functional changes also occur.

TABLE 14-2. CARDIOVASCULAR CHANGES WITH AGING

	Structural Change	Performance Change
Heart	Decreased number and size of cardiac muscle cells	Loss of cardiac muscle strength; reduction in stroke volume
	Increased fat deposition on surface of heart	Reduced oxygen supply to body
	Thickening of heart valves which become sclerotic	Incomplete closure of valves; occurrence of murmurs
	Replacement of pacemaker cells in SA node and AV node by fibrous and connective tissue	Ectopic activity
Vascular system	Reduced elastin content and increased collagenous connective tissue in arterial walls	Decreased elasticity, with reduced ability to rebound after being stretched; increased systolic pressure
	Accumulation of lipids on internal arterial walls	Decreased lumen diameter
	Increased connective tissue and calcium deposits in walls of veins	Thickened veins; incompetent valves

The left ventricle is unable to pump large volumes of blood; thus the total cardiac output per minute is lower. Because of the delay in nerve transmission and the thickening of the cardiac muscles, more time is required to complete the cardiac cycle. With the diminished cardiac output, a greater percentage of the total blood flow is sent to the brain and coronary arteries. Muscles and viscera may receive inadequate blood supplies when there is an increased demand for blood flow (144, 244).

Vascular System. Structural and functional changes also occur in the vascular system. The elastin content of arterial walls is reduced, and collagenous connective tissue increases. This causes a reduction in the elasticity of the walls. Larger arteries are especially affected. In addition, the internal diameter of arteries decreases because of a gradual accumulation of lipids within their walls; changes in the aorta, coronary arteries, and carotid arteries are apparent in some individuals as early as age 40. Veins also undergo structural and functional changes. The walls of veins become thicker as a result of an increase in connective tissue and calcium deposits; this causes decreased distensibility and elasticity. Valves in large veins may become incompetent; varicose veins are common (29, 102, 244).

Respiratory System

Changes produced by aging affect both internal and external respiration; the older adult has difficulty taking oxygen from the atmosphere and delivering it to internal organs and tissues.

The lungs and rib cage undergo structural changes. There is calcification of the chest wall; the rib cage becomes less mobile; the elasticity of the lung tissue decreases; and the alveolar ducts enlarge. In addition, there is an increase in the size and a decrease in the flexibility of the trachea and central airways. The structure and function of the respiratory muscles gradually decline; these changes decrease the strength of the muscles used in breathing. In some older adults calcification of vertebral cartilages and kyphosis can cause additional impairment to respiration. The ability to cough is impaired because of decreased muscle tone and decreased sensitivity to stimuli. In addition, cilia are lost, and the effectiveness of the ciliary mechanism decreases. Both of these factors interfere with effective clearing of the respiratory tract. Since less oxygen is delivered from the outside air to the arterial blood, the arterial oxygen pressure decreases. The lungs remain hyperinflated even on exhalation, and the proportion of dead air space increases, causing a decrease in the ventilation/perfusion ratio and in the vital capacity (29, 102, 149, 244).

Musculoskeletal System

The major age-related change in the skeletal system is the loss of calcium from bone. Bone loss is accelerated with the loss of gonadal function at menopause. Therefore bone loss is greater in females than in males. Some studies have shown that by the age of 70 a woman's skeletal frame may have lost 30% or more of its calcium. With this change in bone composition comes a gradual decrease in height. As the vertebrae collapse from loss of calcium and normal aging, the individual becomes shorter. Height is also affected by curvature of the thoracic spine, which frequently occurs in older adults. In addition to the decrease in height, bone strength is progressively lost because of loss of bone mineral content. Osteoporosis (which is discussed later) is seen as the extreme version of the universal process of adult bone loss (29, 102, 141).

Decreased sensorimotor functions affect postural stability. Increased body sway is associated with reduced visual acuity, tactile sensitivity, vibration sense, joint position sense, ankle dorsiflexion strength, quadriceps muscle strength, and increased reaction time. Peripheral sensation ability is also a factor in sway and maintenance of postural stability (156). These factors must be considered for safety during mobility and fall prevention.

Maintaining upright posture and balance is a complex task. As postural control mechanisms deteriorate with disease and age, the person is more susceptible to falls. Standing on one leg and tandem walking become more difficult. The center of pressure tends not to approach the edges of the base of support as closely as in younger years. One way to determine stability is to measure **functional reach,** *the maximum distance one can reach beyond arm's length while maintaining a fixed base of support in standing position.* Height and age affect reach, but the general ability to reach and the length of reach are related to ability to maintain stability when walking (68).

The older adult experiences a gradual loss of muscular strength and endurance. Muscle cells atrophy, and lean muscle mass is lost. Studies have shown a 30% loss in muscle fiber between the ages of 30 and 80. In addition, as the elastic fibers in the muscle tissues decrease, the muscles become less flexible, and stiffness is noted more frequently (29, 102, 244).

Changes in body weight also occur in the older adult. These changes follow definite patterns. Men usually exhibit an increase in weight until their middle fifties and then gradually lose weight. Women continue to gain weight until their sixties before beginning a gradual reduction in weight. The most significant weight loss occurs near 70 years of age and is probably due to decreased number of body cells, changes in cell composition, and decreased amounts of body tissue (29, 102, 244).

Urinary System

As with the other body systems, major changes in structure and function of the urinary system are associated with aging. The kidneys, bladder, and ureters are all affected by the aging process.

Kidney. A number of structural and functional changes occur within the kidneys. There is a decrease in the thickness of the connective tissue capsule that surrounds the organ, a decrease in the thickness of the cortical region, and atrophy of cells within the organ. Nephron units are lost in the kidneys, and the remaining units undergo degenerative changes, causing a decrease in the glomerular filtration rate (29, 51, 102, 244). By the age of 70 or 80, the glomerular filtration rate is approximately one half the rate of a 30-year-old. Because of the impaired filtration rate, urea nitrogen, creatinine, uric acid, and even drugs are excreted more slowly. The tubular cells have decreased resorption and selection abilities, causing a loss of water and electrolytes. The kidneys respond more slowly to the antidiuretic hormone, decreasing their ability to concentrate urine. The kidneys also need more time to correct alkalosis, acidosis, and or or electrolyte disturbances. When both renal and respiratory functions are impaired, protection against shifts in blood pH is decreased (29, 51, 102, 244).

Bladder. Some muscle tone loss occurs in the bladder and urethra. This loss may cause incomplete emptying of the bladder and increase the risk of retention and bladder infection in the older adult. The bladder capacity gradually decreases, and the older adult experiences frequent urination and nocturia. Older women may develop incontinence when relaxation of the pelvic muscles occurs (244).

Gastrointestinal System

Changes occur throughout the gastrointestinal system.

Mouth. The oral mucosa atrophies; the connective tissue becomes less elastic; vascular tissue becomes calcified and fibrotic; and nerve cells diminish in number. Tooth decay, loss of teeth, degeneration of the jaw bone, progressive gum recession, and increased resorption of the dental arch interfere with the older adult's ability to chew food. Saliva becomes more alkaline as the salivary glands secrete less ptyalin and amylase. All of these changes alter the digestive process at the onset (182).

Gastrointestinal Tract. Because of decreased stimuli from the autonomic nervous system, peristalsis is slowed the entire length of the gastrointestinal tract. Emptying of the esophagus and stomach is delayed. The gastric mucosa shrinks, causing decreased secretion of pepsinogen and hydrochloric acid, which delays digestion. Digestion is decreased further by the reduction in pancreatic enzymes. Bile tends to be thicker, and the gallbladder empties more slowly. These changes result in a decreased absorption of nutrients and drugs by the gastrointestinal tract. In addition, some older adults do not have enough intrinsic factor and develop pernicious anemia (29, 102).

Elimination of waste products is of equal importance to gastrointestinal function in the aged. Elimina-tion depends on fluid intake, muscle tone, regularity of habits, culture, state of health, and adequate nutrition—all of which interrelate. Alterations in many of these areas occur with aging. Daily routines change, activity may be slowed, illness may deplete vital reserve, and diet habits may be more erratic. The changes in the cell, and therefore in tissue structure, and the loss of muscle tone may decrease intestinal mobility. Poor nutrition and lack of exercise add to the problem.

In the majority of persons over age 65 there is some degree of immobility—either physical, social, or environmental. Physical changes in the tissues combine with this immobility to produce constipation or fecal impaction under circumstances that might not so affect a younger person.

Teach the importance of increased fluid intake, of roughage in the diet if possible, and exercise within the person's physical limitations to maintain bowel function. Increasing fluid intake, especially drinking warm water or coffee early in the morning, and having adequate intake of fruits, bulky vegetables, and cereals should be adequate to keep bowel movements normal. Offering daily prune juice and teaching the importance of a regular time for defecation often prevent later problems in the inactive person. (Note that normal bowel function is defined as the passage of soft stool without difficulty, as opposed to having a bowel movement every day.) Often the older person has self-administered laxatives for years; gastrointestinal muscle tone is then so low that the person may have to take a mild stool softener or laxative daily. Prevention, from early adulthood on, through hydration and eating of bulky foods is important.

Endocrine System

During aging the ability of endocrine glands to synthesize hormones appears to remain within normal limits. However, the number or sensitivity of hormonal receptors may lessen. This means that, even though blood levels remain adequate, there is a lack of response to some hormones; this is especially true of the hormones produced by the adrenal and thyroid glands. Failure to respond to these hormones decreases the individual's ability to respond to stress (244).

Beta-cell activity of the pancreas appears altered with age, although the extent varies among people. Aging is associated with elevated glucose levels after ingestion of glucose under that standard conditions of oral glucose tolerance testing. After ingestion of more physiologically mixed meals, a mild degree of postprandial hyperglycemia and hyperinsulinemia can still be demonstrated in the elderly compared with young adults. Postprandial elevations in glucose and insulin levels, however, are much less after mixed meals compared with that observed during the standard glucose tolerance test. Increased circulating glucose and insulin levels are accompanied by a detectable elevation in hemoglobin A₁ concentration. These modest abnormalities, sustained over many years, may contribute to the development of atherosclerosis or other manifestations of aging (29, 102).

Growth hormone, estrogen, and testosterone blood levels do decrease in later maturity. Because of the decrease in estrogen levels after menopause, the breasts of the female have more connective tissue and fat and less glandular tissue. The breast tissues lose elasticity and begin to sag. The lack of estrogen causes the uterus and fallopian tubes to decrease in size. The fallopian tubes also become less motile. The decline of testosterone secretion is not abrupt like that of estrogen. Therefore the changes are less obvious. However, the gradual decline of hormone does increase the incidence of benign prostatic hypertrophy in the older adult male and affects physical reserves since testosterone has a nitrogen-conserving effect (29, 102, 141, 244).

Immune System

During the aging process the thymus gland starts to involute and degenerate; the total number of circulating lymphocytes decreases by approximately 15% and antibody-antigen reactions decline. In addition, lymphoid tissue decreases, and a general decline occurs in immune responses, including both cell-mediated and humoral immunity. All of these changes result in a delayed immune response to infection and a delayed or inadequate response to the stress of infection in older adults. Because these factors alter the normal inflammatory response, the signs and symptoms of an infection may be masked. For example, in the older adult, the white blood count does not become as elevated in response to infection as it does in the middle-aged adult (29, 102).

Hematopoietic System

There are minor changes in the blood components of the older adult; the hemoglobin level, red blood cell count, and circulatory blood volume are not significantly changed. Most of the changes that occur are related to specific pathologic conditions instead of normal aging (29, 102, 244).

Reproductive System and Changes That Influence Sexual Function

Although the male and female experience some common changes as a result of aging, it is well to consider them separately because of certain particular physiologic changes relating to sexual response and vigor.

Male Changes. The production of testosterone continues throughout the man's lifetime, and this hormone is available longer and at a higher level than its counterpart, estrogen, in the woman. As the concentration of the male hormone diminishes, the testes become smaller and softer; the testicular tubes thicken and begin to degenerate; and the sperm production decreases or is inhibited. In addition, the prostate gland enlarges, contractions weaken, the force of ejaculation decreases, and

there is a reduction in the volume and viscosity of seminal fluid (141, 182, 244).

In 1970 Masters and Johnson found that as a sexual partner, the older male experiences reduction in the frequency of intercourse, the intensity of sensation, the speed of attaining erection, and the force of ejaculation. Excitement builds more slowly, and erection takes longer to attain; with diminished vasoconstriction of the scrotum, there is less elevation of the testes. The plateau phase preceding orgasm lasts longer, the orgasmic phase is of shorter duration, and the expulsion of the seminal fluid is usually completed with one or two contractions as compared to four or more in the young male. In the resolution stage loss of erection may take seconds as compared to the young man's minutes or hours (166).

Female Changes. In the older adult woman there is a decline in the blood level of estrogen. This reduction in hormone causes the vaginal wall to shrink and thin and the vaginal secretions to diminish and become more acid. These changes may produce **dyspareunia** (*pain on intercourse*), which can restrict sexual activity. In addition, the size of the clitoris is slightly smaller, and the lubrication from the Bartholin glands decreases. With the loss of subcutaneous body fat, the vulva and external genitalia shrink (183, 244).

Female sexual performance in later maturity reveals no reduction in sexual desire or excitability with advancing age. Regular sexual stimulation and activity seem to overcome the effects of estrogen starvation. Studies reveal an increase in masturbation for relief of sexual tension in postmenopausal women into their sixth and seventh decades and for men over age 65. There may be an increased level of sexual desire among women after hysterectomies, indicating that there is no connection between fertility and libido. Studies have indicated that women who have been exclusively homemakers and mothers have a greater difficulty in meeting the advancing physiologic changes than women who have combined the role of homemaker with a career (153).

Yet neural and hormonal changes can combine to affect her sexual activity. In coitus the thinning vaginal walls, inelasticity of the vagina, and diminished lubrication may make penetration difficult. Burning and frequency of urination may follow intercourse since the atrophic bladder and urethra are not adequately protected. Thus the sex act may become less satisfying and even painful. A number of diseases and some medications can cause impotence. See references 131 and 166.

Sexuality. It is well known that stress, hormonal activity, general health, and aging can each be assessed according to measurable standards. The data are sufficient to infer that psychologic influences can be exerted to produce physiologic change in young and old alike. Because of the relationships between the mind and body and the interdependence of all body systems, the societal attitudes regarding the characteristics and needs of older citizens are crucial to their quality of life.

There is no doubt that normal aging of the reproductive system produces a decreased efficiency and a lengthened time for response for both men and women, but unlike other organ systems that perform more specific functions, the reproductive system extends far beyond procreation. It is deeply tied to the need for interpersonal communication, and it involves that warmth and comfort found only in body contact. When one is old, the yearning for intimacy, security, and belonging becomes intensified as other privations are felt keenly: loss of friends, job status, active participation in parenting or career, and decision making.

The older person is not a nonperson sexually. Research about sexuality in people between the ages of 60 and 91 years indicates the following:

1. Ninety-seven percent like sexual activity.
2. Seventy-five percent think intercourse feels as good now, or better, than it did when they were young.
3. Seventy-two percent are satisfied by their sexual experiences.
4. Ninety percent think sexual activity is good for their health.
5. Women are more satisfied with activities such as sitting close to someone and talking and saying and hearing endearments if sexual intercourse is not a choice.
6. Men are more satisfied with reading or watching erotic materials and caressing another person's body if sexual intercourse is not a choice.

The person's sense of self-worth and the partner's physical health status are positively related to the continuance of sexual intercourse (72, 168, 206).

As our medical technology proliferates and the life span continues to lengthen, we will have an increasing number of elderly, healthy, and alert persons who will demand a greater share of a high quality of life and an opportunity to exercise their capacity for abiding, close relationships with the opposite sex in whatever role seems suited to their needs as individuals. Fig. 14–3 summarizes physical and physiologic changes in later maturity.

Nutritional Needs

Special problems exist in the nutrition of older people. Factors that affect nutrition and their clinical manifestations are shown in Table 14–3. Although caloric requirements may be lower than in earlier life, the elderly require somewhat greater amounts of some of the vitamins and trace elements. *Basic to good nutrition* in any age group is an adequate intake of quality protein, fat, and carbohydrate. There must be enough vitamin coenzymes to ensure metabolism of these three nutrients and absorption of enough bulk elements to main-

tain a balance of sodium, potassium, calcium, magnesium, and other trace-element cofactors for metabolic needs. Because foods today are subjected to many refinement processes with the loss of some vitamins and essential elements, supplements are often recommended. The traditional food groups are the foundation of a balanced diet for the elderly as in any life stage. Assuring enough protein in the diet each day is probably the greatest dietary problem in meal planning for the elderly person who lives alone, for he or she often wants foods that can be prepared and chewed easily, and he or she may seldom eat meat. Milk products may be poorly tolerated, especially in dark-skinned people, because of decreased lactase, the enzyme for digesting lactose. Fermented products such as cheese, yogurt, and buttermilk may be tolerated well and supply needed calcium (111, 280).

The aging process causes an atrophy of olfactory organs and a loss of taste buds. Usually salt and sweet buds are lost first; bitter and sour taste buds remain intact. Two thirds of taste depends on smell. This may contribute indirectly to abnormalities of absorption, motility, or intermediary metabolism, and a concomitant lack of desire for food. Loss of taste is compounded by gum disease and poor teeth or dentures. Fifty percent of the elderly have lost their teeth; 90% who have their natural teeth have periodontal disease. Both loss of teeth and periodontal disease are preventable through good nutrition, oral and dental hygiene, and dental therapy. Food served attractively and at proper temperature is important. The person may find eating each food separately, rather than mixing foods, helps him or her to taste each food better. Food with different textures and aromas should be served in the meal.

Sufficient water or other fluid intake is essential. Fluid intake is often reduced in seniors for several reasons:

1. The aging process reduces the thirst sensation.
2. The senior who has incontinence problems limits fluid intake to reduce output.
3. Fewer meals are eaten; opportunity for fluid intake is less apparent.
4. The senior who takes a diuretic wrongly assumes fluid intake should be reduced.

At least six or seven glasses (8 ounces) of water should be ingested daily to (1) soften stools; (2) maintain kidney function; (3) aid expectoration; (4) moisturize dry skin; and (5) aid absorption of medications, bulk laxatives, and high-fiber foods.

Nursing responsibility begins with the tray that may be served from the kitchen of a person's home or an institution. You can help make mealtime pleasant for the older person. Offer food in a comfortable setting; open cartons and food packets of various sorts and help season the food; and keep the tray attractive, neat, and uncluttered to ensure an appetizing appearance. Make sure

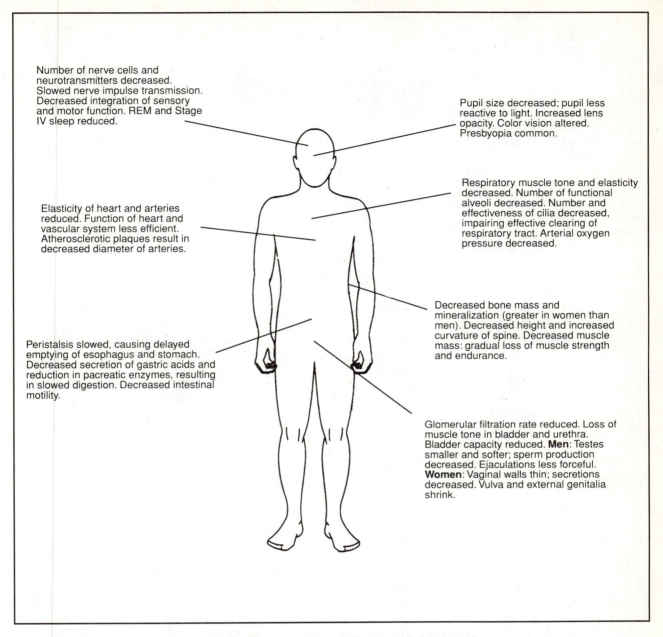

Number of nerve cells and neurotransmitters decreased. Slowed nerve impulse transmission. Decreased integration of sensory and motor function. REM and Stage IV sleep reduced.

Pupil size decreased; pupil less reactive to light. Increased lens opacity. Color vision altered. Presbyopia common.

Elasticity of heart and arteries reduced. Function of heart and vascular system less efficient. Atherosclerotic plaques result in decreased diameter of arteries.

Respiratory muscle tone and elasticity decreased. Number of functional alveoli decreased. Number and effectiveness of cilia decreased, impairing effective clearing of respiratory tract. Arterial oxygen pressure decreased.

Decreased bone mass and mineralization (greater in women than men). Decreased height and increased curvature of spine. Decreased muscle mass: gradual loss of muscle strength and endurance.

Peristalsis slowed, causing delayed emptying of esophagus and stomach. Decreased secretion of gastric acids and reduction in pacreatic enzymes, resulting in slowed digestion. Decreased intestinal motility.

Glomerular filtration rate reduced. Loss of muscle tone in bladder and urethra. Bladder capacity reduced. **Men**: Testes smaller and softer; sperm production decreased. Ejaculations less forceful. **Women**: Vaginal walls thin; secretions decreased. Vulva and external genitalia shrink.

Figure 14-3.   Physical and physiologic changes in later maturity.

dentures and eyeglasses are clean and in place at mealtime instead of in the drawer or in the bedside table. Oral hygiene is important and contributes to a greater enjoyment of food. Mouth care also promotes healthy tissues in the mouth, thereby keeping the first part of the alimentary canal intact and functional.

Adequate treatment of problems at mealtimes is necessary to determine whether or not a poor appetite is caused by poor-fitting dentures, a sore mouth, individual or cultural preferences in food, or some physical or psychologic deterrent to enjoyment of food. The elderly

are denied many pleasures, and food should not be one of them. Consult with other members of the health team, especially the dietician and the physician, if there are problems. The family must be included, too, and can often be of great help when there are cultural, religious, or ethnic reasons for a poor appetite. Often the most important member of the team, the client, is not consulted enough; he or she should be the first one involved in planning nutritional needs if at all possible. These same principles can be used as a basis for helping the elderly maintain good nutrition in the home, where, as the com-

TABLE 14-3. FACTORS THAT MAY AFFECT NUTRITION IN LATER MATURITY

Factor and Process	Effect	Clinical Manifestation
Ingestion		
Loss of teeth; poor dentures; atrophy of jaws	Improper mastication; deletion of important foods from diet	Irritable bowel syndrome; constipation; malnutrition
Dietary habits	Overeating; eccentric diets	Obesity; malnutrition
Psychologic losses and changes; changes in social environment; lack of socialization	Poor appetite	Anorexia; weight loss
Reduced income; difficulty with food preparation and ingestion	Excessive ingestion of carbohydrates	Obesity; malnutrition
Decreased fluid intake	Dry feces	Impacted stools
Digestion and Absorption		
Decreased secretion of hydrochloric acid and digestive enzymes	Interference with digestion	Dietary deficiencies
Hepatic and biliary insufficiency	Poor absorption of fats	Fat-soluble vitamin deficiency; flatulence
Atrophy of intestinal mucosa and musculature	Poor absorption; slower movement of food through intestine	Vitamin and mineral deficiencies; constipation
Decreased secretion of intestinal mucus	Decreased lubrication of intestine	Constipation
Metabolism		
Impaired glucose metabolism and use	Diabetic-like response to glucose excesses	Hyperglycemia; hypoglycemia
Decrease in renal function	Inability to excrete excess alkali	Alkalosis
Impaired response to salt restriction	Salt depletion	Low-salt syndrome
Decline in basal metabolic rate	Lower caloric requirements but same amount of food eaten	Obesity
Changes in iron and calcium (phosphorus, magnesium) metabolism	Iron deficiency; increased requirements for calcium	Anemia; demineralization of bone; osteoporosis
Changes in vitamin metabolism	Deficiency in vitamins K and C especially	Peripheral neuropathy, sensorimotor changes; easy bruising and bleeding tendencies

munity health nurse or primary care practitioner, you may need to make careful assessment of the home situation when problems of poor nutrition exist. Determine whether the problem stems from lack of funds, physical handicaps, family structure, cultural barriers, or any combination of similar unmet needs. Often you will be the one who helps the client contact community agencies, family, church, and whatever other means may be available.

Elderly persons living alone and unable to shop or to prepare food may need the assistance of a home health aide—available through some community agencies—to shop for them and assist with other routines of living. You might arrange to have meals sent in from agencies designed to give this type of service. These programs are discussed more fully later in this chapter under "community planning."

The whole area of client teaching is affected by the changing needs of the older adult. Adapt your nutrition teaching to these changes and keep in mind the altered responses associated with the aging nervous system.

Rest and Sleep

Rest is of importance. Though older adults may not sleep as many hours as they once did, frequent rest periods and sensible pacing of activities will provide the added energy for a full and active life. Rest may consist of lis-

tening to soft music, reading, thinking of happy experiences, napping, or merely lying with eyes closed. Some older adults have several 15- to 60-minute naps during the daylight hours.

With so much diversity among the individuals in this age group, it is difficult to state how many hours of *sleep* are recommended. Older adults in reasonably good health probably do not require any more sleep than was required during their middle adulthood.

Aging affects the process of sleep in three areas: length of sleep, distribution of sleep during the 24-hour day, and sleep stage patterns. The older adult requires a somewhat longer period to fall asleep, and sleep is lighter, with more frequent awakenings. The total amount of daily sleep declines as the spontaneous interruption of sleep increases. The older adult may actually spend more time in bed but sleep less, waking with the feeling of inadequate sleep. The time spent in Stage IV, the deepest sleep period, and rapid eye movement (REM) sleep decreases. This also contributes to feelings of fatigue (34, 75).

Sleep apnea, described in Chapter 12, occurs in many elderly adults. Persons with sleep apnea are more sleepy during the day than nonapneic individuals; apnea during sleep has a detrimental effect on the well-being of elderly adults, even if oxygen desaturation is mild or moderate. Greater levels of depression and cognitive impairment are seen in sleep apneic elders (19).

Insomnia is a common problem in the older adult. Many factors contribute to this. You can determine the person's usual sleeping patterns, the amount and type of daily activity, and the existence of disturbing environmental conditions. Assess the presence of pain, fear, anxiety, lack of exercise, or depression.

Exercise and Activity

Physical activity that is sensibly paced and gradually increased will promote and maintain health. In a longitudinal study of more than 1700 Caucasian adults over 80 years old, one third had no difficulty walking $\frac{1}{4}$ mile; lifting 10 pounds; climbing 10 steps without resting; or stooping, crouching, or kneeling. Fifty percent of the women and 42% of the men remained healthy over a 5-year study period. Physical ability was associated with never having had cardiovascular disease or arthritic complaints, few fractures, a body mass less than 75th percentile, and 13 years or more of education. These results indicate that even the oldest-old can participate in preventive exercise programs and postpone disability (104).

Physical exercise also contributes to improved mood and self-confidence, and when exercise is a group activity, it promotes socialization. Exercise, especially of the low-impact aerobic type such as dance improves cardiorespiratory endurance, general strength and endurance, body agility, flexibility, weight control, and balance. Exercise training appears to produce greater improvements among elderly with concomitant physical or emotional impairments and apparently is a better predictor for physiologic than for psychologic or cognitive well-being (22, 77, 118).

One group of active people is farmers, and farmers age 65 or older generally enjoy better health than city or small-town dwellers of the same age. They have fewer medical conditions and excel at performing tasks. Farmers may be healthier because of their life-style, and 70% are married. If you are looking for a 75-year-old who still works, that person is more likely to farm than do anything else; 61% of farmers say they do not expect to stop working (257).

Even if the individual has a decreased exercise tolerance, with supervision a plan can be developed to help him or her achieve higher levels of physical fitness. It is important, however, that the older adult not start an exercise program without consulting the physician who would be aware of any needed limitations.

For the individual who is not especially interested in planned exercise programs, you can suggest walking, bowling, golf, swimming, dancing, games such as shuffleboard and horseshoes, and home and garden chores. All of these activities can improve the well-being of the older adult (Fig. 14–4).

An exercise program regularly followed may bring a dimension of dynamic fitness to life that helps him or her move vigorously and live energetically as long as possible. Histories of vigorous persons in their eighties

Figure 14-4. Older adults can help maintain health and prevent illness by participating in regular exercise. (From Berger, K.J., and M.B. Williams, *Fundamentals of Nursing: Collaborating for Optimal Health.* Norwalk, Conn: Appleton & Lange, 1992, p. 317.)

and nineties and even over age 100 show that the majority have been physically and mentally active throughout their earlier lives (34).

Health Promotion and Health Protection

Male and female differences in longevity result from hormones, genetic makeup, natural immunity, and life-style behavior. Because of the immunity effects of estrogen, women, statistically, develop heart disease 10 years later than men. In the past, life-style choices of women also gave them a biologic advantage—less drinking of alcoholic beverages, less cigarette smoking, more attention to personal health care, and less exposure to risks at work and play. However, as women are changing their life-styles, the gap between the genders in health status and longevity is narrowing (71).

The focus of health care for individuals in this period of life should be on the prevention of disease and the promotion of health. Although numerous body changes occur with aging, many older adults live active, productive lives. Thorough assessment is essential. Several references are useful to you (33, 34, 75, 131).

Immunizations

Since older adults are more susceptible to acute illnesses, they should be encouraged to avail themselves of recommended immunizations against communicable diseases. Individuals who garden and participate in other outdoor activities should receive tetanus immunization as indicated. Immunization for influenza and pneumococcal pneumonia is usually recommended for older adults, especially those with chronic respiratory and cardiovascular diseases. Adults at risk for hepatitis should receive hepatitis B vaccination (268).

Safety Promotion and Accident Prevention

Older people have a disproportionate share of accidents that cause body injury or death. This is especially true for accidents that occur in the home. Many of these accidents are directly related to physiologic changes that result from normal aging. Older adults are also particularly vulnerable to fraudulent sales pitches and seemingly honest requests for help by strangers (see Box 14–2) (164).

Visual Changes. Changes in visual acuity produce numerous hazards for the older adult. The older adult's problems with color interpretation, light intensity, and depth perception should be considered in the home and hospital environment. Older adults need a higher light intensity than younger persons, and providing room light may reduce restlessness and confusion, especially at night. Direct lights, exposed light bulbs, white surfaces, waxed floors, and glossy furniture all produce glare that interferes with the vision of older persons. Lights should be arranged so that they are not directed down from the ceiling. This creates pools of light that may distort the individual's vision. However, with certain ocular conditions, the person may see better in dim light. Sharply contrasting colors for door facings and walls, brightly colored doors, stripes of contrasting color along the bottom of a wall, or a yellow or red strip at the edge of each step can help the individual distinguish colors and gauge depths (26, 34, 75, 108, 145).

The environment should be kept free of hazards—no articles on the floor, no furniture with sharp edges, no scatter rugs. The baseboards should be painted a darker color than the walls. Signs should be prepared

---

■ BOX 14-2.
Safety in the Home: Do Not Be a Victim of the Con Game

- **Carpet cleaner:** Ad offers very low price to clean carpeting in one or more rooms of your house. Workers flood room, ruin carpet, and scheme to charge more than quoted to replace damaged material.
- **City inspector:** "Inspector" says he or she needs to check plumbing, furnace, heater, wiring, trees, or whatever. Once inside, he or she may rob you or insist something needs repair and charge excessively for the job.
- **Home repair or inspection:** "Contractor" offers, for example, to repair, inspect, or remodel your home, exterminate pests, or check for radon or offers work with leftover materials from another job in area. The person will find unnecessary work, resulting in unnecessary expense.
- **Product demonstration:** Agent offers to describe only (not sell) new product if you will sign paper "for my boss" proving he or she did it. Once inside the house, anything can happen.
- **Contest winner:** You are told you have won vacation, auto, or other prize but must send $5 for postage or registration or call 800 number for details.
- **Lottery:** Person offers to sell you winning lottery ticket he or she cannot cash because "I'm an illegal immigrant," or "I'm behind in my child-care payments"; or "law firm" says anonymous donor has bequeathed a winning lottery ticket to you, but first you must send $20 for a computer search to verify your identity.
- **Land sale:** You are promised cheap land or complete retirement and recreational facilities in sunny gorgeous site. The land may not exist, even if you paid for it.
- **Credit or phone card:** Person asks for your credit- or phone-card number to send you a product, check unauthorized charges, verify insurance, and so on. They can then use your number to charge items.
- **Government service:** Official-sounding firm (e.g., with "Social Security" in name) offers Social Security service that is "required" (e.g., plastic-coated identification cards), "critically needed" (e.g., to help keep agency solvent), or useful (e.g., earnings form). The money sent obtains no service.
- **Mail-order health care or laboratory tests:** You are promised medical care by mail or laboratory screening for AIDS, cholesterol, cancer, hair, and so on. The results are likely to be phony if received at all for the money you sent.
- **Medical products:** You buy health, beauty-care, or "cure" product by mail, or you are sent newspaper clipping extolling magic diet with note scribbled across it, "It works—try it!" Signed "J."
- **900 number:** Products are offered through special 900 number. (Such numbers are common and legitimate.)
- **Obituary:** You are recently widowed; COD. box arrives for product "your husband or wife ordered."
- **Pigeon drop:** Person offers to share "found" money with you if you will put up some of your own money "to show good faith."
- **Need help:** Man says his wife is sick, his car has been impounded, he has run out of gas, or some such tale; he needs just $10 or $20, promises to pay it back, and shows extensive identification.
- **Unknown callers:** Woman with child knocks on door and asks for some favor requiring entrance.
- **Travel club:** Firm offers bargain airfare or hotel package in glamorous foreign locale. You may never get where you are going or find the accommodations listed.

Modified from Marklein, M., Con Games Proliferate: New Threats Haunt City Folks, *AARP Bulletin,* 32, no. 2 (1991), 1, 16–17.

with dark backgrounds and light lettering. Blues and greens on signs should be avoided. Numbers on doors, elevators, and telephones should be large enough for the older adult to see (26, 108). Encourage use of a magnifying glass for close vision work and a small flashlight to illuminate dim areas, and having properly fitted and cared for eyeglasses. Teach proper care of contact lenses.

Television should be viewed with normal room illumination and at a distance at least 6 feet from the screen. Some persons with impaired vision may have to sit closer. Glasses correcting distance vision should be worn while watching television, and the set should be adjusted as clearly as possible.

Some signs and symptoms that indicate the need for appropriate referral to an ophthalmologist include:

1. Pain in and around eyes.
2. Headaches, especially at night or early morning.
3. Mucous discharge from eyes.
4. Obvious inflammation or irritation of the eyes and surrounding tissue.
5. Avoidance of activities requiring sight.
6. Glasses not being worn, missing, or not fitting properly.
7. Change of previous visual habits (requiring different light or reading distance).

When you are caring for a blind person, follow the guidelines in Box 14–3.

Hearing Impairment. Changes in hearing acuity may predispose the person to accident risks. Many elderly persons have been diagnosed as being mentally ill, whereas in reality they were suffering from a gradual loss of hearing. If one is unable to hear clearly, it is easy to imagine one is being talked about or ignored. This leads to a feeling of depression, and then behavior often is categorized as irrational, suspicious, or hostile. This produces isolation and further frustrations, and the vicious cycle that ensues may in the end cause real paranoia to develop.

Refer to Box 14–4 for suggestions on effective communication with the hearing impaired person. Encourage the hearing impaired person to consult with a physician about use of a hearing aid rather than going to a nonqualified practitioner.

Tactile Changes. Changes in *temperature regulation* and the inability to feel pain also produce safety problems. The elderly usually *feel cold* more easily and may require more covering when in bed; a room temperature somewhat higher than usual may be desirable. Most hospitals and nursing homes do not have thermometers that register body temperatures below 94° F (35° C). Therefore statistics are not available on how many elderly persons suffer and die from hypothermia, but a figure of 25,000 deaths per year has been cited. Mildly cool temperatures of 60° F (15.5° C) to 65° F (18.3° C) can trigger hypothermia. A nighttime room temperature of 66° F (18.3° C) can be too low for an aged person.

■ **BOX 14-3.**
Guidelines for Helping the Blind Person

- Talk to the blind person in a normal tone of voice. The fact that he or she cannot see is no indication that hearing is impaired.
- Be natural when talking with a blind person.
- Accept the normal things that a blind person might do such as consulting the watch for the correct time, dialing a telephone, or writing his or her name in longhand without calling attention to them.
- When you offer assistance to a blind person, do so directly. Ask, "May I be of help?" Speak in a normal, friendly tone.
- In guiding a blind person, permit him or her to take your arm. Never grab the blind person's arm, for he or she cannot anticipate your movements.
- In walking with a blind person, proceed at a normal pace. You may hesitate slightly before stepping up or down.
- Be explicit in giving verbal directions to a blind person.
- There is no need to avoid the use of the word *see* when talking with a blind person.
- When assisting a blind person to a chair, simply place his or her hand on the back or arm of the chair. This is enough to give location.
- When leaving the blind person abruptly after conversing with him or her in a crowd or where there is a noise that may obstruct hearing, quietly advise that you are leaving so that he or she will not be embarrassed by talking when no one is listening.
- Never leave a blind person in an open area. Instead, lead him or her to the side of a room, to a chair, or some landmark from which he or she can obtain direction.
- A half-open door is one of the most dangerous obstacles that blind people encounter.
- When serving food to a blind person who is eating without a sighted companion, offer to read the menu, including the price of each item. As you place each item on the table, call attention to food placement by using the numbers of an imaginary clock. ("The green beans are at 2 o'clock.") If he or she wants you to cut up the food, he or she will tell you.
- Be sure to tell a blind person who the other guests are so that he or she may know of their presence.

The victim may not be aware of the extreme loss of body heat, especially when supine and relatively inactive.

Clues to *hypothermia* risk or presence follow:

1. Medications to treat anxiety or depression, hypothyroidism, vascular disease, alcoholism, and immobility reduce the body's response to cold.
2. Living alone or anything that increases nighttime accidents can increase risk, as do poverty and poor housing.
3. The elder may insist he or she is comfortable in a cool environment; the person is unaware of temperature of surroundings.

■ **BOX 14-4.**
Guidelines for Communicating With the Hearing Impaired Person

- When you meet a person who seems inattentive or slow to understand you, consider the possibility that hearing, rather than manners or intellect, may be at fault. Some hard-of-hearing persons refuse to wear a hearing aid. Others wear aids so inconspicuous or clearly camouflaged that you may not spot them at first glance. Others cannot be helped by a hearing aid.
- Remember the hard-of-hearing may depend to a considerable extent on reading your lips. They do this even though they may be wearing a hearing aid, for no hearing aid can completely restore hearing. You can help by trying *always to speak in a good light* and by facing the person and the light as you speak.
- When in a group that includes a hard-of-hearing person, try to carry on your conversation with others in such a way that he or she can watch your lips. Never take advantage of the disability by carrying on a private conversation in his or her presence in low tones that cannot be heard.
- Speak distinctly but naturally. Shouting does not clarify speech sounds, and mouthing or exaggerating your words or speaking at a snail's pace makes you harder to understand. On the other hand, try not to speak too rapidly.
- Do not start to speak to a hard-of-hearing person abruptly. Attract his or her attention first by facing the person and looking straight into the eyes. If necessary, touch the hand or shoulder lightly. Help him or her grasp what you are talking about right away by starting with a key word or phrase, for example, "Let's plan our weekend now," "Speaking of teenagers. . . ." *If he or she does not understand you, do not repeat the same words.* Substitute synonyms: "It's time to make plans for Saturday," and so on.
- If the person to whom you are speaking has one "good" ear, always stand or sit on that side when you address him or her. Do not be afraid to ask a person with an obvious hearing loss whether he or she has a good ear and, if so, which one it is. The person will be grateful that you care enough to find out.
- Facial expressions are important clues to meaning. Remember that an affectionate or amused tone of voice may be lost on a hard-of-hearing person.
- In conversation with a person who is especially hard-of-hearing, do not be afraid occasionally to jot down

key words on paper. If he or she is really having difficulty in understanding you, the person will be grateful for the courtesy.
- Many hard-of-hearing persons, especially teenagers, who hate to be different are unduly sensitive about their disability and will pretend to understand you even when they do not. When you detect this situation, tactfully repeat your meaning in different words until it gets across.
- Teach the family to avoid use of candles. Electric light will give the person a better chance to join the conversation because he or she can see the lips during conversation. Similarly, in choosing a restaurant or night club, remember that *dim lighting may make lipreading difficult.*
- Teach family members that they do not have to exclude the hard-of-hearing person from all forms of entertainment involving speech or music. Concerts and operas may present problems, but movies, plays, ballets, and dances are often just as enjoyable to people with a hearing loss as to those with normal hearing. (Even profoundly deaf persons can usually feel rhythm, and many are good and eager dancers.) For children, magic shows, pantomimes, and the circus are good choices.
- When sending a telegram to someone who does not hear well, instruct the telegraph company to deliver your message, not telephone it.
- The speech of a person who has been hard-of-hearing for years may be difficult to understand since natural pitch and inflection are the result of imitating the speech of others. To catch such a person's meaning more easily, watch the face while he or she talks.
- Do not say such things as "Why don't you get a hearing aid?" or "Why don't you see a specialist?" to a person who is hard-of-hearing. Chances are he or she has already explored these possibilities, and there is no need to emphasize the disability.
- *Use common sense* and tact in determining which of these suggestions apply to the particular hard-of-hearing person you meet. Some persons with only a slight loss might feel embarrassed by any special attention you pay them. Others whose loss is greater will be profoundly grateful for it.

4. The person is not thinking clearly or acting as usual.
5. Low body temperature, irregular or slow pulse, slurred speech, shallow respirations, hypotension, drowsiness, lack of coordination, and sluggishness may be present—singly or in combination.
6. Coma may occur and is probable when the body temperature is 90° F (32.2° C) or less.

Severe hypothermia can cause complications of

kidney, liver, or pancreatic disorders, ventricular fibrillation, and death. Recovery depends on severity and length of exposure and previous health and on the rewarming treatment (34, 75).

Teach the elderly person the following measures to *prevent hypothermia* in cold weather (34, 75):

1. Stay indoors as much as possible, especially on windy, wet, and cold days.

2. Wear layered clothing, and cover the head when outdoors.
3. Eat high-energy foods such as some fats and easily digested carbohydrates and protein daily.
4. Keep at least one room warm at 70° F (20° C) or above.
5. Use extra blankets, caps, socks, and layered clothing in bed.
6. Have contact with someone daily.
7. Avoid drinking alcoholic beverages.

Perception of and reaction to *painful stimuli* may be decreased with age. Because pain is an important warning device serving the safety of the organism, use caution when applying hot packs or other hot or cold applications. The elderly person may be burned or suffer frostbite before being aware of any discomfort. More accurate assessment of physical signs and symptoms may be necessary to alleviate conditions underlying complaints of pain such as abdominal discomfort or chest pain, which may be more serious than the older person's perception indicates.

Dulling of *tactile sensation* occurs because of a decrease in the number of areas of the body responding to all stimuli and in the number and sensitivity of sensory receptors (102). There may be clumsiness or difficulty in identifying objects by touch. The person may not respond to light touch but needs to be touched. Because fewer tactile cues are received from the bottom of the feet, the person may get confused about position and location. These factors, combined with sensitivity to glare, poorer peripheral vision, and a constricted visual field, may result in disorientation, especially at night when there is little or no light in the room (34). Because the aged person takes longer to recover visual sensitivity when moving from a light to a dark area, night lights and a safe and familiar arrangement of furniture are essential. Sensory alterations may require modification of the home environment and extra orientation to new surroundings. Simple explanations of routines, location of the bathroom, and the way the signal cord works in the hospital are just a few examples of information the older client needs. Objects in a familiar environment should not be moved. Use touch, if acceptable to the person. Increased hairbrushing or combing, back rubs, hugs, and touch of shoulders, arms, or hands increase tactile sensation.

Understand that some of the changed behavior, discussed later under psychologic concepts, is directly related to physical changes in nerve and sensory tissue and influences nursing practice, whether you are giving physical care, establishing a relationship, providing a safe environment, or planning recreational needs. Research indicates that hand, foot, and eye preference becomes more right-sided and ear preference becomes more left-sided with advancing age. Adapt nursing care measures to accommodate these changes (207). The whole area of client teaching is also affected, because you must understand the altered responses and the changing needs of the elderly before beginning their health education.

Common Health Problems: Prevention and Treatment

The health problems of the older adult may be associated with the aging process, a disease state, or both. Yet more than 90% of the elderly need no help with activities of daily living (278). You should consider all of the aspects of aging before deciding on a course of action. As you care for the older adult, refer to Appendices III and IV for a schedule of health-screening measures. Refer to a medical-surgical nursing text for in-depth information on all of the following health problems. Other references will also be useful (26, 34, 45, 55, 75, 91, 95, 109, 117, 147, 163, 213).

Table 14–4 summarizes common neurologic and respiratory diseases, blood dyscrasias, and genitourinary and skeletal diseases. Cardiovascular, endocrine-metabolic, sexual function diseases, and substance abuse are also presented in overview (34, 117, 280).

Cardiovascular Disease

Cardiovascular disease is common in the aged. **Congestive heart failure (CHF)** is a condition of *altered cardiac function in which there is not enough cardiac output to meet demands of tissue metabolism; consequently, sodium and body water are retained*. Often arteriosclerotic heart disease and hypertension are precursors. The person may complain of difficulty with breathing in any position other than sitting or standing, especially after exertion and at night. There may be ankle swelling, and the person may void much more frequently at night. Fluid retention will show as weight gain. The neck veins may be distended, and rales may be auscultated in the lungs. The heart may beat rapidly and display a "gallop rhythm."

When the diagnosis is established and other conditions are ruled out, the goal is to improve cardiac function and renal excretion. A low-sodium diet is recommended (usually 85 mEq/day). High blood pressure must be corrected with medication if lesser measures do not succeed. Rate and rhythm of heartbeat are regulated with a digitalis preparation, and oral diuretics may be used to increase urinary output. The person should be followed closely until the condition has stabilized (34, 117).

Chronic occlusive arterial disease of the extremities is diagnosed when, because of *partial or complete occlusion of one or more of the peripheral blood vessels*, there is a *decreased blood flow to one or more of the extremities*. Often this condition is associated with diabetes. Depending on the site of the occlusion, the person may experience the following: a cramping pain in the muscles during exercise that is relieved by rest, although cramping may occur at night; the extremity involved may feel cool and pulses may be de-

TABLE 14-4. COMMON HEALTH PROBLEMS IN LATER MATURITY

Problem	Definition	Symptoms/Signs	Prevention/Treatment
Neurological Diseases			
Herpes zoster (shingles)	Caused by same virus that causes chickenpox. Involves dorsal root ganglia	Unilateral vesicular eruption that follows dermatomes of affected nerve root. Severe pain; rash that progresses from macules to crusting pustules	Analgesics; cool soaks; acyclovir (Zovirax). Investigation of underlying immunologic problems
Parkinson's disease	Slowly progressive degenerative disorder of nervous system	Resting tremor; masklike face; shuffling gait; forward flexion; muscle weakness; rigidity	Symptomatic; medicine to correct depleted dopamine and rid excessive acetylcholine
Alzheimer's disease	Presenile dementia or neural atrophy	Cognitive, physical, and emotional deterioration	Treatment extremely varied, depending on areas affected. Much support and understanding needed from families and caretakers; in turn, families and caretakers need support
Respiratory Diseases			
Chronic obstructive pulmonary disease	Consists of three components: bronchitis, bronchoconstriction, and emphysema	Three components: (1) bronchitis—excessive mucous and sputum production with inflammation of the bronchi; (2) bronchoconstriction—narrowing airways; (3) emphysema—irreversible destruction of distal air space. Shortness of breath, sputum production, wheezing, tachypnea, hyperinflation	Smoking cessation; increased fluids; yearly influenza vaccine; one-time pneumonia vaccine; bronchodilator; expectorants as necessary; avoidance of sedatives and cold, wet weather; postural drainage; antibiotics if infection. General attention to proper nutrition, rest, and hygiene
Blood Dyscrasias			
Pernicious anemia	Progressive megaloblastic microcytic anemia that results from lack of intrinsic factor essential for absorption of vitamin B_{12}	Weakness, numbness, tingling of extremities; fever, pallor; anorexia, weight loss	Vitamin B_{12} injections; folic acid and iron medications
Secondary anemia	Reduced hemoglobin, hematocrit, and red blood cell counts, resulting from nutritional deficiency, blood loss, and primary problem	Fatigue, shortness of breath, lightheadedness, skin pallor; sometimes arrhythmia	Iron preparation or perhaps blood transfusion; maintenance or stable activities of daily living; attention to primary issue
Chronic lymphocytic leukemia	Neoplasm of blood-forming tissue	Characterized by small, long-lived lymphocytes, chiefly B cells in bone marrow, blood, liver, and lymphoid tissue	Complexity of disease dictates seeking medical-surgical text
Hodgkin's disease	Malignant disorder	Characterized by painless progressive enlargement of lymphoid tissue	Complexity of disease necessitates seeking medical-surgical text
Genitourinary			
Benign prostatic hypertrophy (BPH)	Overall enlargement of prostate gland via enlargement of fibrous and muscular tissue	Difficulty in stopping and starting urinary flow; voiding frequent small amounts. Diffuse enlargement of prostate; landmarks preserved	No medical treatment; possible surgical intervention; rule out cancer
Skeletal Disease			
Osteoporosis	Absence of normal quantity of bone. Predisposes to fracture	Loss of normal cortisol thickness; increased porosity in cortical bone; thinning, fragmentation and loss of trabeculae in cancellous bone	Prevention: diet in earlier years containing adequate calcium, vitamin D, phosphorus, protein, and fluoride
Osteoarthritis	Degeneration of articular cartilage and hypertrophy of bone	Pain and stiffness, mainly in weight-bearing joints and dorsal interphalangeal joints of fingers	Exercise to improve stiffness; rest to help pain; heat, antipyretic, adequate nutrition, physical therapy

creased; and the skin may appear shiny with loss of normal skin hair. Appropriate laboratory studies are helpful in ruling out diabetes and blood lipid problems.

After diagnosis, the person should be evaluated for revascularization. General treatment measures include practicing good skin care, avoiding excess heat or cold, and avoiding smoking and caffeine ingestion. Drugs have not proved beneficial in this condition (34, 117).

Stasis ulcer of the lower extremity results in a *chronic ulcerative skin lesion caused by venous stasis and consequent poor circulation*. In contrast to an arterial problem, the person will have intact peripheral pulses in the extremity involved. There may be **pitting edema** (*induration remains after pushing in skin and tissue with a finger*) or **brawny edema** (*thickened and hardened skin*) around the ulcer cite.

Treatment involves rest and elevation of the involved leg, once or twice daily cleaning with povidone-iodine (Betadine) or hydrogen peroxide solution, and occasionally application of moist heat or Unna's paste boat, a protective device. Healing can be slow and difficult, and the person's extremity must be watched for widening of the lesion and cellulitis (34, 117).

Directly related to cardiovascular integrity are such concepts as the maintenance of fluid balance, adequate aeration, and relief of undue strain on the aging circulation. These goals can be a basis for planning nursing care in a variety of ways such as providing enough fluids to ensure sufficient blood volume, guarding against the possibility of circulatory stasis by proper positioning, and encouraging mobility whenever possible. Simple precautions such as not keeping a backrest up too long, thereby preventing pooling of blood in the pelvis or extremities, may be extremely important when the circulation is impaired. Prolonged sitting in a chair should be avoided to prevent dependent edema of the lower extremities. Straining to defecate may cause undue strain on the right side of the heart as the blood is suddenly poured through the vena cava after pressure is decreased in the thorax; therefore a regimen to ensure easy defecation will indirectly protect the heart from overwork.

The elderly person is prone to experience orthostatic hypotension and should be assisted out of bed slowly to prevent a sudden drop in the blood supply to the brain with resultant vertigo. Allowing him or her to sit for a moment on the side of the bed before standing will help circulation to adjust to postural changes. The aged person normally has a higher blood pressure; thus hypotension may occur, even though the blood pressure level appears at the textbook range of normal.

Endocrine-Metabolic Disorders

Hormonal changes are significant to health since a wide variety of physiologic processes are regulated by the endocrine glands. Cellular metabolism, fluid and electrolyte balance, diameter of small blood vessels, and consequently the supply of blood to various tissues are among the body functions mediated by endocrine regulation.

The chemical composition of fluids surrounding body cells must be closely regulated, and when analysis of blood shows alterations in blood volume, acidity, osmotic pressure, or protein and sugar content, older adults require a longer time to recover internal chemical equilibrium. Insulin, secreted by cells in the pancreas, normally accelerates the removal of sugar from the blood. In older adults given intravenous insulin with extra glucose, the glucose is removed from their bloodstreams at a slower rate than in younger people because of poorer hormone production. Stress intensifies glucose intolerance. Elderly persons undergoing the stress of surgery, illness, or injury or emotional stress may manifest diabetic symptoms; the elevated blood and urinary glucose usually returns to normal when the stressor subsides (34, 117, 280).

Certain physiologic changes in the elderly may be caused by these subtle alterations in the chemical composition of body fluids. "Diseases of adaptation" are largely caused by derailments of the stress defense mechanism. Overproduction of the defense hormones in response to bacterial infection, injury, psychologic, and other stresses can alter body metabolism enough to have a harmful or even fatal effect on body systems.

Diabetes mellitus is the most common of the endocrine-metabolic disorders in the elderly. It takes its heavy toll because it contributes to inadequately nourished tissues and can lead to retinitis or severe peripheral vascular disease. It patently interferes with normal healing processes and thus precludes optimum recovery from illness or after surgery. This disease has been summarized in other chapters.

Diseases That Affect Sexual Function

Health problems associated with the *sexual changes* of aging are of concern to the older adult. Certain diseases in the elderly female have been linked to estrogen deficiency. There is a statistical rise in atherosclerosis attacking the coronary arteries in aged females (and in younger women who have had ovaries removed); women treated with estrogen therapy have had fewer myocardial infarctions. Although there is no clear-cut case for a cause-and-effect relationship, the female hormones apparently are crucial to the enzymatic system in the metabolism of fats and proteins.

Factors that contribute to *sexual dysfunction* are essentially the same as those that affect performance at any age: disease or mutilating surgery of the genitourinary tract, diverse systemic diseases, and emotional disturbance coupled with societal attitudes. Treatment of the aged for a physical complaint often contributes to widespread use of drugs. Tranquilizers can give way to excessive use of alcohol or marijuana. They weaken erection, reduce desire, and delay ejaculation. Many of the metabolic disorders are overlooked and go untreated; anemia, diabetes, malnutrition, and fatigue may negatively affect the quality of life and cause impotence. Obesity may impose a hazard for cardiac and vascular integrity and at best is damaging to a healthy self-image.

Many older persons are under the false impression that any sexual activity will increase the danger of illness or even death because of stress on heart or blood pressure. In truth, oxygen consumption, heart rate, and blood pressure increase only moderately during intercourse and may actually afford a distinct therapeutic and preventive measure. In persons with arthritis, for example, the increase in adrenal corticosteroids during sexual activity relieves some of the symptoms. The present-day practice of prescribing exercise for cardiac patients attests that sexual intercourse need not be considered dangerous for anyone able to walk around a room.

Radical surgery or dysfunction of the genitourinary tract produces the most devastating effects on sexual capacity and libido. Extensive resectioning due to malignancy may make intercourse difficult if not impossible. Although a decline in desire and capacity for climax may follow hysterectomies, they are by no means inevitable. The loss of childbearing ability and the lack of an ejaculation are for some women and men psychologically traumatic, and these clients may need some support and guidance in adjusting to change.

Nursing care involves first a reexamination of one's own bias about sex and sexuality in the aged. Human sexuality covers a wide spectrum, and the pattern for each individual is a product of prenatal development and postnatal learning experiences coupled with one's inherent sense of personal identity within a sex classification. This basic pattern is not altered simply by age. It continues to mediate one's capacity for involvement in all life activities.

With this in mind, nursing care planning for the elderly can be made most effective. Realizing the need for sexual expression in some form or other, nurses can be open and nonjudgmental when clients display a desire for warmth, close contact, and companionship. Touch is particularly important to the older person who has been bereft of family ties, perhaps for many years. Some people require more relief from sexual tension than others. If incidents arise that seem unduly unorthodox such as open masturbation or unusual behavior with the opposite sex, the nurse can be a support person if there is a sincere desire to be available for counseling. An atmosphere of trust must prevail in which the nurse focuses on the person and not on any specific act.

Exploring alternate life-styles with persons who are single, alone, and old may be a way for the nurse to assist. Teaching that includes information about therapy available such as estrogen replacement when there are emotional or physiologic problems associated with the climacteric can help the elderly woman to choose treatment. A thorough knowledge of anatomy and the physiology of normal aging is essential for the nurse who cares for the elderly. Only then can information be accurate and teaching effective. The nurse has a responsibility to communicate also to the families and friends of the older client and to colleagues information that will help in dealing with their inability to understand the sexual needs of the aged.

Intervention can include the following:

1. Becoming better educated about sexuality
2. Increasing self-awareness
3. Discussing openly sexuality with peers, staff, and students
4. Attempting to manipulate the environment of the aged client to provide a healthier milieu in which relationships can be a source of comfort
5. Evaluating own behavior in terms of intimacy, touch, friendships, and interest in the aged
6. Above all, accepting the challenge ourselves to live fully and to assist the aged in our care to do the same

Substance Abuse

Approximately 10% to 15% (more than 2 million) of elderly Americans suffer from alcoholism, and an increasing number are abusing not only prescription drugs, but also heroin, LSD, marijuana and cocaine. Contrary to popular opinion, they can be successfully treated.

There are two types of elderly alcoholics: those who began alcohol abuse in their youth (approximately two thirds of the elderly) and those whose minimum drinking habits increased in old age as a reaction to and way to cope with various problems and losses. Widowers comprise the largest proportion of late-onset elderly alcoholics (242).

Because alcohol is a central nervous system depressant, there are some adverse effects of alcohol abuse. With low blood levels the person may feel relaxed and comfortable. With increased blood levels, the person may feel a sense of stimulation, but in reality the brain centers lose ability to check belligerent or antisocial behavior. Alcohol also interacts with various drugs, either through potentiation of or interference with medication action, as shown in Table 14–5. Other effects such as loss of coordination, slower reflex reaction time, slower mental response cause the person to be accident prone, which may in turn cause injury, fractures, or death. Excess alcohol intake and as a result poor dietary intake, malabsorption, and progressive liver damage cause hypomagnesemia and hypocalcemia, resulting in osteoporosis and avitaminosis, causing various deficiency states. Esophagitis, erosive gastritis and ulcer formation, pancreatitis, and liver cirrhosis are serious diseases that may hasten death. Cancer of the mouth, pharynx, and esophagus is more common in the alcoholic. Finally, excessive alcohol intake may cause pneumonia, respiratory failure, or cardiac failure and death.

As a nurse your acceptance of, listening to, and assessment of the elderly person in various health care

TABLE 14-5. ALCOHOL INTERACTIONS WITH MEDICATIONS

Alcohol Taken With Medication	Effect on Person
Antidiabetic agents	Increased hypoglycemia; increased effects of alcohol
Anticoagulants	Increased effect; possible hemorrhage
Barbiturates	
Tranquilizers	
Narcotics	
Antidepressants	Increased central nervous system depression, oversedation
Antihistamines	
Anesthetics	
Antibiotics	Inhibition of antimicrobial action

sites can be critical for diagnosis and treatment. You are a liaison between the client and other professionals and can facilitate treatment of the alcoholism and prevention or treatment of various complications. Further, your education of and support to the family and client can foster their acceptance of the diagnosis and pursuit of treatment. See reference 187 for additional information on alcohol and drug abuse. signs and symptoms, treatment, and nursing care.

PSYCHOLOGIC CONCEPTS

The psychologic and socioeconomic concepts of aging are significant for all who work with the aged, and you will find older people concerned and needing to talk about the many changes to which they must adjust. Knowledge of the crises in this life stage is necessary if you are to aid clients and families in the attainment of developmental tasks, in meeting the crises, and in the early or appropriate treatment of these crises.

Cognitive Development

One universal truth that concerns the process of aging is that its onset, rate, and pattern are singularly unique for each person. Especially is this true in psychologic and mental changes, which generally have a later and more gradual onset than physical aging. Many factors must be considered when assessing the intellectual functioning of older people: (1) sociocultural influences; (2) motivation; (3) interest; (4) sensory impairments that interfere with integration of sensory input into proper perception; (5) educational level; (6) the time since school learning; (7) isolation from others; (8) deliberate caution; (9) using more time to do something, which others may interpret as not knowing; and (10) the adaptive mechanism of conserving time and emotional energy rather than showing assertion. The initial level of ability is important: a bright, 20-year-old will be a bright 70-year-old. Overall, mental ability it incremental (65, 231).

The elder demonstrates **crystallized intelligence,** *knowledge and cognitive ability maintained over the lifetime, dependent on sociocultural influences, life ex-*
periences, and broad education, which involve the ability to perceive relationships, engage in formal operations, and understand the intellectual and cultural heritage. Crystallized intelligence is measured by facility with numbers, verbal comprehension, general information, and integrative and interpretive ability. It is influenced by the amount the person has learned, the diversity and complexity of the environment, the person's openness to new information, and the extent of formal learning opportunities. Self-directed learning opportunities and educational opportunities to gain additional information increase crystallized intelligence after 60 years of age.

A decline occurs in many people after the late seventies. The loss of biologic potential is offset by acquired wisdom, experience, and knowledge. In contrast, **fluid intelligence,** *independent of instruction, social or environmental influences, or acculturation and dependent on genetic endowment, is less apparent. It consists of ability to perceive complex relationships, use of short-term or rote memory, creation of concepts, and abstract reasoning.* Fluid intelligence is measured by ability to do tasks of memory span, inductive reasoning, and figural relations. (The fluid intelligence actually begins to decrease in middle age.) However, there is no uniform pattern of age-related changes for all intellectual abilities, nor is there a consistent decline in all elders (231).

Decrease in reaction time or the speed of response in the sixties and thereafter is central in origin rather than the result of changes in sensory or motor end organs. The central organization of material, if hurried, will result in decreased quality and quantity of response (279).

The senior performs certain cognitive tasks more slowly for several reasons: (1) decreased visual and auditory acuity; (2) slower motor response to sensory stimulation; (3) loss of recent memory; (4) divided attention; (5) greater amount of prior accumulated knowledge and learning that must be scanned and appropriately placed mentally; (6) perceived meaninglessness of task; and (7) changed motivation. He or she may be less interested in competing in timed intellectual tests. Further, an apparently shorter duration of alpha rhythm in the brain wave affects the timing of response. Reaction time is also slower when the person suffers significant environmental or social losses, is unable to engage in social contact, and is unable to plan daily routines. The person who is ill often endures environmental and social losses by virtue of being in the client role. Thus he or she may be slower responding to your questions or requests (34, 170, 200, 231).

Studies of intelligence in the aged have shown that, although some decline occurs in the sixth decade of life, persons in later decades show little change when tested. (Results of intelligence quotient tests may reflect the stress of having to cope with the test more than actual intelligence.) Overall, general and verbal intelligence, problem solving, coordination of ideas and facts, judgment, creativity, and other well-practiced cognitive skills and wisdom are maintained even into old age if there is no deterioration caused by extensive physical or neurologic changes (54, 61, 124). Further, *memory can be improved* with skills training and motivational incentives (115).

Studies indicate that elderly adults are equivalent to young adults in cue use, encoding, specificity, decision-making speed, design recognition, and spatial memory or awareness of location, especially when distinctive cues are available. Other studies indicate that cognitive performances of young and old adults are comparable when the task is divided or attention has not been interrupted, on assessing contents and products of memory, and on recall and recognition of factual information (61, 236).

In recall of sets of items or letter sequences, the older person usually is less accurate in memory and slower because he or she uses a limited number of strategies for remembering (4). **Episodic memory,** *recall on demand of specific learned facts,* does decline. However, when the older person deliberately uses memory or encoding strategies such as rehearsal, he or she does as well as the young adult (9, 61).

Older women excel over men in verbal ability and speed of reaction. Older people are able to tolerate very extensive degenerative changes in the central nervous system without serious alteration of behavior if their social environments are sufficiently supportive. If their environment was restricted in early life, however, learning is inhibited in later life. Mental functions, especially vocabulary and other verbal abilities, do not deteriorate appreciably until 6 to 12 months before death (153, 220, 277).

Usually the capacity to learn, relearn, synthesize, and problem solve continues into old age, even though difficulty in the ordering of time sequences of more recent events and in immediate recall of new learning may exist. Test scores on spatial perception and decoding tasks decrease, possibly because of sensory and coordination changes. Tasks that appear meaningless and require making analogies or new learning that is in con-

flict with prior learning and novel situations are more difficult. In addition, older people are apprehensive about new learning, especially in competitive situations, and ask for more details and more specific directions because they anticipate difficulty in learning new tasks (48, 57, 162, 170).

The older person is favored over the younger person if tasks require redundant information or inference processing. Associations between words and events that are logically related and habitual behavior become strengthened throughout life by the continual accumulation of information and adaptation of the person. The person seems more concrete in thinking because he or she strives to be functional or practical. Previously reinforced ways of doing things take precedence over new behavior. But he or she takes longer to react. This slowing of response affects not only learning but also contributes to accident proneness (48, 57).

Cognition and intellectual development are part of maturity. Maturity involves the achievement of an efficiently organized psychic growth predicated on the integration gained from solving environmentally stimulated conflicts and a variety of situations. It is in the last half of life that the person best draws on cumulative experiences to establish social, moral, and ethical standards; render decisions; assist in planning; erect social guideposts; and establish pacific relationships between oncoming generations. The judgmental functions of the mind are most highly developed after midlife (78, 130, 153).

In your care of the older person and in teaching about cognitive characteristics of later maturity, recognize that the normal aging brain, free of disease, may function as effectively and efficiently as the normal young adult brain except for speed and recent memory. Significant cognitive impairment is related to disease, not normal aging. Alzheimer's disease may represent a final common pathway for a variety of causative factors—ranging from genetic predispositions to environmental forms, nutritional deficiencies, infectious agents, or a combination of them. These factors, combined with the person's life-style, inactivity, and lifelong experiences, may be responsible for what we consider aging brain changes. Just as a cognitive decline predicts mortality, low-level performance on certain tests may predict dementia two or three decades later since the pre-symptom phase may be extended. Such test results, plus the known chromosomal loss that occurs with dementia (human chromosomes can be counted by using the lymphocytes), would allow ample time for intervention and prevention (124).

Adapt activities such as obtaining proper nutrition, preoperative or discharge teaching, or the learning of new content or techniques such as insulin injections and colostomy care to the changes in the aging nervous system, other physiologic changes, and cognitive and emotional changes. Use the following suggestions as you teach:

1. Always approach the teaching situation in a way that enhances the person's self-concept and self-confidence.
2. Keep in mind and assess the elder's experiences, current knowledge, needs, interests, questions, health status, and developmental level as you plan and implement teaching.
3. Minimize distracting noise; have a comfortable setting.
4. Tell the person that you are planning a teaching session, state the general topic, and emphasize its importance. Get the person's attention and increase anticipation.
5. Arrange for the person to be near the teacher, the teaching aids, or demonstration.
6. Consider the aged person's difficulty with fine movement and failing vision when you are using visual aids.
7. Provide adequate lighting without glare; do not have the person face outdoor or indirect light.
8. Use sharp colors with a natural background and large print to offset visual difficulties.
9. Explain procedures and directions with the person's possible hearing loss and slowed responses in mind.
10. Use a low-pitched, clear speaking voice; face the person so he or she can lip read if necessary.
11. Teach slowly and patiently, with sessions not too long or widely spaced and with repetition and reinforcement.
12. Mentally "walk through" or imagine a task through verbal explanation before it is to be done to enhance recall.
13. Material should be short, concise, and concrete; present material in a logical sequence; summarize often.
14. Break complex tasks or content into smaller and simpler units; focus on a single topic to promote concentration.
15. Match your vocabulary to the learner's ability and define terms clearly and as frequently as needed.
16. Give the aged person time to perceive and respond to stimuli, to learn, to move, to act.
17. Help the person make associations between prior and new information and emphasize abilities that remain constant to enhance recall and application.
18. Have the person actively use several sensory modalities to make motions and repeat the content aloud verbally while seeing or hearing it.
19. Plan extra sessions for feedback and return demonstrations and extra time for these sessions.
20. Whenever possible, include a significant other in the teaching session to ensure further interpretation and support in using the information.

These measures, combined as necessary, allow for comprehension and appropriate response and compensate for decline in perception, memory, and slower formation of associations and concepts.

Emotional Development

Erikson (79), describing the eight stages of man, states the developmental or psychosexual task of the mature years is ego integrity versus despair. A complex set of factors combines to make the attainment of this task difficult for the elderly person.

Ego integrity is the *coming together of all previous phases of the life cycle* (79). Having accomplished the earlier tasks, the person accepts life as his or her own and as the only life for the self. He or she would wish for none other and would defend the meaning and the dignity of the life-style. The person has further refined the characteristics of maturity described for the middle-aged adult, achieving both wisdom and an enriched perspective about life and people. Even if earlier development tasks have not been completed, the aged person may overcome these handicaps through association with younger persons and through helping others resolve their own conflicts. The historical situation, family environment, marital status, and individual development all influence the integrity achievement (78, 153).

Use the consultative role to enhance ego integrity. Ask the person's counsel about various situations that relate to him or her personally or to ideas about politics, religion, or activities current in the residence or institution. Although you will not burden the person with your personal problems, the senior will be happy to be consulted about various affairs, even if his or her advice is not always taken. Acting as a consultant enhances ego integrity. Having the person reminisce also promotes ego integrity, and reintegration and recasting of life events put traumatic events into perspective.

The person who has achieved ego integrity remains creative. Decrement in achievement is rarely so substantial that the person becomes devoid of creativity at life's end. Even an octogenarian can expect to produce many notable contributions to any creative activity, as has been witnessed with artists, composers, and statesmen. Creativity in the late years depends on initial creative potential, but creativity may lie dormant during the demanding young adult years. The older adult has many of the necessary qualities for creativity: time, accumulated experience, knowledge, skills, and wisdom. Often the changes mandated by retirement and late life trigger new creative levels, including those in ordinary people (239).

Without a sense of ego integrity, the person feels a sense of **despair** and **self-disgust.** *Life has been too short and futile. The person wants another chance to redo life.* If life has not been worth the struggle, death is fearsome. The person becomes hypercritical of others, disengages, and projects self-disgust, inadequacy, and anger onto others. Such feelings are enhanced by society's emphasis on youth, the mass media's extolling beauty, and enforced retirement. Ultimately, the people around him or her help the aged person feel either a sense of importance or a feeling of being a burden, too slow, and worthless (79). Feelings of despair and disgust about self are compounded by the relationship losses suffered and the consequent loneliness and hopelessness that may occur. Having no confidant or companion and physical health status are both related to the emotional status (25, 41, 78, 272). Suicidal thoughts or attempts may result; this is a growing problem (174). Jung (130) believed the old person could not face death in a healthy manner without some image of the hereafter. He believed the unconscious has an archetype of eternity that wells up from within the person as death nears.

Nursing care for the person in despair involves use of therapeutic communication and counseling principles, use of touch, and being a confidant so that the person can work through feelings from the past and present ones of sadness and loneliness. The maintenance phase of the nurse-client relationship is important since the person needs time to resolve old conflicts and learn new patterns of thinking and relating. The person can move to a sense of ego integrity with the ongoing relating of at least one caring person—a person who listens; meets physical needs when the person cannot; nurtures and encourages emotionally; brings in spiritual insights; validates the senior's realistic concerns, fears, or points of anguish; and listens to the review of life, patching together life's experiences. Other references furnish more detail (187).

Personality Development and Characteristics

No specific personality changes occur as a result of aging; values, life orientation, and personality traits remain consistent from at least middle age onward. *The older person becomes more of what he or she was.* The older person continues to develop emotionally and in personality but adds on characteristics instead of making drastic changes (130, 159, 190, 230). If he or she were physically active and flexible in personality and participated in social activities in the young years, these characteristics will continue appropriate to physical status and life situation. If the person was hard to live with when younger, he or she will be harder to live with in old age. The garrulous, taciturn person becomes more so, and problems of control and dominance are common. Stereotypes describe the older person as rigid, conservative, opinionated, self-centered, and disagreeable to be with. Such characteristics are not likely to be new; rather they are an exaggeration of lifelong traits that cannot be expressed or sublimated in another way.

Personality Types

Studies of large samples of seniors reaffirm their uniqueness, but researchers have categorized the variety of their behaviors.

Four personality types were described by Neugarten (190, 191): the integrated, defended, passive dependent, and disintegrated.

The *integrated personality* type is characteristic of most elderly. These people function well and have a complex inner life, intact cognitive abilities, and competent ego. They are flexible, open to new stimuli, and mellow. They adjust to losses and are realistic about the past and present. They have a high sense of life satisfaction. The integrated group is made up of three subtypes: the reorganizers, focused, and disengaged. The *reorganizers* engage in a wide variety of activities; when they lose old roles and related activities, they substitute new ones. They are as active after retirement as before. The *focused* are selective in their activities; they devote energy to a few roles that are important to them rather than being involved in many organizations. The *disengaged* are well-integrated persons who have voluntarily moved away from role commitments. Activity level is low but not because of external losses or physical deficits. They are self-directed and interested in the world but have chosen the rocking-chair approach to life without guilt. They are calm, aloof, but contented. Thus Neugarten defines the disengaged person differently from Cummings and Henry (190, 191).

The *defended personality* is seen in ambitious, achievement-oriented persons who have always driven themselves hard and who continue to do so. They have a number of defenses against anxiety and a tight control over impulses. This "armored" group has medium to high life satisfaction. The defended group is made up of two subtypes: those who hold on and the constricted. The *holding on* persons have a philosophy of, "I'll work until I drop." So long as they can keep busy, they can control their anxieties and feel worthwhile. The *constricted* are preoccupied with their losses and deficits. They have always shut out new experiences and have had minimum social interactions. Their caution continues as they try to defend themselves against aging. Nevertheless, they are satisfied with life, possibly because they know nothing different (190, 191). Most seniors are resourceful and psychologically healthy.

The *passive-dependent personality* type is divided into two patterns: the succorance-seeking and the apathetic. The *succorance-seeking* have strong dependency needs and seek help and support from others. They manage fairly well as long as they have one or two people on which to lean. They have medium levels of activity and medium life satisfaction. The *apathetic* have an extremely passive personality. They engage in few activities and little social interaction. They have little interest in the world around them. They believe that life has been and continues to be hard and that little can be done about it. They have low satisfaction with life (190, 191).

The *disintegrated* or *disorganized personality* type is found in a small percentage of elderly who show gross defects in psychologic functions and deterioration in thought processes. They may be severely neurotic or psychotic. Yet these elderly are not necessarily institutionalized. They may manage to live in the community because of the forbearance or protection of others around them.

Personality and Life-Style Types

These types were categorized extensively for women and men in one longitudinal study. Results of the study showed a diversity of behavior in seniors. No correlations existed between personality and life-style, and spouses did not show similar personality types. Health status strongly influenced life-style and personality characteristics; healthy people were more active and involved in life roles. Evidence supports the general hypothesis that personality characteristics in old age are highly correlated with early life characteristics. Although early adult life-styles are more likely to continue into old age for men than for women, the early life personality of women is more likely to continue into old age than the early personality type of men (159).

Although the popular stereotype is that women cannot cope effectively, this study revealed that *all* women, even those who were more rigid in ego defenses, were higher in ability to cope than in ego disorganization and women were more adaptable than men. Whenever defensiveness or ego disorganization does occur, it is related to general personality predisposition throughout life, outlook on life, and physical health (159).

Personality problems in old age are related to problems in early life. Even when the younger years are too narrowly lived or painfully overburdened, the later years may offer new opportunities. Different ways of living can be developed as the social environment changes and as the person also changes. Later maturity can provide a second and better chance at life (78, 159).

Authors cite personality trends that are commonly found in the elderly. Some difference is noted between the earlier and later decades of later maturity.

Young-Old Personality

In the *young-old* person (65 to 75 or 80 and sometimes beyond) (153), the personality is frequently flexible, shows characteristics commonly defined as maturity, and is less vulnerable to the harsh reality of aging. The person manifests self-respect without conceit; tolerates personal weakness while using strengths to the fullest; and regulates, diverts, or sublimates basic drives and impulses instead of trying to suppress them. He or she is guided by principles but is not a slave to dogma; maintains a steady purpose without pursuing the impossible goal; respects others, even when not agreeing with their behavior; and directs energies and creativity to master the environment and overcome the vicissitudes of life (30, 32).

Motivations change; the senior wants different things from life than he or she did earlier. Concerns about appearance, standards of living, and family change. Stronger incentives, support, and encouragement are needed to do what used to be eagerly anticipated. He or she avoids risks or new challenges and is increasingly introspective and introverted.

The elderly are tough; they often endure against great physical and social odds. Experience has taught the senior to be somewhat suspicious since he or she is likely to be a victim of "borrowings," a fast-sell job for something he or she does not need, thievery, or physical attacks.

Yet generosity is a common trait of the elderly; the person gives of self fully and shares willingly with people who are loved and who seem genuinely interested in him or her.

The elderly person hopes to remain independent and useful as long as possible, to find contentment, and to die without being a burden to others. Increasingly, dependency may undermine self-esteem, especially if the person values independence.

Personality characteristics differ for men and women, especially in relation to assertiveness. The man becomes more dependent, passive, and submissive and more tolerant of his emerging nurturant and affiliative impulses. The woman becomes more dominant and assertive and less guilty about aggressive and egocentric impulses. Perhaps the reversal in overt behavior is caused by hormonal changes. Perhaps the man can be more open to his long-unfulfilled emotional needs when he is no longer in the role of chief provider and no longer has to compete in the work world. Perhaps the woman reciprocates in an effort to gratify needs for achievement and worth; she expresses more completely the previously hidden conflicts, abilities, or characteristics (191).

Old-Old Personality

Old-old age (80 or 85 years and beyond) (153) is a time for meditation and contemplation, not camaraderie. Camaraderie is for young people who have energy and similarities in background, development, and interest. Old-old people may be friendly and pleasant, but they are also egocentric. Egocentricity is a physiologic necessity, a protective mechanism for survival, not selfishness. Life space shrinks. When old-old people get together, certain factors block camaraderie, even if they want to be sociable: varying stages of deafness and blindness, other faulty sense perceptions, and the fact that they may have little in common other than age and past historical era. Old-old people are even more unique in the life pattern than young-old people because they have lived longer. Further, they have less energy to deal with challenging situations, and relating to a group of oldsters can be challenging (30, 32). There is increased interiority in the personality (192).

The person in later maturity, especially in old-old age, may be called childish. Rather, the person is childlike; he or she pays attention to quality in others. He or she senses when another is not genuine or honest—as a person or in activities. The old-old person reacts with sometimes exasperating conduct because he or she sees clearly through the facade and lacks the emotional energy to be as polite as earlier. Self-control, will power, and intellectual response are less effective in advanced age. Many of the negative emotional characteristics ascribed to the elderly may be based on this phenomenon. Only the very simple, those who have not grappled with the complexities of life, or the very ill and regressed will be infantile.

The old-old have greater need than ever to hold onto others. They are often perceived as clingy, sticky, demanding, loquacious, and repetitious. This often causes the younger person to want to be rid of the senior, which causes a vicious circle of increased demand and increased rejection.

Preoccupation with the body is a frequent topic of conversation, and other elderly people respond in kind. The behavior is analogous to the collective monologue and parallel play of young children. The talk about the body satisfies narcissistic needs, and it is an attempt magically to relieve anxiety about what is happening. This pattern alienates the young and the young-old, and they tend to avoid or stop conversing with the aged.

Old-old persons intensely appreciate the richness of the moment, the joys or the sorrows. They realize the transience of life, and they are more likely to start each day with a feeling of expectancy, not neutrality or boredom. Their future is today. As a result, they become more tolerant of others' foibles, more thrilled over minor events, and more aware of their own needs, even if they cannot meet them.

Irritating behavior of the old-old person is frequently related to the frustration of being dependent on others or helpless and the fear that accompanies dependency and helplessness. The tangible issue at hand—coffee too hot or too cold, visitors too early, too late or not at all, or the fast pace of others—is often not really what is irritating, although the person attaches complaints to some thing that others can identify. The irritability is with the self, loss of control, lost powers, and present state of being.

Perhaps the most frequent error in assessing the elderly is the diagnosis of senility. Conditions labeled as such may actually be the result of physiologic imbalances, depression, inadequacy feelings, or unmet affectional and dependency needs. Psychologic problems in the elderly are often manifested in disorientation, poor judgment, perceptual motor inaccuracy, intellectual dysfunction, and incontinence. These problems are frequently not chronic and may respond well to supportive therapy. Just as few young adults reach complete maturity, few older persons attain an ideal state of personality integration in keeping with their developmental stage.

Nursing needs a strong commitment to assist the elderly in maintaining adaptive mechanisms appropriate to this period of life, although each person will accomplish them in his or her unique way, pertinent to life experiences and cultural background. Cooper's study (53) of concentration camp survivors illustrates the impact of the experience on the person's adaptation.

Carry out principles of care previously described to meet emotional and personality needs of the elderly. For further detail about normal emotional development and related nursing functions to maintain emotional health in later maturity, see *Psychiatric/Mental Health Nursing: Giving Emotional Care* (187).

Adaptive Mechanisms

Persons in their older years are capable of changes in behavior but find changing difficult. As new crises develop from social, economic, or family restructuring, new types of ego defenses may be needed. At the same time, the need to change may interfere with developing a sense of ego integrity.

Changing adaptive mechanisms must be developed for successful emotional transition in these later years. They help the person maintain a sense of self-worth and control over external forces, which in turn promotes a higher level of function (107, 153). Peck (199) lists three developmental tasks related to adaptation, and they serve to show not only the tasks involved but also the mechanisms undergoing change as the older personality strives to become integrated.

Ego differentiation *versus work-role preoccupation is involved in the adaptation to retirement, and its success depends on the ability to see self as worthwhile not just because of a job but because of the basic person he or she is.* **Body transcendence** *versus body preoccupation requires that happiness and comfort as concepts be redefined to overcome the changes in body structure and function,* and consequently, in body image and the decline of physical strength. The third task is **ego transcendence** *versus ego preoccupation, the task of accepting inevitable death.* Mechanisms for adapting to the task of facing death are those that protect against loss of inner contentment and help to develop a constructive impact on surrounding persons (199).

Certain adaptive or defensive mechanisms are used frequently by the aged. **Regression,** *returning to earlier behavior patterns,* should not be considered negative unless it is massive and the person is incapable of self-care. A certain amount of regression is mandatory to survival as the person adapts to decreasing strength, changing body functions and roles, and often increasing frustration. Regression is an adaptive mechanism used by the older adult who is dying, and it is manifested differently than in younger years. The regression is a complex of behaviors not associated solely with a return to former levels of adaptation.

To integrate into self-concept and handle the anxiety created by a complex of losses, changes, and adaptation related to aging and dying, the older person behaves in a way that may be confused with dementia or drug reactions. Careful assessment is needed, using history of the person's normal patterns and history of illness (153).

The dying elderly person may express regression in any or all of the following behaviors (34, 75, 153):

1. Massive denial and projection
2. Misuse of words, confusion about familiar concepts, fragmentation of speech, misinterpretation
3. Preoccupation with minutiae, impaired ability to deal with simple abstractions
4. Awkward childlike thinking

The dying elderly person will invest little emotionally into goal setting and care planning. Any goal must be short term. Caregivers, including family, must provide physical and emotional support, recognizing the dying person's need to disengage from self-care and significant others. During the care process you must support the family caregivers and encourage them to talk about perceptions and feelings and to explain behavioral changes and needs of the dying person.

Other commonly used adaptive mechanisms are described in Table 14–6 (153, 187). McCrae (169) found in a study that controlled for types of stress that older persons did not consistently differ from younger ones in using 26 of 28 coping mechanisms, including rational action, expression of feelings, and seeking help. Middle-aged and older persons were less likely than younger ones to use immature and ineffective mechanisms of hostile responses and escapist fantasy. Health threats in all ages elicit wishful thinking, faith, and fatalism. Using **insight** (*intellectual understanding*) and reminiscing is also adaptive (153). Resilience is also a part of adaptation. Characteristics of the successfully adjusted older woman include the following (270):

1. **Equanimity,** *a balanced perspective of one's life and experiences*
2. **Perseverance,** *persistence despite adversity or discouragement*
3. **Self-reliance,** *belief in oneself and one's abilities*
4. **Meaningfulness,** *realization that life has purpose and the value of one's contribution*
5. **Existential aloneness,** *realization that each person's path is unique and some experiences must be faced alone*

The following are components for an adaptive old age (75, 78):

1. High mental status
2. Absence of organic brain damage or disease

TABLE 14-6. ADAPTIVE MECHANISMS USED BY THE OLDER ADULT

Mechanism	Description
Isolation	*By repressing the emotion associated with a situation or idea while intellectually describing it,* the person can cope with very threatening situations and ideas such as personal and another's disease, aging, and death and can begin to resolve the associated fears. Thus the aged can appear relatively calm in the face of crisis.
Compartmentalization	*Narrowing of awareness and focusing on one thing at a time* so that the aged seem rigid, repetitive, and resistive.
Denial	*Blocking a thought or the inability to accept the situation* is used selectively when the person is under great stress and aids in maintaining a higher level of personality integration.
Rationalization	*Giving a logical sounding excuse for a situation* is often used to minimize weakness, symptoms, and various difficulties or to build self-esteem.
Somatization	*Complaints about physical symptoms and preoccupation with the body* may become an outlet for free-floating anxiety. The person can cope with vague insecurities and rapid life changes by having a tangible physical problem to deal with, especially since others seem more interested and concerned about disease symptoms than feelings about self.
Counterphobia	*Excessive behavior in an area of life to counter or negate fears about that area of life* is observed in the person who persists at activities such as calisthenics or youthful grooming or fashion to retain a youthful appearance.
Rigidity	*Resisting change or not being involved in decision making* is a common defense to help the person feel in control of self and life. A stubborn self-assertiveness is compensatory behavior for the person who has been insecure, rigid, and irritable.
Sublimation	*Channeling aggressive impulses into sociably acceptable activity* can be an effective defense to meet old age as a challenge and maintain vigor and creativity. Often the elderly desire to live vicariously through the younger generation, and they become involved with the young through mutual activities and listening or observing their activities.
Displacement	*Expressing frustration or anger onto another person or object that is not the source of the feelings* provides a safe release and disguises the real source of anxiety. The elder may blame another for his or her deficiencies, bang furniture, throw objects, or unjustly criticize family or health care workers.
Projection	*Attributing personal feelings or characteristics, usually negative, to another* allays anxiety, releases unpleasant feelings, or elevates self-esteem and self-concept. Projection is done unconsciously, usually to those closest to the person; a milieu free of counteraggression helps the person feel secure.

3. High morale
4. Counterphobic rather than passive-dependent behavior
5. Denial of aging
6. Vitality, interest, and enjoyment
7. Adequate income
8. Relatively good health
9. Personal adaptability
10. Available family
11. Psychosocial stimulation
12. Maintenance of meaningful goals
13. Acceptance of death
14. Sense of legacy

Acute illness at any age influences behavior, affective responses, and cognitive function. These aspects of the person are also affected by chronic illness, but their effects and adaptive mechanisms used are less well known.

Body-Image Development

Physical changes discussed earlier have both private and public components and combine to change the appearance and function of the older individual and thereby influence the self-image (186). In one study healthy elderly, when compared to healthy young adults, were more conscious of external physical appearance, possibly because of societal attitudes about youth and beauty. They also self-evaluated higher body competence; perhaps this was a result of their health status or a denial of aging. Both young and older adults revealed no differences in private body consciousness (222). However, as the person ages, loss of muscle strength and tone are reflected through a decline in the ability to perform tasks requiring strength. The old-old or frail person sees self as weakened and less worthwhile as a producer of work either in actual tasks for survival or in the use of energy for recreational activities.

The loss of skin tone, although not serious in itself, causes the aged in a society devoted to youth and beauty to feel stigmatized. Changing body contours accentuate sagging breasts, bulging abdomen, and the dowager's hump caused by osteoporosis. These changes all produce a marked negative effect. This stigma can also affect the sexual response of the older person because of perceived rejection by a partner.

Loss of sensory acuity causes alienation from the environment. Full sensory status cannot be regained once it is loss through aging. Although eyeglasses and better illumination are of great help in fading vision, the elderly recognize their inability to read fine print and to do handwork requiring good vision for small objects. The danger of injury caused by failure to see obstacles in their paths because of cataracts, glaucoma, or senile macular degeneration make the elderly even more insecure about the relationship of their body to their environment. They often seek medical help too late because they do not understand the implications of the diagnosis or the chances for successful correction.

Hearing loss, the result of degeneration of the central and peripheral auditory mechanism and increased rigidity of the basilar membrane, is likely to cause even more negative personality changes in the older person than loss of sight (34). Behavior such as suspiciousness, irritability, and impatience and paranoid tendencies may develop simply because hearing is impaired. Again the person may fear to admit the problem or to seek treatment, especially if he or she is unaware of the possibilities of help, either through the use of hearing aids or corrective surgery.

Often the elderly view the hearing aid as another threat to body image. Eyeglasses are worn by all age groups and hence are more socially acceptable, but a hearing aid is conceived as overt evidence of advanced age. Adjustment to the hearing aid may be difficult for many people, and if motivation is also low, the idea may be rejected.

Be especially alert as you assess visual and auditory needs of the elderly. One of the modern medical miracles is lens implant surgery for those with cataracts. Seeing the senior before and after surgery allows you to share the joy of blindness-to-sight and to do necessary teaching. Surgery and discharge are usually the same day.

Hearing needs may not be met as easily, but astute observation can change the situation quickly. Consider the elderly woman who returned to her home after colostomy surgery. Although she had been pleasant and cooperative in the hospital, always nodding "Yes," she had failed to learn her colostomy irrigation routine. The visiting nurse learned, through being in the home and getting information from the family, that the client was nearly deaf. The client covered her loss by nodding pleasantly. Slow, distinct instructions allowed her to grasp the irrigation techniques, and within several days she was managing well. The nurse also had an opportunity to refer the woman for auditory assessment. Kopac (147) and Hayter (108) give a number of specific ways to modify the environment for persons with sensory impairments.

Jourard (129) speaks of *spirit-titre*. He thinks the way we perceive our body determines the degree to which our self-structure can be organized for optimum body defense against loss of energy. Jourard suggests that the term *spirit* be used to express the *titre*, or concentration of purpose, which may be encouraged in the aged to produce a well-integrated "personality-health."

Helping the senior keep an intact, positive body image will raise his or her *spirit-titre*, Encourage the senior to talk about feelings related to the changing body appearance, structure, and function. Provide a mirror so that he or she can look at self to integrate the overt changes into his or her mental image. Photographs can also be useful in reintegrating a changing appearance. Help the senior to stay well groomed and attractively dressed, and compliment efforts in that direction. Touch and tactile sensations are important measures to help the person continue to define body boundaries and integrate structural changes.

Moral-Spiritual Development

The elderly person with a mature religious outlook and philosophy still strives to incorporate broadened views of theology and religious action into the thinking. Self-transcendence is related to lower loneliness scores and to mental and spiritual health (216). Because the elderly person is a good listener, he or she is usually liked and respected by all ages. Although not adopting inappropriate aspects of a younger life-style, he or she can contemplate the fresh religious and philosophic views of adolescent thinking, thus trying to understand ideas previously missed or interpreted differently. Similarly, others listen to him or her. The elderly person feels a sense of worth while giving experienced views. He or she is concerned about moral dilemma and conflict and offers suggestions on ways to handle them. Basically he or she is satisfied with living personal beliefs, which can serve as a great comfort when he or she becomes temporarily despondent over life changes, changes in the family's life, or when confronting the idea of personal death.

Life experience that is meaningful has a spiritual quality. Four themes give life meaning and promote spiritual well-being (263):

1. Concern for the welfare of others
2. Opportunity to be helpful or useful as needed
3. Becoming involved in activity that is useful to someone else
4. Maintaining positive feelings about self and others

Religious belief and participation are important for most elders, regardless of ethnicity. However, different ethnic groups vary in how they participate, and they differ in the role religion plays in providing a resource for coping with adversities of aging. Nonorganizational religious participation includes reading religious materials, watching or listening to religious programs, prayer, and requests for prayer. Demographics, religious denomination, and health disability factors influence participation in these and organizational activities (188, 253).

The elderly person who has not matured religiously or philosophically may sense a spiritual impoverishment and despair as the drive for professional and economic success wanes. An immature outlook provides no solace, and, if a church member, he or she may become bitter. The person may believe that the church organization to which he or she gave long and dedicated service has forgotten since he or she has less stamina for organizational work. The person may feel cast aside in favor of the young who have so many activities planned for them. This person needs help to arrive at an adequate spiritual philosophy and to find some appropriate reli-

gious or altruistic activities that will help him or her gain feelings of acceptance, self-esteem, and worth.

Nursing Care to Meet Spiritual Needs

Care of clients' spiritual needs is an essential part of holistic care. This includes talking with the elderly, listening to statements that indicate religious beliefs or spiritual needs, and reading scriptures of praying with the person when indicated or requested. Giving spiritual care to the elderly person may involve providing prompt physical care to prevent angry outbursts and accepting apologies as the person seeks forgiveness for a fiery temper or sharp tongue. Quoting or reading favorite scripture verses, saying a prayer, providing religious music, or joining with the person in a religious song may calm inner storms. Acknowledging realistic losses and feeling with those who weep can provide a positive focus and hope. Helping the aged person remain an active participant in church, religious programs, or bible study in the nursing home can maintain his or her self-esteem and sense of usefulness. Finally, in dying and near death, the religious person may want to practice beloved rituals and say, or have quoted, familiar religious or scriptural verses.

Developmental Tasks

The following developmental tasks are to be achieved by the aging couple as a family and by the aging person living alone. You can assist the elderly person to meet these tasks (45, 70, 78, 105):

1. Recognize the aging process, define instrumental limitations, and adjust to societal views of aging.
2. Adjust to decreasing physical strength and health changes.
3. Decide where and how to live out the remaining years; redefine physical and social life space.
4. Continue a supportive, close, warm relationship with the spouse or significant other, including a satisfying sexual relationship.
5. Find a satisfactory home or living arrangement and establish a safe, comfortable household routine to fit health and economic status.
6. Adjust living standards to retirement income and reduced purchasing power; supplement retirement income if possible with remunerative activity.
7. Maintain culturally assigned functions and tasks.
8. Maintain maximum level of health; care for self physically and emotionally by getting regular health examinations and needed medical or dental care, eating an adequate diet, and maintaining personal hygiene.
9. Maintain contact with children, grandchildren, and other living relatives, finding emotional satisfaction with them.
10. Establish explicit affiliation with members of own age group.

CASE SITUATION: Later Maturity

Mrs. Bertini, 78 years old, has been a widow for 20 years. She and her husband had no children, but two nieces and a nephew who live in another state visit occasionally. Mrs. Bertini has coped with arthritis for many years and with the help of a home health agency and friends, has been able to remain in her home after suffering a broken hip. She has taken medication for cardiac disease and hypertension since experiencing a mild heart attack 10 years ago.

Despite increasing physical disability, Mrs. Bertini has maintained close ties with three female friends, two of whom had worked with her in a hat factory when they were young. These friends and their husbands were also friends of her husband. The four couples often played cards and attended social functions together.

Mrs. Bertini has begun to find it increasingly difficult to do her housework and shopping. Although the neighborhood pharmacy still delivers medication, the family-owned grocery on the block where she has lived for 20 years recently closed, and she cannot manage the 4-block walk to the bus stop. She has admitted to her friends that she needs assistance, but on her limited income of a small pension from her husband and the minimum amount from social security, she cannot afford to hire help.

Although Mrs. Bertini had occasionally considered entering a nursing home, the decision is forced when her landlord announces a rent increase of $90.00 monthly. With great reluctance, she asks her closest friends to take her to several nursing homes in her area of the city. As a devout Catholic, her decision is immediate; she feels most comfortable with the home operated by The Sisters of the Poor. It is accredited, looks homey, and is clean. The sisters and other workers are friendly and kind. Her friends help her sell her furniture and move to the nursing home. She takes her television and stand, her favorite chair and footstool, and her most treasured mementos and clothes with her.

The first few days in the nursing home are eventful as Mrs. Bertini meets new people and attends the planned activities. Then she begins to feel confined by having only a small room. She misses her independence and occasionally feels lonely. In her own home she used to sleep until 9 A.M., but now if she wants breakfast, she must be in the dining room no later than 8 A.M. Although mobility is painful, slow, and possible only with aid of a walker, Mrs. Bertini makes a point to attend the activities given in the home and accepts invitations from her friends to go out to eat at favorite restaurants. She looks forward to the letters, gifts, and holiday visits from her nieces and nephews and writes short notes to keep in touch with them. She also attends chapel services weekly. She tells her visitors that she is not afraid of death; her only wish is that she does not suffer long.

11. Maintain interest in people outside the family and in social, civic, and political responsibility.
12. Pursue alternate sources of need satisfaction and new interests and maintain former activities to gain status, recognition, and a feeling of being needed.
13. Find meaning in life after retirement and in facing inevitable illness and death of oneself, spouse, and other loved ones.
14. Work out values, life goals, and a significant philosophy of life, finding comfort in a philosophy or religion.
15. Reassess criteria for self-evaluation.
16. Adjust to the death of spouse and other loved ones.

McCoy (167) describes similar developmental tasks for this era:

1. Disengage from paid work.
2. Reassess finances.
3. Be concerned with personal health care.
4. Search for new achievement outlets.
5. Manage leisure time.
6. Adjust to more constant marriage companion.

7. Search for meaning of life.
8. Adjust to single state.
9. Problem solve.
10. Manage stress accompanying change.
11. Be reconciled to death.

Brown (30) refers to different developmental tasks for the young-old and old-old persons since the changing life situations necessitate different attitudes, efforts, and behaviors. The tasks are listed as follows for each age group.

The *young-old:*

1. Prepare for and adjust to retirement from active involvement in the work arena with its subsequent role change (especially for men).
2. Anticipate and adjust to lower and fixed income after retirement.
3. Establish satisfactory physical living arrangements as a result of role changes.
4. Adjust to new relationships with one's adult children and their offspring.

5. Learn or continue to develop leisure time activities to help in realignment of role losses.
6. Anticipate and adjust to slower physical and intellectual responses in the activities of daily living.
7. Deal with the death of parents, spouses, and friends.

The *vulnerable old or old-old:*

1. Learn to combine new dependency needs with the continuing need for independence.
2. Adapt to living alone in continued independence.
3. Learn to accept and adjust to possible institutional living (nursing and/or proprietary homes).
4. Establish an affiliation with one's age group.
5. Learn to adjust to heightened vulnerability to physical and emotional stress.
6. Adjust to loss of physical strength, illness, and approach of one's death.
7. Adjust to losses of spouse, home, and friends.

These developmental tasks coincide with the Standards for Geriatric Nursing Practice developed by the American Nurses' Association. These standards address themselves to the following nursing actions, which summarize those discussed in this chapter (26):

1. Observing and interpreting signs and symptoms of normal aging and pathologic changes and intervening appropriately
2. Differentiating between pathologic social behavior and the usual life-style of the aged person
3. Demonstrating an appreciation for the heritage, values, and wisdom of older persons
4. Supporting and promoting physiologic functioning in the aged
5. Providing protective and safety measures and supporting the aged during stressful situations
6. Using methods to promote effective communication and socialization of aged persons with individuals, family, and others, thus increasing sensory stimulation
7. Helping the older person adapt to the physical and psychosocial limitations of the environment, yet fulfill needs
8. Assisting with the obtaining and use of helpful mechanical devices for improving function
9. Resolving personal attitudes about aging, dependency, and death to provide assistance in meeting these crises with dignity and comfort.

SOCIOECONOMIC CONCEPTS

Retirement

Age, gender, health status, family background, ethnicity, type of job or profession, lifetime work experience, and economic incentives all influence when the person voluntarily or involuntarily ceases the career or job. As corporations reduce their work force numbers, the older worker is most likely to be released because of salary and pension costs and despite job-discrimination legislation. Yet keeping the older worker may be less costly because of retraining costs and lower turnover and absenteeism. He or she is loyal and committed to the company, is flexible about accepting new assignments, and often is a better salesperson. Many people are living longer but are working shorter careers; yet the proportion of young to old people is diminishing. After the turn of the century, it is likely that more older people will be needed in the workplace to relieve the labor shortage (74).

Retirement affects all the other positions the person has held and the relationships with others. Retirement is a demotion in the work system. It will, for many people, mean a reduction in income, or the person may seek a new job, either part-or full-time, for financial reasons but also for emotional and socialization reasons. Inability to keep up with the former activities of an organization or group may result, and a change in status may require a changing social life (24, 152, 219, 227, 288).

Retirement Planning

Prior planning will help in the transition from worker to retiree. Nurses are often with persons nearing retirement and may be asked directly or through nonverbal cues and disguised statements to help them sort out their feelings as they face this adjustment. Although some persons who disliked their jobs, have an adequate income, and participate in a variety of activities eagerly look forward to a pleasurable retirement, many seniors would prefer and are able to work past 65 years.

Despite much work in recent years at both the national and local levels to develop comprehensive programs for the aged, few business organizations have recognized the many ways in which they might assist the potential retiree. Private organizations with large numbers of employees are, for the most part, the only ones having effective retirement preplanning programs. The federal government offers little in retirement planning for its employees, and this is true for almost all state and local governments as well. Those programs offered usually include lectures and discussions on financial security, health insurance, legal matters, Social Security benefits, company pension and retirement policies, and health maintenance information.

The retiree may be faced with these questions: Can I face loss of job satisfaction? Will I feel the separation from people close to me at work? If I need continued employment on a part-time basis to supplement social security payments, will the old organization provide it, or must I adjust to a new job? Shall I remain in my present home or seek a different one because of easier maintenance or reduced cost of upkeep? Might a different climate be better and, if so, will I miss my relatives and neighbors?

Whatever the elderly person's need, your role will

be supportive. Advocate retirement planning. Recommend agencies that may be useful in making plans, and provide current information on Social Security benefits and Medicare coverage. Unless you are able to discuss these areas of concern and to answer questions, the needs of the person approaching retirement cannot be met. One of the most helpful resources is the large supply of government publications available at little or no cost from the Superintendent of Documents of the Government Printing Office in Washington, D.C. Current lists of material pertinent to health and social programs may be obtained directly from the National Clearing House on Aging, U.S. Department of Health and Human Services, 330 Independence Avenue, S.W., Washington, D.C. 20201.

Use of Leisure

The constructive use of free time is often a problem of aging. What a person does when he or she no longer works is related to past life-style, continuous core activities, accumulated experiences, and the way in which he or she perceives and reacts to the environment (138).

Leisure time, *having opportunity to pursue activities of interest without a sense of obligation, demand, or urgency,* is an important aspect of life satisfaction, expression of self, and emotional and social development. Leisure activity is chosen for its own sake and for the meaning it gives to life, but it involves both physical or mental activity and participation. It is a way to cope with change. Adults value most the leisure activity that involves interaction with others and/or a pet, promotes development, or is expressive and maintains contact with the broader community. Most people have a core of activity that they enjoy (138). Reading and viewing television are popular pastimes; interestingly, television preferences are similar for older and younger adults, but reading preferences vary strongly with age and gender (185).

Use of leisure time by volunteering is rewarding but constrained by household income, education, and age. In a study of elders in Minnesota, 52% of them did volunteer work that could be classified as formal or informal, regular or occasional, and with either people, objects, or community system (85). Older Americans participate in many unpaid productive activities at levels commensurate to those reached by young and middle-aged adults (114). Elders who have been self-reliant and have always worked hard are more likely to incorporate service to others into their leisure and volunteer time (3, 114).

The elder can contribute in many ways to the community and society after his or her retirement:

1. Through volunteer or part-time work with any hospital, community agencies, or social, welfare, or conservation organization of choice
2. Through a friendly visitor program to other old or homebound people
3. Through a telephone reassurance program (calling the same person at the same time each day to determine the status)
4. Through foster grandparent programs in nurseries, with failure-to-thrive children, and in preschool or day-care settings, homes for abused or orphaned children, or juvenile detention centers
5. To homes for battered women or children, providing mothering or fathering skills
6. To shelters for the homeless, providing counseling, teaching for General Education Development (GED) certification, or socializing
7. To churches and church-related organizations in many capacities
8. To Habitat for Humanity, an organization that builds or remodel homes for poor people in various rural and urban areas of the United States and in other underdeveloped nations
9. As a volunteer for a crisis hot line: suicide, drug use, child care, prayer line
10. Through collaboration with police, clergy, or community leaders, working to create drug free and gun free neighborhoods and schools

Box 14–5 lists questions to consider before assuming the volunteer role or questions the senior should ask key people in an agency that is being considered for a volunteer role. Explore these questions with the person.

Because Americans live in a society that has a high work priority, more training for leisure in middle age and earlier or more opportunity for continued employment in old age must be provided through public policy.

■ BOX 14–5.
Questions to Consider Before Volunteering

- Do you have the time to give?
- Do you make punctuality a habit?
- Do you take responsibility seriously?
- Can you give reasonable advance notice if you must cancel plans or appointments?
- Do you consistently follow through on projects?
- Do you work well with others?
- Do you adhere to an organization's policies and procedures?
- Do you accomplish tasks that have been assigned?
- Would you receive orientation or training you want or need?
- Do you understand and agree with the details of the position and the demands it will place on you?
- Would you have enough responsibility or authority to challenge you if you desired the challenge?
- Is the organization respected in your community?
- Does the organization respect its volunteers' time?
- Are the current volunteers dedicated to the organization or cause?
- Would you be able to use your experience or educational background?

The American Association of Retired Persons (AARP) is studying the potential impact on people as America moves from an industrialized mass society into a more technologically complex but fragmented society. Older people will be retained as consultants in the work place. All people will need an education for a life of ceaseless change, for new activities, and for new roles with passing years. Older people can lead in creating a better society for all generations (122).

Materialism and productivity have been key American values. As population shifts occur and society becomes more technologically complex, causing earlier retirement for some workers, the definition of productivity must be changed from that which involves exchange of money. Toffler has coined the word **prosumers,** *people who produce goods and services for their families and friends but not for monetary gain.* Family roles are also likely to change, with an older family adopting or nurturing a younger family, giving assistance with child care or other tasks. The elderly will be needed as caregivers across family lines as home care becomes an important aspect of the health care system, and the caregiving role can give added meaning to life (122).

Federal Planning for the Aged in America

The United States is not alone in having to consider ways to provide care for the dependent elderly. Many countries throughout the world are experiencing a growing aging population. Some of the issues and approaches are similar across nations; some differences reflect basic national ethics and beliefs about how human services should be rendered. Kane and Kane (132) examine themes that transcend boundaries. We present issues related only to the United States.

Administration on Aging

In 1958 government interest in the older citizen inspired the formation of the President's Council on Aging, which later expanded and became the Administration on Aging (AOA). The AOA was established by the Older Americans Act of 1965 and operated as the central agency for assistance to the aged under the U.S. Department of Health and Human Services (DHHS).

The focus of AOA has been to identify the needs, concerns, and interests of older persons and to carry out the programs of the Older Americans Act. It was the principal agency for promoting coordination of the federal resources available to meet the needs of the elderly. Federal grants to state agencies on aging have been administered by AOA. The state agencies then acted as advocates and assisted in the establishment of comprehensive, coordinated service systems for older Americans at the community level. State agencies, in turn, designated and funded area agencies, county or municipal, which then served the aged within their own communities. The various social and nutritional services were planned and managed by these local area agencies. Direct grants to

Indian tribal organizations have been made by AOA for social and nutritional services to older American Indians. AOA has awarded grants for research, educational demonstrations, and manpower development projects. It has operated the National Information and Resource Clearinghouse for the Aged.

The Older Americans Act has promoted research to improve or expand social or nutritional services. It has also supported education of individuals working with aging. Multidisciplinary centers of gerontology established under AOA developed, employed, and disseminated models for teaching and training, conducted research, and operated experimental model service community laboratories in the areas of policy and program significance.

Under the amended Domestic Volunteer Service Act of 1973, special programs more geared to the development of a greater, more significant role in the society for older Americans were begun so that they could participate more fully in the life of their communities and the nation. One of them, the Foster Grandparents Program, had a dual purpose: (1) to provide part-time volunteer service opportunities for low-income persons age 60 and over and (2) to give supportive, person-to-person assistance in health, human services, and educational and related agencies to help alleviate the physical, mental, and emotional problems of children having exceptional needs. Through grants, AOA provided the recruitment and training of the volunteers. The participants worked 4 hours a day, 5 days a week and received a stipend equal to the federal minimum hourly wage. Everyone gained in this program: the elderly earned much-needed income along with a sense of dignity and achievement and the children blossomed in the warmth of personal attention (34).

The following are examples of projects developed under this program: work in a juvenile prison helping youth gain education, guidance, and companionship; work with severely burned children in whom the warmth and personal attention seemed to promote healing; assisting autistic children with basic tasks and encouraging performance through praise; providing care to infants while unwed mothers attend basic education classes; and helping teenagers prepare to move out of a mental health institution into a community setting such as a group home or foster home. In Babylon, New York, 10 mildly to moderately mentally retarded persons who were formerly institutionalized later served as foster grandparents themselves. Not only did they gain a feeling of self-worth, but the institutional cost to the public was eliminated.

Another program sponsored by AOA, the Retired Senior Volunteer Program (RSVP), afforded out-of-pocket expenses to persons over 60 who wished to participate in locally organized volunteer projects. The local service organization, the RSVP sponsor, developed a wide variety of service opportunities in the community in hospitals, courts, schools, day-care centers, libraries, and other volunteer setting. Grants were used primarily for travel expenses of the volunteers. The advantage in this program was that many older persons could participate as volunteers whose income might otherwise have limited their eligibility.

Knowing about the programs available to the elderly is helpful to nurses in several ways. In counseling, health teaching, and giving support, the nurse will find this knowledge useful as older clients demonstrate a need for guidance in seeking help. Often the answer to loneliness is participation in a program to help others. In addition, the nurse may have occasion through an employing health agency to apply for federal grant money either for supportive services or for research relevant to aging.

For more information about functions of state and local Area Agencies on Aging, see local AOA representatives.

Social Security

Under the Social Security Act were grouped Old Age Survivors Insurance, Medicare, and Supplemental Security Income for the Elderly.

Old Age Survivors Insurance provides a consistent monthly income to men 65 and older and to women 62 and older. Family payments are made to various dependents: wives 62 and older; dependent children; wives younger than 62 caring for dependent children; dependent husbands or widowers 62 or older; and dependent parents 62 or older after the death of the insured worker. Payments are made also to persons certified to be disabled (75).

The *Supplemental Security Income* program was begun as part of the Social Security Amendments of 1972. It guarantees that the annual income of an older or a disabled person will not fall below a minimum level. This redirected the responsibility for the aged, blind, and disabled poor from the states to the federal government. The program is administered by the Social Security Administration and had one standard for eligibility: low assets and specified low income.

Of public concern in our age is the ultimate viability of the Social Security system. Originally it was assumed that our expanding population and labor force would provide adequately for continued growth as an increasing wage base would provide greater taxes. On the contrary, zero population growth, decline of productivity, and inflation threaten the system. The problem is whether or not a diminishing work force of young and middle-aged persons will be willing to support the steadily growing numbers of retired persons. Population aging has created a concern that the projected number of elderly persons in the future will represent a crushing burden on the working population.

The general mandatory retirement age will continue to be raised in the future. Federal and some other sec-

tors have already increased mandatory retirement age to 70. According to the Social Security Amendments of 1983, the general retirement age will be gradually raised to 67 from 65 in two stages. A major argument for raising the retirement age is that life expectancy at age 65 has been increasing over the years and is expected to continue to rise in the future. It will be difficult to determine how much to raise the retirement age. Many would consider it unfair to expect that all the years of life expectancy gained should be spent working. At the same time, it is probably unreasonable to expect that all the additional years of life expectancy should be spent in leisure (34). Even if retirement ages are postponed, the number of dependent elderly will continue to increase, and it will do so quite substantially around the end of the first quarter of the twenty-first century.

Although increasing longevity is also a factor, population aging during the first quarter of the next century primarily will result from (1) high birthrates from mid-1940s to mid-1960s and (2) subsequent declining birthrates in the 1970s and beyond. As fewer children are born, the age structure of the population changes: the young segment becomes a smaller and the old larger. Decreased morbidity accompanies increased longevity; the elderly of the future could remain in or reenter the work force to compensate for the relatively smaller labor force in the traditional age groups. Then paying Social Security benefits could be postponed. Changes in the work environment, however, are the prerequisites for keeping older persons in the work force (42).

Understanding the problems that are developing in the Social Security system is important for all who care for the elderly. The elderly will need support when their fears arise, and they will benefit from the help of an informed nurse, one who has taken the time, through the use of the media and numerous government publications, to keep abreast of the changing scene regarding Social Security.

Medicare

The federally financed health insurance program in the United States is called Medicare. It provides benefits to persons over age 65 who paid into Social Security, and since 1972 it has extended care to the disabled and some chronically ill persons. There are two parts to Medicare: Part A, hospital insurance, and for those who choose to have a nominal monthly fee deducted from their Social Security checks, Part B, medical insurance.

Under Part A, most hospital costs and costs for a specified period in a skilled nursing facility or home are covered after an annual deductible is met by the insured. Part B of Medicare covers 80% of allowable costs for physicians' services and outpatient care. If the charges for services rendered exceed that which Medicare Part A or B deems reasonable and proper for the particular service, the enrollee must pay the difference, although prospective payment regulations are changing this. Insurance programs specific for supplement to Medicare payments are available.

January 1992 marked the start of a new nationwide fee schedule for physicians who see Medicare clients. They cannot charge more than 20% of what Medicare allowed to charge clients (39).

As with Social Security, the nurse must be conversant with current public announcements and other information to help and assure the elderly who may have great concern when they are ill about their security and care under this program. The Social Security representative available in all cities and most hospitals can help the nurse in planning for any problems arising in the areas of either Social Security or Medicare. Inform elders, if necessary, of the Medicare Catastrophic Insurance Act, which provides extra coverage.

Federal Role in Health Promotion

The major federal role in the area of health has been that of the Public Health Service, under the DHHS. All planning for health care has been filtered through the state, county, and city health departments. Under the U.S. Public Health Service are countless agencies with programs that include health services to veterans, control of food and drugs, construction of health facilities, medical services for retired civil service employees, rent supplements, and provision of public housing.

As part of the ongoing federal concern for the aged, the third decennial White House Conference on Aging was held in Washington, D.C., in November to December of 1981. Whereas the first conference in 1961 produced the concept of Medicare and the second in 1971 helped yield the Older Americans Act, this next conference was more general in its recommendations. The conference empowered older persons to speak their minds. There was a positive stand taken on residents' rights in nursing homes, the need for staff training, and the upgrading of nursing assistants. Although no definitive policy was forthcoming, the conference of 1981 reflected a concern by the elderly for continued improvement and expansion of services, both in long-term care facilities and in the community.

As a nurse, your influence can be felt in these areas through your work and community activities and in civic affairs by participation in your professional organization.

Community Planning

As people become older, infirm, and less mobile, a battery of community services is needed, not only to provide social activities and a reason to remain interested in life, but also to enable them to live independently. Most of the federal programs operate at the local level in actual practice, but, in addition, there is much that each community can do to provide needed services, which are available through the local Council on Aging. In small communities these services may be limited, but

further information is available through any county public health agency.

Community Services

Supportive services may include the following:

1. Referral services
2. Visiting and telephone-reassurance programs, sometimes offered through churches or private organizations
3. Services that provide shopping aides
4. Portable meals, sometimes known as "Meals on Wheels" for those who cannot shop for or prepare their own food
5. Transportation and handy-person services, including home upkeep
6. Day-care or foster home placement for the elderly (patterned after services for young children but modified for older adults)
7. Recreation facilities geared to the older person
8. Senior-citizen centers that provide recreation and a place for the lonely to belong
9. Respite services so that the family can get relief from caregiving while the elderly person receives needed care (The AARP offers numerous benefits socially and financially through insurance and other programs.)

All of these services can be used to promote health, prevent dysfunction, enhance a sense of independence, and aid family caregivers. Adult day-care services allow the person to remain at home and avoid institutionalization; the elder has daytime supervision and care, and the family member can continue employment (Fig. 14–5). Box 14–6 provides criteria to use in selecting adult (elder) day care. Home health care prevents lengthy hospitalization, assists families and the elder with the tasks of care, and permits respite for the family.

Another helpful community service for elders is the senior center. Senior centers are found in almost all communities and are based in a variety of settings. Some are operating in buildings built for this purpose, but most are housed in facilities originally planned for other purposes: church halls, community buildings, old schools, mobile-home park clubhouses, and the like. Their programs are federally funded to some extent but rely heavily on community support. A small staff is maintained, and most of the help with programs, maintenance, and materials comes from volunteers among the older persons who attend the center. Programs include activities such as crafts, social events from cards to dancing, exercise classes, and a full meal served at noon most weekdays. Other services may be daily telephone calls to homebound elderly, information and referral services, home-delivered meals, minor profit-making endeavors, and discount programs in cooperation with local merchants.

Several approaches are being tried in various com-

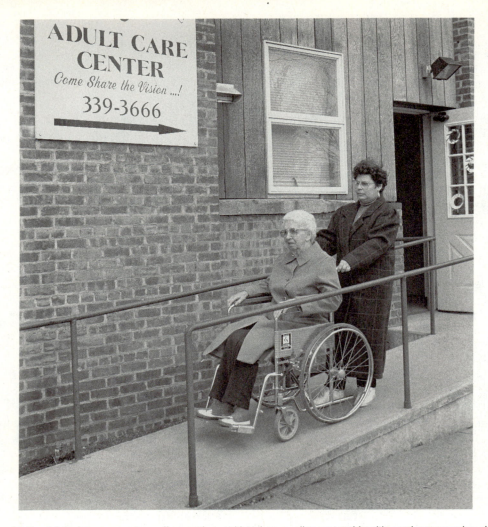

Figure 14-5.   Adult day-care centers offer meals, nutritional counseling, mental health services, exercise classes, physical therapy, and social activities to elders. (From Berger, K.J., and M.B. Williams, *Fundamentals of Nursing: Collaborating for Optimal Health.* Norwalk, Conn: Appleton and Lange, 1992, p. 1717.)

munities based on the principle that before helping maintain heath in the aged or contributing toward restoration of health, those working with community health must understand this age group. Toward this end, many persons enrolled in educational programs for the health professions are carrying out visiting programs with the elderly. Most nursing students are exposed to elderly persons through visits to geriatric centers or by interviewing experiences designed to sharpen communication skills and afford opportunities to gain insight into the needs of older persons.

Group work among the aged has been done with much success in a number of communities and in a variety of settings. Some of this work has been initiated in centers operated for the elderly and has been used not only to encourage the individual to participate in a group activity, but also to carry out health teaching. Many types of groups can be developed for the elderly; some are described in reference 187.

As a citizen of the community, you can be active in

initiating and supporting local programs such as those described above and in Table 14–7.

Extended Care Facility or Campus

The concept of long-term care for the elderly has broadened to be less custodial, more homelike, more holistic, and community focused. The names for the institutions vary: extended care facility or campus or senior health care center. The term *nursing home* is used less frequently. The facility must be approved for skilled nursing, although it may have both skilled and intermediate care levels for residents. Criteria are set by Medicare as to what constitutes a person who needs skilled versus intermediate care. Medicare pays for 100 days of care when a client has been discharged directly from the hospital; Medicare does not pay for intermediate care. The person who needs intermediate care either will pay individually, or if he or she has a minimum amount of financial income or savings, Medicaid will pay for these services (289).

■ **BOX 14-6.**
Criteria for Selecting Elder Day Care

- Is agency certified or licensed? (Forty-two states now regulate elder day care.) Who sponsors the agency?
- Is the agency designed in space, furniture, decor and color, equipment, and safety features for the elderly, including frail but ambulatory elderly and the cognitively impaired?
- What meals are served? Are special diets served? Ask the attendees about food.
- Are nurses and social workers employed? Physical therapists? Occupational therapists? Are attendants certified? Professionals should be available to the extent that the agency enrolls elders with physical or cognitive problems. Staff-client ratio should be no more than 1:8, with fewer clients if they are impaired.
- Is transportation provided? Some agencies have van service to pick up and deliver the senior home—within a certain mile radius and at certain hours—for a nominal fee.
- How do staff members handle medical or psychiatric emergencies? What is the policy if the elder becomes ill during the day?
- What is the schedule for the day? Are a variety of activities available? Are trips taken to the community? Are there activities of interest to and for participation by individuals and groups?
- What is the cost per day? Is financial aid available? Are there extra fees for activities? For clients with special physical or cognitive problems?
- How do staff members interact with clients and families?
- What are the appearance and interaction of the clients? Talk with them. Are they satisfied?

Certification of a nursing care facility is by a representative from the State Department of Aging who also represents standards set by the federal government. The main concern is the quality of care given. (The federal government may send out inspectors to check not only the nursing care facilities but also the state inspectors [289].)

Licensing of a care facility is done by each state. For example, in South Carolina the organization is the Health and Education Council. The main concern is adequacy of the building and equipment (289).

The extended care facility may serve as a transitional stop between hospital and home (generally for those over 65; in some cases, however, the stay is permanent.

The goals of the modern-day facility are to provide continuous supervision by a physician, 24-hour nursing services, hospital affiliation, written client care policies, and specialized services in dietary, restorative, pharmaceutical, diagnostic, and social services. Unfortunately, these are sometimes hollow goals, even though the

physical plant is new, licensing is current, and government funds are being used. Often the homes are operated for profit by those outside the nursing or medical profession. The residents are not always physically or mentally able to protest if care is poor, and often families of the residents do not monitor the care. National exposure of blatant neglect in some of the facilities has awakened public and government consciousness; perhaps this exposure will correct the most glaring problems and alert other facilities to their obligation to follow prescribed goals. If standards are met, the nursing home provides an excellent and needed service to society because the elderly must be discharged from expensive acute care hospital beds as soon as possible. Prolonged hospitalization can foster confusion, helplessness, and the hazards of immobility. Further, some elderly cannot care for self. There are ways to individualize care, give holistic care, and prevent neglect or abuse to residents in long-term care settings (20, 121, 135, 202, 203, 237).

Selecting a Care Facility. When you help the family or senior select a nursing home, the following questions should be asked:

1. What type of home is it, and what is its licensure status?
2. What are the total costs, and what is included for the money?
3. Is the physical plant adequate, clean, and pleasant? How much space and furniture are allowed for each person?
4. What safety features are evident? Are fire drills held?
5. What types of care are offered (both acute and chronic)?
6. What is the staff-resident ratio? What are the qualifications of the staff? What are staff attitudes toward the elderly?
7. What are the physician services? Is a complete physical examination given periodically?
8. What therapies are available?
9. Are pharmacy services available?
10. Are meals nutritionally sound and the food tasty? Is food refrigerated, prepared, distributed, and served under sanitary conditions? Is eating supervised or assisted?
11. Are visitors welcomed warmly?
12. Are residents aware of their Bill of Rights (see Box 14–7)?
13. Do residents appear content and appropriately occupied? (Observe on successive days and at different hours.) Are they treated with dignity and warmth by staff? Is privacy afforded during personal care?
14. Has the local Better Business Bureau received any complaints about this facility?
15. Does the administrator have a current state license?
16. Is the home certified to participate in government or

TABLE 14-7. COMMUNITY RESOURCES FOR OLDER PEOPLE

Resource	Service
Adult Congregate Living Facilities (ACLF)	Room, board, and personal services for elderly who would benefit from living in a group setting but do not require medical services; no nursing or medical services available.
Adult Day Care	Provision of comfortable, safe environment for functionally impaired adults, especially frail elderly, moderately handicapped, or slightly confused, who need care during the day, either because they live alone and cannot manage, or because family needs relief from the care to keep the elderly in the home
Adult Foster Care	Provision for continuous care to a functionally impaired older person in a private home with people who provide all services needed by the elderly individual
After Care	Posthospitalization rehabilitation such as cardiac or respiratory rehabilitation, occupational, or physical therapy
American Association of Retired Persons (AARP)	Nationwide organization for people over 50 that offers discount drug purchases, health and auto insurance, publications, and other activities
Area Agency on Aging	Federal agency that provides information, referral services, planning, and coordination, but not direct or health care services, on a regional or country-wide basis
Congregate Nutrition Sites	Free or low-cost meals, social activities, and nutrition or health education provided in local churches or senior centers
Congregate Living Facility	Apartment complex that provides meals and social programs for older people
Elderhostel	An on-campus educational experience, living on campus for duration of the course that includes opportunity for new knowledge, travel to various campuses and national and international geographic areas, new experiences, meeting new people
Foster Care	Placement of nonrelated elderly person in private residence for care
Foster Grandparents	Federal program paying people with low income who are over 60 a modest amount for working more than 20 hours a week with mentally or physically handicapped children
Friendly Visiting	Organized visiting services staffed by volunteers who visit homebound elderly once or twice weekly for companionship purposes if there are no relatives or friends available
Gray Panthers	Nationwide politically oriented organization that works to raise awareness about issues affecting older people and to advocate and lobby on these issues in local, state, and national government
Home Health Services	Agency providing intermittent nursing, social work, physical, occupational, and speech therapies, and other related services in the home via qualified health care professional or para-professionals to home-bound person
Homemaker/Chore Services	Agency providing help with light housekeeping, laundry, home chores, meal preparation, shopping for older people meeting income and other eligibility requirements
Hospice	Continuum of care systems for persons suffering from terminal disease and for their family, including home care, pain management, respite care, counseling, family support delivered in the home through outpatient and inpatient care—all within the same licensed program (It is medically directed, nurse coordinated, autonomously administered, and provides care for the physical, emotional, spiritual and social needs of client and family, using an interdisciplinary team approach.)
Long-Term Care Ombudsman Committees	Citizen committees appointed by the Governor who volunteer their time to investigate and resolve grievances or problems of people in nursing homes and ACLFs
Meals on Wheels	Provision of hot or cold nutritious meals to a homebound elderly person, brought by another person or agency
Medicaid	Governmental coverage of health care and nursing home costs for older people with limited incomes who are eligible (People who receive Supplemental Security Income or Aid to Families of Dependent Children are automatically eligible.)
Medicare	National health insurance program for people age 65 and older or disabled, or in some special cases under 65, that is administered by the Social Security Administration (Part A is hospital insurance; Part B covers diagnostic tests, physician fees, outpatient and ambulance costs. Dental, vision, hearing, and preventive services are excluded.)
Protective Services	Constellation of social services that assist older, noninstitutionalized people who manifest at least some incapacity to manage their money or their daily living or assist those who need protection of life or property
Respite Care	Agency providing relief for specified hours, a weekend, or a week, for family caregivers, allowing time for the caregiver to shop, have the time for other reasons, or vacation while care is given to functionally impaired person residing in the home setting
Senior Center	Program providing a combination of services; designed to be open 3 or more days a week, with meal, recreational, educational, and counseling services available (Sometimes medical services are provided.)
Senior Corp of Retired Executives	Agency of retired executives who volunteer their counseling services to small businesses and companies on request
Supplemental Security Income (SSI)	Minimum monthly income to blind, disabled, and aged persons whose income falls below a specified level (Personal effects, household goods, and home ownership are not counted as assets, although savings, stocks, jewelry, or car would be.)
Telephone Reassurance	Daily telephone calls to people who live alone, including the aged and disabled, or telephone crisis and information services provided by an agency

BOX 14-7.
Bill of Rights for Residents of Extended Care Facilities

- To choose your own doctor and help plan your course of treatment
- To be free of physical or mental abuse and from any restraints not medically required
- To use pharmacologic drugs by prescription and only for the symptoms for which they are prescribed
- To have privacy
- To be assured of confidentiality of records
- To have services tailored to individual needs and to be given notice before room or roommate is changed
- To voice grievances
- To organize and participate in resident groups
- To participate in social, religious, and community activities
- To examine the most recent survey of the facility and plans to correct deficiencies
- To obtain any other rights established by the Secretary of the Department of Health and Human Services

other programs that provide financial assistance when needed?

17. Is an ombudsman available to investigate complaints of residents or family?

Translocation. The elderly person who is moved to a nursing home or long-term care facility (often rest-of-the-lifetime care facility) or who is moved from one room to another within the same facility undergoes a crisis called **translocation syndrome,** *physical and emotional deterioration as a result of changes or movement.* A move may be made because of changes in health, in staffing, or in the residents or because families desire it. Such a move may be life threatening, however.

People at greater risk are those who are depressed, highly anxious, severely ill, intermittently confused, or over 85 years of age. People who need structure, who cannot stand changes, or who deny problems or feelings are also more likely to experience difficulty.

Reducing relocation's impact begins with enlisting the resident's understanding of the need for the move and participation. The person should be prepared for the move. When he or she can make decisions about the move and predict what will happen, the person maintains a sense of control, which diminishes the move's impact. Moving to a similar environment also reduces the problems. The ability to express fears, concerns, and anger help. If the person to be moved to an institution is relatively young, had good morale, and had an opportunity to select and then felt satisfied with the new surroundings, the translocation syndrome may be minimum (178).

One way to reduce the crisis of admission to a nurs-

ing home or long-term care center or to reduce translocation shock is to have preschool or school children visit in the home. Both generations benefit from the exchange of affection. The youngsters bring stimulation to the elderly generation, the older generation can demonstrate stability, wisdom, and coping with adversities, and the qualities of ego-integrity.

Elderly persons living alone or only with a spouse were, in one study, more likely than those who lived with a child, relative, or friend to prefer moving to an alternate setting such as a nursing home or senior housing when they were unable to care for self (16).

Taking one's frail loved one to a nursing home is not easy at that point in life when he or she can no longer care for self and home, at that point when the person has lost about everything that was precious and gave life meaning. Many family members have given poignant accounts of the pain for the elder and for the family and how the elder works to retain personal integrity and dignity in spite of the emotional assault.

Other Living Arrangements

For those elderly who want to live at home but need some degree of care, there are alternatives. A Florida agency is helping more than 10,000 persons stay out of institutions by delivering meals to them at home or shuttling them to community dining centers. Through the program the elderly can hire helpers to wash windows or rake lawns and homemakers to shop or do light housekeeping. Transportation is provided to doctors' offices. Fees are based on ability to pay. The state of Florida estimates it saved 9.5 million dollars in the past year by assisting these persons to live at home.

Senior day-care centers provide another alternative. The charges are reasonable per day, and they cater to persons not as able as those who may avail themselves of the usual senior center (see Box 14–6).

Some communities have set up centers to match roommates. Two persons may function better than alone, and the costs are shared. A Boston group has sponsored a project that arranges intergenerational living: 14 people ages 30 to 80 share a nineteenth-century townhouse. Everyone takes part in the chores and pays a nominal rent for their own room. Extended families have been created in some cities. A retired hospital administrator with arthritis now shares her four-bedroom home with a young couple and their newborn daughter, and each generation learns from the other.

Remotivation

Many health care providers are doing group work in extended care facilities to combat the effects of institutionalization in the elderly.

Remotivation is *one form of group therapy that can be conducted in a hospital, nursing home, or senior center for disengaged or regressed elderly.* The training materials for instructing employees in remotivation techniques are available from the American Psychiatric Association's central office in Washington, D.C. Although it originated in the psychiatric setting, the technique is now used nationwide in a variety of settings—old-age facilities, general and chronic-disease hospitals, and schools for the retarded. The content used is easily adaptable for the type of people in each group.

The goal of this therapy is to remotivate the unwounded areas in the personality of the older adult. The techniques can be used by the average employee—nurse or ancillary—who is closest to the client or resident for most of the day. It is designed to stimulate self-respect, self-reliance, and self-value in the older person who has become disengaged (94, 187, 261).

Remotivation encourages the person to focus attention on the simple, objective aspects of everyday life. As the client is helped toward resocialization, the nurse-client relationship is also strengthened. Staff members display a greater interest in the client as an individual than they did before the use of this technique; they begin to recognize the therapeutic value of their presence in meeting the needs of clients.

The method consists of a series of meetings, usually around 12, led by a person who has received instruction in the technique. No more than 15 clients comprise the group, and the sessions last approximately an hour each. The leader guides the group in a discussion through five specific steps (94, 212):

1. *Creating a climate of acceptance* (5 minutes) through greeting each person by name, expressing pleasure at his or her presence, and making remarks that encourage replies such as comments on the weather, a familiar incident, or the person's apparel.
2. *Creating a bridge to the world* (15 minutes) by relating a current event or referring to a topic of general interest and then encouraging each one to comment. The central topic—a recipe, a familiar quotation, a newspaper item—differs according to the backgrounds of the group members.
3. *Sharing the world we live in* (15 minutes) by expanding step 2 and developing the subject further through the use of appropriate visual aids.
4. *Appreciating the work of the world* (15 minutes) through discussion of jobs, how a certain commodity is produced, how a job many be done quickly and efficiently, or the type of work the clients have done in the past.
5. *Creating a climate of appreciation* (5 minutes), expressing pleasure in their attendance and their contributions. Plans are made for the next meeting, providing continuity and something to look forward to.

You may use this technique as an adjunct to other nursing interventions, for the principles of remotivation technique can be modified for work with other client groups, to establish initial rapport, or to establish a nurse-client relationship. Remotivation increases communication and strengthens contact with everyday features of the world for the person who may be advanced in years and perhaps is physically debilitated but still has many areas of intact personality.

Group Action Among Older Citizens

Interest in civic, social, political, and economic issues is shown in various action groups that have been organized among older citizens through community projects. The Gray Panthers is a well-known organization, as is AARP, but there are other groups as well.

Older persons can help isolated elderly persons in their community. A survey of community services can determine which services are most and least used, which are inadequate, what changes are needed, and what sort of problems the elderly in the area have to face. In one community a one-to-one visiting service was needed; it brought joy and met needs of the isolated elderly. It also provided the elderly visitors with a sense of independence, social acceptability, recognition, status, and a sense of meaning in their lives at a time when losses of one sort or another had left them vulnerable.

Action groups have been formed in many of our major cities in recent years. Their members are elderly persons who are concerned about the needs of their peers and who believe that group action is effective in bringing about legislative change, especially in the area of financial assistance to meet rising costs. Many of these groups have sent representatives to the White House Conference on Aging and have exerted a considerable influence on federal and local planning. Such issues as tax relief, transportation, medical care, and nutrition are of vital interest to many concerned elderly citizens who still feel responsible for themselves and their community.

You may have the opportunity to work with action groups in either an advisory, consultative, or direct participation role.

Retirement Communities

Along with our increased life span and the development of social planning for retirement has come the emergence of a distinct social phenomenon: the retirement apartment complex community.

Apartment complexes are financed privately, by religious organizations, or by the government. The senior must be able to maintain self, although visiting nurse services are acceptable. These complexes may include a central dining room, a nurse and doctor on call, planned social events, transportation services, and religious services. Essentially all living needs are within easy access. Additionally, the seniors have the company of each other if they so desire.

In many cities hotels have been converted to residence facilities for the elderly. Reminiscent of old-style rooming houses, they provide more supervision and services such as meals, laundry facilities and shopping. In most of these residences each person is responsible for his or her own room, laundry, and breakfast.

Many couples opt for continuous care facilities. An example of this style of living is the type of community that has been built by the Life Care Services Corporation. Since 1961 this nonprofit organization has built 30 retirement communities in 17 states. One- or two-bedroom apartments or cottages are available for a one-time endowment and a monthly fee for two persons. Services include one meal a day, maid service, all utilities, including local telephone bill, full maintenance, a full recreational and social program, and many extras. The residents have at their disposal a fully equipped health center with 24-hour nursing care service as long as needed in the intermediate or long-term care sections of the nursing home facility.

In many regions of the United States, especially in Florida, the desert Southwest, and California, planned communities have been built that are specifically designed for and restricted to those persons over 55. Some are carefully planned miniature cities of low cost with simply designed homes built around clubhouse activities, golf courses, and swimming and therapy pools. Activities such as bingo games, dance instruction, foreign-language study, crafts, or bridge lessons are offered. Other communities are mobile-home parks in which often-elaborate coaches cost as much as and are set up as permanent homes.

One sociologic aspect of these communities bearing such names as "Sun City," "Leisure World," and "Carefree Village" is the life-style adopted by the residents as they try to establish a secure base in a new life that is often far removed from family, former friends, and familiar patterns of living. They show concern for the safety, health, and well-being of each other by watching to see that lights are on at accustomed hours in each other's homes, signifying all is well. Celebration of birthdays with special parties and remembrances, entertaining for visiting friends and relatives of one's neighbors, visiting the sick members, and providing food and transportation to the hospital for the spouse of a sick resident all become part of the new life. The residents participate in activities that are either completely new or have not been indulged in for many years such as golf, bicycle riding, hiking, and dancing. Even clothes become gayer for both sexes, and the popularity of casual dress provides for the members of the snowbird set—those who have moved to a warm climate—a new freedom and a chance to try bright colors and styles they may not have worn in a former setting.

This phenomenon gives you insight into the needs for security, a sense of maximum personal effectiveness and belonging, and a feeling of self-actualization felt by older persons, especially when old patterns are put aside either by choice or because of circumstances mediated by health or socioeconomic conditions. Further, the older adult needs a suitable place to live, supportive

relationships, a sense of community, financial security, and a sense of setting and achieving goals.

See Box 14–8 for guidelines on selecting a retirement community.

Impact of the Able Elderly

The emergence of a population group identified as the well elderly is the result of social and demographic progress in the industrial world. More people are living longer, and poverty, frailty, and dependence are not the common characteristics of most of these older people. In the future there will be more healthy elderly who are better educated and physically and emotionally capable. Our society can already use the elderly population's capabilities; in the future we shall have a rich human resource in larger numbers.

The elderly often give financial support and other kinds of assistance to their younger family members; most old people are not a drain on the family. An aging society offers expanding opportunities for family life. Four types of new potentials are present because of recent demographic change: (1) increased complexity of social networks, (2) increased duration of relationships, (3) prolonged opportunities to accumulate experience,

---

■ **BOX 14-8.**
Guidelines for Selecting a Retirement Community

- Check climate and cultural and recreational facilities in relation to your preferences and life-style.
- Visit the facility; talk with residents; eat a meal. Is it an active, lively community?
- Call state regulators, Chamber of Commerce, and Better Business Bureau to check track record of the developer or owner(s).
- Ask what insurance or bonding instruments will protect you in case the facility experiences financial difficulty. Get copies.
- Review all documents you are asked to sign and seek competent legal advice before signing.
- Ask about lease termination policies. How much notice must the owner give? What are the refund policies?
- Get terms of the deposit in writing. If it is refundable, how and at what percentage? Will interest be applied; if so, at what rate?
- Determine if monthly fees are tied to an index. If so, which one? Ask for a history of increases to date, and check the index at a library.
- If it is a lifetime or continuing care community, are nursing home costs prepaid? If not, what are the additional costs?
- Ask about restrictions and policies about visitors (overnight, for how long), parking a recreational vehicle, parking more than one car in the driveway, use of facilities by visitors.
- Take your time to decide. Visit different facilities.

and (4) new chances to complete or change role assignments.

The elder's accumulated shared experience builds family bonds but also helps others deal with a changing historical context. As the elderly leaves certain roles behind, he or she can pick up new ones—whether it is as a grandparent; in a second career; activity in the political, social, or community arena; as a decision maker; as an advocate for ethical and moral actions; or participating in policy making or creative pursuits in the arts. Hagestad (101) and Hudson (119) describe the contributions that well elderly are and will be making to society and the importance of perceiving the well older person as a contributing resource.

Outlook for the Future

The current generation of older persons is where we shall all be one day; therefore planning for them is planning for all of us. Areas such as health care delivery, distribution of income over a long life span, sustaining adequate social involvement, coping with organizational systems, and use of leisure are all problems of now and the future. Intervention that seems costly now may be, in the long run, the most economical in terms of tax dollars.

In the face of increasing shortages that raise the cost of living and the change in age and sex distribution by that time, future planning for the elderly will include employment and the attendant problems usually associated with younger persons. Our society will need the experience and wisdom of the senior generation. If persons are employed as late as age 75, health maintenance programs, industrial planning, and awareness of safety needs are just a few of the necessary considerations.

For the older less active persons of the future, Burnside (34) suggests intervening in loneliness through listening, exploring what may be significant to the seniors, and helping them to compensate in some way for personal losses. In addition, she suggests that nurses record the experiences of the elderly for posterity. Day schools for the elderly might encourage research projects, family therapy, and the study of successful aging.

Thus you, the nurse of the future, will be challenged to be the innovator. You will be called on to devise and use new treatment methods so that the elderly will function more effectively in society. It is your goal to help them (1) use the potential they have developed throughout life, (2) pass through the years of late maturity with ego intact and satisfying memories, and (3) leave something of their philosophy for posterity.

Nursing Applications

Assessment and Nursing Diagnoses

Your role in caring for the elderly person or couple has been described throughout the chapter. Assessment, using knowledge presented about normal aging changing versus pathology in the elderly, provides the basis for *nursing diagnoses*. Nursing diagnoses that may be applicable are listed in Box 14–9.

Interventions

Interventions may involve direct care, the use of verbal and nonverbal skills, availability of self and therapeutic relationship, support, counseling, education, spiritual care, use of remotivation techniques, or referral as you assist the person in later maturity to meet physical, emotional, cognitive, spiritual, or social needs.

You represent a whole cluster of psychologic potentials for the elderly person; you become the supportive figure, interpreter of the unknown, symbol of the people close to him or her, and possessor of important secrets or privileged information. You become guide and companion. All this occurs if an empathic regard for the elderly person is reflected in your attitude and actions, even though your initial image of him or her may have been that of punitive parent. Of prime importance is your willingness to listen, explain, orient, reassure, and comfort the elderly person. Your role is crucial, for you are the one who is most likely to maintain personal contact with the client either in an institutional setting or in a community agency.

Involve the person's family if possible. The interest of a family member does much to increase motivation on the part of the elderly. Determine family attitudes and evaluate relationships during teaching-learning or visiting sessions at which the family is present. This procedure helps the family members alter their attitudes to a more realistic acceptance of their relative's health needs. Social support of family and friends is critical for maintaining life-style behaviors, emotional and physical health, and coping skills, including for the frail elderly (20, 89, 204, 221, 232, 256).

The cognitive and emotional needs of the elderly person can be met in many ways. Adequate environmental conditions to overcome sensory impairment and clearly defined communication, including explanations of procedures and the necessity for them, are vital. Demonstration and written instructions along with the verbal message, divided into small units, are very effective for teaching skills related to self-care and should be combined with practice sessions. The older person seems to learn more easily when stimuli are logically grouped and sequential, when a larger amount of data is given rather than isolated bits, and when the essential information is relevant to needs, interests, and life experience. He or she is likely to recall this information when necessary. When planning for a new task is overlapped with the execution of a previous one, the older person works slowly and with care. The real situation should be simulated as much as possible so that essential steps of the task can be clearly perceived and the teaching can be adapted to the individual's pattern and ability. Allow the

---

■ **BOX 14-9.**
Selected Nursing Diagnoses Related to Person in Later Maturity[a]

Pattern 1: Exchanging

Altered Nutrition: More Than Body Requirements
Altered Nutrition: Less Than Body Requirements
Hypothermia
Hyperthermia
Stress Incontinence
Potential for Injury
Potential for Trauma
Potential for Disuse Syndrome
Potential Impaired Skin Integrity

Pattern 2: Communicating

Impaired Verbal Communication

Pattern 3: Relating

Impaired Social Interaction
Social Isolation
Altered Role Performance
Sexual Dysfunction
Altered Family Processes
Altered Sexuality Patterns

Pattern 4: Valuing

Spiritual Distress

Pattern 5: Choosing

Ineffective Individual Coping
Impaired Adjustment
Defensive Coping
Ineffective Denial
Ineffective Family Coping: Disabling
Ineffective Family Coping: Compromised
Family Coping: Potential for Growth
Decisional Conflict
Health Seeking Behaviors

Pattern 6: Moving

Impaired Physical Mobility
Fatigue
Potential Activity Intolerance
Sleep Pattern Disturbance
Diversional Activity Deficit
Impaired Home Maintenance Management
Altered Health Maintenance
Bathing/Hygiene Self-care Deficit
Dressing/Grooming Self-care Deficit

Pattern 7: Perceiving

Body Image Disturbance
Self-Esteem Disturbance
Chronic Low Self-esteem
Situational Low Self-esteem
Sensory/Perceptual Alterations
Unilateral Neglect
Hopelessness
Powerlessness

Pattern 8: Knowing

Knowledge Deficit
Altered Thought Processes

Pattern 9: Feeling

Pain
Chronic Pain
Dysfunctional Grieving
Anticipatory Grieving
Post-trauma Response
Anxiety
Fear

[a]Other of the NANDA diagnoses related to physiologic phenomena are applicable to the ill individual in this group.
From North American Nursing Diagnosis Association, *NANDA Nursing Diagnosis Taxonomy I* (Rev.). St. Louis: North American Nursing Diagnosis Association, 1990.

---

person ample time to respond to a task. Your understanding attitude is important if you are to prevent discouragement and depression.

As in all communication, false assurance can only inhibit the person's ability to develop a trusting attitude and suggest paternalism. The display of genuine interest and a receptive attitude will show the older person that he or she is not alone and will help immeasurably in allaying fear. Candor helps decrease anxiety, and the person's fear of death, the dark, or the unknown may be overcome to a great degree through your presence.

Encourage the senior to reminisce; it is an effective intervention for many reasons. Reminiscence helps the older person, through discussion or use of photographs, music, or literature, to do the following (34, 75, 92, 175, 214, 228, 271):

1. Maintain a sense of identity and self-worth
2. Stay oriented
3. Remain aware of his or her environment
4. Relive memorable times
5. Acknowledge and explore changes in life
6. Find meaning in relationships and life-cycle events
7. Facilitate grieving for losses
8. Think in a logical fashion
9. Socialize with others

10. Work through previously unresolved conflicts
11. Manage current stresses with validation of the past
12. Reaffirm the worth of life
13. Gain a new perspective on life and personal accomplishments
14. Refine a sense of ego integrity

Ask questions about his or her early years, work experience, family, special events, travel, and hobbies. Listen as the person shares life philosophy and gives counsel. Look at family photographs and treasured objects with him or her. You may wish to establish a group of seniors whose main goal is to reminisce (34, 137).

Loneliness is an outgrowth of age-related losses and psychologic changes in the elderly (272). It implies a need to assess carefully situations to determine the signs as described in the following case study:

> An elderly man living alone made no complaint of loneliness, but the astute community health nurse found his home in deplorable untidiness and unsafe clutter, his diet extremely limited, and his personal hygiene poor. After a homemaker was sent in to help him clean the house, sit with him during meals, and provide a chance for a trusting relationship with another person, he became receptive to suggestions for modifying his living habits and eventually began to visit a senior-citizen group regularly and to make new friends. He came to realize that adaptation to isolation had been unsafe. Interest and patience showed by others restored the feeling of being a valued and accepted human being again.

The authors know of other individuals who would not modify living habits but chose to remain (from a health care viewpoint) in unsafe and unsanitary conditions. Yet instead of giving the person up as a "hopeless case," the nurses continued to foster a relationship of trust, listened to reasons for remaining in the present situation, and helped the person live out the remaining life on his or her own terms.

Helping the elderly person to remain in contact with the environment may be as simple as providing devices such as clocks, watches, and calendars and letting him or her be the one who winds the clock and turns the calendar page each day. If a hearing aid is worn, check its effectiveness. Sudden moves, even within the same institution, increase mortality rates and psychologic and physical deterioration. The person should be permitted to remain in familiar territory and with the desired clutter. If a move is essential, he or she should have some choice in the decision, an opportunity to keep valued possessions, and time to adjust to the idea. The person needs to have a personal lounging chair or specific place in the dining room. Room furniture should be arranged for physical safety and emotional security. Privacy must be respected.

Darkness is a cause of confusion. Night lights should be left on and call bell, tissues, and water placed within easy reach. In the hospital room contact should be available to the client through frequent, quietly made rounds at night. Sometimes a client remains oriented more easily if the room door is open so that he or she can see the nurses' station and be reassured of not being alone.

The use of touch is very beneficial, for the older person has little physical contact with others. The need for contact comfort is great in the human organism, and you can satisfy this need to a degree, provided you remember that touch is a language and has a special power. In giving medications, physical care, and in doing treatments, touching is a crucial encounter. Often the person will pay close attention to instructions and cooperate more in his or her care when you use touch on the hand or shoulder while speaking. The success of this aid depends on what your hands are saying.

To the elderly, all things connected with food service have psychologic implications. Food represents life—it nurtures. Mealtime is thought of as a time of fellowship with others and a sharing of pleasure, and this attitude should be retained as much as possible for older people. Making the food more attractive, talking with the person, comforting and touching, cajoling if need be, may help, especially if food is being refused. Appetizers and special drinks have been successfully used as an aid to therapy.

The overall loss of physical capacity, decreased resilience, and lowered capacity to resist stress cause most elderly people to view any illness as a potential major crisis in life. Although it may not be obvious, fear is ever present, and death seems to wait in the wings. Unfamiliar surroundings cause apprehension, and either temporary or permanent loss of contact with those who could give support—spouse, friends, relatives—may cause anxiety. Such anxiety can reduce recuperative powers and is sometimes more distressing than the illness itself.

During any crisis in which the organism is under stress, there are several alternatives: exhaustion, recuperation through the help of others, or despondency and dependency. Through the second alternative you may work toward resolution of the crisis. Share the following suggestions with the person:

1. Acknowledge the sadness, anger, guilt, and other feelings that are a part of the loss. It is not a sign of weakness to have those feelings.
2. Allow self to express the feelings; cry alone or talk and cry with someone who is understanding. If you have always been stoic, it is all right to show feelings. Others may feel more comfortable with you.
3. Indulge self constructively. Feelings of fatigue, confusion, and even depression occur with grief. Pay attention to basic needs of nutrition, sleep, and exercise. Do something pleasurable for yourself. Resist artificial consolers such as alcohol, sleeping pills, other drugs, and cigarettes.
4. Ask for support and accept it. Determine wishes,

needs, and wants. It is all right to ask for help. You have done your share of nurturing; now is your time to allow others to help you.

5. Say "No" to major stressors. Take your time in making major decisions. Do not undertake too many life-changing events at once.

6. Move beyond regret—the "if only" or "I should have." Do what is needed in the situation. Learn from mistakes. Forgive self and others.

7. Affirm your power to heal the wounds. Life will not be the same after a loss. However, life can go on. Talk to others. Call forth inner reserves and spiritual strength. Imagine the person is present. State aloud or in a letter or tape to the person that which was left unsaid.

8. Focus memory on the valued or favorite times, the happy scenes, and the pleasant instead of the disease, death, or the traumatic.

The fine line between independence and dependence is difficult to maintain with clients of any age, but especially in the elderly because of society's view of them. Expectations of those around us generally foster behavior to match. Conflict between independent and dependent feelings can be avoided, usually first by assuming a firm control based on professional competence and then later by relaxing and allowing the client to emancipate self.

Working with the elderly person may be very rewarding if you are able to suspend youth-directed attitudes and not measure the person against standards that are inappropriate and perhaps too demanding. As with other age groups and in all our relationships, acceptance of the other person as he or she is, not as you wish him or her to be, is extremely important.

REFERENCES

1. Achenbaum, W., and J. Levin, What Does Gerontology Mean? *Gerontologist,* 29, no. 3 (1989), 393–399.

2. Adamchak, D., et al., Elderly Support and Intergenerational Transfer in Zimbabwe: An Analysis by Gender, Marital Status, and Place of Residence, *Gerontologist,* 31, no. 4 (1991), 505–513.

3. Allen, K., and V. Chin-Sang, A Lifetime of Work: The Context and Meanings of Leisure for Aging Black Women, *Gerontologist,* 30, no. 6 (1990), 734–740.

4. Allen, P., and A. Coyne, Are There Age Differences in Chunking? *Journal of Gerontology: Psychological Sciences,* 44, no. 6 (1989), P181–P183.

5. Andresen, G., A Fresh Look at Assessing the Elderly, *RN Magazine,* 52, no. 6 (1989), 28–40.

6. Atchley, C., *The Social Forces in Later Life* (3rd ed.). Belmont, Calif: Wadsworth Publishing, 1980.

7. Balin, A., and A. Kligman, eds., *Aging and the Skin*. New York: Raven Press, 1988.

8. Baltes, M., H. Wahl, and U. Furstoss, The Daily Life of Elderly Germans: Activity Patterns, Personal Control,

and Functional Health, *Journal of Gerontology: Psychological Sciences,* 45, no. 4 (1990), P173–P179.

9. Batz, J., The Growing Old, *Universitas,* 15, no. 4 (1990), 5–10.

10. Barusch, A., and W. Spaid, Gender Differences in Caregiving: Why Do Wives Report Greater Burden? *Gerontologist,* 29, no. 5 (1989), 667–676.

11. Bass, D., and K. Bowman, The Transition From Caregiving to Bereavement: The Relationship of Care-Related Strain and Adjustment to Death, *Gerontologist,* 3, no. 1 (1990), 35–42.

12. Basteda, E., Sex-Typed Age Norms Among Older Hispanics, *Gerontologist,* 27, no. 1 (1987), 59–65.

13. Bates, B., *A Guide to Physical Examination and History Taking* (4th ed.). Philadelphia: J.B. Lippincott, 1987.

14. Bearon, L., No Great Expectations: The Underpinnings of Life Satisfaction for Older Women, *Gerontologist,* 29, no. 6 (1989), 772–778.

15. Beers, M., et al., Screening Recommendations for the Elderly, *American Journal of Public Health,* 81, no. 9 (September 1991), 1131–1139.

16. Beland, F., Living Arrangement Preferences Among Elderly People, *Gerontologist,* 27, no. 6 (1987), 797–803.

17. Berliner, H., Aging Skin, *American Journal of Nursing,* 86, no. 10 (1986), 1138–1141.

18. ———, Aging Skin: Part Two, *American Journal of Nursing,* 86, no. 11 (1986), 1259–1262.

19. Berry, D., Geriatric Sleep Apnea Syndrome: A Preliminary Description, *Journal of Gerontology: Medical Sciences,* 45, no. 5 (1990), M169–M174.

20. Bitzan, J., and J. Kruzich, Interpersonal Relationships of Nursing Home Residents, *Gerontologist,* 30, no. 3 (1990), 385–390.

21. Blank, T., Social Psychology, Contexts of Aging and a Contextual World View, *International Journal of Aging and Human Development,* 29, no. 3 (1989), 225–239.

22. Blumenthal, J., et al., Long-Term Effects of Exercise on Psychological Functioning in Older Men and Women, *Journal of Gerontology: Psychological Sciences,* 46, no. 6 (1991), P352–P361.

23. Bodde, E., Raising Your Children's Children, *New Choices* (March 1991), 18–21.

24. Bosse, R., et al., How Stressful is Retirement? Findings From the Normative Aging Study, *Journal of Gerontology: Psychological Sciences,* 46, no. 1 (1991), P9–P14.

25. Bowling, A., and P. Browne, Social Networks, Health and Emotional Well-Being Among the Oldest-Old in London, *Journal of Gerontology: Social Sciences,* 46, no. 1 (1991), S20–S32.

26. Bozian, M., and H. Clark, Counteracting Sensory Changes in the Aging, *American Journal of Nursing,* 80, no. 3 (1980), 473–476.

27. Braithwaite, V., Old Age Stereotypes: Reconciling Contradictions, *Journal of Gerontology,* 41, no. 3 (1986), 353–360.

28. Brody, E., et al., Caregiving Daughters and Their Local Siblings: Perceptions, Strains, and Interactions, *Gerontologist,* 29, no. 4 (1989), 529–538.

29. Brookbank, J., *The Biology of Aging*. New York: Harper & Row, 1990.

30. Brown, M., *Readings in Gerontology*. St. Louis: C.V. Mosby, 1978.

31. Bryant, S., Neighbors Support of Older Widows Who Live Alone in Their Own Homes, *Gerontologist,* 25, no. 3 (1985), 305.

32. Buhler, C., The Developmental Structure of Goal Setting in Group and Individual Studies, In Buhler, C., and F. Massarik, eds., *The Course of Human Life*. New York: Spring, 1968.

33. Burggraf, V., and B. Donlon, Assessing the Elderly, *American Journal of Nursing,* 85, no. 9 (1985), 974–984.

34. Burnside, Irene, ed., *Nursing and the Aged,* (3rd ed.). New York: McGraw-Hill, 1988.

35. Burris, K., Recommending Adult Day Care Centers, *Nursing and Health Care,* 1, no. 3 (1981), 437–441.

36. Callahan, J., Elder Abuse: Some Questions for Policymakers, *Gerontologist,* 28, no. 5 (1988), 453–458.

37. Campbell, R., and E. Brody, Women's Changing Roles and Help to the Elderly, *Gerontologist,* 25, no. 6 (1985), 584–592.

38. Carmack, B., and D. Fila, Animal-Assisted Therapy: A Nursing Intervention, *Nursing Management,* 20, no. 5 (1989), 96, 97, 100–104.

39. Carson, E., Enrollees Gain Under Fee Shift, *AARP Bulletin,* 33, no. 1 (1992), 6.

40. Chapman, N., and M. Neal, The Effects of Intergenerational Experiences on Adolescents and Older Adults, *Gerontologist,* 30, no. 6 (1990), 825–832.

41. Chappell, N., and M. Badger, Social Isolation and Well-Being, *Journal of Gerontology: Social Sciences,* 44, no. 5 (1989), S169–S176.

42. Chen, Y.P., Making Assets Out of Tomorrow's Elderly, *Gerontologist,* 27, no. 4 (1987), 410–416.

43. Chiriboga, D., Adaptation of Marital Separation in Later and Earlier Life, *Journal of Gerontology,* 37, no. 1 (1982), 109–114.

44. Choi, N., Racial Differences in the Determinants of Living Arrangements of Widowed and Divorced Elderly Women, *Gerontologist,* 31, no. 4 (1991), 496–504.

45. Clark, M., and B. Anderson, *Culture and Aging*. Springfield, Ill: Charles C Thomas, 1967.

46. Clipp, E., and L. George, Caregiver Needs and Patterns of Social Support, *Journal of Gerontology: Social Sciences,* 45, no. 3 (1990), S102–S111.

47. Cohen, E., and A. Kruschwitz, Old Age in America Represented in Nineteenth and Twentieth Century Popular Sheet Music, *Gerontologist,* 30, no. 3 (1990), 345–354.

48. Colarusso, C., and R. Nemeroff, *Adult Development*. New York: Plenum Press, 1981.

49. Collinsworth, R., and K. Boyle, Nutritional Assessment of the Elderly, *Journal of Gerontological Nursing,* 15, no. 12 (1989), 17–21.

50. Connidis, I., and L. Davies, Confidants and Companions in Later Life: The Place of Family and Friends, *Journal of Gerontology: Social Sciences,* 45, no. 4 (1990), S141–S149.

51. Conway, J., The Aging Kidney, *Journal of Urological Nursing,* 8, no. 3 (1989), 704–707.

52. Cooney, T., Co-Residence With Adult Children: A Comparison of Divorced and Widowed Women, *Gerontologist,* 29, no. 6 (1989), 779–784.

53. Cooper, R., Concentration Camp Survivors: A Challenge for Geriatric Nursing, *Nursing Clinics of North America,* 14, no. 4 (1979), 621–627.

54. Cornelius, S., Classic Pattern of Intellectual Aging: Test Familiarity, Difficulty, and Performance, *Journal of Gerontology,* 39, no. 2 (1984), 201–206.

55. Cowling, W., and V. Campbell, Health Concerns of Aging Men, *Nursing Clinics of North America,* 21, no. 1 (1986), 77–84.

56. Crabtree, D., and L. Antrim, Promoting A Healthy Aging Brain: Changing the Influence of Maturational and Behavioral Factors on the Functional Integrity of the Aging Brain, *Health Values,* 13, no. 5 (1989), 21–25.

57. Cross, K.P., *Adults as Learners*. San Francisco: Jossey-Bass, 1981.

58. Cumming, E., and W.E. Henry, *Growing Old: The Process of Disengagement*. New York: Basic Books, 1961.

59. Curb, J., et al., Health Status and Life Style in Elderly Japanese Men With a Long Life Expectancy, *Journal of Gerontology: Social Sciences,* 45, no. 5 (1990), S206–S211.

60. Dail, P., Prime-Time Television Portrayals of Older Adults in the Context of Family Life, *Gerontologist,* 28, no. 5 (1988), 700–706.

61. Denney, N., et al., An Adult Developmental Study of Contextual Memory, *Journal of Gerontology: Psychological Sciences,* 46, no. 2 (1991), P44–P50.

62. Depner, C., and B. Ingersoll-Dayton, Conjugal Social Support: Patterns in Later Life, *Journal of Gerontology,* 40, no. 6 (1985), 761–766.

63. deSimone, E., The Hospitalized Elderly: A Nursing Perspective, *Recent Advances in Nursing,* 23 (1989), 36–44.

64. DeVos, S., Extended Family Living Among Older People in Six Latin American Countries, *Journal of Gerontology: Social Sciences,* 45, no. 3 (1990), S87–S94.

65. Doka, K., and M. Mertz, The Meaning and Significance of Great-Grandparenthood, *Gerontologist,* 28, no. 2 (1988), 192–197.

66. Doress, P., and D. Siegel, *Ourselves, Growing Older*. Boston: Simon & Schuster, 1987.

67. Duckett, S., ed., *The Pathology of the Aging Human Nervous System*. Philadelphia: Lea & Febiger, 1991.

68. Duncan, P., et al., Functional Reach: A New Clinical Measure of Balance, *Journal of Gerontology: Medical Sciences,* 45, no. 6 (1990), M192–M197.

69. Dura, J., E. Haywood-Niler, and J. Kiecolt-Glaser, Spousal Caregivers of Persons With Alzheimer's and Parkinson's Disease Dementia: A Preliminary Comparison, *Gerontologist,* 30, no. 3 (1990), 332–336.

70. Duvall, E., and B. Miller, *Marriage and Family Development* (6th ed.). Philadelphia: J.B. Lippincott, 1984.

71. Dworetzky, J., and N. Davis, *Human Development: A Lifespan Approach*. St. Paul: West Publishing, 1989.

72. Dychtwald, K., *Age Wave: The Challenges and Opportunities of an Aging America*. New York: Jeremy Torcher, 1989.

73. Dye, C., Memory and Aging: A Nursing Responsibility, *Recent Advances in Nursing,* 23, (1989), 53–65.

74. Easterlin, R., C. Macdonald, and D. Macunovich, Retirement Prospects of the Baby Boom Generation: A Different Perspective, *Gerontologist,* 30, no. 6 (1990), 776–783.

75. Ebersole, P., and P. Hess, *Toward Health Aging: Human Needs and Nursing Response* (3rd ed.). St. Louis: C.V. Mosby, 1990.

76. Eliopoulos, C., *Health Assessment of the Older Adult*

(2nd ed.). Menlo Park, Calif: Addison Wesley Nursing, 1990.

77. Emery, C., and J. Blumenthal, Perceived Change Among Participants in an Exercise Program for Older Adults, *Gerontologist,* 30, no. 4 (1990), 516–521.

78. Erikson, E., *Adulthood.* New York: W.W. Norton, 1978.

79. ——, *Childhood and Society* (2nd ed.). New York: W.W. Norton, 1963.

80. Evans, W., I. Rosenberg, and J. Thompson, *Biomarkers: 10 Determinants of Aging You Can Control.* New York: Simon & Schuster, 1991.

81. Feldman, R., Shared Parenting: When Grandparents Help Out, *New Choices* (February, 1991), 32–35.

82. Fidel-Girgis, M., Family Support for the Elderly in Egypt, *Gerontologist,* 23, no. 6 (1983), 589–592.

83. Field, D., Continuity and Change in Personality in Old Age—Evidence From Five Longitudinal Studies: Introduction to a Special Issue, *Journal of Gerontology: Psychological Sciences,* 46, no. 6 (1991), P271–P274.

84. ——, and R. Millsap, Personality in Advanced Old Age: Continuity or Change? *Journal of Gerontology: Psychological Sciences,* 46, no. 6 (1991), P299–P308.

85. Fischer, L., D. Mueller, and P. Cooper, Older Volunteers: A Discussion of the Minnesota Senior Study, *Gerontologist,* 31, no. 2 (1991), 183–194.

86. Fitzgerald, D., The Aging Ear, *American Family Physician,* 31, no. 2 (1985), 225–332.

87. 5% of People Over 65 Live in Nursing Homes, *Nation's Health* (July 1987), 9.

88. Franzke, A., The Effects of Assertiveness Training on Older Adults, *Gerontologist,* 27, no. 1 (1987), 13–16.

89. Fried, H., and H. Waxman, Stockholm's Cafe 84: A Unique Day Program for Jewish Survivors of Concentration Camps, *Gerontologist,* 28, no. 2 (1988), 253–255.

90. Gaynor, S., The Long Haul: The Effects of Home Care on Caregivers, *Image,* 22, no. 4 (1990), 208–212.

91. Gelein, J., Aged Women and Health, *Nursing Clinics of North America,* 17, no. 1 (1982), 179–185.

92. Gerace, L., Using Family Photographs to Explore Life Cycle Changes, *Nursing and Health Care,* 10, no. 5 (1989), 245–249.

93. Gerber, J., et al., *Lifetrends: The Future of Baby Boomers and Other Aging Americans.* New York: Macmillan, 1989.

94. Gershowitz, S., Adding Life to Years: Remotivating Elderly People in Institutions, *Nursing and Health Care,* 3, no. 3 (1982), 141–145.

95. Gioiella, E., Give the Older Person Space, *American Journal of Nursing,* 80, no. 5 (1980), 898–899.

96. Goldl, E., ed., *Aging and the Immune Response: Cellular and Humoral Aspects.* New York: Dekker, 1987.

97. Goldstein, M., S. Schuler, and J. Ross, Social and Economic Forces Affecting Intergenerational Relations in Extended Families in a Third World Country: A Cautionary Tale From South Asia, *Journal of Gerontology,* 38, (1983), 716–724.

98. Goodman, C., Natural Helping Among Older Adults, *Gerontologist,* 24, no. 2 (1984), 138–143.

99. Greenberg, J., and M. Becker, Aging Parents as Family Resources, *Gerontologist,* 28, no. 6 (1988), 786–791.

100. Hagberg, B., et al., Stability and Change of Personality in Old Age and Its Relation to Survival, *Journal of Geron-*
tology: Psychological Sciences, 46, no. 6 (1991), P285–P291.

101. Hagestad, G., Able Elderly in the Family Context: Changes, Chances, and Challenges, *Gerontologist,* 27, no. 4 (1987), 417–421.

102. Hampton, J., The Biology of Human Aging. San Luis Obispo, Calif: Wm. C. Brown, 1991.

103. Hardy, M., A Pilot Study of the Diagnosis and Treatment of Impaired Skin Integrity: Dry Skin in Older Persons, *Nursing Diagnosis,* 1, no. 2 (1990), 57–63.

104. Harris, T., et al., Longitudinal Study of Physical Ability in the Oldest-Old, *American Journal of Public Health,* 79, no. 6 (1989), 698–702.

105. Havighurst, R., *Developmental Tasks and Education* (3rd ed.). New York: David McKay, 1972.

106. ——, A Social-Psychological Perspective on Aging. In Sze, W., ed., *Human Life Cycle.* New York: Jason Aronson, 1975, 627–635.

107. Hayslip, B., Personality-Ability Relationships in Aged Adults, *Journal of Gerontology: Psychological Sciences,* 43, no. 3 (1988), P79–P84.

108. Hayter, J., Modifying the Environment to Help Older Persons, *Nursing and Health Care,* 4, no. 5 (1983), 265–269.

109. Hazard, M., and R. Kemp, Keep the Well Elderly Well, *American Journal of Nursing,* 83, no. 4 (1983), 567–569.

110. Hazzard, W., et al., *Principles of Geriatric Medicine and Gerontology* (2nd ed.). New York: McGraw-Hill, 1990.

111. Hegarty, V., *Decisions in Nutrition.* St. Louis: Times Mirror/Mosby College Publishing, 1988.

112. Henig, R., Take 2 Poodles and Call Me, *AARP News Bulletin,* 29, no. 11 (1988), 2.

113. Henri, J., An Alternative to Institutionalization, *Gerontologist,* 20, no. 4 (1980), 418–420.

114. Herzog, A., et al., Age Differences in Productive Activities, *Journal of Gerontology: Social Sciences,* 44, no. 4 (1989), S129–S138.

115. Hill, R., M. Storandt, and C. Simeone, The Effects of Memory Skills Training and Incentives on Free Recall in Older Learners, *Journal of Gerontology: Psychological Sciences,* 45, no. 6 (1990), P227–P232.

116. Hirst, S., and J. Miller, The Abused Elderly, *Journal of Psychosocial Nursing,* 24, no. 10 (1988), 28–34.

117. Hoole, A., R. Greenberg, and C. Glenn Pickard, *Patient Care Guidelines for Nurse Practitioners* (3rd ed.). Boston: Little, Brown, 1988.

118. Hopkins, D., et al., Effect of Low-Impact Aerobic Dance on the Functional Fitness of Elderly Women, *Gerontologist,* 30, no. 2 (1990), 189–192.

119. Hudson, R., Tomorrow's Able Elders: Implications for the State, *Gerontologist,* 27, no. 4 (1987), 405–409.

120. Hultsch, D.F., and D. Deutsch, *Adult Development and Aging, A Life Span Perspective.* New York: McGraw-Hill, 1981.

121. Hutchinson, C., and R. Buhr, Types and Meanings of Caring Behaviors Among Elderly Nursing Home Residents, *Image,* 23, no. 2 (1991), 85–88.

122. Imaging the Future, *AARP News Bulletin,* 28, no. 11 (December 1987), 2, 10.

123. Jackson, J., *Minorities and Aging.* Belmont, Calif: Wadsworth, 1980.

124. Jarrik, L., Aging of the Brain: How Can We Prevent It? *Gerontologist,* 28, no. 6 (1988), 739–747.

125. Jenkins, E.H., Homemakers: The Core of Home Health Care, *Geriatric Nursing,* 5, no. 1 (1984), 28–30.

126. Johnson, C., Active and Latent Functions of Grandparenting During the Divorce Process, *Gerontologist,* 28, no. 2 (1988), 185–191.

127. ——, and B. Baner, Families and Networks Among Older Inner-City Blacks, *Gerontologist,* 30, no. 6 (1990), 726–733.

128. Johnston, L., and S.H. Gueldner, Using Mnemonics to Boost Memory in the Elderly, *Journal of Gerontological Nursing,* 15, no. 8 (1989), 22–25.

129. Jourard, S.M., *The Transparent Self.* Princeton, NJ: D. Van Nostrand, 1964.

130. Jung, C., Psychological Types. In Adler, G., et al., eds., *Collected Works of Carl G. Jung,* Vol. 6. Princeton, NJ: Princeton University Press, 1971.

131. Kain, C., N. Reilly, and E. Schultz, The Older Adult: A Comparative Assessment, *Nursing Clinics of North America,* 25, no. 4 (1990), 833–848.

132. Kane, R., and R. Kane, Delivering Long-Term Care: Lessons From the Developed World, *Aging,* 2, no. 4 (1990), 337–345.

133. ——, et al., Adult Foster Care for the Elderly in Oregon: A Mainstream Alternative to Nursing Homes? *American Journal of Public Health,* 81, no. 9 (1991), 1113–1120.

134. Kapp, M., Health Care Decision Making by the Elderly: I Get By With a Little Help From My Family, *Gerontologist,* 31, no. 5 (1991), 619–623.

135. Kayser-Jones, J., The Environment and Quality of Life in Long-Term Care Institutions, *Nursing and Health Care,* 10, no. 3 (1989), 125–130.

136. Keith, P., and F. Lorenz, Financial Strain and Health of Unmarried Older People, *Gerontologist,* 29, no. 5 (1989), 684–691.

137. ——, et al., Confidants and Well Being: A Note on Male Friendship in Old Age, *Gerontologist,* 24, no. 3 (1984), 318–320.

138. Kelly, J., M. Steinkamp, and Janice Steinkamp, Late Life Leisure: How They Play in Peoria, *Gerontologist,* 26, no. 5 (1986), 531–537.

139. Kendig, H., and D. Rowland, Family Support of the Australian Aged: A Comparison with the United States, *Gerontologist,* 23, no. 6 (1983), 643–649.

140. Kennedy, G., College Students' Expectations of Grandparent and Grandchild Role Behaviors, *Gerontologist,* 30, no. 1 (1990), 43–48.

141. Kent, B., and R. Butler, *Human Aging Research: Concepts and Techniques.* New York: Raven Press, 1988.

142. Kidd, J.R., *How Adults Learn.* Englewood Cliffs, NJ: Cambridge Books, 1988.

143. Kivett, V., Centrality of the Grandfather Role Among Older Rural Black and White Men, *Journal of Gerontology: Social Sciences,* 46, no. 5 (1991), S250–S258.

144. Kohen, J., Old But Not Alone: Informal Social Supports Among the Elderly by Mental Status and Sex, *Gerontologist,* 23, no. 1 (1983), 57–63.

145. Kolanowski, A., Restlessness in the Elderly: The Effect of Artificial Lighting, *Nursing Research,* 39, no. 3 (1990), 181–183.

146. Kongable, L., K. Buckwalter, and J. Stolley, The Effects of Pet Therapy on the Social Behavior of Institutionalized Alzheimer's Clients, *Archives of Psychiatric Nursing,* 3, no. 4 (1989), 191–198.

147. Kopac, C., Sensory Loss in the Aged: The Role of the Nurse and the Family, *Nursing Clinics of North America,* 18, no. 2 (1983), 373–384.

148. Kra, S., *Aging Myths: Reversible Causes of Mind and Memory Loss.* New York: McGraw Hill, 1986.

149. Krumpe, P., et al., The Aging Respiratory System, *Clinics in Geriatric Medicine,* 1, no. 1 (1985), 143–173.

150. Kuhlman, G., et al., Alzheimer's Disease and Family Caregiving: Critical Synthesis of the Literature and Research Agenda, *Nursing Research,* 40, no. 6 (1991), 331–337.

151. Lambert, D., M. Dellmann-Jenkins, and D. Fruit, Planning for Contact Between the Generations: An Effective Approach, *Gerontologist,* 30, no. 4 (1990), 553–556.

152. Lee, G., and C. Shehan, Retirement and Marital Satisfaction, *Journal of Gerontology: Social Sciences,* 44, no. 6 (1989), S226–S230.

153. Lidz, T., *The Person: His and Her Development Throughout the Life Cycle* (2nd ed.). New York: Basic Books, 1983.

154. Liptzin, B., M. Grob, and S. Eisen, Family Burden of Demented and Depressed Elderly Psychiatric Inpatients, *Gerontologist,* 28, no. 3 (1988), 397–401.

155. Litvin, S., Status Transitions and Future Outlook as Determinants of Conflict: The Caregiver's and Care Receiver's Perspective, *Gerontologist,* 32, no. 1 (1992), 68–76.

156. Lord, S., R. Clark, and I. Webster, Postural Stability and Associated Physiological Factors in a Population of Aged Persons, *Journal of Gerontology: Medical Sciences,* 46, no. 3 (1991), M69–M76.

157. Lowenthal, M., M. Thurnher, and D. Chiriboga, *Four Stages of Life.* San Francisco: Jossey-Bass, 1976.

158. Lubben, J., P. Weiler, and I. Chi, Health Practices of the Elderly Poor, *American Journal of Public Health,* 79, no. 6 (1989), 731–734.

159. Maas, H., and J. Kuypers, *From Thirty to Seventy.* San Francisco: Jossey-Bass, 1974.

160. Maddox, G.L., Disengagement Theory: A Critical Evaluation, *Gerontologist,* 4, (1974), 80–83.

161. Malcolm J., Creative Spiritual Care for the Elderly. *Journal of Christian Nursing,* 4, no. 1 (Winter 1987), 24–26.

162. Manton, K., I. Siegler, and M. Woodburg, Patterns of Intellectual Development in Later Life, *Journal of Gerontology,* 41, no. 4 (1986), 486–499.

163. Markides, K., and D. Lee, Predictors of Health Status in Middle-Aged and Older Mexican Americans, *Journal of Gerontology: Social Sciences,* 46, no. 5 (1991), S243–S249.

164. Marklein, M., Con Games Proliferate: New Threats Haunt City Folk, *AARP Bulletin,* 32, no. 2 (1991), 1, 16–17.

165. Mason, J., and M. McGinnis, Healthy People 2000: An Overview of the National Health Promotion and Disease Prevention Objectives, *Public Health Reports,* 105, no. 5 (1990), 441–446.

166. Masters, W., V. Johnson, and R. Kolodny, *Masters and Johnson on Sex and Human Loving.* Boston: Little, Brown, 1988.

167. McCoy, V., Adult Life Cycle Tasks/Adult Continuing Ed-

ucation Program Response, *Lifelong Learning in the Adult Years* (October 1977), 16.

168. McCracken, A., Sexual Practice by Elders: The Forgotten Aspect of Functional Health, *Journal of Gerontological Nursing,* 14, no. 10 (1988), 13–18.

169. McCrae, R., Age Differences in the Use of Coping Mechanisms, *Journal of Gerontology,* 37 (1982), 454–460.

170. McDowd, The Effects of Age and Extended Practice on Divided Attention Performance, *Journal of Gerontology,* 41, no. 6 (1986), 764–769.

171. McElmurry, B., and S. LiBrizzi, The Health of Older Women, *Nursing Clinics of North America,* 21, no. 1 (1986), 161–171.

172. McKenna, M., Twice in Need of Care: A Transcultural Nursing Analysis of Elderly Mexican Americans, *Journal of Transcultural Nursing,* 1, no. 1 (1989), 46–52.

173. Mead, G., Mind, Self, and Society. In Strauss, A., ed., *George Herbert Mead: On Social Psychology.* Chicago: University of Chicago Press, 1964.

174. Meehan, P., L. Saltzman, and R. Sattin, Suicides Among Older United States Residents: Epidemiologic Characteristics and Trends, *American Journal of Public Health,* 81, no. 9 (1991), 1198–1200.

175. Merriam, S., The Structure of Simple Reminiscence, *Gerontologist,* 29, no. 6 (1989), 761–767.

176. Merry, A., Take Your Assessment All the Way Down to the Toes, *RN Magazine,* 51, no. 1 (1988), 60–63.

177. Miller, S., and J. Cavanaugh, The Meaning of Grandparenthood and Its Relationship to Demographic, Relationship, and Social Participation Variables, *Journal of Gerontology: Psychological Sciences,* 45, no. 6 (1990), P244–P246.

178. Mirotznik, J., and A. Ruskin, Inter-Institutional Relocation and Its Effects on Psychosocial Status, *Gerontologist,* 25, no. 3 (1988), 263–270.

179. Morgan, D., Adjusting to Widowhood: Do Social Networks Really Make It Easier? *Gerontologist,* 29, no. 1 (1989), 101–107.

180. Morgan, D., T. Schuster, and E. Butler, Role Reversals in the Exchange of Social Support, *Journal of Gerontology: Social Sciences,* 46, no. 5 (1991), S278–S287.

181. Moritz, D., S. Kasl, and L. Berkman, The Health Impact of Living with a Cognitively Impaired Elderly Spouse: Depressive Symptoms and Social Functioning, *Journal of Gerontology: Social Sciences,* 44, no. 1 (1989), S17–S27.

182. Morley, J., Z. Glick, and L. Rubenstein, eds., *Geriatric Nutrition: A Comprehensive Review.* New York: Raven Press, 1990.

183. Morrison-Beedy, D., and L. Robbins, Sexual Assessment and the Aging Female, *Nurse Practitioner,* 14, no. 12 (1989), 35–45.

184. Muller, R., and J. Donnemeyer, Age, Trust, and Perceived Safety from Crime in Rural Areas, *Gerontologist,* 25, no. 3 (1985), 237–242.

185. Mundorf, N., and W. Brownell, Media Preferences of Older and Younger Adults, *Gerontologist,* 30, no. 5 (1990), 685–691.

186. Murray, R., Body Image Development in Adulthood, *Nursing Clinics of North America,* 7, no. 4 (1972), 625–630.

187. ——, and Marilyn Huelskoetter, *Psychiatric/Mental Health Nursing: Giving Emotional Care* (3rd ed.). Norwalk, Conn: Appleton & Lange, 1991.

188. Nelson, P., Ethnic Differences in Intrinsic/Extrinsic Religious Orientation and Depression in the Elderly, *Archives of Psychiatric Nursing,* 3, no. 4 (1989), 199–204.

189. Neufeld, A., and H. Hobbs, Self-Care in a High-Rise for Seniors, *Nursing Outlook,* 33, no. 4 (1985), 298–301.

190. Neugarten, B., Grow Old Along With Me! The Best is Yet to Be, *Psychology Today,* 5, no. 7 (1971), 45ff.

191. ——, Adult Personality: A Developmental View. In Charles, D., and W. Looft, eds., *Readings in Psychological Development Through Life.* New York: Holt, Rinehart & Winston, 1973, 356–366.

192. ——, Adaptation and the Life Cycle, *Counseling Psychologist,* 6, no. 1 (1976), 16–20.

193. Norris, R., Commonsense Tips for Working With Blind Patients, *American Journal of Nursing,* 89, no. 3 (1989), 360–361.

194. Ogburn-Russell, L., and J. Johnson, Oxygen Saturation Levels in the Well Elderly: Altitude Makes a Difference, *Journal of Gerontological Nursing,* 16, no. 10 (1990), 26–30.

195. Oktay, J., and P. Volland, Foster Home Care for the Frail Elderly is an Alternative to Nursing Home Care: An Experimental Evaluation, *American Journal of Public Health,* 77, no. 2 (1987), 1505–1510.

196. Okun, M., J. Melichar, and M. Hill, Negative Daily Events, Positive and Negative Social Ties, and Psychological Distress Among Older Adults, *Gerontologist,* 30, no. 2 (1990), 193–199.

197. Palmone, E., The Effects of Aging on Activities and Attitudes, *Gerontologist,* 8 (1968), 259–263.

198. Passath, P., and F. Cook, Effects of Television Viewing on Knowledge and Attitudes About Older Adults: A Critical Re-Examination, *Gerontologist,* 25, no. 1 (1985), 69–77.

199. Peck, R.C., Psychological Development in the Second Half of Life. In Neugarten, B., ed., *Middle Age and Aging.* Chicago: University of Chicago Press, 1968.

200. Perlmutter, M., and L. Nyquist, Relationships Between Self-Reported Physical and Mental Health and Intelligence Performance Across Adulthood, *Journal of Gerontology: Psychological Sciences,* 45, no. 4 (1990), P145–P155.

201. Phillips, L., Age: A Truly Confounding Variable, *Western Journal of Nursing Research,* 11, no. 2 (1989), 181–195.

202. Pietrukowicz, M., and M. Johnson, Using Life Histories to Individualize Nursing Home Staff Attitudes Toward Residents, *Gerontologist,* 31, no. 1 (1991), 102–106.

203. Pillemer, K., and D. Moore, Abuse of Patients in Nursing Homes: Findings From a Survey of Staff, *Gerontologist,* 29, no. 3 (1989), 314–319.

204. Ploeg, J., and S. Faux, The Relationship Between Social Support, Lifestyle Behaviors, Coping, and Health in the Elderly, *Canadian Journal of Nursing Research,* 21, no. 2 (1989), 53–65.

205. Pollick, M., Abuse of the Elderly: A Review, *Holistic Nursing Practice,* 1, no. 2 (1987), 43–53.

206. Poorman, S., *Human Sexuality and the Nursing Process.* New York: Appleton & Lange, 1987.

207. Porac, C., S. Coven, and P. Duncan, Life-Span Age Trends in Laterality, *Journal of Gerontology,* 35, no. 3 (1983), 715–721.

208. Pratt, C., V. Schmall, and S. Wright, Ethical Concerns of Family Caregivers to Dementia Patients, *Gerontologist,* 27, no. 5 (1987), 632–638.

209. Profiles of Centenarians, *Statistical Bulletin,* 68, no. 1 (1987), 2–7.

210. *A Profile of Older Americans.* Long Beach, Calif: American Association of Retired Persons, 1988.

211. Pruchno, R., and N. Resch, Husbands and Wives as Caregivers: Antecedents of Depression and Burden, *Gerontologist,* 29, no. 2 (1989), 159–165.

212. Pullinger, W., F., Jr., A History of Remotivation, *Hospital and Community Psychiatry,* 18, no. 1 (1967), 35–39.

213. Rantz, M., and K. Egan, Reducing Death From Translocation Syndrome, *American Journal of Nursing,* 87, no. 10 (1987), 1351.

214. Rattenbury, C., and M. Stones, A Controlled Evaluation of Reminiscence and Current Topic Discussion Groups in a Nursing Home Context, *Gerontologist,* 29, no. 6 (1989), 768–771.

215. Rebensen, M., The Physiologic Changes That Occur With Aging, *Critical Care Nursing Quarterly,* 12, no. 1 (1989), 1–14.

216. Reed, P., Self-Transcendence and Mental Health in Oldest-Old Adults, *Nursing Research,* 40, no. 1 (1991), 5–11.

217. Reichel, W., ed., *Clinical Aspects of Aging.* Baltimore: Williams & Wilkins, 1989.

218. Revicki, D., and J. Mitchell, Strain, Social Support, and Mental Health in Rural Elderly Individuals, *Journal of Gerontology: Social Sciences,* 45, no. 6 (1990), S267–S274.

219. Richardson, V., and K. Kilty, Retirement Intentions Among Black Professionals: Implications for Practice with Older Black Adults, *Gerontologist,* 32, no. 1 (1992), 7–16.

220. Riegel, K., and R. Riegel, Development, Drop, and Death, *Developmental Psychology,* 6, no. 2 (1972), 306–319.

221. Riffle, K., J. Yoho, and J. Sams, Health Promoting Behaviors, Perceived Social Support, and Self-Reported Health of Appalachian Elderly, *Public Health Nursing,* 6, no. 4 (1989), 204–211.

222. Roos, N., and B. Havens, Predictors of Successful Aging: A 12 Year Study of Manitoba Elderly, *American Journal of Public Health,* 81, no. 1 (1991), 63–68.

223. Rosenbaum, J., Cultural Care of Older Greek Canadian Widows Within Leininger's Theory of Culture Care, *Journal of Transcultural Nursing,* 2, no. 1 (1990), 37–47.

224. Ross, M., et al., Age Differences in Body Consciousness, *Journal of Gerontology: Psychological Sciences,* 44, no. 1 (1989), P23–P24.

225. Rubenstein, R., Never Married Elderly as a Social Type: Re-Evaluating Some Images, *Gerontologist,* 27, no. 1 (1987), 108–112.

226. ——, et al., Key Relationships of Never Married, Childless Older Women: A Cultural Analysis, *Journal of Gerontology: Social Sciences,* 46, no. 5 (1991), S270–S277.

227. Ruhm, C., Why Older Americans Stop Working, *Gerontologist,* 29, no. 3 (1989), 294–299.

228. Rybarczyk, B., and S. Auerbach, Reminiscence Interviews as Stress Management Interventions for Older Patients Undergoing Surgery, *Gerontologist,* 30, no. 4 (1990), 522–528.

229. Sargis, N., J. Jennrich, and K. Murray, Housing and Health, *Nursing and Health Care,* 8, no. 6 (1987), 334–339.

230. Schaie, K., The Hazards of Cognitive Aging, *Gerontologist,* 29, no. 4 (1989), 484–493.

231. ——, and S. Willis, Adult Personality and Psychomotor Performance: Cross-Sectional and Longitudinal Analysis, *Journal of Gerontology: Psychological Sciences,* 46, no. 6 (1991), P275–P284.

232. Schank, M., and M. Lough, Profiles of Frail Elderly Women, Maintaining Independence, *Journal of Advanced Nursing,* 15, no. 6 (1990), 674–682.

233. Schneider, E., and J. Rowe, eds., *Handbook of the Biology of Aging* (3rd ed.). San Diego: Academic Press, 1990.

234. Schroots, J., J. Birren, and A. Svanborg, eds., *Health and Aging: Perspectives and Prospects.* New York: Springer, 1988.

235. Seccombe, K., and M. Ishii-Kuntz, Perceptions of Problems Associated with Aging: Comparisons Among Four Older Age Cohorts, *Gerontologist,* 31, no. 4 (1991), 527–533.

236. Sharp, M., and E. Gollin, Aging and Free Recall for Objects Located in Space, *Journals of Gerontology: Psychological Sciences,* 43, no. 1 (1988), P8–P11.

237. Shulman, M., and E. Mandel, Communication Training of Relatives and Friends of Institutionalized Elderly Persons, *Gerontologist,* 28, no. 6 (1988), 797–799.

238. Sill, J., Disengagement Reconsidered: Awareness of Finitude, *Gerontologist,* 20, no. 4 (1980), 457–462.

239. Simonton, D., Creativity in the Later Years: Optimistic Prospects for Achievement, *Gerontologist,* 30, no. 5 (1990), 626–631.

240. Smeeding, T., and L. Straub, Health Care Financing Among the Elderly: Who Really Pays the Bills? *Journal of Health Politics, Policy and Law,* 12, no. 1 (1987), 35–52.

241. Sohngen, L., The Experience of Old Age as Depicted in Contemporary Novels: A Supplementary Bibliography, *Gerontologist,* 21, no. 3 (1981), 303.

242. Soloman, K., Geriatric Substance Abuse Clinic Opens, *Insight* (April 18, 1991), 4.

243. Speake, D., M. Cowart, and K. Pellet, Health Perceptions and Lifestyles of the Elderly, *Research in Nursing and Health,* 12, no. 2 (1989), 93–100.

244. Spence, A., *Biology of Human Aging.* Englewood Cliffs, NJ: Prentice Hall, 1989.

245. Spencer, G., Commentary: Dramatic Growth of Centenarian Population, *Statistical Bulletin,* 68, no. 1 (1987), 8–9.

246. Stenchever, M., and G. Aagaard, eds., *Caring for the Older Woman.* New York: Elsevier, 1991.

247. Stevens, J., Aging and Spatial Acuity of Touch, *Journal of Gerontology: Psychological Sciences,* 47, no. 1 (1992), P35–P40.

248. Stone, R., G. Cafferta, and J. Sangl, Caregivers of the Frail Elderly: A National Profile, *Gerontologist,* 27, no. 5 (1987), 616–626.

249. Strong, C., Stress and Caring for Elderly Relatives: Inter-

pretations and Coping Strategies in an American Indian and White Sample, *Gerontologist*, 24, no. 3 (1984), 251–255.

250. Sung, K., A New Look at Filial Piety: Ideals and Practices of Family Centered Parent Care in Korea, *Gerontologist*, 30, no. 5 (1990), 610–617.

251. Swisher, K., ed., *The Elderly: Opposing Viewpoints*. San Diego: Greenhaven Press, 1990.

252. Talbott, M., The Negative Side of the Relationship Between Older Widows and Their Adult Children: The Mother's Perspective, *Gerontologist*, 30, no. 5 (1990), 595–603.

253. Taylor, R., and L. Chatters, Nonorganizational Religious Participation Among Elderly Black Adults, *Journal of Gerontology: Social Sciences*, 46, no. 2 (1991), S103–S111.

254. Tennstedt, S., J. McKinlay, and L. Sullivan, Informal Care for Frail Elders: The Role of Secondary Caregivers, *Gerontologist*, 29, no. 5 (1989), 677–683.

255. Terpstra, T., et al., As Young As You Feel: Age Identification Among the Elderly, *Journal of Gerontological Nursing*, 15, no. 12 (1989), 4–10.

256. Tesch, S., M. Nehrke, and S. Whitbourne, Social Relationships, Psychosocial Adaptation, and Intrainstitutional Relocation of Elderly Men, *Gerontologist*, 29, no. 4 (1989), 517–523.

257. Tevis, C., The Old Tigers! Gray Haired, But Still Scratching, *Successful Farming*, 86, no. 12 (1988), 22–26.

258. Thomas, J., Predictors of Satisfaction With Children's Help for Younger and Older Elderly Parents, *Journal of Gerontology: Social Sciences*, 43, no. 1 (1988), P9–P14.

259. Thompson, M., and W. Forbes, The Various Definitions of Biological Aging, *Canadian Journal on Aging*, 9, no. 2 (1990), 91–91.

260. Timiras, P., ed., *Physiological Basis of Geriatrics*. New York: Churchill Livingstone, 1990.

261. Tolbert, B.M., Reality Orientation and Remotivation in a Long-Term Care Facility, *Nursing and Health Care*, 5, no. 1 (1984), 40–44.

262. Trends in Longevity after Age 65, *Statistical Bulletin*, 68, no. 1 (1987), 10–17.

263. Trice, L., Meaningful Life Experience to the Elderly, *Image*, 22, no. 4 (1990), 248–251.

264. Troll, L., New Thoughts on Old Families, *Gerontologist*, 28, no. 5 (1988), 586–591.

265. Uhlenberg, P., and M.A. Myers, Divorce and the Elderly, *Gerontologist*, 21, no. 3 (1981), 276–282.

266. U.S. Department of Commerce, *Statistical Abstract of the United States: 1990* (110th ed.). Washington, DC: Bureau of the Census, 1990.

267. ——, *USA Statistics in Brief: 1990. A Statistical Abstract Supplement*. Washington, DC: Bureau of the Census, 1990.

268. U.S. Department of Health and Human Service, New Recommended Schedule for Active Immunization of Normal Infants and Children, *Morbidity and Mortality Weekly Report*, 35, no. 37 (September 19, 1986), 577–579.

269. Vaillant, G., The Association of Ancestral Longevity With Successful Aging, *Journal of Gerontology: Psychological Sciences*, 46, no. 6 (1991), P292–P298.

270. Wagnild, G., and H. Young, Resilience Among Older Women, *Image*, 22, no. 4 (1990), 252–255.

271. Wallace, J., Reconsidering the Life Review: The Social Construction of Talk About the Past, *Gerontologist*, 32, no. 1 (1992), 120–125.

272. Walton, C., et al., Psychological Correlates of Loneliness in the Older Adult, *Archives of Psychiatric Nursing*, 5, no. 3 (1991), 165–170.

273. Ward, R., The Never-Married in Later Life, *Journal of Gerontology*, 34, no. 6 (1979), 861–869.

274. ——, Informal Networks and Well-Being in Later Life: A Research Agenda, *Gerontologist*, 25, no. 1 (1985), 55–61.

275. Weissert, W., et al., Models of Adult Day Care: Findings From a National Survey, *Gerontologist*, 29, no. 5 (1989), 640–649.

276. Wentowski, G., Older Women's Perceptions of Great Grandparenthood, *Gerontologist*, 25, no. 6 (1985), 593–596.

277. White, N., and W. Cunningham, Is Terminal Drop Pervasive or Specific? *Journal of Gerontology: Psychological Sciences*, 43, no. 6 (1988), P141–P144.

278. Wiener, J., et al., Measuring the Activities of Daily Living: Comparisons Across National Surveys, *Journal of Gerontology: Social Sciences*, 45, no. 6 (1990), 229–237.

279. Wilkinson, R., and S. Allison, Age and Simple Reaction Time: Decade Differences for 5,325 Subjects, *Journal of Gerontology: Psychological Sciences*, 44, no. 2 (1989), P29–P35.

280. Williams, S.R., *Nutrition and Diet Therapy* (6th ed.). St. Louis: Times Mirror/Mosby, 1989.

281. Winkler, A., et al., The Impact of a Resident Dog on an Institution for the Elderly: Effects on Perceptions and Social Interactions, *Gerontologist*, 29, no. 2 (1989), 216–223.

282. Wister, A., Environmental Adaptation by Persons in Their Later Life, *Research on Aging*, 11, (1989), 267–291.

283. Worach-Kardas, H., The Polish Family Tradition, *Gerontologist*, 23, no. 6 (1983), 593–596.

284. Worobey, J., and R. Angel, Functional Capacity and Living Arrangements of Unmarried Elderly Persons, *Journal of Gerontology: Social Sciences*, 45, no. 3 (1990), S95–S101.

285. Yurick, A.G., et al., *The Aged person and the Nursing Process* (3rd ed.). East Norwalk, Conn: Appleton & Lange, 1989.

286. Zarit, S., P. Todd, and J. Zarit, Subjective Burden of Husbands and Wives as Caregivers: A Longitudinal Study, *Gerontologist*, 26, no. 3 (1986), 260–266.

287. Zopf, P., Jr., *America's Older Population*. Houston: Cap & Gown, 1986.

288. Zsembik, B., and A. Singer, The Problem of Defining Retirement Among Minorities: The Mexican Americans, *Gerontologist*, 30, no. 6 (1990), 749–757.

INTERVIEW

289. Alverson, P., Jr., Nursing Home Administrator, March 15, 1992, Greenwood, S.C.

Chapter 15

Death, the Last Developmental Stage

Death is universal, but there is no universal meaning to death. Meaning comes from a merging of philosophical, spiritual, emotional, sociocultural, historical and geographical factors.
—Ruth Beckmann Murray

KEY TERMS

Death	Near-death experience
Euthanasia	Closed awareness
Active	Suspicious awareness
Passive	Mutual pretense
Living will	Open awareness
Durable power of attorney	Predilection to death
for health care	

OBJECTIVES

Study of this chapter will enable you to:

1. Explore personal reactions to active and passive euthanasia and the right-to-die movement versus extraordinary measures to prolong life. Contrast home or hospice care to hospital or nursing home care.
2. Contrast the child's, adolescent's, and adult's concept of death.
3. Discuss personal feelings about death and the dying person.
4. Discuss the stages of awareness and related behavior as the person adapts to the crisis of approaching death.
5. Discuss sequence of reactions when the person and family are aware of terminal illness.
6. Talk with another about how to plan for eventual death.
7. Assess reactions and needs of a dying client and family members with supervision.
8. Plan and give care, with supervision, to a client based on understanding of his or her awareness of eventual death, behavioral and emotional reactions, and physical needs.
9. Intervene appropriately to meet needs of family members of a dying person.
10. Evaluate the effectiveness of care given.

Death has been avoided in name and understanding. There may be no harm in saying "he passed" instead of "he died." There is harm in suddenly facing a client's death without sufficient emotional preparation.

ISSUES RELATED TO DYING AND DEATH

Definitions of Death

The aged differ from persons in other life eras in that their concept of future is realistically limited. The younger person may not live many years into the future but generally thinks of many years of life ahead. The older person knows that, despite medical and technical advances, life is limited.

Death is the last developmental stage. It is more than simply an end process—it can be viewed as a goal and as fulfillment. If the person has spent his or her years unfettered by fear, if he or she has lived richly and productively, and if he or she has achieved the developmental task of ego integrity, he or she can accept the realization that the self will cease to be and that dying has an onset long before the actual death.

If death is considered the last developmental phase, it is worth the kind of preparation that goes into any developmental phase, perhaps physically, certainly emotionally, socially, philosophically, or spiritually.

Until this century death usually occurred in the home, but at present more than 70% of deaths in American cities occur in institutions so that death has become remote and impersonal.

Because of technologic advances, the determination of **death** is *changing from the traditional concept that death occurs when the heart stops beating. Newer definitions of death refer to brain death, established by a flat encephalogram (EEG), usually for a duration of 24 to 48 hours, lack of reflex activity, and pupil dilation.* Vital organs can be kept alive by machines for use in transplants, even though the client is essentially dead, showing no brain activity (72, 78).

The sophisticated machinery has caused some to ask questions such as, "If we declare someone entirely dead when the brain is 'dead,' even though most of the body remains alive with the help of life supports, then doesn't that body lose its sanctity and become the object of transplant organ harvesting?" The opposition might answer, "Without the present life-support systems, this person would certainly have been dead. Why not take the opportunity to save another person's life with the needed organ(s)?"

The current issue is not only "When is someone dead?" but "Who decides when to turn off the machines?" Is it the client, medical personnel, a lawyer, the clergy, or the courts?

The family, more than anyone else, must live with the memories of their loved ones and the events surrounding death. It is a violation of the family's dignity to rush death. Even though a lesser involved person might say, "Why don't they turn the machines off!" this person should be ignored until all those closely involved with the client can say with acceptance and assurance, "Now is the time" (38). Increasingly, the *person* is saying that he or she has a right to decide how long machines should maintain personal life or that of a loved one. There are several plausible death concepts: those related to flow of body fluids (heart and lung oriented), integrating capacity (whole brain oriented), or experiential and social interaction (neocostically oriented).

Kellmer (47) discusses historical, social, and ethical perspectives of resuscitation and use of life-support technology and court cases that have set precedents in determining who is declared competent or incompetent to make decisions about right to refuse treatment. She discusses approaches that can be used by hospitals and health care agencies to arrive at decisions about orders not to resuscitate and the importance of policies that have been formulated collaboratively by all departments that are involved in care of clients.

Euthanasia

Euthanasia is *legally defined as the act or practice of painlessly putting to death persons suffering from incurable or distressing diseases.*

Although maintaining life beyond all reason is an ethical dilemma for the nurse, an equally taxing ethical dilemma occurs when the doctor deliberately hastens the client's death by increasing the dose of a narcotic analgesic such as morphine to the point of lethality. The issues and suggested ways to handle them are discussed by a hospital nurse, hospice nurse, pastor, and physician in an article by Janet Fuller (28). Brown (5) also distinguishes between passive and active euthanasia and the moral, ethical, and legal problems with the concept of euthanasia. He emphasizes the need of responsible, moral caregivers who will promote quality of life and right to die with dignity. If each human life is seen as of infinite value, it will be worth the efforts to ease pain and help the person find meaning in the current situation.

Euthanasia is not new. It was practiced in Greece. African bushmen and North American primitive tribes abandoned their infirm elderly to die; there was insufficient food for anyone who could not produce his or her own food. Eskimo tribal elders cut a hole in the ice and disappeared when they became burdensome.

Most Western countries consider **active euthanasia,** *deliberately hastening death,* as first-degree murder. On the other hand, court decisions have been inconsistent about *omission of care or inaction to prolong life,* which results in **passive euthanasia.**

The development of Judeo-Christian law from the beliefs of St. Augustine and St. Thomas Aquinas held that suicide was a sin and against natural law. In the past in American institutions, physiologic aspects only were considered in prolonging life. Today sociologic and economic aspects are also being considered. The value or

quality of life when the person is kept alive by artificial support systems is considered. Costs to client, family, and society are being considered. Ordinary care is the prevailing standard, not extraordinary means, although what constitutes ordinary care is debated.

Euthanasia is based on two fundamental legal premises: the right to privacy and the right to refuse treatment when informed. The competent client may decline treatment for religious reasons, fear of pain or suffering, exhaustion of finances, and unlikelihood of recovery. The incompetent client is not allowed the right to refuse in similar situations for fear of an irrational choice. Medical practice defers to wishes of the family. Those who are disabled, elderly, retarded, or insane may not receive the treatment ordinarily given to others.

Right-to-Die Movement

Another increasingly publicized facet with moral and ethical aspects is the right-to-die movement, which was first begun in England, Holland, and Scandanavian countries and which has gained momentum in the United States. Originally the Right-to-Die Society and the movement insisted that people should have the last word about their own lives, either to maintain or discontinue treatment when ill or dying. The District of Columbia and many states have adopted living-will laws (also known as right-to-die or natural death laws) that permit mentally competent adults to declare, before they are ill, that they do not want life prolonged artificially or by heroic measures. In states with no formal legislation, living wills have been upheld in courts. Many states have brain-death laws that allow withdrawal of respirators when a client no longer shows signs of brain activity. In the case of a lingering, comatose, incompetent person, the relatives, hospital ethics committee, or the courts must make decisions about not instituting or withdrawing life-prolonging measures; or the person may have designated someone to have durable power of attorney, available in all states, who can make decisions about health care, finances, property in the event of incapacity.

The Patient Self-Determination Act became effective in December 1991. All health care institutions receiving Medicare or Medicaid funds are required to give clients written information about these rights under state law to allow them to make decisions about medical care. Various types of treatment directives that a person must consider are (1) the **Living Will** (Fig. 15–1), which *states what medical treatment a person chooses to omit or refuse in case he or she cannot make a decision at the time of the illness* and which indicates that the person would rather die than be kept alive by artificial or heroic measures if there is no reasonable expectation of recovery; (2) a **durable power of attorney for health care** (Fig. 15–2); (3) a medical directive (Fig. 15–3); or (4) a declaration of desire for a natural death (Fig. 15–4).

Anyone interested in having a living will drawn up can request the free forms appropriate to his or her state from Choice in Dying—The National Council for the Right to Die, 200 Varick St., New York, NY 10014, (212) 366-5540.

Physicians fear indictment for homicide or aiding suicide even when following the living will, although these laws in all states grant immunity to health care professionals who comply with the declaration. Further, in some states there is a penalty if the physician does not comply. Relatives may sue the physician and/or hospital that refuses to follow the client's wishes reflected in the living will. (Legally, the physician may be charged with battery.)

ADVANCE DIRECTIVE
Living Will and Health Care Proxy

D eath is a part of life. It is a reality like birth, growth and aging. I am using this advance directive to convey my wishes about medical care to my doctors and other people looking after me at the end of my life. It is called an advance directive because it gives instructions in advance about what I want to happen to me in the future. It expresses my wishes about medical treatment that might keep me alive. I want this to be legally binding.

If I cannot make or communicate decisions about my medical care, those around me should rely on this document for instructions about measures that could keep me alive.

I do not want medical treatment (including feeding and water by tube) that will keep me alive if:
- I am unconscious and there is no reasonable prospect that I will ever be conscious again (even if I am not going to die soon in my medical condition), <u>or</u>
- I am near death from an illness or injury with no reasonable prospect of recovery.

I do want medicine and other care to make me more comfortable and to take care of pain and suffering. I want this even if the pain medicine makes me die sooner.

I want to give some extra instructions: [*Here list any special instructions, e.g., some people fear being kept alive after a debilitating stroke. If you have wishes about this, or any other conditions, please write them here.*]

The legal language in the box that follows is a health care proxy.
It gives another person the power to make medical decisions for me.

I name _____, who lives at _____

_____, phone number _____,

to make medical decisions for me if I cannot make them myself. This person is called a health care "surrogate," "agent," "proxy," or "attorney in fact." This power of attorney shall become effective when I become incapable of making or communicating decisions about my medical care. This means that this document stays legal when and if I lose the power to speak for myself, for instance, if I am in a coma or have Alzheimer's disease.

My health care proxy has power to tell others what my advance directive means. This person also has power to make decisions for me, based either on what I would have wanted, or, if this is not known, on what he or she thinks is best for me.

If my first choice health care proxy cannot or decides not to act for me, I name _____

_____, address _____,

phone number _____, as my second choice.

(continued on other side)

Figure 15-1. Living will declaration. (Reprinted by permission of Choice in Dying [formerly Concern for Dying/Society for the Right to Die], New York.)

(continued)

I have discussed my wishes with my health care proxy, and with my second choice if I have chosen to appoint a second person. My proxy(ies) has(have) agreed to act for me.

I have thought about this advance directive carefully. I know what it means and want to sign it. I have chosen two witnesses, neither of whom is a member of my family, nor will inherit from me when I die. My witnesses are not the same people as those I named as my health care proxies. I understand that this form should be notarized if I use the box to name (a) health care proxy(ies).

Signature _____

Date _____

Address _____

Witness' signature _____

Witness' printed name _____

Address _____

Witness' signature _____

Witness' printed name _____

Address _____

Notary [to be used if proxy is appointed] _____

Drafted and distributed by Choice In Dying, Inc.—the national council for the right to die. Choice In Dying is a national not-for-profit organization which works for the rights of patients at the end of life. In addition to this generic advance directive, Choice In Dying distributes advance directives that conform to each state's specific legal requirements and maintains a national Living Will Registry for completed documents.

CHOICE IN DYING, INC.—
the national council for the right to die
(formerly Concern for Dying/Society for the Right to Die)
200 Varick Street, New York, NY 10014   (212) 366-5540

5/92

Figure 15-1. Continued

Nurses are increasingly having to face questions of conscience, ethics, morals, and legalities in relation to what to say to the client and relatives and what to do in relation to whether to assist with initiating heroic measures when it is known that the client does not want them or whether to disconnect life-support machines.

It is possible to buy manuals on how to commit suicide. These books are becoming increasingly in demand as the public realizes it is illegal for doctors to practice euthanasia and that often doctors feel forced to prolong life, in whatever condition. The manuals argue against suicide when the problem is a distortion of judg-

STATE OF NORTH CAROLINA

COUNTY OF CATAWBA

HEALTH CARE POWER OF ATTORNEY

NOTICE: This document gives the person you designate your health care agent broad powers to make health care decisions for you, including the power to consent to your doctor not giving treatment or stopping treatment necessary to keep you alive. This power exists only as to those health care decisions for which you are unable to give informed consent.

This form does not impose a duty on your health care agent to exercise granted powers, but when a power is exercised, your health care agent will have to use due care to act in your best interests and in accordance with this document. Because the powers granted by this document are broad and sweeping, you should discuss your wishes concerning life-sustaining procedures with your health care agent.

I,

being of sound mind, hereby execute this Health Care Power of Attorney as follows:

1. Designation of Health Care Agent. I hereby appoint:

    Name:

    Home Address:

    Home Telephone No.

    Work Telephone No.

as my health care attorney-in-fact (herein referred to as my "Health Care Agent") to act for me and in my name (in any way I could act in person) to make health care decisions for me as authorized in this document.

If the person named as my Health Care Agent is not reasonably available or is unable or unwilling to act as my Agent, then I appoint the following persons (each to act alone and successively, in the order named), to serve in that capacity:

    A. Name:

    Home Address:

    Home Telephone No.

    Work Telephone No.

    B. Name:

    Home Address:

    Home Telephone No.

    Work Telephone No.

Each successor Health Care Agent designated shall be vested with the same power and duties as if originally named as my Health Care Agent.

2. Effectiveness of Appointment. ***Notice:*** **This Health Care Power of Attorney may be revoked by you at any time in any manner by which you are able to communicate your intent to revoke to your Health Care Agent and your attending physician.**

Absent revocation, the authority granted in this document shall become effective when and if the physician (or physicians) designated below determine that I lack sufficient understanding or capacity to make or communicate decisions relating to my health care and will continue in effect during my incapacity, until my death. This determination shall be made by the following physician (or physicians). (You may include here a designation of your choice, including your attending physician, or any other physician. You may also name two or more physicians, if desired, both of whom must make this determination before the authority granted to the Health Care Agent becomes effective.)

    A. First Physician's Name:

    Address:

    Work Telephone No.

    Home Telephone No.

    B. Second Physician's Name:

    Address:

    Work Telephone No.

    Home Telephone No.

3. General Statement of Authority Granted. I hereby grant to my Health Care Agent named above full power and authority to make health care decisions on my behalf.

My Health Care Agent is authorized in my Health Care Agent's sole and absolute discretion to exercise the powers granted herein relating to matters involving my health and medical care. In exercising such powers, my Health Care Agent should first try to discuss with me the specifics of any proposed decision regarding my medical care and treatment if I am able to communicate in any manner, however rudimentary. My Health Care Agent is further instructed to give, withhold or withdraw consent to any medical treatment for me based upon any treatment choices that I have expressed while competent, whether under this document or otherwise. If my Health Care Agent cannot determine the treatment choice I would want made under the circumstances, then my Health Care Agent should make such choice for me based upon what my Health Care Agent believes to be in my best interests.

My Health Care Agent shall have the following powers and authority:

    A. To request, review, and receive any information, verbal or written, regarding my physical or mental health, including, but not limited to, medical and hospital records, and to consent to the disclosure of this information.

    B. To employ and discharge medical personnel including physicians, psychiatrists, dentists, nurses, and therapists as my Health Care Agent shall deem necessary for my physical, mental and emotional well-being, and to pay them (or cause to be paid to them) reasonable compensation.

    C. To consent to and authorize my admission to and discharge from a hospital, nursing or convalescent home, or other institution.

    D. To give consent for, to withdraw consent for, or to withhold consent for x-ray, anesthesia, medication, surgery, and all other diagnostic and treatment procedures ordered by or under the authorization of a licensed physician, dentist or podiatrist. This authorization specifically includes the power to consent to measures for relief of pain.

Figure 15-2. Health care power of attorney.

E. To authorize the withholding or withdrawal of life-sustaining procedures when and if my physician determines that I am terminally ill, permanently in a coma, suffer severe dementia, or am in a persistent vegetative state. Life-sustaining procedures are those forms of medical care that only serve to artificially prolong the dying process and may include mechanical ventilation, dialysis, antibiotics, artificial nutrition and hydration, and other forms of medical treatment which sustain, restore or supplant vital bodily functions. Life-sustaining procedures do not include care necessary to provide comfort or alleviate pain.

> **I DESIRE THAT MY LIFE NOT BE PROLONGED BY**
> **LIFE-SUSTAINING PROCEDURES IF I AM TERMINALLY**
> **ILL, PERMANENTLY IN A COMA, SUFFER SEVERE**
> **DEMENTIA OR AM IN A PERSISTENT VEGETATIVE STATE.**

F. To exercise my right of privacy and my right to make decisions regarding my medical treatment even though the exercise of my rights might hasten my death or be against conventional medical advice.

G. To consent to and arrange for the administration of pain-relieving drugs of any kind or other surgical or medical procedures calculated to relieve my pain, including unconventional pain-relief therapies which my Health Care Agent believes may be helpful, even though such drugs or procedures may lead to permanent physical damage, addiction or hasten the moment of (but not intentionally cause) my death.

H. To exercise any right I may have to make a disposition of any part or all of my body for medical purposes, to donate my organs, to authorize an autopsy, and to direct the disposition of my remains.

I. To take any lawful actions that may be necessary to carry out these decisions, including the granting of releases of liability to medical providers.

4. Special Provisions and Limitations. *Notice:* **The above grant of power is intended to be as broad as possible so that your Health Care Agent will have authority to make any decisions you could make to obtain or terminate any type of health care. If you wish to limit the scope of your Health Care Agent's powers, you may do so in this section.**

In exercising the authority to make health care decisions on my behalf, the authority of my Health Care Agent is subject to the following special provisions and limitations: (Here you may include any specific limitations you deem appropriate such as your own definition of when life-sustaining treatment should be withheld or discontinued, or instructions to refuse any specific types of treatment that are inconsistent with your religious beliefs, or unacceptable to you for any other reason)

_____

_____

_____

5. Guardianship Provision. If it becomes necessary for a court to appoint a guardian of my person, I nominate my Health Care Agent acting under this document to be the guardian of my person, to serve without bond or security.

6. Reliance of Third Parties on Health Care Agent.

A. No person who relies in good faith upon the authority of or any representations by my Health Care Agent shall be liable to me, my estate, my heirs, successors, assigns, or personal representatives, for actions or omissions by my Health Care Agent.

B. The powers conferred on my Health Care Agent by this document may be exercised by my Health Care Agent alone, and my Health Care Agent's signature or act under the authority granted in this document may be accepted by persons as fully authorized by me and with the same force and effect as if I were personally present, competent, and acting on my own behalf. All acts performed in good faith by my Health Care Agent pursuant to this Power of Attorney are done with my consent and shall have the same validity and effect as if I were present and exercised the powers myself and shall inure to the benefit of and bind me, my estate, my heirs, successors, assigns, and personal representatives. The authority of my Health Care Agent pursuant to this Power of Attorney shall be superior to and bind upon my family, relatives, friends and others.

7. Miscellaneous Provisions.

A. I revoke any prior health care Power of Attorney.

B. My Health Care Agent shall be entitled to sign, execute, deliver, and acknowledge any contract or other document that may be necessary, desirable, convenient, or proper in order to exercise and carry out any of the powers described in this document and to incur reasonable costs on my behalf incident to the exercise of these powers; provided, however, that except as shall be necessary in order to exercise the powers described in this document relating to my health care, my Health Care Agent shall not have any authority over my property or financial affairs.

C. My Health Care Agent and my Health Care Agent's estate, heirs, successors and assigns are hereby released and forever discharged by me, my estate, my heirs, successors, and assigns and personal representatives from all liability from and all claims or demands of all kinds arising out of the acts or omissions of my Health Care Agent pursuant to this document, except for the willful misconduct or gross negligence.

D. No act or omission of my Health Care Agent, or of any other person, institution, or facility acting in good faith in reliance on the authority of my Health Care Agent pursuant to this Health Care Power of Attorney shall be considered suicide, nor the cause of my death for any civil or criminal purposes, nor shall it be considered unprofessional conduct or as lack of professional competence. Any person, institution, or facility against whom criminal or civil liability is asserted because of conduct authorized by this Health Care Power of Attorney may interpose this document as a defense.

8. Signature of Principal. By signing here, I indicate that I am mentally alert and competent, fully informed as to the contents of this document, and understand the full import of this grant of powers to my Health Care Agent.

_____   _____ (SEAL)

Date

Figure 15-2. Continued

9. Signature of Witnesses. I hereby state that the Principal, _____ being of sound mind, signed the foregoing Health Care Power of Attorney in my presence, and that I am not related to the principal by blood or marriage, and I would not be entitled to any portion of the state of the principal under any existing will or codicil of the principal or as an heir under the Intestate Succession Act, if the principal died on this date without a will. I also state that I am not the principal's attending physician, nor an employee of the principal's attending physician, nor an employee of the health facility in which the principal is a patient, nor an employee of a nursing home or any group care home where the principal resides. I further state that I do not have any claim against the principal.

_____   _____ (SEAL)
Date   Witness

_____   _____ (SEAL)
Date   Witness

STATE OF NORTH CAROLINA

COUNTY OF MECKLENBURG

CERTIFICATE

I, _____ , a Notary Public for Mecklenburg County, North Carolina, hereby certify that _____ appeared before me and swore to me and to the witnesses in my presence that this instrument is a Health Care Power of Attorney, and that she willingly and voluntarily made and executed it as her free act and deed for the purposes expressed in it.

I further certify that _____ and _____ , witnesses, appeared before me and swore that they witnessed _____ sign the attached Health Care Power of Attorney, believing her to be of sound mind; and also swore that at the time they witnessed the signing (i) they were not related within the third degree to her or her spouse, and (ii) they did not know nor have a reasonable expectation that they would be entitled to any portion of her estate upon her death under any will or codicil thereto then existing or under the Intestate Succession Act as it provided at that time, and (iii) they were not a physician attending her, nor an employee of an attending physician, nor an employee of a health facility in which she was a patient, nor an employee of a nursing home or any group-care home in which she resided, and (iv) they did not have a claim against her. I further certify that I am satisfied as to the genuineness and due execution of the instrument.

This the _____ day of _____ , 1991.

(NOTARY SEAL)

_____
Notary Public
My Commission expires: _____

NOTICE: A copy of this form should be given to your Health Care Agent and any alternate named in this Power of Attorney and to your physician and family members.

I, _____ agree to act as Health Care Agent for _____ pursuant to this Health Care Power of Attorney.
This the _____ day of _____ , 1991.

_____ (SEAL)
Health Care Agent

I, _____ agree to act as Health Care Agent for _____ pursuant to this Health Care Power of Attorney.
This the _____ day of _____ , 1991.

_____ (SEAL)
Health Care Agent

I, _____ agree to act as Health Care Agent for _____ pursuant to this Health Care Power of Attorney.
This the _____ day of _____ , 1991.

_____ (SEAL)
Health Care Agent

Figure 15-2. Continued

MEDICAL DIRECTIVE

I, _____ being of sound mind, make this statement as a directive to be followed if I am ever unable to participate in decisions regarding my medical care. Should I become mentally incompetent because of a medical condition like a coma or persistent vegetative state or severe dementia and my doctors do not expect me to recover, I direct the following treatment decisions be made in my behalf. These directions express my legal right to refuse treatment.

	YES	NO	UNSURE
1. **CPR:** Use drugs, electric shock and artificial breathing to bring me back to life when my heart stops.	____	____	____
2. **Mechanical breathing:** Use a machine to do my breathing for me when I cannot breathe unaided.	____	____	____
3. **Artificial nutrition:** Give me food through a tube in my vein or my stomach.	____	____	____
4. **Artificial hydration:** Give me liquid through a tube in my vein.	____	____	____
5. **Hospitalization:** Move me from home or hospice or nursing home to a hospital.	____	____	____
6. **Major surgery:** Operate on something like a blockage in my stomach or remove my gall bladder.	____	____	____
7. **Kidney dialysis:** Have a machine do the work of my kidneys—cleansing my blood—when they stop working on their own.	____	____	____
8. **Chemotherapy:** Give me drugs to fight cancer.	____	____	____
9. **Minor surgery:** Operate on something minor like an infected toe.	____	____	____
10. **Major tests:** Do tests like heart catheterization or colonoscopy to see what's wrong inside me.	____	____	____
11. **Blood:** Transfuse blood or blood products into me if I am in need of them.	____	____	____
12. **Antibiotics:** Give me drugs to fight diseases like pneumonia or a kidney infection.	____	____	____
13. **Minor tests:** Do an x-ray or a blood test to see what's wrong with me.	____	____	____
14. **Pain medication:** Give me enough medication so that I am not in pain.	____	____	____
15. **Home:** Move me from the hospital so that I can die at home.	____	____	____
16. **Other:** _____			

I provide this directive in addition to my living will.

Signed _____   Date _____

Witness _____

Witness _____

Figure 15-3.   Medical directive.

ment or a psychiatric disorder but give a factual guide about the least painful and most effective measures. Violent methods such as shooting, jumping, or hanging are counseled against because they are too traumatic for the survivors.

In contrast, the Samaritans, an international suicide prevention group and professionals who work in hospice care and the medical association of each country have been sharply critical of such manuals, believing that they may pressure terminally ill, depressed, or elderly people to exit early because they believe they are a burden and unwanted. It is as if society fosters rejection instead of seeking solutions to the problem.

For more information on the types of euthanasia and the moral-ethical issues, see the references at the end of this chapter (3, 5, 11, 15, 17, 26, 28, 34, 38, 41, 42, 47, 48, 52–55, 60, 64, 78, 81). Many other references are available, for much has been written about dying and death. This chapter gives only an overview of the subject.

Withholding food and water or discontinuing a feeding tube and intravenous fluids to the chronically or terminally ill or those in a persistent vegetative state is a form of passive euthanasia and is of growing ethical concern for nurses. The nurse is taught to be an advocate for the client—a very special charge and a difficult but committed kind of caring related to client's needs and rights.

Several legal cases concerning clients in a persistent vegetative state surviving solely because of the use of

DECLARATION OF A DESIRE FOR A NATURAL DEATH

I, _____ being of sound mind, desire that, as specified below, my life not be prolonged by extraordinary means or by artificial nutrition or hydration if my condition is determined to be terminal and incurable or if I am diagnosed as being in a persistent vegetative state. I am aware and understand that this writing authorizes a physician to withhold or discontinue extraordinary means or artificial nutrition or hydration, in accordance with my specifications set forth below:

(Initial any of the following as desired):

          If my condition is determined to be terminal and incurable, I authorize the following:

_____   My physician may withhold or discontinue extraordinary means only.

            In addition to withholding or discontinuing extraordinary means if such means are necessary, my physician may withhold or discontinue either artificial nutrition or hydration, or both.

          If my physician determines that I am in a persistent vegetative state, I authorize the following:

_____   My physician may withhold or discontinue extraordinary means only.

            In addition to withholding or discontinuing extraordinary means if such means are necessary, my physician may withhold or discontinue either artificial nutrition or hydration, or both.

This the _____ day of _____ , 1991.

I hereby state that the Declarant, _____ being of sound mind, signed the above Declaration in my presence and that I am not related to the Declarant by blood or marriage and that I do not know or have a reasonable expectation that I would be entitled to any portion of the estate of the Declarant under any existing Will or Codicil of the Declarant or as an heir under the Intestate Succession Act if the Declarant died on this date without a Will. I also state that I am not the Declarant's physician, or an employee of any health facility in which the Declarant is a patient or an employee of a nursing home or any group-care home where the Declarant resides. I further state that I do not now have any claim against the Declarant.

WITNESS our hands and seals this the _____ day of _____ , 1991.

_____(SEAL)
Witness

_____(SEAL)
Witness

CERTIFICATE

I, _____ , Notary Public for Mecklenburg County, North Carolina, hereby certify that _____ the Declarant, appeared before me and swore to me and to the witnesses in my presence that this instrument is her Declaration of a Desire For a Natural Death, and that she had willingly and voluntarily made and executed it as her free act and deed for the purposes therein expressed.

I further certify that _____ and _____ , witnesses, appeared before me and swore that they witnessed _____ the Declarant, sign the attached Declaration, believing her to be of sound mind; and also swore that at the time they witnessed the Declaration (i) they were not related within the third degree to the declarant or to the Declarant's spouse, and (ii) they did not know or have a reasonable expectation that they would be entitled to any portion of the estate of the Declarant upon the Declarant's death under any Will of the Declarant or Codicil thereto then existing or under the Intestate Succession Act as it provides at that time, and (iii) they were not a physician attending the Declarant or an employee of an attending physician or an employee of a nursing home or any group-care home in which the Declarant resided, and (iv) they did not have a claim against the Declarant. I further certify that I am satisfied as to the genuineness and due execution of the Declaration.

This the _____ day of _____ ,

(Notary Seal)

_____
Notary Public for Mecklenburg
County, North Carolina

My Commission expires: _____

Figure 15-4.   Declaration of a desire for a natural death.

respirators and tube feeding have come before the courts, beginning with the Karen Quinlan case in 1977. At least two thirds of the court rulings in these cases have allowed the removal of the life-support equipment. Many of these people were chronically ill. The cases of Nancy Cruzan and Christine Busalacchi in Missouri are two recent cases involving discontinuance of feeding and hydration. Nancy Cruzan died in 1990, 12 days after a Missouri judge ruled that her feeding tube be discontinued since three previous coworkers testified that she had said she "never wanted to live life as a vegetable." In 1991 the Missouri legislature began to study bills that would legalize euthanasia for an expanded group of physically and chronically ill clients. These bills include the Durable Power of Attorney, Health Care Surrogate, and Health Care Consent bills. The Hemlock Society believes people should be allowed to die. In fact, the society advocates lethal injection as more humane with less suffering. The International Anti-Euthanasia Task Force believes such action is the forerunner for outright killing of sick, disabled, and vulnerable people, rather than having a society and professionals committed to caring for these people. The questions to decide concern who will die when and who will decide (40).

When caring for such ill clients, the clients and the nurses often see meaning in the person's life; to terminate that life would be against what nursing represents. What will be the effects on the nurse of carrying out euthanasia orders? What if the nurse refuses? Nursing is a caring profession. Can caring nurses be educated to participate in planned killing?

The nursing profession has a great deal at stake, and the members of the American Nurses' Association (and the nurses who are not members) need to speak out. Nurses must decide the meaning of being a nurse and how that meaning applies to caring for the seriously, chronically, terminally, or vegetatively ill. Further, nurses must:

1. Listen carefully to clients and families about their concerns.
2. Educate society to think and act rationally.
3. Act on spiritual convictions about the sanctity of life and health.
4. Engage in research about the life-promotion effects of imagery, faith, prayer, anointing with oil, and other spiritual or emotional methods of healing.
5. Publicize healing events, including the "miracles" so that clients and families can be encouraged and believe in remission and recovery.
6. Let live and let die, discerning when the fight must be for life and when death is inevitable, acceptable, and natural; discerning when to engage in life extension and when to continue life support.

CASE SITUATION: Issues in Death and Dying

Mrs. Morton is a 94-year-old widow who has resided in the same farmhouse since her marriage in the early 1920s. She has had a history of cardiac disease for approximately 45 years. She now has a pacemaker and daily takes medication for her heart. She has had a bilateral modified mastectomy but has had no further recurrence of cancer. Several times she has been hospitalized, and during the last two hospitalizations she required resuscitation after suffering cardiac arrest.

Mrs. Morton is a very determined, devout, Christian woman, and each time she has been gravely ill, she has proclaimed her faith and has been discharged to her home. She firmly refused admittance to a senior residence center after the last hospitalization, insisting that if she had a visiting nurse and continued help from her grandson, she could live alone in her farm home. Her grandson, who has shopped for her for the last 10 years, agreed to do more tasks as necessary. Reluctantly, her physician agreed and ordered home health aide and nurse services. Because of her grave condition and inability to walk except for a few steps, the physician also made occasional home visits.

Mrs. Morton is chronically ill. In fact, her cardiovascular condition is so grave that she is considered terminally ill. According to the euthanasia movement, she should have been allowed to die the last time she required resuscitation. *How wrong that perspective would have been.*

In the 9 months since her discharge, Mrs. Morton has regained her strength, and her circulation has improved. She now walks in her home with a walker and cooks meals for herself and her grandson. She does receive help with bathing and vacuuming. Thus she contributes to the employment of several people. Recently her divorced granddaughter, Jean, and two great-grandchildren have come to live with her because Jean is on welfare and cannot pay the rent and other expenses.

Mrs. Morton acknowledges that having three more people in her home is stressful but says she believes she must help them. She has loaned, or given, considerable money from her farm income and Social Security check to all three of her grandchildren and several of her great-grandchildren. Thus she contributes to the economic support of three, and sometimes more, people. She doubts that anyone will ever repay her.

Because Mrs. Morton is very alert, friendly, indeed very wise, she is a joy to visit. When her many friends come to visit, she shares a piece of cake she has baked and chats about local news. She reminisces some, but not excessively. She seldom complains, even briefly. Although her physical condition is marginal, her mental health is excellent. Possibly because of those healthy components, her physical condition has improved. Mrs. Morton is very much alive and looking forward to her ninety-fifth birthday. It is fortunate the emergency team responded by resuscitating Mrs. Morton during her last hospitalization. Indeed, many people would have felt the loss.

It is important for you to struggle with the values and issues of death—accidental death, long-term dying, active or passive euthanasia, and right-to-die choices— and consequently the issues and values of life. You will often be asked about your thoughts and beliefs; it is impossible to be valuefree, but you can be nonjudgmental and accepting of another's values. How you proceed with nursing care of the chronically ill or dying person will be influenced by your beliefs. Do not force your beliefs and values on another, but often the client will appreciate your open sharing of values and beliefs. Such sharing may even give him or her energy to continue to live—with quality of life—against overwhelming odds. *Certainly do all possible so that the person does not face dying and death alone.*

DEVELOPMENTAL CONCEPTS OF DEATH

To understand how adults and aged persons perceive death, a review is given here of how the child, adolescent, and adult perceive death. The concept of death is understood differently by persons in the different life eras because of general maturity, experience, ability to form ideas, and understanding of cause and effect.

Children's Concepts of Death

Nagy (63) found three stages in the child's concept of death: (1) death is reversible—until age 5 years; (2) death is personified—ages 5 to 9; and (3) death is final and inevitable—after age 9 or 10.

The child less than 5 sees death as reversible, a temporary departure like sleep, being less alive, very still, or unable to move. There is much curiosity about what happens to the person after death. The child connects death with funerals, with cemeteries, and absence. He or she thinks dead persons are still capable of growth, that they can breathe and eat and feel, and that they know what is happening on earth. Death is disturbing because it separates people from each other and because life in the grave seems dull and unpleasant. Fear of death in the child of this age may be related to parental expression of anger; presence of intrafamily stress such as arguing and fighting; physical restraints, especially during illness; or punishment for misdeeds. At times the child feels anger toward the parents because of their restrictions and wishes they would go away or be dead. Guilt feelings arising from these thoughts may add to the fear of death (56, 63).

The child from ages 5 to 9 accepts the existence of death as final and not like life. He or she thinks of death as a person such as an angel, a frightening clown, or monster who carries off people, usually bad people, in the night. Personal death can be avoided; he or she will not die if he or she runs faster than Death, locks the door, or tricks Death unless there is bad luck. Parental

disciplining techniques inadvertently add to this belief if they threaten that bad things will happen to the child. Traumatic situations also can arouse fear of death (63).

The child after ages 9 or 10 realizes that death is inevitable, final, happens according to certain laws, and will one day happen to him or her. Death is the end of life, like the withering of flowers or falling of leaves, and results from internal processes. Death is associated with being enclosed in a coffin without air, being slowly eaten by bugs, and slow rotting unless cremation is taught. The child may express thoughts about an afterlife, depending on ideas expressed by parents and other adults and their religious philosophy (56, 63, 73).

Death is an abstract concept, and Nagy's stages offer a guide. However, not all children's thinking about death fits into those stages. Children (and adults) may have a concept of death that contains ideas from all three stages. The ability to think abstractly is acquired slowly and to varying degrees by different people. Usually the child is unable to understand death until he or she is preadolescent or in the chum stage, for until then he or she has not learned to care for someone else as much as for self.

The child's ideas and anxiety about separation and death and the ability to handle loss are influenced by many factors: experiences with rejecting or punitive parents; strong sibling rivalry; violence; loss, illness, or death in the family; the reaction and teaching of adults to separation or death; and ability to conceptualize and assimilate the experience (18).

The child may think of the parent's death as deliberate abandonment for which he or she is responsible and expect death to get him or her next. The child may fear death is catching and for that reason avoid a friend whose parent has just died. If the child perceives death as sleep, he or she may fear sleep to the point of being unable to go to bed at night or even to nap. He or she may blame the surviving parent for the other parent's death, a feeling that is compounded when the surviving parent is so absorbed in personal grief that little attention is given to the child. The child may use magical thinking, believing that wishing to have the parent return will bring the parent back (18).

The child's fascination with and fear of death may be expressed through the games he or she plays or concern about sick pets or a dead person. Short-lived pets such as fish or gerbils help the child deal with death. Parents should handle these concerns and the related questions in a relaxed, loving manner (75).

Self-Knowledge of Death

Can the sick child realize personal approaching death? Waechter's study (79) showed that despite widespread efforts by adults to shield sick children from awareness of their diagnosis of cancer and the inevitability of death, the school-aged children in her study knew of their impending death, although they might not say so directly to their parents. The evasiveness and false cheerfulness of the adults, either parents or staff, did not hide their real feelings from the child.

Often children know more about death than adults may realize. Children are harmed by what they do not know, by what they are not told, and by their misconceptions. Parents should monitor the child's television viewing carefully, for programs often give an unrealistic impression of death, for example, cartoons and movies that show that death is reversible (or that there is survival or no harmful effects after obviously lethal injuries).

Children's Attendance at Funerals

There are age-based guidelines for a child's involvement in a funeral. Children from 2 to 3 can view the body or be given a brief explanation, depending on their level of understanding and relationship to the deceased. But 3- to 6-year-olds benefit from a short private funeral home visit or the service itself. Seven- to 9-year-old children should attend the funeral unless they resist. Eleven- and 12-year-olds should be included in making the arrangements and the funeral service itself. In the teen years friends of the adolescent should be encouraged to share the grief, and all should be treated as adults.

Suggestions for discussing death with children are presented in Box 15–1.

Other research is finding similar results about children and the subject of death (12, 18, 24, 26, 27, 29, 30, 43, 49, 56, 82). Although it is not easy for adults to talk with children about death, the book, *Talking About Death: A Dialogue Between Parent and Child,* by Grollman (34) is a helpful reference.

Adolescents' Concept of Death

The adolescent is concerned about a personal future and is relatively realistic in thinking, but because of dependency-independency conflicts with parents and efforts to establish individuality, he or she has a low tolerance for accepting death. The healthy young person seldom thinks about death, particularly as something that will happen to the self. He or she fears a lingering death and usually views death in religious or philosophic terms. He or she believes death means lack of fulfillment; there is too much to lose with death (24, 43, 56).

Because of inexperience in coping with crisis and the viewpoints of death, the adolescent may not cry at the death of a loved one or parent. Instead he or she may continue to play games, listen to records, withdraw into seclusion or vigorous study, or go about usual activities. If the young person cannot talk, such activities provide a catharsis. Mastery of feelings sometimes comes through a detailed account of the parent's death to a peer or by displacing grief feelings onto a pet. Also, the adolescent may fantasize the dead parent as perfect or

---

■ BOX 15-1.
Dos and Don'ts for Discussing Death With Children

Do

- Ask the child what he or she is feeling. Bring up the subject of death naturally in the context of a dead pet, a book character, television show, movie, or news item.
- Help the child have a funeral for a dead pet.
- Help the child realize he or she is not responsible for the death.
- Tell the child what has happened on his or her level (but not in morbid detail).
- Explain the funeral service briefly beforehand; attendance depends on the child's age and wishes.
- Answer questions honestly, with responses geared to the child's age.
- Remember that expressions of pain, anger, loneliness or aloneness do not constitute symptoms of an illness but are part of a natural process of grieving.
- Help the child realize that the adults are also grieving and feel upset, anger, despair, and guilt.

Do not

- Admonish the child not to cry; it is a universal way to show grief and anxiety.
- Tell a mystical story about the loss of the person; it could cause confusion and anxiety.
- Give long, exclusively detailed explanations beyond the level of understanding.
- Associate death with sleep, which could result in chronic sleep disturbances.
- Force the child to attend funerals or ignore signs of grieving in the child.

---

feel much the way a child would about loss of a parent. Often the adolescent's behavior hides the fact that he or she is in mourning. Be attuned to the thoughts and feelings of the adolescent who has faced death of a loved one so that you can be approachable and helpful.

Adult Concepts of Death

The adult's attitudes toward and concept about dying and death are influenced by cultural and religious backgrounds. A number of references can provide information (1, 7, 10, 16, 24, 40, 44, 50, 53). The adult's reactions to death are also influenced by whether the death event is sudden or has been anticipated. Fear of death is often more related to the process of dying than to the fact of death—to mutilation, deformity, isolation, pain, loss of control over body functions and one's life, fear of the unknown, and permanent collapse and disintegration. Premonitions about coming death, sometimes correct, may occur.

Anticipation of Death

There are four responses to viewing death: positivist, negativist, activist, and passivist. Fear of death is less in the person who believes that most of the valued goals have been attained. This person is likely to reflect positively on present activities and death as an aspect of the future and is referred to as a *positivist*. If the person believes that the time left is short, fears loss of ego integration, wishes that he or she could relive part of life, and fears death, the person is referred to as a *negativist*. A person may perceive death as diminishing the opportunity for continued fulfillment of goals. The achieved goals do not offset the fear of death. Death as a foreclosing of ambition is more distasteful than the prospect of loss of life. A person with such an attitude is referred to as an *activist*. Finally, the person may not view death with concern or fear but as a respite from disappointments of life because attempts to attain life goals may have been so overshadowed by failure. Death may be accepted as a positive adjustment to life. Such a person is referred to as a *passivist* (46).

Keith (46) researched changes in four life areas—change in marital status, health, church involvement, and informal family and friend contacts—in relation to perceptions of life and death. In this study women were more likely to be positivists, and men were more likely to be negativists. Persons with lower incomes were more likely to be passivists and negativists than persons with higher incomes. Married men were more likely to be activists and positivists, although change in marital status was not associated with women's perceptions. Men who experienced change in health tended to be negativists, whereas women whose health had deteriorated were as likely to be positivists as negativists. Women who experienced continuity in health remained positivists. Continuity in church involvement gave no assurance of fostering positive attitudes toward death in men; but women who participated regularly were likely to be positivists, deriving comfort from their religion. Persons with continuous support from social participation more often had positive attitudes toward life. Persons who experienced discontinuity in life were more likely to be negativists or passivists. Women often expressed acceptance of death and less death anxiety than men. Women were more likely to perceive death as another beginning, and men perceived death as an end. In the low-income family in which care of an ill spouse is undertaken by the family, death may be perceived as a release.

Women are more likely to integrate widowhood than are men, and greater stability of friendships through the life cycle eases adaptation to loss of spouse. The widow is likely to seek intimacy with same-sexed friends, who replace family ties in late life.

The importance of will to live, or lack of it, has been recognized by nurses and others for many years.

The person may not be terminally ill yet, because of loss of a loved one, loss of feelings of self-worth and usefulness, boredom, or disillusionment with life, may lose the will to live and rapidly decline and die. Often there are few or no causes for death apparent on autopsy. Some individuals, despite impending death, maintain hope and endurance and apparently refuse to die and live beyond the time of expected death. A person can program, through unconscious or conscious will, onset of illness, recovery from severe illness, or the time of death. A strong will to live is often associated with the person's being interested, involved, or active in life or having a loved one, spouse, or dependent whom he or she desires to be with or for whom he or she feels responsible. For some the death month is related to the birth month in that some people postpone death to witness their birthdays or another important holiday. The person with excessive fear of death may be unable to die until able to express and work through conscious fears or phobias (46).

Meaning of Death

To the adult facing death because of illness, particularly the elderly, death may have many meanings. Death may convey some positive meanings: a teacher of transcendental truths uncomprehended during life; an adventure; a friend who brings an end to pain and suffering; or an escape from an unbearable situation into a new life without the present difficulties. The great destroyer who is to be fought, punishment and separation, or a means of vengeance to force others to give more affection than they were willing to give in the past are examples of negative meanings (24).

The person who is dying may have suicidal thoughts or attempt suicide. Suicide is a rebellion against death, a way to cheat death's control over him or her.

One woman who had breast cancer spent 15 months planning her suicide. She wrote a book on her right to die when and as she wished, made a videotape, and collected her mementos for preservation after her death. Her last meal before she took a lethal dose of medicine included champagne and special sharing with her husband and son. This approach is repulsive and anti-Christian to some; see *The Illusion of Rational Suicide* published by the Hastings Center Report, December 1982, for a counterattack.

Cox (14) writes a poignant account of how one person made a choice about where and how he would die—making his death and the events leading to it a triumph—in a society in which society and health care professionals believe that the system is more important than the individual. She writes also of her feelings and beliefs and the ethical decision-making process involved in ensuring that his choice was carried out.

The time comes in an illness or in later life when both the person and the survivors-to-be believe death would be better than continuing to suffer. The client has the conviction that death is inevitable and desirable and works through feelings until finally he or she has little or no anxiety, depression, or conflicts about dying. The body becomes a burden, and death holds a promise. There is little incentive to live.

Recently in the United States the concept of death has been investigated by adults who are not necessarily facing immediate death of themselves or their loved ones. The stigma that formerly caused people to use euphemisms has been replaced with research involving attitudes toward death and classes on dying and death. For example, one study concluded that highly creative artists and scientists who believe they have successfully contributed their talents to society have little fear of death. Another example involves a religion professor who for several years has taught courses on death at two universities and has had to limit class size because of the subject's popularity. The students face their own concepts and fears about death, study various religious views and myths surrounding death, examine the possible stages of dying, and interview a dying person.

A phenomenon that has gained public interest through Moody's publication *Life After Life* (61) is the **near-death experience (NDE)** of *"coming back to life" after just being declared clinically dead or near dead.* The stories (those told to Moody and those heard before and since) have a sameness, although details and interpretation depend on the personality and beliefs of the person (61, 65, 66, 67, 83).

There is additional publicity about men and women of a wide range of age, education, background, religious and nonreligious belief, and temperament who came close to death or had a near-death experience and who, when recalling what had happened to them after they returned to consciousness, describe a sense of comfort, beauty, peace, and bliss. The person experienced being outside or separated from the body, communicating with deceased loved ones, gliding down a dark tunnel toward a bright light, and reaching a threshold but drawing back because of a sense of responsibility for others. The person longed to remain in this bliss, and the intensity of the experience affected the person's life thereafter in the earthly world. Most were convinced they had been in Paradise or in Heaven or in the presence of a Supreme and Loving Power and had a glimpse of life to come, regardless of prior religious beliefs. Death is no longer feared. Life is seen as precious and meaningful.

Researchers Michael Sabon, a cardiologist at Emery University, Kenneth Ring, Bruce Greyson, and Ian Stevenson, all psychiatrists, Fred Shoenmaker, physician in charge of Cardiovascular Services at St. Luke's Hospital in Denver, and Dr. Raymond Moody, Jr., have accumulated several thousand case studies to verify near-death experiences. Anesthesia, drugs, hallucinations, or wishful fantasies do not account for these experiences. Clinical death has been recorded by absence of electric ac-

tivity in the brain for 3 to 30 minutes in hundreds of subjects, although at times adequate brain function continued when heart function stopped. Often the person describes exactly what happened when the medical team was working to revive him or her as if the person were looking on from above. See also Orne's article (66).

Papowitz (67) describes near-death experiences that have been recounted by various people. She describes guidelines for caring for the person who is being resuscitated in light of the fact that the person may be able to hear and see what is happening. She describes ways to help the person talk about the near-death experience if it is recalled and the importance of listening and taking the necessary time to allow the person to express emotions. Respect that some people view this as a religious experience; some do not. Ask for permission to share the account with family members as a way to enrich their understanding.

This trend toward talking about, investigating, and studying death points to a willingness to confront finally an absolute fact: Each of us will die.

There is evidence of life after death. Each person must integrate this information and come to terms with it in his or her own life.

BEHAVIOR AND FEELINGS OF THE PERSON FACING DEATH

When death comes accidentally and swiftly, there is no time to prepare for death. However, death is a normal, expected event to the old, and studies show that most old people anticipate death with equanimity and without fear. The crisis is not death but where and how the person will die. Studies show that old persons living in their own homes or having adjusted to living in an institution do not fear death. Those who are close to death and are on a waiting list for admission to an institution score the highest for fear of death. The prospect of dying under nonnormal, unexpected circumstances creates the crisis (58).

Widowhood is more expected after age 65; thus women who are over 65 show less mental or physical illness or immediate mortality than widows who are under 65 years. Mental illness in the widow is associated with self-blame, reports of having missed opportunities and having failed to live up to potentials, and with unexpected death of spouse (58). When the person approaches death gradually by virtue of many years lived or from a terminal illness, he or she will go through a predictable sequence of feelings and behavior.

Awareness of Dying

Glaser and Strauss (37) describe the stages of awareness that the terminally ill or dying person may experience, depending on the behavior of the health team and family, which, in turn, influences interaction with others. He or she may not be aware of the prognosis, may respect approaching death, or may be totally aware of diagnosis and prognosis.

Closed Awareness

Closed awareness *occurs when the person is dying but has neither been informed nor made the discovery*. He or she may not be knowledgeable about the signs of terminal illness, and the health team and family may not want the person to know for fear that "he will go to pieces."

Hospitals are designed to keep information from the client. Even other clients who know are likely to keep the information from him or her. The doctor and nursing staff spend less time with this client than other clients; topics of conversation are brief, direct, superficial, and about the present.

Maintaining closed awareness is less likely to occur if the dying person is at home. In the hospital it is maintained primarily to protect the health team and the family; yet the burden of keeping the prognosis a secret from the client becomes an ever-increasing strain. The only person who really is protected is the doctor, for the nurses who are with this client throughout the day find being deceitful increasingly difficult. The family may continue to pretend, but they are robbed of the opportunity to express openly and share the burden of grief with their loved one and helpful others. The client and family cannot support each other, nor can the staff fully support the client. The client and family have no opportunity to review their lives, plan realistically for the family's future, and close life with the proper rituals. Even legal and business transactions of the client may suffer as he or she tries to carry on life as usual, starts unrealistic plans, and works less feverishly on unfinished business than he or she would if the prognosis were known.

However, in spite of intentions and efforts of the health team and family, the client may become increasingly aware. He or she has a lot of time to observe the surroundings, even when very ill. Clients no doubt spend more time assessing the personnel and environment than the staff spends assessing them. He or she has time to think about the nonverbal cues and indirect comments from the staff, the inconsistent answers, the new and perplexing symptoms that do not get better in spite of reassurance that they will improve. Privileges that were previously denied are granted, and the client is subjected to a barrage of diagnostic and treatment procedures. At times the staff may relax their guard when they think he or she does not understand and say something about the prognosis that is understood. All these things help the person formulate the conclusion that he or she is very sick and perhaps even dying. Of course, if the person is kept sedated, as much to relieve the staff from having to face the client as to relieve the client's suffering, he or she may be less aware of the external cues.

Suspicious Awareness

Suspicious awareness *develops for the reasons previously described. The person may or may not voice suspicions to others, and they are likely to deny his or her verbal suspicions*. A contest for control develops, with the client on the offensive and the staff on the defensive.

The client watches more closely for signs to confirm suspicions. The changing physical status; the nonverbal and verbal communications of others, with their hidden meanings; the silence; the intensity of or challenges in care; and the briskness of conversation usually will inadvertently tell or imply what he or she suspects.

Now deceitfulness has fully developed. The client knows that he or she is dying but realizes that others do not know he or she knows.

Mutual Pretense

Mutual pretense *occurs when staff and family become aware that the client knows he or she is dying, but all continue to pretend otherwise*. There is no conversation about impending death unless the client initiates it, although on occasion staff members may purposely drop cues because they believe the client has a right to know.

Although the client now knows and can plan for the remaining life, this measure of dignity is offset because intimate relationships are denied. There is no one to talk with honestly, although all persons involved could benefit. Neither anticipatory grieving nor other preparation for death can be accomplished very well.

Open Awareness

Open awareness *exists when the person and family are fully aware of the terminal condition, although neither may realize the nearness nor all the complications of the condition and the mode of death*.

With the certainty of death established, the person may plan to end life in accord with personal ideas about proper dying, finish important work, and make appropriate plans for and farewells with the family. He or she and the family can talk frankly, make plans, share grief, and support each other. The anguish is not reduced but can be faced together.

The health team in the hospital has ideas, although not always verbalized, about how the person ought to die morally and stylistically. These ideas may conflict with or differ from the ideas of the client and family. The wishes of the client and the family should always have priority, particularly when they ask that no heroic measures be taken to prolong life. Extra privileges, special requests, or the client's discharge to the family can be granted. Most people wish to die without pain, with dignity, in privacy, and with loved ones nearby. Often dying in the hospital precludes both privacy and dignity, and the health team should continuously work to provide these rights.

But how? Research physicians, students, and other team members hover over the client as they attempt to learn more and to develop future treatments. Clients sometimes feel more like experimental animals than dignified human beings. Do you follow orders to prolong life with gadgetry or to hasten death with a lethal dose of medication? How do you decide what the client's rights are? What if they conflict with the doctor's orders? Does the health team work together on these matters?

One way to work through feelings, clarify ideas, and collaborate with other health-team members would be to suggest a seminar, or series of them, on the topic of death, to be attended by the team. Certain general guidelines could be set, based on the premise that the client should be granted the right to die as he or she wishes.

Sequence of Reactions to Approaching Death

When the person becomes aware of the diagnosis and prognosis, whether he or she is told directly or learns by advancing through the stages of awareness discussed previously, he or she and the family usually go through a predictable sequence of reactions described by Kübler-Ross (51).

Denial and Isolation

Denial and isolation are the initial and natural reactions when the person learns of terminal illness: "It can't be true. I don't believe it's me." The person may go through a number of rituals to support this denial, even to the point of finding another doctor. He or she needs time to mobilize resources. Denial serves as a necessary buffer against overwhelming anxiety.

The person is denying when he or she talks about the future; avoids talking about the illness or the death of self or others; or when he or she persistently pursues cheery topics. Recognize the client's need, respond to this behavior, and let him or her set the pace in conversation. Later the person will gradually consider the possibility of the prognosis; anxiety will lessen; and the need to deny will diminish.

Psychologic isolation occurs when the client talks about the illness, death, or mortality intellectually but without emotion as if these topics were not relevant. Initially the idea of death is recognized, although the feeling is repressed. Gradually feelings about death will be less isolated, and the client will begin to face death but still maintain hope.

If the client continues to deny for a prolonged time in spite of advancing symptoms, he or she will need much warmth, compassion, and support as death comes closer. Your contacts with the client may consist of sitting in silence, using touch communication, giving meticulous physical care, conveying acceptance and security, and looking in on him or her frequently. If denial is extensive, he or she cannot grieve or face the inevitable

separation. Yet Kübler-Ross (51) found that few persons maintain denial to the end of life.

Anger

The second reaction, anger, occurs with acknowledgment of the reality of the prognosis. It is necessary for an eventual acceptance of approaching death. As denial and isolation decrease, anger, envy, and resentment of the living are felt. In America direct expression of anger is unacceptable, so this stage is difficult for the client and others. Anger is displaced onto things or people: "The doctor is no good"; "the food is no good", "the hospital is no good"; "the nurses are neglectful"; and "people don't care." The family also bears the brunt of the anger.

Anger results when the person realizes life will be interrupted before he or she finishes everything planned. Everything reminds the person of life while he or she is dying, and he or she feels soon-to-be-forgotten. He or she may make angry demands, frequently ring the bell, manipulate and control others, and generally make the self heard. He or she is convincing self and others that he or she is not yet dead and forgotten.

Do not take the anger personally. The dying person whose life will soon end needs empathy. The person who is respected, understood, and given time and attention will soon lower the angry voice and decrease demands. The person will realize he or she is considered a valuable person who will be cared for and yet allowed to function at maximum potential as long as possible. Your calm approach will lower anxiety and defensive anger.

Bargaining

The third reaction, bargaining, occurs when the person tries to enter into some kind of agreement that may postpone death. He or she may try to be on the best behavior. He or she knows the bargaining procedure and hopes to be granted the special wish—an extension of life, preferably without pain. Although the person will initially ask for no more than one deadline or postponement of death, he or she will continue the good behavior and will promise to devote life to some special cause if he or she lives.

Bargaining may be life promoting. As the person continues to hope for life, to express faith in God's willingness to let him or her live, and to engage actively in positive, health-promoting practices, the body's physical defenses may be enhanced by mental or emotional processes yet unknown. This process may account for those not-so-uncommon cases in which the person has a prolonged, unexpected remission during a malignant disease process. Hope, which is involved in bargaining and which you can support, gives each person a chance for more effective treatment and care as new discoveries are made.

Depression

Depression is the fourth reaction and occurs when the person gets weaker, needs increasing treatment, and worries about mounting medical costs and even necessities. Role reversal and related problems add to the strain. Depression about past losses and the present condition; feelings of shame about the illness, sometimes interpreted as punishment for past deeds; and hopelessness enshroud the person and extend to the loved ones.

Depression is normal. The family and staff need to encourage the person by giving realistic praise and recognition, letting him or her express feelings of guilt, work through earlier losses, finish mourning, and build self-esteem. You will need to give more physical and emotional help as the person grows weaker. He or she should stay involved with the family as long as possible.

Preparatory Depression

Preparatory depression is the next stage and differs from the previous depression. Now the person realizes the inevitability of death and comes to desire the release from suffering that death can bring. He or she wishes to be a burden no more and recognizes that there is no hope of getting well. The person needs a time of preparatory grief to get ready for the final separation of impending loss—not only are loved ones going to lose him or her, but the person is losing all significant objects and relationships. The person reviews the meaning of life and searches for ways to share insights with the people most significant to him or her, sometimes including the staff. Often the fear that he or she cannot share aspects of life or valued material objects with people of his or her own choosing will cause greater concern than the diagnosis of a terminal illness or the knowledge of certain death. As the person thinks of what life has meant, he or she begins to get ready to release life, but not without feelings of grief. Often he or she will talk repetitiously to find a meaning in life.

The family and health team can either inhibit the person during this stage or promote emotional comfort and serene acceptance of death. The first reaction to depressed, grieving behavior and life review is to cheer him or her. This meets your needs but not those of the client. When the person is preparing for the impending loss of all love objects and relationships, behavior should be accepted and not changed. Acceptance of the final separation in life will not be reached unless he or she is allowed to express a life review and sorrow. There may be no need for words if rapport, trust, and a working nurse-client relationship have been previously established. A touch of the hand and a warm accepting silence are therapeutic. Too much interference with words, sensory stimuli, or burdensome visitors hinders rather than helps emotional preparation for death. If the person is ready to release life and die and others expect him or her to want to continue to live and be concerned about things, the person's own depression, grief, and turmoil are increased. He or she wishes quietly and gradually to disengage self from life and all that represents life. He or she may request few or no visitors and

modifications in the routines of care and repeatedly request no heroic measures to prolong life.

Honor the client's requests but at the same time promote optimum physical and emotional comfort and well-being. Explain the feelings and needs of the client to the family and other members of the health team so that they can better understand his or her behavior. The family should know that this depression is beneficial if the client is to die peacefully and that it is unrelated to their past or present behavior.

Acceptance

The final reaction, acceptance or a kind of resolution, comes if the person is given enough time, does not have a sudden, unexpected death, and is given some help in working through the previous reactions. He or she will no longer be angry or depressed about the fate and will no longer be envious or resentful of the living. He or she will have mourned the loss of many people and things and will contemplate the end with a certain degree of quiet expectation. Now the ultimate of ego integrity described by Erikson (23) becomes evident. Acceptance is difficult and takes time. It depends in part on the client's awareness of the prognosis of illness so that he or she can plan ahead—religiously, philosophically, financially, socially, and emotionally. This last stage is almost devoid of feeling.

The healthy aged person will also go through some aspects of the reactions discussed previously, for as the person grows old, he or she contemplates more frequently personal mortality and begins to work through feelings about it.

Whereas Kübler-Ross looks at the dying *person* with the family implied, Giacquinta (33) looks at the *family* with the dying person implied. Table 15–1 outlines the four main stages and the 10 phases that the family will experience from the time of diagnosis through the postdeath period.

Both the Kübler-Ross (50, 51) and the Giacquinta (33) models are helpful. They are built on observations of hundreds of dying persons and families, but you must not stereotype responses into these stages. Do not assume that everyone is experiencing each stage as the research results describe. Sometimes the person or family will not go through every one of these stages, and the stages will not always follow in this sequence. The person or family may remain in a certain stage or revert to earlier stages. Feelings related to several of the researched stages may exist; the person who has been told he or she has cancer and a limited time to live feels fear, loss of control over destiny, a discontinuity in life goals, a sense of future time being meaningless, and a sense of isolation. A magazine subscription is chosen 1 year at a time; the 20,000-mile guarantee on tires seems more appropriate than the 40,000-mile guarantee. Friends may react out of fear of disease contagion. Professional colleagues, relatives, and friends avoid talking about the

TABLE 15-1. FAMILY'S RESPONSE TO DYING AND DEATH

Four Main Stages	Family Experiences:	Nurse Can Foster:
Living With Terminal Illness Person learns diagnosis, tries to carry on as usual, undergoes treatment.	*Impact:* emotional shock, despair, disorganized behavior	
	Functional disruption: much time spent at hospital (if traditional surgery or treatment chosen), ignoring of home tasks and emotional needs, weakening of family structure, emotional isolation	Hope as different treatment methods are used, communication, seeking helpful resources, family cohesiveness
	Search for meaning: questioning why this happened; casting blame on various persons, deity, institutions, habits; realization that "Someday I will die too"	Security
	Informing others (family and friends): ascent from isolation, with moral and practical support—or feeling of rejection: others do not understand, do not care, or are afraid; possible need to retreat again into emotional isolation	Courage, reliable help, understanding of why some people cannot help
	Engaging emotions: beginning grieving, fearing loss of emotional control, assumption of roles once carried by dying person	Problem solving; idea that life will change but will be ongoing
Living—Dying Interval Person ceases to perform family roles, is cared for either at home or hospital. Person needs to come to terms with accomplishments and failures and to find renewed meaning in life.	*Reorganization:* firmer division of family tasks	Cooperation instead of competition; analysis to see if new role distribution is workable
	Framing memories: reviewing life of dying person—what he or she has meant and accomplished, new sense of family history, relinquishment of dependency on dying member	Focus on life review rather than only on what person is now
Bereavement Death occurs	*Separation:* absorption in loneliness of separation as person becomes unconscious	Intimacy among family members; release of grief as normal
	Mourning: guilt, "Could I have done more?"	
Reestablishment	*Expansion of the social network:* overcoming feelings of alienation and guilt	Looking back with acceptance and forward to new growth and socialization with a reunited, normally functioning family

condition, and the person does not bring up the subject out of deference not to burden them—or that may be all friends or relatives seem to want to discuss. Priorities change; family and close friends become more important. Gradually the person is able to plan for the not-too-far future. Money is less important. Negative friends are avoided. The person must adjust to fatigue, changes in body function or structure, effects of chemotherapy or radiation, the continuing treatment appointments, and the loss of control. Do not convey that the client or family should be in a certain stage or reacting a certain way. Avoid social and religious clichés. Rather, be a caring, concerned, available person, willing to do nondramatic, simple, but helpful tasks such as bringing the family member something to drink, watering the flowers sent by a friend, or offering to call a significant person. Equally important will be doing physical care procedures in a thorough but efficient manner so that visiting family members can spend as much time with their dying loved one as possible. Listen to feelings when the person wants to talk but do not probe. Megerle (58) writes a personal account of the difficulties of terminal illness and death for the surviving family members and makes suggestions how health care professionals can help.

Anniversary Reaction and Emotionally Invested Deadlines

The classic anniversary reaction is a psychodynamic pattern in a child who is sensitized by some emotional event—most severely by the death of the parent of the same sex when the child is between the ages of 2 and 16. The specific age of this child at the time of trauma is the key time marker. When the traumatized child grows into adulthood and has a child the same age as he or she was when originally traumatized, the stressful reaction occurs. This reaction also typically involves the age of the parent at the time the event occurred, and the exact date (day, month, year) of the event—these factors function as related emotionally invested markers. For example, a 54-year-old man who suffered a coronary occlusion after apparent good health, revealed that when he was 18 his 54-year-old father had died of a heart attack.

He had experienced hostilities toward his father, describing him as having a vicious temper and being responsible for the family's poverty. Now he was 54 and had an 18-year-old son. He blamed his heart attack on the hatred and tension between himself and his relatives. In short, this man had repeated the experience of his father and perhaps subconsciously brought it on himself through his unresolved feelings toward his father (25).

Emotionally invested deadlines are the result of the emotional investment of the individual into specific dates, events, and anniversaries. When such an emotionally invested date is reached, the person may react with varying degrees of psychologic stress, ranging from illness to death. Emotionally invested occasions are unique for each person, yet a characteristic in common is that all these dates and events have long-standing emotional meaning for these individuals. The choice of the date or event for the time of death seems fitting to the uniqueness of the person (25). For example, two of the first four presidents died on July 4, undoubtedly an emotionally invested event for them. The person appears to have psychologic vulnerability on an emotionally charged occasion; it is well known and accepted that an emotionally depressed or brooding client is a poor surgical risk.

Although anniversary reaction is classically seen in the middle-aged or aging person, emotionally invested deadlines may be seen at any age. Both phenomena, however, tend to increase with age as one accumulates more and more emotionally charged experiences.

Predilection to Death

The phenomenon of **predilection to death** is *seen in people who, although lacking any signs of emotional conflict, suicidal tendencies, severe depression, or panic, correctly anticipate their own deaths* (14). These persons are firmly convinced of their impending death yet feel no depression or anxiety toward it, regarding it as completely appropriate. Such clients are resigned to death—to fight against it is unthinkable, for death is a release from the burden of their life or body. It is significant that predilection clients experience a lack of close human relationships and emotional isolation from significant others during their terminal period. Death holds more appeal than life because it promises either a reunion with lost love, resolution of long conflict, or respite from anguish. Death is perceived as a release from continuing in a world in which there are no longer any emotional bonds; thus there is no fear, anxiety, or depression regarding its approach, but rather a distinctly eager and expectant attitude toward its swift occurrence. Research shows that death comes to the predilection clients just as they have anticipated it would, although

medically their condition does not warrant such a quick demise or in some cases, any death at all (6, 11, 18, 25, 52, 55, 60, 80).

"Scared to Death" (Death by Autosuggestion)

Unlike the predilection client, who, convinced of impending death, anticipates it, the scared-to-death individual does not see death as appropriate (2, 8, 20, 70, 71). He or she believes self the victim of a curse or prediction and therefore cannot be saved by anyone or by any means. Psychic death is said to occur when a person is convinced of and accurately predicts his or her own death when no medical cause for death exists. Autosuggestion is the most accurate description for the cause of psychic death; it implies that the person responded in such a way as to convince self of imminent death. A synonym for autosuggestion might be "self-hypnosis." Death without any apparent organic cause has been documented to have occurred as a result of belief in voodoo, curses, predictions (fortune tellers, psychics, clairvoyants), premonitions, and dreams predicting death. Two types of behavior are exhibited by persons who are scared to death: (1) in some individuals after a suggestion of impending death, a panic reaction occurs, and they literally die of fright; or (2) the person may take the suggestion calmly, believe it to be useless to resist, give up, and simply die. Death by fright or autosuggestion can occur at any age; Baker (2) cites the case of a 3-year-old boy who died of fright after being caught in a rainstorm.

Fear is one of the strongest of emotions and has very definite and demonstrable effects on body homeostasis, particularly the cardiovascular and endocrine systems, which prepare the body to defend itself physically or escape. Several physiologic causes have been suggested for voodoo and other deaths resulting solely from the conviction of death. Cannon (8), one of the first researchers of voodoo death, proposed that death was the result of a state of shock due to persistent overactivity of the sympathicoadrenal system, with continuous outpouring of adrenaline and rapid depletion of the adrenal corticosteroid hormones. Cannon reviewed voodoo deaths in primitive cultures in South America, Africa, Australia, New Zealand, Haiti, and some Pacific Islands. Richter (71) and Engel (20) assumed such deaths were the result of complete surrender and loss of hope, the expectation of death, the giving up–given up phenomenon with parasympathetic system failure. Rahe and Romo (70) have correlated illness and death with overwhelming life events. Sudden deaths do not occur only in primitive societies. They occur in more developed societies as the result of acute or accumulating stress after rejection, separation, or loss and the consequent feelings of hopelessness and helplessness. Beliefs may be planted by family or culture during the formative years and later in life as posthypnotic suggestions that are acted out. Removal of support systems and the violation of shared belief systems may cause a sense of rejection, abandonment, and hopelessness, with death as the consequence. Immaturity, suggestibility, infantile dependency, external locus of control, and fatalistic orientation are individual variables observed in relation with sudden death. Sudden death may be the result of a complex of psychologic, social, and biologic factors (20, 71). Richter (71) proposed that death from autosuggestion resulted from overstimulation of the parasympathetic, rather than the sympathetic, autonomic nervous system and that cardiac arrest had resulted from excessive stimulation of the vagus nerves. Rigidity is one of the first human responses to fear; hence intense panic could lead to a state of body rigidity, with cessation of respiration leading to cerebral anoxia, cardiac arrest, and death (2).

Be aware that voodoo, premonitions, dreams, and predictions are taken seriously by some people and are practiced as a part of health care in some cultures. Do not discount the impact of such phenomenon. Listen carefully to what the client and family say and do.

Legal Planning for Death

While the person is still healthy and capable of making the many decisions in relation to death, he or she can do much to relieve worries and take the burden of those decisions off others. You are in a position to give the following information to others as indicated.

Although not legally binding, the Living Will (see Fig. 15–1) is being used by increasing numbers of people (see "Right-to-die Movement" section in this chapter).

Representatives from some nursing and funeral homes and cemeteries are educating people to keep a folder, revised periodically, of all information that will be used by those making arrangements at the time of death. Such a folder might include names of advisors such as attorney, banker, life-insurance broker, and accountant. Personal and vital information should be included such as birth certificate, marriage license, military-discharge papers, and copies of wills, including willing of body parts to various organizations. Financial records (or a copy of those held in a safety deposit box), estimated assets and liabilities, and insurance and social security information should be there. Personal requests and wishes, listing who gets what, should be written along with funeral arrangements and cemetery deeds.

Having this information written assumes that the person has made a legal will, has some knowledge of the purposes and functions of probate court, has access to Social Security information, and has decided on a funeral home and burial plot.

Knowledge of matters such as how to claim survivor's benefits from Social Security and how to claim the government burial allowance for honorably discharged veterans can ease the loved one's confusion at time of death.

These are intellectual preparations. They cannot ease the sense of loss in the living, but they can foster peace of mind, realizing that the deceased's wishes were carried out.

Nursing Applications

Death is an intensely poignant event, one that causes deep anguish, but one you may frequently encounter in client care.

Self-Assessment

Personal assessment, being aware of and coping with your personal feelings about death, is essential to assess accurately or intervene helpfully with the client, family, or other health care providers. How do you protect yourself from anxiety and despair resulting from repeated exposure to personal sufferings? The defenses of isolation, denial, or "professional" behavior are common in an attempt to cope with feelings of helplessness, guilt, frustration, and ambivalence about the client's not getting well or the secret wish for the client to die. It takes courage and maturity to undergo the experience of death with clients and families and yet remain an open, compassionate human being. You are a product of the culture as much as is the client and the family and hence will experience many of the same kinds of reactions. Religious, philosophic, educational, family experiences and general maturity also affect your ability to cope with feelings related to death.

You may see, consciously or unconsciously, yourself in the dying person. The more believable the identification with the person or family, the more devastating the experience will be as you are forced to recognize personal vulnerability to death. The client may remind you of your grandfather, aunt, or friend, and you may react to the dying client as though he or she were that person.

The dying client may seek an identification and partnership with someone, and often this person is the nurse. You may be unwilling to share the relationship or respond to the dying client. The sense of guilt that results may be as burdensome as the actual involvement.

Dying in the hospital has become so organized and care so fragmented that you are not necessarily vulnerable to personal involvement in the client's death. However, you are more likely to be personally affected by and feel a sense of loss from the client's death if an attachment has been formed to the client and family because of prolonged hospitalization and if the death is unexpected. Also, if you perform nursing measures you believe might have contributed to the client's death, if you have worked hard to save a life, or if the client's social or personal characteristics are similar to your own, you will feel the loss (1, 12, 16, 19, 22, 31, 36, 40, 74).

Glaser and Strauss (36) describe how the nurse judges a client's value according to social status and responds accordingly. The client's death is considered less a social loss and is therefore less mourned by the nursing staff if he or she is elderly, comatose, or confused, of a lower socioeconomic class or a minority group, poorly educated, not famous, or unattractive. The dying client in these categories is likely to get less care or only routine care. The client with high social value, whose death is mourned, and who receives optimum care by the nursing staff is the person who is young, alert, or likeable, has prominent family status, has a high-status occupation or profession, is from the middle or upper socioeconomic class, or is considered talented or pretty.

If the client's death is very painful or disfiguring, you may avoid the client because of feelings of guilt or helplessness. In addition, you may be aware of the callous attitudes of other health team members or of the decision of the family and doctor about prolonging life with heroic measures or not prolonging life. These situations can provoke intense negative reactions if you disapprove of the approaches of other members of the health team.

You must attempt to deal with the various pitfalls of working with the dying: withdrawal from the client, isolation of emotions, failure to perceive own feelings or feelings of client and family, displacing own feelings onto other team members, "burning out" from intense emotional involvement, and fearing illness and death.

Support for Nurses

The nurse should be able to say, "I need help in dealing with my feelings about this dying client" just as easily as she or he would say, "I need help in starting this respirator."

A support system should be available. Specific times should be set aside for staff members to share emotional needs related to a specific dying client or to learn specifics of the dying process. Often nurses can help each other, but there should also be a specialist with whom to confer: a nurse with additional training, a religious leader, a nun, a psychologist, or a psychiatrist. The specialist should also be available for spontaneous sessions.

The administration may also encourage and sponsor the nurses in taking courses other than in nursing (sociology, philosophy, religion) to gain different perspectives, joining professional organizations in which they can share problems or solutions and gain support, changing departments either temporarily or permanently to feel the accomplishment of working with those who recover, and arranging for two primary care nurses (if that is the system) to work together so that they can share emotions and support each other.

If you work with cancer clients exclusively, you may also need special assistance. Although cancer does not always cause death, many people still equate cancer

with death. Optimism and logical thinking must be encouraged in the client and maintained in yourself. The cause(s) of cancer is(are) not definitely known, and some people still worry about "catching cancer." You may hear many opinions about helpful treatment, both inside and outside the medical establishment; and you may see that some of the established treatments have unpleasant side effects. The question comes: why must the client endure so much?

If you can think of death as the last stage of life and as fulfillment, you can mature and learn from the client as he or she comes to terms with personal illness. The meaning of death can serve as an important organizing principle in determining how the person conducts his or her life, and it is as significant for you as for the client. With time and experience, you will view the role of comforter as being as important as that of promoting care. Then the client who is dying will be less of a personal threat.

Vachon (76, 77) summarizes some guidelines for the nurse working with dying clients:

1. Individual staff members should be encouraged to gain personal insight and acknowledge their own limits. One's limits vary over time, and extra support or time off may be necessary when staff members are under a high degree of stress. However, the needs of clients deserve priority; if certain staff members constantly require considerable support, they may be encouraged to seek employment elsewhere.
2. A healthy balance must be maintained between work and an outside life. Although this type of work demands considerable personal involvement, there must be times when staff is totally off call and left to pursue own life-affirming activities.
3. The individual must be careful when the "need to be needed" becomes too great and he or she attempts to be everything to everyone. This work is probably best accomplished by a team.
4. The individual must maintain a support system at work and outside the work setting. Hospice units must make provision for ongoing staff support through the use of visitation, psychiatric consultants for the staff, weekly staff support meetings, or other models that seem appropriate to a given unit. In addition, individuals should be encouraged to seek relationships outside the work setting for additional support.
5. For those working in isolation, it may be wise to consider seriously on-going contact with an outside consultant and therapist who can offer guidance as needed and provide support as well.

Two books are useful in helping you become aware of and to work through your feelings, either alone or with colleagues (12, 22).

Assessment of Client and Family

Assessment of the client and family is done according to the standard methods of assessment. The total person (physical, intellectual, emotional, social, and spiritual needs and status) must be assessed to plan effective care. Learn what the client and family know about the client's condition and what the doctor has told them, to plan for a consistent approach.

Recognize also that people differ in the way they express feelings about dying and death. Mourning may be private or public. Listen to the topics of conversation the person discusses, observe for rituals in behavior, and learn of typical behavior in health from him or her or the family to get clues of what is important. The routines that are important in life may become more important now, and they may assist in preparation for death. Observe family members for pathologic responses—physical or emotional—since grief after loss from death increases the risk of mortality for the survivor, especially for the male spouse or relative who is in late middle age or older.

Nursing Diagnoses

Box 15–2 lists nursing diagnoses that may be pertinent to the dying person and are related to assessment and need for holistic care.

■ BOX 15-2.
Nursing Diagnoses Related to the Dying Person[a]

Pattern 1: Exchanging

Altered Nutrition: Less than body requirements
Potential for Infection
Ineffective Thermoregulation
Constipation
Diarrhea
Bowel Incontinence
Altered Patterns of Urinary Elimination
Altered (Specify Type) Tissue Perfusion
Potential for Injury
Impaired Tissue Integrity
Impaired Skin Integrity
Potential Impaired Skin Integrity

Pattern 2: Communicating

Impaired Verbal Communication

Pattern 3: Relating

Impaired Social Interaction
Social Isolation
Altered Role Performance
Altered Family Processes
Altered Sexuality Patterns

Pattern 4: Valuing

Spiritual Distress

Pattern 5: Choosing

Ineffective Individual Coping
Impaired Adjustment
Defensive Coping
Ineffective Denial
Ineffective Family Coping: Disabling
Ineffective Family Coping: Compromised

Family Coping: Potential for Growth
Decisional Conflict
Health Seeking Behaviors

Pattern 6: Moving

Impaired Physical Mobility
Activity Intolerance
Fatigue
Potential Activity Intolerance
Sleep Pattern Disturbance
Diversional Activity Deficit
Impaired Home Maintenance Management
Altered Health Maintenance
Bathing/Hygiene Self-care Deficit
Dressing/Grooming Self-care Deficit
Toileting Self-care Deficit

Pattern 7: Perceiving

Body Image Disturbance
Self-esteem Disturbance
Sensory/Perceptual Alterations
Hopelessness
Powerlessness

Pattern 8: Knowing

Knowledge Deficit

Pattern 9: Feeling

Pain
Chronic Pain
Anticipatory Grieving
Anxiety
Fear

[a]Other NANDA diagnoses are applicable to the dying person.
From North American Nursing Diagnosis Association, *NANDA Nursing Diagnosis Taxonomy I* (Rev.). St. Louis: North American Nursing Diagnosis Association, 1990.

Intervention with the Family

The family will be comforted as they see compassionate care being given to their loved one. Your attitude is important, for both family members and clients are very perceptive about your real feelings, whether you are interested and available, giving false reassurance, or just going about a job. Family members often judge your personal relationship with the loved one as more important than your technical skill. Being interested and available takes emotional energy. Without this component in your personality, perhaps you should not be in the profession of nursing.

Try to help the relatives compensate for their feelings of helplessness, frustration, or guilt. Their assisting the client with feeding or grooming or other time-consuming but nontechnical aspects of care can be helpful to them, the client, and the nursing staff. The family may be acting toward or caring for the client in a way that seems strange or even nontherapeutic to the nursing staff. Yet these measures or the approach may seem fine to the client because of the family pattern or ritual. It is not for you to judge or interfere unless what the family is doing is unsafe for the client's welfare or is clearly annoying to the client. In turn, recognize when family members are fatigued or anxious and relieve them of responsibility at that point. Encourage the family to take time to rest and to meet needs adequately. A lounge or other place where the family can alternately rest and yet be near the client is helpful.

Show acceptance of grief. By helping the family members express their grief and by giving support to them, you are helping them, in turn, to support the client.

Prepare the family for sudden, worsening changes in the client's condition or appearance to avoid shock and feelings of being overwhelmed.

The crisis of death of the loved one may result in a life crisis for the surviving family members. The problems with changes in daily routines of living, living arrangements, leisure-time activities, role reversal and assuming additional responsibilities, communicating with other family members, or meeting financial obligations can seem overwhelming. The failure of relatives and friends to help or relatives and friends who insist on giving help that is not needed are equally problematic. Advice from others may add to rather than decrease the burdens. The fatigue that a long illness causes in a family member may remain for some time after the loved one's death and may interfere with adaptive capacities. You can help by being a listener, exploring with the family ways in which to cope with their problems, and making referrals or encouraging them to seek other persons or agencies for help. Often your willingness to accept and share their feelings of loss and other concerns can be enough to help the family mobilize their strengths and energies to cope with remaining problems.

The most heartbreaking time for the family may be the time when the client is disengaging from life and from them. The family will need help to understand this process and recognize it as normal behavior. The dying person has found peace. His or her circle of interests has narrowed, and he or she wishes to be left alone and not disturbed by any news of the outside world. Behavior with others may be so withdrawn that he or she seems unreachable and uncooperative. He or she prefers short

■ Research Abstract

Constantino, R., Comparison of Two Group Interventions for the Bereaved, Image, *20, no. 2 (1988), 83-87.*

Approximately 5% of the population in the United States is widowed. This group includes more women than men since women outlive men by 7 or 8 years and usually marry men older than themselves.

This experimental study sought to test the helpfulness of two types of group interventions, a bereavement crisis intervention and a social adjustment intervention, in reducing depression and increasing socialization among widows aged 50 to 79 years. The Beck Depression Inventory, the Depression Adjective Check Test, and the Revised Social Adjustment Scale were used to test two experimental groups and a control group. Participants were randomly assigned to each type of group. Levels of depression and socialization were tested initially and at 6 weeks, 5 months, 9 months, and 12 months after the group interventions.

In the bereavement crisis intervention group the leader was active in leading discussion, planned a theme for discussion, gave mental health education, and provided insight into each member's plight. The group lasted 6 weeks, with $1\frac{1}{2}$ hour sessions weekly. In the social adjustment group the leader was an inactive person, a timekeeper, gathering the group weekly for 6 weeks for a social activity. The group was task oriented, discussing current problems and planning an outing for each week. Each leader was a doctoral student and was prepared to do group leading.

The participants (44 in crisis group, 36 in social group, and 37 in control group) had been widowed from less than 1 year to 29 years. Causes of husbands' death included accidents, acute and chronic illness, and suicide. A two-way repeated measures analysis of variance (ANOVA) test was used to analyze the changes in level of depression over time. The mean score for depression decreased over time in the crisis group and remained the same in the social and the control groups. The results in social adjustment were similar.

The implications are that 6 weeks of group bereavement crisis intervention are effective in lowering depression and increasing social adjustment. However, the results are greatest while the group is being conducted, according to test scores. Thus group intervention for widows should be longer and in two stages: (1) to deal with the crisis of loss and emerging physical, emotional, and social problems and reactions; and (2) to continue a support program focusing on education and reorientation to the internal and external resources.

visits and is not likely to be in a talkative mood. The television set remains off. Communication is primarily nonverbal. This behavior can cause the family to feel rejected, unloved, and guilty about not doing enough for the client. They should understand that the client can no longer hold onto former relationships as he or she accepts the inevitability of death. The family needs help in realizing that their silent presence can be a very real comfort and shows that he or she is loved and not forgotten. Concurrently, the family can learn that dying is not a horrible thing to be avoided.

News of impending or actual death is best communicated to a family unit or group rather than to a lone individual to allow the people involved to give mutual support to each other. This should be done in privacy so they can express grief without the restraints imposed by public observation. Stay and comfort the person facing death, at least until a religious leader or other close friends can come.

Requests by an individual or family to see the dead person should not be denied on the grounds that it would be too upsetting. The person who needs a leave taking to realize the reality of the situation will ask for it; those for whom it would be overwhelming will not request it.

Sometimes the survivor of an accident may ask about people who were with him or her at the time of the accident. The health team should confer on when and how to answer these questions; well-timed honesty is the healthiest approach; otherwise the person cannot adapt to the reality of the accidental death. The person's initial response of shock, denial, and tears or later grief will neither surprise nor upset the medical team who understand the normal steps in resolving crisis and loss. Cutting off the person's questions or keeping him or her sedated may protect the staff, but it does not help the survivor.

The parents who grieve for their dying child must be respected, be given the opportunity to minister to the child when indicated, and be relieved of responsibilities at times. Encourage the parents to share feelings, and work to complement, not compete with, the parents in caring for the child. Also, remember that grandparents, siblings, peers, and sometimes the babysitter will need understanding in their grieving.

Intervention for the Dying Person

Care of the dying client falls primarily on the nurse. You have sustained contact with the client and understand dying and the many needs of the dying person. You know the value of compassionate service of mind and hands. You can protect the vulnerable person and understand some of the distress felt by client and family. You have an opportunity to help the client bring life to a satisfactory close, truly to live until he or she dies, and to promote comfort. The client needs your unqualified

interest and response to help decrease loneliness and make the pain and physical care or treatment bearable.

You will encounter frustrations during the care of the dying person for many reasons. There is the challenge of talking with or listening to the client. Will he or she talk about death? Pain may be constant and difficult to relieve, causing you to feel incompetent. He or she may be demanding, nonconforming to the client role, or disfigured and offensive to touch or smell. The family may visit so often and long that they interfere with necessary care of the client. Accusations from the client or family about neglect may occur or be feared. It is no wonder that in spite of good intentions, religious convictions, and educational programs, you may avoid the dying client and family. They are left to face the crisis of death alone. As you rework personal feelings about crisis, dying, and death and become more comfortable with personal negative feelings and emotional upset, you will be able to serve more spontaneously and openly in situations previously avoided. You will be able to admit, without guilt feelings, personal limits in providing care, to use other helpers, and yet to do as much as possible for the client and family without showing shock or repugnance about the client's condition.

Physical care of the dying person includes providing for nutrition, hygiene, rest, elimination, and relief of pain or other symptoms. Castles and Murray's *Dying in an Institution,* "Strategies of Care," published by Appleton-Century-Crofts in 1980, includes care of the mouth, nose, eyes, skin, and peripheral circulation, positioning, and environmental considerations. Hospital personnel should not focus exclusively on the client's complaints of pain or other physical symptoms or needs to avoid the subject of death. Complaints may be a camouflage for anxiety, depression, or other feelings and covertly indicate a desire to talk with someone about the feelings. Analgesics and comfort measures to promote rest can be used along with crisis therapy. Spend sufficient time with the client to establish a relationship that is supportive. Provide continuity of care. Try to exchange information realistically within the whole medical team, including client and family, to reduce uncertainty and feelings of neglect. Clients can withstand much pain and distress as long as they feel wanted or believe their life has meaning.

Thorough, meticulous physical care is essential to promote physical well-being but also to help prevent emotional distress. During the prolonged and close contact physical care provides, you can listen, counsel, and teach, using principles of effective communication. But let the client sleep often, without sedation if possible. The many physical measures to promote comfort and optimum well-being can be found in texts describing physical care skills. Nursing care is not less important because the person is dying.

Avoid too strict a routine in care. Let the client make some decisions about what he or she is going to do as long as safe limits are set. Modify care procedures as necessary for comfort. Through consistent, comprehensive care you tell the client you are available and will do everything possible for continued well-being.

During care conversation should be directed to the client. Explain nursing procedures, even though the client is comatose since hearing is the last sense lost. Response to questions should be simple, encouraging, but as honest as possible. Offer the person opportunities to talk about self and feelings through open-ended questions. When the client indicates a desire to talk about death, listen. There is no reason to expound your philosophy, beliefs, or opinions. Focus your conversation on the present and the client. Help the client maintain the role that is important to him or her. Convey that what he or she says has meaning for you. You can learn by listening to the wisdom shared by the client, and add to feelings of worth and generativity. Recognize when the client is unable to express feelings verbally, and help him or her reduce tension and depression through other means—physical activity, crying, or sublimative activities.

If the client has an intense desire to live and is denying or fearful of death, be accepting but help him or her maintain a sense of balance. Do not rob the person of hope or force him or her to talk about death. Follow the conversational lead; if the topics are concerned with life, respond accordingly.

Encourage communication among the doctor, client, and family. Encourage the client to ask questions and state needs and feelings instead of doing it for him or her, but be an advocate if the person cannot speak for self.

Explore with family members the ways they can communicate with and support the client. Explain to the family that since the comatose client can probably understand what is being said, they should talk in ways that promote security and should avoid whispering, which can increase the person's fears and suspicions.

Psychologic care includes showing genuine concern, acceptance, understanding, and promoting a sense of trust, dignity, or realistic body image and self-concept. Being an attentive listener and providing for privacy, optimum sensory stimulation, independence, and participation in self-care and decision making are helpful. You will nonverbally provide a feeling of security and trust by looking in frequently on the client and using touch communication.

Spiritual needs of the dying person, regardless of the spiritual beliefs, can be categorized as follows (13):

1. Search for meaning and purpose in life and in suffering, including to integrate dying with personal goals and values, to make dying and death less fearful, to affirm the value of life, and to cope with the frustration caused by anticipated death.
2. Sense of forgiveness in the face of guilt about unful-

filled expectations for self, accepting nonfulfillment or incompleteness and making the most of remaining life, acts of omission or acts of commission toward others, resolving human differences.
3. Need for love through other's words and acts of kindness and silent, compassionate presence; if family and friends are not present, the nurse may be the primary source of love.
4. Need for hope, which connotes the possibility of future good. Concrete hope consists of objects of hope within the person's experience such as freedom from pain or other symptoms, ability to perform certain tasks, or to travel. Abstract hope or transcendent hope is characterized by distant and abstract goals and incorporates philosophic or religious meanings. Hope may be expressed as belief about afterlife, reunion with deceased loved ones, and union with God, a superior alternative to present existence. If there is no belief in the afterlife, hope may be expressed as belief about transfer of physical energy from the deceased body, belief about contributing to another's life through an organ donation, or belief in leaving a legacy in his or her children or community or organizational contributions.

You may assist with meeting the person's spiritual needs if requested and if you feel comfortable in doing so. Certainly you should know whom to contact if you feel inadequate. The religious advisor is a member of the health team. If the client has no religious affiliation and indicates no desire for one, avoid proselytizing.

Consider the social needs of the client until he or she is comatose or wishes to be left alone. Visitors, family, or friends can contribute significantly to the client's welfare when visiting hours are flexible. If possible, help the client dress appropriately and groom to receive visitors, go out of the room to a lounge, meet and socialize with other clients, or eat in a client's dining room or the unit.

Community health nurses have found two distinct attitudes in families of dying clients. The first attitude is, "If he is going to die soon, let's get him to the hospital!" For these families the thought of watching the actual death is abhorrent. They feel personally unable to handle the situation and feel comforted by the thought of their loved one's dying in a place where qualified professionals can manage all the details. If possible, these families should have their wishes met.

The second attitude is, "I want her to die at home. This is the place she loved. I can do everything that the hospital personnel can do." This attitude can be supported by the visiting nurse. The visiting nurse can usually coordinate community resources so that a home health aide, homemaker services, proper drug and nutrition supplies, and necessary equipment can be available in the home. Even the comatose client who requires a hospital bed, tube feedings, catheter change and irrigation, daily bed bath, feces removal, and frequent turning can be cared for in the home if the health team, family, and friends will share efforts. The families who desire this approach and who are helped to carry out their wishes seem to derive a great satisfaction from giving this care.

In one study one half of the clients and one half of the family members interviewed selected the home as the place of care in the terminal stages of disease and as the place to die. Being with family and friends and living in their own home was a high priority for clients. Home represented their life's work and helped to maintain a sense of dignity, identity, and control over dying. They realized at home they would not have to battle extraordinary measures. The family wanted the client at home because it was his or her wish and because they believed they would desire to be at home if they were dying. In this study clients and families who chose the hospital as the place of death believed clients would receive better care there. Clients did not want to burden families. Families were concerned about their loved one's comfort (69).

Age, diagnosis, length of illness, and presence of children in the home were not factors influencing choice of home or hospital in a sample of 441 male client/female family pairs at a Veterans Administration Hematology-Oncology Clinic. However, the longer the diagnosis had been known, the more likely was the family member to want to keep the client at home. The older the family member, the more likely she or he was to want to keep the client in the hospital. The most important anticipated services at home by clients were pain control and the availability of someone to assist day or night if needed. Family members expressed need for equipment, help with the client's physical care, and assurance that emergency measures could be obtained if necessary (69).

The *hospice* is an institution and a concept that gives the dying person homelike care either at home with the help of an interdisciplinary team or in an institution with a homelike atmosphere and special attention to the needs of the dying and their families. The hospice concept is indeed a "care system" that coexists with a "cure system." In the United States the definition of what constitutes hospice care varies from region to region; the goal, however, is essentially the same. The hospice concept originated in the Middle Ages; St. Christopher's Hospice in England has been the most famous to date. In some hospitals one unit is designated as the hospice area. A modern, freestanding hospice was opened in 1980 in Branford, Connecticut. Connecticut was the first state to regulate the licensing of hospices. In other states licensing depends on the types of facilities and services a hospice provides (57). More information about hospice care, especially ways that physical pain and other common symptoms can be relieved and ways to work with the psychologic aspects of late stage cancer, is found in Geltman and Paige (32), McPherson (57), and Gates (31).

Most hospice care programs enable the family to care for the dying person through a team approach: (1) a visiting nurse does multiple interventions, (2) home health aides do morning household chores, (3) a family physician enables pain control through effective use of medications, (4) a physical therapist helps the person maintain mobility and later teaches the family various transfer techniques, (5) a music therapist brings diversion and suggests exercise to music, and (6) the clergy and church choir visit the home.

At times the client needs to be alone, either at home or in the hospital, as he or she goes through the preparatory depression discussed by Kübler-Ross and is disengaging self from life, loved ones, and all that has been important to him or her. For you to impose yourself at these times might complicate the emotional tasks near the end of life. You should not, however, abandon the client; give the necessary care but go at his or her pace in conversation and care.

Although most people who are about to die have made peace with themselves, some bargain or fight to the end. Accept this behavior, but do not encourage the client to fight for life when the last days are near with no chance for continuing life. Instead, let him or her know that accepting the inevitable is not cowardly. Remember that fear of death is often found more in the living than in the dying and that this fear is more for the impending separation of intimate relationships than of death itself.

After the death of the client, your relationship with the family need not end immediately. Explore with them how they will manage. Follow-up intervention in the form of a telephone call or home visit by a nurse, minister, social worker, or nursing care coordinator would be a way of more gradually terminating a close relationship and performing further crisis intervention as needed. Use this opportunity to evaluate the effectiveness of care given to the family throughout the client's terminal care period.

Evaluation

Throughout intervention with the dying client or his or her family you must continually consider whether your intervention is appropriate and effective, based on their needs rather than yours. Observation alone of their condition or behavior will not provide adequate evaluation. Ask yourself and others how you could be more effective, whether a certain measure was comforting and skillfully administered, and how the client and family perceived your approach and attitude. Assigning a person unknown to the client and family to ask these questions will help obtain an objective evaluation. Because of your involvement, you may be told only what people think you want to hear. If you and the client have established open, honest communication that encompasses various aspects of dying and if the client's condition warrants it, perhaps you will be able to interview the dying to get evaluation answers. You might ask if and how each member of the health team has added physically, intellectually, emotionally, practically, and spiritually to the person's care. You may also ask how each member of the health team has hindered in these areas.

Through careful and objective evaluation you can learn how to be more skillful at intervention in similar situations in the future.

REFERENCES

1. Aries, P., *Western Attitudes Toward Death*. Baltimore: Johns Hopkins University Press, 1974.
2. Baker, J.C., *Scared to Death, An Examination of Fear—Its Cause and Effects*. London: Frederick Muller 1968.
3. Beauchamp, J., Euthanasia and the Nurse Practitioner, *Nursing Digest*, 4, no. 5 (Winter 1976), 83–85.
4. Bergman, A., Psychological Aspects of Sudden Unexpected Death in Infants and Children, *Pediatric Clinics of North America*, 21, no. 1 (February 1974), 115–121.
5. Brown, H., Euthanasia: Drawing New Distinctions, *Journal of Christian Nursing*, 3, no. 4 (Fall 1986), 10–14.
6. Burgess, K., The Influence of Will on Life and Death, *Nursing Forum*, 15, no. 3 (1976), 238–258.
7. Butler, R., The Roman Catholic Way in Death and Mourning. In Grollman, E., ed., *Concerning Death: A Practical Guide for the Living*. Boston: Beacon Press, 1974, 101–118.
8. Cannon, W., Voodoo Death, *Psychosomatic Medicine*, 19 (1957), 182.
9. Carpenito, L., *Handbook of Nursing Diagnosis* (4th ed.). New York: J.B. Lippincott, 1991.
10. Cassini, N., Care of the Dying Person. In Grollman, E., ed., *Concerning Death: A Practical Guide for the Living*. Boston: Beacon Press, 1974, 13–48.
11. Cate, S., Death by Choice, *American Journal of Nursing*, 91, no. 7 (1991), 33–34.
12. Caughill, R., ed., *The Dying Patient: A Supportive Approach*. Boston: Little, Brown, 1976.
13. Conrad, N., Spiritual Support for the Dying, *Nursing Clinics of North America*, 20, no. 2 (1985), 415–426.
14. Cox, C., The Choice, *American Journal of Nursing*, 81, no. 9 (1981), 1627–1628.
15. Coyle, N., The Last Four Weeks of Life, *American Journal of Nursing*, 90, no. 12 (1990).
16. Davis, A., and P. Slater, U.S. and Australian Nurses' Attitudes and Beliefs About the Good Death, *Image*, 21, no. 1 (1989), 34–39.
17. Devich, L., B. Fields, and R. Carlson, Supportive Care for the Hopelessly Ill, *Nursing Outlook*, 36, no. 3 (1990), 140–142.
18. Dunton, H., The Child's Concept of Death. In Schoenberg, B., et al., eds., *Loss and Grief*. New York: Columbia University Press, 1970, 355–361.
19. Eakes, G., Grief Resolution in Hospice Nurses, *Nursing and Health Care*, 11, no. 5 (1990), 243–248.
20. Engel, G., Sudden and Rapid Death During Psychological Stress: Folklore or Folk Wisdom? *Annals of Internal Medicine*, 74 (1971), 771–792.
21. ——, Psychological Stress, Vasodepressor (Vasovagal) Syncope, and Sudden Death, *Annals of Internal Medicine*, 89 (1978), 405–412.
22. Epstein, C., *Nursing the Dying Patient*. Reston, Va: Reston, 1975.
23. Erikson, E.H., *Childhood and Society* (2nd ed.). New York: W.W. Norton, 1963.
24. Feifel, H., ed., *The Meaning of Death*. New York: McGraw-Hill, 1959.
25. Fischer, H.K., and B.M. Dlin, Man's Determination of His Time of Illness or Death, *Geriatrics*, 26, no. 7 (1971).
26. Foy, N., A Good Birth—A Good Life—Why Not a Good Death? *Nursing Digest*, 4, no. 2 (1976), 24.
27. Fronn, S., Coping With a Child's Fatal Illness: A Parent's Dilemma, *Nursing Clinics of North America*, 9, no. 1 (March 1974), 81–87.
28. Fuller, J., Lethal Dose: Should a Nurse Resist Doctor's Orders, *Journal of Christian Nursing*, 3, no. 4 (Fall 1986), 4–8.
29. Gartley, W., and M. Bernascini, The Concept of Death in Children, *Journal of Genetic Psychology*, 110 (1967), 71.
30. Gartner, C., Growing Up to Dying: The Child, The Parents, and The Nurse. In Caughill, R., ed., *The Dying Patient: A Supportive Approach*. Boston: Little, Brown, 1976, 159–190.
31. Gates, M.F., Transcultural Comparison of Hospital and Hospice as Caring Environments for Dying Patients, *Journal of Transcultural Nursing*, 2, no. 2 (Winter 1991), 3–15.
32. Geltman, R., and R. Paige, Symptom Management in Hospice Care, *American Journal of Nursing*, 83, no. 1 (1983), 78–85.
33. Giacquinta, B., Helping Families Face the Crises of Cancer, *American Journal of Nursing*, 77, no. 10 (October 1977), 1585–1588.
34. Gianelli, D., Would Aiding in Dying Make MDs Hired Killers? *American Medical News* (February 16, 1990), 1.
35. Gifford, B., and B. Cleary, Supporting the Bereaved, *American Journal of Nursing*, 90, no. 2 (1990), 49–53.
36. Glaser, B., and A. Strauss, The Social Loss of Dying Patients, *American Journal of Nursing*, 64, no. 6 (1964), 119ff.
37. ——, *Awareness of Dying*. Chicago: Aldine Publishing, 1965.
38. Griffin, J., Family Decision, *American Journal of Nursing*, 75, no. 5 (May 1975), 795–796.
39. Grollman, E., *Talking About Death: A Dialogue Between Parent and Child* (3rd ed.). Boston: Beacon Press, 1990.
40. Gyulay, J., The Forgotten Grievers, *American Journal of Nursing*, 75, no. 9 (1975), 1476–1479.
41. Henderson, M., Beyond the Living Will, *Gerontologist*, 30, no. 4 (1990), 480–485.
42. Herter, F., The Right to Die in Dignity, *Archives of the Foundation of Thanatology*, 1, no. 3 (October 1969), 93–97.
43. Hogan, N., and D. Balk, Adolescents' Reactions to Situational Death: Perceptions of Mothers, Fathers, and Teenagers, *Nursing Research*, 39, no. 2 (1990), 103–106.
44. Jordon, M., The Protestant Way in Death and Mourning.

In Grollman E., ed., *Concerning Death: A Practical Guide for the Living.* Boston: Beacon Press, 1974, 81–100.

45. Kaprio, J., M. Koskenvao, and H. Rita, Mortality After Bereavement: A Prospective Study of 95,647 Widowed Persons, *American Journal of Public Health,* 77, no. 3 (1987), 283–287.

46. Keith, P., Life Changes and Perceptions of Life and Death Among Older Men and Women, *Journal of Gerontology,* 34, no. 6 (1979), 870–878.

47. Kellmer, D., No Code Orders: Guidelines for Policy, *Nursing Outlook,* 34, no. (1986), 179–183.

48. Killian, W., Knowledge of Living Will Laws Essential, *American Nurse* (July, August 1990), 33.

49. Koocher, G., Talking With Children About Death, *American Journal of Orthopsychiatry,* 44, no. 3 (1974), 404–411.

50. Kübler-Ross, E., ed., *On Death and Dying.* New York: Collier-Macmillan, 1969.

51. ———, *Death, the Final Stage of Growth.* Englewood Cliffs, NJ: Prentice-Hall, 1975.

52. Levy, N.B., Self-Willed Death, *Lancet* (September 1, 1973).

53. Lieberman, M., Social Setting Determines Attitudes of Aged to Death, *Geriatric Focus,* 6, no. 16 (November 1, 1967), 1ff.

54. Lippman, H., After Cruzan: Right to Die, *RN,* no. 1 (1990).

55. Maguire, D., *Death by Choice.* Garden City, NY: Doubleday, 1973.

56. McIntire, M., C. Angle, and L. Struempler, The Concept of Death in Midwestern Children and Youth, *American Journal of Diseases of Children,* 123 (June 1972), 527–532.

57. McPherson, J., Principles of Hospice Care, *Clinical Medicine,* 24, no. 1 (1981), 243–250.

58. Megerle, J.A., Surviving, *American Journal of Nursing,* 83, no. 6 (1983), 892–894.

59. Miles, M., Emotional Symptoms and Physical Health in Bereaved Parents, *Nursing Research,* 34, no. 2 (1985), 76–81.

60. Montalvo, B., The Patient Chose to Die: Why? *Gerontologist,* 31, no. 5 (1991), 700–703.

61. Moody, R.A., *Life After Life.* New York: Bantam Books, 1975.

62. Murphy, S., Preventive Intervention Following Accidental Death of a Child, *Image,* 22, no. 3 (1990), 174–179.

63. Nagy, M., The Child's View of Death. In Fietel, H., ed., *The Meaning of Death.* New York: McGraw-Hill, 1959.

64. Oleson, M., Subjectively Perceived Quality of Life, *Image,* 22, no. 3 (1990), 187–190.

65. Olson, M., The Out-of-Body Experiences and Other States of Conscious, *Archives of Psychiatric Nursing,* 1, no. 3 (1987), 201–207.

66. Orne, R., Nurses' View of NDE, *American Journal of Nursing,* 86, no. 4 (1986), 419–420.

67. Papowitz, L., Life/Death/Life, *American Journal of Nursing,* 86, no. 4 (1986), 416–418.

68. Philips, D.P., Deathday and Birthday: An Unexpected Connection. In Tanur, J.M., et al., eds., *Statistics: A Guide to the Unknown.* San Francisco: Holden-Day, 1972.

69. Putnam, S., et al., Home as a Place to Die, *American Journal of Nursing,* 80, no. 8 (1987), 1451–1453.

70. Rahe, R., and M. Romo, Recent Life Changes and the Onset of Myocardial Infarction and Sudden Death in Helsinki. In Gunderson, E., and R. Rahe, eds., *Life, Stress, and Illness.* Springfield, Ill: Charles C Thomas, 1974, 105–120.

71. Richter, G., On The Phenomenon of Sudden Death in Animals and Man, *Psychosomatic Medicine,* 19 (1959), 191.

72. Rosner, F., The Definition of Death, *Archives of the Foundation of Thanatology,* 1, no. 3 (October 1969), 105–107.

73. Schoenberg, B., Management of The Dying Patient. In Schoenberg, B., et al., eds., *Loss and Grief.* New York: Columbia University Press, 1970, 238–260.

74. Stephany, T., A Death in the Family, *American Journal of Nursing,* 90, no. 4 (1990), 54–56.

75. Sugar, M., Normal Adolescent Mourning, *American Journal of Psychotherapy,* 22 (1968), 258–264.

76. Vachon, M.L.S., Motivation and the Stress Experienced by Staff Working With the Terminally Ill, *Death Education,* (Winter 1978), 12–15.

77. ———, W. Lyall, and S. Freeman, Measurement and Management of Stress in Health Professionals Working With Advanced Cancer Patients, *Death Education* (Spring 1978), 10–13.

78. Van Ora, L., Terminal Is a Relative Term, *Nursing and Health Care,* 10, no. 2 (1989), 97–100.

79. Waechter, E., Children's Awareness of Fatal Illness, *American Journal of Nursing,* 71, no. 6 (1971), 1168–1172.

80. Weisman, A., and T. Hackett, Predilection to Death, *Psychosomatic Medicine,* 23, no. 3 (1961).

81. West, J., Civilized Societies Don't Kill Coma Victims, *San Francisco Chronicle,* January 9, 1989.

82. White, A., The Needs of Dying Children and Their Families, *Health Visitor,* 62, no. 6 (1989), 176–178.

83. Zentner, R., Personal Story of Life After Life, March 1971.

Part V

Health Promotion Principles and Strategies

Chapter 16

Basic Considerations in Health and Illness

All work together: physical fitness, positive attitude, and the spiritual fitness.
—Kenneth Cooper, M.D.

KEY TERMS

Wellness	Physiologic	Daily hassles	Stage of exhaustion
Health-wellness	Libidinal	Eustress	Anxiety
Disease-illness	Ego developmental	Local adaptation syndrome	Mind-body relationship
Biopsychosocial/holistic health	Intelligence	General adaptation syndrome	Psychosomatic or psychophysiologic
Aerobics	Personality hardiness	Alarm stage	Somatopsychic
Health	Self-concept	Stage of resistance	Psychoneuroimmunology
Behavior	Stress	Protective factors	
Human needs	Stressors		
	Distress		

OBJECTIVES

Study of this chapter will enable you to:

1. Define *health, holistic health,* and *illness* and explain the development of these concepts and the meaning of the health-illness continuum.
2. Identify factors that influence development of health and illness.
3. Identify needs that influence behavior and that must be met to maintain health.
4. Describe the external environmental and internal variables that affect behavior and health.
5. Differentiate between stress and anxiety and describe physiologic, cognitive, emotional, and behavioral reactions to stress responses in each stage of the general adaptation syndrome.
6. Differentiate levels of anxiety and physical, cognitive, emotional, and behavioral manifestations at each level.

"Al, are you ill?"

"No. Why?"

"Your face looks a little puffy."

Al, who thought he was well, suddenly decides he has not had his usual energy for several weeks. He thinks he will make an appointment to see the physician.

"I wish I knew what you meant by being sick. Sometimes I feel so bad I could curl up and die, but I have to go on because the kids have to be taken care of. Besides, we don't have money for the doctor. Some people can go to bed most anytime with anything, but most of us can't take time to be sick— even when we need to be."

These expressions immediately portray the difficulty in defining health and illness. Each person's definition is affected by cultural concepts, economic level, the value system of self and others, ethnic background, customs, and past experiences.

As a nurse, your concern, knowledge, and skill are directed to the health needs of persons from many different kinds of backgrounds and in various settings. It is essential therefore to understand the physical, mental, emotional, spiritual, and social aspects of wellness and illness; the factors influencing health and illness; and the basic regulatory mechanisms in the human body that normally maintain a state of health. The use of this information will assist you in helping others to maintain and regain health.

DEFINITIONS OF HEALTH AND ILLNESS

Working definitions of *health* and *illness,* although generalized, can give perspective. Traditionally they have been defined as opposites. Although *health* and *illness* are subjective and relative terms, Jourard believes that such qualities as hope, purpose, and direction in life can produce and maintain wellness, even in the presence of stress. Similarly, demoralization through daily struggle for existence can help produce illness (38).

Wellness is a *process of moving toward greater awareness of and satisfaction from engaging in activities that move the person, at any age, with others, toward fitness, a positive nutritional state, positive relations, management of stress, a life purpose, a consistent belief system, commitment to self-care, and environmental sensitivity and comfort.* The wellness process can be pursued to prevent illness, for rehabilitation, or to enhance the quality of life and maximize potential, whether ill, dying, or overcoming disability, in any setting. Differentiation of self occurs so that a clear boundary develops between the emotional and intellectual subsystems of a whole person, leading to enhanced problem solving, flexibility in behavior, intimacy in interpersonal relationships, and a higher level of wellness. If the person is not clear about values, a pseudoself exists and is at the whim of the emotional system of others. A solid sense of self increases as consistency between beliefs, feelings, and actions is realized through the value clarification process. Environment is external to the person; it is a changing field that is continuous and contiguous with whole persons. Environment can be modified by, as well as modify, the whole person (9).

Health-wellness and **disease-illness** are now thought of as *complex, dynamic processes on a contin-*

uum that includes physical, psychologic (emotional, cognitive, and developmental), spiritual, and social components and adaptive behavioral responses to internal and external stimuli. Health depends on genetic, environmental, sociocultural, and spiritual influences that either help or hinder an individual in actively fulfilling the basic needs and reaching the highest health potential (21, 63). The emotionally healthy person generally shows behavior congruent with events within or around him or her. Key concepts in health-wellness include homeostasis, adaptation, dynamic nature of health-illness continuum, influence of internal and external environment, state of harmony with nature and people, comfort, safety, social relationships, and prevention of disease, disability, and social decay.

In nursing we are concerned about **biopsychosocial** or **holistic health** because the term refers to a *high level and total view of health, the unity of body, mind and spirit, and the person's interrelatedness with others and the environment* (2). **Holistic health** *focuses on acceptance and harmony between one's body, feelings, attitudes, and beliefs; on being open to relationships and change; and on being responsible for one's health and behavior.* A holistic philosophy means viewing people and their wellness and illness from every possible perspective and using natural, cultural, or nontraditional methods and medical means to treat the person—not the disease (2).

Webster (98) describes the need to define health from a holistic view for women and to be sensitive to specific health needs of women in the home, workplace, and health care setting. It is important to gain an understanding of the woman's personal experience from her rather than making assumptions or acting on traditional biases. The nurse can assist the woman to feel empowered, to feel that she is capable of responsibility for her health. Interdependence, caring, cooperation, experience as a base for knowledge, and responsibility are valued by women, and the nurse can convey to the woman that these values can be enacted in the health care system. With social roles in transition, poverty, single parenthood, role conflict, and other sources of stress, the nurse and other members of the health care system must focus on the specific individual or family to provide the maximum care possible.

Wellness is a part of holistic health. Ardell defines **wellness** as *an ever-changing process focusing on health enrichment and promotion.* **Wellness** is the *ability to adapt, to relate effectively, and to function at near maximum capacity and includes self-responsibility, nutritional awareness, physical fitness, stress management, environmental sensitivity, productivity, expression of emotions, self-expression in a variety of ways, creativity, personal care, and home and automobile safety* (9, 21).

The wellness movement in the United States was, at least in part, begun by the physician Kenneth Cooper in the late 1960s. He is known as the Father of Aerobics.

Aerobics is the *type of exercise that demands large amounts of oxygen for long periods.* Cooper (12) emphasized six factors as necessary for total well-being:

1. Proper diet and weight
2. Proper exercise (Running or jogging more than 15 miles weekly does not add to cardiovascular health but does add to musculoskeletal injury.)
3. Elimination of tobacco use
4. Control of alcohol and elimination of habit-forming drugs
5. Stress management, emotional balance, spiritual development
6. Periodic wellness examinations

Further, with the current mass media campaigns about health and illness control in the Western world, people have become more health conscious and knowledgeable. Health behavior thus has been influenced, as shown by changes in trends related to a decreased incidence of cardiovascular disease in North America (60).

As used in this book, **health** is a *state of well-being in which the person is able to use purposeful, adaptive responses and processes, physically, mentally, emotionally, spiritually, and socially, in response to internal and external stimuli (stressors) to maintain relative stability and comfort and to strive for personal objectives and cultural goals.*

Table 16–1 summarizes a historical review of definitions or concepts of health developed by various theorists, including nursing theorists and leaders.

Factors That Influence Definitions of Health and Illness

The **health care system** and **national health policy** of any nation are instrumental in defining health and illness for the people of that nation, and each of these factors influences the other. The insurance industry adds to the influence of national health policy.

Since the 1974 Canadian Lalonde Report (45), the best national plans for health progress have emphasized disease prevention and health promotion. In this report the Canadian health care system was acknowledged as equal to or better than any other in the world, but other health determinants were also cited: human biology, environment, and life-style.

In 1974 the U.S. Department of Health, Education, and Welfare published a 5-year projection for health programs and prevention (96). In 1976 the government of the United Kingdom published a document, *Prevention and Health: Everybody's Business,* emphasizing prevention (15). In 1978 the U.S. Centers for Disease Control (CDC) placed greater emphasis on prevention, listing 31 preventable health problems in the fields of environment, life-style, and medical services. The CDC produced the often-cited observation that 50% of premature mortality in the United States is due to life-style, 20% to human biology, and 10% to health care—or lack

TABLE 16-1. DEVELOPMENT OF CONCEPTS AND DEFINITIONS OF HEALTH

Era/Date	Theorist	Concept/Definition
1000 AD		English word, **hoelth,** meaning safe, sound, whole of body. Physical wholeness essential for social acceptance. Persons with malformations or disease ostracized because conditions represented lack of harmony with nature or being unclean.
Late 1800s		Concept of mental health originated as opposed to mental illness, which meant unpredictable, hostile behavior, being a lunatic and thereby ostracized. Causation attributed to evil spirits, satanic powers.
1900		Health—freedom from disease; disease caused by microbes.
1940s		Health included physical and mental status; concept received impetus from experience with psychologic trauma in World War II.
		Mental health manifested in ability to withstand environmental stresses; mental illness occurred when person succumbed to life stresses and was unable to carry out activities of daily living.
		Dichotomy between physical and mental illness remains.
	Harry Stack Sullivan	**Mental health** is interpersonal adjustive success. Basic or intrinsic direction of the person is forward or toward mental health. **Mental disorder** is a pattern of inadequate or inappropriate interpersonal processes inadequate to the situation, an ineffectiveness of behavior.
1950s	Halbert Dunn	**High-level wellness** is integrated functioning oriented to maximizing person's potential, which requires that person maintain a balance through purposeful activity and direction within the environment. The result is a forward direction toward higher or more mature function throughout the life cycle amid a constantly changing environment.
	L. Aubrey	**Health** is structural wholeness in which sensory processes are intact and function so that balance and adaptability characterize the person. **Mental health** is separate from physical health and is characterized as emotional stability, integration, and adaptation to surroundings so person remains viable in spite of changing conditions. The healthy person experiences contentment, performs functions of human existence and societal living, and manifests cognitive efficiency.
	T. Parsons	**Health** is effective performance of valued roles and tasks for which person has been socialized. Health status determined by ability currently to maintain normal standards of adequacy and future role and task performance.
1960s	René Dubois	**Health** is a state or condition that enables person to adapt to internal and external stresses that arise in the environment. Health is a physical and mental state free of discomfort and pain that permits person to function effectively as long as possible within the environment. Optimum health is a mirage because of an unpredictable environment.
	H. Hayman	**Health** is optimum personal fitness for full creative living; a dynamic process involving interaction of heredity, environment, and behavior to result in vigor, vitality, zest, meaning in life and fulfillment.
1970s	Myra Levine	**Health** is a state characterized by balance between input and output of energy and in which structural, personal, and social integrity exist.
	Dorothea Orem	**Health** is a state characterized by soundness or wholeness of human structures and body and mental functions. **Well-being** is a state characterized by experiences of contentment, pleasure, and happiness, by spiritual experiences, by movement to fulfilling self-ideal, by achieving human potential.
	I. Bermosk and S. Porter	**Health** is an integration of mind, body, spirit, and environment; person is responsible for own health and evolution to greater levels of zest and well-being, to healing self, to expanding consciousness.
	M. Newman	**Health** is the totality of life process, evolving to an expanded consciousness, a fusion of disease and nondisease, a manifestation of a unique pattern, a greater frequency of energy exchange.
1974	World Health Organization	"**Health** is a state of complete physical, mental and social well-being and not merely absence of disease and infirmity." Health is an ideal. Definition reflects person as a total being rather than sum of parts, that health is related to environment and equated with productive and creative living.
1980s	Dorothy Johnson	**Health** or **wellness** is a balance and stability among the following behavioral systems: affiliative or attachment, dependency, ingestive, eliminative, sexual, aggressive, and achievement, which results in efficient, effective, goal-directed predictable behavior.
	Betty Neuman	**Health** and **wellness** is a condition in which all subsystems—physiologic, psychologic, and sociocultural—are in balance and in harmony with the whole of man; a state of energy saturation in which the person is free of disruptive needs, forces, or noxious stressors that create disharmony and expend energy. The healthy person has considerable resistance to disequilibrium.
	J. Smith	**Health** is characterized by four models; (1) clinical—presence or absence of disease; (2) role performance—extent to which social roles can be performed; (3) adaptive—adaptation to or isolation from the environment; and (4) eudaemonistic—exuberant well-being versus languishing debility.
	Sister Callista Roy	**Health** is a state and process of successful adaptation through modes that promote being and becoming an integrated whole model, with completeness, unity, and freedom from ineffective coping attempts. The four modes are physiologic self-concept, interdependence, and role performance.
	J.K. Dixon and J.P. Dixon	**Health** is a condition in which positive viability emotions such as acceptance, usefulness, optimism, and clarity about life are present and result in psychologic comfort, productive behavior, normal physiologic function, and self-maintenance behavior. Health is evolutionary and is related to extent to which person contributes to stability and survival of the social group(s).

(continued)

TABLE 16-1. DEVELOPMENT OF CONCEPTS AND DEFINITIONS OF HEALTH (Continued)

Era/Date	Theorist	Concept/Definition
1980s (cont.)	T. Tripp-Reimer	**Health** has two dimensions: etic, or disease-nondisease state; and emic, or wellness-illness, the subjective perception of person or group. Focus on normality or homeostasis as medically defined; some cultures do not focus on medical disease states.
	Nola Pender	**Health** is the actualization of inherent and acquired human potential through goal-directed behavior, knowledgeable and competent self-care, constructive amelioration of barriers to growth, and satisfying interpersonal relationships while adjustments are made to maintain structural integrity, harmony with the environment, and positive change over time.
	L. Wright and M. Leahey	**Family health** is characterized by stability and integrity of structure, adaptability, mastery of developmental tasks leading to progressive differentiation and transformation to meet changing requisites for survival.
	C. Petze	**Family health** is characterized by a functional and productive network, a sense of togetherness that promotes capacity for change, a balance between mutual and independent action among the members, and adaptation to life events.
	G. Smilkstein	**Family health** is characterized by availability of cohesiveness, nurturance, and resources for members growth and sustenance in face of life's challenges.
	Jeanette Goeppinger	**Community health** is the meeting of collective needs through problem identification and management of interactions within the community and between the community and the larger society, considering status, structure, and process dimensions.
	Catherine Tinkham, Elizabeth Voorheis, and N. McCarthy	**Community health** is the process, activities, and concerns designed to enhance the quality of life and promote well-being of the total population of the community.
	Sarah Archer, C. Kelly, and S. Bisch	**Community health** is characterized by openness to energy exchange, interdependence among community groups, hierarchical organization, self-regulation, dynamic activity, goal-directedness, and synthesizing process of wholeness.

of it. This observation began anew the work on the current national health objectives (68). By this time (1977) the World Health Organization (100) had declared its goal that by the year 2000 all citizens of the world would have a level of health that would permit them to lead a socially and economically productive life. During the 1980s in the United States, the Surgeon General's report on health promotion and disease prevention became the basis for services to infants, children, youth, adults, and the elderly. There were 226 quantifiable objectives; one half could be achieved in the 1990s, one fourth would not be achieved, and one fourth could not really be measured (61, 96). *Healthy People, 2000,* the latest U.S. guide, presents three goals: (1) to increase the healthy life span, (2) to reduce health disparities, and (3) to achieve universal access to preventive services. In the United States a national health program is needed to achieve equity in access to health care for the individual and family (27, 88).

In the United States the medical costs rose 117% from 1980 to 1989, a time when many programs to reduce health costs were being implemented. In 1990 the cost of health care was estimated at $600 billion or 12% of the gross national product. During this period many surgeries were changed to an outpatient or 1-day status, and in-hospital days were reduced. But the cost of the new 1-day surgery centers and the rising cost of outpatient surgery ballooned the cost in shifted areas. Canceling insurance or not allowing for preexisting conditions

is a problem that adds people to the rosters of the noninsured. Thus climbing costs for fewer insured people create yet more problems (27, 54).

Various groups have developed proposals to address the problems of the U.S. health care system, among them, a congressional committee, the American Medical Association, the American Nurses' Association, the insurance industry, Physicians for a National Health Plan, and social workers. The plans vary from mostly privately sponsored to completely public-sponsored programs, with variations of both segments. Health Maintenance Organizations (HMOs) and Preferred Provider Organizations (PPOs), along with the traditional private and public health approaches, are seeking to gain inroads into being an ongoing part of the system.

A list of seven "musts" have been outlined for a feasible health care system future (27, 88):

1. The health care system must be restructured to create incentives to save money.
2. Business (that provides health care through insurance) must become a demanding buyer.
3. Business must have better data on cost and effectiveness and must use those providers that perform best.
4. Business must demand more stringent management—from both HMOs and PPOs.
5. Business must accept the government mandate to provide insurance but only with *demands* for specific results.

6. Business must, in exchange for setting up insurance, get cost-containment tools.

7. The government must fulfill its responsibilities to insure and educate the poor.

The health care systems in Canada, Australia, and New Zealand, although national health care programs, are also financially troubled. One complaint is that the Canadian system is lulled by "high-tech" emergency approaches, which are very expensive, as opposed to more emphasis on reducing accidents through education and preventive behaviors (22).

Another way of looking at the health care system is through nonallopathic approaches, some of which have ancient roots from various parts of the world. They include chiropractic, homeopathy, herbalism, naturopathy, aromatherapy, reflexology, acupuncture, hypnosis, biofeedback, and stress reduction. All alternative medicine is based on the principle that the body has a natural healing ability and that practitioners simply help the process along. Thus the practitioners work primarily at preventive medicine. For example, homeopathy is a system of medicine based on two laws: "like cures like," and "less is more." Like cures like means that remedies are chosen according to the client's symptoms, not the disease. Less is more means that the less there is of a remedy, the more potent its effect. Homeopathy should be used in conjunction with the care of a regular physician and is not for anyone who has a high temperature (53). Acupuncture, biofeedback, and other stress management techniques are discussed in Chapter 17. Often these approaches are not covered by traditional insurance payments.

Culture and historical era define health and illness. Thus there are many definitions of health and illness since each family interprets the culture to the child.

Health is *perceived uniquely by the person* and may vary from day to day and even within a day. According to Third Force theorists, described in Chapter 5, health and illness are defined differently by each person, although the definitions are generally in line with cultural definitions. Health in all of its components is dynamic in that it includes the degree of fitness and adaptation that varies from one time period to another. Interaction between the physical, mental, spiritual, and social components is continual (55).

Men and women are socialized to define health and illness differently. Statistics show that women in the United States report more illnesses and disabilities, visit the physician more, and are hospitalized more often, including for emotional illnesses. Physicians are also more likely to prescribe drugs for women than for men, especially the mood-changing drugs (34). Often the physician does not take a complete history or learn of underlying problems that can be corrected other than through use of medication. Yet women have longer life expectancies than men, and there is no difference between men and women in the incidence of psychosis. Perhaps

the seeking of more health care by women reflects (1) a different perception of illness or disability; (2) different cultural norms about health care behavior for men and women; (3) sex-role conflicts for women, which result in more illness; and (4) differences in diagnostic and treatment services for men and women. All these factors may be operating. The longer life expectancy of women may be the result of early diagnosis and treatment of disease, of inherent sex-linked resistance to disease, or of different exposure or response to noxious physical and social stressors (55, 90).

A person's *age* influences the definition of health. Children define health as feeling good and being able to participate in desired activities. Children's ideas about health progress from a specific, concrete concern for health practices to future-oriented interests in optimum development and societal problems. Six-year-olds view health as completely different from illness and as a series of specific health practices such as eating nutritional foods, getting exercise, and keeping clean. Nine-year-olds are less concerned with specific health practices and are more concerned with total body states such as feeling good or being "in shape." To them, health means being physically fit to do the activities of daily living; it is impossible to be partly healthy and partly unhealthy. Twelve-year-olds view health as long-term feeling good, not being sick, participating in desired activities, and as including both mental and physical components. Some children include a fit environment as part of health. In contrast, adults typically define health as a state enabling them to perform at least minimum daily activities and include physical, mental, spiritual, and social components (56). The adult's perception and life situation influence the definition of health.

VARIABLES THAT AFFECT BEHAVIOR AND HEALTH

The nursing profession focuses on health, not just disease. An ecologic view, realizing multiple causation in many situations that threaten health and for many diseases, is essential. What causes many diseases, even cardiovascular disease, remains unknown because of the many variables that contribute to any disease. Some people will do all of the right things and die young. Some will break all the health rules and live a long life. As health professionals we must not blame the person for becoming ill—whatever the causes—although we should share our knowledge about risk factors (49).

Basic Needs

Behavior is the *observable response to environmental stimuli, including verbal reports about emotional state, perceptions, and thoughts.* The primary purpose of behavior is to meet the needs of the person or the group.

Research Abstract

McAuley, E., K. Courneya, and J. Lettunich, Effects of Acute and Long-Term Exercise on Self-Efficacy Responses in Sedentary, Middle-Aged Males and Females, Gerontologist, 31, no. 4 (1991), 534–542.

Exercise has been suggested as the single health practice most strongly associated with health and longevity among the aged, and low physical activity has been implicated as a major risk factor in all-cause mortality, cardiovascular disease, and cancer. Older people make substantial physiologic gains as a result of regular exercise, but psychologic gains are less well known. Self-efficacy, a situation-specific sense of control or a power to produce intended results, is concerned with the person's beliefs in his or her capability to execute necessary actions to satisfy demands. Self-efficacy mediates behavioral change, including health-related behaviors, and may influence thought processes and affective reactions. Perceptions of personal efficacy are influenced by postperformance accomplishments. Coping successfully with the past creates confidence that influences effort, persistence, and affect in future behavioral attempts.

The purpose of this study was to examine the effects of a graded exercise test and a long-term structured exercise program with sedentary middle-aged adults on perceptions of personal efficacy with respect to physical capabilities and enhanced cognitions. The study also sought to determine whether men and women have different perceptions about themselves, as research has reported that healthy men have more positive perceptions of their physical capacities than women, although there are relatively few differences in physical capabilities between them.

The sample comprised 103 (53 female, 50 male) middle-aged adults; only 81 were available for postexercise program testing. Subjects were divided into four age groups: 45 to 49, 50 to 54, 55 to 59, and 60 to 64 years. The average age was 54 years; 80% were married, and 67% had some college education.

Efficacy was studied in relationship to sit-ups, bicycling, and walking-jogging capabilities at baseline and after 20 weeks. Physical fitness was assessed in relation to cardio-respiratory and vascular functions, abdominal strength, body composition, and total blood serum cholesterol. Subjects participated in a 20-week structured exercise program, three times weekly for 1 hour, led by trained instructors.

Results on physiologic measures were analyzed by multivariate analysis of variance (MANOVA). Gender differences were shown in cardiorespiratory responses; men took longer to reach 70% of predicted heart rate maximum. Blood pressure was decreased by exercise, but women had a lower systolic and diastolic blood pressure than men over the course of the program. Both weight and percentage of body fat were reduced by exercise; men were leaner and heavier than women. Abdominal strength was increased through sit-ups and was greater in men than in women. Total blood cholesterol decreased as a result of the exercise in both men and women. Subjects showed significant gains in self-efficacy from before the exercise program to after it, indicating that acute bouts of exercise can affect cognitions. Further, successful mastery experiences related to perception about one type of physical activity produced success with other types of physical activity. Women had significantly lower perceptions of physical capabilities than did men before the exercise program; men and women increased similarly in their efficacy after exercise.

Implication of this research is that sedentary middle-aged adults can make significant health-related gains through exercise, even through a relative low-impact activity such as walking. Further, success in exercise activities can increase perceptions of effectiveness and efficacy in relation to personal behavior.

Human needs are *those aspects of the individual that must be satisfied for life to continue and that can be divided into three broad categories: physiologic, libidinal (sensual and affectional), and ego developmental.* **Physiologic needs** are *cyclic, perpetual, and imperative for survival.* They include the *need for oxygen, water, food, elimination, sleep, temperature control or shelter, safety, or movement* (50).

Libidinal needs refer to *sensual-sexual and affectional-emotional needs. Sensual-sexual* needs are not uniformly rhythmic in humans, although hormonal rhythms of the menstrual cycle are correlated with affective and behavioral changes in some women. The basis of sensual-sexual needs is organic, but these needs take on psychologic meanings. *Affectional-emotional* needs are constant and are at the core of normal psychic dependence. The person must be given love, security, approval, respect, support, care, and protection for emotional and physical development (84).

Ego developmental needs refer to the *need for cognitive, perceptual, and memory development (training and education).* The person must have opportunity for and help with mastery of age-adequate behaviors, including motor coordination; emotional autonomy, independence, and self-identity; social skills; communication skills (speech, reading, writing, nonverbal); adaptive mechanisms, moral development; control of drives; problem solving; work skills; and the opportunity for development of creative and self-actualization behavior (84).

Libidinal and ego developmental needs emerge together; they influence each other and are equally significant for psychic and physical well-being. Ego development proceeds from mastery of simple to complex tasks (84).

Humans are very adaptable in meeting their needs, but adaptive potentials are not unlimited. In prehistoric evolution humans met many stresses, but their genetic constitutions were able to adapt over time. Now humans face threats created by modern technology that have no precedent in their evolutionary past. The rate of biologic evolution is too slow to keep up with the effects of technologic and social changes (17). Thus certain needs may not be met as well; other needs may be created. Unmet needs affect health status.

In countries where the population continues to increase rapidly, there is a strain on all social and human resources, including economic and educational development, and many people will have unmet needs. In such countries health promotion is an ideal; preventing starvation and providing shelter are already consuming the resources of many nations. When physiologic needs are not met, the other needs previously described cannot be met. It is a challenge to international nursing to foster the meeting of basic needs, disease prevention, and health in the people of all nations.

Health in the Third World's developing countries could be improved and mortality and morbidity rates reduced by several not-too-costly measures that are available to developed countries (52):

1. Measles vaccination for each child (for approximately the cost of a pack of cigarettes)
2. Proper diet, vitamin and mineral supplementation to prevent blindness, complications from communicable diseases and diarrhea, malnutrition, and death at cost of pennies per day
3. Education to local populations about early signs and symptoms of specific diseases and measures to reduce their impact and local resources for help
4. Education for and assistance with prenatal care to all women
5. Education about and assistance to local populations in the areas of sanitation and food production

External Environmental Variables

The external environment includes all stimuli, objects, and people impinging on the person.

The *physical environment* contains a wide variety of potential stimuli: gravity, light and sound waves, and meteorologic stimuli such as temperature variation, wind velocity, atmospheric pressure, humidity, solar radiation, air pollutants, ozone, oxygen, carbon dioxide and carbon monoxide levels, electromagnetic fields, day-night and seasonal periodicity, and infectious microorganisms. The physical environment such as housing and sanitation facilities affects health.

Cities are perceived as hostile environments because of the numerous barriers to physical and social good health. Urban environments may increase the severity of many illnesses or at least interfere with comfort, safety, and health. In any year the average urban dweller faces a 9% greater chance of dying than a suburban dweller and a 15% greater chance than a rural dweller. The Clean Air Act of 1970, amended in 1977, was revised in 1989. The revisions emphasized urban pollution associated with automobile fuel and technology, trace air pollutants related to industrial emissions, and acid rain associated with power plant emissions. Incidence of cancer is related directly or indirectly to air and other pollutants.

Smog in Los Angeles and other cities is associated with death from malignancy, pulmonary and cardiac disease, impaired breathing, cardiac problems, sensory irritation, and interference with well-being. Lead poisoning has a direct relationship to environmental pollution found in urban areas: airborne lead emitted by motor vehicles, chipped and peeling lead-based paint, and lead in soil as a result of vehicular traffic. Lead is still a threat to 3 to 4 million children. Social health problems are also higher in urban areas, including a higher incidence of low-birthweight infants, infant mortality, inadequate prenatal care, unplanned pregnancies, tuberculosis, and violence. The rates are one to three times higher in poverty areas than in higher income areas. Underclass communities are plagued by massive joblessness, flagrant and open lawlessness, and low-achieving students from the schools. Unemployment, hunger, homelessness, and poverty continue to increase, and there has been a significant increase in the number of the working poor (83).

The *workplace* can be hazardous to health; approximately one in every 11 workers suffers from illness or injury that is due to hazards in the workplace. The National Safety Council estimates that 11,500 injuries and 50,000 to 70,000 deaths occur annually in the United States as a result of work-related exposure to toxic substances (83).

The *indoor physical environment* also can affect health. Asbestos is associated with lung and other disease in workers in asbestos plants and in residents and schoolchildren who are in buildings in which asbestos is used for insulation. Cigarette smoke is a form of indoor pollution. Maternal smoking increases the risk of ectopic pregnancy and low birthweight and of respiratory infection and asthma in the child. Nonsmokers who are chronically exposed to cigarette smoke in the workplace have pulmonary function similar to that of light smokers and poorer than nonsmokers in a smokefree environment. Lung cancer is increased in nonsmoking wives of heavy smokers. Nonsmoking persons seated adjacent to smoking environments are exposed to similar levels of carbon monoxide and show similar physiologic reactions as the smoker. Migrants moving from one environment to another develop the cancer pattern of the new geographic area. Mortality rates from cancer and other disease differ according to geographic region. See Chapter 2 and other references for more information (9, 10, 21, 24, 35, 44, 63, 95).

Meteorologic stimuli are mediated primarily by the thermoregulatory centers of the hypothalamus and the autonomic nervous system. Seasonal variations affect every physiologic system. In winter calcium, magnesium, and phosphate blood levels are lowered; thyroid and adrenocorticoid activities are elevated; hemoglobin levels are increased; and gastric acid secretion is high. These changes are gradual and reflect the thermostatic properties of the hypothalamus in conserving heat and energy during cold winter months (9, 26).

Daily variations in *thermal stimuli* simultaneously affect the person. Responses to an approaching cold front include diuresis without increased fluid intake, increased thyrotropin production, elevated leukocyte and thrombocyte levels, elevated hemoglobin, lowered erythrocyte sedimentation rate, and increased fibrinolysis. The opposite changes occur during a heat wave. Any extreme fluctuation in environmental conditions results in a temporary disruption of internal environment and requires more energy to restore physiologic adaptation (9, 26).

Sociocultural attributes of climate and weather are reflected in the person's life-style, the kind of clothing worn, the food eaten, or the activities engaged in. The sedentary life-style produces a negative effect on health and eventually adds to health care costs and costs in the work setting (39).

Psychologic attributes of climate and weather relate to personal preference and symbolic interpretation. Some people perform optimally in cold weather, others in warm weather. Some people associate fog and rain with depression; to others such weather symbolizes security.

Although weather and climatic conditions affect the person in a given geographic setting, the *immediate physical environment* also provides multiple sensory stimuli. Room design and color, combinations of light and sound, and the arrangement of objects and persons in the room all form a *gestalt,* a whole pattern that may be perceived as either pleasant or unpleasant. One is sensitive to the physical and chemical stimuli in the environment that are of sufficient intensity and interest; some stimuli will not be perceived.

The *psychologic environment* surrounding someone is difficult to ascertain because it has a specific meaning to that person; the person's perception of the environment is a major determinant of behavior. The reactions of others contribute to the development of self-concept and self-esteem, foster support to and involvement with the person, stimulate maturity, and convey limits on behavior. A part of the psychologic environment is holiday time, and holidays such as Christmas, Hanukkah, Thanksgiving, or birthdays can be stressors and create great sadness and remembrance of losses in relation to past happy times. Thus the suicide rate and clinical depression are higher at such times (7).

To remain emotionally healthy, it is necessary to be with people who are healthy and in a group climate that contributes to developing one's optimum potential. Emotional health implies the capacity to love, learn, live fully, and share with others in the adventure of life. The emotionally ill person comes from an environment in which there is excessive tension, a barrier to emotional communication, and an isolation between people and in which emotional and social needs are not met. The emotional illness of one person in the family or group spills over so that all members are unhealthy to some degree.

Married and unmarried persons differ in their health status. Married men and women have lower morbidity rates for physical illness, use health services less frequently, and live longer than unmarried people. Although married women have a higher incidence of emotional illness than married men, single women have less incidence of emotional illness than single men. Married, employed women exhibit fewer physical and psychiatric symptoms than married, nonemployed women. Single men are at a greater risk for both physical and emotional illness. Sex-role expectations, lifestyle, and resultant emotional stress may be factors behind these statistics (36, 67).

Today more women, married and unmarried, are employed than ever before. Many working women also bear the major responsibility of child care. Women are exposed to the same physical and emotional hazards of the work environment as men plus the pressures created by multiple roles and conflicting expectations. The long-term health consequences of these complex changes are generally unknown; however, the National Institutes of Health report increased incidence of stress-related illnesses as a result of these changes (6, 36, 63, 67).

The *sociocultural environment* includes the historical era, family, and other people and groups; social institutions such as government, schools, and church; all sorts of social events; and shared values and moral, ethical, and religious beliefs. All groups have developed rules and regulations that assist an individual in the specific historical time in the process of becoming a useful and valued member of the group and that serve to constrain certain behaviors. Society helps an individual decide on the rules applicable in a particular situation, but it also grants the privilege of ignoring the rule if he or she so chooses. Punishment will be established for deviancy by the group if the rule is essential for the group's survival. Rules, values, and beliefs are fairly stable and resistant to change, thus giving the person variety with a basis for predicting outcome. However, change occurs so rapidly in our society that old values and relationships no longer have the same importance or meaning. Social instability produces conflict and alienation between groups, creates lack of direction for members, and contributes to illness (32, 67).

Migration and *resettlement* present special stresses and changes for the person and family, including grief over loss of and disruption in the environment and lifestyle, loss of relationships and country of birth, and the stress of novelty, culture shock, language and occupation changes, and a subordinate role in the new land. Stress is lessened when the person believes he or she is mastering the new environment (5).

The *family* contributes not only to genetic predisposition but also to the actual cause of specific diseases through lack of hygiene measures, nutritional imbalance, transmission of social values, the socialization process of the child, and the family pattern of daily living and behavior. Most dual-earner families experience a moderate level of family stress, especially when there are preschool children. Income, satisfaction with income, satisfaction with child care, flexibility in vacation scheduling, and age of parents and children are all factors affecting the stress levels of such families; and stress levels affect physical and emotional health (90). The family may also contribute to long-term health problems in its members through physical or emotional abuse or through sexual assault or incest.

Population density affects social behavior in animal studies and parallels human behavior in crowded conditions. Studies on small mammals show that uncontrolled population growth causes specific behaviors as population density increases: aggression, confusion as the number of social roles in the animal colony decreases, social withdrawal and avoidance of other animals, and loss of interest in tending young.

Socioeconomic class, occupation, and social roles influence behavior at various times of the day, preventive health measures practiced, and susceptibility to disease (24, 67, 94). Socioeconomic level influences health care accessibility. More affluent urban people can afford housing, food, and regular medical examinations that can promote health. Yet more affluent people may also be in executive positions or occupations or social roles that are highly stressful or that encourage overeating or social use of drugs or alcohol, thus predisposing the person to chemical dependency. The poorer rural person may not have an annual physical examination but may eat a diet composed primarily of simple carbohydrates, fish, and homegrown fruits and vegetables, which will contribute to health. Social roles are significant to health because they place various demands on the person and call for shifts and flexibility in attitude and behavior, which may be demanding to the point of illness. The occupational role is important. Whether the person is a farmer, nurse, coal miner, physician, executive, or clerk predisposes to different stressors and illnesses. The worker in an industrial plant may be exposed to carcinogenic materials. The miner living in poverty develops respiratory disease; he may realize his work is making him sick, but he is financially unable to change jobs or geographic locations. The middle-class person may work in a clean office, have conveniences to assist with housework, and see the dentist twice yearly for a checkup. The higher the socioeconomic class and occupational position, the greater is the variety of behavioral choices available to specific goals. For example, a study of 1000 professional executive women revealed, in comparison to an age-, gender-, and education-matched group of working women, greater life satisfaction, stronger social support, excellent health status, and higher satisfaction with personal and professional or work lives (46).

When availability of resources becomes restricted because of age, ethnic, economic, or geographic reasons, life-style and behavior are restricted.

Minority persons, including the elderly, often do not receive adequate health care because of (1) preference for informal help systems; (2) lack of accessibility to services; (3) lack of minority service providers or providers specialized in gerontology; (4) negative stereotyping or lack of knowledge held by nonminority mental health professionals; (5) Medicare limits on reimbursement and other financial constraints; and (6) fragmentation of services at the local, state, and national level. Minority elderly and persons from the lower socioeconomic class tend to somatize their emotional problems and to accept accompanying discomforts and are more likely to be seen in primary than in mental health care settings. For example, Chinese medical theory encourages this practice because the vocabulary is deficient in psychologic terms and diagnoses and treats somatic and psychosomatic illness identically. Puerto Ricans are likely to associate physical symptoms with psychosocial causes (23).

Neglect of the health of individuals, families, and the public at large—children, women, workers; the poor, the financially less secure, the elderly—costs far more in money, lives, and lost potential than is at first observable (54).

Internal Variables

Genetic inheritance influences the physical characteristics, innate temperament, activity level, and intellectual potential of the person. Physical characteristics include sex and features such as skin and eye color, hair color and degree of curl, facial structure, and height. The physical characteristics influence the response of others and the persons's response to the environment. The positive reinforcement and the interaction from the environment that a child or adult with desirable physical characteristics receives affect that person's self-concept development and relationship to others.

Intelligence, the *ability to deal with complex, abstract material,* is influenced by inheritance, environment, and sociocultural influences. The test score reflecting intelligence is influenced by many factors: motivation at the time of testing, what the test means to the person, level of anxiety, cultural and social class background of the person, physical environment of the testing situation, and the race and other characteristics of the tester.

Circadian and psychobiologic rhythms are part of the internal processes of the person, are interdependent with the time-space aspects of the environment, and help to organize behavior. They are discussed further in Chapter 12.

Gender of the person affects disease susceptibility; certain genetic and acquired diseases are more common in one sex than the other. One author believes that women, because of their unique biology and socialization, are subject to more physical and psychologic stresses than men (12, 99). *Sexual identity,* determined embryologically and molded through the influences of sociocultural environment, affects patterns of behavioral responses developed by that person. Cross-cultural studies show that division of labor is made on the basis of sex, although not all cultures designate home and child care as female functions. The environment makes distinctions in the expected and valued behaviors for each sex and indicates which sex is more valuable.

Age and developmental level influence illness susceptibility and behavior. Response patterns and capabilities are minimum for the first few years of life and near the end of life. The infant has few response patterns available because of two factors: lack of experience and a state of physiologic and psychologic immaturity. The old-old person has limited responses because of declining sensory-perceptual monitoring of the environment and declining physical abilities; the aged perceive their health as worse than that of middle-aged adults (48). The periods of greatest availability of responses to environmental and social demands are in young and middle adulthood; the peak years vary with each person and with occupational groups. Athletes peak earlier than physicians, for example.

Race of the person is related to cultural and ethnic experiences, values, and attitudes and to the responses of others to the person. Behavioral patterns may vary with the race, as does susceptibility to illness. Descendants of African and Mediterranean people, for instance, are more prone to sickle cell trait and sickle cell anemia.

Personality of the individual affects stress response, and stressors affect personality development. **Personality hardiness** is the *personality predisposition that functions as a mediator variable to mitigate effects of stressful events.* Hardiness involves three dimensions: (1) sense of commitment to self and work, (2) perception of control over one's environment, and (3) ability to approach life changes as challenges rather than threats (41). Staff nurses with higher hardiness scores indicated less of a sense of burnout or stress response on the job (71). The person with higher self-actualization scores tends to interpret stress more positively. The events that promote the feelings that are part of self-actualization may mediate against stressful life experiences or the perception of stress itself (65). The type A personality (competitive, hard-driving, aggressive, time-pressured, impatient) has been linked to cardiovascular and other disease (12). Less research has been done on type B personality (calm, relaxed). Individuals with type B personalities experience less stress as a result of dysfunction and feel less pressured by responsibility. They are more likely than individuals with type A personality to view life as a joy and to express fewer concerns about

the meaning of life (92). The type A personality may be made rather than born, for it may be the result of culture and socialization (e.g., the life-style, pace, and stresses in the United States tend to produce a high number of type A personalities). This personality type is rare or unknown in some cultures. Even in the United States, type A workers reverted to type B after 1 year of retirement in one study (33).

Self-concept is the *person's perception of self physically, emotionally, and socially, based on the internalized reactions of others to self.* The self-concept, self-expectations, perceived abilities, values, attitudes, habits, and beliefs affect how that person will handle situations and relate to others. How the person behaves depends on whether he or she feels positively or negatively and on how the person believes others expect him or her to behave in a specific situation. Additionally, the person discloses different aspects of self in various situations, depending on personal needs, what is considered socially acceptable, how others react, and past experience with self-disclosure. Thus the hospitalized client's behavior may be different from the usual pattern; the person may behave according to others' expectations instead of how he or she desires. These variables also affect health practices and treatment sought. The incidence of cancer has been linked to geographic and environmental factors, for example. In the United States, Seventh Day Adventists and rural Mormons in Utah have a lesser incidence of cancer, apparently because of their life-style, which is related to their religion.

The feelings of the person may be related to internal neuroendocrine processes, but they are also related to events in the external environment, including stressful events. A sense of hopelessness, despair, or extreme fear may cause death as well as disease. Many human and animal studies confirm this fact, and the death that results from a hex being placed on a member is documented in various societies. When the person becomes an outcast and has nothing to live for or feels hopeless, physiologic processes stop and death occurs (51).

Feelings are often related to the person's perception of the event. *The Social Readjustment Rating Scale (Life Change Scale)* was devised to assess perceptions of the amount of adjustment required by 43 life events involving personal, social, occupational, and family changes (Table 16–2). The scale has validity for various cultural groups (42, 69). Certain life events, especially undesirable ones, are perceived by most people as stressful or as crises because of the amount of change or extent of readjustment required. Scales have also been devised for different age levels (Table 16–3) (11) and for Spanish-speaking individuals (93). Because change is stressful and stress is a causative factor in illness, a relationship exists between the amount of recent change, number of crises encountered, and onset of illness (32, 70). Stressful events may even hasten death (32, 51).

TABLE 16-2. SOCIAL READJUSTMENT RATING SCALE[a]

Rank	Life Event	Mean Value
1	Death of spouse	100
2	Divorce	73
3	Marital separation	65
4	Jail term	63
5	Death of close family member	63
6	Personal injury or illness	53
7	Marriage	50
8	Fired at work	47
9	Marital reconciliation	45
10	Retirement	45
11	Change in health of family member	44
12	Pregnancy	40
13	Sex difficulties	39
14	Gain of new family member	39
15	Business readjustment	39
16	Change in financial state	38
17	Death of close friend	37
18	Change to different line of work	36
19	Change in number of arguments with spouse	35
20	Mortgage over $10,000	31
21	Foreclosure on mortgage or loan	30
22	Change in responsibilities at work	29
23	Son or daughter leaving home	29
24	Trouble with in-laws	29
25	Outstanding personal achievement	28
26	Wife begins or stops work	26
27	Begin or end school	26
28	Change in living conditions	25
29	Change in personal habits	24
30	Trouble with boss	23
31	Change in work hours or conditions	20
32	Change in residence	20
33	Change in schools	20
34	Change in recreation	19
35	Change in church activities	19
36	Change in social activities	18
37	Mortgage or loan less than $10,000	17
38	Change in sleeping habits	16
39	Change in number of family get-togethers	15
40	Change in eating habits	15
41	Vacation	13
42	Christmas	12
43	Minor violations of the law	11

Life Crisis Categories and LCU Scores[a]

No life crisis	0–149
Mild life crisis	150–199
Moderate life crisis	200–299
Major life crisis	300–or more

[a]The LCU score includes those life event items experienced during a 1-year period.
From Holmes, T. H., and R. H. Rahe, The Social Readjustment Rating Scale, *Journal of Psychosomatic Research,* 11, no. 8(1967), 213–217.

TABLE 16-3. LIFE EVENT SCALES FOR CHILDREN

Rank	Life Event	Life Change Units
Preschool Age Group		
1	Beginning nursery school	42
2	Increase in number of arguments with parents	39
3	Change in parents' financial status	21
4	Birth of a brother or sister	50
5	Decrease in number of arguments between parents	21
6	Change of father's occupation requiring increased absence from home	39
7	Death of grandparent	30
8	Outstanding personal achievement	23
9	Serious illness requiring hospitalization of parent	51
10	Brother or sister leaving home	39
11	Serious illness requiring hospitalization of brother or sister	37
12	Mother beginning to work	47
13	Change to a new nursery school	33
14	Change in child's acceptance by peers	38
15	Decrease in number of arguments with parents	22
16	Increase in number of arguments between parents	44
17	Serious illness requiring hospitalization of child	59
18	Loss of job by a parent	23
19	Death of a close friend	38
20	Having a visible congenital deformity	39
21	Addition of third adult to family	39
22	Marital separation of parents	74
23	Discovery of being an adopted child	33
24	Jail sentence of parent for 30 days or less	34
25	Death of parent	89
26	Divorce of parents	78
27	Acquiring a visible deformity	52
28	Death of brother or sister	59
29	Marriage of parent to stepparent	62
30	Jail sentence of parent for 1 year or more	67
Elementary Age Group		
1	Beginning another school year	27
2	Outstanding personal achievement	39
3	Beginning school	46
4	Move to a new school district	46
5	Increase in number of arguments with parents	47
6	Change in parents' financial status	29
7	Death of a grandparent	38
8	Decrease in number of arguments between parents	25
9	Mother beginning to work	44
10	Becoming a full-fledged member of a church	25
11	Brother or sister leaving home	36
12	Serious illness requiring hospitalization of parent	55
13	Decrease in number of arguments with parents	27
14	Change in father's occupation requiring increased absence from home	45
15	Change in child's acceptance by peers	51
16	Increase in number of arguments between parents	51
17	Death of a close friend	53
18	Birth of a brother or sister	50
19	Pregnancy in unwed teenage sister	36

(continued)

TABLE 16-3. LIFE EVENT SCALES FOR CHILDREN (Continued)

Rank	Life Event	Life Change Units	Rank	Life Event	Life Change Units
20	Serious illness requiring hospitalization of brother or sister	41	34	Fathering an unwed pregnancy	76
21	Loss of job by a parent	38	35	Acquiring a visible deformity	83
22	Failure of a grade in school	57	36	Jail sentence of a parent for 30 days or less	50
23	Divorce of parents	84	37	Death of a brother or sister	71
24	Suspension from school	46	38	Unwed pregnancy of child	95
25	Addition of third adult to family	41	39	Discovery of being an adopted child	70
26	Marital separation of parents	78	40	Jail sentence of a parent for 1 year or more	76
27	Serious illness requiring hospitalization of child	62		**Senior High Age Group**	
28	Marriage of parent to stepparent	65	1	Breaking up with boy or girlfriend	53
29	Having a visible congenital deformity	60	2	Increase in number of arguments with parents	47
30	Acquiring a visible deformity	69	3	Beginning senior high school	42
31	Death of a brother or sister	68	4	Beginning to date	51
32	Discovery of being an adopted child	52	5	Outstanding personal achievement	46
33	Becoming involved with drugs or alcohol	61	6	Becoming involved with drugs or alcohol	76
34	Jail sentence of parent for 30 days or less	44	7	Brother or sister leaving home	37
35	Jail sentence of parent for 1 year or more	67	8	Not making an extracurricular activity he or she wanted to be involved in	55
	Junior High Age Group		9	Decrease in number of arguments with parents	26
1	Outstanding personal achievement	45	10	Decrease in number of arguments between parents	27
2	Breaking up with a boyfriend or girlfriend	47	11	Change in parents' financial status	45
3	Increase in number of arguments with parents	46	12	Death of a close friend	63
4	Beginning junior high school	45	13	Increase in number of arguments between parents	46
5	Beginning to date	55	14	Death of grandparent	36
6	Brother or sister leaving home	33	15	Mother beginning to work	26
7	Decrease in number of arguments between parents	29	16	Suspension from school	50
8	Suspension from school	54	17	Becoming a full-fledged member of a church	31
9	Not making an extracurricular activity he or she wanted to be involved in	24	18	Serious illness requiring hospitalization of parent	55
10	Becoming a full-fledged member of a church	28	19	Change in child's acceptance by peers	67
11	Death of a grandparent	35	20	Move to a new school district	56
12	Death of a close friend	65	21	Change in father's occupation requiring increased absence from home	38
13	Increase in number of arguments between parents	48	22	Failure of a grade in school	56
14	Becoming involved with drugs or alcohol	70	23	Serious illness requiring hospitalization of brother or sister	41
15	Mother beginning to work	36	24	Loss of job by a parent	46
16	Decrease in number of arguments with parents	29	25	Being accepted at a college of his or her choice	43
17	Change in parents' financial status	40	26	Pregnancy in unwed teenage sister	54
18	Move to a new school district	52	27	Birth of a brother or sister	50
19	Serious illness requiring hospitalization of parent	54	28	Marital separation of parents	69
20	Serious illness requiring hospitalization of brother or sister	44	29	Serious illness requiring hospitalization of child	58
21	Failure of a grade in school	62	30	Divorce of parents	77
22	Change in child's acceptance by peers	68	31	Fathering an unwed pregnancy	77
23	Change in father's occupation requiring increased absence from home	42	32	Addition of third adult to family	34
24	Pregnancy in unwed teenage sister	60	33	Marriage of parent to stepparent	63
25	Loss of job by a parent	48	34	Unwed pregnancy of child	92
26	Birth of a brother or sister	50	35	Having a visible congenital deformity	62
27	Divorce of parents	84	36	Getting married	101
28	Addition of third adult to family	34	37	Death of parent	87
29	Serious illness requiring hospitalization of child	59	38	Discovery of being an adopted child	64
30	Marital separation of parents	77	39	Death of a brother or sister	68
31	Marriage of parent to stepparent	63	40	Jail sentence of a parent for 30 days or less	53
32	Death of a parent	94	41	Acquiring a visible deformity	81
33	Having a visible congenital deformity	70	42	Jail sentence of a parent for 1 yr or more	75

STRESS RESPONSE

Adaptation Syndrome

Stress is a *physical and emotional state always present in the person, one influenced by various environmental, psychologic, and social factors but uniquely perceived by the person and intensified in response when environmental change or threat occurs internally or externally and the person must respond.* The manifestations of stress are both overt and covert, purposeful, initially protective, maintaining equilibrium, productivity, and satisfaction to the extent possible (76, 79, 80, 81).

The person's survival depends on constant mediation between environmental demands and adaptive capacities. Various self-regulatory physical and emotional mechanisms are in constant operation, adjusting the body to a changing number and nature of internal and external stressors, agents, or factors causing intensification of the stress state. **Stressors** (*stress agents*) include cold, heat, radiation, infectious organisms, disease processes, mechanical trauma, fever, pain, imagined events, and intense emotional involvement. A moderate amount of stress, when regulatory mechanisms act within limits and few symptoms are observable, is constructive. The exaggerated stress state occurs when stressors are excessive or intense, limits of the steady state are exceeded, and the person cannot cope with the stressor's demands. **Distress** is *negative, noxious, unpleasant, damaging stress* that results when adaptive capacity is decreased or exhausted (79, 80). **Daily hassles** are the *repeated and chronic strains of everyday life.* Daily hassles have a negative effect on both somatic health and psychological status (14). **Eustress** is the *stress that comes with successful adaptation and that is beneficial or promotes emotional development and self-actualization.* It is *positive stress,* an optimum orientation to life's challenges coupled with the person's ability to regulate life and maintain optimum levels of stress for a growth-promoting life-style (79, 80).

Responses to stress are both local and general. The **local adaptation syndrome,** typified by the inflammatory response, is the *method used to wall off and control effects of physical stressors locally.* When the stressor cannot be handled locally, the *whole body responds to protect itself and ensure survival in the best way possible through the* **general adaptation syndrome.** The general body response augments body functions that protect the organism from injury, psychologic and physical, and suppresses those functions nonessential to life. The general adaptation syndrome is characterized by alarm and resistance stages and, when body resistance is not maintained, an end stage, exhaustion (80, 81).

General Adaptation Syndrome

The **alarm stage** is an *instantaneous, short-term, life-preserving, and total sympathetic–nervous system response* when the person consciously or unconsciously perceives a stressor and feels helpless, insecure, or biologically uncomfortable. This stage is typified by a "fight-or-flight" reaction (79). Perception of the stressor—the alarm reaction—stimulates the anterior pituitary to increase production of adrenocorticotropic hormone (ACTH). The adrenal cortex is stimulated by ACTH to increase production of glucocorticoids, primarily hydrocortisone, or cortisol, and mineralocorticoids, primarily aldosterone. Catecholamine release triggers increased sympathetic nervous system activity, which stimulates production of epinephrine and norepinephrine by the adrenal medulla and release at the adrenergic nerve endings. The alarm reaction also stimulates the posterior pituitary to release increased antidiuretic hormone (76, 79, 80). Generally the person is prepared to act, is more alert, and is able to adapt (Fig. 16–1).

Physiologically, the responses that occur when the sympathetic nervous system is stimulated are shown in Fig. 16–2 (72, 76, 77, 79–81).

To complicate assessment, there are times when *parts* of the parasympathetic division of the autonomic nervous system are inadvertently stimulated during a stressful state because of proximity of sympathetic and parasympathetic nerve fibers. With intensification of stress, opposite behaviors are then observed. They are shown in Fig. 16–3 (76–81).

The **stage of resistance** is the *body's way of adapting, through an adrenocortical response, to the disequilibrium caused by the stressors of life.* Because of the adrenocortical response, increased use of body resources, endurance and strength, tissue anabolism, antibody production, hormonal secretion, and changes in blood sugar levels and blood volume sustain the body's fight for preservation. Body response eventually returns to normal.

If biologic, psychologic, or social stresses, single or in combination, occur over a long period of time without adequate relief, the stage of resistance is maintained. With continued stressors, the person becomes distressed and manifests objective and subjective emotional, intellectual, and physiologic responses, as shown in Fig. 16–4 (77–81).

Protective factors *modify, ameliorate, or alter the person's response to stressors and to a potentially maladaptive outcome.* They include factors such as positive temperament; intelligence; ability to relate well to others; participation in achievements; success in school or the job; family support, closeness, and safe family environment; and extended family, friends, and teachers (74).

Be aware of these signs and symptoms (Figs. 16–2

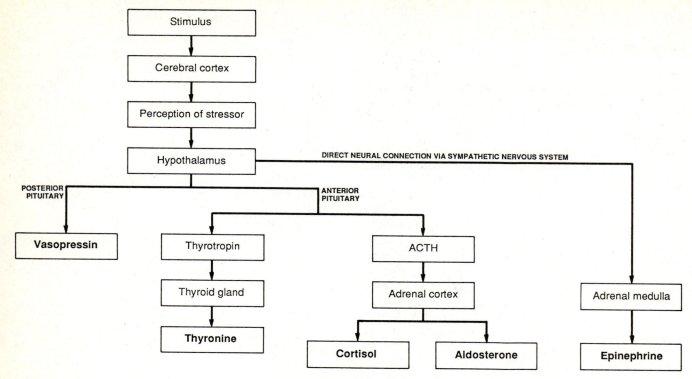

Figure 16-1. Neuroendocrine response to stress.

to 16–4) in yourself and in clients. You will encounter considerable stress in the work of nursing. Identify stressors, especially in situations in which your sense of self is threatened or in which you are made to feel incompetent. Share your feelings and talk about your work experiences with someone whom you trust and who will offer feedback about your coping skills. You will need someone who values you as a person, not just as a worker, who sees you as more than nurse, job, position, or nurturer, and who can help you put stressful work situations into perspective. Strive to develop a sense of being master of your own life and circumstances, a feeling that you can exert some control over what happens to you by the way you view yourself and adjust your behavior. When you can cope with your own work-related and other stressors, you can help clients and their families to adapt.

Stress is additive. The repeated or chronic exposure to stress, even when the stressors are of widely differing kinds, including other people and their feelings, ultimately takes a toll on the individual. Reserves of adaptability are used that cannot be replaced. Developmental milestones and tasks are less likely to be achieved. Some experience with stressors may aid coping with stress and be protective against stress-induced disease. Certain coping methods, feeling in command of the situation, and strong family and social ties can help a person to suffer less deleterious effects of stress. Breaking ties by separating from the group or a loved one, divorce, mobility, or death, and the resultant sense of loss, rejection,

and loneliness predispose to disease and death (55, 78, 79).

The **stage of exhaustion** occurs when the *person is unable to continue to adapt to internal and external environmental demands*. Physical or psychic disease or death results because the body can no longer compensate for or correct homeostatic imbalances. Manifestations of this stage are similar to those of the alarm stage except that all reactions first intensify and then diminish in response and show no ability to return to an effective level of function. Frequent or prolonged general adaptation syndrome response triggers disease through adrenocortical hypertrophy, thymolymphatic atrophy, elevated blood glucose, ulceration of the gastrointestinal tract, reduced tone and fibrosis of tissues, and vasoconstriction (79, 80).

Health care providers are concerned with promoting the resistance stage and preventing or reversing the exhaustion stage, whether through drugs, bed rest, medical treatments, crisis intervention, psychotherapy, or social action. Ideally you should identify potential stressors that the person might encounter and determine how to alter the stressors or best support the person's adaptive mechanisms and resources physically, emotionally, and socially, for the person will respond as an entity to the stressors. The relationship of stress to life crises or changes must be considered whenever you are doing health promotion measures or intervening with the ill person (55).

Although responses to stressful situations vary, anx-

Headache from neck & shoulder tense muscles.

Anti-inflammatory responses increase from glucocorticoid production. Defenses against inflammation/infection high for short time.

Thymus and lymph nodes atrophy if stage prolonged.

Respiratory rate/depth increased as bronchi dilate, due to increased epinephrine; allows adequate oxygenation.

Hyperglycemia from glucagon secretion in pancreas causing glycogenolysis; for energy demands after initial hypoglycemia. Increased glucocorticoid production results in gluconeogenesis in liver; body cells have sufficient glucose for stress response. Protein catabolism due to conversion of protein to glucose.

Gastric glandular acid and volume secretion increased; less essential functions such as digestion and excretion reduced. Intestinal smooth muscle relax, reducing motility. Sphincters contract. Anorexia, constipation, or flatulence may occur.

Adrenals enlarge, hyperactive, discolor. Salt and water retained by kidneys bolster intravascular blood volume due to increased antidiuretic hormone and aldosterone production and peripheral vasoconstriction; fuller blood pressure, less urinary output, and hemoconcentration result. Sodium chloride in extracellular fluid reduced; potassium levels rise. Hypochloremic.

Muscle tonus increased by epinephrine production; activities may be better coordinated, or rigidity and tremors may occur. Metabolic alterations in muscles with glycogenolysis and reduced use of glucose. Blood lactate and glucose increase.

Metabolic changes in adipose tissue; lipolysis and release of free fatty acids for use by muscles. Glycerol converted to glucose. depletion of corticolipids in adrenal cortex.

Pupils dilate, use maximum light for vision. Vision initially sharp, later blurred.

Myocardial rate, strength, and output increased by greater epinephrine production; more blood available throughout body as pulse rate and strength increase. Palpitations or arrhythmias may occur.

Blood pressure rises when increased norepinephrine produces peripheral vasoconstriction.

Increased blood clotting due to catecholamine stimulation of increased production of clotting factors. Increased blood viscosity may result in stasis and thrombosis if Alarm Stage persists.

Disappearance of blood eosinophiles.

In urinary bladder, detrusor muscle relaxes and trigone sphincter contracts; micturition inhibited. Or person voids only small amounts but feels urgency.

Blood supply shunted to brain, heart, and skeletal muscles rather than to periphery due to peripheral vasoconstriction. Skin pale, ashen, cool. Vasoconstriction stimulated by increased secretion of renin by kidney with reduced blood supply to kidney. Renin secretion stimulates production of plasma angiotensinogen; in turn, production of angiotension I and II causes vasoconstriction and increased blood pressure in vital organs.

Tissue Catabolism.

Metabolism increased up to 150%, providing immediate energy and producing more heat due to catecholamine release. Body temperature may rise. Perspiration. Mild dehydration from increased insensible fluid loss. (Dry lips and mouth occur.) If metabolism remains high, tissue catabolism, insomnia, fatigue, and signs of dehydration such as dry skin, weight loss, and decreased urinary output occur.

Immune responses initially suppressed.

Figure 16-2. Alarm stage, general adaptation syndrome: physiologic responses to sympathetic nervous system stimulation. (From Murray, R., and M.M. Huelskoetter, *Psychiatric/Mental Health Nursing: Giving Emotional Care* (3rd ed.). Norwalk, Conn.: Appleton & Lange, 1991, p. 336.)

iety is a common one. **Anxiety,** a *state of mental discomfort or uneasiness related to a feeling of helplessness or threat to self-image,* occurs in everyone, well or ill. Often there is no objective cause. The ill or hospitalized person may experience anxiety because of environmen-

tal changes. The individual exhibits signs of anxiety about the unknown: the outcome of surgery, the stability of job and family income, and possible death. The anxious person may experience the physical and behavioral effects that are described in Table 16–4. Other re-

Syncope may result

Respirations may become difficult because of constricted bronchi. If considerable carbon dioxide has been exhaled earlier with deep respirations, hyperventilation with accompanying tremors, syncope, and dizziness may occur.

Sphincters have diminished tone. Gastrointestinal secretion and propulsion increase, so that the person may have involuntary defecation or diarrhea. Urinary sphincter tone reduced; involuntary urination or frequency may result.

Muscle tonus may relax, so that incoordination results. Increased blood flow through muscles affects alterness and cognition and may cause syncope.

Pupil dilation may become fixed causing blurred vision, or constriction may occur, reducing acuity.

Cardiovascular output may diminish causing slow, thready pulse and a drop in blood pressure.

Blood supply does not remain shunted to vital organs but returns to periphery, causing flushed, hot skin and feelings of faintness.

Elevated body metabolism uses much energy; body reserves of glycogen may be depleted, and the person feels nauseated and hungry when hypoglycemia occurs.

Figure 16-3. Alarm stage, general adaptation syndrome: physiologic responses to parasympathetic nervous system stimulation. (From Murray, R., and M.M. Huelskoetter, *Psychiatric/Mental Health Nursing: Giving Emotional Care* (3rd ed.). Norwalk, Conn: Appleton & Lange, 1991, p. 337.)

sponses to stress include grief, mourning, and denial. These concepts are referred to in Chapter 13. Should the felt mental, emotional, or even physical disequilibrium become severe, mental or physical illness may result. Therefore the health of persons is directly related to and affected by their reactions to both the internal and external environment. You must be observant of the response that may indicate psychologic stress.

People use various behaviors to cope with anxiety or to attempt to change a stressful situation. Redistribution of energy is often not consciously recognized; thus a person may be unaware of any behavioral shifts, although others notice them. Certain behavioral changes may be the best the person can do at the time, although they seem inadequate to an objective observer.

Table 16–4 summarizes manifestations of the various levels of anxiety (8, 55, 64, 72).

Mind-Body Relationship

The **mind-body relationship,** the *effect of emotional responses to stress on body function and the emotional reactions to body conditions,* has been established

through research and experience. Emotional factors are important in the precipitation or exacerbation of nearly every organic disease and may increase susceptibility to infections. Stress and emotional distress, including depression, may influence function of the immune system via central nervous system and endocrine mediation, which is related to incidence of cancer, infections, and autoimmune diseases. Apparently adrenocortical steroid hormones are immunosuppressive. Recurring or chronic emotional stress has a cumulative physiologic effect and eventually may produce chronic dysfunction such as hypertension or gastric ulcers (26). The dynamics involve repression of certain feelings such as rage or guilt, fooling the mind into thinking the feelings have disappeared. But the body's physiologic functions respond to the feelings or perception of the effect (stressor) (52, 72, 78, 80, 84). *When physical or organic symptoms or disease result from feeling states, the process is called* **psychosomatic** *or* **psychophysiologic.** *The opposite process, feeling states of depression or worry in response to physical states, is called* **somatopsychic.**

The new field of **psychoneuroimmunology** *focuses on the links between the mind, brain, and immune system.* This is a newer perspective of the mind and body relationship in psychophysiologic causation of illness. Research shows that the immune system responds to the mind. The immune system is a very complex system consisting of approximately 1 trillion cells called lymphocytes and approximately 100 million trillion molecules called antibodies. The immune system has a special capability that allows it to patrol the body and guard its health (25, 26, 84).

Studies have correlated the levels of one immune substance in saliva (immunoglobulin A [IgA] and defense against respiratory infection for individuals with different motivational styles. People driven by an inhibited power motivation have lower IgA levels than those who form warm, close relationships. Studies show that, although not everyone reacts the same consciously to caring and loving, their bodies react by secreting more IgA. Salivary IgA increases even in people who intensely dislike the caring healer. These findings support the premise that it is not necessary to believe in the healer (placebo effect) to benefit. At the unconscious level something in the person will respond to the healer. Increased salivary IgA secretion occurs when the person feels an affiliative connection with the person who is trying to help or is involved in a friendly relationship (26).

Studies also show that type A behavior and an inhibited power motive are connected with the increased secretion of catecholamines, which suppress some aspects of the immune function. Too much of the catecholamine norepinephrine is associated with decline in immunoglobulin A, which makes the body less able to fight off certain viruses (26).

Psychoneuroimmunology provides a first step to-

Preoccupied. Forgetful. Disoriented. Confused. Low tolerance for ambiguity. Errors in judgment in relation to work, distance, grammar, or mathematics. Misidentification of people. Inability to concentrate, to solve problems, or to plan. Inattention to detail or instructions. Reduced fantasy, creativity, and preceptual field.

Lacks initiative; less interest in usual activities, future, or people.

Headache and neckache from tense trapezius muscle. Lower self-esteem, negative self-concept. Decreased awareness to external stimuli.

Sleep patterns irregular; nightmares.

Stomach muscles tight. Eating and elimination patterns irregular—increased or decreased. Emesis. Diarrhea. Flatulence.

Adrenal cortex hypertrophy Hyperchloremia.

Skeletal muscles tight, causing aches, trembling, tics, tremors. Restless. Agitated movements. Easily startled.

Immune system changed
Natural killer cell activity.

Susceptibility to disease and accidents increased.

Free-floating anxiety. Overreaction to most events. Regressive behavior.

Irritable. Impatient. Angry. Withdrawn. Suspicious. Depressed. Crying. Stuttering. High-pitched voice or laughter. States feelings of worthlessness, criticism of others, helplessness. Rumination about past. Grinding of teeth. Dry mouth.

Vital signs remain elevated, but lower than in Alarm Stage. Palpitations. Chest muscles tight, causing dyspnea, shortness of breath. Hemodilution.

Pain in body, including lower back or limbs.

Premenstrual tension or missed menstrual periods.

Urinary frequency. Sexual dysfunction.

Inefficient movement; lowered productivity. Inefficient use of work or leisure time.

Tissue anabolism initially.

Posture slumps. Weakness. Feeling of fatigue constant.

Increased use of medications. Increased smoking. Alcohol and drug addiction. Emotional instability. Neurotic behavior. Psychosis.

Strained relations with others. Impaired ability to love.

Stage of Exhaustion occurs if Stage of Resistance cannot be maintained.

Aggressive behavior. Impulsive.

Figure 16-4. Stage of resistance, general adaptation syndrome: signs of emotional, intellectual, and physiologic distress. (From Murray, R., and M.M. Huelskoetter, *Psychiatric/Mental Health Nursing: Giving Emotional Care* (3rd ed.). Norwalk, Conn: Appleton & Lange, 1991, p. 338.)

ward an affirmative science that makes quality of life as important as traditional sciences have made extension of life.

Simonton (84), a radiation oncologist, believes that just as we participate in our illness, so we participate in our health. His program involves a frank, honest ap-

praisal of the stresses in life before illness, why they were stressful, benefits derived from the illness, and methods to achieve an honest, relatively stressfree, positive attitude about life-style and illness. Often the client finds that before illness, the stresses did have the person's full participation. The person may have had a

TABLE 16-4. MANIFESTATIONS AND LEVELS OF ANXIETY

Level	Type	Effect
Mild	Physiologic	Tension of needs motivates behavior.
		Adaptive to variety of internal and external stimuli.
	Cognitive	Attentive, alert, perceptive to variety of stimuli, effective problem solving.
	Emotional	No intense feelings; self-concept not threatened.
		Use of ego adaptive mechanisms minimal, flexible.
		Behavior appropriate to situation.
Moderate	Physiologic	Some symptoms may be present.
	Cognitive	Perceptual field narrows; responds to directions.
		Tangible problems solved fairly effectively, at least with direction and support.
		Selective inattention—focus is on stimuli that do not add to anxiety.
	Emotional	Impatient, irritable, forgetful, demanding, crying, angry.
		Uses any adaptive mechanism (e.g., rationalization, denial, displacement) to protect from feelings and meaning of behavior.
		(Physiological, cognitive, and emotional changes of alarm and resistance stages. Individual functions in normal pattern but may not feel as healthy physically or emotionally as usual. Illness may result if feeling persists.)
Severe	Physiologic	Alarm stage changes intensify, and stage of resistance may progress to stage of exhaustion.
	Cognitive	Perceptual field narrows; stimuli distorted, focus is on scattered details.
		Selective inattention prevails.
		Learning and problem solving ineffective.
		Clarification of restatement needed repeatedly.
		Misinterprets statements.
		Unable to follow directions or remember main points.
		Unable to plan or make decisions; needs assistance with details.
		Disorganized.
		Consciousness and lucidity reduced.
	Emotional	Self-concept threatened; sense of helplessness; mood changes.
		Behavior erratic, inappropriate, regressive, inefficient; may be aware of inappropriate behavior but unable to improve.
		Many ego defense mechanisms used; dissociation and amnesia may be used.
		Disorientation, confusion, suspicion, hallucinations, and delusions may be present.
		(Psychoses or physical illness or injury may result.)
Panic	Physiologic	Severe symptoms of exhaustion stage may be ignored.
	Cognitive	Sensory ability and attention reduced so that only object of anxiety noticed.
		May fail to notice specific object of concern or disastrous event but will be preoccupied with trivial detail.
	Emotional	Self-concept overwhelmed.
		Ego defense mechanism used, often inappropriately and uncontrollably.
		Behavior focused on finding relief; may scream, cry, pray, thrash limbs, run, hit others, hurt self.
		Often easily distracted; cannot attend or concentrate.
		No learning, problem solving, decision making, or realistic judgments.
		May become immobilized, assume fetal position, become mute, or be unresponsive to directions.
		Needs protection.
		(Psychoses may occur.)

stressor because of failure to confront, to express anger, to grieve, or to trust intuitive feelings or because of unrealistic expectations or lack of courage of personal convictions. Current stressors are analyzed and resolved. An important part of the program is to use mental imagery or visualization, in which natural body defenses are combined with medical treatment to overcome malignant cells by visualizing the body's white cells in overcoming cancer cells. The client switches from a passive to active role, which enhances the body's immune system. Physical exercise, counseling, and mental imagery are used to overcome feelings about the disease, to set realistic goals, to find an inner advisor to talk and listen to, and to list steps to wellness. The hopelessness and helplessness feelings are removed. The person gains a sense of control by participating actively in the recovery process. Positive, hopeful messages are sent to the limbic system, stimulating the immune system.

REFERENCES

1. Abraham, I., and H. van Koss Krowchuk, Unemployment and Health: Health Promotion for the Jobless Male, *Nursing Clinics of North America,* 21, no. 1 (1986), 39–50.
2. Alster, K., *The Holistic Health Movement.* Tuscaloosa: University of Alabama Press, 1989.
3. Archer, S., C. Kelly, and S. Bisch, *Implementing Change in Communities: A Collaborative Process.* St. Louis: C.V. Mosby, 1984.

4. Arling, G., Strain, Social Support and Distress in Old Age, *Journal of Gerontology,* 42, no. 1 (1987), 107–113.

5. Aroian, K., A Model of Psychological Adaptation to Migration and Resettlement, *Nursing Research,* 39, no. 1 (1990), 5–10.

6. Aubrey, L., Health as a Social Concept, *British Journal of Sociology,* 4 (June 1953), 115.

7. Baier, M., The "Holidays Blues" as a Stress Reaction, *Perspectives in Psychiatric Care,* 24, no. 2 (1987/1988), 64–68.

8. Carson, R., J. Butcher, and J. Coleman, *Abnormal Psychology and Modern Life* (8th ed.). Glenview, Ill: Scott, Foresman, 1988.

9. Clark, C. *Wellness Nursing: Concepts, Theory, Research, and Practice.* New York: Springer, 1986.

10. Clemen-Stone, S., D. Eigsti, and S. McGuire, *Comprehensive Family and Community Health Nursing* (3rd ed.). St. Louis: C.V. Mosby, 1991.

11. Coddington, R., The Significance of Life Events as Etiologic Factors in the Diseases of Children, *Journal of Psychosomatic Research,* 16 (1972), 7–18, 205–213.

12. Cooper, K., *The Aerobic Program for Well-Being.* New York: Bantam Books, 1982.

13. Coste, J., N. Job-Spiro, and H. Fernandez, Increased Risk of Ectopic Pregnancy With Maternal Cigarette Smoking, *American Journal of Public Health,* 81, no. 2 (1991), 199–201.

14. De Longis, A., S. Folkman, and R. Lazarus, The Impact of Daily Stress on Health & Mood: Psychological and Social Resources as Mediators, *Journal of Personality and Social Psychology,* 54 (1988), 486–495.

15. Department of Health and Social Security, *Prevention and Health: Everybody's Business.* London: Her Majesty's Stationary Office, 1976.

16. Dixon, J.K., and J.P. Dixon, An Evolutionary-Based Model of Health and Viability, *Advances in Nursing Science,* 6, no. 3 (1984), 1–8.

17. DuBois, R., *Man Adapting.* New Haven: Yale University Press, 1965.

18. ———, Man Overadapting, *Psychology Today,* 4, no. 9 (1971), 50 ff.

19. Dunn, H., High Level Wellness for Man and Society, *American Journal of Public Health,* 49 (1959), 789.

20. ———, What High Level Wellness Means, *Canadian Journal of Public Health* (November 1959), 447.

21. Edelman, C., and C. Mandel, *Health Promotion Throughout the Life Span* (2nd ed.). St. Louis: C.V. Mosby, 1990.

22. Fangham, P., and D. Flagel, Medical Intervention and Effectiveness of the Health Care Delivery System: A Canadian Perspective, *Holistic Nursing Practice,* 5, no. 3 (1991), 77–84.

23. Fellin, P., and T. Powell, Mental Health Services and Older Adult Minorities: An Assessment, *Gerontologist,* 28, no. 4 (1988), 442–447.

24. Goeppinger, J., Community as Client: Using the Nursing Process to Promote Health. In Stanhope, M., and J. Lancaster, eds., *Community Health Nursing: Process and Practice for Promoting Health.* St. Louis: C.V. Mosby, 1984.

25. Groër, M., Psychoneuroimmunology, *American Journal of Nursing,* 91, no. 8 (1991), 33.

26. Guyton, A.C., *Basic Human Physiology: Normal Function and Mechanisms of Defense* (7th ed.). Philadelphia: W.B. Saunders, 1986.

27. Haddon, R., An Economic Agenda for Health Care, *Nursing and Health Care,* 11, no. 1 (1990), 21–30.

28. Hall, B., and J. Allan, Sharpening Nursing's Focus by Focusing on Health, *Nursing and Health Care,* 7, no. 6 (1986), 315–320.

29. Hall, L., and A. Farel, Maternal Stresses and Depressive Symptoms: Correlates of Behavior Problems in Young Children, *Nursing Research,* 37, no. 3 (1988), 156–161.

30. Hayman, H., Our Modern Concept of Health, *Journal of School Health* (September 1962), 253.

31. Higginson, J., A Hazardous Society? Individual Versus Community Responsibility in Cancer Prevention, *American Journal of Public Health,* 66, no. 4 (1976), 359–366.

32. Holmes, T.H., and R.H. Rahe, The Social Readjustment Rating Scale, *Journal of Psychosomatic Research,* 11, no. 8 (1967), 213–217.

33. Howard, J., et al., Change in Type A Behavior a Year After Retirement, *Gerontologist,* 26, no. 6 (1986), 643–649.

34. Howell, M., *National Women's Health Network Newsletter* (Fall 1982), 1–4.

35. Humble, C., et al., Passive Smoking and 20-Year Cardiovascular Disease Mortality Among Nonsmoking Wives, Evans County, Georgia, *American Journal of Public Health,* 80, no. 5 (1990), 599–601.

36. Jacobson, S., Psychosocial Stresses of Working Women, *Nursing Clinics of North America,* 17, no. 1 (1982), 137–144.

37. Johnson, D., The Behavioral System Model for Nursing. In Riehl, J., and C. Roy, eds., *Conceptual Models for Nursing Practice* (3rd ed.), Norwalk, Conn: Appleton & Lange, 1988.

38. Jourard, S., *The Transparent Self.* New York: D. Van Nostrand, 1971.

39. Keeler, E., et al. The External Costs of a Sedentary Lifestyle, *American Journal of Public Health,* 79, no. 8 (1989), 975–981.

40. King, I., *A Theory for Nursing: Systems, Concepts, Processes.* New York: Wiley, 1981.

41. Kobasa, S., The Hardy Personality: Toward a Social Psychology of Stress and Health. In Suls, J., and G. Sanders, eds., *Social Psychology of Health and Illness.* Hinsdale, NJ: Erlbaum, 1982.

42. Kamaroff, A., M. Masuda, and T. Holmes, The Social Readjustment Rating Scale: A Comparative Study of Negro, Mexican, and White Americans, *Journal of Psychosomatic Research,* 12 (1968), 121–128.

43. Krick, J., and J. Sobel, Relationship Between Health Protective Behaviors, *Journal of Community Health,* 15, no. 1 (1990), 19–34.

44. Kristiansen, C., Smoking, Health Behavior, and Value Priorities, *Addictive Behaviors,* 10, no. 1 (1985), 41–44.

45. Lalonde, M., *New Perspective on the Health of Canadians.* Ottawa, Ontario: Information Canada, 1974.

46. LaRosa, J., Executive Women and Health: Perceptions and Practices, *American Journal of Public Health,* 80, no. 12 (1990), 1450–1454.

47. Levine, M., *Introduction to Clinical Nursing* (2nd ed.). Philadelphia: F.A. Davis, 1973.

48. Levkoff, S., P. Cleary, and T. Wetle, Differences in the Appraisal of Health Between Aged and Middle Aged Adults, *Journal of Gerontology,* 42, no. 1 (1987), 114–120.

49. Marantz, P., Blaming the Victim: The Negative Consequence of Preventive Medicine, *American Journal of Public Health,* 80, no. 10 (1990), 1186–1187.

50. Maslow, A., *The Further Reaches of Human Behavior.* New York: Viking Press, 1971.

51. Miller, J., and M. Powers, Development of an Instrument to Measure Hope, *Nursing Research,* 37, no. 1 (1988), 6–10.

52. Miller, T., Advances in Understanding the Impact of Stressful Life Events on Health, *Hospital and Community Psychiatry,* 39 (1988), 625.

53. Montague, K., Let Like Cure Like, *Nursing Mirror,* 160, no. 21 (May 22, 1985), 30–33.

54. Montgomery, P., At Risk: The Hidden Cost of Neglecting Public Health, *Common Cause Magazine* (March-April 1989), 29–33.

55. Murray, R., M.M. Huelskoetter, and D. O'Driscoll, *Psychiatric/Mental Health Nursing: Giving Emotional Care* (3rd ed.). Norwalk, Conn: Appleton-Lange, 1991.

56. Natapoff, J., Children's View of Health: A Developmental Study, *American Journal of Public Health,* 68, no. 10 (1978), 995–999.

57. Neugarten, B., Time, Age, and the Life Cycle, *American Journal of Psychiatry,* 136 (1979), 887–894.

58. Neuman, B., *The Neuman System's Model: Application to Nursing Education and Practice* (2nd ed.). Norwalk, Conn: Appleton & Lange, 1989.

59. Newman, M., *Theory Development in Nursing.* Philadelphia: F.A. Davis, 1980.

60. Niknian, M., C. Lefebvre, and R. Carleton, Are People More Health Conscious? A Longitudinal Study of One Community, *American Journal of Public Health,* 81, no. 2 (1991), 203–205.

61. Office of Assistant Secretary for Health and Surgeon General, *Healthy People.* Washington, DC: U.S. Government Printing Office, 1979.

62. Orem, D., *Nursing: Concepts of Practice* (3rd ed.). New York: McGraw-Hill, 1986.

63. Pender, N., *Health Promotion in Nursing Practice* (2nd ed.). E. Norwalk, Conn: Appleton & Lange, 1987.

64. Peplau, H., *Interpersonal Relations in Nursing.* New York: G.P. Putnam's Sons, 1952.

65. Petosa, R., Eustress and Mental Health Promotion, *Health Values and Achieving High Level Wellness,* 9, no. 1 (1985), 3–7.

66. Petze, C., Health Promotion for the Well Family, *Nursing Clinics of North America,* 19, no. 2 (1984), 229–237.

67. Polan, K.C., Determinants of Health-Promotive Behaviors: A Review of Current Research, *Nursing Clinics of North America,* 26, no. 4 (1991), 815–832.

68. Program and Policies Advisory Committee, *Recommendation for a National Strategy for Disease Prevention.* Atlanta: Centers for Disease Control, 1978.

69. Rahe, R., Multi-Cultural Correlations of Life Change Scaling: America, Japan, Denmark, and Sweden, *Journal of Psychosomatic Research,* 13 (1969), 191–195.

70. Rahe, R., and R. Arthur, Life Change Patterns Surrounding Illness Perception, *Journal of Psychosomatic Research,* 11, no. 3 (1968), 341–345.

71. Rich, V., and A. Rich, Personality Hardiness and Burnout in Female Staff Nurses, *Image,* 19, no. 2 (1987), 63–66.

72. Robinson, L., Stress and Anxiety, *Nursing Clinics of North America,* 25, no. 4 (1990), 935–943.

73. Roy, C., *Introduction to Nursing: An Adaptation Model* (2nd ed.). Englewood Cliffs, NJ: Prentice-Hall, 1984.

74. Rutter, M., Resilience in the Face of Adversity: Protective Factors and Resistance to Psychiatric Disorder, *British Journal of Psychiatry,* 147 (1985), 598–611.

75. Samet, J., New Effects of Active and Passive Smoking on Reproduction, *American Journal of Epidemiology,* 133, no. 4 (1991), 348–350.

76. Seyle, H., Stress Syndrome, *American Journal of Nursing,* 65, no. 3 (1965), 97–99.

77. ———, *Stress Without Distress.* Philadelphia: J.B. Lippincott, 1974.

78. ———, Implications of Stress Concept, *New York State Journal of Medicine* (October 1975), 2139–2145.

79. ———, Forty Years of Stress Research: Principal Remaining Problems and Misconceptions, *Canadian Medical Association Journal,* 115 (July 3, 1976), 53–56.

80. ———, *The Stress of Life* (rev. ed.). New York: McGraw-Hill, 1976.

81. ———, Stress and the Reduction of Distress, *Primary Cardiology,* 5, no. 8 (1979), 22–30.

82. ———, The Stress Concept Today. In Kutash, I.C., and L. B. Schlesinger, eds., *Handbook on Stress and Anxiety.* New York: Jossey-Bass, 1980, 127–144.

83. Shannon, I., Urban Health: Challenges and Opportunities, *Henry Ford Hospital Journal,* 38, nos. 2 and 3 (1990), 144–147.

84. Simonton, O.C., et al., *Getting Well Again: A Step-by-Step Self-Help Guide to Overcoming Cancer for Patients and Their Families.* New York: Bantam, 1982.

85. Smilkstein, G., The Cycle of Family Functions: A Conceptual Model for Family Medicine, *Family Practitioner,* 11 (1980), 223.

86. Smith, J., *The Idea of Health: Implications for the Nursing Profession.* New York: Teachers College Press, 1983.

87. Sorochan, W., Health Concepts as a Basis for Orthobiosis. In Hart, E., and W. Sechrist, eds., *The Dynamics of Wellness.* Belmont, Calif: Wadsworth, 1970.

88. Stoto, M., and J. Durch, National Health Objectives for the Year 2000: The Demographic Impact of Health Promotion and Disease Prevention, *American Journal of Public Health,* 81, no. 11 (1991), 1456–1465.

89. Sullivan, H.S., *The Interpersonal Theory of Psychiatry.* New York: W.W. Norton, 1953.

90. Sund, K., and S. Ostwald, Dual-Earner Families' Stress Levels and Personal and Life-Style–Related Variables, *Nursing Research,* 34, no. 6 (1985), 357–361.

91. Survey Shows Improvements and Setbacks in Healthy Habits, *Nation's Health,* 21, no. 7 (1991), 9.

92. Thomas, S., A Descriptive Profile of Type B Personality, *Image,* 18, no. 1 (1986), 4–7.

93. Timmreck, T., and L. Stratton, The Schedule of Recent Events: A Measure of Stress Due to Life Change Events Translated for the Spanish-Speaking, *Journal of Psychosocial Nursing and Mental Health Services,* 16, no. 8 (1978), 20–30.

94. Tinkham, C., E. Voorheis, and N. McCarthy, *Community Health Nursing: Evolution and Process in the Family and Community* (3rd ed.). Norwalk, Conn: Appleton-Century-Crofts, 1984.

95. Tripp-Reimer, T., Reconceptualizing the Concept of Health: Integrating Emic-Etic Perspectives, *Research in Nursing and Health,* 7 (1984), 101–109.

96. U.S. Public Health Service, *Promoting Health, Preventing Disease. Objectives for the Nation.* Washington, DC: U.S. Government Printing Office, 1980.

97. Walker, S., et al., A Spanish Language Version of the Health Promoting Lifestyle Profile, *Nursing Research,* 39, no. 5 (1990), 268–273.

98. Webster, D., Changing Definitions; Changing Times, *Nursing Clinics of North America,* 21, no. 1 (1986), 87–97.

99. Witkin-Lanoil, G., *The Female Stress Syndrome: How to Recognize and Live With It.* Berkeley, Calif: Berkeley Press, 1985.

100. World Health Organizations, *Global Strategy for Health by All by The Year 2000.* Geneva: World Health Organization, 1981.

Chapter 17

Health Promotion Strategies

Over 99 percent of us have been healthy and made sick as a result of personal misbehavior and environmental conditions.
—*John H. Knowles*

Life is not a matter of holding good cards but of playing a poor hand well.
—*Robert Louis Stevenson*

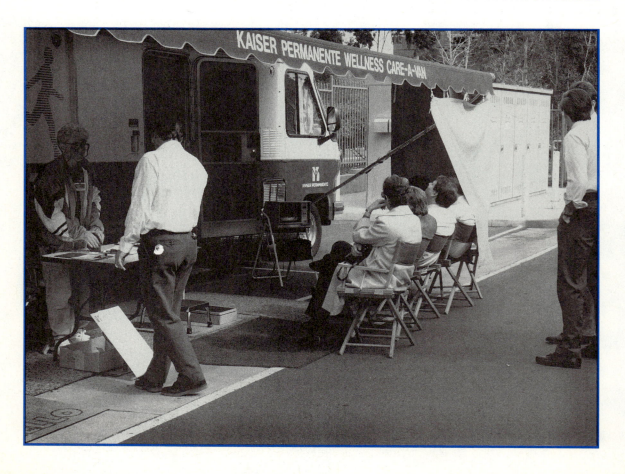

KEY TERMS

Health promotion	Human Ecologic Model	Teaching	Biofeedback
Health protective behavior	Model of Multiple Risk Factor Behavior	Education	Massage
Primary prevention		Health education	Yoga
Secondary prevention	Nurse-client relationship	Self-care	Autogenics
Tertiary prevention	Initial or orientation phase	Quack	Thought stopping
Health behaviors	Identification phase	Health screening	Self-talk
Illness behavior	Working phase	Progressive relaxation	Coping skills training
Health Belief Model	Maintenance phase	Acupuncture	Centering
Health Promotion Model	Termination phase	Acupressure	Assertiveness
Resource Model of Preventive Health Behavior	Learning	Shiatsu	Guided imagery
		Reflexology	Plus factor

OBJECTIVES

Study of this chapter will enable you to:

1. Discuss the concept of health promotion and its application to holistic nursing.
2. Define terms related to health promotion and illness prevention.
3. Compare and contrast models of health promotion and illness prevention.
4. Assess health promotion behaviors or life-style, using a selected instrument.
5. Differentiate between a social and helpful nurse-client relationship.
6. Describe guidelines for a therapeutic nurse-client relationship.
7. List and describe the phases of the nurse-client relationship and the effect of the nurse's and client's feelings on each phase.
8. Describe methods of therapeutic communication and the rationale for each method.
9. Discuss ways to modify a communication approach to be effective with clients who have communication disorders.
10. Explore how use of effective communication methods is basic to nursing care and contributes to health promotion.
11. Define *health education* and *self-care*.
12. Compare methods of teaching with various ages, including individual and group approaches, and predict when each might be appropriate.
13. Identify the varied opportunities for teaching health promotion.
14. List the characteristics of a medical quack and discuss how you can help people avoid hazards of medical quackery.
15. Describe health screening procedures that should be done at various ages.
16. Describe the importance of and recommendations for adequate nutrition.
17. Describe the benefits of a well-planned exercise schedule and the balance of exercise and rest for health.
18. Review methods to prevent illness and injury such as immunizations, infection control, safety promotion, control of environmental hazards, and measures to eliminate hazards destructive to life.
19. Describe and practice various methods of relaxation or physical methods for stress management.
20. Discuss stress management measures that will assist the person or family to adapt to or cope with internal or external changes (physical, emotional, social, cultural).
21. Discuss groups in your area whose health promotion needs are not adequately met and ways that could be implemented to improve their health care.
22. Discuss nursing measures that are conducive to health promotion–wellness, considering factors that influence preventive health behavior.

Health promotion and maintenance and disease prevention are not new roles in nursing, although holistic health promotion roles are given increasing emphasis in the nursing process. The knowledge and theories pertinent to health promotion and maintenance are diverse and broad and relate to physical, psychologic, cognitive, social, and spiritual or moral dimensions of the person or family, as shown in Table 17–1.

Health promotion measures are described in each chapter as appropriate to the content of the chapter. For example, assessment and intervention for health promotion of people of various cultures and religions are described in Chapters 1 and 3, respectively, based on knowledge of cultural and religious or spiritual concepts. Chapter 2 describes health promotion measures in response to environmental contaminants and in the occupational setting. General strategies to promote health of the family unit are described in Chapter 4. The importance of and measures for health promotion for the de-

TABLE 17-1. EXAMPLES OF HEALTH PROMOTION STRATEGIES TO DIMENSIONS OF THE WHOLE PERSON

Physical/Physiologic	Emotional	Cognitive	Social	Spiritual/Moral
Proper nutrition/fluid balance Balance of exercise-rest Immunizations Safety measures Temperature control Prevention of environmental hazards and pollution Cessation of habits destructive to health (smoking, alcohol or drug abuse, overeating) Health screening	Consistent warm, tender, nurturing of offspring Effective communication Effective guidance/discipline Promotion of self-esteem, self-confidence, security Anxiety reduction measures Play, use of toys, leisure activities Crisis resolution	Promotion of curiosity and learning Coping methods Visualization Imagery Health education	Socialization processes Family, friend, peer relations Group associations and processes Maintenance of cultural ties	Values clarification Acknowledgment of meaning and purpose of life Establishment of belief system Establishment of moral and ethical behaviors

veloping embryo and fetus and for the woman in the prenatal period are described in Chapter 6. Health promotion and safety measures are described for each developmental era, infancy through later maturity, in Chapters 7 through 14. These various measures or strategies are referred to later in this chapter for purposes of integration and synthesis.

Application of knowledge of developmental theories, as described in Chapter 5, facilitate emotional and mental or cognitive health. For example, Erikson's theory can help parents understand normal developmental needs and behavior of their offspring and themselves. Ways to promote a sense of trust, autonomy, initiative, industry, identity, intimacy, generativity, and ego integrity are discussed in Chapters 7 through 14, respectively, and are pertinent to nurses and other health care providers and to families and parents. Duvall's theory can help parents understand developmental tasks of offspring and the family unit. With such information they can contribute better to the emotional and mental health of offspring, middle-aged and elderly family members, and the total family unit. Understanding of Piaget's theory can assist nurses, teachers, and parents in facilitating intellectual and cognitive development and health of the child. Piaget's theory is discussed in Chapters 7 through 11. Behavioral theories are frequently applied by families in discipline of the child. Understanding the importance of reinforcement and modeling of behavior is useful to nurses, other health care professionals, teachers, and parents and the family unit. Application of behavioral theories are described in Chapters 7 through 14 as appropriate to the developmental era. Behavioral, psychodynamic, family, and humanistic theories all assist in understanding aspects of socialization, social development, and development of language and communication abilities.

This chapter focuses primarily on health promotion strategies not previously described.

HEALTH PROMOTION: WHAT IS IT?

The nursing profession must focus on health and not just the disease model (125). An ecologic view, realizing multiple causation in many situations that threaten health, is essential. Further, an ecologic view can be useful in health promotion and wellness nursing, resulting in a total or holistic approach and looking at all aspects of the person.

Wellness nursing focuses on joint assessment with the client, including body, mind, and spirit interaction and integration and historical, social, and cultural factors; application of theory to the specific needs and goals of the person; promoting whole-person healing and self-healing; self-care measures; and evaluation of the movement toward wellness. The person evolves toward wellness by learning: (1) to manage life experiences, (2) to seek challenges, (3) to relate to others flexibly and assertively, (4) to use self-care strategies, (5) to examine and readjust beliefs and practices to maintain goal-directed wholeness, and (6) to develop coping strategies that reduce stress. Clark (20) believes that Wellness Theory is a broad base for practice that can unite nurses in their practice, especially health promotion practice. Wellness Theory can increase cohesiveness among nurses and should reduce arguments about the purpose of nursing. Further, theory on wellness can be explained as a basis for action when members of other disciplines challenge the nurse's practice. Lastly, Wellness Theory can help nurses work with clients to improve their quality of life. From the client's view, a wellness focus is more in harmony with the perceived needs, sense of autonomy, and life-style. A shift in the allocation of governmental funds and services and private insurance programs reinforces the emphasis in use of Wellness Theory and practice and working with the self-care movement.

The use of Wellness Theory is applicable to holistic

nursing (defined in Chapter 16), which can be practiced in any setting. In holistic nursing you view the client as more than just a collection of body parts. In addition to biologic aspects, you also address psychologic, social, cultural, and spiritual aspects of care. Nurses and physicians have a complementary relationship. The physician focuses on body system pathology; the nurse focuses on the whole person, well or ill, and the response to illness, in addition to the technology of the specialty. Caring for a client holistically means being part of a team that includes the client and his or her family, nurses, doctors, physical therapists, respiratory therapists, dieticians—anyone who can contribute to the recovery and well-being of the person. For example, in working with persons who have chronic pain, the most important thing is to help them realize that their situation is not hopeless—that in addition to more traditional medical treatments, there are many self-help therapies to which they can turn such as acupressure, exercise, relaxation training, and imagery. A staff of nurses, physicians, psychologists, and physical, occupational, and family therapists work with each person to teach him or her how best to manage the pain and the response to it (2).

Various models are proposed to understand better health promotion and illness prevention behaviors.

DEFINITIONS

Until recently most of the focus, and therefore the definitions, in health care was on disease and death. Now more emphasis is placed on how to achieve, measure, or maintain health. The goal of health promotion is to raise the levels of wellness in individuals, families, and communities. Wellness and illness may exist simultaneously within each of us; you must relate to both aspects of the person.

Concepts of health promotion, health protection, and illness prevention are different, although they are used interchangeably. Definitions for health promotion and primary, secondary, and tertiary prevention follow.

Health promotion consists of *activities that increase the levels of health and well-being and actualize or maximize the health potential of individuals, families, groups, communities, and society.* Health promotion is multidimensional in nature: individual, family, community, environment, and society. The person, family, or community moves toward a positively valued state of better health. Avoiding illness is not a significant motive for health promotion behavior. Frequently former patterns of behavior are diminished as new patterns of behavior are learned (101).

Health protective behavior is any *behavior performed by a person, regardless of the perceived or actual health status, to protect, promote, or maintain health,* whether or not that behavior is actually effective (54). *It is the process of guarding or defending a person, family, or group against specific illness or injury. The goal is removal or avoidance of anything that may prevent optimum health* (12).

Health promotion behaviors also focus on prevention or reduction of illness. **Primary prevention** consists of *activities that decrease the probability of occurrence of specific illness or dysfunction in an individual, family, group, or community and reduce incidence of new cases of disorder in the population by combating harmful forces that operate in the community and by strengthening the capacity of people to withstand these forces* (20, 93, 101).

Secondary prevention consists of *early diagnosis and treatment to the pathologic process, thereby shortening disease duration and severity and enabling the person to return to normal function as quickly as possible* (20). By shortening the duration of existing cases, the prevalence of disorder is reduced. Early case finding and prompt intervention are emphasized.

Tertiary prevention focuses on *restoring the person to optimum function through rehabilitation and within the constraints of the problem when a defect or disability is fixed, stable, or irreversible* (20, 93, 101). *There is a reduction of the rate of residual defects that are sequel to disorder in the affected population.* Tertiary prevention seeks to ensure that people who have recovered from disorders will be hampered as little as possible by their past illness in returning to full participation in the occupational and social life of the community.

Health behaviors are *activities in which the person engages to enhance health, prevent illness, or detect illness.* **Illness behavior** includes *actions an individual who feels ill takes to obtain a diagnosis, prevent complications, and restore health* (101).

MODELS RELATED TO HEALTH PROMOTION AND ILLNESS PREVENTION

Health Belief Model

The **Health Belief Model** is a *paradigm used to predict and explain health behavior based on the Value-Expectancy Theory and Lewin's Theory. Beliefs, attitudes, values, and knowledge contribute to motivation and underlie any decisions to change behavior.* Lewin conceptualized that some regions of the person's life space have negative value or valence, others have positive valence, and others are neutral. Disease has a negative valence and is expected to exert a force to move the person toward health behaviors (101).

The Health Belief Model, developed in the early 1950s, (1) explains why some people who are well take action to avoid illness but others fail to do so; (2) predicts persons who will use preventive measures; and (3) presents interventions that might increase participation in health-protecting or prevention behaviors (113).

The Health Belief Model states that the client's perception of health states and risk of disease and the person's probability for taking appropriate health care actions depend on the person's value of health, perceptions about disease, perceived threat of disease, perceptions about the medical team and therapy plans, past experience, contact with risk factors, level of participation in regular health care, life aspirations, and various motivating factors in the environment. The model does not specify which interventions to use to improve the likelihood of someone following health care and preventive actions. The provider and client negotiate which interventions are appropriate (101). Becker (7, 8) modified the model. He believed perceptions about the susceptibility to illness and about seriousness of the illness affect whether the person denies illness, engages in primary prevention, or seeks early treatment. Perceptions are modified by (1) demographic variables of age, sex, race, and ethnicity; (2) sociopsychologic variables of personality, social class, or peer pressure; and (3) structural variables such as knowledge about the disease and personal contact with the disease. Action to prevent illness and the perceived way to treat disease are also affected by cues to action, including the mass media campaigns, advice from others, reminder postcards from health care professionals, illness of a family member or friend, and newspaper or magazine articles. This model is directed to health protection behavior rather than health promotion. It is assumed that the higher the level of readiness to act, the lower will be the intensity of cues, internal or external, needed to trigger preventive behaviors. Benefits minus barriers determine the likelihood of taking recommended preventive health action. Beliefs about the effectiveness of recommended preventive actions are also an important determinant of health protecting behaviors. The lower the chance of recovery, the longer people may wait before seeking medical attention. Barriers such as cost, inconvenience, unpleasantness of procedures, extent of life change required, and fear of pain have great power to prevent the person from engaging in preventive behaviors.

Health Promotion Model

The **Health Promotion Model** *developed by Pender derives from Social Learning Theory, which emphasizes the importance of cognitive mediating processes in the regulation of behavior.* Determinants of health promotion behavior are categorized into cognitive-perceptual factors, modifying factors, and variables affecting the likelihood of actions. Cognitive-perceptual factors include (1) the individual's perceptions, (2) the importance of health, (3) the perceived self-efficacy or conviction that one can carry out behavior to achieve desired

outcome, (4) the definition of health, (5) the perceived health status, (6) the perceived benefits of health promoting behavior, and (7) the perceived barriers to health promotion actions. These factors are the primary motivational factors for initiating and maintaining health promotion behavior. Modifying factors that influence health promotion behavior to varying degrees include the following (101):

1. Demographic variables—age, gender, race/ethnicity, education, income
2. Biologic characteristics— weight, size
3. Interpersonal influences—expectations of significant others, family patterns of health care, interactions with health professionals
4. Situational factors—access to health promotion services and alternatives, environmental constraints in health behavior
5. Behavioral factors—previous experience with behaviors that promoted well-being, gaining of necessary knowledge or skill

Cues to action or variables affecting the likelihood of the person's initiating or maintaining health behaviors may be of internal or external origin. Important internal cues are personal awareness of the potential of growth or increased feelings of well-being from beginning health promotion efforts. External cues include conversations with others about their efforts and resulting success; support of significant others; mass media problems about health; family health status; and environmental variables on the level of readiness of the person, family, or group to follow health promotion activity.

Resource Model of Preventive Health Behavior

The **Resource Model of Preventive Health Behavior** has been proposed by Kulbok (77). *The model hypothesizes that people act in ways to maximize their "stock in health." The greater the social and health resources of the person, the more frequent is the performance of preventive behaviors.* Social resources are education level and family income. Health resources are (1) health status, (2) energy level, (3) concern about health, (4) feelings about independence in caring for self, (5) participation in social groups and religious services, (6) number and closeness of friends and relatives, and (7) general psychologic well-being. Preventive health behaviors include diet, physical activity, sleeping, dental hygiene, use of seatbelts, and use of professional services. The model explains some preventive health behaviors.

Human Ecologic Model

Shaver (118) describes the components of the **Human Ecologic Model** in explaining health-wellness status. She uses a biopsychosocial approach. Personal factors that affect health include life-style, stress management, affiliation with others, and involvement in healthful activities. Sense of well-being, mood state, and cognitive performance can affect personal behaviors. Environmental factors such as social support, cultural norms, space, time perspectives, energy exchange, and life events affect and are affected by personal behaviors and health status. Host factors such as personality, gender, age, cognitive ability, and physiologic regulation affect and are affected by personal behaviors and health status. Activities of daily living, signs and symptoms of disease, and sense of personal control influence host factors and environmental factors. Thus *all biopsychosocial components are interrelated and interdependent.* This integrated, holistic view has considerable implications for the nursing process and if applied, would contribute to greater service to and with the client.

Model of Multiple Risk Factor Behavior

A **Model of Multiple Risk Factor Behavior** proposed by Kar, Schmitz, and Dyer (70) is a *multidimensional psychosocial model of determinants of risk-taking behavior.* The model proposes that in populations with comparable ethnicity, socioeconomic, and biologic status, risk-taking behavior is dependent on the following variables: (1) behavioral intentions, (2) social support from significant others, (3) accessibility of information and services, (4) personal autonomy, and (5) action situations. The model is based on the Systems Theory: behavioral intentions and personal autonomy are internal variables; the other variables are system or external influences. The model has transcultural applicability.

INSTRUMENTS TO ASSESS HEALTH PROMOTION AND ILLNESS PREVENTION BEHAVIORS

Various instruments have been developed to assess the behaviors and life-styles of the person or family to determine intent or activity directed to either health promotion or illness prevention.

Cox (27) has developed the *Health Self-Determinism Index,* which measures motivation in health behavior. Four subscales in the Index are (1) self-determined health judgments, (2) self-determined health behaviors, (3) perceived competency in health matters, and (4) internal-external cue responsiveness. This tool, with further research, should be useful in determining client motivation and how various interventions affect motivation for specific health behaviors.

Clark (20) has devised a *Wellness Belief Scale,* based on Rotter's concepts of internal locus of control, to help clients examine wellness beliefs and their sense of responsibility for wellness.

Clark (20) has also developed a self-assessment tool for wellness, which the client uses to determine state of wellness in areas of nutrition, exercise and fitness, cop-

ing with stress, relationships with others, and interaction with the environment. The tool also helps the person determine what areas are important and whether or not a change of behavior is desired in a specific aspect of life. Commitment to wellness is also determined.

Walker, Sechrist, and Pender (134) developed the *Health-Promoting Lifestyle Profile,* which measures six dimensions that indicate a healthy life-style: self-actualization, health responsibility, exercise, nutrition, interpersonal support, and stress management. The tool enables researchers to investigate patterns and determinants of a healthy life-style and the effects of interventions to alter life-style. A Spanish language version has been developed (135).

Pender (101) has designed an extensive assessment tool to help an individual formulate a health protection–promotion plan. The form reviews present physical and stress status, self-care strengths of the person, health goals, areas for self-improvement, family health status, family values, family self-care patterns, family health goals, areas for improvement in family health, and evaluation of progress toward goals (101).

One format for an adult health history is suggested by Pender. The history can be administered by the nurse, or a self-administered questionnaire format that clients can use for self-assessment could be developed. Techniques are also described for both adult and pediatric health histories in *A Guide to Physical Examination and History Taking* by Barbara Bates (6). Kopf, Salamon, and Charytan (75) describe a preventive health history form designed to obtain medical and psychosocial information for older adults.

Any health history is incomplete if it does not include items concerning sexuality. A sexual history can be obtained most comfortably within the context of a comprehensive health history. In Pender's adult health history form (101), sexuality questions have been placed in the sections on psychosocial history and review of the genitoreproductive system. Information on obtaining a sexual history can also be obtained from Hogan (58).

Sometimes the assessment tool may be very specific such as the one shown in Figure 17–1, which can be used to gather data about eating habits as a basis for assessing nutritional status and nutritional health promotion.

FACTORS THAT INFLUENCE HEALTH PROMOTION AND ILLNESS PREVENTION BEHAVIORS

Why do some people engage in activities to promote health or prevent illness and others who appear equally in need for such activities do not? Many forces are in play as a person decides for or against what has been defined as health promotion or illness prevention behavior. Internal (personality), external (environmental),

---

Record all foods and drinks that you had during the day and during the night.

Day of Week   (Circle   Mon   Tues   Wed   Thurs   Fri   Sat   Sun)

Breakfast
Foods/Amounts (cup, tbsp)   Drinks/Amounts (cup, glass)

Lunch
Foods/Amounts (cup, tbsp)   Drinks/Amounts (cup, glass)

Dinner
Foods/Amounts (cup, tbsp)   Drinks/Amounts (cup, glass)

Snacks
Time   Foods or Drinks   Amount (cup, glass, Tbsp, or pieces)

Do you take vitamin or mineral supplements?   Yes ___   No ___
If yes, please list kind and how many per day.

Do you take any other nutritional supplement? (e.g., yeast, protein bran)
If yes, please list and describe.   Yes ___   No ___

Figure 17-1.   Form for assessing eating habits and nutritional state.

and various knowledge and emotional forces, some unknown to the person, all contribute. *Health behavior* is related to subjective ideas about vulnerability and present health state, the value placed on health and early detection of illness, and the sense of internal versus external control.

Influences on Healthful Behaviors

Understanding the person's perception of health assists in understanding how health behaviors influence appraisal of symptoms, perceived vulnerability, and decisions to seek treatment. Perceptions of health are related to a number of factors already mentioned plus: (1) cultural norms of activity and inactivity, (2) continuation of rewarding roles and activities, (3) participation in social life, and (4) levels of psychologic well-being.

A study by the Penders (102) indicated that persons at highest risk for health crises may be the least likely to engage in positive health habits. Subjective personal norms about exercise, weight, or diet affected intention to change behavior more than did health teaching or professional guidance. Behavioral change and continued health behavior were influenced positively by family or group support.

People with high self-esteem who perceive their social support as very adequate maintain more positive health practices than do those with lower levels of self-esteem and social support. Individuals who take better care of themselves are more likely to attract supportive relationships, and good social support predisposes one to engage in good self-care. Those with more self-esteem would be likely to consider it worthwhile to enhance their health status. Those not needing to expend their time and energy protecting and defending what little self-esteem they have would have more resources available to maintain or improve their health (35, 92, 108).

There is a direct effect of gender on self-esteem, social support, and life-style. The typical woman is more emotionally involved in relationships than is the average man. Women generally take better care of themselves than do men. It may be that a way to influence health behaviors is through education about interpersonal and intrapersonal factors and how they can effect health behaviors. The holistic approach to health care is to blend the social and psychologic factors in maintaining the physical self (92, 108).

Findings from Alexy's study (1) suggest that setting goals for illness risk-reduction can be effective in changing behavior. However, results provided no indication that client participation in setting goals was superior to a directive approach. The provider goal-setting group made significant changes in exercise levels, alcohol intake, and seatbelt usage. The control group, which did their own goal-setting, made significant changes in exercise. The provider-client collaborative goal-setting group also changed significantly in exercise and weight reduction. Overall changes in this group were sufficient to make significant differences in life expectancy and potential life expectancy increase. Although significant change occurred in exercise levels and weight reduction in the collaborative group and change occurred in exercise levels in the provider goal-setting and control groups, such change may be related to the current emphasis on these factors in modern culture. The higher level of success with the provider goal-setting group may indicate that individuals prefer specified programs. Interventions focusing on intermediate behavior change (daily or weekly goals) rather than outcome criteria might represent a more successful strategy with most clients (1).

Illness Prevention Attitudes and Behavior

Sometimes people are unaware of the illness hazards to which they are exposed unless you teach and help them pursue alternate behaviors. Sometimes exposure occurs unwittingly or is unavoidable. For example, neurologic and endocrine conditions, spontaneous abortions, and congenital anomalies are increasing perhaps as a result of applications of pesticide malathion in the food-growing sectors of the United States (49). Sometimes exposure to health hazards is the result of unpredictable, unpreventable environmental conditions such as volcanic eruption or earthquake and cannot be avoided. However, increased awareness may encourage action to prevent additional complications or future exposure. Increased awareness may also encourage citizen activity that can change national policy, enforce established standards or create more effective standards, or change practices by the offending parties. A consideration may be the person's or family's perception of the effectiveness of an activity versus the difficulty in implementing it. Your most effective intervention may be to teach and counsel, guide and persuade so that the difficulty of the preventive care or the necessary medical treatment regi-

men is perceived as low and the effectiveness of it is perceived as at least moderately, if not highly, effective (117).

Four factors contribute to the perceived seriousness of any given health problem: (1) degree of threat or personal vulnerability; (2) overt visibility of illness or disability; (3) degree of interference with a person's lifestyle, family, or occupational roles; and (4) communicability of disease to others. The person's concern for the welfare of others may be greater than for personal health. Thus preventive measures more likely will be followed for communicable diseases than for those that affect only the individual (20, 24, 29, 38, 101).

The person chooses the preventive services that are perceived as being most effective in lowering the threat of illness. The higher the educational or socioeconomic levels, the more will people be aware of the entire range of preventive health alternatives available (29, 101, 108).

The person who feels powerless or unable to control the environment is not likely to try preventive health behavior. The person who feels able to control the self internally perceives self as less vulnerable to ill health and usually takes preventive health actions (35, 101, 108, 114).

Several key factors influence the decision to seek preventive care services. First, the person's decision, is influenced by the belief about health, whether or not it is possible to influence direction of health or illness progression and whether the necessary changes are worth the effort (29). Second, the person may seek health care because of family encouragement. Third, patterns of using preventive services are learned in the family. The level of the mother's education correlates highly with preventive practices because the mother is often the decision maker in this area. Fourth, expectations of friends are powerful motivators to seek preventive health care, for parents especially want to fulfill the expectations of peers, neighbors, or friends about what "good parents should do." Fifth, information and respectful care from health care professionals also increase the readiness to engage in preventive health behavior, especially if the health care professional is seen as knowledgeable and caring. The small-group approach to giving information is more effective than teaching only one person. However, knowing what is healthful is no guarantee that the person will follow healthful patterns of living (101).

Situational determinants that influence the decision to practice preventive measures include cultural values on health and prevention, group norms and pressures, and information from mass media (101, 108).

Yet various barriers impede a person's action even after the decision to take action: high costs, inconvenience, unpleasantness of treatment measures or facilities, pain, fear of findings from early detection measures, inability to decide which course of action would be best, psychologic needs that are fulfilled by the illness, or perceived changes in life-style that are prescribed as undesirable.

HEALTH-PROMOTING RELATIONSHIPS

All people need relationships with others to remain healthy physically and psychologically. How you relate to the client will contribute to the health status and may determine whether the person maintains and continues health practices.

Differences Between a Social and a Helpful Relationship

Establishing a helpful relationship is one of the unique functions separating nursing from other health services.

The **nurse-client relationship** is a *helpful, purposeful interaction over time between an authority in health care, the nurse, and a person or group with health care needs, with the nurse focusing on needs of the client while being empathic and using knowledge.* Through this process the nursing process is put to use, and it must be differentiated from mere association. Social contact with another individual, verbal or nonverbal, may exercise some influence on one of the participants and needs may be met. But inconsistency, nonpredictability, or partial fulfillment of expectations often results. Characteristics of *social relationships* are as follows:

1. The contact is primarily for pleasure and companionship.
2. Neither person is in a position of responsibility for helping the other.
3. No specific skill or knowledge is required.
4. The interaction is between peers, often of the same social status.
5. The people involved can, and often do, pursue an encounter for the satisfaction of personal or selfish interests.
6. There is no explicit formulation of goals.
7. There is no sense of accountability for the other person.
8. Evaluation of interactions does not concern personal effectiveness in the interaction.

A nurse-client relationship is established *when the person's or family's needs are met consistently and unconditionally.* A working nurse-client relationship is, by definition, good, helpful, and therapeutic. There is no such thing as a poor nurse-client relationship; there are only poor or unsatisfactory experiences that prevent establishing the relationship. Interactions moving toward a relationship occur whenever direct client care, health teaching, listening, or counseling are done or when the person's or family's activities are directed or modified in some way.

The following types of interactions are *not helpful* to the person because needs are met inconsistently or conditionally:

1. Automatic, in which there is no meaning to either person
2. Impersonally helpful, in which a service is expertly given but no personal interest or empathy is displayed
3. Involuntary, in which "carrying out orders" is done as a duty, often the result of the nurse's perception of work as just a job to be done
4. Inconsistent (that which is conditional in nature), assisting the client only when the situation is interesting or when it fulfills the nurse's needs

The nurse-client relationship is one in which the person's real complaint is uncovered. The focus is on the client's needs rather than on your own. The person is not a social buddy. There is a giving of self in an objective way to the person and family; yet you do not identify with (feel the same as), pity, or reject the one seeking help. Neither do you believe you are the only person who can help the client. You use the resources that a team can offer whenever doing so is beneficial to the person or family.

Effect of Feelings on the Relationship

Only through mutual striving for self-awareness and appreciation of the other person's reactions can a nurse-client relationship grow to maturity. Knowing that each person has needs to be met gives meaning to this relationship. You must expect both positive and negative feelings in yourself and in the other, and you must realize that both can be expressed either overtly or covertly.

The client's positive feelings may be those relating to a sincere desire to cooperate in his or her own care and may include a polite manner toward others. The feelings may be a result of educational, religious, or cultural background or a combination of these factors. In any event you are in a position to capitalize on such positive feelings to establish rapport and a sense of trust as a foundation for the nurse-client relationship. Additionally, make every effort to learn the person's negative feelings. Insecurity; distrust of unfamiliar persons, routines, and treatments; or helplessness or hostility because of a lack of control over his or her own responses—all may be present.

The positive feelings that you may have toward the client are strongly bound to your commitment to nursing as a way of life. They cannot develop if you are merely doing a job because the negative feelings we all possess can overpower the positive and interfere with the nurse-client relationship. Negative feelings, which may at times be expressed in your reactions, will provoke inappropriate behavior. Talking out your negative feelings with the staff is better than unloading them on the client or family.

Effect of Behavior on the Relationship

To develop an awareness of the feelings that you take with you to the client, examine your behavior to determine whether it is modified for some people in a helping way and for others in a manner that hinders your effectiveness. Modification of your behavior with, or approach to, different persons is a valuable tool. Surely you would behave differently toward the child than toward the aged person. But behaving differently because a person is rich or poor, African-American or Caucasian, quiet or boisterous, grateful or ungrateful, in agreement or disagreement with your value system may prevent you from meeting that person's needs.

Remembering that all behavior has meaning will help you to sharpen and improve those qualities you possess that produce a positive response in others. When inappropriate reactions do occur, analyze them in terms of what preceded them and of what happened after the incident. Search for clues to establish the meaning of feelings. Using the process recording format, you might record the event by writing the conversation and the nonverbal responses of both you and client for closer analysis. Discussing the incident with objective persons, perhaps in team conference, may help. Become familiar with your own coping mechanisms; seek to understand their relative value and the ways in which you use them in your approach to nursing care. Take sufficient care of your personal needs outside the nursing setting so that you can give your best professional care to the person or family or group.

Although the relationship with a client is a reciprocal experience, the responsibility for establishing it and for making appropriate changes in it rests with you, not with the client. The relationship is based on each person's perceiving the other as a unique individual without stereotyping. Help the person *not* to see you as the command officer or the "angel in white," and avoid seeing the client as a "gallbladder" or a room number.

Carrying out the person's planned regimen for health maintenance or restoration will be accomplished more easily because of the nurse-client relationship, for it will naturally foster the tangible and the intangible aspects of your care. Above all, keep expectations mutual and remember that the major characteristic of the nurse-client relationship is that the *nursing needs of the individual or family are met in an emotional climate of warmth, support, and mutual trust* (131, 132).

Guidelines for the Nurse-Client Relationship

If you consider your behavior an influence on the person's or family's behavior, you will be in a better position to advise specific approaches for bringing about change. You will want to develop characteristics of a helpful, humanistic relationship. These characteristics include being:

1. *Respectful*—feeling and communicating an attitude of seeing the client as a unique human being, filled with dignity, worth, and strengths, regardless of outward appearance or behavior; being willing to work at communicating with and understanding the client because he or she is in need of emotional care.
2. *Genuine*—communicating spontaneously, yet tactfully, what is felt and thought, with proper timing and without disturbing the client, rather than using professional jargon, facade, or rigid counselor or nurse role behaviors.
3. *Attentive*—conveying rapport and an active listening to verbal and nonverbal messages and an attitude of working with the person.
4. *Accepting*—conveying that the person does not have to put on a facade and that the person will not shock you with his or her statements; enabling the client to change at his or her own pace; acknowledging personal and client's feelings aroused in the encounter; to "be for" the client in a nonsentimental, caring way.
5. *Positive*—showing warmth, caring, respect, and agape love; being able to reinforce the client for what he or she does well.
6. *Strong*—maintaining separate identity from the client; withstanding the testing behavior of the client.
7. *Secure*—permitting the client to remain separate and unique; respecting his or her needs and your own; feeling safe as the client moves emotionally close; feeling no need to exploit the other person.
8. *Knowledgeable*—having an expertise based on study, experience, and supervision; being able to assist the client in formulating goals.
9. *Sensitive*—being perceptive to feelings; avoiding threatening behavior, responding to cultural values, customs, norms as they affect behavior; using knowledge that is pertinent to the client's situation.
10. *Empathic*—looking at the client's world from his or her point of view; being open to his or her values, feelings, beliefs, and verbal statements; stating your understanding of his or her verbal or nonverbal expressions of feelings and experiences.
11. *Nonjudgmental*—refraining from evaluating the client moralistically or telling the person what to do.
12. *Congruent*—being natural, relaxed, trustworthy, and dependable and demonstrating consistency in behavior and between verbal and nonverbal messages.
13. *Unambiguous*—avoiding contradictory messages; using purposeful communication.
14. *Creative*—viewing the client as a person in the process of becoming, not being bound by the past, and viewing yourself in the process of becoming or maturing as well (112).

Other features that correlate highly with being effective in a helping relationship are being open instead of closed in interaction with others, perceiving others as friendly and capable instead of unfriendly and incapable, and perceiving a relationship as freeing instead of controlling another (104–106).

Establishing and maintaining a relationship or counseling another does not involve putting on a facade of behavior to match a list of characteristics. Rather, both you and the client will change and continue to mature. As the helper you are present as a total person, blending potentials, talents, and skills while assisting him or her to come to grips with needs, conflicts, and self (93, 104–106).

Working with another in a helping relationship is challenging and rewarding. You will not always have all the characteristics just described; at times you will be handling personal stresses that will lower your energy and sense of involvement. You may become irritated and impatient while working with the person. Accept the fact that you are not perfect; remain as aware as possible of your needs and behavior and your effect on the other. Remember that the most important thing you can share with another is your own uniqueness as a person. As you give of yourself, you will in return be given to—rewarded with warmth and sharing from the client.

Phases of the Nurse-Client Relationship

Unless the encounter is brief, the feelings between you and the client and the family and the work jointly done evolve through a sequence of phases. The phases are not sharply demarcated, and they vary in duration. They can be compared to human developmental stages because of the degree of dependency-independency and feelings of trust involved: the orientation phase is comparable to infancy, identification to childhood, the working phase to adolescence, and termination to adulthood (104–106). This author observes that in long-term care another phase of the relationship is evident—the maintenance phase (93).

Orientation Phase

The **initial** or **orientation phase** of the relationship *begins when you first meet the person or family*. You might carry out intervention measures shortly thereafter as you function in the role of technical expert, counselor, teacher, referral person, or substitute mother. Your main tasks during this phase, however, are to become oriented to the other's expectations, health needs, and goals through assessment while orienting the person to your role and health care goals and his or her role in the health care system. You formulate a tentative care plan. Establishing rapport and showing acceptance are vital for assessing and orienting the other person. Be aware of how you are affecting the person and how he or she is affecting you. During this period the person clarifies the health status and its meaning through your exploration of the many factors affecting him or her. Essential to this phase is caring for the person or family in such a way that a sense of trust and confidence in you is established (104–106).

Identification Phase

The second phase, the **identification phase,** *marks the time when the person has become better acquainted with you, places trust in your decisions and actions, works closely with you, follows your suggestions, and at times imitates your behavior*. He or she sees you as "his or her nurse." You continue the nursing process, actively guiding him or her but also providing opportunities for participation in self-care. You accept dependency without fostering it excessively (104–106).

Working Phase

The third, the **working phase,** is the *time when the client is becoming more independent, actively using all services and resources offered by the health team*. He or she becomes more assertive and no longer relies so heavily on you. By now he or she is usually regaining physical and emotional health—optimum function—so that behavior begins to change as he or she becomes more involved in decision making about certain aspects of the situation. Although the person seems more independent and even self-centered, you can now work as equal partners in meeting health goals. The client is preparing for convalescence and discharge from your services (104–106).

Maintenance Phase

Often the nurse who works in an acute care setting does not really experience the rewards of a relationship with the client. The short stay typical of hospitalization or even the few visits given by a home health nurse allow nothing more than establishing rapport, if that.

The **maintenance phase** in the relationship is *only possible in the setting in which a client is followed by the same nurse over a period of time* (e.g., in a rehabilitation center, nursing home, senior residence, or psychiatric-mental health agency). Also, the nurse in independent practice or in an ambulatory care clinic may see the same clients over a period of years.

In this phase termination does not occur for a long time. Often termination only comes with the geographic move or death of the person. The active, working, therapeutic stage goes on until the person has reached his or her potential. In this situation the person has reached a plateau at which support and maintenance are essential for daily living. He or she may live at home, following your directions for health promotion measures, and may call on you for assistance only when chronic illness becomes uncontrolled or when a new condition of pathology or aging arises; or he or she may be in an institution and need maximum or minimum assistance with daily physical care. What characterizes this phase is that you must actively pursue intervention to maintain emotional and social well-being. The reward will be the gratification of seeing a person reassert a will to live, become creative in coping with problems or making "ends meet," and remain independent.

Termination Phase

The last phase, **termination,** is *marked by the person's becoming as fully independent as possible, leaving the health care system to return to the community.* Together you plan the management of the health situation after discharge, especially if the client requires any special life-style modifications such as in exercise, hygiene, or diet. This is a time of separation, and both you and the person must work through feelings about separation—sometimes both past and present situations. Mutual attachment develops between you and someone you take care of for a long time, and either one or both of you may feel uncertain about the person's ability to manage without you. Together you need to talk about feelings about separation and your confidence in the ability to be independent and remain healthy. Avoid increasing dependency on you at this time to meet your needs. When the client leaves the health care system, each of you should feel no regret about the termination. On the other hand, if there is need for follow-up visits after discharge, your interest and concern in the person or family extend to this ongoing care (104–106).

Without the nurse-client relationship, the person's needs are not met, and the nursing process is not in force. Mechanical tasks become an end in themselves, and the person is not helped to prevent or adapt to his or her illness.

There may be people with whom you cannot form a helpful relationship and situations in which it would be best for the client if someone else were to work with him or her. You must be aware of your own feelings of discomfort with him or her, and you should be able to accept the fact that you cannot work with certain people. Often the reasons will be obscure; you may want to work through the reasons with an instructor or supervisor for your own personal growth (104–106). Reference 93 gives more information on barriers to an effective nurse-client relationship.

COMMUNICATION TO PROMOTE HEALTH

The ability to communicate should not be taken for granted; it is not a simple process but rather a complex system by which the world's work gets done.

Communication is the matrix for all thought and relationships between persons and is bound to the learning process. Early sensory experiences shape subsequent learning abilities in speech, cognition, and symbol recognition and in the capacity for maturing communication. Perception of the self, the world, and one's place in it results from communication. Verbal and nonverbal communication is learned in a cultural setting; if the person does not communicate in the way prescribed by the culture, many difficulties arise, for that person cannot conform to the expectations of society. Disordered thinking, feeling, and actions result, along with mental anguish and perhaps even physical illness.

Communication is the heart of the nursing process, for it is one of the primary methods used to accomplish specific and general goals with many different kinds of people. It is used in assessing and understanding the client and family and in nursing intervention. Communication helps people express thoughts and feelings, clarify problems, receive information, consider alternate ways of coping or adapting, and remain realistic through feedback from the environment. Essentially the client learns something about the self, how to identify health needs, and if and how he or she wishes to meet them.

Analysis of your communication pattern will help you improve your methods. Realize that you cannot become skilled in therapeutic communication without supervised and thoughtful practice. As you talk with another, however, do not get so busy thinking about a list of methods that you forget to focus on the person. Your keen interest in the other person and use of your personal style are essential if you are to be truly effective. To be effective while communicating with the person or family, use simple, clear words geared to the person's intelligence and experience. Develop a well-modulated tone of voice. Be attuned to your nonverbal behavior. Several authors have described principles, attitudes, and methods essential in therapeutic communication that are useful with individual persons and with groups (4, 62, 84, 93, 104–106, 130, 131).

Effective Methods

The following methods are basic for conducting purposeful, helpful communication with a person along with their rationale.

Using Thoughtful Silence to Encourage the Person to Talk. Silence gives you and the person time to organize thoughts. It directs the person to the task at hand but allows him or her to set the pace, aids consideration of alternative courses of action and delving into feelings, conserves energy during serious illness, and gives time for contemplation and relaxation. There is a time not to talk. Always focus on the person you are talking with, especially during silence.

Being Accepting. This is a difficult task at times. Realize that *all* behavior is motivated and purposeful. Indicate that you are following the person's trend of thought. Encourage the person to continue to talk while you remain nonjudgmental, although not necessarily in agreement.

Helping the Person Strengthen Self-Identification in Relation to Others. Always use *you, I,* and *we* in their proper context. Do not say "We can take a bath now" but rather "You can take a bath now."

Suggesting Collaboration and a Cooperative Relationship.
Offer to share and work together with the person; offer to do things *with* and not *for* or *to* him or her. Encourage participation in identifying and appraising problems and involvement as an active partner in treatment. Tell the person you are available to help. "I'll stay with you" or "I'm interested in your comfort" are examples of statements that can help to reassure that you will stay and care regardless of the person's behavior.

Stating Open-Ended, Generalized Leading Questions.
Use these questions to encourage the person to take the initiative in introducing topics and to think through problems. Examples include "Is there something you'd like to talk about?" "Tell me about it." "Where would you like to begin?" "Go on." "And what else?" "Would you like to talk about yourself now?" "After that?" Avoid conventional pleasantries after initial greetings because they constrict the person's expression of feelings and ideas. It is important for the person to talk about his or her mental and emotional distress and turmoil and questions, for often he or she cannot cope with feelings until the feelings are stated.

Stating Related Questions.
Do not let a subject drop until it is adequately explored. Peripheral or side questions help the person work through larger issues and engage in problem solving. Explore by delving further into the subject or idea without seeming to pry. Many clients deal superficially with a topic to test if you are truly interested. Avoid questions that call for a yes or no answer. Explorative questions call for answers that elaborate, thereby helping the person to increase understanding and do further problem solving or clarifying.

Placing Events Described in Time Sequence.
To clarify relationships associated with a given event, determine how it happened, place it in perspective, determine the extent to which one event led to another, and seek to identify recurrent patterns or difficulty or significant cause-and-effect relationships. Ask such questions as "What happened then?" or "What did you do after that?"

Stating Observations That You Perceive About the Person.
Statements such as "You appear . . . ," "It seems to me that . . . ," "I notice that you are . . . ," and "It makes me uncomfortable when you . . . " encourage mutual understanding of behavior. Such observations offer a basis on which the person can respond without your having to probe, and they call attention to what is happening to help him or her notice or clarify personal behavior. Using this technique, you and the other person can compare observations and you can encourage a description of self-awareness. In addition, when you openly acknowledge that another's efforts at a task or behavior are appropriate to the situation, you reinforce the behavior and add to the person's self-esteem.

Encouraging Description of Behavior or Observation.
Through statements such as "What did you feel?" "Tell me what you now feel," "What does the voice seem to be saying?" and "What is happening?" you can better understand the person when you observe matters as they seem to him or her. There is no need to act out impulses and feelings if the person feels free to state them.

Restating or Repeating the Main Idea Expressed.
Doing this will convey that the idea was communicated to you effectively, thereby encouraging the person to continue. Restate the idea until the person does clarify. Reformulating certain statements and using different words bring out related aspects of material that might otherwise have escaped the client's (or your) attention.

Reflecting by Paraphrasing Feelings, Questions, Ideas, and Key Words.
This will encourage further talking. Indicate that the person's point of view is important; acknowledge the right to personal opinions and decisions. Encourage the person to accept personal feelings and ideas. Show interest in hearing as much as the person wishes to tell you. Emphasize the word *you* while conversing, as in "*You* feel . . . ," to reflect what the person has said. (However, do not just mindlessly parrot his or her words.)

Verbalizing the Implied.
State the implied or what the person has hinted or suggested to make the discussion less obscure, to clarify the conversation, and to show that you are listening and interested and that you accept what is said. Questions can be used as a subtle form of suggestion. As an example, you might ask, "Have you ever told your wife how you feel?" or "Have you ever asked your boss for a raise?" Regardless of the answer, you have indicated that such an act is conceivable, permissible, and perhaps even expected.

Attempting to Translate Feelings into Words.
Sometimes what the person says seems meaningless when taken literally. Hidden meanings of verbal expressions and their actual content must be considered and can be explored by describing the implicit feelings.

Clarifying.
Clarify when necessary through statements such as "I don't understand what is troubling you" or "Could you explain that again?" The person is usually aware if he or she is not being understood and may withdraw or cease to communicate. It is not necessary to understand everything stated as long as you are honest about it and do not pretend to understand when you do not. Attempting to discover what the person is talking about can help him or her become clearer to self.

Reintroducing Reality.
State reality by voicing doubt or by calmly presenting your own perceptions of the facts in the situation when the person is being unrealistic. Indicate an alternate line of thought for consideration; do not attempt to convince him or her of error by arguing. Such action only provokes resistance and a determination to maintain the idea. Encourage the person to rec-

ognize that others do not necessarily perceive events as he or she does or draw the same conclusions. Encourage reconsideration and reevaluation (even though doing so may not change his or her mind) through statements such as "What gives you that impression?" "Isn't that unusual?" and "That's hard to believe." Expressing doubts may reinforce doubts the person already has but has discounted because no one else shared them before. A doubting tone of voice can be as effective as any specific statement.

Offering Information. Make facts available whenever the person needs or asks for them. Well-timed teaching builds trust, orients, and gives additional knowledge from which to make decisions or draw realistic conclusions. Inappropriate, excessive, or partial information or advice may cause alarm or needlessly suggest problems to the person. Give the person information about what can be expected and what he or she can do to help self. At times it may be appropriate for you to disclose briefly your own thoughts, feelings, or experiences; do not elaborate on yourself.

Seeking Consensual Validation. Search for mutual understanding; words should mean the same thing to both of you. Therapeutic communication cannot take place if both you and the other person attach autistic (private) meanings to the words you both use. Always ask yourself if what you heard could have a meaning other than what you think. As a person defines self for the listener, he or she also clarifies what is meant. Avoid words and phrases that are easily misinterpreted or misunderstood and encourage the person to ask whenever there is doubt about what you mean.

Encouraging Evaluation of the Situation by the Person. Help the person to appraise the quality of the experience, to consider people and events in relation to personal and others' values, to evaluate the way in which people affect him or her personally, and to understand how he or she affects others. A simple query may help the person understand feelings in connection with what happened and refrain from uncritically adopting the opinions and values of others.

Encouraging Formulation of a Plan of Action. Do this by asking the person to consider examples of behavior likely to be appropriate in future situations. The person can then plan how to handle future problems or how to carry out necessary self-care.

Summarizing. Summarize important points of discussion and give particular emphasis to progress toward greater understanding. Summarizing encourages both you and the person to part company with the same ideas in mind, provides a sense of closure at the end of discussion, and promotes a grasp of the significance of what was said.

The quality of any response depends on the degree of mutual trust in the relationship. Techniques can be highly successful or they can misfire or be abused, depending on how they are used, your attitude at the time, and the other's interpretation. There must be a feeling of caring, of safety and security in your company, and a feeling that you want to help the person help himself or herself. The more important or highly personal a feeling or idea is, the more difficult it is to say. This situation causes hesitancy in revealing thoughts, feelings, or intimate needs. By using therapeutic principles such as those previously listed, you will help the person and his or her family identify you as someone to whom ideas and feelings can be safely and productively revealed.

Communicating With the Client Who Has Communication Difficulties

You will need to gather data from clients with sensory impairments. When you interview a person with hearing impairment, inability to speak the language, or visual impairment, the basic principles still apply, although the specific condition will necessitate some adaptations. The guidelines presented in Boxes 14–2 and 14–4 will be helpful. For anyone with a communication disorder, develop rapport and a trust relationship slowly to overcome the reticence or suspicion that might be present. Introduce yourself and your purpose. Use appropriate nonverbal behavior to convey ideas. Use an intermediary such as a family member or interpreter if available and necessary, but *not* to the exclusion of talking with the client.

Other Considerations

The first communication problem that you must control is that of personal emotions in the nurse-client-family relationship. Because the main barrier to communication is emotion, you must develop skill in building bridges over this barrier. The basic bridge to effective communication is feeling. Everyone seeks *warmth, security, assurance,* and *appreciation.* When these qualities are present, tough problems can be taken in stride, especially when commitment is combined with skillful use of the methods described in this chapter.

Study yourself to discover those points at which you could be responsible for blocking communication through your own shortcomings. Know your likes and dislikes; recognize them for what they are; and keep them under control. To accept another person, you must first accept yourself. You must be aware of your own needs to help another meet personal needs.

Cultivate an understanding of the part played by body language in human interactions and be as aware of what you are saying with your body movements as you are of what others say with theirs. Feelings are frequently expressed by gestures, attitudes, gait and body posture, and facial expressions.

To make full use of therapeutic communication, the person must feel safe with you, respected by and trusting of you. Revealing one's innermost thoughts and feelings to someone one scarcely knows is difficult for any individual, even when help is needed and expected. Use of communication techniques in counseling makes no attempt to influence the speed or direction of the person's problem-solving efforts; be a facilitator instead of a doer or a teller.

The nurse is in a key position to apply an understanding of the communication process and to carry out therapeutic communication methods in nursing while conducting routine procedures, teaching, and counseling or giving support. Thus you can enable the person and family to achieve optimum wellness and prevent future health problems. In addition, through communication, you will learn of the effectiveness of care you have given.

Application to Daily Living

Although this section centers around nurse-client-family interaction, the discussions of the communication process, of interviewing, and of techniques and blocks to communication apply equally to associations with your colleagues and other health care team members. In fact, application of all information in this chapter to your everyday relationships with family and friends will promote an increasingly appropriate, harmonious living pattern. The smoother the communication system, the smoother all other systems will function.

Appropriate, realistic, constructive communication between persons is a basic step toward mental, emotional, and, indirectly (but no less significantly), physical health. Communication patterns that block or resist the other person reduce feelings of autonomy and equality and increase feelings of being misunderstood. The resultant emotions—frustration, anger, depression, and the like—will eventually affect the relationship between the persons involved and the physiologic functioning of the body.

As a nurse you will find yourself refining your personal pattern of communication, practicing therapeutic communication with others, and teaching others patterns of communication that promote health individually, within the family, and within community social groups.

HEALTH EDUCATION

Teaching and learning are important at any stage of the wellness-illness continuum, but recently more emphasis has been placed on health promotion and early prevention.

Definitions

Learning is the *process of acquiring wisdom, knowledge, or skill; an overt change in behavior may be observed.* **Teaching** is the *process of sharing knowledge*

and insight or facilitating another to learn knowledge, insight, and skills (28, 73). These definitions are deceptively simple. Popular magazines, textbooks, and library shelves are full of theories and explanations about how these processes take place. Yet no one can say learning will always take place under certain conditions or teaching will never take place under certain conditions. In spite of myriads of information, people with their unique minds and personalities are always modifying the existing theories.

In actuality, teaching and learning cannot be separated, for while a person is teaching, learning is also taking place or at least should be. Perhaps the substandard use of *learn,* as in the sentence "I'm going to learn you something" has more accuracy than people have thought. Both terms connote a lifelong process, an internalization (learning) of thoughts, attitudes, facts, and a consequent externalization (teaching) of those thoughts, attitudes, and facts. Teaching and learning can be conscious and formal, as in the announced situation "Today we are going to learn about the digestive system"; or they can be unconscious and informal, as when a mother frowns and says with a certain tonal emphasis "What is that smell?" The listening and watching child combines a certain smell with a negative mental attitude.

The word **education** *has traditionally meant a process that transmits the culture.* But the word originally came from a Latin word meaning "to draw out." Although we are more familiar with education as a cramming full of facts and information, the other side of the definition is to draw out the mysterious hidden qualities within a person. The amount of education a person has gained and retained has long been measured by intelligent quotient (IQ) tests. But many qualities cannot be measured this way. The IQ test cannot measure how much creative imagination a person has, how much ambition, perseverance, or willingness to cooperate (97). These qualities are significant although previously not often considered or given priority. Thus a balanced definition of education is the continuing process of using immeasurable inner resources to gain external information.

Health education *specifically transmits information, motivates the inner resource of the person, and helps people adopt and maintain healthful practices and life-styles.* It is also concerned with the environment, professional training, and research to maintain and evaluate the process. Traditionally health education focuses on what the professional thinks is good for the client. A positive reinforcement approach is more effective than an approach emphasizing fear (65).

Self-care, increasingly popular in recent years, *focuses on what the learner perceives as needs and goals to maintain or enhance health and well-being.* It is generally undertaken before illness rather than in response to disease. For example, a health clinic can be established in a geriatric residential setting to help the elders remain functional and independent (91). Health educators should shift their emphasis from pathology that has never been experienced to things the person has done and enjoyed and will be unable to continue to do if healthier behavior is not implemented. Further, the person who is involved in self-help is more likely to feel greater self-control, higher self-esteem, and be more socially involved (11).

Assessment

With a wellness orientation, you work with the client where he or she is—culturally, socially, developmentally, physiologically, mentally, emotionally, and spiritually—for previously the average lay person did not place health on the same level as did the health care professional. The lay person generally takes action only when he or she believes the susceptibility to a health threat could have serious effects on the person's life, when he or she knows what actions to take to reduce the health threat, and when the health threat is greater than the action threat. Several references present guidelines to assist you in thorough assessment as a basis for intervention (20, 38, 101, 129).

Teaching possibilities should be assessed starting at first contact, whether that be in a group meeting, on admission to the hospital, or in an industrial health work setting. Thereafter teaching ought to take place at every opportunity, be it mealtime, medicine time, or when talking about family life.

Realistic teaching goals should be set, keeping in mind the basic skills or knowledge you wish to convey. The family should be constantly assessed for its help or hindrance in the process.

Intervention

Some techniques are best suited for teaching on an individual basis whereas others are best for large groups or several subgroups.

Individual Teaching

Individual teaching can be provided through programmed learning, reading material, audiovisual materials, and one-to-one instruction. *Programmed learning* provides material in carefully planned sequential steps that lead the person to a mastery of the subject. The material is presented through program instruction books or a teaching machine, a simple manually operated machine or a complex computer. One frame of information is presented at a time. The learner then tests his or her grasp of the information in the frame by writing, or in the case of a computer, keying, a response to a question, usually a multiple-choice type. The book or machine then gives the correct response. If the learner's response was incorrect, the program presents (or, in the case of a book, directs him or her to turn to) a repetition of the information or a more detailed explanation, de-

pending on the program and his or her response. The advantages of programmed learning include logical presentation, active learner participation, immediate disclosure of correct response, reinforcement of material, and individual pacing. Interactive computer and regular computer and videotaped instruction are increasingly available and popular for health education.

Another method of giving individual instruction is by providing factual material. Many health organizations provide preventive health teaching *literature* as part of their programs. Evaluating the benefits gained from these materials is difficult because people who receive the material often do not respond to the organization's request for feedback, even when given a stamped answer form. The tendency of upper-class persons to read better and to respond more readily to scientific health teaching than lower-class persons must be considered when using literature.

Other factual reading materials include *autobiographies* of persons with certain disease processes and "how-to" books by persons who have experienced certain health problems directly or indirectly and want to pass along suggestions to others. Fiction also provides valuable insights into physical and mental illness.

With the constant introduction of more sophisticated *audiovisual* equipment into the teaching-learning area, you can get and adapt these devices to individual learning. A recorder and cassettes explaining preventive measures, disease processes, or specific instructions can be loaned to the client. He or she can stop the cassette at any point and replay necessary portions until satisfied with the learning. "Talking Books" is a program that records information for the visually impaired. Closed-circuit television or videotape setups allow the person to hear and view material. You can be involved in producing teaching cassettes and television or VCR programs.

These methods of individual instruction are only individual to a certain point. Only when the client can check learning with a *resource person,* ask further questions as necessary, and have help in making personal applications will learning become more significant. That process involves you. The person does not learn from a machine alone. These discussions with the person need not be long. The important point is to be available when they do have questions and to convey that any question or problem is worthy of your consideration. Realize, also, that excessively detailed explanations can raise rather than lower anxiety.

Group Teaching

Group teaching can meet the person's need to achieve status or security through being a group member. Client groups provide a channel through which feelings and needs can be expressed and met, especially if the people have similar problems such as colostomy or diabetes. Thus you can use the group process to enhance health teaching or for therapy to aid coping with problems (Fig. 17–2). You may also have opportunity to work with a group that has formed to accomplish some specific goal such as losing weight, promoting research to find a cure for cancer, or providing guidance to parents with mentally retarded children. In some cases information is not enough. Social support is also necessary, especially when engaging in a lesser-valued activity—such as not eating sugar when society says that dessert is the best part of the meal.

Clients who participate in a small group session the night before surgery can discuss their concerns and fears and learn what to expect and how to aid in their convalescence. Such clients may be more difficult to assemble, however, with the current greater emphasis on one-day surgery.

One minister who had visited hundreds of clients on the night before surgery said,

> Fear of the unknown is what I continually find. I don't necessarily mean about the outcome of the surgery, although that is involved. I mean they don't even know about the recovery room process. Instead of giving spiritual help, I find myself telling them many details which the nursing staff should have taught. With these important details at their command, I can see their anxiety lessen.

Small group sessions could reduce these fears.

If you work with a group, you should initially set a working social climate. People do not automatically start revealing their problems and supporting and helping each other. You must use some introductory technique that focuses on the individual and his or her personality strengths and resources rather than on a disease or problem. (The person already knows why he or she is there.) Each person can introduce self if the group is small. If the group is large (25 or more), you can break it up into subgroups of five each and allow each subgroup at least

20 minutes to plan a presentation. One technique is the inquiring reporter: one person in each group (or subgroup) is chosen to compose a feature story about the personalities and resources of group members. The person then presents the story to the total group in 3 minutes. This method produces immediate ego involvement, creates an atmosphere conducive to participative learning and sharing of problems and resources, and starts the spirit of creative inquiry. You can think of other introductory techniques for your particular group situation.

Special Concerns in Client Teaching

Most health care agencies post a list of *client's rights*. You can be instrumental in teaching clients about their right to health care and rights within a health care agency (Boxes 17–1 and 17–2). Palmer and Deck (96) describe specific assertive communication techniques that the clients can be taught to ensure obtaining their rights.

Teaching to Prevent Quackery Within the Health Care System

Standards are set by professional organizations, among them the American Medical Association and the American Nurses' Association. However, the "incompetent" or careless doctor has been ignored or "unseen" until recently. Published findings revealing unnecessary operations and fatal reactions from inappropriate antibiotics are making people more aware of their need to use certain standards for choosing and using a doctor. Additionally, self-styled health care providers and "quacks" are also offering services. The self-styled health care provider may emphasize certain herbs for healing or a special "hand-me-down" formula and does not rely on professionally set standards. A **quack,** *one who makes*

Figure 17-2. Group teaching provides an opportunity to provide health teaching to individuals with similar health concerns and problems. (From Berger, K.J., and M.B. Williams, *Fundamentals of Nursing: Collaborating for Optimal Health.* Norwalk, Conn: Appleton & Lange, 1992, p. 181.)

■ **BOX 17-1.**
Patient's Bill of Rights

- The patient has a right to considerate and respectful care.
- The patient has a right to obtain from his physician complete current information about his diagnosis, treatment, and prognosis in terms the patient can be reasonably expected to understand.
- The patient has a right to receive from the physician information necessary to give informed consent to the start of any procedure and/or treatment.
- The patient has a right to refuse treatment to the extent permitted by law.
- The patient has a right to every consideration of privacy concerning personal medical care program.
- The patient has a right to expect that all communications and records pertaining to care should be treated as confidential.
- The patient has a right to expect that, within its capacity, a hospital must make reasonable response to the request of a patient for services.
- The patient has a right to obtain information as to any relationship of the hospital to other health care and educational institutions insofar as care is concerned.
- The patient has a right to be advised if the hospital proposes to engage in human experimentation affecting care or treatment the right to refuse to participate in such research projects.
- The patient has a right to expect reasonable continuity of care.
- The patient has the right to examine and receive an explanation of the bill, regardless of source of payment.
- The patient has the right to know what hospital rules and regulations apply to conduct as a patient.

Reprinted with permission of the American Hospital Association, copyright 1972.

■ **BOX 17-2.**
Teaching Guide for Client's Rights

Dos

- When you call the nurse or secretary for an appointment, state your request or problem so that the appropriate appointment time can be scheduled.
- Organize thoughts about your present health status or illness and write them down so you can present pertinent facts to the physician. They will aid him or her in giving a thorough examination or in making a diagnosis.
- Cooperate during the physical examination and allow the physician to be complete. Do not tell the physician to skip certain procedures.
- Ask your physician about proper diet, work load, exercise, and rest to help you maintain maximum health. Ask about realistic limitations. If ill, ask your physician questions about cost of treatment, medication, diagnosis, causes of conditions, chances for recovery, or whatever you want to know related to the situation. If you have more questions after you leave, write them down and call back for answers. If hospitalized, continue to ask questions about drugs and ongoing treatment.
- Follow instructions after health promotion plan is established. After time, effort, and money are spent, you are the only loser if you refuse to follow suggestions or directions.

Don'ts

- Unless an emergency arises, do not take up extra, unplanned-for time. For example, do not say, "Oh, while I'm here for my ear infection, why don't you do my complete physical."
- Do not lie to yourself or to the physician. Do not let fear cause you to ignore a situation that may need immediate but minimum treatment.
- Do not tell the physician to give you pills. Do not feel cheated if you do not get medication; many illnesses are minor and self-limiting. Your own observance of a health-promotion regimen may be all you need.
- Do not ask for unnecessary hospitalization for x-ray examinations or for tests because the insurance will pay or because grandma is burdensome. Talk with your physician about alternate plans that will promote long-range health for everyone involved.
- Do not leave the physician's office dissatisfied. At least express and explain your feelings. The physician needs to understand your point of view. Maybe a change can be made or perhaps you need additional information to understand a suggestion or decision.

pretentious claims about the ability to treat others with little or no foundation, may be found representing any health profession. The quack raises false hopes and causes loss of money and time—often money and time that could be better used for proven treatment (132).

Why do people go to quacks? Probably the main reason is *fear:* fear of mutilation from surgery, of pain, of dying. Some may go out of ignorance. Some may go to seek a miracle cure. Others may go because they lack patience with the traditional, approved treatment methods. Some have tried everything else—the quack is the "last resort."

You can help people avoid quacks by helping them set realistic health goals and by helping them recognize the following typical behaviors of the false practitioner:

1. Claims use of a special or secret formula, diet, or machine
2. Promises an easy or quick cure

3. Offers only testimonials as proof of healing power
4. Claims one product or service is good for a variety of illness
5. States that he or she is ridiculed or persecuted by traditional health professionals

6. Promotes products through faithhealers, door-to-door health advisors, or sensational ads
7. Refuses to accept proven methods of research
8. Claims the treatment is better than any prescribed by a physician

You can identify quackery victims in need of counseling by asking the person the following questions:

1. Is anything taken to combat fatigue, headaches, inability to sleep, bowel or bladder problems, or muscle or backaches? If so, what?
2. Is anything taken to aid digestion, to lose or gain weight, to improve appetite, or as a food supplement of any kind?
3. What home remedies are used to alleviate the problem under treatment?
4. Ask about foreign travel and uses of alternative therapies if the person has cancer; diabetes; arthritis; or other major chronic diseases.

The following guidelines can be followed if the person asks about quack cures:

1. Answer without sarcasm or antagonism.
2. Explain that promises in the advertisements are not necessarily true.
3. Offer to check the remedy if you are not familiar with it to give more information.
4. Attempt to discredit the false claims by citing studies that disprove the miracle cure.
5. Inform other members of the health care team of any alternate therapies or quack methods being used by the person.

You should be aware of quackery in your community. Examine the claims of the quack against standard treatment plans. Be willing to compare approaches with the client. Do not ridicule the person who has gone the nontraditional route. Above all, this person needs your listening ear and understanding guidance. Remember that people think in terms of having symptoms and eradicating them. If the latter takes place to their satisfaction, they will place their trust in the health care provider who was responsible for their improvement, regardless of his or her credentials. What you call a *hoax* others may call *hope*. Refer people who have been a victim of a quack to their local Better Business Bureau, local medical society and nursing organization, and The National Council Against Health Fraud, P.O. Box 1276, Loma Linda, CA, 92354, (714) 824-4690.

Use of Health Education Literature

Health care literature is published for consumers in many countries. For example, in the United States many baby formula and food companies such as Ross Laboratories print booklets on prenatal, postnatal baby, and child care. In London, England, Domestos Hygiene Advisory Service prints pamphlets under the title *Areas of Risk,* and others such as *The Domestic Safe Houses Book.* The pamphlets are colorful, easy to read, and contain the main health promotion and disease prevention points of the subject. Other literature is also available (50 Upper Brook Street, London).

The journal *Health Link* was first printed in 1985 in the United States. It is published quarterly by the National Center for Health Education, 30 East 29th Street, New York City, 10016, to inform and link professionals and volunteers who are engaged in health education. It is written for practitioners in health care, education, public health, social services, and business, and presents timely information and current resources.

Health education and promotion are considered important for every country, not just for the United States. In 1976 the Health Departments of Great Britain and Northern Ireland prepared a booklet, *Prevention and Health, Everybody's Business* (32), to present a historical discussion on contributions of prevention toward solution of health problems, to suggest ways to advance disease prevention and health promotion, and to present the costs, benefits, and resources available.

A text, *Promoting Health: A Practical Guide to Health Education* (45), published in England in 1985, was at that time the only basic guide in England for professionals that presented theory and practice of health education. More publications will follow, just as more health promotion texts are being published in the United States.

At least 20% of people in the United States and approximately 50% of health care clients are not able to read materials written at a fourth- or fifth-grade level; they are functionally illiterate. Most client education materials are written at at least an eighth-grade level. Thus most health education via the booklet, pamphlet, or written material is not comprehended (30, 81, 128). Further, Streif's study (128) found that the client's reading level could not be accurately estimated from their reported last grade completed in school. The Wide Range Achievement Test (WRAT) apparently is an accurate assessment tool to determine comprehension of written materials and could be incorporated into initial assessment. Thus more appropriate educational aids could be selected, and clients with low reading skills could be encouraged to contact local resources for reading instruction. Dixon and Park (33) present helpful guidelines for improving health education materials and health education. Information presented at the fifth-grade reading level yields better comprehension (87).

Evaluation

Evaluation is judging how effective teaching has been. Evaluation is sometimes difficult because clients cannot always be followed long enough to see the results of teaching and human behavior is so complicated that true changes are hard to measure. However, a starting point is to review your objectives (37) and to document everything you teach so that you can recall exactly what you attempted.

Evaluation can be informal or formal. Informal judgments are made constantly. A client compliments or complains. You react to these judgments. You observe how well a client dresses a wound, irrigates a catheter, or cooks a meal after your demonstration. You write evaluation notes on the learning ability. By questioning the person's understanding, you are evaluating your teaching. If he or she has learned appropriately—can give explanations and can perform the activities that were taught—the teaching has been adequate. Clients can evaluate their own learning, whether goals were met, and your teaching by using a rating scale or checklist, which further assists your evaluation process.

Every person connected with a teaching-learning program should be involved in evaluating the program. Depending on the specific situation and program, these people might include the participants (clients and teachers); the program director and staff, who can see the program as a whole; the directing committee, who establish objectives and policy; and outside experts, who can be totally objective. Community representatives can supply valuable evaluative information when the teaching is aimed at serving the general public (28, 73).

HEALTH SCREENING

Health screening, *assessing present health status regularly through periodic health examinations,* including dental checkups, and participating in mass screening programs in the community, is essential. Learning preventive measures and warning signals of disease such as those published by the American Cancer Society, American Heart Association, and Diabetic Association assists in keeping up to date. Further, such literature provides useful education for the average citizen.

Regular health assessments are essential for two reasons: (1) the person remains cognizant of practices that will contribute to ensure health, and (2) early detection of health problems—potential or actual—is possible.

Refer to the section on physical assessment in Chapters 7 through 14 on how to screen effectively for specific conditions through the life span.

Refer to Appendix III, Review of Systems: Physical Assessment and Health History, at the end of the text, which presents health promotion and disease prevention factors to consider for each body system.

Refer to Appendix IV, Health Maintenance Procedures, at the end of the text for a list of screening procedures that should be regularly implemented from birth to 17 years and a list of procedures that should be regularly implemented from ages 18 to 80 or beyond. In addition, provide the following:

1. Glaucoma testing for all adults over age 40
2. Electrocardiograms for all adults over age 40 as part of routine examination
3. Dental screening for caries and preventive care to teeth and gums from age $2\frac{1}{2}$ to 3 years throughout the life span
4. Mammogram every 1 or 2 years for adults after their mid-thirties
5. Proctosigmoidoscopic examination every 3 to 5 years after 50.

Many people engage in self-screening practices; in fact, some types of self-examination practice to detect breast, testicular, skin, or mouth cancer are effective in early detection of disease and thereby prevent serious results or death. However, the person cannot do an accurate Papanicolaou (Pap) smear or rectal examination of self. Self-screening for hypertension requires the right kind of equipment and the correct procedure.

Many kinds of self-examination kits are available. Warn the client that self-screening for some conditions may not be preferable to examination by a nurse practitioner, nurse-midwife, or physician. Many of the self-test kits, whether for diabetes, pregnancy, or blood in the stool, that are bought over the counter have questionable accuracy. Even reliable kits give a false positive or false negative result if the procedure is not accurately done.

Risk factors to consider when appraising the person's health status include:

1. Genetic factors
2. Age
3. Congenital conditions
4. Past illness and injury
5. Family history such as presence of illness or causes of death in parents, siblings, grandparents, or other relatives and history of abuse or incest in family
6. Environmental threats such as economic deprivation, occupational hazards, unsafe conditions of home or neighborhood
7. Life-style considerations such as daily eating and sleeping patterns, work and leisure habits, use of tobacco, alcohol, or drugs, and stress management practices
8. Personal health habits such as nutritional practices, mouth and dental care, exercise and sleep patterns, immunizations, and periodic physical examinations
9. Life stresses or changes that have occurred in the past 2 years

A specific format for risk appraisal for cardiovascular disease, breast, lung, cervical, colorectal, uterine or ovarian, and skin malignancy, automobile accidents, diabetes, and suicide is presented by Pender (101).

Risk appraisal for illness alone is unlikely to result in better health. In fact, even if a risk score is high, that specific person may not develop a specific disease for uniquely individual reasons, although population studies indicate that statistically the person has a greater chance of disease development. Further, it is meaningless and unethical to do an appraisal or tell a person of risk without providing education, support, or resources to encourage behavior change that could prevent the risk occurrence. Risk appraisal must be done carefully and with the individual's personality status and needs in mind. The person should indicate a desire for such information before your spontaneously giving such information. Predictions about disease occurrence or shortened life expectancy may cause anxiety and depression, a giving-up, and fewer efforts at health promotion, especially in older adults who believe it is too late to change risk status. Risk predictions may create a sense of guilt and hypochondrial complaints that are not given sufficient attention by the physician, which could further the chance of disease development (31, 65).

NUTRITIONAL RECOMMENDATIONS

You have an important role in teaching the client and can act as a role model for healthy nutrition. Encourage the person to maintain essential nutrition and stay within 10 pounds of normal body weight. Refer to Chapters 11 and 12 about the hazards of obesity. Nutritionists, in general, agree that the best diet is high in fiber, moderate in protein and fat, and low in sugar, and salt. High-fiber foods include bran and other whole grains, raw fruits, and vegetables. These fruits prevent constipation and apparently other gastrointestinal diseases, including cancer. Red meat should not be the main source of protein. Sources of saturated fats such as red meat, butter, or whole milk should be limited because they impair the body's ability to reverse cholesterol buildup. Processed foods should not be the mainstay of the diet. Coffee, tea, and cola intake should be limited, for excessive caffeine intake has been linked to feelings of increased stress. Cooking with herbs or using lemon juice, vinegar, or other condiments can decrease the need to use salt as a flavoring.

Maintaining normal nutrition is basic to promoting health. Although recommended daily allowances have been established for the average person, it is unknown whether the daily nutritional recommendations are adequate for the man who is 6 foot, 6 inches tall; for the person who weights 225 pounds; for the person who works hard 16 hours a day; for the athlete; or for the person who is under excessive stress. Extra protein, calories, and fluids are needed for all of these people; it is likely that extra vitamins and minerals are also needed.

Refer to Chapters 7 through 14 for descriptions of nutritional needs and requirements for each age group. Refer also to Appendix I at the end of the text for Recommended Daily Dietary Allowances for infants, children, adult males and females, and pregnant and lactating women. Refer to Appendix II, Major Sources and Functions of Primary Nutrients, at the end of the text for a list of nutrients, their major sources, and their major functions. Herron (57) describes strategies for promoting healthy dietary intake.

EXERCISE, MOVEMENT, AND REST RECOMMENDATIONS

Refer to Chapters 7 through 14 for information about normal sleep, rest, and exercise needs throughout the life span. Play and leisure as a part of movement and exercise are discussed in each chapter as well. Normal adult sleep cycles are described in Chapter 12.

Edmunds (39) describes strategies to promote physical fitness, including warm-up, aerobic exercises, cool-down, floor work, and a final cool-down session. The interaction of exercise and diet augments weight loss and physical toning. Encourage the client to maintain a regular, moderate exercise program to enhance physical and emotional health. The exercise should involve large muscle groups in dynamic movement for approximately 20 minutes 3 or more days a week and should require 60% or more of a person's cardiorespiratory capacity. The exertion should be within limits appropriate to the physical status and needs of the person and should also be accompanied by a sense of excitement, flexibility, strength, and energy. At the end of exercise the person should feel replenished rather than bored, burned out, or excessively fatigued. Aerobic exercise to increase pulse rate and induce perspiration also boosts maximum oxygen use and increases blood flow through the body. Furthermore, the personal need to increase exercise to the point of competitive winning or achievement of maximum physical performance may contribute to eventual anatomic, physiologic, and psychologic breakdown (14, 39, 80).

There is no evidence that running is better than other aerobic physical exercise such as fast walking, swimming, bicycling, or dancing. The benefits of running are that it allows for psychomotor expression without the hazards of contact sports and is adaptable to a wide range of weather or geographic conditions, time schedules, personalities, and body types. Running can be social or asocial or organized or unorganized as an activity. Of equal importance to other exercise is regular flexibility exercises done slowly and gently to maintain range of joint motion (20, 38, 39, 101).

Running, or any strenuous physical exercise, also has some hazards. It can become addicting because release of endorphins in the body causes the person to feel euphoric and oblivious to pain or injury while running and very anxious when the exercise is omitted or delayed (23). The person who engages in intense exercise may engage in other health promotion measures or may feel invulnerable to disease and death. That myth of invulnerability may prevent his or her engaging in other health promotion measures. The long-term effects on joints and organs of regular, long-distance running is currently unknown; some orthopedic physicians report musculoskeletal damage resulting from the "pounding" effects. Some physicians also report that breast tissue is damaged if inadequately supported by a brassiere, and pelvic organs in women may suffer prolapse from excessive long-distance running. Other physicians disagree (13, 25, 80).

Emphasize to clients the importance of avoiding extreme stress, fatigue, or exhaustion, providing for adequate relaxation, rest, and sleep, and using relaxation techniques if necessary. Effectiveness of relaxation techniques has been demonstrated. These techniques are discussed in this chapter.

The two major obstacles to overcome in undertaking and keeping at an exercise program are making exercise part of a life-style and avoiding injury. Suggestions for making exercise a safe part of a life-style include the following:

1. Start in small increments and keep it fun.
2. Avoid exercising for 2 hours after a large meal and eating for 1 hour after exercising.
3. Include at least 10 minutes of warm-up and cooldown exercises in an exercise program (Fig. 17–3).
4. Use proper equipment and clothing when exercising.
5. Post goals, pictures of the ideal self, and notes of encouragement in a readily seen place for self-encouragement.
6. Use visualization daily to picture successful attainment of exercise benefit (e.g., looking toned or graceful, ideal weight).
7. Keep records of weekly measures of weight, blood pressure, and pulse.
8. Focus on the rewards of exercise; keep a record of feelings and compare differences in relaxation, energy, concentration, and sleep patterns.
9. Work with a peer or join a structured exercise class, running club, or fitness center. Spend more time with people dedicated to wellness.
10. Stop exercising or at least slow down and consult with a practitioner if any unusual, unexplainable symptoms occur.
11. Reward self for working toward exercise goals and for attaining them. For example, after a month in an exercise program, buy a new pair of running shoes or treat yourself to a special wish (13, 20, 30, 39).

Various theories and methods have been proposed to improve health through exercise and movement. They are based on a variety of concepts, including evolutionary development, dance, physical therapy techniques, and brain and endocrine function. Nulls and Cohen (95) propose a developmental movement theory that the body teaches the brain; certain movements are

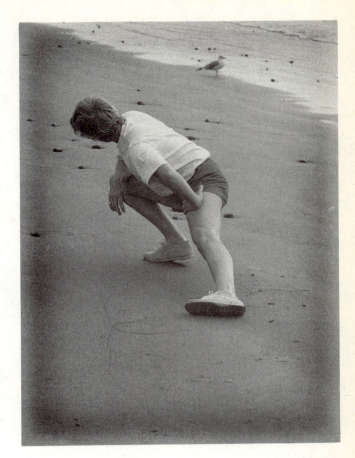

Figure 17-3. Stretching is an important element of any exercise program. (From Berger, K.J., and M.B. Williams, *Fundamentals of Nursing: Collaborating for Optimal Health.* Norwalk, Conn: Appleton & Lange, 1992, p. 1422.)

proposed to strengthen certain body parts. One theory and method is Feldenkrais' Awareness Through Movement Theory (46). His technique is to increase range of motion through increments of small, smooth, slow movements of the body in the direction of balance with gravity and with rhythmic breathing and centering on using imagery with the movement. Kurtz and Prestera (78) propose a body message theory, which focuses on muscular patterns and movements related to feelings. Aerobic exercise, with sustained rhythmic activity of large muscle groups, entails using large amounts of oxygen and increases heart rate, stroke volume, respiratory rate, and relaxation of blood vessels. Cardiovascular fitness and increased stamina are the goals. Body fat is also reduced. Aerobic exercises include running, jogging, brisk walking, swimming, aquadynamics, and aerobic dance. Correct posture, proper shoes, and strengthening abdominal muscles are helpful to enhance effects of aerobic exercise and reduce risks of injury. Increasingly a walk-jog program or brisk walking only is being recommended (139).

Refer to the references by Edmunds (39), Nulls and Cohen (95), Feldenkrais (46), Kurtz and Prestera (78),

Bloch and Graves (13), Cooper (25), Lally (80), Jones (66), Jordan (67), and Yanker (139) for more information about various exercise techniques and precautions. Clark (20) also furnishes a detailed description of various techniques. Clark also describes exercises for bedridden individuals and for those in a wheelchair.

Exercise such as walking, jogging, or swimming can reduce anxiety, tension, anger, depression, and pain perception because exercise serves to increase endorphin levels in the body. However, meditation, arts and crafts activities, and diversion have similar effects, and these methods could be used with individuals who are antagonistic to an exercise program.

PREVENTION OF ILLNESS AND INJURY

Immunizations

Teach clients the importance of securing necessary immunizations for the children and adults in the family, especially with outdoor exercise and athletic programs, wide travel, and resurgence of communicable diseases. Refer to Chapters 7 through 14 for information about immunization recommendations for each age group. Bigbee and Jansa (12) discuss individual, family, and community strategies for effective immunization programs.

Infection Control

Refer to Chapters 7 through 14 for information about common infections for each age group and basic preventive or treatment measures. Teach clients basic hygiene—hand washing, covering mouth when sneezing, avoidance of spitting, avoidance of close contact with others if contagion is possible—as one way to prevent spread of infection. Suggest measures that will help him or her prevent, when possible, and attend to any infection that occurs. First aid measures can be obtained from the Red Cross or can be found in a medical-surgical nursing text. Refer the person to a first aid course taught by the Red Cross.

Caring for the body functions, including those factors affecting the skin, mucous membranes, teeth, elimination, and sensory organs, also prevents infection.

Safety Promotion Measures

Teach safety measures to prevent injury and emergency treatment to avoid excessive or unnecessary tissue damage if an accident or illness occurs. A Red Cross course can be useful to the client. Mayhew (86) describes strategies for promoting safety and preventing injury from motor vehicle accidents, unintentional injuries in the home environment, occupational hazards, and violent and abusive behavior. These strategies are for young, middle-aged, and old adults.

For example, everyone should know how to do the Heimlich maneuver, named for the physician who developed it. This technique is done if the person is an adult and the airway is blocked by food or an object. First, ask the person if he or she can speak. If the person cannot, stand behind the person, place your arms around the waist slightly above the belt line, and make a fist with your right hand. Place your fist with the thumb side against the victim's abdomen. Allow the person's head, arms, and upper torso to hang forward on your arm. Grasp your right fist with the other hand and press rapidly and forcefully several times into the victim's abdomen, slightly above the navel and below the rib cage, with a quick upward thrust. This reverse bearing pushes up on the diaphragm, compresses the air in the lungs, and expels the object blocking the respiratory tract. Repeat several times if necessary. If the victim is sitting, stand behind the victim and perform the maneuver in the same way (Fig. 17–4).

Other important measures are to use sunscreening lotions and avoid excessive exposure to sun and heat (to avoid heat exhaustion or heat stroke) or cold weather (to avoid frostbite). Drinking plenty of fluids and wearing cool clothing are important in extreme summer temperatures. Wearing several layers of warm clothing, covering the head, and avoiding the vasoconstricting effects of alcohol, nicotine, and fatigue are ways to prevent frostbite.

Many states require the use of seatbelts for the driver and front passengers or all passengers in the car. Reinforce to the client the importance of using safety measures or devices such as seatbelts in cars, safety equipment in power machines, and sturdy ladders to prevent injury.

Using principles of body mechanics can prevent injury (Box 17–3) (20, 101, 109). Injury is also prevented by using the proper chair in the workplace. The back of the chair should be high enough to come approximately

Figure 17-4. Heimlich maneuver. (From Berger, K.J., and M.B. Williams, *Fundamentals of Nursing: Collaborating for Optimal Health.* Norwalk, Conn: Appleton & Lange, 1992, p. 1296.)

HEALTH PROMOTION STRATEGIES

BOX 17-3.
Principles of Body Mechanics

1. The wider the base of support and the lower the center of gravity, the greater is the stability of the object.
2. The equilibrium of an object is maintained as long as the line of gravity passes through its base of support.
3. When the line of gravity shifts outside the base of support, the amount of energy required to maintain equilibrium is increased.
4. Equilibrium is maintained with least effort when the base of support is broadened in the direction in which movement occurs.
5. Stooping with hips and knees flexed and the trunk in good alignment distributes the work load among the largest and strongest muscle groups and helps to prevent back strain.
6. The stronger the muscle group, the greater is the work it can perform safely.
7. Using a larger number of muscle groups for an activity distributes the work load.
8. Keeping center of gravity as close as possible to the center of gravity of the work load to be moved prevents unnecessary reaching and strain on back muscles.
9. Pulling an object directly toward (or pushing directly away from) the center of gravity prevents strain on back and abdominal muscles.
10. Facing the direction of movement prevents undesirable twisting of spine.
11. Pushing, pulling, or sliding an object on a surface requires less force than lifting an object since lifting involves moving the weight of the object against the pull of gravity.
12. Moving an object by rolling, turning, or pivoting requires less effort than lifting the object since momentum and leverage are used to advantage.
13. Using a lever when lifting an object reduces the amount of weight lifted.
14. The less the friction between the object moved and surface on which it is moved, the smaller is the force required to move it.
15. Moving an object on a level surface requires less effort than moving the same object on an inclined surface because the pull of gravity is less on a level surface.
16. Working with materials that rest on a surface at a good working level requires less effort than lifting them above the working surface.
17. Contraction of stabilizing muscles preparatory to activity helps to protect ligaments and joints from strain and injury.
18. Dividing balanced activity between arms and legs protects the back from strain.
19. Variety of position and activity helps maintain good muscle tone and prevent fatigue.
20. Alternating periods of rest and activity helps prevent fatigue.

2 inches above the lower tip of the shoulder blades and should tilt backward 10 degrees. The back of the seat should be 3 degrees higher than the front edge. This will place you forward a bit so that you can lean back to maintain balance, thus putting your body in a good natural position. The depth of the seat should be such that the front edge comes to within 1 inch of the back of your knee, allowing your thighs to rest on it without putting pressure on your knees or calves. Feet should rest on the floor. The person should be advised not to cross knees, which interferes with circulation. The aches and strains that develop in workers who sit or stand in poor posture daily can finally result in feeling ill and even in injury. Teach these same body mechanics principles to your clients.

Control of Environmental Hazards

Chapter 2 gives a comprehensive description of environmental hazards to health and ways to control these hazards. Teach the client and family about ways to protect self from (1) air pollution (indoor and outdoor); (2) water pollution and soil pollution, including pesticides and herbicides; (3) food contaminants; (4) excess noise; (5) surface pollution; or (6) other hazards related to various occupations.

Cessation of Habits Destructive to Health

Smoking

The hazards of smoking are well publicized; refer to Chapter 2 for description of effects of smoking and to Chapter 6 for effects of smoking in the fetus. More than 60 carcinogens and tumor initiators have been identified in tobacco and tobacco smoke. Involuntary smokers receive the same chemical mix as smokers, only less of it. Children of smoking parents are more likely to have slower expansion of lungs and more respiratory problems and disease than are children of nonsmoking parents (133). Nonsmoking persons married to smokers have a twofold increased risk of lung cancer. Lung cancer risk in persons who never smoked increased with duration of exposure to a smoking spouse (61).

Nurses in the past often worked in a smoke-filled environment—sitting in the nurse's station or lounge or the supervisor's office, lighting the cigarettes of psychiatric clients, being in the clients' lounge when clients were smoking. Nurses' associations have worked with hospitals and other health care agencies to set up standards that reduce the amount of tobacco smoke in the environment. Nurses can be leaders in promoting smoking cessation and smoking prevention programs in their communities. Nurses can lead public education campaigns about the hazards of smoking for the smoker and nonsmoker, pregnant women, and children. Nurses who smoke themselves need to join smoking cessation programs so that they can serve as role models for others. The success of antismoking campaigns and smoking

Research Abstract

Magnee, C., Perceived Well-Being of Persons Quitting Smoking, Nursing Research, *40 no. 4 (1991), 200–203.*

Effects of smoking cessation are complex, including nicotine withdrawal, disruption of existing coping patterns, and a new set of stresses and strains, which have an impact on smoking cessation. Changing a behavior can create new demands for which a person might not have readily available responses. The theoretic basis for this study was Lazarus' stress-coping theory, which defines *stress* as the result of a person's transactions with environment. Current models of health behavior suggest that stress is an aspect of health behavior. The Health Belief Model and Health Promotion Model both suggest that conflicting forces may prevent adoption of a behavior that is perceived as healthy.

The purpose of this study was to investigate the effect of smoking cessation on well-being and whether a negative effect on well-being contributes to relapse in cessation efforts. The sample consisted of 240 people: 75 nonsmokers, 74 smokers, and 92 people who were quitting smoking (114 men and 126 women). The average age was 33 years; a wide range of income and education levels were represented.

A modified version of the Daily Hassles Scale, Bradburn Morale Scale, Physical Symptoms Survey, and Symptoms Checklist 10 were instruments used in this study. One-way analysis of variance and chi-square analysis indicated no difference on any demographic characteristics or on any well-being measures between subjects from the two sampling sites.

Findings revealed that smokers, nonsmokers, and persons quitting smoking differed in education, marital status, and age. Smokers were from a lower socioeconomic group than nonsmokers. The subjects differed in intensity of daily hassles experienced. Persons who quit smoking had lower levels of well-being than either smokers or nonsmokers and experienced more than effects of nicotine withdrawal. Apparently the process of quitting smoking negatively affects well-being; the person experiences more stress.

cessation programs is documented (3, 21, 47, 69, 72, 103, 107).

Box 17–4 provides suggestions for smoking cessation. A recent intervention for smoking cessation is the use of nicotine gum. Although originally considered a panacea, recent research shows it is most effective when used in combination with other approaches. Nicotine chewing gum is suggested primarily for smokers who are heavily addicted to nicotine (40, 94, 133).

Alcohol and Drug Abuse

Health teaching and counseling of the client who abuses alcohol and/or drugs could include information from Chapter 6 (effects in fetus and pregnant woman and on men), from Chapter 11 (effects of drug abuse), and from Chapter 12 (effects of alcohol). Reference 93 gives more information.

The excessive intake of most drugs, alcohol, and food is linked to various diseases. Excessive or inappropriate use of prescribed or over-the-counter drugs frequently has serious consequences. A major problem involves overuse and inappropriate prescription of antibiotics, resulting in resistant strains of microorganisms and inadequate treatment of infections. The excessive and careless prescribing of mood-changing drugs can result in loss of behavioral control and even in physical and psychologic addiction. Taking a combination of many prescribed or unprescribed drugs can result in interactive effects that are toxic to the body. Alcohol is a major cause of many accidental injuries and deaths and of other diseases. Excessive caffeine consumption has also been linked to breast cancer and other diseases.

Emphasize the importance of not using tobacco, of limited alcohol use, and of moderate to, preferably, limited caffeine use.

STRESS MANAGEMENT

Stress management involves not only a variety of techniques, but also knowing the stress level at which response is harmful; avoiding excess stress; and seeking involvement with other people and groups.

Assessment

Stressful life events interfere with health promotion and precede many health problems. Assessment of stress encounters in life and the potential impact on health can be done by using several instruments: the *Social Readjustment Rating Scale* (see Table 16–2), developed by Holmes and Rahe (59); the *State-Trait Anxiety Inventory,* developed by Spielberger (126); and the *Signs of Distress,* developed by Everly and Girdano (44). Modified forms of the life-change index are available for different age and ethnic groups. Holmes and Rahe found that life changes predict the possibility of becoming ill. If enough changes occur within a 2-year period, the chances of becoming ill are increased. The State-Trait Anxiety Inventory consists of 20 items that pertain to anxiety the person currently feels (state) and 20 items that pertain to anxiety the person generally feels (trait). A high level of state and trait anxiety indicates that the person may suffer physiologic effects of anxiety, which may result in disease (126).

You may have the person do a stress-charting exercise, listing all the stressors presently occurring and the area of life in which the stressors occur (e.g., spouse, children, relatives, friends, work or the profession, personal health effects, finances, social concerns, recreation or leisure, church, other organizational activity, or other areas). Then each stressor should be rated as to the im-

■ **BOX 17-4.**
Smoking Cessation Suggestions

- Keep a notebook of current and past successes. Use the list as a reminder of your ability to succeed in new ventures.
- Identify a personal reason for quitting smoking other than because "It's bad for me."
- Make a list of things that are personally pleasurable; choose one as a reward (instead of a cigarette) when feeling uncomfortable or bored.
- Make a list of reasons smoking began and compare it with a list of current reasons for smoking.
- Keep a log of each cigarette lit, including the purpose; focus on smoking the cigarette and sensations occurring during and after smoking.
- Put cigarettes in an unfamiliar place.
- Every time a cigarette is reached for, ask "Do I really want this cigarette?," "Do I really need a cigarette?," "What can I do instead of smoking this cigarette?"
- Develop and prepractice responses to peer pressure to smoke, including: "Come on, one won't hurt," "Smoking makes you independent, like an adult," "Here, have one," "Are you a sissy?" Take an assertiveness course if necessary to develop the skill of saying "No."
- Smoke with the opposite hand from the one usually used.
- Buy cigarettes only by the pack, not by the carton.
- Buy different brands of cigarettes and avoid smoking two packs of the same brand in a row.
- Stay away from friends who smoke and from places where people smoke.
- End all meals with foods not associated with smoking (e.g., a glass of milk or half a grapefruit rather than a cup of coffee or a drink).
- Switch to noncaffeinated coffee or tea or bouillon.
- When using cigarettes as an energizer, substitute six small high-protein meals, sufficient sleep, a glass of milk, a piece of fresh fruit, fruit or vegetable juice, exercise or movement, or a relaxation exercise.
- Have carrot sticks, celery, or sunflower seeds ready to chew instead of smoking a cigarette.
- Eat more foods that leave the body alkaline such as vegetables, seeds, and fruits and reduce the urge to smoke.
- Write a list of stress enhancers; learn structured relaxation and stress reduction approaches to deal with each stressor.
- Use affirmations such as, "I no longer smoke," "I can quit," "It's getting easier and easier to quit smoking," or "It's getting easier and easier to think about quitting smoking." Tell six people.
- Use deep breathing or breath for centering when the urge for a cigarette appears.
- Work with a peer who can be called for positive feedback when the urge for a cigarette occurs. Be sure the peer is positive about ability to quit and does not nag or induce guilt.
- Ask friends and coworkers not to leave cigarettes around or offer them.
- When the urge for a cigarette occurs, picture the word "STOP" in big red letters.
- Ask for a hug instead of having a cigarette.
- Choose a time to stop smoking when peak mental or physical performance is not expected.
- Write a contract and sign it with a trusted person so continuing to smoke will prove embarrassing or will result in great loss.
- Read articles and books by people who have successfully quit smoking or helped others to do so.
- When feeling depressed, talk with people who have successfully quit smoking and ask for information about why they are glad they quit.

pact it is having, using a scale of 1 to 5, with the number 5 indicating severe impact. Awareness gained from this exercise may motivate the person in use of stress management and relaxation techniques.

Pender (101) has developed the Life Style and Health Habits Assessment, which is divided into 10 sections:

1. Competence in self-care
2. Nutritional practices
3. Physical or recreational activity
4. Sleep patterns
5. Stress management
6. Self-actualization
7. Sense of purpose
8. Relationships with others
9. Environmental control
10. Use of health care system

After the person has completed the form, you can use responses as a basis for health teaching.

Intervention

Strategies for adaptation to stressors include biologic mechanisms, psychologic adaptive mechanisms, and coping behaviors. There are intrapsychic, interpersonal, and system or institutionalized ways of coping with stressors. You will assist clients to develop and use these strategies through (1) direct care, (2) exploration with the person, (3) teaching or counseling of the person, or (4) creating changes in the person, family, group, health care agency, or the client's environment. Approach intervention from a *holistic* philosophy; mind, body, and culture are a fully unified system. A variety of approaches can be used to prevent or treat illness.

Biologic coping mechanisms and responses of the

endocrine, neurologic, cellular, and biochemical regulatory systems occur in the alarm stage and help the person to maintain the resistance stage, recover from disease, and have the energy level necessary to maintain other adaptive strategies. These responses were described in Chapter 16.

Scandrett and Uecker (116) include self-hypnosis, biofeedback, autogenics, and meditation under the rubric of relaxation therapy and suggest it as an appropriate intervention for the following nursing diagnoses: anxiety, activity intolerance, ineffective breathing pattern, comfort alterations in pain, ineffectual coping, fear, impaired physical mobility, powerlessness, and sleep disturbance.

Physical Methods of Relaxation/Stress Management

Relaxation and stress management techniques can be used with people of any age. Even school-age children can learn relaxation training to reduce anxiety and cope with stress which may enhance subsequent stress management (15, 82).

Progressive Relaxation. **Progressive relaxation** was developed by Jacobson in 1938 and *involves tightening and relaxing muscle groups* of the body for 5 to 7 seconds each, beginning with the hand and moving to the upper and lower arm, the forehead and face, neck, upper back, abdomen, buttocks, thigh, calf, and foot. The person is encouraged to check for relaxation before moving to the next major muscle group. In a relaxation session you and the individual can agree that if he or she is tense, the index finger of the right or left hand will be raised when relaxation is felt (20, 30, 38, 101).

The person may be able to relax through breathing techniques that use deep, slow inhalation and full exhalation, with the person focusing mentally on the body part to which the inhalation is directed. Rapid, shallow breathing is often induced by stress. Thus concentration on proper breathing can help relieve stress, especially with the use of abdominal breathing. Music can be used with the breathing exercises (10).

A careful assessment of the person is essential before using relaxation techniques. Baseline and posttreatment vital sign measures will validate physiologic changes associated with relaxation. Essential components of the pretreatment interview include assessing:

1. Client's identification of the most bothersome symptom(s), including onset, duration, and full description.
2. Family history of similar complaints.
3. Client interventions and description of the results, including use of current and recent medications, including over-the-counter drugs.
4. Physical limitations or illnesses.

5. Previous experience with relaxation training.
6. Use of alcohol or mind-altering drugs to relax.
7. Dietary patterns, especially use of caffeine and sugar, and foods that connote relaxation and are eaten at stressful times.
8. Sleep and exercise patterns.
9. Overview of daily routine, including stressors.
10. Psychiatric history, including screening for major depressive or psychotic disorders.
11. Willingness to learn techniques and to practice at home (20, 30, 38, 101).

Although progressive relaxation has proved effective in most studies, precautions should be taken for persons described in the following:

1. Depressed or withdrawn persons: relaxation may cause further withdrawal.
2. Persons who are experiencing hallucinations and delusions: they may lose reality contact.
3. Persons with cardiac conditions; they should use nontensing relaxation exercises since tightly tensing muscles can increase blood pressure.
4. Persons on medications: the toxic effects of some medications can be increased by the relaxation state.

Acupuncture. **Acupuncture** is a *treatment method based on the Chinese philosophy that all life is a microcosm of a vast, constantly changing flowing circle of energy,* without beginning or end, that flows through the karma (fate) of our lives. This circle is divided into a rising energy, *yang,* seen as positive and male, and a descending energy, *yin,* seen as negative and female. Yet yang and yin are symbolic rather than superior or inferior to each other. The body can reach a balanced state only if both forces are flowing smoothly. The energy of yin and yang together is called *qi* (chee), and in the body is called *true qi.* Illness occurs when the flow of true qi around the 12 main channels or meridians of body is impeded or blocked and energy balance becomes disturbed. The 12 meridians are named after 12 organs as defined by Chinese acupuncturists: lung, large intestine, pericardium, bladder, small intestine, triple warmer, stomach, heart, gallbladder, spleen, kidney, and liver (2, 14).

Acupressure. **Acupressure** is the *predecessor of acupuncture.* The term is applied to a *number of techniques of applying pressure to stimulate acupuncture points on the body.* Acupressure releases tension and relieves pain. It is a preventive treatment used to balance energy by applying pressures to specific points (2, 14, 20).

Shiatsu. **Shiatsu** is an *ancient, simple treatment method whereby a form of manipulation is administered by the thumbs, fingers, and palms, without any use of instruments,* mechanical or otherwise, to apply pressure to the human skin, correct internal malfunctioning, promote and maintain health, and treat specific disease. Shiatsu is a fusion of the ancient Japanese manipulation therapy, anma, and the Chinese concept of acupuncture; however, no needles are used, only pressure. The philosophy is similar to that of Chinese acupuncture. Illness occurs as a result of excess or deficiency of yin and yang energy or a block of true qi. Gentle pressure along the meridian lines restores the balance (2, 4, 120).

Reflexology. **Reflexology** is a *technique based on the premise that body organs have corresponding reflex points on other parts of the body.* The reflex points are believed to be up to 20 times more sensitive than the corresponding organs. The foot is viewed as one of the scanner screens that records body functions. Working the reflexes in the feet helps rebalance organs by releasing blocks that impede the smooth flow of body energy. Other areas have reflex points (wrist, hand, ear, neck, abdomen, face, head, arms, legs, nose, and iris), but the feet are the most effective. The act of reflexology is a giving and receiving, a sharing of communication resulting in confidence and mental calming. Together, healer and client call on the healing energy of the universe to surround, uplift, and permeate; the use of affirmations and the projection of a positive healing environment are a spiritual act of being of service to others (2, 20, 120).

Biofeedback. **Biofeedback** is a *means of receiving feedback or a message from the body about internal physiologic processes, using specific techniques or equipment.* It involves use of instruments to develop the ability to read tension in various body systems and to learn ways of releasing the tension when cues of stress response are identified.

Biofeedback permits a person to become familiar with internal functions such as a moving index of body temperature or a reading of brain waves. As with externally directed behavior, the person is able with practice to learn how to control internal behavior (20). Most people have experienced the physician's interpreting for them, in an illness-wellness context, the results of physiologic tests. If the person is able to read the same information as it is occurring within him or her, he or she is using biofeedback.

Biofeedback has two aspects: (1) the actual use of biomedical devices capable of taking a reading of one's physiologic activity such as temperature or heart rate and (2) the training in which one learns what to do with the devices. The client is linked to the instruments, which are modified to display the body information as visual or auditory signals, by delicate wires or tubes connected to special sensing materials taped to the skin. The body information is carried back to the devices, which continually read the signals reflecting the constantly changing activity within. As the person continues

to work with biofeedback instrumentation, an association develops between changes in body signals and various subjective feelings that are either consciously or subconsciously recognized. The monitor gives information about the degree of success. Dependence on the instrumentation is temporary. Eventually the person should be able to monitor the fluctuations and thereby exercise some conscious control over physiologic adaptation. Once learned, control over a physiologic function is retained in the person's memory for a long time (2, 20, 120). Biofeedback has been used successfully to treat tension headaches, migraine headaches, hypertension, insomnia, peptic ulcers, colitis, muscle spasms or pain, epilepsy, asthma, anxiety states, panic disorders, phobic reactions, stuttering, and teeth grinding.

A directory of certified feedback practitioners is available from the Association for Applied Psychophysiology and Biofeedback, 10200 44th Ave., Suite 304, Wheat Ridge, CO, 80033.

Massage. Massage has had a long and checkered history. It has been alternately extolled and rejected as a therapeutic procedure. Its popularity is increasing because the public is disillusioned with modern depersonalized clinical practices that emphasize surgery and medications rather than personal contact and self-responsibility or preventive maintenance.

The effects of massage are psychologic, mechanical, physiologic, and reflexive. **Massage** is an art (a unique way of communicating without words and showing caring) and a science; a *systematic manipulation of the body tissue* produces beneficial effects on the nervous and muscular systems, local and general circulation, the skin, viscera, and metabolism (2, 120).

During massage the hands stimulate the sensory receptors of the skin and subcutaneous tissues, causing a series of reflex effects, including capillary vasodilation or constriction, relaxation or stimulation of voluntary muscle contraction, and possible sedation or stimulation of pain in an area remote from the area being touched, depending on the type of massage or stroking movements (2, 20, 120).

Yoga. The word **yoga** means *to unite, implying the balance or harmony that can exist within the individual.* Yoga is an Indian philosophic system that emphasizes the practice of special techniques to attain the highest degree of physical, emotional, and spiritual integration. Hatha-yoga is the branch that emphasizes physical postures and breathing practices to attain body-mind balance.

Studies of the effects of hatha-yoga have shown it especially beneficial to optimum functioning of the endocrine, circulatory, musculoskeletal, respiratory, and nervous systems. Yoga reduces blood pressure, lowers pulse rate, reduces serum cholesterol, regulates menstrual flow and thyroid function, increases range of motion in joints, reduces joint pain, and increases feeling of well-being (2, 20).

Autogenics. **Autogenics** is a *form of self-hypnosis that allows the person to induce the feeling of warmth and heaviness associated with a trance state.* The method was developed by Johannes H. Schultz, a Berlin psychiatrist. Autosuggestion with some yoga techniques was developed into a system of autogenic training. The system is effective in treatment of disorders of the respiratory and gastrointestinal tracts and of the circulatory and endocrine systems and for anxiety and fatigue. The exercises can be used to increase resistance to stressors, reduce or eliminate sleep disorders, and modify pain reactions. Autogenic therapy is not recommended for children less than 5 years old or for adults who lack motivation or have severe emotional disorders. Those with diabetes, hypoglycemic conditions, or heart conditions should discuss the use of the method with their physicians. Occasionally, a client experiences a sharp rise or drop in blood pressure when doing the exercises; blood pressure should be taken to ensure the exercises are useful. The exercises can be completed in a comfortable sitting or lying position in which the person assumes an attitude of passive concentration. It may take up to 10 months to master the six exercises. Ninety-second sessions five to eight times a day are recommended for mastery. Clark (20) describes in detail the technique to follow.

Krieger's Theory of Therapeutic Touch

Dolores Krieger (76) draws on Eastern beliefs and literature in her theory of therapeutic touch. She theorizes that *prana* (Sanskrit term for energy) is transferred in the healing act; the source of prana in Eastern thinking is the sun. Eastern thinking contends that well people have an excess of prana; Western physiology texts state there is a great deal of energy in the human body. Krieger pictures the healer as a person with excess prana or energy who has a strong sense of commitment and intention to help people. Healing entails channeling of this energy flow by the healer for the well-being of the sick individual. Healers do not become depleted of energy, however, because they are in a constant state of energy input. Healers become depleted of energy only if they draw on their own energy rather than being a channel of energy. Healers are thought to accelerate the healing process by giving the client an extra boost to his or her recuperative system.

Krieger presents physiologic data to support her theory. There is evidence that therapeutic touch raises hemoglobin levels and influences electroencephalogram (EEG) patterns. The healer's EEG changes to a high-amplitude beta state, indicative of deep concentration similar to meditation, and the person's brain waves are typically low-amplitude alpha waves, correlated with a state of calmness and well-being. The person experiences

slower, deeper respirations and a sense of warmth and relaxation.

According to Krieger, therapeutic touch works well with all stress-related diseases, having a significant effect on the autonomic nervous system and reducing nausea, dyspnea, tachycardia, pallor, and peristalsis. Use of therapeutic touch has also been successful with children and with the terminally ill person.

The healer centers and uses the hands (placed 2 to 3 inches from the person's skin) to move quickly over the body, reading signals of illness or blockage of energy flow. The feeling of pressure sensed in the hands when congestion or blockage is present is explained biophysically; as the healer moves the hands over the body, positive ions are sensed. Positive ions are associated with feelings of lethargy, headache, irritability, and inflammations of the mucosal tissues. Negative ions are noted when the person has a feeling of well-being (76, 110).

Krieger (76) refers to the pressure as a "ruffling in the field"; the healer can move the positive ions by shaking or wiping the hands. When the healer's hands are placed in the area of a "ruffle" and the hands are moved away from the body in a sweeping gesture, the pressure is reduced, and the feeling of energy flow is sensed; this is called "unruffling the field." The unruffling motion can be used to soothe babies or reduce pain and tension. A 2- to 3-minute treatment is sufficient for children or the debilitated. With others the healer stops when the body feels balanced (62, 76, 110).

The object of therapeutic touch is to balance the healer's "field" so that symmetry of energy flow is restored. With practice the hands begin to move toward areas of unbalanced energy flow as they become more sensitive to changes in the field of another person's body. Therapeutic touch can raise hemoglobin levels, reduce anxiety, relieve headache, and promote other physical well-being and healing by redirecting energy fields and enabling the sick person to mobilize personal healing powers (55, 76, 110).

The spiritual implications of therapeutic touch are discussed by two nurses, Wuthnow (138) and Miller (89). Wuthnow (138) believes that the technique can be used by nurses of all faiths who are trained in the technique and that it can be used with or without Christian beliefs. Miller (89) believes that Christian nurses cannot use the technique because it represents a wrong relationship with the Holy Spirit and assumes a manipulating role of God. (This same argument is used by some Christian nurses against use of guided imagery, visualization, and other cognitive techniques for healing.)

Clark (20) describes in detail various touch and healing interventions that can be used by the nurse, including: (1) behavioral kinesiology interventions, (2) therapeutic touch interventions, (3) yoga interventions, (4) massage interventions, (5) acupressure interventions, and (6) reflexology interventions. A number of books are also available to explain these therapies in detail.

COGNITIVE METHODS OF COPING, RELAXATION, AND STRESS MANAGEMENT

Both you and your clients need to take time for play, leisure, or diversional activities and spiritual pursuits that (1) are rewarding emotionally, (2) are done voluntarily rather than out of obligation, (3) are outside of ordinary life routines, (4) absorb attention, (5) are not necessarily productive in earnings, and (6) have definite time and space boundaries. Laughter, pleasant thoughts, and relaxing activities stimulate production of endorphins and enkephalins, chemical pain relievers. Adrenalin and other hormones are also produced, stimulating body function. The body's production of immune cells increases. Arteries and muscles relax, reducing blood pressure.

Thought Stopping

Thought stopping is a *behavioral modification technique useful when nagging, repetitive thoughts interfere with behavior and wellness.* Unwanted thoughts are interrupted with the command "Stop." An image of the letters of the word *stop,* a loud noise, (e.g., a buzzer or bell), or a negative stimulus such as wearing a rubber band around the wrist and snapping it when the unwanted though occurs is used with the command. Then a thought that is positive, healthful, or desirable is substituted. Thought stopping may work because (1) distraction occurs, (2) the interruption behaviors serve as a punishment, (3) an assertive response can be followed by reassuring or self-accepting comments, and (4) a chain of negative and frightening thoughts leading to negative and frightening feelings is interrupted, thus reducing the stress level. Regular practice for 3 to 7 days is necessary for the person to learn to interrupt quickly a negative thought with a positive, constructive alternative thought (16, 20).

Refuting Irrational Ideas

People engage in almost continuous self-talk during waking hours. **Self-talk** is the *internal language used to describe and interpret the world.* When self-talk is accurate and realistic, wellness is enhanced; when irrational and untrue, stress and emotional disturbance occur.

Albert Ellis (41, 42) developed a system to attack irrational ideas or beliefs and replace them with more realistic interpretations and self-talk. Irrational self-talk includes statements that "awfulize" experience, that is, make catastrophic, nightmarish interpretations of events. An irrational self-thought leads to unpleasant emotions. Rational self-talk leads to pleasant feelings and a positive interpretation of experiences. Rational thought is based on the idea that events occur and people experience these events (16, 41, 42).

The kinds of statements that Ellis (41) considers irrational include the following:

1. External events cause most human misery; people simply react as events trigger their emotions.
2. People must always be competent and perfect in all endeavors.
3. Happiness can be achieved by inaction, passivity, and endless leisure.
4. It is easier to avoid than to face life's difficulties and responsibilities.
5. The past determines the present.
6. It is horrible when people and things are not the way you want them to be.
7. Unfamiliar or potentially dangerous situations always lead to fear and anxiety.
8. People are helpless and have no control over what they experience or feel.
9. People are fragile and cannot be told the truth.
10. Rejection and abandonment are the result if one does not always try to please others.
11. There are a perfect love and a perfect relationship.
12. A person's worth is dependent on achievement and production.
13. Anger is bad and destructive.
14. It is bad and wrong to go after what you want and need.

Refusing irrational ideas is a skill and requires practice in the following nine steps (41):

1. Write down the facts of the event, including only the observable behaviors.
2. Write down self-talk about the event, including all subjective value judgments, assumptions, beliefs, predictions, and worries.
3. Note which statements are classified by Ellis as irrational.
4. Focus on the emotional response to the event, using one or two words such as angry, hopeless, felt worthless, afraid.
5. Select one irrational idea to refute.
6. Write down all evidence that the idea is false.
7. Write down the worst outcome that could happen if what is feared happens or what is desired is not attained.
8. Write down positive results that might occur if what is feared happens or if what is desired is not attained.
9. Substitute alternative self-talk to focus on positive statements.

Coping Skills Procedures

Coping skills training *grew out of relaxation and systematic desensitization procedures* that were expanded and refined by Meichenbaum and Cameron (88). The procedures include a combination of progressive relaxation and stress-coping self-statements that are used to replace the defeatist self-talk called forth in stressful situations. Coping skill procedures can be used to rehearse via the imagination for real life events deemed stressful. First, a stressful situation is called forth. Next, progressive relaxation is practiced. Finally, coping skills statements are repeated until the situation can be thoroughly completed in rehearsal without feelings stressed. The procedures are effective in the reduction of tension, anxiety, phobias, insomnia, and hypertension. Coping skills procedures can be mastered in approximately 1 week once progressive relaxation has been learned (16, 41, 48, 88).

Centering

Centering refers to *separating or differentiating from others so that there is an inner reference or thought of stability, calm, and self-awareness; a sense of self-relatedness, a place of quietude within self where one can feel integrated, unified, and focused.* As a result, you can communicate more openly and listen to self and others more effectively (76).

Centering reduces fatigue, stress, depression, or anger when working with a client. Centering takes little time once the idea is mastered and can be helpful to use before any anxiety-provoking situation in the hospital, at home, in social situations, or at work. Centering can also be taught to people to help them gain self-control. Centering can be achieved while standing or sitting, but beginning efforts produce the best results in a sitting position. The method is as follows:

1. Sit in a comfortable chair with feet flat on the floor and hands resting quietly in your lap; close your eyes.
2. Check out your body for tension spots and relax these areas as you exhale.
3. Inhale easily, filling your body with relaxation.
4. Exhale, moving your breathing to your center, about the level of your navel.
5. Continue breathing in this matter until you feel calm, integrated, unified, and focused.
6. (Optional) Picture the body surrounded by a protective shield that allows positive energy in but keeps negative energy out. The shield may be conceived as a color, light source, or spiritual sense (20).

Assertive Communication or Behavior

Assertiveness means *to be able to express personal thoughts, feelings, and desires, defining and making known personal rights that are reasonable, while being respectful to the other person and of his or her rights.* Expression of honest feelings, being willing to act on rational thoughts and controlled feelings to achieve a goal, and taking responsibility for consequences are a part of assertive communication and behavior. Stating "I . . ." messages to express feelings and ideas rather than

"You make me feel . . . " or "You should . . . " will increase self-confidence, enhance relationships with others, reduce anxiety and stress, and control fear and anger (16, 20, 48, 120).

Assertive communication comes with practice with another, in a group, in front of a mirror, and/or using a tape recorder. Assertiveness includes paying attention to facial expression, voice tone, posture, use of gestures, congruity between words and appearance, and the way statements are phrased.

Various techniques are useful in assertive communication and behavior. You can use them in your personal and professional life and can teach them to clients. A summary of several techniques follows:

1. *Acknowledgment:* When you are criticized, you acknowledge the comment of the other, the feeling implied, and whatever of the criticism is applicable to you. Avoid giving excuses or apologies.

   "Yes, I was late to work this morning. I punched in the time clock 10 minutes after 7:00, so I was 10 minutes late."
   "Yes, I overlooked carrying out the garbage last night, and I can appreciate your sense of frustration."

2. *Clouding:* When you are given a nonconstructive, manipulative criticism with which you disagree, you can stand your ground, implying that there could be other reasons for your action, while continuing to listen and communicate. You agree to the part of the criticism that is true without agreeing to any specific action plan.
   a. *Agreeing in part:*

Parent:	"You always have an excuse to get out of work around home."
Teen:	"I do have a lot of school and church group responsibilities."
Parent:	"You don't seem to care anything about your family."
Teen:	"You're right. I guess it does seem that way."

   b. *Agreeing in probability:*

Parent:	"You're putting on a lot of weight."
Teen:	"I may have gained a few extra pounds."
Parent:	"You'd better go on a diet."
Teen:	"Perhaps it is time for starting a diet."

   c. *Agreeing in principle:*

Parent:	"If you don't study more, you're not going to pass this semester."
Teen:	"You're right. If I don't study, I will fail."

3. *Probing:* This response can determine whether criticism is constructive or manipulative and clarifies unclear comments. First you isolate the part of the criticism that is most bothersome to the other and

then ask what specifically is bothersome about the behavior.

Assertive Probing:

Supervisor: "Your work is not satisfactory."

Nurse: "What about my work bothers you?"

Supervisor: "Everyone else works overtime when necessary; you always leave on time."

Nurse: "What is it about my leaving on time that bothers you?"

Supervisor: "It's not right that you work only by the clock when the rest of us work overtime. None of us likes to work overtime, but the work has to be done."

Nurse: "What bothers you about me working by the clock?"

Supervisor: "When you leave, someone else has to finish your work. The rule here is that no one leaves until the shift's work is done."

4. *Broken record:* This technique can be used when another is not listening to you, when it is necessary to clarify limits about what should be done, or when explanation would provide the other with an opportunity to continue a pointless discussion. The steps are:

a. Give a short, specific statement about what is desired, without giving excuses.

b. Use body language that shows you are calm and in control of your feelings: stand or sit erect, maintain eye contact, keep hands and arms quiet at the side.

c. Calmly and firmly repeat the chosen statement as many times as necessary until the other person realizes there is no negotiation possible. Ignore the other's excuses, ramblings, curses, or false accusations.

Situation: Driver A pulls out of a parking place, very fast, with a too sharp turn, managing to pull loose the back bumper of the car in the next parking place (Driver B), which is parked right on the line. Driver A pulls forward into the parking place, gets out of the car, and proceeds toward Driver B. Driver B stays in the car. Driver A stands by the car door, yelling how stupid Driver B is to park on the line.

Driver B: Rolling down the window slightly, "Yes, you are right; I am parked on the line."

Driver A: Continues to accuse Driver B, yelling invectives.

Driver B: Maintains eye contact, every 1 minute rolls down the window slightly and says, "When you are ready, I'll talk about what can be done about the bumper." This is repeated for approximately 10 minutes.

Driver A: Begins to calm down, finally smiles, and says, "OK, what do you want."

Driver B: "I want you to pay for repair of my ripped bumper."

Driver A: "OK." Proceeds to give telephone number, with an adequate down payment (in cash) toward bumper repair, and promises to pay more if cost is greater. "I just don't want my insurance company to get hold of this. Call if it costs more."

5. *Content to process shift:* When focus of conversation drifts from the original topic, conversation can be purposefully shifted from the subject (content) being discussed to the feelings between the two speakers (process). The statement should be made with a calm voice and demeanor, defusing anger that has arisen. Attack is avoided.

"We're off the subject; let's get back to what we agreed to discuss."

"I'm feeling uncomfortable about the drift of our conversation, and I notice we both appear tense."

"We seem to be getting into a battle. I sense we are both talking about the same thing but are coming from a different perspective."

6. *Momentary delay:* When a situation is compelling or another gives a command or implies an answer right away, it is important not to be swayed by the emotion of the moment. After a deep breath and a moment of delay, the comment could be:

"I'll need more information before I can act."

"There may be something to what you say, I need a few minutes to think about this."

"I can understand your feeling. I need a minute to sort out what you are saying."

7. *Time out:* If the conversation is important but has reached an impasse because of angry feelings or bias, conversation can be delayed and continued later by setting a near-future time to continue talking when both parties are more calm.

"We've been talking about this for quite a while, and I don't think we're getting anywhere. I'd like to sleep on it and talk more with you about it tomorrow morning. Let's meet to talk at 8:30 A.M."

(Designate a mutually neutral place if possible.)

8. *Joining and circling the attacker:* This technique is derived from the martial art of akido, in which the attacked person accepts and turns with the attack, then lets the attacker pass on. The focus of the intervention is to resolve conflict, restore harmony, and problem solve. There are four alternative responses:

a. *Do nothing.* This is a conscious choice, not a response of fear, when (1) the attack makes no sense, (2) the attacked does not want to dignify the attack by reacting, and (3) more information is needed to determine the reason for the attack

b. *Use humor or deflection*. Give an absurd reason or a surprise line as a reason for not accomplishing something that should have been done.

c. *Joining the attacker*. The attack is not taken personally and the attacker agrees, then moves to resolve the problem.

> "I don't blame you for feeling the way you do."
> "My job is to work with you. If you think we can work together, I want to hear your complaints."

d. *Parley*. This technique is useful if you have been engaged in a no-win situation; the other person has defined the encounter as a competition or contest.

Laughter, Humor, Play, Tears

Laughter, humor, play, and tears are natural ways of handling stress and releasing tension. The psychologic effects of a deep laugh or of a playful attitude works against the stress response: muscles in the face, diaphragm, abdomen, and blood vessels relax; blood pressure lowers; respirations normalize; the brain releases endorphins; and the immune system is strengthened. Tears and nasal secretions, excreted during both laughter and crying, contain hormones, steroids, and toxins that accumulate in the body during stress when there are feelings of anger, fear, frustration, sadness, and tedium. When these substances are secreted, the negative effects of the General Adaptation Syndrome are counteracted.

Emotionally and cognitively, humor, comedy, cartoons, and playing games help us to develop another perspective, to see the absurdity of a situation, to clarify the situation and be better able to think clearly, to problem-solve, and to cope. Laughing at personal foibles and mistakes enables others to laugh with us, not at us. Inanimate objects such as computers can be safe targets for humor about peoples' behavior and life's ironies. The catharsis that comes with both laughter and tears brings not only emotional release, but a sharing of feelings and consequent support from others. Without crying, healing cannot occur. Without laughter, forgiveness, and thereby healing, is impossible (17, 26, 36, 81, 122, 123).

Norman Cousins (26) conquered his own illness and pain through comedy, humor, and laughter. Sometimes people have to cry before they can laugh. There is no way to force either. In some cultures the value is to be stoic; the person may not cry in front of others, and a cheerful countenance is practiced. In other cultures if you do not cry with the person during troubled times, you are considered unfeeling, uncaring—not a friend.

Nurses can integrate laughter and tears appropriately into nursing care. To do so means that the nurse must integrate them into self. Hutchinson (63) found that humor was a self-care strategy that facilitated other strategies of assertion, catharsis, cultivating relationships by offering help to others, and withdrawal—becoming aloof and rising above the situation or resigning self to it. These are strategies nurses use to handle job stress; these strategies can also be taught to clients to handle their stress. Buxman (17) presents details about how to use humor and laughter for client recovery, staff morale, and hospital regulation. She lists specific resources for a "humor room," including books, magazines, newsletters, audiocassettes, movies, and videocassettes. Further, she describes how to establish a humor room administratively so that clients, families and staff can use the resources.

Clients, especially those suffering the greatest pain or fear, often express a joke, a sarcastic remark, a flippant line, a pun, cynicism, or dry humor. Acknowledge these statements. Be prepared to both laugh and cry with the person since the need for both may be implied.

Guided Imagery

Guided imagery can be defined as *focused attention on an inner, mental picture or a statement of belief of what the individual wants to accomplish by being open to and responding to the language of the unconscious or the deeper body levels.* Other terms are used for imagery such as imagination, visualization, autosuggestion, mental programming, or self-hypnosis. The term *imagination* or *visualization* is not totally descriptive of guided imagery. The term *self-hypnosis* is frightening to some. Thus the term that is used in the literature and is effective with clients is *guided imagery, imagery,* or *use of imaging.*

Imagery is not new. Some people say, without diminishing God the creator, that the first record of what could be considered a mental image producing results is written in Genesis with the creation. God said, "Light, be," and there was light. There are a number of accounts in the Old and New Testaments of the *Bible* of how people accomplished what was mentally visualized. For example, records of the fall of the walls of Jericho and the miracles of Jesus convey the power of the mental image. Whenever faith is involved, for example, in the healings of today, the person visualizes what is to be before it comes.

Guided imagery is not the same as a trance, play acting, use of fantasy or denial, the raising of false hope, or the claim to working of miracles. Rather, it is the purposeful use of a technique that requires time and effort to accomplish a purpose.

Physiologic Mechanisms Involved In Imagery. Much is still unknown about the private physiologic mechanisms that occur during private processes that allow for the manifestation of various results.

Imagery is a covert process whose characteristics, while observed, must be inferred. Imaging activity apparently is a complex blend of receptive-perceptual processes and efferent activity. Imagery can be conditioned under certain circumstances; it can show properties of skill learning; it is responsive to motivation; and it has properties of passive receptivity similar to those of reverie, dreams, and hypnosis (43, 119, 121, 124).

Muscle activity changes occur in response to the content of the image. For example, images of lifting an object were associated with increased activity in the arm muscles that would be involved in the actual movement, although the magnitude of the muscular changes are less during imagery than they would be during the overt movement (119, 121, 124). Imagery can reduce muscular tension as measured by electromyographic recording from the frontalis muscles on the forehead.

Images of moving objects are associated with greater oculomotor activity than images of stationary objects. Skin conduction responses during vividly imagined stressful scenes are more frequent, of greater magnitude, and slower to habituate than are skin conduction responses of nonvivid imagers. Different levels of activity of facial muscles have been measured during imagery of different emotional states, representational of changes that actually occur with different emotional states in real life (43, 119, 121, 124).

Studies using physiologic measures of imagery have used a wide range of measures. They are heart rate, respiration, EEG, alpha activity, skin temperature, electromyograph (EMG) activity in a number of different muscle groups, diastolic and systolic blood pressure, salivation, eye movements and pupillary responses, vasomotor responses, and measure of electrodermal activity such as the galvanic skin response (GSR), skin conductance, and skin resistance. Furthermore, significant effects have been reported, at least sometimes, for each measure that has been used. In general, it appears that heart rate is the most sensitive measure in that changes in heart rate associated with imagery have been the most consistently reported. Studies also show an increase in thymosin and white blood count with imagery (43, 121, 124).

Images, especially those without external representation, are apparently processed by the right hemisphere, which has a passive-receptive quality to the type of function it sustains. Right brain hemisphere function is concerned with intuition, visual and spatial events, imagination, and emotion. Receptive, representational, and spatial imagery is linked to right hemisphere functioning. The right hemisphere mediates analogic thinking and perceives the whole experience or "gestalt." In contrast, the left brain is logical and reasoning; it breaks down experience into sequential units, compartmentalizes and interprets information, and deals with verbal images. The right brain is stimulated by and receptive to imagery and in turn promotes release of chemicals and enzymes in the body that result in relaxation, healing, and well-being. Positive feelings release endorphins, which promote well-being and healing. Brain wave changes occur when the person is in a relaxed state (34, 43, 119, 121, 124). When these physiologic changes are facilitated regularly and over time, changes occur in body tissues, individual feelings and reactions, cognition, and life patterns.

Technique of Guided Imagery. First, a rapport and a climate of trust must be established between the client and you, the nurse or therapist. After initial assessment and exploration of the problem and often after trying other techniques, guided imagery is proposed to the client as another way to promote healing or change. An explanation is given of what is involved: (1) sitting in a quiet, comfortable environment without distractions; (2) beginning with a technique to obtain total body relaxation; (3) envisioning a peaceful, soothing scene that can maintain relaxation and a positive attitude; (4) focusing attention on what is desired or to be accomplished; (5) telling the therapist what thoughts or feelings come to mind, answering questions, describing the healing; and (6) repeating the process regularly three or four times a day for 15 or 20 minutes. In that way the body learns to respond to the mind.

The nature of the instructions presented to the client appears to have an important impact on the response. Instructions must be clear, suggestive, and encouraging. Instructions that emphasize involvement of the person in the experience and the goals to obtain facilitate the process. Imagery works best when the person is motivated to try the technique, when there is confidence in the nurse or therapist, and when there is expectation of success. Some people need more time to relax and to engage in the imagery process. The person should feel it is acceptable if he or she is unable initially to use imagery. However, if you suggest success, the person likely will be able to image. Use fun imagery exercises initially to help the person realize that he or she can engage in imagery. Then if the person believes that he or she wants to try imagery further as a method, continue with more introduction to and use of the technique.

As the person purposefully sets aside negative or sick images and images the positive, the healthy, the desired results while in a relaxed state, he or she is told that changes within the body and mind have been activated, which will be seen externally.

It may take some time for the person to gain an image of the desired goal. During that time have the person talk about the problem as imaged (e.g., physical, emotional, interpersonal, job) and the feelings and thoughts that come spontaneously and then allow the mind (the deep unconscious) to tell him or her what it would take to correct, heal, or overcome the problem—and thus to reach the goal. It may take a number of sessions to get to this point. At times you may suggest a way for the person to image relief from a symptom.

Before the initial session is ended, emphasize that this technique is totally under the control of the person and therefore can be used in the home or office at will. Encourage regular daily use of imaging, following the same routine each time. The imaging can be combined with prayer, devotional reading, or meditation. This method frees the person to make choices, to accomplish goals, to have a sense of mastery. The person is not under the control of the therapist. One time of full explanation and going through the method with the client may be enough to have the person successfully continue this on his or her own, or it may take several times. Thus the method may be useful if you have only one contact with the person; or this method may be repeated in following sessions with the person, especially if there is a deep-seated or long-term problem.

In guided imagery use of the *inner advisor* after relaxation and a comfortable mental peace have been achieved can be helpful. It is a way of gaining access to the feelings, anxiety, guilt, and intuitions in the right hemisphere of the brain or the unconscious. The inner advisor is an imaginary creature drawn from the person's subconscious mind that can be questioned about physical and emotional feelings and through which dialogue can be continued that can resolve conflicts and aid decision making. The inner advisor may be expressed as the Holy Spirit or a religious figure; it may be a parent or spouse (living or dead), or it may be a friend, relative, or work colleague. Some people have a pet or favorite animal such as a squirrel, dog, cat, or pony (50).

Guided imagery can be used alone or with other therapies, whether these therapies involve use of medication, surgery, biofeedback, or individual counseling. Tapes, records, cassettes, disks, posters, and board games that can be used to create a background or an environment for relaxation, meditation, imagery, or just a peaceful mood can be obtained from Music Design, 207 E. Buffalo Street, Milwaukee, WI 53202. The catalogue is available on request and features many artists and a variety of selections in type of music and instrumentation. Other such catalogues are also available.

Clinical Application of Imagery. If the person believes and participates regularly in the process of guided imagery, there would be a point at which there may be no need for other relaxation therapies.

Guided imagery can be used to promote emotional health by (1) building self-awareness; (2) helping the person to face issues and facilitating mood change; (3) clarifying the meaning of the situation; (4) assisting in dyadic communications and expression of feelings; (5) promoting a sense of strength and self-control, including overcoming phobias; (6) overcoming negative attitudes about self; and (7) increasing coping resources by releasing unconscious energies (85, 98).

Research increasingly shows that the body responds to our mental picture of it. The body may develop a full-blown infection, remain ill or less functional, or return to a healthy or normally functioning state, de-

pending on the mental image we hold and what we continue to say about the body to self or others. Imagery can be used to enhance healing either by using a general image or by picturing what the impaired or diseased area would look like if it were normal. Table 17–2 describes universal and specific images that can be used for various conditions after the person becomes relaxed. These are only suggestions. Each person can produce the image that is uniquely applicable and possible to achieve. Both universal and specific images can be held by the person in relation to a body part. Guided imagery can be used to promote physical health by:

1. Reducing the intensity of the stress response.
2. Assisting in control of various body symptoms.
3. Reducing and controlling pain symptoms.
4. Promoting weight loss in the obese person.
5. Helping the person to control or stop habits of smoking, alcohol or drug abuse.
6. Promoting healing after surgery or from cancer or various chronic conditions.
7. Increasing mobility and reducing tension, such as in arthritic conditions (85, 98, 119, 121, 123, 124, 127).

Guided imagery can be used to help the person gain cognitive control—to make choices, to make decisions, to change life pattern and behavior, to respond to a situation by imaging and portraying a role, to reduce anxiety and fear, and to reduce depression. Box 17–5 lists how imagery can be used to cope with or find solutions to a problem. Allow sufficient time, free of distractions, to carry out the process (85, 98, 121, 123, 124).

When you have experienced guided imagery and used it with yourself and others under supervision of someone who knows how to use the technique and when you believe in the results, you will see results.

You may wish to ask the client to verbalize the process by which healing was enhanced or may allow the person to complete the process without verbalizing unless he or she wishes to do so. The verbalization does not aid in the process for the client but can give clues about his or her ability to visualize and further issues with which you can be of assistance.

A major asset of imagery as a nursing intervention is that the person or group member need not expose situations that may be anxiety provoking or embarrassing or discuss the problem. Additionally, imagery interventions allow you to work with clients who are unable or unwilling to establish an open, working relationship. Imagery works best in nursing situations when the nurse gives the broadest directions, allowing the person to develop his or her own images.

Plus Factor. Norman Vincent Peale (99), the first person to advocate the concept of positive thinking (which became the basis for the concept and practice of imagery), has formulated the concept of the "plus factor." According to Peale, the **plus factor** is a *power within*

TABLE 17-2. USE IMAGERY TO PROMOTE HEALTH AND HEALING

Symptom/Disorder	Universal Image	Specific Image
Sore throat	Image of cool air or moisture flowing over throat	Image of normally pink throat color; that normal color overtaking red, inflamed area
Fever	Image of coolness	Image of cool breeze, waterfall, fountain around self, with overall environment a comfortable temperature; image of self standing erect and feeling strong, invigorated, comfortable
Upper chest congestion; asthmatic attack	Image of cool throat and warm chest	Image of cool, normally pink throat and respiratory tree; lung sacs and bronchi expanding; air flow (seen as arrows, bubbles, streams of clouds) moving in and out (Hold image while breathing in relaxed manner.)
Chronic sinus problem	Image of tubes opening and draining	Image of sinus compartment as a sink, that you pulled the plug, and that draining is occurring: if persistent congestion, picture of self like a plunger at top of sinus compartment, pushing down the drainage through open drain pipe
Headache	Image of hole in head in area of headache; on exhalation, pain goes through hole as a color	Image of pain shooting out of head like a volcano with each exhalation and of a color that denotes calmness setting in and taking over the brain and head area
Itch or pain	Image of coolness to area	Image of ice cube on the area; as ice melts, itch or pain melts away; depending on location, may picture pain or itch as sliding off the body area
Low back pain	Image of heavy spine	Image of pain dropping down to the floor and walking away from it; image of self as erect, strong, active as pain is dropping away
Tight, tense muscle area	Image of muscles in area getting wider and longer, unknotting	Image that with deep, slow inhalation, breath is directed to the muscle area, that breath soaks up the tension, and tension is removed with exhalation; picture of muscle stretching and smoothing out; picture of self in a calm, relaxing environment such as being surrounded by flower beds, the ocean, a lake, and meadow and that the body is stretched out, a relaxed, happy mood
Fatigue	Image of energy flow entering the body area	Image of self as light in weight; image of self surrounded by warmth, color, and music that represents happiness, energy, joy; picture of self as full of joy and dancing or skipping lightly in a meadow, lane, by the seashore
Stiff, painful joint; arthritis	Image of warmth	Image of self in warm sunlight at a relaxing place (seashore, field of grass or flowers) and moving freely; image of rising sun with warm rays aimed at joint or total body; picture of joint as normal in size; picture of self as light, moving at desired pace
Diarrhea, colitis	Image of coolness, control	Image of intestine as a tube that is set, firm, not moving and smooth, without bumps, rough areas, irritation; picture of self at activities and being in control; image of intestine as a pipe with plug firmly in place at lower end
Infection, cancer	Image of white cells carrying off abnormal cells	Image of white cells surrounding infectious area or cancer growth, eating up the abnormal area; image of area of infection or growth becoming smaller and smaller; image of antibiotic, chemotherapy, or radiation as an arrow piercing infectious or cancer area and causing abnormal cells to fall apart and be excreted by body; image of medication like Pacman, gobbling up the abnormal cells
Anger, resentment	Image of peace or harmony	Image of feeling as a ball of color; place it in front of you, kick it away; picture of self in control and solving the problem that is creating anger; picture of self in an area that was the happiest or most pleasant or most relaxing place you were ever in (vacation area, favorite childhood spot, most comfortable chair in your home, lovely garden area); soak up the calm and beauty and feel anger drain away; image of calming music—see yourself relaxed, light, dancing

the person that can transform and create a stronger, more confident, better balanced, more energetic and resilient, and more capable individual. It is a special manifestation of the life force that animates everything in the universe. Attitudes and actions that are important to activate the plus factor and develop its power are faith, positive thinking, persistence, confidence, positive imaging, prayer, affirmation, belief, love, and work. Box 17–6 lists several principles of the plus factor (99).

Larson (83) echoes these ideas as he talks about conquering fears and anxieties and the inevitable insecurities that humans encounter and in turn find meaning in life and values by which to live. Siegel (122) also affirms them as he writes of the power of love and faith and their importance in healing.

Time Management

Symptoms of inappropriate time management include chronic rushing, fatigue, listlessness with many slack hours of nonproductive activity, vacillation between unpleasant alternatives, missing of deadlines, insufficient time for rest or personal relationships, and the sense of being overwhelmed by demands and details (30).

——— CASE SITUATION: COMBATING THE STRESSES OF DISABILITY ———
—BECOMING A SURVIVOR

Until her car was wrecked in a snowstorm, Marlene was a healthy, divorced 37-year-old woman who led an active and rewarding life. Almost immediately after the accident she noticed difficulty using her hands but discounted this as "nerves." The car was hit on the driver's side at 50 mph, and although Marlene experienced severe pain in the neck and upper back area, she conscientiously returned to work as a medical secretary within a few days after the accident.

The back pain and weakness in Marlene's arms and hands continued to worsen, but nothing specific showed on the x-rays films. She consulted with an orthopedist, neurologist, rheumatologist, physical therapist, and internist; none was able to make a specific diagnosis related to the increasing pain and weakness.

After a year of misdiagnosis Marlene was becoming unable to live independently. She could not use her arms for preparing food, shopping, or doing laundry and was barely able to dress herself or comb her hair. At the age of 38, Marlene was afraid that she would have to move into a nursing home. Finally, after a year of frustration and despair she requested referral to a Pain Management Program (PMP). She had decided that if the physicians could not cure the problem, she would have to learn to live with it. That was when life began to turn around for her.

At PMP Marlene's pain and dysfunction were identified as probable results of the whiplash injury, which caused thoracic outlet syndrome, soft tissue injury in the cervical area, and chronic myofascial pain. The PMP team's opinion was that surgery was not a viable option.

Marlene was taught stress-reduction strategies such as relaxation techniques, biofeedback, and guided imagery. But most important, she learned to listen to her body and set appropriate limits on what she could make it do. Since the pain was not always constant and did not immediately follow action but sometimes occurred as much as 2 hours later, it became necessary to set limits and not do things that would increase pain.

Pacing and/or setting appropriate limits to accommodate the lack of physical strength was and remains the hardest thing Marlene had to learn. It was like living on a very strict budget of physical energy. If she expended too much energy in the morning, nothing was left for the rest of the day. It meant taking breaks, conserving energy, avoiding long shopping trips, resting up for big days, taking into consideration barometric changes, and practicing pain-management techniques. She had to do a tremendous amount of planning, negotiating, and compromising.

One of the greatest causes of stress, especially for persons with chronic pain and/or various physical limitations, is created from feeling like a victim of life. Marlene felt powerless over much of her life—as if she were controlled by everyone and everything around her. When she learned how to control some of the physical problems, she felt she had more control of life and felt less like a victim. She made it a point to join organizations that could provide information and find people who could share areas of her disabilities. She found this was extremely rewarding. She learned she could not afford to waste energy on emotional problems from the past. Resolving them was necessary so that all available energy could be used with current physical problems. Becoming mentally healthy made a big difference in the quality of her life, although the past problems were not the cause of the disabilities.

Continued typing work as a secretary would eventually have caused Marlene to lose the use of her arms and hands, so she gave up her job of 8 years and started over at age 39. Fortunately, Marlene had been doing self-help counseling on a volunteer basis before the auto accident. She could not tolerate doing nothing and decided to enroll in school for a graduate degree in counseling. (One of the most important methods of controlling pain is keeping the mind occupied.) Her physical abilities were limited, but her brain and mouth still functioned with no impairment. To stay within her physical limitations, she was able to take only 6 graduate hours per semester. It took 4 years to complete a 2-year graduate curriculum in counseling services.

Marlene has had to discover and develop new and different ways of living, to change totally her previous methods of dealing with life, to accept her limitations, and to move beyond those limits. She had to learn not be a victim of chronic illness and the value of sharing and caring for others. She has developed the following program for recovery and survival:

1. Let reality sink in slowly. Acceptance of disability is necessary before one can find happiness.
2. Expect a time of anger and denial.
3. Learn to use anger constructively rather than destructively. Fight for personal rights.
4. Let yourself experience the grief; do not be afraid to cry. It hurts in many, many ways. Tears are healing.
5. Become determined to accept the past and make the best of the present. Live 1 day at a time.
6. Be good to yourself and do not forget to pace activities. Try to look forward to a new future and new interests.
7. Learn to be flexible and trust in yourself. Do not let the world pass by; get more active in a personally satisfying way.

— **CASE SITUATION:** (Continued) ——————————————

8. Start taking charge of small areas of life. Feeling in control is extremely important.

9. Find a support group and use it. Do not stand on the outside looking in. Participate.

10. Develop regular phone contacts, which will help you as others are helped.

11. Create meaning in life, develop new interests, and stay mentally active. Find goals that are consistent with limitations.

12. Look outward instead of inward. It is impossible to feel hateful and grateful at the same time.

Author: Marlene Cannady, M.A.

Most methods of time management include these steps:

1. Keep a detailed log of each activity and time spent on each for 5 days.

2. Establish priorities about what to accomplish.

3. Eliminate low-priority tasks.

4. Write specific goals for 1 month and 1 year.

5. Learn to make and follow through with decisions.

Effective time management is effective in minimizing anxiety and job fatigue. To avoid being overwhelmed by goals, priorities, and decisions, work on one at a time (20, 30).

Other rules also help for making time (20, 30):

1. Learn to say "no"; remind yourself that this is your life and your time to spend as best befits you. Only when your boss asks should you spend time on bottom-priority items.

2. Build time into your schedule for unscheduled events, interruptions, and unforeseen occurrences.

3. Set aside several time periods during the day for structured relaxation; being relaxed allows you to use the time you have more efficiently.

4. Keep a list of tasks that can be done in a few minutes any time you are waiting or are between other tasks.

5. Learn to do two things at once; plan dinner while driving home or organize an important letter or list while waiting in line at the bank.

6. Delegate low-priority tasks to others, if possible.

7. Get up 15 to 30 minutes earlier every day than in the past to have a time for meditation or a hobby.

8. Allow no more than 1 hour of television watching for yourself daily. Use it as a reward for your accomplishing high-priority items.

■ **BOX 17-5.**
Using Imagery to Solve Problems

• Find a quiet place and sit in a relaxed position; close the eyes.
• Clearly and succinctly define the problem; picture telling the problem to a friend.
• Mentally ask, "Am I ready to solve this problem?" If yes is the inner answer, proceed.
• Place the clearly defined problem in a frame or a box.
• Visualize the situation you desire and place it in a frame or box.
• Visualize the steps that will be necessary to achieve the solution. Differentiate each step; continue to think until each step is clearly pictured.
• Any barriers that come to mind in relation to any step of the solution can be looked at and then moved from the pathway to be cast off into space or to be placed in a locked box. Do this for each barrier that presents itself. Take a deep breath to relax as you do this so that you feel fully in control of handling barriers.
• Mentally review each step that moves to a solution and picture yourself with the final desired solution. Hold the image.
• Slowly open the eyes.
• In the days or weeks that follow, repeat this process as necessary with your moving toward the goal or solution. See yourself with the solution or goal at hand in the frame or box. If certain intermediary steps have already been finished, omit them from the mental picture.

NOTE: Imagery can also be used quickly for an immediate situation with which you must cope or which must be mastered. The preceding method would be done in one sitting.

■ **BOX 17-6.**
Positive Thinking/Plus Factor Principles to Turn Setbacks into Comebacks

• Expect and image good health. See yourself as vigorous and energetic.
• Develop spirit and soul health.
• Don't let a sense of guilt or anger fester in you.
• Stand up to your fear. Faith is bigger and stronger than fear.
• Think positively, especially when you feel the lowest. In the setback may be the answer to your comeback.
• Remind yourself that you are bigger than anything that can happen to you.
• Keep elasticity in your attitude. Change occurs, and you need to change also. Don't abandon basic principles, but listen to different points of view.
• Live one day at a time. See each day as precious. See opportunity.

Part of time management is the ability to make decisions. Procrastination is the great time robber. Procrastination can often be overcome by:

1. Recognizing the unpleasantness of doing a task versus the unpleasantness of putting it off; analyzing the cost and risks of delay.
2. Examining the payoffs you receive by procrastinating (e.g., you will not have to do the task; you will not have to face the possibility of failure; you can be taken care of by others; you can gain attention; examining payoffs for finishing the task; building a special reward for completing an unpleasant task.
3. Exaggerating whatever you are doing to put off the decision; keeping it up until you are bored and making the decision seems more attractive than procrastination.
4. Taking responsibility for your delaying tactics by writing down how long each delay took; writing down how long it took to actually complete the task; comparing.
5. When making unimportant decisions, using a formula to choose—south or east over north or west, left over right or smooth over rough, easiest, shortest, or closest, the one that comes first alphabetically; then deciding a formula for making major decisions.
6. Taking small steps toward a major decision; listing each step; crossing it off the list as it is accomplished.
7. Avoiding beginning a new task until you have completed a predecided segment of the current one; allowing yourself to experience fully the reward of finishing something (20, 30).

In summary, based on your assessments and related nursing diagnoses such as those listed in Box 17–7, you can practice some of the following ways to adapt to stress and teach these methods to others:

1. Identify stressful aspects of your life-style to reduce frequency of the stress response or to avoid stressors when possible.
2. Analyze what is making you tense or anxious and try to lessen the stressfulness of the situation.
3. Develop spiritual and philosophic resources by talking to others who are wiser than you and by using literature and prayer.
4. Keep something as the central core of your life and being, as your shelter or haven (e.g., a religious, philosophic, moral, or ethical belief; a special place in your home to relax; a specific time for doing certain pleasurable activities; or a person who is a confidant and friend).
5. Try to slow your hectic pace. Do one thing at a time.
6. Use temporary avoidance of identified stressors at times for regaining strength, energy, and ideas about fun in order to cope.

 BOX 17-7.
Selected Nursing Diagnoses Related to Stress Management[a]

Pattern 1: Exchanging

Altered Nutrition: Less than body requirements
Altered Nutrition: Potential for more than body requirements

Pattern 2: Communicating

Impaired Verbal Communication

Pattern 3: Relating

Impaired Social Interaction
Social Isolation
Potential Altered Parenting
Altered Family Processes
Altered Sexuality Patterns

Pattern 4: Valuing

Spiritual Distress

Pattern 5: Choosing

Ineffective Individual Coping
Impaired Adjustment
Defensive Coping
Ineffective Denial
Family Coping: Potential for growth
Decisional Conflict
Health Seeking Behaviors

Pattern 6: Moving

Activity Intolerance
Fatigue
Potential Activity Disturbance
Sleep Pattern Disturbance
Diversional Activity Deficit
Impaired Home Maintenance Management
Altered Health Maintenance

Pattern 7: Perceiving

Body Image Disturbance
Self-esteem Disturbance
Sensory/Perceptual Alterations
Hopelessness
Powerlessness

Pattern 8: Knowing

Knowledge Deficit
Altered Thought Processes
Pain
Chronic Pain
Dysfunctional Grieving
Post-trauma Response
Anxiety
Fear

[a]Other NANDA diagnoses may be applicable to the individual.
From North American Nursing Diagnosis Association, *NANDA Nursing Diagnosis Taxonomy I* (Rev.). St. Louis: North American Nursing Diagnosis Association, 1990.

7. Assume a more passive attitude toward irritating or frustrating events. Consciously work to remain calm or avoid the problem until you are in a better emotional condition to cope with it.

8. Determine ways to enjoy selected stressors as a challenge by adjusting personal philosophy or behavior patterns.

9. Accept love and support and encouragement and suggestions from others; be willing to receive help.

10. Set aside time for relaxation each day. You may want to try relaxation techniques such as transcendental meditation, yoga, biofeedback, or the relaxation response or seek sources of joy and humor.

11. Talk about your feelings with friends, family, or a counselor to gain objectivity about the problem, validate ideas and possible solutions, and affirm what you need and want to do.

12. Accept things you cannot change. Do not expect too much from others. Accept your own normal irritation, anger, or crying.

13. Try to correct aspects of your life that cause stress or worry or change a role that does not suit you.

14. Do not push yourself beyond your limits of achievement or expect too much of yourself. Be satisfied with less while you do your best.

15. Use physical exercise and recreation to work off the energy of anxiety and to relieve tension. Find a fulfilling hobby or try doing something helpful for someone. Books and audiotapes are available describing relaxation techniques and recreational activities or hobbies.

16. Use visualization, imagery, or faith to affirm the answer to the problem until the solution is reached.

17. Use conscious cognitive coping responses such as those described in this chapter.

18. Seek psychotherapy if stress keeps you from functioning at your full capacity.

19. Carry out health promotion measures described in each chapter.

20. Realize that stressors are inevitable and can be handled and that some are necessary for survival, learning, development, and self-actualization.

Lafferty (79) lists a number of suggestions that contribute to physical, intellectual, spiritual, emotional, and social health and to a healthy life-style:

1. Intellectual health is stimulated by (a) decreasing the amount of time spent in watching television except for educational or scientific programs, (b) developing a daily routine for study, reading, or adding a vocabulary word, and (c) attending special lectures and programs when available.

2. Spiritual health is promoted through (a) daily meditation, prayer, and devotional reading, (b) discussing spiritual or religious topics with another person, (c) identifying the weakest personal characteristic to work on overcoming it, and (d) reaffirming personal values and strong personal characteristics as a guide to life and behavior.

3. Emotional health is enhanced by (a) recognizing and constructively expressing positive and unhappy or angry feelings, (b) identifying personal strengths and limits and working to overcome limits, (c) dealing appropriately with feelings toward the opposite sex, and (d) seeking professional help with serious adjustment problems or crises.

4. Social health is promoted by (a) showing affection rather than directing criticism to friends and family, (b) working to overcome prejudices or fears of people of another race, the opposite sex, or persons in authority, (c) fulfilling responsibilities to others, and (d) communicating verbally and nonverbally in a way that is honest and clear.

SITES FOR HEALTH PROMOTION NURSING AND WELLNESS PROGRAMS

Traditionally the main health concerns for employees in the workplace were safety and accident prevention. A yearly physical examination was also included in many industries.

Today industries and some hospitals and other work settings are adding programs for their employees that generally include emphasis in four areas: stress reduction, exercise, smoking cessation, and nutritional and weight guidance, particularly for obesity and sodium and cholesterol reduction. Some industries have also established employee assistance programs to help the chemically dependent employee reduce alcohol or drug intake and remain a safe, dependable worker. Some settings offer day care for workers with young children—to reduce the worker's stress related to child care. Others have stress management programs for their employees and their clients. Facilities may boast nearly 24-hour availability of a fully equipped exercise room, gymnasium, handball court, and whirlpool baths or, for example, a rough running track that has been measured out around a furniture factory in rural North Carolina. In some cities the employer uses existing exercise facilities in various clubs or organizations such as the local chapter of the American Heart Association for screening or teaching programs.

A variety of services can be implemented in housing projects, in nutrition sites, or in other sites by a Visiting Nurses Association to keep the well-elderly healthy. These services could include a biweekly coffee hour to bring free counseling, nutrition and health education, health assessment, referrals, home visits after hospital discharge, and assistance with drug and diet prescriptions. Flexible times for services and easy accessibility would encourage the seniors to come to the nurse-operated health maintenance clinics. That entry into the health care system is often the way to encourage the senior to obtain necessary medical care and to continue health promotion practices.

Various authors propose the following ways to promote and maintain high-level wellness in a community (20, 22, 101):

1. Improvement of family living and community life conditions
2. Education to assist the person or family in applying healthful behavior
3. Education to assist the person or family to apply principles of human relations
4. Development of high-level wellness among individuals in leadership positions so that they can carry out their roles responsibly and effectively
5. Maintenance of open information channels and free access to information for intelligent decision making in the community and family
6. Enhancement of opportunities for creative expression
7. Promotion of caring relationships and concern for others' welfare
8. Education about concepts of maturity and its achievement
9. Extension of the life span, with the mature person sharing potentials for the benefit of society

Health protection or preventive measures in the environment can be used by governmental and other agencies, industries, and communities to protect people from harm of disease, including implementation of:

1. Toxic agent control.
2. Occupational safety and health measures.
3. Accident prevention and injury control.
4. Water fluoridation and dental health.
5. Surveillance and control of infectious disease.
6. Mass screening programs (101).

The seventy-fifth session of the World Health Organization (WHO) executive board, meeting in Geneva in 1985, emphasized the important role the nursing profession can and must play in the "Health for All" movement. The organization recommended reorientation and training of nurse educators, managers, and nursing leaders in primary health care. Using nursing in the "Health for All" strategy requires a commitment to change on the part of the nursing profession; nurse leaders could serve as activists, stimulating change and pushing for action. The changing role of nurses in the "Health for All strategy demands a sound grasp of nursing and the ability to relate with other health personnel and the community in need of health care. The director-general of WHO, Dr. Halfdan T. Mahler, said it was evident that the nursing profession was infinitely more ready for change than other professional groups. He pointed out that to practice primary health care one needed love for one's fellow travellers, and he considered that nurses had great potential for that kind of love. He stated that it was time

that nurses were brought in much more than hitherto as leaders and managers of the primary health care "Health for All" team (136).

NEW HORIZONS IN HEALTH PROMOTION: THE NURSE ENTREPRENEUR

The nurse entrepreneur spirit is changing the future of health care. Entrepreneurial opportunities are available for those with foresight and a desire to apply nursing skills in a different fashion. Nurse entrepreneurs are now writing about their role development (60).

One definition of a **nurse entrepreneur** is someone who has a big enough ego to think that he or she could do anything and a small enough ego to do anything to accomplish that goal, including being financially dependent on parents, spouse, or others.

The health care field does not encourage entrepreneurial behavior, but there are numerous agencies available to assist those with innovative ideas. The Small Business Administration has a packet of information available by mail that will help one get started. Some community colleges offer courses ranging from 1 day to several weeks. These courses cover various aspects of starting a business. Internal Revenue Service offers a no-charge 1-day workshop quarterly that assists with various government reports such as state and federal taxes and employment security requirements.

To become an entrepreneur, one must be motivated by achievement rather than power or affiliation. Some characteristics of an entrepreneur are persistence, optimism, resourcefulness, self-confidence, and not being afraid to follow personal convictions.

Several special qualities are essential: positive self-expectancy, self-direction, self-image, self-awareness, self-projection, self-perception, self-control, self-esteem, and self-discipline. An entrepreneur is not one who depends on other sources for any of the above.

Nurses have skills that are applicable to business. Problem-solving skills are taught and nurtured in nursing. Nurses have learned to delegate responsibilities and make excellent use of their time. They know how to motivate, teach, and gain confidence.

To do well in business, one must become a part of the business community. Join the local Chamber of Commerce and business organizations. Take personal responsibility when things do not work well. Let people know you care. Test your ideas and develop marketing skills. Be alert for business opportunities and learn how to "operate on a shoestring." Learn how to compute cash flow and conduct budget analysis. It is essential to learn how to charge enough, but not too much, for your services or product. You must be convinced that you are the best in your field. Be alert for opportunities. Timing is essential. An entrepreneur is not necessarily a risk taker since he or she is always analyzing the situation and minimizing risks.

Among the factors causing a need for nurse entrepreneurs is the change in the public attitudes and values and growing emphasis on prevention. The present trend of reducing hospital use and curtailing Medicare and Medicaid is presenting a need for more cost-effective health care providers. Nurses have been geared to total health care, the best possible care, and high quality care regardless of cost. We must now learn how to encompass these ideas with increased productivity and more efficiency and define nursing care as a product.

Nurse entrepreneurs are doing well in several areas. One nurse practitioner in North Carolina has a business providing health care for industries. She employs another nurse practitioner, several parttime registered nurses, a part-time physician, and a parttime health educator. The firm provides whatever is needed in health care, from screenings to primary health care and care of chronic problems, with a great emphasis on wellness and preventive programs. Another nurse has a business in southern California providing acute hemodialysis service. Yet another nurse started a business in Florida providing a day-care center for children with medical problems.

These are only a few examples. Each state differs in the legal authority, reimbursement practices, and the prescription authority given to nurses in advanced practice. These factors greatly influence how much of an entrepreneur a nurse can be. A 1991 survey found that 40 states have some degree of legislative prescription authority for nurse practitioners. In 25 states nurse practitioners can receive third-party reimbursement (100).

Because of change and uncertainty, a whole new set of career opportunities is available. The future belongs to those who are able to respond to new demands and who have the courage to follow their convictions.

REFERENCES

1. Alexy, B., Goal Setting and Health Risk Reduction, *Nursing Research,* 34, no. 5 (1985), 283–288.
2. Alster, K., *The Holistic Health Movement.* Tuscaloosa, Ala: University of Alabama Press, 1989.
3. Altman, D., et al., Sustained Effects of an Educational Program to Reduce Sales of Cigarettes to Minors, *American Journal of Public Health,* 81, no. 7 (1991), 891–893.
4. Arnold, E., and K. Boggs, *Interpersonal Relationships: Professional Communication Skills for Nurses.* Philadelphia: W.B. Saunders, 1989.
5. Aroian, K., A Model of Psychological Adaption to Migration and Resettlement, *Nursing Research,* 39, no. 1 (1990), 5–10.
6. Bates, B., *A Guide to Physical Examination and History Taking* (4th ed.). Philadelphia: J.B. Lippincott, 1987.
7. Becker, M., ed., *The Health Belief Model and Personal Health Behavior.* Thorofare, NJ: Charles B. Slack, 1974.
8. ———, et al., Selected Psychosocial Models and Correlates of Individual Health-Related Behaviors, *Medical Care,* 15 (1977), 27-46.
9. Benson, H., *Beyond the Relaxation Response.* New York: Times Books, 1988.
10. ———, and W. Proctor, Your Maximum Mind. New York: Avon, 1989.
11. Berkowitz, M., R. Waxman, and L. Yaffe, The Effects of a Resident Self-Help Model in Control, Social Involvement, and Self-Esteem Among the Elderly, *Gerontologist,* 28, no. 5 (1988), 620–624.
12. Bigbee, J., and N. Jansa, Strategies for Promoting Health Protection, *Nursing Clinics of North America,* 26, no. 4 (1991), 895–913.
13. Bloch, G., and D. Groves, Stretching: The Truth, *Health* (June, 1990), 34–37.
14. Box, D., Putting on the Pressure, *Nursing Mirror,* 60, no. 21 (May 22, 1985), 28–29.
15. Brenner, A., *Helping Children Cope With Stress.* Lexington, Mass: D.C. Heath, 1985.
16. Burns, D., *The Feeling Good Handbook: Using the New Mood Therapy in Everyday Life.* New York: William Morrow, 1989.
17. Buxman, K., Make Way for Laughter, *American Journal of Nursing,* 91, no. 12 (1991), 46–51.
18. Byrd, R., Positive Therapeutic Effects of Intercessory Prayer in a Coronary Care Unit Population, *Southern Medical Journal,* 81, no. 7 (1988), 126–129.
19. Champion, V., Instrument Development for Health Belief Model Constructs, *Advances in Nursing Science,* 6, no. 3 (1984), 73–85.
20. Clark, C., *Wellness Nursing: Concepts, Theory, Research, and Practice.* New York: Springer, 1986.
21. Clark, J., S. Haverty, and S. Kendall, Helping People to Stop Smoking: A Study of the Nurse's Role, *Journal of Advanced Nursing,* 15, no. 3 (1990), 357–363.
22. Clemen-Stone, S., D. Eigsti, and S. McGuire, *Comprehensive Family and Community Health Nursing* (3rd ed.). St. Louis: C.V. Mosby, 1991.
23. Colt, C., S. Wardlow, and A. Frantz, The Effect of Running on Plasma Endorphins, *Life Science,* 28 (1981), 1637–1640.
24. Conn, V., Self-Care Actions Taken by Older Adults for Influenza and Cold, *Nursing Research,* 40, no. 3 (1991), 176–181.
25. Cooper, K., *The Aerobic Program for Well-Being.* New York: Bantam Books, 1982.
26. Cousins, N., *The Anatomy of an Illness as Perceived by the Patient's Reflections on Healing and Regeneration.* New York: Bantam, 1983.
27. Cox, C., The Health Self-Determinism Index, *Nursing Research,* 34, no. 3 (1985), 177–183.
28. Cross, P., *Adults as Learners.* San Francisco, Calif: Jossey-Bass, 1981.
29. Damroch, S., General Strategies for Motivating People to Change Their Behavior, *Nursing Clinics of North America,* 26, no. 4 (1991), 833–843.
30. Davis, M., M. McKay, and E. Eshelman, *The Relaxation and Stress Reduction Workbook* (2nd ed.). Oakland, Calif: New Harbinger, 1982.
31. Dawson, D., G. Henderson, and B. Bloom, Trends in Routine Screening Examinations, *American Journal of Public Health,* 77, no. 8 (1987), 1004–1005.

32. Department of Health and Social Security, *Prevention and Health: Everybody's Business*. Kent, England: Health Departments of Great Britain and Northern Ireland, 1976.

33. Dixon, E., and R. Park, Do Patients Understand Written Health Information? *Nursing Outlook,* 8, no. 6 (1990), 278–281.

34. Dossey, B., Awakening the Inner Healer, *American Journal of Nursing,* 91, no. 8 (1991), 31–32, 34.

35. Duffy, M., Determinants of Health Promotion in Midlife Women, *Nursing Research,* 37, no. 6 (1988), 358–362.

36. Dugan, D., Laughter and Tears: Best Medicine for Stress, *Nursing Forum,* 24, no. 1 (1989), 18–26.

37. Durbach, E., et al., Instructional Objectives in Patient Education, *Nursing Outlook,* 35, no. 2 (1987), 82–83, 88.

38. Edelman, C., and C. Mandle, *Health Promotion Throughout the Lifespan* (2nd ed.). St. Louis: C.V. Mosby, 1990.

39. Edmunds, M., Strategies for Promoting Physical Fitness, *Nursing Clinics of North America,* 26, no. 4 (1991), 855–866.

40. Eells, M., Strategies for the Promotion of Harmful Substance Avoidance, Nursing Clinics of North America, 26, no. 4 (1991), 915–927.

41. Ellis, A., *A New Guide to Rational Living.* Englewood Cliff, NJ: Prentice-Hall, 1978.

42. ——, *The Practice of Rational Emotive Therapy (RET).* New York: Springer, 1987.

43. Epstein, G., *Healing Visualization.* New York: Bantam, 1989.

44. Everly, G., and D. Girdano, *The Stress-Mess Solution.* Bowie, Md: Robert J. Brady, 1981.

45. Ewles, L., and I. Simnett, *Promoting Health: A Practical Guide to Health Education.* Sussex, England: John Wiley, 1985.

46. Feldenkrais, M., *Awareness Through Movement.* New York: Harper & Row, 1977.

47. Flay, B., et al., One Year Follow-Up of the Chicago Televised Smoking Cessation Programs, *American Journal of Public Health,* 79, no. 10 (1989), 1377–1380.

48. Grainger, R., Anxiety Interrupters, *American Journal of Nursing,* 90, no. 2 (1990), 14–15.

49. Grether, J., et al., Exposure to Aerial Malathion Application and the Occurrence of Congenital Anomalies and Low Birthweight, *American Journal of Public Health,* 77, no. 8 (1987), 1009–1010.

50. Griffin, M., In the Mind's Eye, *American Journal of Nursing,* 86, no. 7 (1986), 804–806.

51. Grossman, J., The Quest for Quiet, *Health* (February 1990), 57–61, 84.

52. Guyton, A., *Textbook of Medical Physiology* (8th ed.). Philadelphia: W.B. Saunders, 1991.

53. Hall, B., and J. Allan, Sharpening Nursing Focus by Focusing on Health, *Nursing and Health Care,* 7, no. 6 (1986), 315–320.

54. Harris, D., and S. Guten, Health Protective Behavior: An Exploratory Study, *Journal of Health and Social Behavior,* 20 (1979), 17–29.

55. Heidt, P., Effect of Therapeutic Touch on Anxiety Level of Hospitalized Patients, *Nursing Research,* 30, no. 1 (1981), 32–37.

56. ——, Openness: A Qualitative Analysis of Nurses' and Patients' Experiences of Therapeutic Touch, *Image,* 22, no. 3 (1990), 190–196.

57. Herron, D., Strategies for Promoting a Healthy Dietary Intake, *Nursing Clinics of North America,* 26, no. 4 (1991), 875–884.

58. Hogan, R., *Human Sexuality: A Nursing Perspective* (2nd ed.). Norwalk, Conn: Appleton-Century-Crofts, 1985.

59. Holmes, J., and R. Rahe, The Social Readjustment Rating Scale, *Journal of Psychosomatic Research,* 11 (1967), 213.

60. *How I Became a Nurse Entrepreneur: Tales From 50 Nurses in Business.* Petaluma, Calif: National Nurses in Business Association, 1989.

61. Humble, C., J. Samet, and D. Pathak, Marriage to a Smoker and Lung Cancer Risk, *American Journal of Public Health,* 77, no. 5 (1987), 598–602.

62. Hutchins, D., and C. Cole, *Helping Relationships and Strategies* (2nd ed.). Belmont, Calif: Brooks/Cole, 1992.

63. Hutchinson, S., Self-Care and Job Stress, *Image,* 19, no. 4 (1987), 192–196.

64. Jarrett, P., Some Mental Aspects of Physical Fitness, *Journal of Florida Medical Association,* 67, no. 4 (1980), 378–389.

65. Job, R., Effective and Ineffective Use of Fear in Health Promotion Campaigns, *American Journal of Public Health,* 78, no. 2 (1988), 163–167.

66. Jones, D., What's Missing in Aerobic Dance? *Wellness News,* 6, no. 3 (1985), 2.

67. Jordan, M.M., Development of a Tool for Diagnosing Changes in Concern About Exercise: A Means of Enhancing Compliance, *Nursing Research,* 34, no. 2 (1985), 103–107.

68. Kabut-Zinn, J., *Full Catastrophe Living: Using the Wisdom of Your Body and Mind to Face Stress, Pain, and Illness.* New York: Delacorte Press, 1990.

69. Kaiserman, M., and B. Rogers, Tobacco Consumption Declining Faster in Canada Than in US, *American Journal of Public Health,* 81, no. 7 (1991), 902–904.

70. Kar, S., M. Schmitz, and D. Dyer, A Psychosocial Model of Health Behavior: Implications for Nutrition Education, Research, and Policy, *Health Values: Achieving High Level Wellness,* 7, no. 2 (1983), 29–37.

71. Keller, E., and V. Bzdek, Effects of Therapeutic Touch on Tension Headache Pain, *Nursing Research,* 35, no. 2 (1986), 101–105.

72. Kilburn, K., and R. Warshaw, Effects of Individually Motivating Smoking Cessation in Male Blue Collar Workers, *American Journal of Public Health,* 80, no. 11 (1990), 1334–1337.

73. Knowles, M., *The Adult Learner: A Neglected Species* (2nd ed.). Houston: Gulf Publishing, 1978.

74. Kobasa, S., *The Hardiness Scale.* Chicago: The Hardiness Institute, 1987.

75. Kopf, R., M. Salaman, and P. Charytan, The Preventive Health History Form: A Questionnaire to Use with Older Patient Populations, *Journal of Gerontological Nursing,* 8, no. 9 (1982), 519–523.

76. Krieger, D., *The Therapeutic Touch.* Englewood Cliffs, NJ: Prentice-Hall, 1979.

77. Kulbok, P., Social Resources, Health Resources, and Preventive Health Behaviors: Patterns and Predictions, *Public Health Nursing,* 2, no. 2 (1985), 67–81.

78. Kurtz, R., and H. Prestera, *The Body Reveals.* New York: Harper & Row, 1984.

79. Lafferty, J., A Credo of Wellness, *Health Education* (September-October 1979), 10–11.

80. Lally, S., The Doctor's Walking Prescription, *Prevention* (March 1990), 67–86.

81. ——, Laugh Your Stress Away, *Prevention* (June 1991), 50–55.

82. Lamontagne, L., K. Mason, and J. Hepworth, Effects of Relaxation on Anxiety in Children: Implications for Coping With Stress, *Nursing Research,* 34, no. 5 (1986), 289–292.

83. Larson, B., Living Beyond Our Fear, *Possibilities* (July-August, 1990), 25–27.

84. MacKinnon, R., and R. Michels, *The Psychiatric Interview in Clinical Practice.* Philadelphia: W.B. Saunders, 1971, pp. 1–64.

85. Mast, D., Effects of Imagery, *Image,* 8, no. 3 (1986), 118–120.

86. Mayhew, M., Strategies for Promoting Safety and Preventing Injury, *Nursing Clinics of North America,* 26, no. 4 (1991), 885–894.

87. Meade, C., J. Byrd, and M. Lee, Improving Patient Comprehension of Literature in Smoking, *American Journal of Public Health,* 79, no. 10 (1989), 1411–1412.

88. Meichenbaum, D., and R. Cameron, Modifying What Clients Say to Themselves. In Mahoney, M., and R. Cameron, eds., *Self-Control Power to the Person.* Monterey, Calif: Brooks-Cole, 1974.

89. Miller, A., Should Christian Nurses Practice Therapeutic Touching? No, *Journal of Christian Nursing,* 4, no. 4 (1987), 15 ff.

90. Miller, J., and M. Powers, Development of an Instrument to Measure Hope, *Nursing Research,* 37, no. 1 (1988), 6–10.

91. Morris, C., and E. Dexter, Taking the Clinic to the Clients: Geriatric Health Care in a Residential Setting, *Gerontologist,* 29, no. 6 (1989), 822–825.

92. Muhlenkamp, A., and J. Sayles, Self-Esteem, Social Support, and Positive Health Practices, *Nursing Research,* 36, no. 6 (1986), 334–338.

93. Murray, R., and M. Huelskoetter, *Psychiatric/Mental Health Nursing: Giving Emotional Care* (3rd ed.). Norwalk, Conn: Appleton-Lange, 1991.

94. National Institute on Drug Abuse, *Life Skills Program.* Kensington, Md: Clearinghouse on Drug Abuse, 1984.

95. Nulls, M., and B. Cohen, *Developmental Movement Therapy,* Amherst, Mass: The School for Body/Mind Centering, 1979.

96. Palmer, M., and E. Deck, Teaching Your Patients to Assert Their Rights, *American Journal of Nursing,* 87, no. 5 (1987), 650–654.

97. Pardue, A., Don't be Frightened by Failure, *Guideposts* (May 1973), 26.

98. Peale, N.V., *Imaging: The Powerful Way to Change Your Life.* Carmel, NY: Guideposts, 1982.

99. ——, *Power of the Plus Factor.* Old Tappan, NJ: Fleming H. Revell, 1987.

100. Pearson, L., 1991–1992 Update: How Each State Stands on Legislative Issues Affecting Advanced Nursing Practice, *Nurse Practitioner,* 17, no. 1 (1992), 14–23.

101. Pender, N., *Health Promotion in Nursing Practice* (2nd ed.). E. Norwalk, Conn: Appleton & Lange, 1987.

102. ——, and A. Pender, Attitudes, Subjective Norms, and Intentions to Engage in Health Behaviors, *Nursing Research,* 35, no. 1 (1986), 15–18.

103. Pentz, M., et al., The Power of Policy: The Relationship of Smoking Policy to Adolescent Smoking, *American Journal of Public Health,* 79, no. 7 (1989), 857–862.

104. Peplau, H., *Interpersonal Relations in Nursing.* New York: G.P. Putnam's Sons, 1952.

105. ——, *Basic Principles of Patient Counseling* (2nd ed.). Philadelphia: Smith, Kline & French Laboratories, 1969.

106. ——, Talking With Patients, *American Journal of Nursing,* 70, no. 7 (1970), 964–966.

107. Pierce, J., P. Macaskill, and D. Hill, Long-Term Effectiveness of Mass Media Led Antismoking Campaigns in Australia, *American Journal of Public Health,* 80, no. 5 (1990) 565–569.

108. Polunk, C., Determinants of Health-Promotive Behavior: A Review of Current Research, *Nursing Clinics of North America,* 26, no. 4 (1991), 815–832.

109. Potter, P., and A. Perry, *Fundamentals of Nursing: Concepts, Process, and Practice* (2nd ed.). St. Louis: C.V. Mosby, 1989.

110. Quinn, J., Therapeutic Touch as Energy Exchange: Testing the Theory, *Advance in Nursing Science,* 42 (1984), 49.

111. Robinson, V., *Humor and the Health Professions* (2nd ed.). Thorofare, NJ: Charles B. Slack, 1991.

112. Rogers, C., *Client-Centered Therapy.* Boston: Houghton Mifflin, 1951.

113. Rosenstock, J., Why People Use Health Services, *Milbank Memorial Fund Quarterly,* 44, (July 1966), 94–127.

114. Rotter, J.B., *Social Learning and Clinical Psychology.* Englewood Cliffs, NJ: Prentice-Hall, 1954.

115. Ruxton, J., Humor Deserves Our Attention, *Holistic Nursing Practice,* 2, no. 5 (1988), 54–62.

116. Scandrett, S., and S. Uecker, Relaxation Training. In Bulechech, G., and M. McCloskey, eds., *Nursing Interventions: Treatment for Nursing Diagnosis.* Philadelphia: W.B. Saunders, 1984.

117. Sennott-Miller, L., and J. Miller, Difficulty: A Neglected Factor in Health Promotion, *Nursing Research,* 36, no. 5 (1987), 270–272.

118. Shaver, J., A Biopsychosocial View of Human Health, *Nursing Outlook,* 33, no. 4 (1985), 186–191.

119. Sheikh, A.A., ed., *Imagination and Healing.* New York: Baywood Press, 1984.

120. Shimer, P., Stress Relief, *Prevention* (August 1990), 100–119.

121. Shorr, G., et al., eds., *Imagery.* New York: Plenum Press, 1980.

122. Siegel, B., *Love, Medicine, and Miracles.* New York: Harper & Row, 1986.

123. Simonton, O.C., S. Matthews-Simonton, and J. Creighton, *Getting Well Again.* Los Angeles: J.P. Tarcher, 1978.

124. Singer, J., Towards the Scientific Study of Imagination. In Shorr, J., et al., eds., *Imagery: Theoretical and Clinical Applications,* Vol. 3. New York: Plenum Press, 1983.

125. Spellbring, A., Nursing's Role in Health Promotion: An Overview, *Nursing Clinics of North America,* 26, no. 4 (1991), 805–814.

126. Spielberger, C.D., et al., *Manual for the State-Trait Anx-*

iety Inventory. Palo Alto, Calif: Consulting Psychologists Press, 1983.

127. Squires, S., Visions to Boost Immunity, *American Health* (July 1987), 56–61.

128. Streif, T., Can Clients Understand Our Instructions, *Image,* 18, no. 2 (1986), 48–52.

129. Tanner, E., Assessment of a Health-Promotive Lifestyle, *Nursing Clinics of North America,* 26, no. 4 (1991), 845–854.

130. Travelbee, J., *Interpersonal Aspects of Nursing.* Philadelphia: F.A. Davis, 1967.

131. ———, *Intervention in Psychiatric Nursing.* Philadelphia: F.A. Davis, 1969.

132. Uretsky, S., and C. Birdsall, Quackery: A Thoroughly Modern Problem, *American Journal of Nursing,* 86, no. 9 (1986), 1030–1032.

133. Van Deusen, D., Kicking the Cigarette Habit: Some Reflections From an Old Pro, *Wellness Newsletter,* 5, no. 2 (1984), 3–4.

134. Walker, S., K. Sechrist, and N. Pender, The Health-Promoting Lifestyle Profile: Development and Psychometric Characteristics, *Nursing Research,* 36, no. 2 (1987), 76–81.

135. ———, et al., A Spanish Language Version of the Health-Promoting Lifestyle Profile, *Nursing Research,* 39, no. 5 (1990), 268–273.

136. WHO Executive Board Emphasizes Key Role of Nurses in Primary Health Care, *WHO* (January 14, 1985), 1.

137. Witten-Lanoil, G., *The Female Stress Syndrome: How to Recognize and Live With It.* Berkeley, Calif: Berkley Press, 1985.

138. Wuthnow, S., Should Christian Nurses Practice Therapeutic Touch? Yes, *Journal of Christian Nursing,* 4, no. 4 (1987), 15 ff.

139. Yanker, G., *The Complete Book of Exercisewalking.* Chicago: Contemporary Books, 1983.

Appendices

Appendix *I*

A. Recommended U.S. Dietary Allowances, Revised 1989

B. Recommended Nutrient Intakes for Canadians

A. Recommended U.S. Dietary Allowances[a], Revised 1989

Category	Age (years) or Condition	Weight[b] (kg)	Weight[b] (lb)	Height[b] (cm)	Height[b] (in)	Protein (g)	Fat-Soluble vitamins Vitamin A (µg RE)[c]	Vitamin D (µg)[d]	Vitamin E (mg α-TE)[e]	Vitamin K (µg)
Infants	0.0–0.5	6	13	60	24	13	375	7.5	3	5
	0.5–1.0	9	20	71	28	14	375	10	4	10
Children	1–3	13	29	90	35	16	400	10	6	15
	4–6	20	44	112	44	24	500	10	7	20
	7–10	28	62	132	52	28	700	10	7	30
Males	11–14	45	99	157	62	45	1000	10	10	45
	15–18	66	145	176	69	59	1000	10	10	65
	19–24	72	160	177	70	58	1000	10	10	70
	25–50	79	174	176	70	63	1000	5	10	80
	51 +	77	170	173	68	63	1000	5	10	80
Females	11–14	46	101	157	62	46	800	10	8	45
	15–18	55	120	163	64	44	800	10	8	55
	19–24	58	128	164	65	46	800	10	8	60
	25–50	63	138	163	64	50	800	5	8	65
	51 +	65	143	160	63	50	800	5	8	65
Pregnant						60	800	10	10	65
Lactating	First 6 Mo					65	1300	10	12	65
	Second 6 Mo					62	1200	10	11	65

[a]The allowances, expressed as average daily intakes over time, are intended to provide for individual variations among most normal persons as they live in the United States under usual environmental stresses. Diets should be based on a variety of common foods to provide other nutrients for which human requirements have been less well defined. See text for detailed discussion of allowances and of nutrients not tabulated.

[b]Weights and heights of reference adults are actual medians for the U.S. population of the designated age as reported by NHANES II. The use of these figures does not imply that the height-to-weight ratios are ideal.

[c]Retinol equivalents. 1 retinol equivalent = 1 µg retinol or 6 µg β-carotene.

[d]As cholecalciferol, 10 µg cholecalciferol = 400 IU of vitamin D.

[e]Tocopherol equivalents. 1 mg d-α tocopherol = 1 α-TE.

[f]1 NE (niacin equivalent) is equal to 1 mg of niacin or 60-mg of dietary tryptophan.

Reprinted with permission from *Recommended Dietary Allowances, 10th Edition,* © 1989 by the National Academy of Sciences. Published by National Academy Press, Washington, D.C.

A. Recommended U.S. Dietary Allowances[a], Revised 1989 (Continued)

	Water-Soluble Vitamins						Minerals						
Vita-min C (mg)	Thia-min (mg)	Ribo-flavin (mg)	Niacin (mg NE)[f]	Vita-min B$_6$ (mg)	Fo-late (µg)	Vita-min B$_{12}$ (µg)	Cal-cium (mg)	Phos-phorus (mg)	Mag-nesium (mg)	Iron (mg)	Zinc (mg)	Iodine (µg)	Sele-nium (µg)
30	0.3	0.4	5	0.3	25	0.3	400	300	40	6	5	40	10
35	0.4	0.5	6	0.6	35	0.5	600	500	60	10	5	50	15
40	0.7	0.8	9	1.0	50	0.7	800	800	80	10	10	70	20
45	0.9	1.1	12	1.1	75	1.0	800	800	120	10	10	90	20
45	1.0	1.2	13	1.4	100	1.4	800	800	170	10	10	120	30
50	1.3	1.5	17	1.7	150	2.0	1200	1200	270	12	15	150	40
60	1.5	1.8	20	2.0	200	2.0	1200	1200	400	12	15	150	50
60	1.5	1.7	19	2.0	200	2.0	1200	1200	350	10	15	150	70
60	1.5	1.7	19	2.0	200	2.0	800	800	350	10	15	150	70
60	1.2	1.4	15	2.0	200	2.0	800	800	350	10	15	150	70
50	1.1	1.3	15	1.4	150	2.0	1200	1200	280	15	12	150	45
60	1.1	1.3	15	1.5	180	2.0	1200	1200	300	15	12	150	50
60	1.1	1.3	15	1.6	180	2.0	1200	1200	280	15	12	150	55
60	1.1	1.3	15	1.6	180	2.0	800	800	280	15	12	150	55
60	1.0	1.2	13	1.6	180	2.0	800	800	280	10	12	150	55
70	1.5	1.6	17	2.2	400	2.2	1200	1200	300	30	15	175	65
95	1.6	1.8	20	2.1	280	2.6	1200	1200	355	15	19	200	75
90	1.6	1.7	20	2.1	260	2.6	1200	1200	340	15	16	200	75

B. Recommended Nutrient Intakes for Canadians: Average Energy Requirements and Summary Examples of Recommended Nutrient Intakes

Age	Sex	Average Height (cm)[c]	Average Weight (kg)[c]	Requirements[a,b]					
				kcal/kg[c,d]	MJ/kg[d]	kcal/day[e]	MJ/day[f]	kcal/cm[g]	MJ/cm[f]
Months									
0–2	Both	55	4.5	120–100	0.50–0.42	500	3.0	9	0.04
3–5	Both	63	7.0	100–95	0.42–0.40	700	2.8	11	0.05
6–8	Both	69	8.5	95–97	0.40–0.41	800	3.4	11.5	0.05
9–11	Both	73	9.5	97–99	0.41	950	3.8	12.5	0.05
Years									
1	Both	82	11	101	0.42	1100	4.8	13.5	0.06
2–3	Both	95	14	94	0.39	1300	5.6	13.5	0.06
4–6	Both	107	18	100	0.42	1800	7.6	17	0.07
7–9	M	126	25	88	0.37	2200	9.2	17.5	0.07
	F	125	25	76	0.32	1900	8.0	15	0.06
10–12	M	141	34	73	0.30	2500	10.4	17.5	0.07
	F	143	36	61	0.25	2200	9.2	15.5	0.06
13–15	M	159	50	57	0.24	2800	12.0	17.5	0.07
	F	157	48	46	0.19	2200	9.2	14	0.06
16–18	M	172	62	51	0.21	3200	13.2	18.5	0.08
	F	160	53	40	0.17	2100	8.8	13	0.05
19–24	M	175	71	42	0.18	3000	12.4		
	F	160	58	36	0.15	2100	8.8		
25–49	M	172	74	36	0.15	2700	11.2		
	F	160	59	32	0.13	1900	8.0		
50–74	M	170	73	31	0.13	2300	9.6		
	F	158	63	29	0.12	1800	7.6		
75 +	M	168	69	29	0.12	2000	8.4		
	F	155	64	23	0.10	1500	6.0		

Pregnancy (additional)[h]

Lactation (additional)[h]

[a]Recommended nutrient intakes for Canadians, 1982—Committee for the revision of the Dietary Standard for Canada, Bureau of Nutritional Sciences, Department of National Health and Welfare. Recommended intakes of energy and of certain nutrients are not listed in this table because of the nature of the variables on which they are based. The figures for energy are estimates of average requirements for expected patterns of activity. For nutrients not shown the following amounts are recommended: thiamin, 0.4 mg/100 kcal (0.48 mg/5000 kJ); riboflavin, 0.5 mg/1000 kcal (0.6 mg/5000 kJ); niacin, 6.6 NE/1000 kcal (7.9 NE/5000 kJ); vitamin B_6, 15 μg, as pyridoxine, per gram of protein intake; phosphorus, same as calcium. Recommended intakes during periods of growth are taken as appropriate for individual representative of the midpoint in each age group. All recommended intakes are designed to cover individual variations in essentially all of a healthy population subsisting on a variety of common foods available in Canada. It is emphasized that these are examples of the application of the RNI to particular classes of individuals and/or particular situations.

[b]Requirements can be expected to vary within a range of ±30%.

[c]Figures rounded to the closest whole number when ≥10 and to the closest 0.5 when <10.

[d]First and last figures are averages of those at the beginning and the end of the 3-month period.

[e]Figures rounded to the nearest 50 when <1000 and to the nearest 100 when ≥1000.

[f]Figures include 2 decimals if value is <1 and 1 decimal if ≥1.

[g]Figures rounded to the nearest 0.5.

[h]Pregnancy: add 100 kcal during the first trimester and 300 for the second and third trimesters; lactation: add 450 kcal/day.

[i]The primary units are grams per kilogram of body weight. The figures shown here are only examples.

One retinol equivalent (RE) corresponds to the biologic activity of 1 μg of retinol, 6 μg of β-carotene or 12 μg of other carotenes.

Expressed as cholecalciferol or ergocalciferol.

Expressed as d-α-tocopherol equivalents, relative to which β- and γ-tocopherol and α-tocotrienol have activities of 0.5, 0.1, and 0.3 respectively.

Expressed as total folate.

Assumption that the protein is from breast milk or is of the same biologic value as that of breast milk and that between 3 and 9 months adjustment for the quality of the protein is made.

For the infant it is assumed that breast milk is the source of iron up to 2 months of age.

Based on the assumption that breast milk is the source of zinc up to 2 months of age.

After menopause the recommended intake is 7 mg/day.

From Bureau of Nutritional Sciences, Department of National Health and Welfare, Ottawa, Canada, 1982. Reproduced with permission of the Minister of Supply and Services, Canada, 1992.

B. Recommended Nutrient Intakes for Canadians: Average Energy Requirements and Summary Examples of Recommended Nutrient Intakes (Continued)

Protein (g/day)[i]	Fat-Soluble Vitamins			Water-Soluble Vitamins			Minerals				
	Vit A (RE/day)[j]	Vit D (μg/day)[k]	Vit E (mg/day)[l]	Vit C (mg/day)	Folacin (μg/day)[m]	Vit B_{12} (μg/day)	Ca (mg/day)	Mg (mg/day)	Fe (mg/day)	I (μg/day)	Zn (mg/day)
11[n]	400	10	3	20	50	0.3	350	30	0.4o	25	2[p]
14[n]	400	10	3	20	50	0.3	350	40	5	35	3
16[n]	400	10	3	20	50	0.3	400	45	7	40	3
18	400	10	3	20	55	0.3	400	50	7	45	3
18	400	10	3	20	65	0.3	500	55	6	55	4
20	400	5	4	20	80	0.4	500	65	6	65	4
25	500	5	5	25	90	0.5	600	90	6	85	5
31	700	2.5	7	35	125	0.8	700	110	7	110	6
29	700	2.5	6	30	125	0.8	700	110	7	95	7
38	800	2.5	8	40	170	1.0	900	150	10	125	6
39	800	2.5	7	40	170	1.0	1000	160	10	110	7
49	900	2.5	9	50	160	1.5	1100	220	12	160	9
43	800	2.5	7	45	160	1.5	800	190	13	160	8
54	1000	2.5	10	55	190	1.9	900	240	10	160	9
47	800	2.5	7	45	160	1.9	700	220	14	160	8
57	1000	2.5	10	60	210	2.0	800	240	8	160	9
41	800	2.5	7	45	165	2.0	700	190	14	160	8
57	1000	2.5	9	60	210	2.0	800	240	8	160	9
41	800	2.5	6	45	165	2.0	700	190	14[q]	160	8
57	1000	2.5	7	60	210	2.0	800	240	8	160	9
41	800	2.5	6	45	165	2.0	800	190	7	160	8
57	1000	2.5	6	60	210	2.0	800	240	8	160	9
41	800	2.5	5	45	165	2.0	800	190	7	160	8
15	100	2.5	2	0	305	1.0	500	15	6	25	0
20	100	2.5	2	20	305	1.0	500	20	6	25	1
25	100	2.5	2	20	305	1.0	500	25	6	25	2
20	400	2.5	3	30	120	0.5	500	80	0	50	6

Major Sources and Functions of Primary Nutrients

Nutrient	Major Sources	Major Functions
Protein	Meat; poultry, fish; dried beans and peas; eggs; nuts; cheese; milk. Whole grain cereals are incomplete and must be combined with animal protein. Animal and vegetable protein combined increase use by body of all amino acids.	Builds, maintains, and repairs body cells; is required for amino acids (eight are essential). Constitutes part of the structure of every cell such as muscle, blood, bones, and ligaments. Supports growth and maintains healthy body cells. Maintains pH balance of blood; acts as buffer system. Regulates osmotic pressure. Constitutes part of enzymes, some hormones, body fluids, antibodies that increase resistance to infection, hemoglobin, plasma proteins. Is source of energy and fuel when inadequate carbohydrate and fat unavailable. Because protein and other nitrogenous compounds are degraded and resynthesized continually, daily intake is needed. Essential for nitrogen balance; excess excreted in urea and urine.
Carbohydrate	Bread; potatoes; pasta; dried beans; corn; rice; fruit; vegetables; sugar; desserts, candy; jam; syrup; honey.	Supplies energy and forms ATP so protein can be used for growth maintenance of body cells, and metabolic processes. Maintains body temperature. Supplies fiber in unrefined products—complex carbohydrates in fruits, vegetables, and whole grains—for regular elimination. Assists in fat utilization.
Fat	Animal fat; shortening; vegetable oil; butter; margarine; salad dressing; mayonnaise; sausages; lunch meats; whole milk and milk products; nuts. No more than 30% of total calories should be from fat. No more than 10% of fat intake should be saturated fat intake.	Provides concentrated source of energy. Constitutes part of the structure of every cell. Helps control cell permeability. Supplies essential fatty acids. Necessary for absorption of (carrier for) fat-soluble vitamins (A, D, E, and K).

Major Sources and Functions of Primary Nutrients (Continued)

Nutrient	Major Sources	Major Functions
		Maintains adipose tissue, which insulates and protects inner organs from trauma. Is component of thromboplastin, used in blood clotting. Adds to food taste, texture, and appearance. Provides reserve supply of phosphate ions. Excess animal fat is linked to cancer of gastrointestinal tract and possibly cancer of breast and prostate.

Vitamins

Nutrient	Major Sources	Major Functions
Vitamin C (ascorbic acid) (water soluble)	Citrus fruits such as orange, grapefruit, lime, lemon, papaya; mango; kiwi; cantaloupe; pineapple; rose hips; strawberries; raspberries; blackberries; black currants; melons; cherries; alfalfa sprouts; watercress; parsley; tomatoes; broccoli; sweet peppers; raw potatoes; raw leafy vegetables; kale; brussel sprouts; cabbage; cauliflower; asparagus; bok choy; thyme; horehound root; celery seed; sarsaparillo root; dandelion root.	Forms cementing substances such as collagen that hold body cells together, thus strengthening blood vessels, hastening healing of wounds and bone fractures, and increasing resistance to infection. Helps develop and maintain healthy bones, teeth, gums; skin, muscles, and blood vessels. Prevents scurvy. Regulates mitochondria and microsomial respiratory cycle. Aids use of iron and folic acid metabolism. Normalizes body cholesterol. Decreases risk of cancer of esophagus and stomach; aspirin prevents absorption.
Thiamine (B_1) (water soluble)	Pork; lean meat; nuts; liver; fish; oysters; crabmeat; dried yeast; milk; whole grains, enriched bread and cereals; pasta; dry beans; peas; lima beans; soybeans; sunflower seeds; brown rice; asparagus; raisins; alfalfa.	Functions as part of coenzyme to promote use of carbohydrate and protein and release of energy. Reduces fatigue and weakness. Promotes normal appetite. Contributes to normal functioning of nervous, muscle, and digestive systems. Prevents beriberi.
Riboflavin (B_2) (water soluble)	Liver and other organ meats; ham; poultry; milk and milk products; yogurt; cottage cheese; egg yolk; green leafy vegetables; lean meat; whole grains; soybeans; peas; beans; nuts; enriched bread and cereal; brewer's yeast; blackstrap molasses; sunflower seeds; wheat germ; alfalfa.	Is component of flavoprotein involved in biologic oxidation. Is essential for building and maintaining body tissues, antibodies, and red blood cells. Functions as part of a coenzyme in the production of energy within body cells. Promotes carbohydrate, fat, and protein metabolism. Maintains nitrogen balance. Is essential for use of oxygen in cells. Promotes healthy skin, eyes, tongue, lips, mucous membranes. Prevents sensitivity of eyes to light.
Niacin (water soluble)	Liver; meat; rabbit; poultry; fish; peanuts; whole grains; brewer's yeast; fortified cereal and bread products, wheat germ; gentian root; licorice root; alfalfa.	Aids use of vitamins B_1 and B_2. Is essential for tissue respiration. Functions as part of a coenzyme in fat synthesis, protein use, glycolysis and use of carbohydrate, and release of energy. Promotes healthy skin, nerves, digestive tract, and blood vessels. Aids digestion and fosters normal appetite. Is required for formation of certain hormones and nerve-regulating substances. Prevents pellagra.
Pyridoxine (B_6) (water soluble)	Liver, meat; fish; poultry; whole grain bread and cereals; wheat germ; brewer's yeast; sunflower seeds; soybeans; nuts; brown rice; bananas; avocado; sweet potato; white potato; corn; white beans; green leafy vegetables; alfalfa.	Is coenzyme in basic reactions of amino acid, fat metabolism, and protein metabolism. Assists antibody hormone and red blood cell formation. Is involved with function of neurotransmitters. Helps maintain balance of sodium and phosphorus and metabolism of iron and potassium.
Cyanocolabalamin (B_{12}) (water soluble)	Organ meats such as liver, kidney, and heart; lean meat; poultry; fish; oysters; clams; sea vegetables (kelp, dulse, komba); eggs; milk; cheese; brewer's yeast; angelica root; alfalfa.	Is essential for all blood cell formation. Is coenzyme for synthesis of materials for nucleus of all cells. Is essential for synthesis of nucleic acids, metabolism of certain amino acids, protein, carbohydrate, fat, and generally normal cell function.

(continued)

Major Sources and Functions of Primary Nutrients (Continued)

Nutrient	Major Sources	Major Functions
		Converts folic acid to folinic acid.
		Is especially important for cells of bone marrow, intestinal tract, and central nervous system.
		Strict vegetarian at risk for deficiency, pernicious anemia.
Folacin (folic acid) (water soluble)	Dark green, leafy vegetables such as collards, mustard greens, turnip greens, kale; organ meats; dried beans; root vegetables; whole grains; brewer's yeast; oysters; salmon; milk; black-eyed peas; lima beans; watermelon; cantaloupe.	Synthesizes nucleic acid and proteins. Acts with B_{12} in making genetic material. Assists metabolism of certain amino acids. Assists in hemoglobin, red blood cell, and protein formation. Is necessary for normal cell division. Prevents anemia.
Vitamin A (retinol) (fat soluble)	Liver; orange-colored fruits; orange, yellow, and dark green vegetables such as carrots, winter squash, sweet potatoes, broccoli, and greens; eggs; fortified milk, butter, margarine, cheese; horehound root; celery seed; dandelion root; red peppers.	Assists formation, maintenance, and repair of normal skin, hair, and mucous membranes that line body cavities and tracts such as nasal passages and intestinal tract, thus increasing resistance to infection. Maintains mitochondrial and liposomal membranes. Functions in visual processes, forms visual purple, thus promoting healthy eye tissue and eye adaptation in dim light or at night. Increases resistance to infection. Decreases risk of cancer of lung, thyroid, esophagus, bladder because it aids in controlling cell differentiation.
Vitamin D (fat soluble)	Fortified milk, butter, margarine; fish liver oil; salmon; tuna; egg yolk; liver; bone meal; sunshine; thyme.	Regulates calcium and phosphorus metabolism; promotes intestinal absorption of calcium and phosphorus. Promotes bone mineralization (prevents rickets) and tooth formation.
Vitamin E (fat soluble)	Vegetable oils; liver; wheat germ; whole grain cereals; rice; oats; brewer's yeast; peanuts; foods high in polyunsaturated fatty acids; eggs; molasses; sweet potatoes; leafy vegetables; lettuce; spinach; asparagus; cauliflower; broccoli; angelica root; horehound root.	Is essential in cellular respiration. Is antioxidant at tissue level; maintains tissue. Prevents abnormal fat breakdown in tissues. Assists in formation of normal red blood cells and muscle. Functions in reproductive system. Prevents buildup of cholesterol plaque and blood clot formation in blood vessels, thus preventing coronary disease. Protects against exposure to radiation.
Vitamin K (fat soluble)	K_1 is found in lean meat; liver; green plants, green leafy vegetables; tomatoes; cauliflower; peas; carrots; potato; cabbage; soybean and safflower oil; egg yolk; blackstrap molasses; wheat germ. K_3 is synthetic therapeutic form. Half of vitamin K in body synthesized by intestinal bacteria as K_2.	Is essential for synthesis of blood-clotting factors: prothrombin (factor I), factors VII, IX, X. Stimulates coagulation proenzymes II, VII, IX, X.
Biotin	Egg yolk; organ meats; fish; brewer's yeast; whole grains; legumes; sardines; most fresh vegetables; lima beans; mushrooms; peanuts; bananas; yogurt.	Is necessary for formation of folic acid. Is necessary for carbohydrate, protein, and fat metabolism. Aids in use of other B vitamins.
Pantothenic acid	Organ meats; lobster; oyster; salmon; brewer's yeast; egg yolk; legumes; whole grains; wheat germ; nuts; soy flour; sunflower and sesame seeds; green leafy vegetables; broccoli; cauliflower; potato; licorice root.	Aids in formation of some fats, hormones. Aids in metabolism and release of energy from carbohydrates, fats, and proteins. Aids in use of some vitamins. Improves resistance to stress and infection.
Choline	Egg yolk; organ meat; fish; salmon; brewer's yeast; wheat germ; soybeans; legumes.	Aids normal nerve transmission. Aids metabolism and transport of fats.
Inositol	Citrus fruits; whole grains; brewer's yeast; molasses; meat; milk; nuts; vegetables; gentian root.	Is necessary for formation of lecithin. Aids hair growth.
Para-aminobenzoic acid (PABA)	Organ meats; wheat germ; yogurt; molasses; green leafy vegetables.	Aids bacteria producing folic acid. Acts as a coenzyme in use of proteins. Aids in formation of red blood cells. Acts as sunscreen.
Pangamic acid	Brewer's yeast; brown rice; sunflower, pumpkin, and sesame seeds.	Helps eliminate hypoxia. Promotes protein metabolism. Stimulates nervous and glandular systems.

Major Sources and Functions of Primary Nutrients (Continued)

Nutrient	Major Sources	Major Functions
Minerals		
Calcium	Milk and milk products; chowder, cream soups, puddings made with milk, custards; yogurt; shellfish; salmon; sardines; bone meal; dark green leafy vegetables; kale; egg yolk; whole grains; legumes; nuts; tofu; molasses; broccoli; tomatoes; chamomille flower; cascara sagrada; angelica root; passion flower.	Works with phosphorus, magnesium, vitamin D, other minerals, and protein to build bones and teeth. Assists blood clotting. Is necessary for nerve transmission, heart function, muscle contraction and relaxation, and cell wall permeability. Activates enzyme ATPase. Intestinal absorption of vitamin D, which decreases with age, necessary for calcium metabolism. Oxylates and phytates in green leafy vegetables, and grains interfere with calcium absorption by combining with calcium and creating insoluble compound. Fiber may combine with calcium and limit absorption. Alcohol intake interferes with metabolism. Caffeine and excess salt intake cause calcium excretion.
Phosphorus	Milk and milk products; meat; liver; seafood; whole grains; wheat germ; nuts; egg yolk; legumes; peas; beans; lentils; brown rice; sunflower seeds; brewer's yeast.	Helps formation of nucleic acids. Works with calcium and vitamin D to build and maintain healthy bones, teeth, and cell membranes. Aids absorption of glucose and glycerol. Transports fatty acids. Acts as buffer system. Aids energy metabolism.
Potassium	Lean meat; chicken; whole grains; bananas; oranges; apricots; dried fruits; potato; vegetables; broccoli; spinach; raw cabbage; swiss chard; okra; legumes; lima beans; sunflower seeds; molasses; wheat germ; skim milk; roasted chestnuts; cascara sagrada; horehound root.	Controls activity of heart, muscles, nervous system, kidneys. Regulates neuromuscular excitability and muscle contraction. Is major intracellular fluid cation. Promotes acid-base balance. Is necessary for glycogen formation and protein synthesis.
Magnesium	Whole grains; cereals; nuts; citrus fruits, figs; green leafy vegetables; swiss chard; dried beans and peas; soybeans; meat; milk; nuts; brown rice; wheatgerm; chamomile flower; passion flower; sevega root.	Promotes healthy nerve and muscle tissue and function. Is component of bones and teeth. Is activator and coenzyme in carbohydrates, fat, and protein metabolism. Acts as catalyst in use of calcium and phosphorus. Is essential intracellular fluid cation.
Iodine	Iodized salt; seafood; kelp; green leafy vegetables.	Is necessary for thyroid gland to control cell activities and metabolism. Synthesizes thyroxine, the thyroid hormones, which regulates cell oxidation. Promotes growth. Prevents goiter.
Sodium	Table salt; fish; seafood; kelp; baking powder and baking soda; milk; cheese; meat; eggs; celery; carrots; beets; spinach; cucumber; asparagus; turnips; stringbeans; coconut; processed foods and cereals; snack foods such as potato chips, pretzels, or salted nuts.	Maintains normal fluid level and osmotic pressure in cells. Is major extracellular fluid cation. Maintains health of nervous, muscular, blood, and lymph systems. Promotes cell permeability and absorption of glucose. Transmits electrochemical impulse in muscle, resulting in contraction. Promotes acid-base balance; acts with potassium, magnesium, chlorine; buffers carbon dioxide and ketones.
Cobalt	Organ meats; oysters; clams; poultry; milk; green leafy vegetables; fruits; supplied by preformed vitamin B_{12}.	Is component of vitamin B_{12}. Is essential for red blood cell formation. Activates a number of body enzymes.
Chlorine	Table salt; seafood; meats; liver; fish; ripe olives; rye flour; soybeans; egg yolks; peanuts; wheat germ.	Regulates acid-base balance and chlorine-bicarbonate shift. Is major extracellular fluid anion. Maintains osmotic pressure. Stimulates production of hydrochloric acid. Helps maintain joints and tendons.

(continued)

Major Sources and Functions of Primary Nutrients (Continued)

Nutrient	Major Sources	Major Functions
Sulfur	Fish; shrimp; eggs; meat; cabbage; brussels sprouts; asparagus; milk; cheese; nuts; legumes; peas; beans; mustard greens; cauliflower; mashed potatoes.	Is component of amino acids and B vitamins. Is essential for formation of body tissues, collagen, skin, bones, tendons, cartilage. Assists in tissue respiration. Required for oxidation-reduction reactions. Activates enzymes. Aids in detoxification reactions.
Fluorine	Natural supply in water in some areas of United States; fluoridated water; seafood; bone meal; tea.	Is deposited in teeth and bones. May reduce tooth decay by discouraging growth of acid-forming bacteria.
Molybdenum	Legumes; whole grain cereals; milk; liver; dark green vegetables.	Acts in oxidation of fat and aldehydes. Aids in mobilization of iron from liver reserves. Assists in conversion of purine to uric acid.
Vanadium	Fish; whole grains; root vegetables; nuts; vegetable oils.	Inhibits cholesterol formation. May assist in tooth and bone formation.
Trace Minerals		
Iron	Organ and red meats; fish; poultry; beef; pork; lamb; dried and canned beans and peas; enriched whole grain breads and cereals; dark green leafy vegetables; mustard and dandelion greens; egg yolk; blackstrap molasses; cherry and prune juice; legumes; nuts; dried fruits (raisins, apricots); chamomile flower; horehound root; sevega root; celery seed.	Is essential for hemoglobin and myoglobin formation. Helps protein metabolism. Is used by cells as component for oxidation of glucose in production of energy. Aids tissue respiration. Promotes growth. Increases resistance to infection. Is more readily used by body when ascorbic acid, copper, folic acid, and vitamin B_{12} available. Excess calcium intake interferes with iron absorption.
Zinc	Organ and red meats; sunflower seeds; oysters; herring; seafood; eggs; mushrooms; brewer's yeast; soybeans; wheat germ.	Is component of insulin, serum proteins, reproductive fluid, bone, muscle, eyes, hair, teeth, and liver. Aids digestion and metabolism of phosphorus. Necessary for adequate respiration and digestion. Important for sensory functioning, normal growth, hair, complexion, sexual function, wound healing. Aids healing and resistance to infection, excess of deficiency interferes with immune function.
Copper	Organ and lean meats; seafood; nuts; legumes; molasses; raisins; bone meal; cocoa; food cooked in copperware.	Absorbs and transports iron and aids in formation of red blood cells. Is component of many enzymes, which, in turn, are necessary for development and maintenance of skeletal, cardiovascular, and central nervous systems. Works with vitamin C to form elastin.
Manganese	Whole grains; green leafy vegetables; legumes; nuts; pineapple; grapefruit; egg yolk; tea; coffee; cascara sagrada; licorice root.	Is enzyme activator for urea formation, protein and fat metabolism, glucose oxidation, and synthesis of fatty acids. Is necessary for normal skeletal formation, brain function. Maintains sex hormone production. May protect against pancreatic cancer.
Chromium	Corn oil; clams; whole grain cereals; meat; liver; wheat germ; brewer's yeast; drinking water in some areas of United States.	Stimulates enzymes in metabolism of energy and synthesis of fatty acids, cholesterol, and protein. Increases effectiveness of action of insulin in cell, which improves glucose uptake by body tissues.
Selenium	Seafood; tuna; herring; organ and red meat; brewer's yeast; wheat germ; bran; asparagus; mushrooms; broccoli; whole grains; bread; cereals; garlic.	Acts as cofactor in cell oxidation enzyme systems. Is constituent of factor III, which acts with vitamin E to prevent fatty liver. Preserves tissue elasticity. Protects against heart disease. May prevent liver, colon, breast cancer.
Water	Water; coffee; tea; milk; soup; fruit juices; flavored gelatin; fruits; vegetables.	Is part of blood, lymph, and body secretions. Aids digestion. Dissolves nutrients and enables them to pass through intestinal wall. Regulates body temperature. Transports body wastes for elimination.

Review of Systems: Physical Assessment and Health History

Constitutional	Health overall; weight gain or loss; fever; fatigue; repeated infections; ability to carry out activities.
Psychologic	Dreams or nightmares; crying; depression; anxiety; insomnia; diagnosed mental illness.
Integument	General skin condition and care. Any changes; rash; itch; nail deformity; hair loss; moles; open areas.
Head, ears, eyes, nose, throat, teeth	Head: aches; evidence of trauma or bumps; hair loss. Eyes: eye care; poor eyesight; double or blurred vision; use of corrective lenses or medications. Ears: hearing acuity; reaction to noise level; tinnitus (ringing in ears); presence of infection or pain. Nose and throat: upper respiratory infections; hoarseness; sore throat; sinusitis; epistaxis (nose bleeds); dysphagia (difficulty swallowing). Teeth: dentures or dental work; caries. Pattern of brushing and use of dental floss. Fluoride application (to 12 years).
Respiratory	History of respiratory infections; self-treatment of colds. Cough and its duration; last chest x-ray examination; tuberculin skin test and results; dyspnea (difficulty breathing) and when (nighttime, with exertion); wheezing; asthma or bronchitis; hemoptysis (coughing or spitting up blood).
Cardiovascular	Exercise pattern to maintain cardiovascular health. Edema; varicose veins; heart sounds, including murmur; chest pains; palpitations; hypertension (high blood pressure); electrocardiogram (ECG) and when.
Gastrointestinal	Dietary pattern; amount of fiber in diet. Heartburn; epigastric pain; abdominal pain; nausea and vomiting; food intolerance; flatulence; diarrhea; constipation; clay-colored, tarry, or bright red stools; hemorrhoids; history of ulcers.
Genitourinary	Nocturia; dysuria; incontinence; resistance; sexual difficulty; venereal disease; history of stones. Men: slow stream; penile discharge; contraceptive use; self-testicular examination (technique and frequency). Women: breast lumps, breast self-examination and how often; menarche; menopause; intermenstrual bleeding; last menstrual period; contraceptive use; last Pap smear.
Musculoskeletal	Exercise pattern. Neck pain or stiffness; joint pain or swelling; incapacitating back pain; paralysis; deformities.
Neurologic	Syncope; stroke; seizures; paresthesia.
Lymphatic and hematologic	Enlarged, tender nodes; easy bruising; anemia; bleeding.
Endocrine	Polydipsia; polyphagia; polyuria; intolerance of heat or cold; weight gain or loss; changes in skin, hair, or nail texture.
Immunologic	Immunization record; what diseases and dates.

Health Maintenance Procedures

Health Maintenance Procedures

Procedure	B[b]	Months 2	4	6	12	15	18	Years 2	3	5	8	11	13	15	17
Complete History	x	x	x	x	x		x	x (or at first visit)	x	x	x	x	x	x	x
Update History (including developmental)		x	x	x	x	x	x	x	x	x	x	x	x	x	x
Complete Physical Examination	x	x		x	x		x	x	x	x	x	x	x	x	x
Height, weight	x	x	x	x	x		x	x		x	x	x	x	x	x
Head circumference	x	x	x	x	x		x	x							
Blood pressure									x	x	x	x	x	x	x
Vision/strabismus[a]		xa	x		x[a]		x[a]	x	x	x	x	x	x	x	x
Hearing		x		x	x				x	x	x	x	x	x	x
Hip, feet, spine	x	x											x		
Language screen							x	x	x	x					
Pap—high risk													x	x	x
Immunizations/Screenings															
Phenylketonuria (PKU)	x														
Hypothyroid (T$_4$)	x														
Silver nitrate drops (AgNO)	x														
Vitamin K injection	x														
DTP/TD		x	x	x			x			x			x		
OPV (polio)		x	x				x			x					
MMR (measles, mumps, rubella)						x									
Laboratory															
Tine test					x				x	x		x		x	
Rubella titer (if not vaccinated)												x			
Hematocrit/hemoglobin					x					x			x		
Urine culture (female)										x	x				
Dental/Mouth Check		x	x	x	x		x	x	x	x	x	x	x	x	x
Fluoride history		x		x											
Counseling—Health Education															
Safety/accidents	x	x	x	x	x		x	x	x	x	x	x	x	x	x
Poison control		x	x	x	x		x	x	x	x	x	x	x	x	x
Nutrition	x	x	x	x	x		x	x	x	x	x	x	x	x	x
Physical care	x	x	x	x	x		x	x	x	x	x	x	x	x	x
Behavior/psychologic/social															
Sex education									x	x	x	x	x	x	x
Tobacco/alcohol use													x	x	x
Safety belt use/driver education													x	x	x

[a]Strabismus checked at 2, 12, and 18 mo.
[b]B denotes at birth.

(continued)

Health Maintenance Procedures (Continued)

Procedure	18	19	20	21	22	23	24	25	26	27	28	29	30	31	32	33	34	35	36	37	38	39	40	41	42
Complete History	x																								
Update History		x	x	x	x	x	x	x	x	x	x	x	x	x	x	x	x	x	x	x	x	x	x	x	x
Health Hazard Appraisal	x																								
Complete Physical Examination	x					x					x					x					x				
Height/weight	x	x	x	x	x	x	x	x	x	x	x	x	x	x	x	x	x	x	x	x	x	x	x	x	x
Blood pressure	x	x	x	x	x	x	x	x	x	x	x	x	x	x	x	x	x	x	x	x	x	x	x	x	x
Vision (Snellen)	x			x			x				x					x				x			x	x	x
tonometry																							x		
Hearing (Gross)	x	x	x	x	x	x	x	x	x	x	x	x	x	x	x	x	x	x	x	x	x	x	x	x	x
audiometry																									
Dental	x	x	x	x	x	x	x	x	x	x	x	x	x	x	x	x	x	x	x	x	x	x	x	x	x
Breast examination	x	x	x	x	x	x	x	x	x	x	x	x	x	x	x	x	x	x	x	x	x	x	x	x	x
Mammography																		x		x		x		x	
Pap—high risk	x	x	x	x	x	x	x	x	x	x	x	x	x	x	x	x	x	x	x	x	x	x	x	x	x
Pap—low risk	x	x		x			x			x			x			x			x			x			
Stool guiac		x					x				x					x						x	x	x	x
Testicular examination	x	x	x	x	x	x	x	x	x	x	x	x	x	x	x	x	x	x	x	x	x	x	x	x	x
Prostate examination		x					x				x					x						x	x	x	x

Hearing audiometry: Influenced by circumstances, especially work/noise environment, and symptoms.

Mammography: Influenced by symptoms and family history.

Hernia examination: Influenced by work/sports demands—part of complete physical examination.

Immunizations	18	19	20	21	22	23	24	25	26	27	28	29	30	31	32	33	34	35	36	37	38	39	40	41	42
TD								x										x							
Influenza	x	x	x	x	x	x	x	x	x	x	x	x	x	x	x	x	x	x	x	x	x	x	x	x	x

Pneumococcal: High-risk persons and certain age groups; one time only.

Hepatitis B: High-risk persons.

Laboratory	18	19	20	21	22	23	24	25	26	27	28	29	30	31	32	33	34	35	36	37	38	39	40	41	42
Chemistry panel, lipid panel, and CBC	x			x			x			x			x			x			x		x		x		x
Urinalysis	x	x	x	x	x	x	x	x	x	x	x	x	x	x	x	x	x	x	x	x	x	x	x	x	x
Tine test		x					x					x					x								

Other Tests

Pulmonary function/ECG: Influenced by symptoms.

Chest x-ray: Influenced by symptoms; if positive tine test; work hazards; heavy smoking history.

Counseling and Health Education	18	19	20	21	22	23	24	25	26	27	28	29	30	31	32	33	34	35	36	37	38	39	40	41	42
Nutritional	x	x	x	x	x	x	x	x	x	x	x	x	x	x	x	x	x	x	x	x	x	x	x	x	x
Behavior/psychologic/social	x	x	x	x	x	x	x	x	x	x	x	x	x	x	x	x	x	x	x	x	x	x	x	x	x
Safety/accident	x	x	x	x	x	x	x	x	x	x	x	x	x	x	x	x	x	x	x	x	x	x	x	x	x
Sexuality	x	x	x	x	x	x	x	x	x	x	x	x	x	x	x	x	x	x	x	x	x	x	x	x	x
Tobacco/alcohol/drugs	x	x	x	x	x	x	x	x	x	x	x	x	x	x	x	x	x	x	x	x	x	x	x	x	x

Complete History: x or at any beginning point.

Health Hazard Appraisal: x or at any beginning point (optional).

Health Maintenance Procedures (Continued)

Procedure	Years 43	44	45	46	47	48	49	50	51	52	53	54	55	56	57	58	59	60	61
Complete History	At any beginning point.																		
Update History	x	x	x	x	x	x	x	x	x	x	x	x	x	x	x	x	x	x	x
Health Hazard Appraisal	At any beginning point (optional).																		
Complete Physical Examination	x					x					x					x			x
Height, weight	x	x	x	x	x	x	x	x	x	x	x	x	x	x	x	x	x	x	
Blood pressure	x	x	x	x	x	x	x	x	x	x	x	x	x	x	x	x	x	x	x
Vision (Snellen)	x	x	x	x	x	x	x	x	x	x	x	x	x	x	x	x	x	x	x
tonometry								x					x					x	x
Hearing (Gross)	x	x	x	x	x	x	x	x	x	x	x	x	x	x	x	x	x	x	x
audiometry	Influenced by circumstances, especially work/noise environment, and symptoms.																		
Dental	x	x	x	x	x	x	x	x	x	x	x	x	x	x	x	x	x	x	x
Breast examination,	x	x	x	x	x	x	x	x	x	x	x	x	x	x	x	x	x	x	x
mammography	x		x	x	x	x	x	x	x	x	x	x	x	x	x	x	x	x	
Pap—high risk	x	x	x	x	x	x	x	x	x	x	x	x	x	x	x	x	x	x	x
Pap—low risk	x		x			x				x			x			x			x
Stool guiac	x	x	x	x	x	x	x	x	x	x	x	x	x	x	x	x	x	x	x
Sigmoidoscopy			x				x				x					x			
Testicular examination	x	x	x	x	x	x	x	x	x	x	x	x	x	x	x	x	x	x	x
Prostate examination	x	x	x	x	x	x	x	x	x	x	x	x	x	x	x	x	x	x	x
Hernia examination	Influenced by work/sports demands—part of complete physical examination.																		
Immunizations																			
TD			x										x						
Influenza	x	x	x	x	x	x	x	x	x	x	x	x	x	x	x	x	x	x	x
Pneumococcal	High-risk persons and certain age groups; one time only.																		
Hepatitis B	High-risk persons.																		
Laboratory																			
Chemistry panel, lipid panel, and CBC		x		x		x		x	x	x	x	x	x	x	x	x	x	x	x
Urinalysis		x		x		x		x	x	x	x	x	x	x	x	x	x	x	x
Tine test	If negative, no need to repeat unless specific situation arises or in high-risk group.																		
Other Tests																			
ECG							x	Baseline, then as needed.											
Pulmonary function	Influenced by symptoms.																		
Chest x-ray	Influenced by symptoms; if positive tine test; work hazards; heavy smoking history.																		
Counseling and Health Education	x	x	x	x	x	x	x	x	x	x	x	x	x	x	x	x	x	x	x
Nutritional	x	x	x	x	x	x	x	x	x	x	x	x	x	x	x	x	x	x	x
Behavior/psychologic/social	x	x	x	x	x	x	x	x	x	x	x	x	x	x	x	x	x	x	x
Safety/accident	x	x	x	x	x	x	x	x	x	x	x	x	x	x	x	x	x	x	x
Sexuality	x	x	x	x	x	x	x	x	x	x	x	x	x	x	x	x	x	x	x
Tobacco/alcohol/drugs	x	x	x	x	x	x	x	x	x	x	x	x	x	x	x	x	x	x	x

(*continued*)

Health Maintenance Procedures (Continued)

Procedure	Years																		
	62	63	64	65	66	67	68	69	70	71	72	73	74	75	76	77	78	79	80
Complete History	At any beginning point.																		
Update History	x	x	x	x	x	x	x	x	x	x	x	x	x	x	x	x	x	x	x
Health Hazard Appraisal	At any beginning point (optional).																		
Complete Physical Examination		x					x					x					x		
Height/weight	x	x	x	x	x	x	x	x	x	x	x	x	x	x	x	x	x	x	x
Blood pressure	x	x	x	x	x	x	x	x	x	x	x	x	x	x	x	x	x	x	x
Vision (Snellen)		x	x	x	x	x	x	x	x	x	x	x	x	x	x	x	x	x	x
tonometry				x	x	x	x	x	x	x	x	x	x	x	x	x	x	x	x
Hearing (Gross)	x	x	x	x	x	x	x	x	x	x	x	x	x	x	x	x	x	x	x
audiometry	Influenced by circumstances, especially work/noise environment, and symptoms.																		
Dental	x	x	x	x	x	x	x	x	x	x	x	x	x	x	x	x	x	x	x
Breast examination mammo-graphy	x	x	x	x	x	x	x	x	x	x	x	x	x	x	x	x	x	x	x
Pap—high risk	x	x	x	x	x	x	x		x	x		x	x	x	x		x	x	x
Pap—low risk		x				x			x			x			x			x	
Stool guiac	x	x	x	x	x	x	x	x	x	x	x	x	x	x	x	x	x	x	x
Sigmoidoscopy		x					x					x					x		
Testicular examination	x	x	x	x	x	x	x	x	x	x	x	x	x	x	x	x	x	x	x
Prostate examination	x	x	x	x	x	x	x	x	x	x	x	x	x	x	x	x	x	x	x
Hernia examination	Influenced by work/sports demands—part of complete physical exam.																		
Immunizations																			
TD				x										x					
Influenza	x	x	x	x	x	x	x	x	x	x	x	x	x	x	x	x	x	x	x
Pneumococcal				x															
Hepatitis B	High-risk persons.																		
Laboratory																			
Chemistry panel and CBC		x		x				x			x			x			x		
Lipid panel			x																
Urinalysis	x		x			x			x		x			x			x		x
Tine test	x			x			x			x			x			x			x
Other Tests																			
ECG	Influenced by symptoms.																		
Pulmonary function	Influenced by symptoms.																		
Chest x-ray	Influenced by symptoms.																		
Counseling and Health Education	x	x	x	x	x	x	x	x	x	x	x	x	x	x	x	x	x	x	x
Nutritional	x	x	x	x	x	x	x	x	x	x	x	x	x	x	x	x	x	x	x
Behavior/psychologic/social	x	x	x	x	x	x	x	x	x	x	x	x	x	x	x	x	x	x	x
Safety/accident	x	x	x	x	x	x	x	x	x	x	x	x	x	x	x	x	x	x	x
Sexuality	x	x	x	x	x	x	x	x	x	x	x	x	x	x	x	x	x	x	x
Tobacco/alcohol/drugs	x	x	x	x	x	x	x	x	x	x	x	x	x	x	x	x	x	x	x

Italicized letters following page numbers indicate tables (*t*), figures (*f*), and boxes (*b*).

Italicized letters following page numbers indicate tables (*t*), figures (*f*), and boxes (*b*).

Italicized letters following page numbers indicate tables (*t*), figures (*f*), and boxes (*b*).

Italicized letters following page numbers indicate tables (*t*), figures (*f*), and boxes (*b*).

Italicized letters following page numbers indicate tables (*t*), figures (*f*), and boxes (*b*).

Italicized letters following page numbers indicate tables (*t*), figures (*f*), and boxes (*b*).

Italicized letters following page numbers indicate tables (*t*), figures (*f*), and boxes (*b*).

Italicized letters following page numbers indicate tables (*t*), figures (*f*), and boxes (*b*).

Upper-upper socioeconomic level, 25–26
Urbanization, family and, 153–154
Urinary system:
  of adolescent, 378
  in elderly, 563*f*
  of elderly person, 559–560
  of infant, 228
  of schoolchild, 331
  of toddler, 260
Urinary tract infection:
  in preschool child, 300*t*
  of schoolchild, 338
Urination, toilet training and, 274
Urticaria, 474*t*

V

Vaccine; *see* Immunization
Vaginitis in adolescent, 402
Value system, 4
Values:
  basic, 14*t*
  comparison of, 9–13, 10*b*, 10*t*
  of dominant culture, 22–23
  in Middle Eastern culture, 21–22
  in United States, 9–13, 10*b*, 10*t*
Valve prolapse, mitral, in young adult, 474*t*
Vanadium, sources of, 712*t*
Varicella, toddler and, 267*t*, 268–269
Vascular system of elderly person, 559
Vascularization, exercise and, 451
Vasectomy, 405*t*
Vasocongestion, 432
Vasomotor instability, 332
Vegetarian:
  lacto-ovo, 96
  young adult as, 441–442
Vehicular accident:
  adolescent and, 397
  schoolchild and, 337
Vernix caseosa, 217
Very low birth weight infant, 243
Vessels:
  of elderly person, 559
  of middle-aged person, 515
Vestibular response in later maturity, 557
Victim of con game, 566*b*
Vietnamese culture, 39
Vinyl chloride, 70*t*
Violence:
  as occupational hazard, 66–67
  preoccupation with, 13
  on television, schoolchild and, 351
  against women, 483–487, 484*b*, 485*b*, 486*b*, 488*t*–489*t*
Vision:
  biological variations in, 37–38
  in later maturity, 557–558, 566–567, 580
  middle-aged person and, 515
  newborn and, 220, 222
  preschool child and, 299
  schoolchild and, 331, 333, 339
  toddler and, 259, 261, 266–267
  of young adult, 430
Vital signs:
  of preschool child, 291
  of schoolchild, 330
  of young adult, 445–446
Vitamins:
  colic and, 227

  in later maturity, 562
  prenatal development and, 183
  sources of, 709*t*–711*t*
Vocalization, by infant, 240
Volunteer work, by young adult, 457
Volunteering, by elderly person, 584*b*
Voodoo, 101
Vulnerable child, 199, 356
Vulvovaginitis in preschool child, 300*t*

W

Waldenses, 98
Walkaway, teen, 394
Walking, as exercise, 451
Walking reflex, 221*t*
Wart:
  genital, 402
  in schoolchild, 340*t*
Waste:
  conservation solutions concerning, 72*b*
  hazardous, 59–60
    disposal of, 62–63
Water:
  conservation solutions concerning, 72*b*
  for infant, 232
  sources of, 713*t*
Water intoxication of infant, 231
Water pollution, 54–57
  air pollution and, 51
Watson, John B., 156
Wax, ear, variations in, 37
Weaning of infant, 234
Wear-and-tear theory of aging, 547
Weather, influence on health of, 641–642
Weight:
  of adolescent, 380–383
  in early childhood, 196
  of infant, 233
  of newborn, 218
  prenatal development and, 182
  of schoolchild, 330
  of young adult, 429–430
Well-baby care, 140–143
Wellness, 636
Wellness Belief Scale, 661
White House Conference on Aging, 587
Widowhood:
  in later maturity, 553
  in middle age, 505–506
Witch in Mexican-American culture, 33
Withdrawal, by family member, 122
Withdrawing reflex, 221*t*
Women; *see* Female
Work:
  circadian rhythm and, 446
  cultural comparisons of, 17*t*
  health and, 641, 643
  of middle-aged person, 524–525, 525*b*
  occupational hazard and, 65–67, 68–70*t*, 74*f*
    pregnancy and, 186, 188
  occupational hazards and, 65–67, 68–70*t*, 74*f*
  suicide and, 481
  young adult and, 453–457
Workaholic, 453
Working mother:
  infant of, 246*b*
  latch key child of, 326–327

Working phase of relationship, 666
Working socioeconomic level, 28–29
World Health Organization, health promotion and, 696

X

X chromosome, 179

Y

Y chromosome, 179
Yoga, 87, 683–684
Yogurt, for colic, 227
Young adult, 426–499
  abortion and, 490–491
  adaptive mechanisms of, 462–463
  alcohol abuse of, 482
  battered woman syndrome and, 483–487, 484*b*, 485*b*, 486*b*, 488*t*–489*t*
  biologic rhythms and, 442–446
  body image of, 463–467
  cognitive development of, 451–453
  developmental tasks of, 470–471, 471*b*
  divorce in, 487, 489–490
  eating disorders of, 482–483, 483*b*
  emotional development of, 457–461, 459*f*
  family of, 428–429
  family planning and, 467–470
  health of, 471–491, 474*t*
    acquired immunodeficiency syndrome and, 472–473, 475–476
    anxiety and, 479*t*
    biofeedback and, 480–481
    dental, 476
    gastrointestinal disorder and, 478
    hepatitis and, 476
    immunizations and, 471–472
    life-style and, 478–480
    malignancy and, 476–478
  leisure of, 456–457
  life-style options of, 467
  mentor to, 526
  moral-spiritual development of, 461–462
  nutrition for, 438–442, 439*t*, 440*t*
  physical characteristics of, 429–430
  physical fitness of, 449–451
  self-concept of, 463
  sexuality of, 430–438
  sleep patterns in, 446–449, 447*f*, 448*b*
  stress and, 481
  suicide of, 481–482
  work of, 453–456
Young-old, 545, 577
  developmental tasks of, 582–583

Z

Zinc:
  as occupational hazard, 70*t*
  prenatal development and, 183
  sources of, 712*t*–713*t*
Zoonoses, 60
Zygote, 179

Italicized letters following page numbers indicate tables (*t*), figures (*f*), and boxes (*b*).